Oculoplastic, Orbital, and Reconstructive Surgery

Volume One. EYELIDS

Oculoplastic, Orbital, and Reconstructive Surgery

Volume One. EYELIDS

ALBERT HORNBLASS, M.D.

Clinical Professor of Ophthalmology,
State University of New York,
Health Science Center at
Brooklyn, New York

Director of Ophthalmic Plastic, Orbital and
Reconstructive Surgery at the
Manhattan Eye, Ear and Throat Hospital, and the
Lenox Hill Hospital, and the
State University of New York,
Health Science Center at
Brooklyn, New York

CARL J. HANIG, M.D.

Assistant Editor
Syracuse, New York

WILLIAMS & WILKINS
Baltimore • Hong Kong • London • Sydney

Senior Editor: Kimberly Kist
Associate Editor: Carol Eckhart
Copy Editor: Elia A. Flanegin
Design: JoAnne Janowiak
Illustration Planning: Lorraine Wrzosek
Production: Raymond E. Reter

Accurate indications, adverse reactions, and dosage schedules for drugs are provided in this book, but it is possible that they may change. The reader is urged to review the package information data of the manufacturers of the medications mentioned.

Printed in the United States of America

Library of Congress Cataloging in Publication Data

Oculoplastic, orbital, and reconstructive surgery.

Includes bibliographies and index.
Contents: v. 1. Eyelids.
1. Adnexa oculi—Surgery. 2. Eye-sockets—Surgery. 3. Eyelids—Surgery. 4. Surgery, Plastic. I. Hornblass, Albert, 1939–■. [DNLM: 1. Eyelids Diseases—therapy. 2. Eyelids—surgery. 3. Orbit—surgery. 4. Surgery, Plastic. WW 168 0209]
RE87.0266 1988 617.7′71059 86-32452
ISBN 0-683-04151-7 (v. 1)

To my late father of blessed memory, who stressed education, honesty, and service, who, along with my mother, taught me compassion, humility, respect, and the love of medicine.

To my dear children, David, Moshe, and Elana, who bring sunshine, innocence, and meaning to my life.

To my dear beloved wife, Bernice, who provides intelligence, love, patience, and purpose of life.

Preface

Several years ago, Dr. Walter Schachet, then consulting editor at Williams & Wilkins and a longtime friend, suggested that I write a book that would be encyclopedic in scope in the field of ophthalmic plastic and orbital surgery. I resisted this temptation for many reasons; the scope seemed awesome and overwhelming. However, I finally agreed to take on the challenge when I realized that the need for such a book existed.

This textbook is modeled after the system of ophthalmology used by Sir Stewart Duke Elder and other major comprehensive ophthalmic textbooks. Although there are numerous excellent books and monographs written on the subject of ophthalmic plastic and orbital surgery, there is no text containing extensive information on a variety of subjects in oculoplastic surgery. This two-volume comprehensive text presents all phases of diseases of the eyelids and the orbit. Major surgical procedures are discussed and illustrated.

Outstanding authorities in the field of ophthalmic plastic surgery have contributed to this textbook. Although attempts have been made to avoid redundancies, some repetition is educationally sound and needed.

The text is divided into two volumes. The first deals with every aspect of diseases and management of the eyelids. The second volume, *Orbit and the Lacrimal System*, focuses on the orbit and the lacrimal system.

Both volumes follow a similar format and are highly referenced for further study by the student.

The first volume contains chapters on anatomy, physiology, anesthesia, instrumentation, and psychological and legal aspects of eyelid surgery. There are nine sections. Section I is an Introduction. Section II presents congenital and developmental anomalies. Section III discusses systemic disorders associated with diseases of the eyelid. Section IV provides a comprehensive compilation of neoplastic disorders of the eyelids. Treatment options for every phase of eyelid tumors, both benign and malignant, are presented. Section V studies the eyebrows and eyelashes, a subject rarely included in conventional oculoplastic textbooks.

In Section VI, acquired eyelid malpositions are thoroughly examined, including recent advances in blepharospasm. Ophthalmologists and general plastic surgeons who have had extensive experience in civilian and military trauma provide thorough discussions in Section VII. In Section VIII, cosmetic oculoplastic surgery, which is commonly performed in the 1980s, is examined in depth in every phase by eminent aesthetic plastic surgeons. The final section deals with reconstruction of the eyelids and conjunctiva.

This text presents the most current methods, diagnosis, and treatment of eyelid, orbital, and lacrimal problems. These techniques include surgery, radiology, radiotherapy, chemotherapy, cryotherapy, immunotherapy, and laser surgery. This book should interest ophthalmologists, plastic surgeons, oculoplastic and orbital surgeons, head and neck surgeons, otorhinolaryngologists, radiologists, dermatologists, internists, and anesthesiologists. Its scope will be informative for the medical student as well as the most advanced oculoplastic and orbital physician.

The field of ophthalmic plastic surgery has exploded in the last 20 years. When the American Society of Ophthalmic Plastic and Reconstructive Surgery was created in 1969, there were only a handful of fully trained surgeons. Today, there are fellowship-trained oculoplastic surgeons in most cities in the United States as well as in Europe and Asia.

My interest in this field was literally sparked in the Vietnam war. From 1969 through 1970, I was stationed at the 71st Evacuation Hospital in Pleiku, South Vietnam. As an ophthalmologist, I treated all aspects of eye and eyelid surgery. To all the wounded whom I treated, I thank you for your confidence and your loyalty. I thank my colleagues at the Walter Reed Army Hospital and, in particular, Col. Frank Lapiana, for their collaborative study in ocular and periorbital war injuries. To the soldiers and civilians who died in combat, may they rest in eternal peace.

Dr. Byron C. Smith was my preceptor and mentor. He continues to be my teacher. Many of the basic precepts in oculoplastic surgery, were formulated by him, and we are all indebted to him. I received support for this project from my former fellows, Drs. Virginia Soarez, Brian Herschorn, David Reifler, Larry G. Kass, Neil D. Gross, and Michael Gingold. Dr. Carl Hanig was a fellow and is assistant editor of the book; he contributed greatly to this book. Dr. Crowell Beard is someone special whom I have admired and respected. Dr. Richard C. Troutman, my former chief, has always encouraged and supported me. Dr. Arthur Wolintz, Chief of Ophthalmology, SUNY Health Sciences Center in Brooklyn, is always there to be counted on as a friend and consultant. I appreciated the advice and friendship of Drs. Robert Coles and Frederick A. Jakobiec. I thank my editors at Williams & Wilkins, Kimberly Kist, Carol-Lynn Brown, and John Gardner, for their encouragement and professionalism. Carol Eckhart, associate editor at Williams & Wilkins, did an outstanding job in supporting this endeavor. My appreciation to my secretary, Sheila Silverstein, for her patience and managerial skills; Rochelle Singer coordinated typing and communication, and I cannot thank her enough for her devotion and loyalty. Meryl Green Solomon provided the excellent medical illustrations.

I am indebted to the hundreds of referring physicians who have had the confidence to refer their interesting and perplexing patients for consultation and treatment. To all the residents and students who continue to stimulate me with their questions and problems, I am most indebted.

To my dear wife Bernice, who had the patience, love, and devotion to help sustain and support me during this project and to my children, David, Moshe, and Elana: I thank you for giving up precious time to allow me to complete this endeavor. To God, who sustained my family and who guides every physician to treat and heal the sick.

"The Education of Today is the Future of Tomorrow"

Contributors

Gary L. Aguilar, M.D.
Assistant Clinical Professor of Ophthalmology, University of California, San Francisco, San Francisco, California; Assistant Clinical Professor of Surgery, Division of Ophthalmology, Stanford University Medical Center, San Francisco, California

Donald I. Altman, M.D.
Irvine, California

Richard L. Anderson, M.D.
Professor, Department of Ophthalmology, Director, Oculoplastic, Orbital, and Oncology Services, University of Utah School of Medicine, Salt Lake City, Utah

Alan D. Andrews, M.D.
Assistant Clinical Professor of Dermatology, Columbia University, College of Physicians and Surgeons, New York, New York

George B. Bartley, M.D.
Consultant in Ophthalmology, Mayo Clinic, Rochester, Minnesota

Henry I. Baylis, M.D.
Clinical Professor and Director, Division of Ophthalmic Plastic and Reconstructive Surgery, Jules Stein Eye Institute, UCLA School of Medicine, Los Angeles, California

Crowell Beard, M.D.
Clinical Professor Emeritus, University of California Medical School, San Francisco, California

Donald J. Bergin, M.D., F.A.C.S.
Southeastern Eye Center, Greensboro, North Carolina

Irving Berlin, M.D.
Director of Anesthesiology, Manhattan Ear, Eye and Throat Hospital, New York, New York

Evalina A. Bernardino, M.D.
Dermatopathologist, American Oncologic Hospital, Philadelphia, Pennsylvania

Vitaliano B. Bernardino, Jr., M.D.
Professor of Ophthalmology, and Associate Professor, Department of Pathology, Jefferson Medical College, Thomas Jefferson University, Philadelphia, Pennsylvania

Charles K. Beyer-Machule, M.D.
Associate Clinical Professor, Department of Ophthalmology, Harvard Medical School, Massachusetts Eye and Ear Infirmary, Boston, Massachusetts

Laszlo Biro, M.D., F.A.C.P.
Clinical Professor of Dermatology, State University of New York, Health Science Center, Brooklyn, New York

Gary E. Borodic, M.D.
Clinical Instructor, Department of Ophthalmology, Harvard Medical School, Massachusetts Eye and Ear Infirmary, Boston, Massachusetts

Stephen L. Bosniak, M.D.
Clinical Assistant Professor of Ophthalmology, State University of New York, Health Science Center, Brooklyn, New York; Assistant Attending Ophthalmologist, Manhattan Eye, Ear and Throat Hospital, New York, New York; Associate Adjunct Surgeon, New York Eye and Ear Infirmary, New York, New York; Attending Ophthalmologist, Catholic Medical Center, Queens, New York.

Bernice Z. Brown, M.D.
Clinical Associate Professor, University of California Medical School, Doheny Eye Foundation, Children's Hospital of Los Angeles, Los Angeles, California

Stuart I. Brown, M.D.
Professor and Chairman, Department of Ophthalmology, University of California, San Diego, La Jolla, California

George F. Buerger, Jr., M.D.
Clinical Associate Professor of Ophthalmology, University of Pittsburgh School of Medicine; Chief, Oculoplastic Service, Department of Ophthalmology, Eye and Ear Hospital of Pittsburgh and Ear Institute of Pittsburgh, Pittsburgh, Pennsylvania

John D. Bullock, M.D., M.S., F.A.C.S.
Professor and Chairman, Department of Ophthalmology, Professor of Plastic Surgery, Wright State University School of Medicine, Dayton, Ohio

John A. Burns, M.D.
Clinical Professor, Department of Ophthalmology, Ohio State University, Columbus, Ohio; Chairman, Department of Ophthalmology, Otolaryngology, and Maxillofacial Surgery, Grant Medical Center, Columbus, Ohio

Kenneth V. Cahill, M.D.
Clinical Associate Professor, Department of Ophthalmology, Ohio State University, Columbus, Ohio

Alston Callahan, M.D., F.A.C.S.
President, Eye Foundation, Inc.; Staff, Eye Foundation Hospital, Birmingham, Alabama

Michael A. Callahan, M.D.
Associate Professor of Clinical Ophthalmology, University of Alabama, The Eye Foundation Hospital, Birmingham, Alabama

Richard P. Carroll, M.D., F.A.C.S.
Clinical Associate Professor, Department of Ophthalmology, University of Minnesota; Consultant, Oculoplastic, Lacrimal, and Orbital Surgery, Minneapolis, Minnesota

Jack Chalfin, M.D.
Chief of Ophthalmology, Cod Hospital, Tufts-New England Medical Center, Hyannis, Massachusetts

Joel Confino, M.D.
Clinical Instructor, Mt. Sinai School of Medicine, New York, New York; Assistant Attending Physician, Overlook Hospital, Summit New Jersey; Co-Director, Cornea and External Disease Clinic, City Hospital, Elmhurst, New York

Philip L. Custer, M.D.
Instructor in Clinical Ophthalmology, Ophthalmic Plastic and Reconstructive Surgery, Washington University School of Medicine, St. Louis, Missouri

Robert M. Dryden, M.D.
Adjunct, Associate Professor, Director, Eye Plastic and Reconstructive Surgery, Department of Ophthalmology, University of Arizona, Tucson, Arizona

Ira Eliasoph, M.D.
Associate Clinical Professor of Ophthalmology, Mt. Sinai School of Medicine; Associate Attending Ophthalmic Surgeon, Manhattan Eye, Ear and Throat Hospital, Beth Israel Hospital, New York, New York

Gil A. Epstein, M.D.
Department of Ophthalmology, Florida Medical Center, Bennett Hospital, Ft. Lauderdale, Florida

Alexander A. Fisher, M.D.
Clinical Professor, Department of Dermatology, New York University Postgraduate Medical School, Woodside, New York

Robert Folberg, M.D.
Associate Professor, Department of Ophthalmology; Director, Eye Pathology Laboratory, University of Iowa Hospitals and Clinics, Iowa City, Iowa

Alan H. Friedman, M.D.
Clinical Professor, Department of Ophthalmology, Mt. Sinai School of Medicine, New York, New York

David W. Furnas, M.D.
Clinical Professor and Chief, Division of Plastic Surgery, California College of Medicine, University of California, Irvine Medical Center, Orange, California

Paul T. Gavaris, M.D.
Assistant Clinical Professor, Georgetown University; Chief, Oculoplastic Section, Washington Hospital Center; Consultant, Naval Hospital, Bethesda, Maryland

Russell S. Gonnering, M.D., F.A.C.S.
Assistant Clinical Professor, Department of Ophthalmology, The University of Wisconsin; Assistant Clinical Professor, Department of Ophthalmology, The Medical College of Wisconsin, Milwaukee, Wisconsin

Neil D. Gross, M.D.
Attending Surgeon, Florida Hospital Center, Orlando, Florida; Florida Eye Clinic, Altamonte Springs, Florida

Hadassah Neiman Gurfein, Ph.D.
Clinical Instructor of Psychiatry, Mt. Sinai School of Medicine, New York, New York

Carl Hanig, M.D.
Clinical Assistant Professor, Department of Ophthalmology, State University of New York Health Science Center; Attending Surgeon, Crouse-Irving Memorial Hospital, Syracuse, New York

John N. Harrington, M.D.
Associate Clinical Professor of Ophthalmology, Director of Ophthalmic Plastic and Reconstructive Surgery, University of Texas Health Science Center, Dallas, Texas

Albert Hornblass, M.D., F.A.C.S.
Clinical Professor of Ophthalmology, State University of New York, Health Science Center at Brooklyn; Director of Ophthalmic Plastic, Orbital, and Reconstructive Surgery, Manhattan Eye, Ear, and Throat Hospital, and Lenox Hill Hospital and the State University of New York, Brooklyn, New York

C. Gary Jackson, M.D., F.A.C.S.
Associate Clinical Professor of Otolaryngology, (Otology/Neurotology), Vanderbilt University Medical Center, Nashville, Tennessee

Glenn W. Jelks, M.D.
Assistant Professor of Plastic Surgery, New York University Medical Center, Attending Surgeon, Bellvue

Hospital, Manhattan Eye, Ear and Throat Hospital, Manhattan Veterans Hospital, New York Eye and Ear Infirmary, New York, New York

David F. Kamin, M.D.
Associate Clinical Professor, Jules Stein Eye Institute, University of California, Los Angeles, Los Angeles, California; Visiting Professor of Ophthalmology, Hebrew University of Jerusalem/Haddasah, University Hospital, Jerusalem, Israel

Roger Kohn, M.D.
Professor, Department of Ophthalmology, Division of Ophthalmic Plastic and Reconstructive Surgery, UCLA School of Medicine, Los Angeles, California

Kenneth H. Kraemer, M.D.
Research Scientist, Laboratory of Molecular Carcinogenesis, National Cancer Institute, National Institutes of Health, Bethesda, Maryland

Burton J. Kushner, M.D.
Clinical Professor, Department of Ophthalmology, Pediatric Ophthalmology, University of Wisconsin Clinical Science Center, Madison, Wisconsin

Steven J. LauKaitis, M.D.
Medical Director, Project Orbis Inc., New York, New York

Robert E. Levine, M.D.
Associate Professor, Clinical Ophthalmology, University of Southern California, School of Medicine, Los Angeles, California

Richard D. Lisman, M.D.
Assistant Clinical Professor of Ophthalmology, Mt. Sinai School of Medicine, Co-Chief of Clinic in the Department of Ophthalmic Plastic Surgery, Manhattan Eye and Ear Hospital, Associate Attending Surgeon, New York Eye and Ear Infirmary, New York, New York

Don Liu, M.D., Ph.D.
Oculoplastic and Orbital Surgery, Department of Ophthalmology, Henry Ford Hospital, Detroit, Michigan

Andrew S. Markovits, M.D.
Chief, Section of Ophthalmology, Department of Ophthalmology, U.S. Naval Aerospace Institute, Medical Institute, Naval Air Station, Pensacola, Florida

Alfred C. Marrone, M.D.
Associate Clinical Professor, Department of Ophthalmology, University of Southern California, Doheney Eye Foundation, Torrance Memorial Hospital Burn Center, Los Angeles, California

Rodney W. McCarthy, M.D.
Assistant Clinical Professor, Department of Ophthalmology and Pathology, Medical College of Ohio, Toledo, Ohio

Clinton D. McCord, M.D., F.A.C.S.
Professor of Ophthalmology and Director of Ophthalmic Plastic Surgery, Emory University School of Medicine, Atlanta, Georgia

John F. Meagher, M.D.
Clinical Instructor, Department of Ophthalmology, University of California San Diego, San Diego, California; Consultant in Ophthalmology, Veterans Administration Hospital, La Jolla, California; Attending Ophthalmology, Little Company of Mary Hospital, Torrance, California

Gary D. Monheit, M.D.
Assistant Professor, Department of Dermatology, University of Alabama, Medical Center at Birmingham, Birmingham, Alabama

Janet M. Neigel, M.D.
Clinical Assistant Professor of Ophthalmology, UMDNJ, New Jersey Medical School, Eye Institute of New Jersey, Newark, New Jersey

Christine Nelson, M.D.
Assistant Professor of Ophthalmology, University of Michigan, Ann Arbor, Michigan

William B. Nolan, M.D., F.A.C.S.
Director of Residency Training, Manhattan Eye, Ear, and Throat Hospital, New York, New York

J. Justin Older, M.D.
Associate Professor of Ophthalmology and Director, Oculoplastic Service, Department of Ophthalmology, University of Southern Florida, College of Medicine, Tampa, Florida

David S. Orentreich, M.D.
Clinical Instructor, Department of Dermatology, Mt. Sinai School of Medicine, New York, New York

Norman Orentreich, M.D.
Clinical Professor of Dermatology, New York University School of Medicine, New York, New York

Michael Patipa, M.D.
General Ophthalmology, Good Samaritan Hospital, St. Mary's Hospital, Humana Hospital of the Palm Beaches, West Palm Beach, Florida

Kevin I. Perman, M.D.
Assistant Clinical Professor, George Washington University Medical Center; Clinical Instructor, Georgetown University; Consultant, Ophthalmic Plastic Reconstruction, Washington Hospital Center, Washington, D.C.

Richard L. Petrelli, M.D.
Assistant Clinical Professor of Ophthalmology and Director, Oculoplastic Service, Department of Ophthalmology, Yale University School of Medicine; Attending Surgeon, Hospital of St. Rafael, New Haven, Connecticut

Ely Price, M.D., F.A.C.P.
Clinical Associate Professor of Dermatology, State University of New York, Health Science Center at Brooklyn, New York

Allen M. Putterman, M.D.
Professor of Clinical Ophthalmology and Chief, Oculoplastic Surgery, Department of Ophthalmology, University of Illinois College of Medicine at Chicago;

Senior Attending Surgeon, and Director, Oculoplastic Surgery, Michael Reese University of Chicago Hospitals, Chicago, Illinois

J. Earl Rathbun, M.D., F.A.C.S.
Clinical Professor of Ophthalmology, University of California, San Francisco; Consultant, Ophthalmic Plastic and Reconstructive Surgery, Ft. Miley Veterans Administration Hospital, San Francisco, California

Thomas D. Rees, M.D., F.A.C.S.
Chairman, Department of Plastic Surgery, Manhattan Eye, Ear and Throat Hospital; Clinical Professor of Plastic Surgery, New York University School of Medicine, New York, New York

Raymond Reich, M.D.
Assistant Professor, State University of New York, Health Science Center at Brooklyn, Brooklyn, New York

David M. Reifler, M.D.
Assistant Clinical Professor, Division of Ophthalmology, Michigan State University, College of Human Medicine (GRAMEC); Attending Surgeon, Blodgett Memorial Medical Center, Butterworth and St. Mary's Hospitals, and the Western Michigan Ambulatory Surgical Center, Grand Rapids, Michigan

Stuart R. Seiff, M.D.
Director of Oculoplastic Surgery, Plastic Surgery, University of California, San Francisco, California

Amiram Shapiro, M.D.
Associate Professor, Hahnemann College, Philadelphia, Pennsylvania

Philip A. Shelton, M.D., J.D., F.A.C.S., F.C.L.M.
Assistant Clinical Professor of Ophthalmic Surgery, University of Connecticut Medical School, Farmington, Connecticut

John D. Sheppard, Jr., M.D.
Research Ophthalmologist, Francis I. Proctor Foundation, University of California, San Francisco, California

William Shields, C.R.A.
Georgetown University Center for Sight, Washington, D.C.

Norman Shorr, M.D., F.A.C.S.
Clinical Professor of Ophthalmology, Division of Ophthalmic Plastic and Reconstructive Surgery, Jules Stein Eye Institute, University of California at Los Angeles, Center for the Health Sciences, Los Angeles, California

Philip Silverstone, M.D.
Attending Physician Milford Hospital, Milford, Connecticut; Attending Physician, Hospital of St. Raphael's, New Haven, Connecticut

Robert G. Small, M.D., F.A.C.S.
Professor, Department of Ophthalmology, University of Oklahoma, Dean A. McGee Eye Institute, Oklahoma City, Oklahoma

Nicolas Tabbal, M.D., F.A.C.S.
Associate Attending Surgeon, Manhattan Eye, Ear and Throat Hospital; Clinical Instructor in Plastic Surgery, New York University Medical Center, New York, New York

Richard R. Tenzel, M.D.
Clinical Professor of Ophthalmology, University of Miami School of Medicine, Chief, Ophthalmic Plastic Surgery Associates, Bascom Palmer Eye Institute, Miami, Florida

Daniel J. Townsend, M.D.
Clinical Instructor, Department of Ophthalmic Plastic Surgery, Harvard Medical School, Massachusetts Eye and Ear Infirmary, Boston, Massachusetts

Hagai Tsur, M.D.
Associate Professor of Plastic Surgery, Sackler School of Medicine, Tel Aviv University; Head, Plastic Surgery Department and Burns Unit, Sheba Medical Center, Tel-Hashomer, Israel

Robert R. Waller, M.D.
Consultant, Department of Ophthalmology, Mayo Clinic and Mayo Foundation; Professor of Ophthalmology, Mayo Medical School, Rochester, Minnesota

Gary S. Weinstein, M.D.
Clinical Professor of Ophthalmology, University of Pittsburgh School of Medicine, Pittsburgh, Pennsylvania

Ralph E. Wesley, M.D.
Director, Ophthalmic Plastic and Reconstructive Surgery, Vanderbilt University Medical Center; Director, Ophthalmic Plastic and Orbital Surgery, Baptist Medical Center; Chief, Ophthalmic Section, Park View Medical Center; Assistant Clinical Professor of Ophthalmology, Meharry Medical College, Nashville, Tennessee

Eugene O. Wiggs, M.D.
Clinical Professor of Ophthalmology and Chief, Oculoplastic Service, University of Colorado Health Sciences Center, Denver, Colorado

Robert B. Wilkins, M.D., F.A.C.S.
Houston, Texas

Stephen S. Winfield, M.D.
Staff Physician, Meriden-Wallingford Hospital, Meriden, Connecticut

Allan E. Wulc, M.D.
Assistant Professor of Ophthalmology, Oculoplastic/Orbital Service, Department of Ophthalmology, University of Pennsylvania, Scheie Eye Institute, Philadelphia, Pennsylvania

Christine L. Zolli, M.D., F.A.C.S.
Clinical Associate Professor, Department of Ophthalmology, University of Medicine and Dentistry of New Jersey, Newark, New Jersey; Chief, Oculoplastic Service, Eye Institute of New Jersey; Assistant Surgeon, Wills Eye Hospital, Philadelphia, Pennsylvania

Contents

SECTION VI. Acquired Eyelid Malpositions

SECTION VII: Trauma

SECTION VIII. Cosmetic Ophthalmic Plastic Surgery

SECTION IX: Reconstruction of the Eyelids

SECTION I

INTRODUCTION

CHAPTER 1

Eyelid and Anterior Orbital Anatomy

GARY L. AGUILAR, M.D.
CHRISTINE NELSON, M.D.

The eyelids and eyebrows are anatomically extraordinarily complex structures whose major function is to aid and protect the visual system. The eyebrows and eyelids function synchronously to regulate the amount of light that enters the pupil and also serve to protect the globe from injury, exposure, and unwanted moisture. The lid brow complex also serves as the single most important distinctive aspect of our facial appearance. It is the first area viewed when people meet. The slant and thickness of the eyebrow, the width and length of the palpebral apertures, and the distribution of anterior orbital fat all participate in the creation of the facies that is unique to each individual. Even small abnormalities in the lid brow complex have a profound effect on appearance. The surgeon who alters the eyelids or eyebrows must have a precise understanding of the structural relationships of these areas to be able to favorably modify their anatomy.

EYELID SKIN

The eyelids act as movable shutters as they protect the eye from excessive light, injury, or dessication. The lids contain glands that produce the mucus, watery, and lipid components of the tear film. The action of the upper lid serves to move foreign material or excessive mucus away from the cornea toward the medial canthus while evenly spreading the tear film across the eye. When excessive tearing occurs, repeated blinking serves to pump the tears from the eye to the nose through the lacrimal excretory system. With the eyelids open the palpebral aperture is an almond-shaped opening that measures approximately 12 mm × 29 mm and slants slightly upward from medial to lateral (Fig. 1.1). The lateral canthus is approximately 1 to 2 mm higher than the medial canthus in Occidentals and often higher than that in Asians. This lateral elevation promotes movement of the tears toward the lacrimal excretory system. The lateral canthus is the junction between the lateral upper and lower lids and is 5 mm from the orbital margin and approximately 1 cm from the frontozygomatic suture. Whereas the lateral canthal angle is acute and in contact with the globe, the medial canthal angle is rounded and away from the globe allowing a small space, the *lacus lacrimalis* (1, 2). The *lacrimal caruncle* is the most medial mucous membrane–covered elevation of the inner canthus. It contains modified sweat glands and sebaceous glands that open into the follicles of very fine soft hairs. Just temporal to it is a pink-colored thickening, the plica semilunaris, thought to be a remnant of the nictitating membrane found in lower animals (Fig. 1.1). The lacrimal papilla is a small elevation in the lid margin approximately 4 mm from the inner canthus and marks the opening into the lacrimal punctum. The lid margins medial to the papillae houses the lacrimal canaliculi and contain no true lashes or tarsus (Fig. 1.1).

The width of the lid margin is approximately 2 mm. The posterior margin is sharp, and just anterior to it are

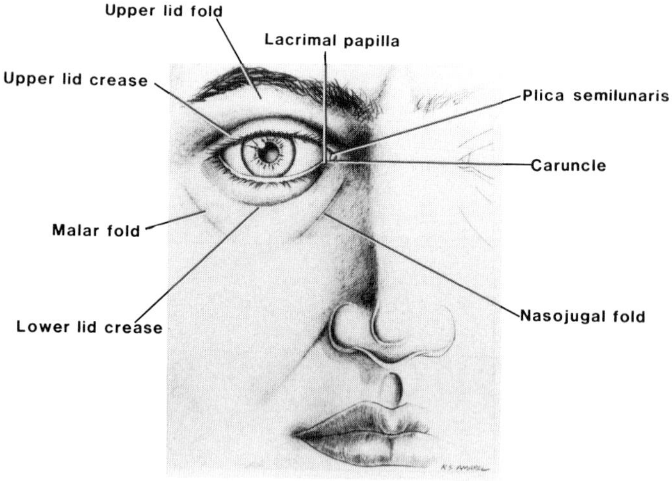

Figure 1.1. Topographical anatomy.

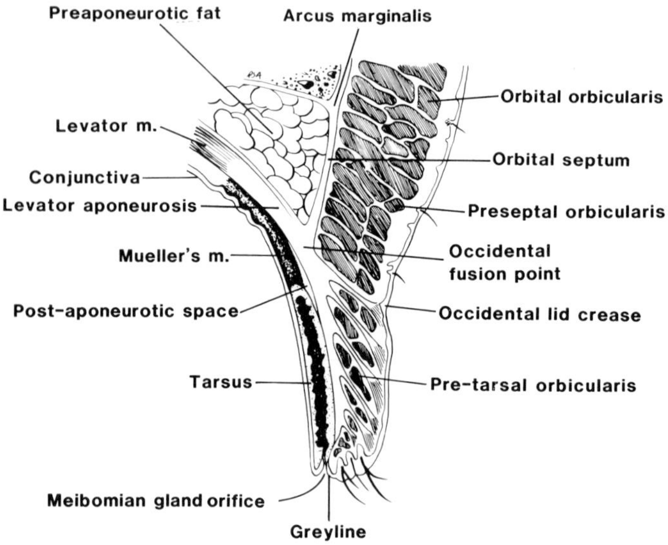

Figure 1.2. Occidental upper lid shows orbital septum fusing with levator above the tarsus.

found the mucocutaneous junction and meibomian gland orifices. Between the orifices and the lashes lies the so-called grey line, which is an often-used landmark in surgical procedures that split the lid into anterior and posterior lamellae. Incisions made here will separate the tarsus from the orbicularis and the orbital septum from the orbicularis (Fig. 1.2).

The eyelid skin is unique in that it is extraordinarily thin and very movable. It is less than 1 mm thick and has a thin epidermis and loose subcutaneous tissue with little fat (3). The nasal portions of the eyelids have finer hairs and more sebaceous glands and are therefore smoother and more oily than temporal eyelid skin (1). The lids can be divided into the loose movable portion that overlies the orbital septum and the portion that overlies the tarsus, which is fixed to the anterior surface of the tarsus by anterior fibers of the levator aponeurosis. The pretarsal skin is demarcated from the preseptal skin at the supratarsal lid crease, 8 to 11 mm from the lid border. It is at the lid crease that the projections of the levator aponeurosis first reach the skin surface and bind the skin to the deeper lid structures (4) (Fig. 1.2). Below the lid crease the levator aponeurosis has anterior projections to the skin and posterior projections to the anterior surface of the tarsus that limit the movement of the pretarsal skin (1, 4; Fig. 1.2). With the eye open the loose preseptal skin overhangs the eyelid crease forming the so-called upper eyelid fold (Fig. 1.1). The distinctive appearance of the Asian eyelid results from a smaller and lower upper lid crease than is seen in Occidentals and a very full and prominent upper lid fold that often hangs over and obliterates the upper lid crease. Doxanas (5, 6) has shown that this results from a more inferior fusion of the orbital septum with the levator aponeurosis. The lid crease is formed by anterior projections of levator fibers as they pass through the lower border of the septum. When this fusion occurs at a lower level, as in Asians, the corresponding lid crease is lower (Fig. 1.3). Preaponeurotic fat is bound by the fusion between the septum and the levator aponeurosis. In Occidentals the fat is therefore confined to the area above the tarsus, where the fusion occurs. In

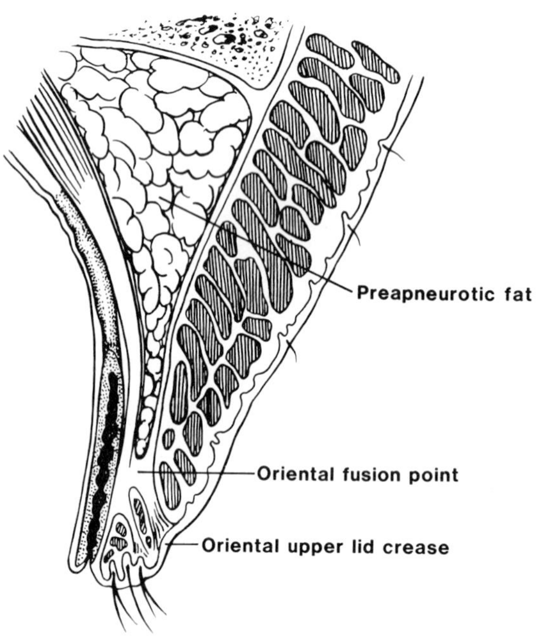

Figure 1.3. Asian upper lid shows orbital septum fusing with levator aponeurosis below the upper edge of tarsus with preaponeurotic fat present anterior to tarsus.

Asians, by contrast, the fat is present more inferiorly and creates a more prominent and upper eyelid fold (5) (Fig. 1.3).

The lower eyelid often has a lid crease formed by the anterior projections of the so-called capsulopalpebral fascia to the skin. The lower lid crease, which is usually present in the young and which often disappears with age, is 3 to 4 mm from the lower lid margin medially and 5 to 6 mm from the lower lid margin laterally (6) (Fig. 1.1).

There is an increase in the thickness of the skin and density of the subcutaneous tissue as one approaches the peripheral margins of the eyelids: the brow superiorly, the lateral orbital rim temporally, and the cheek inferiorly. The margins of the lower lid extend beyond the lower orbital rim to the nasojugal and the malar folds, which are thought to be created by fascial attachments of skin to underlying periosteum and the facial musculature (Fig. 1.1).

ORBICULARIS AND POSTERIOR ORBICULAR FASCIA

The orbicularis oculi is the most superficial muscle of the eyelids and extends beyond the orbital margins to overly the frontalis, temporalis, and the cheek musculature. It is separated from the eyelid skin by a thin layer of delicate connective tissue that is devoid of fat. Between the fourth and sixth week of embryonic life the orbicularis migrates from the area just beneath the ear toward the eyes (the orbicularis and all superficial facial muscles are derived from the second branchial arch). It grows in a horseshoe manner, with the upper arm growing toward the upper eyelid and the lower arm growing toward the lower lid (3). The migration is complete by the 12th week (Fig. 1.4).

For descriptive and functional purposes the orbicularis may be somewhat arbitrarily divided into three portions: *orbital, preseptal* and *pretarsal* (3, 7) (Fig. 1.5). The orbital portion seems to be under entirely voluntary control while the preseptal and pretarsal orbicularis are under voluntary and involuntary control (3). The orbicularis muscles function as protectors of the lid and both consciously and unconsciously serve to help close the lids and protect the globe (Fig. 1.5).

The *frontalis* muscle terminates without a bony insertion in the undersurface of the orbicularis under the eyebrow. Medially, fibers from the frontalis give rise to two muscle groups that are important in facial expression: the *corrugator superciliaris* and the *procerus*. The corrugator superciliaris develops from a slip of frontalis fibers that turn underneath the main body of the muscle and curve medially to attach to the superomedial orbital margin (Fig. 1.5). Contraction of this muscle pulls the eyebrow medially and slightly downward, reflecting disappointment, anger, or sorrow. The procerus muscle develops from a medial bend of vertically oriented frontalis muscle that attaches to the nasal bone. Its action depresses the medial portion of the brow, and it acts synergistically with the corrugator (3, 7).

The outer orbital orbicularis extends beyond the orbital margins superficial to the frontalis, temporalis, and cheek muscles. Superomedially, its terminal fibers interdigitate with the frontalis, corrugator supraciliaris, and procerus muscles before inserting into the orbital rim medial to the supraorbital notch. The fibers then sweep without interruption over the lateral orbital margin to insert inferomedially into the frontal process of the maxillary bone medial to the infraorbital foramen (3, 5) (Fig. 1.5).

The preseptal orbicularis overlies the upper and lower orbital septa. Superomedially, it inserts into the medial canthal tendon with posterior extensions to the lacrimal diaphragm, as well as the posterior lacrimal crest (3, 7). Its fibers then sweep over the upper orbital septum and lateral canthus, giving rise to the lateral palpebral raphe. This is not a true raphe but merely an interdigitation of continuously sweeping muscle bundles. The fibers then continue inferomedially to insert both onto the lower portion of the medial canthal tendon as well as the lacrimal diaphragm and the posterior lacrimal crest.

The pretarsal orbicularis is penetrated by anterior projections from the levator aponeurosis, which also has firm attachments posteriorly to the tarsus (4, 8) (Fig. 1.2). These aponeurotic bands firmly anchor the orbicularis in this area to the anterior surface of the tarsus. The upper and lower pretarsal orbicularis give rise laterally to the lateral canthal tendon, which inserts at the lateral orbital tubercle just inside the lateral orbital rim (Fig. 1.6). Medially, the pretarsal orbicularis muscles give rise to the medial canthal

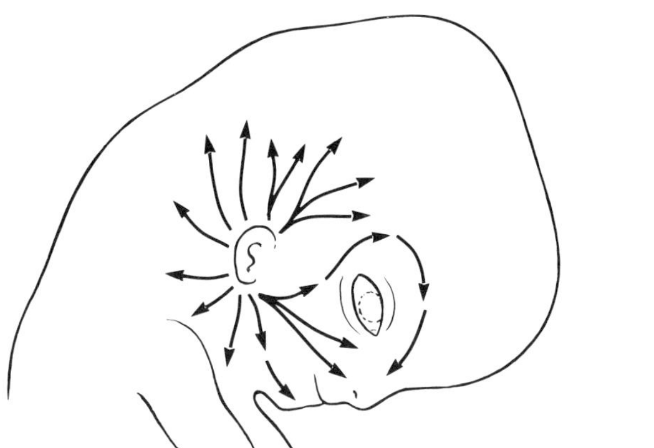

Figure 1.4. Migration of preorbicularis mesenchyme from second branchial arch in a horseshoe manner around orbit.

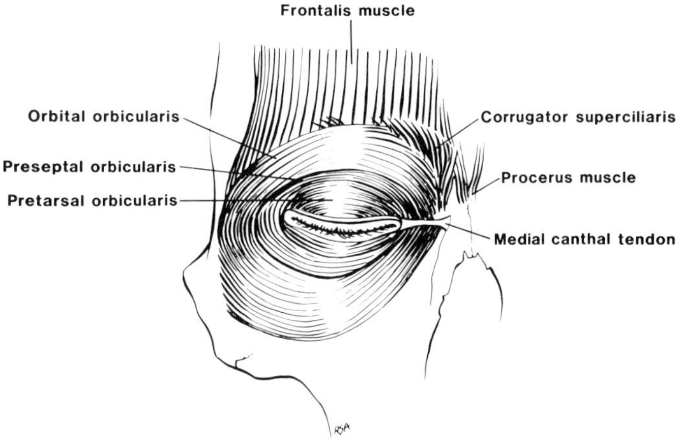

Figure 1.5. Eyelid musculature. Orbicularis muscle overlies frontalis muscle. Superomedially, the orbicularis and frontalis muscles have been cut away to reveal the corrugator superciliaris, which derives from a slip of frontalis muscle that turns medially under the frontalis to insert in the superomedial orbital rim (see text).

Figure 1.6. Pretarsal orbicularis gives rise to the medial and lateral canthal tendons. Superior support for the medial canthal tendon is shown (see text).

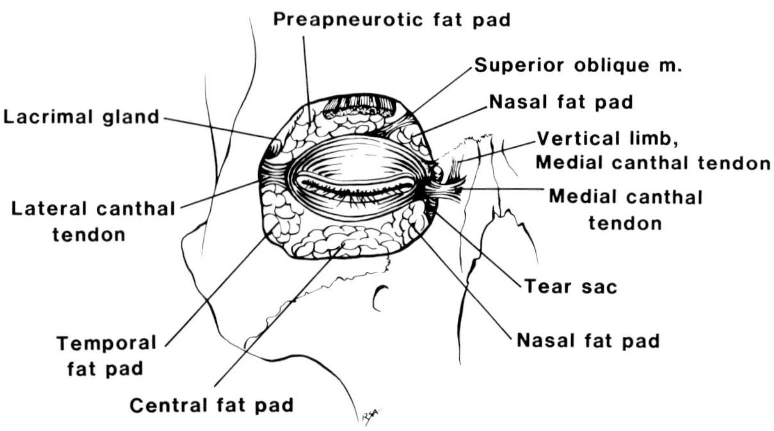

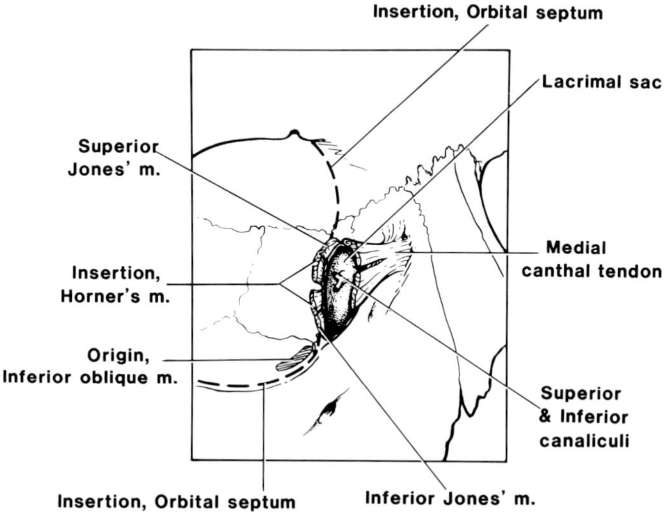

Figure 1.7. Medial canthal tendon surrounding tear sac. Both pretarsal and preseptal orbicularis muscles have projections anterior to, overlying, and posterior to the tear sac. The posterior projection of the pretarsal orbicularis is Horner's tensor tarsi muscle. The posterior projection of the preseptal orbicularis is Jones's muscle. Horner's and Jones's muscle are not easily separated but act as a single muscle sheet that inserts into the posterior lacrimal crest (see text).

tendon, whose superficial and deep heads surround the tear sac (1) (Fig. 1.7). The larger superficial head inserts at and anteriorly to the anterior lacrimal crest on the frontal process of the maxillary bone. Anderson (9) claims that there is a superior attachment of the superficial head that inserts into the maxillary process of the frontal bone, preventing telecanthus after medial canthal tendon disinsertion (Fig. 1.6). The deep head of the medial canthal tendon inserts onto the posterior lacrimal crest and onto the lacrimal diaphragm. In addition to the tendon, the deep head has muscle elements, the *tensor tarsi*, (Horner's muscle), which insert into the posterior lacrimal crest (10) (Fig. 1.7). Thus both the preseptal and pretarsal orbicularis have insertions anterior to, posterior to, and overlying the tear sac. This arrangement may be necessary for tear elimination. With each blink the lacrimal portion of the eyelid moves medially and the lacrimal diaphragm is pulled away from the lacrimal fossa. Thus tears are propelled medially along the canaliculus and aspirated into the tear sac by the negative pressure from expansion of this hollow viscus. A cessation of the blink releases the traction on the lacrimal diaphragm and allows it to collapse, propelling the tears down the nasolacrimal duct toward the nose (1).

Beneath the orbicularis there is a fairly dense fascial layer, the *posterior orbicular fascia*, to which the orbicularis firmly adheres (4). Small peripheral facial nerve fibers pass vertically through the lid in this layer. The posterior orbicular fascia overlies the orbital septum above the tarsus and the levator aponeurosis anterior to the tarsus. There is no separation between the posterior orbicular fascia and the septum except in the region of the superior orbital rim. Here the eyebrow fat pad may extend a short distance inferiorly between the posterior orbicular fascia and the orbital septum into the superior orbit (10) (Fig. 1.8).

DEEP ANATOMY OF THE UPPER EYELID

ORBITAL SEPTUM

The orbital septum is the thin fascial barrier of the true anatomic orbit that underlies the posterior orbicular fascia. It is thinner medially as it is perforated by the lacrimal, supraorbital, supratrochlear, and infratrochlear vessels and nerves. This attenuation of the septum medially allows the prolapse of preaponeurotic fat, which may often be seen in the elderly (1). Clinically, the septum often acts as a barrier and may prevent the intraorbital spread of a "preseptal cellulitis." It arises from the *arcus marginalis*, which is the firmly adherent periosteum of the orbital rim. The arcus marginalis marks the junction between the firmly attached periosteum of the frontal bone and the loose periorbita of the orbit (Fig. 1.8). The orbital septum of the upper lid fuses with the levator aponeurosis at, or just above, the eyelid crease 2 to 3 mm above the upper edge of the tarsus (4) (Fig. 1.2). In the lower lid the septum fuses with the capsulopalpebral fascia, the retractor of the

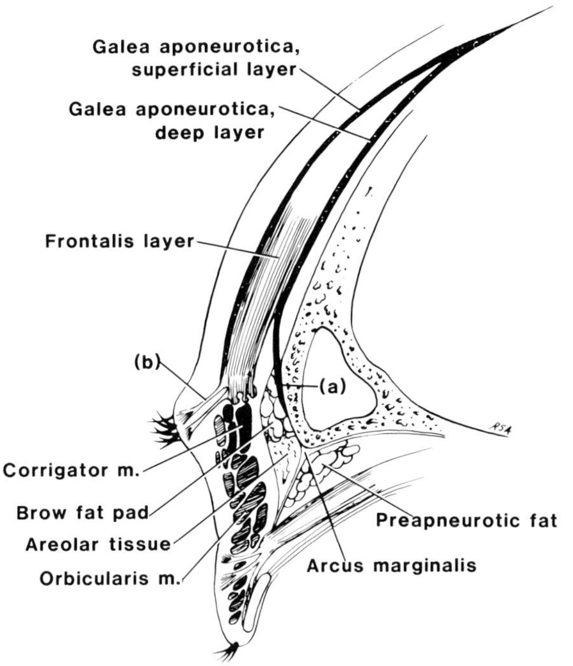

Figure 1.8. Eyebrow showing a large brow fat pad extending between the posterior orbicular fascia and the orbital septum into the superior orbit. *A,* Deep galea aponeurotica attaching along supraorbital ridge. *B,* Superficial galea aponeurotica inserting with frontalis into the undersurface of the brow.

lower lid, approximately 5 mm beneath the lower border of the tarsus. Superior to this fusion a single fascial layer then proceeds upward toward the lower tarsal edge (11, 12) (Fig. 1.11). The peripheral orbital septum follows the orbital margin closely, deviating only to follow the superior medial orbital margin inferiorly toward the posterior lacrimal crest behind Horner's muscle. Its attachments then cross the lacrimal diaphragm to the anterior lacrimal crest, whereupon the orbital septum again follows the orbital rim closely deviating only 1 to 2 mm onto the anterior orbital surface along the inferotemporal portion of the rim (1, Fig. 1.7). The septum dips beneath the lateral orbital rim over the lateral canthal tendon and fuses with the tendon and the lateral horn of the levator aponeurosis. The septum can serve as a useful surgical landmark. When little preaponeurotic fat exists, there may be a confusion between the septum and the levator in the upper lid or capsulopalpebral fascia in the lower lid. Traction on the septum will reveal a firm band of attachment to the orbital rim, whereas if levator or capsulopalpebral fascia is grasped, no such band will be found.

Directly beneath the orbital septum are found two fat compartments in the upper lid and three in the lower lid (Fig. 1.6). The preaponeurotic fat pad and nasal fat pads of the upper lids are separated by a thin fascial barrier that passes between the peritrochlear fascia and the orbital septum. The nasal, central, and temporal fat pads of the lower lid are separated respectively by thin fascial sheaths between the inferior oblique and the orbital septum and the capsulopalpebral fascia and the orbital septum (6) (Fig. 1.6). The upper and lower nasal fat pads can be easily identified by their distinct pale-yellow color, which contrasts with the bright-yellow color of the remainder of the anterior orbital fat. This is especially valuable in blepharoplasty surgery. The preaponeurotic fat of the upper lid is bound posteriorly by the levator aponeurosis and inferiorly by the fusion of the levator aponeurosis and the orbital septum. A large pocket of preaponeurotic fat can give a very full appearance to the upper lid. A small pocket of preaponeurotic fat may give a hollow appearance to the upper eyelid. With disinsertion and retraction of the levator aponeurosis, as is often seen in the elderly, the orbital septum and preaponeurotic fat retract into the upper orbit, with the receding aponeurosis causing a characteristic "high lid fold" and a hollowing of the upper eyelid (Fig. 1.9). Eyelid elevation, however, can still be demonstrated because of the attachment of Muller's muscle between the levator muscle and the top of the tarsus.

LEVATOR APONEUROSIS

The levator aponeurosis is the anatomically unique tendon responsible for delivering the force of a horizontally acting muscle, the levator palpebrae superioris, into the vertical and posterior motion of lid elevation. This is done by a unique fascial condensation of levator muscle and tendon, *Whitnall's ligament*.

The levator muscle arises just above the annulus of Zinn from the lesser wing of the sphenoid in the apex of the orbit. It lies immediately above the superior rectus muscle, which supplies its motor nerve and with which it functions synergistically. It passes anteriorly in the orbit, and as it approaches the superior transverse ligament of Whitnall it loses its horizontally oriented muscular elements and becomes aponeurotic (Fig. 1.10).

Whitnall's ligament is a condensation of the muscle sheath of the levator and is suspended in the superior orbit by nasal and temporal attachments so that the levator aponeurosis which hangs vertically below this area is "suspended" from the superior orbit. The fascial condensation of Whitnall's ligament begins in the muscular levator 14 to 20 mm above the tarsus in the adult, and it broadly overlies the zone of transition of muscular levator to aponeurosis (4). Below Whitnall's ligament the levator is entirely aponeurotic with few or no muscle elements. Whitnall's ligament attaches nasally to the fascia of the trochlea and superior oblique tendon (7). Temporally it attaches through the orbital lobe of the lacrimal gland to the superior portion of the inner orbital wall 10 mm above the lateral orbital tubercle. It also sends branches to the medial nd lateral retinacula. Anderson (14) has shown that Whitnall's ligament acts more as a suspensory ligament of the lid than as a check ligament. Upper lid elevation is more restricted by the firm attachments of the medial and lateral levator horns to the medial and lateral ocular retinacula than by the immobility of Whitnall's ligament.

The levator aponeurosis emerges from the lower border of Whitnall's ligament and splits anteriorly into the levator aponeurosis and posteriorly into Muller's muscle. Muller's muscle then travels inferiorly closely bound to the conjunctiva to insert on the top of the tarsus (Fig. 1.2). The

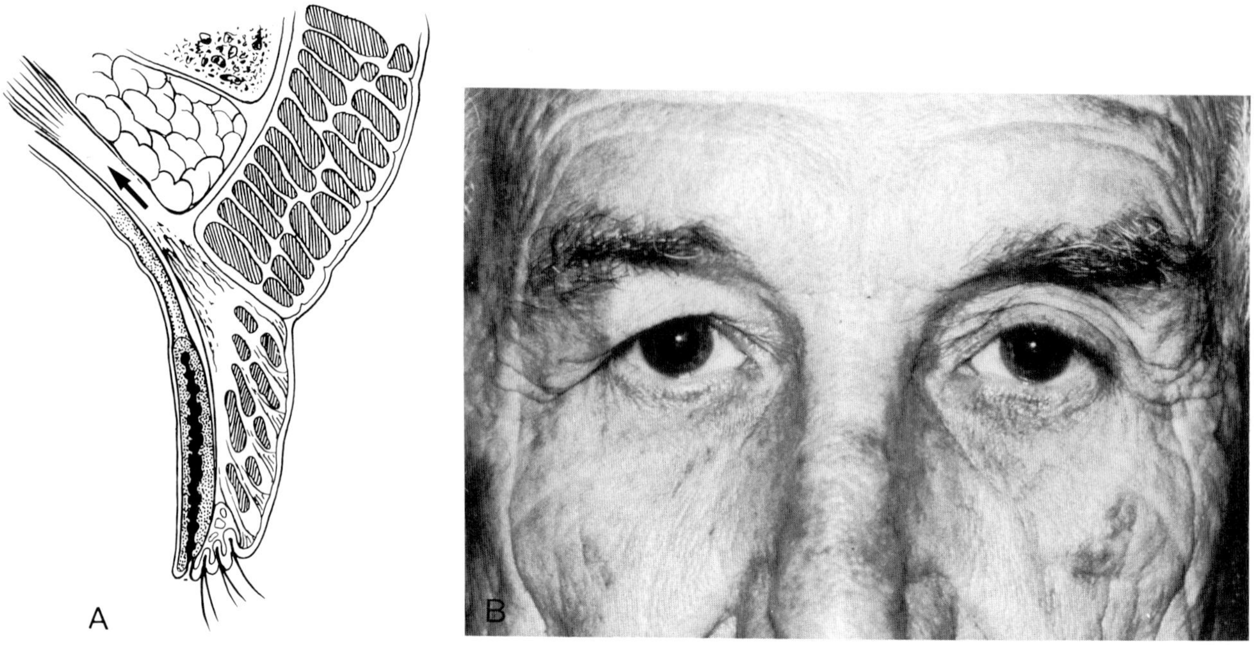

Figure 1.9. *A,* Disinsertion of levator aponeurosis from anterior tarsal surface. Orbital septum and acutaneous attachments to levator persist, causing the lid fold to be pulled superiorly. A high and hollow lid fold is created from retraction of orbital septum and preaponeurotic fat with receding levator aponeurosis into upper orbit. *B,* Patient demonstrating levator disinsertion with ptosis and a high and hollow upper lid fold.

Figure 1.10. Whitnall's ligament and levator aponeurosis.

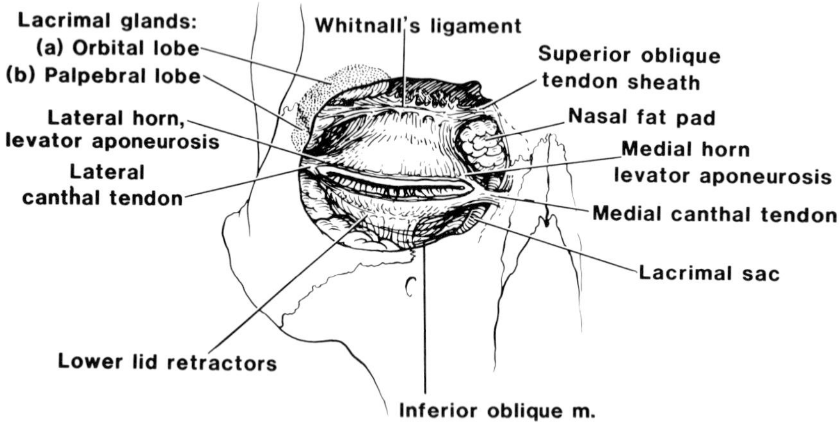

levator aponeurosis fans broadly across the eyelid attaching temporally to the lateral canthal tendon by the firm lateral horn of the levator. It attaches medially to the area of the posterior lacrimal crest, where it blends with fibers from the orbital septum. This medial horn of the levator is much thinner and weaker than the lateral horn (15, Fig. 1.10).

As the broad levator aponeurosis passes inferiorly, it fuses with the orbital septum at the upper eyelid crease, 1 to 3 mm above the tarsus in Occidentals (Fig. 1.2) and 3 to 4 mm below the upper edge of the tarsus in Asians (Fig. 1.3). Below this area of fusion, aponeurosis fibers branch both anteriorly and posteriorly. The aponeurosis' anterior attachments to the orbicularis create the upper eyelid crease and the firm attachment to the pretarsal orbicularis to the tarsus. Posteriorly, the aponeurosis attaches initially to the anterior surface of the tarsus approximately 3 mm above the upper edge of the tarsus. Below that the aponeurosis attaches across the entire anterior surface of the tarsus, being most firmly attached 3 mm above the lid margin (15, Fig. 1.2) (30).

The levator aponeurosis is loosely adherent to Müller's muscle posteriorly, the so-called postaponeurotic space. Within this space temporally is found the accessory palpebral lacrimal gland and the secretory ducts from the lacrimal gland (6). Also in this space just above the tarsus passes the peripheral arterial arcade (1,3). The superior 2 or 3 mm of tarsus is not firmly bound to the levator aponeurosis thereby creating the so-called pretarsal space, a useful surgical landmark in exploration of the levator aponeurosis from the conjunctival surface (16) (Fig. 1.2).

MÜLLER'S MUSCLE

The superior tarsal, or Müller's muscle, is a smooth muscle under cervical sympathetic control. It arises from the area of the posterior terminal fibers of the levator muscle as that muscle is becoming aponeurotic. No direct connections exist, however, between Müller's and levator muscle (17–19). Müller's muscle then descends for 8 to 10 mm as individual fibers mixed with connective tissue, fat, and blood vessels. It adheres closely to the conjunctiva as it inserts onto the top of the tarsus, with a few fibers inserting onto the conjunctiva itself. Innervation of Müller's muscle, while uncertain, is felt by some to travel with the peripheral arterial arcade (4). Loss of innervation to Müller's muscle, as in Horner's syndrome, causes 1 to 2 mm of upper lid ptosis (Fig. 1.2).

TARSUS

The upper and lower tarsi are composed of dense connective tissue and form the posterior, firm "skeleton" of the eyelids. The tarsi extend from just beneath the punctum nasally to within 4 mm of the lateral canthal angle. The upper tarsus is 9 to 10 mm wide in the central lid and tapers toward the nasal and temporal canthi. The lower tarsus averages 3.7 mm in maximal width and likewise tapers away from the center of the lid (20). There are 30 to 40 parallel holocrine sebaceous glands (the meibomian glands) in the upper lid and 20 to 30 in the lower eyelid (3). Nasally and temporally, the tarsi merge with less dense connective tissue that fuses with the medial and lateral canthal tendons. Posteriorly, the tarsi are so firmly attached to the conjunctiva that no cleavage plane can be dissected without destroying the conjunctiva.

CONJUNCTIVA

The conjunctiva follows the globe away from the eye (bulbar conjunctiva) toward the conjunctival fornix. Here it changes direction to descend on the posterior portion of the eyelid (palpebral conjunctiva). In the upper eyelid the fornix is maintained in its position by fibroelastic attachments between the common sheaths of the levator muscle and the superior rectus. In the lower lid, as in the upper, the palpebral conjunctiva is firmly attached to projections of the capsulopalpebral fascia, the lower eyelid retractor (1). Thus the upper fornix is pulled superiorly on upgaze and the lower fornix is pulled inferiorly on downgaze, prevents prolapse of the conjunctiva in these gaze positions.

LACRIMAL GLAND

The lacrimal gland consists of two lobes, the orbital and palpebral, which is partly separated by the lateral horn of the levator aponeurosis. The orbital lobe is located in a shallow depression in the superior temporal orbit just inside the orbital rim, the lacrimal fossa. Its four to six excretory ductules pass through the palpebral lobe, which is smaller. The palpebral lobe is located anteriorly and inferiorly to the orbital lobe and is between the levator aponeurosis and the conjunctiva. It is firmly adherent to the conjunctiva, and its six to eight excretory ductules empty with the ductules from the orbital lobe into the temporal conjunctival sac 4 to 5 mm above the tarsus. The orbital lobe of the gland is supported by the lateral orbital attachments of Whitnall's ligament and by the lateral horn of the levator aponeurosis, as well as by a fine plexus of connective tissue between the periorbita of the roof of the lacrimal fossa (*Soemmering's ligament*) and the connective tissue surrounding the orbital lobe (21). The palpebral lobe is less well supported. Its attachments include the excretory ductules from the orbital lobe, the conjunctival attachments, and its support from the lateral horn of the levator aponeurosis (Fig. 1.10).

DEEP ANATOMY OF THE LOWER EYELID

ORBITAL SEPTUM AND ANTERIOR ORBITAL FAT

Similar to the upper eyelid, the posterior surface of the orbicularis of the lower lid is bound by the posterior orbicular fascia, which is continuous posteriorly with the orbital septum. Only with meticulous dissection can the posterior orbicular fascia be separated from orbital septum. Also as in the upper eyelid, the orbital septum of the lower eyelid is firmly attached to the orbital margin at the arcus marginalis. As the lower eyelid septum rises toward the tarsus, it fuses approximately 5 mm below the lower tarsal edge with the fascia of the lower lid retractor, the capsulopalpebral fascia. A single fascial sheath then proceeds upward to insert on the lower tarsal edge (11, Fig. 1.11). Posterior to the septum, the anterior orbital fat is bound superiorly by the capsulopalpebral fascia and inferiorly by the periorbita of the orbital floor.

CAPSULOPALPEBRAL FASCIA

The capsulopalpebral fascia (CPF) is a structure of the lower lid that is comparable with the levator aponeurosis. Its anatomy, however, differs in important respects. Whereas the levator of the upper lid is a true and distinct striated muscle with a tendon, the CPF is a fibroelastic extension of the inferior rectus muscle with no striated muscle elements. It serves only to transmit inferior rectus muscle pull to the lower lid and conjunctival fornix on downgaze. The capsulopalpebral head arises from the inferior rectus near the junction of the muscle and tendon. At the origin, smooth muscle elements of the inferior tarsal muscle are absent. They appear a short distance beyond (11). Within a short distance of its origin, the capsulopalpebral head splits into a larger superior and a smaller inferior portion that surround the inferior oblique muscle. These portions re-fuse anteriorly to the inferior oblique muscle, contributing Lockwood's ligament (Fig. 1.11). Anterior to Lockwood's ligament the retractor fascia is called "the capsulopalpebral fascia." It proceeds anteriorly and superiorly to fuse with the orbital septum approximately 5 mm below the lower tarsal edge, and above that a single fascial sheath passes upward to attach onto the lower border of the tarsus. Disinsertion of this layer may cause congenital (22) or acquired entropion (23, 24) or ectropion (25). Additional fascial strands from the CPF pass anteriorly and insert into the orbital septum, and others pass inferiorly to insert in the periorbita of the orbital floor. Additionally, the CPF has projections to the conjunctiva that blend with Tenon's capsule, as well as

Figure 1.11. Lower eyelid capsulopalpebral head is derived from inferior rectus muscle and splits to surround inferior oblique, then rejoins as the capsulopalpebral fascia contributing to Lockwood's ligament (see text).

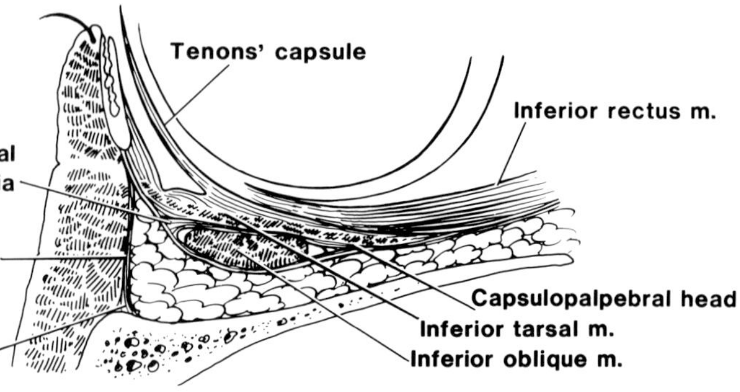

projections to the conjunctival fornix that act as a suspensory ligament (Fig. 1.12).

The CPF inserts onto the lower border of the tarsus as well as onto its posterior and anterior surfaces (11). Projections from it penetrate the preseptal orbicularis to insert subcutaneously and create the lower eyelid crease. Dryden and associates (26) maintained that, as with the levator aponeurosis of the upper lid, projections of the CPF insert subcutaneously in the pretarsal area, binding the skin to the anterior surface of the tarsus.

LOCKWOOD'S LIGAMENT

Support for the globe is provided by the inferior transverse ligament, which is called Lockwood's ligament. Unlike the superior transverse ligament of Whitnall, which has few attachments to the medial and lateral retinacula, Lockwood's ligament's major support comes from these retinacula. The fascial confluences that occur as the inferior oblique muscle passes through the CPH provide the major contribution to Lockwood's ligament (Figs. 1.10 and 1.11). In addition, Lockwood's ligament has contributions from the intermuscular septum, the inferior tarsal muscle and the medial and lateral check ligaments (7).

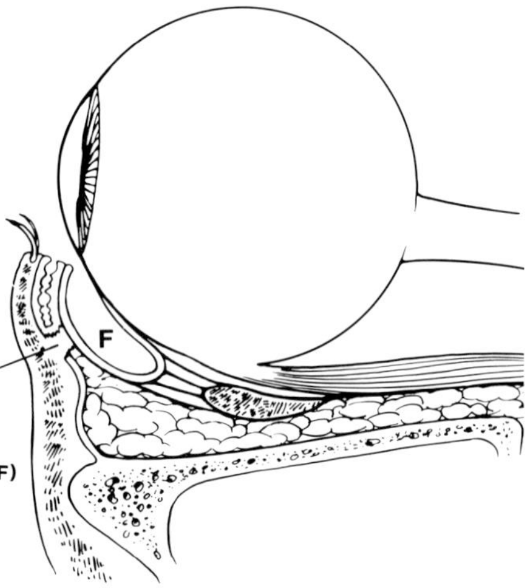

Figure 1.12. Lower eyelid entropion with disinsertion of lower eyelid retractors from lower tarsal edge. Projections from the capsulopalpebral fascia shown inserting into Tenon's capsule and the conjunctival fornix.

INNERVATION

Sensory innervation of the upper eyelid and anterior orbit is provided by branches of the first, ophthalmic division of the fifth cranial nerve. The second, maxillary division of the fifth cranial nerve provides sensory innervation for the lower eyelid.

Behind the orbit in the anterior aspect of the cavernous sinus the ophthalmic division of the trigeminac nerve divides into three branches: the lacrimal, frontal, and nasociliary nerves. The lacrimal nerve enters the orbit through the superior orbital fissure and passes anteriorly along the upper border of the lateral rectus muscle. Posterior to the orbital lobe of the lacrimal gland it may be joined by an anastomotic branch from the zygomaticotemporal nerve. This branch carries post–ganglionic parasympathetic secretomotor fibers to the lacrimal gland, which control its secretion. The lacrimal nerve passes through the lacrimal gland and penetrates the orbital septum to supply sensation to the lateral aspect of the upper eyelid (Fig. 1.13).

The frontal nerve passes into the orbit through the superior orbital fissure and travels anteriorly between the levator muscle and the periorbita. It divides into the supraorbital and supratrochlear nerves. The supraorbital nerve exits the orbit through the supraorbital notch and innervates the central portion of the upper eyelid, the eyebrow, and the forehead and scalp. The supratrochlear nerve penetrates the septum superiomedially and courses upward to supply the medial upper eyelid, eyebrow, and central forehead (Figs. 1.13 and 1.14).

The nasociliary division of the ophthalmic nerve enters the orbit through the annulus of Zinn and sends several sensory branches to the globe. One branch passes without synapsing through the ciliary ganglion; two long posterior ciliary branches innervate the globe without passing through the ciliary ganglion. The nasociliary nerve then passes anteriorly, giving off the anterior ethmoidal nerve to supply the sinuses and other structures. Finally, the nasociliary nerve, as the infratrochlear nerve, penetrates the orbital septum to supply sensation to the medial aspect of the upper eyelid and the side of the nose.

The maxillary nerve leaves the cranium through the foramen rotundum and then enters the pterygopalatine fossa. Here, the nerve divides into the infraorbital, zygomatic, and inferior alveolar nerves. The infraorbital nerve passes anteriorly along the infraorbital groove and then exists at the infraorbital foramen, where it provides sensation to the lower eyelid. The zygomatic nerve receives parasympathetic lacrimal secretomotor fibers from the sphenopalatine ganglion in the pterygoid fossa. The zygomatic nerve then enters the orbit through the inferior orbital fissure and divides into the zygomaticotemporal and zygomaticofacial nerves. The zygomaticotemporal nerve passes along the lateral wall of the orbit and then exits the orbit through the foramen of the same name and provides sensation to the lateral aspect of the forehead. Before exiting the orbit, however, the zygomaticotemporal nerve gives off the parasympathetic fibers that pass anteriorly and then join the lacrimal gland directly or join the lacrimal gland via the lacrimal nerve (Fig. 1.13).

The zygomaticofacial nerve passes anteriorly along the inferolateral orbital wall and exits through a foramen of the same name. It provides sensation to the lateral lower eyelid and cheek.

VASCULARIZATION

The arterial supply of the upper eyelid and brow is derived principally from the internal carotid artery through its ophthalmic artery branches. The lower lid is supplied principally by the external carotid artery through its facial, maxillary, and superficial temporal branches. Numerous anastomoses exist between the arteries of the upper and lower lids and thus between the internal and external carotid arteries.

The branches of the ophthalmic artery that supply the upper lid include the lacrimal, supraorbital, supratrochlear, dorsonasal, and medial palpebral. The lacrimal artery arises from the ophthalmic artery posteriorly in the orbit as it ascends to pass over the optic nerve. It travels anteriorly between the lateral rectus and superior rectus. It gives off the zygomaticofacial and zygomaticotemporal branches, which exit the orbit laterally through foramina of the same name to supply the lateral aspect of the orbit and forehead. The lacrimal artery penetrates and supplies the lacrimal gland and then pierces the orbital septum to end in the two lateral palpebral arteries. These arteries pass inferiorly, one to the upper lid and one to the lower lid, and then course medially across the eyelids to anastomose with the medial palpebral arteries and thereby create the arterial arcades of the upper and lower lids (1, Fig. 1.15).

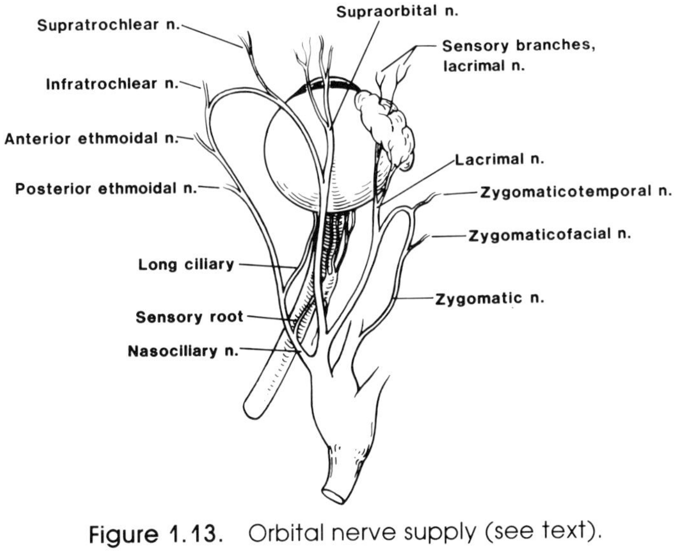

Figure 1.13. Orbital nerve supply (see text).

The supraorbital artery arises from the ophthalmic artery posteriorly in the orbit and passes anteriorly, with the supraorbital nerve between the levator and the periorbita. It exits with the nerve through the supraorbital foramen to supply the upper lid, the eyebrows, and the forehead.

The supratrochlear and dorsonasal arteries are the terminal branches of the ophthalmic artery. The supratrochlear artery pierces the orbital septum in the medial aspect of the upper lid, and it proceeds superiorly to supply the scalp and forehead. The dorsonasal artery pierces the orbital septum just below the supratrochlear artery and proceeds inferiorly to anastomose with the facial artery; creating the angular artery, which supplies the medial canthal area, the lacrimal sac, and the central forehead.

The medial palpebral arteries arise as two branches from the ophthalmic artery below the trochlea. The superior branch passes to the upper lid; the inferior branch passes to the lower lid. Both branches then travel laterally along the lids to anastomose with the corresponding lateral palpebral arteries and form the arcades. The marginal arcades are located between the orbicularis and the tarsus 4 mm above the lid margin in the upper lid and 2 mm below the margin in the lower lid. The peripheral arcades are found at the top and the bottom of their respective tarsi.

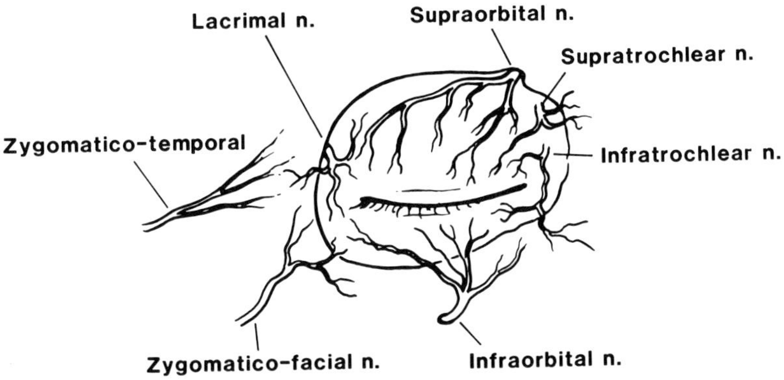

Figure 1.14. Cutaneous branches of sensory nerves (see text).

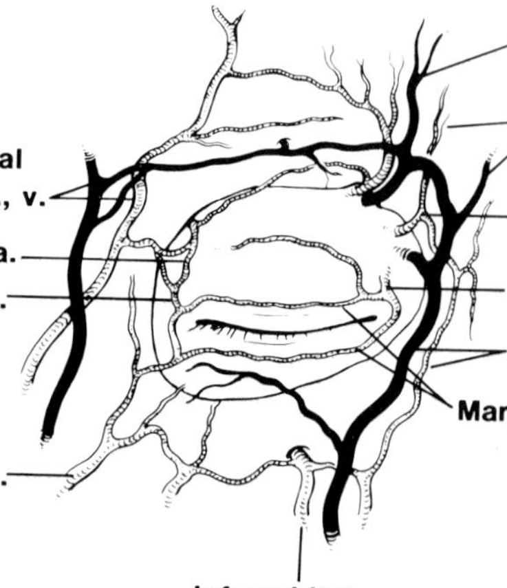

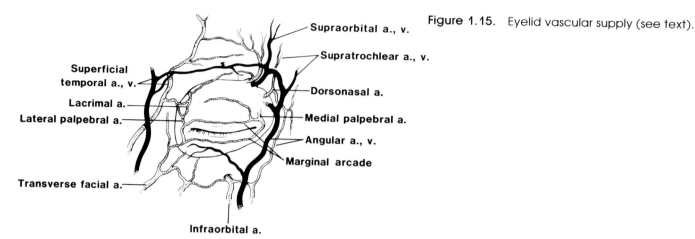

Figure 1.15. Eyelid vascular supply (see text).

The facial, superficial temporal and maxillary branches of the external carotid artery provide the principal blood supply to the lower lid. The facial artery passes superomedially across the face towards the medial canthal area where it is called the angular artery.

The superficial temporal artery gives rise to the transverse facial artery which supplies the lateral lower lid and which anastomoses with the infraorbital artery. The infraorbital artery is derived from the external carotid artery through the maxillary branch in the pterygopalatine fossa. From here the infraorbital artery enters the orbit through the infraorbital fissure and follows the nerve of the same name anteriorly in the infraorbital groove. It exits the orbit through the infraorbital foramen and supplies the lower lid and upper cheek area.

EYEBROWS

Eyebrows represent a specialized area of the forehead that functions as an integral part with the eyelids and muscles of the face to communicate emotions and facial expressions. The eyebrows function closely with the eyelids to protect and maintain the globe. They are morphologically part of the scalp, originating within the galae aponeurotica, which is connected to the occipitalis muscle posteriorly. The eyebrows may also serve as an important indicator of both localized and systemic disease processes.

The eyebrows are formed by the characteristic hair distribution, underlying muscle layer, connective tissue and fat, as well as by the galea aponeurotica and supraciliary ridge of the frontal bone. The color, size, hair density, shape of hair distribution, and brow position are typically symmetric and distinctive in each individual. Poliosis, or a whitening of the hair of the eyebrows and eyelashes, occurs most commonly in the elderly. It is seen also in the Vogt-Koyanagi-Harada syndrome, Waadenburg's syndrome, albinism, and leprosy. An abnormally coarse hair density of the eyebrows may be a normal variation or consistent with Hurler's syndrome (MPS I), Hunter's syndrome (MPS II), Sanfilippo's syndrome (MPS III), Rubinstein-Tayki syndrome, or congenital hypothyroidism (cretinism) (28). A low eyebrow position is usually associated with a straight brow, whereas a brow above the superior orbital rim is typically curved convexly upward. This latter shape and position is more common in females; most commonly the intersupraciliary region, or glabella, is hairless. When the brows are confluent and meet in the midline without interruption, the condition is called *synophrys.* Synophrys may be a variation of normal or a part of the following syndromes: Cornelia de Lange, Waadenburg, basal cell nevus, or Trisomy 13 (28).

Three types of eyebrow hairs exist: fine vellus hairs, pigmented medium sized terminal hairs and large supracilia. The male hair is usually heavier, but even in the bushiest eyebrow, over one-half of the hair population is made of the fine small vellus hairs (29). These fine hairs are closely spaced and form an effective moisture barrier deflecting liquids such as sweat from the eyes. Though rarely necessary for surgery, the brows may be clipped or shaved and the hairs will regrow. The large hairs of the brow are the first to develop embryologically, and these supracilia hair follicles do not have arrectores pilorum (29). The pattern of hair growth is generally directed laterally or upward, but in the most nasal portion they may grow medially. Hair growth is parallel to the supraorbital rim, and in the lateral aspect, the supracilia are often pointed downward. The direction of hair growth is important in positioning the scalpel blade when making incisions through the brow. The correct angle of the blade follows the hair shafts and avoids transecting them. The hairs of the eyebrow have extensive sensory innervation, such that any tactile stimulation to the eyebrow or forehead results in reflex closure of the eyelids to protect the eye.

The skin of the eyebrow is thicker than that of the eyelid and similar to skin of the upper face (29). There are no sweat glands present in the skin of the brow area; therefore, the numerous sebaceous glands create an oily secretion that coats the hairs of the brow, adding a hydrophobic film that enhances the moisture barrier and gutter mechanism for deflecting liquids from the eyes. The skin of the brow has a high degree of mobility, primarily because of numerous elastic muscle slip insertions from the frontalis muscle and superior orbital portion of the orbicularis. In addition, the subcutaneous tissue contains fibrous tissue that firmly binds the muscle layer to the skin, enhancing the mobility of the brow.

The eyebrows may be raised, lowered, or drawn towards the midline in conjunction with movements of the scalp, and may be elevated or depressed with changes in the direction of vision.

The muscle layer includes the frontalis muscle, the orbicularis, the obliquely oriented corrugator muscle lying between these first two muscles, and the procerus. The frontalis muscle arises from the epicranial aponeurosis about midway between the coronal suture and superior orbital margins. It inserts in the skin of the eyebrow and has no bony attachments (Fig. 1.8). It functions to aid in elevating the eyelid a maximum of an additional 3 to 5 mm, thereby acting as a synergist to the levator palpebrae superioris. The frontalis muscle is the antagonist muscle of the orbicularis muscle. These two muscles exhibit reciprocal innervation patterns; one muscle relaxes while the other relaxes. There is an interdigitation of the orbicularis muscle with the terminal fibers of the frontalis muscle at the superior orbital rim.

Medially, the corrugator supracilii muscle attaches to the superomedial orbital rim and inserts through the frontalis-orbicularis interdigitation into the cutaneous part of the eyebrow (Fig. 1.5). The action of the corrugator is to pull the brow downward and medially, creating vertical folds in the glabellar area, such as while frowning. The corrugator muscle is assisted in pulling the eyebrows medially by the procerus muscle, which has a bony attachment at the nasal bones. All four muscles interdigitate extensively in the eyebrow region, making distinct dissection difficult. The epicranial muscles are all innervated by the temporal branches of the seventh cranial nerve. The nerves enter each muscle on its deep surface near its lateral border.

Embryologically, the orbicularis oculi, corrugator supraciliaris, and procerus muscle develop from the infraorbital lamina; the frontalis muscle develops from the temporal lamina. These lamina interdigitate just above the eye forming the muscular component of the brow at the 37 mm embryo stage (10).

The eyebrow fat pad separates the frontalis-orbicularis layer anteriorly from the galea aponeurotica layer posteriorly. This posterior layer continues anteriorly into the upper lid as orbital septum. The eyebrow fat pad space continues just anterior to the septum into the upper lid as a filmy areolar tissue that may variably contain fat (Fig. 1.8). If the brow fat extends lower into the lid than usual, this may occasionally be mistaken for the preaponeurotic space and fat beneath the septum. With age there may be a decrease in the brow fat pad, allowing greater mobility of the brow. The deep bony fat pad attachments would then act as the check ligament medially.

The galea aponeurotica is divided into deep and superficial layers, which surround the frontalis and orbicularis muscle as a sheath. The deep galea forms the anterior boundary of the eyebrow fat pad and attaches along the medial two-thirds of the supraorbital ridge (Fig. 1.8). The muscle layer has little attachment laterally, which accounts for more severe brow ptosis occurring in this lateral area. Posteriorly, the galea is attached to the occipitalis muscle (10).

The prominence of the eyebrows is formed by the transverse elevation of the supraciliary ridge of the frontal bone over which the brow lies. It extends over the frontal sinuses nasally and to the zygomaticofrontal suture temporally. The supraciliary ridge is less prominent in females.

The facial nerve nucleus receives bilateral cortical innervation; therefore, the eyebrow muscles remain largely unaffected by supranuclear lesions, while the lower facial muscle will be completely involved. However, a peripheral facial nerve palsy will cause the ipsilateral frontalis muscle to loose tone and the brow to become ptotic. In the patient with a third nerve palsy causing levator dysfunction and lid ptosis, the brow will be typically arched and elevated more by the action of the frontalis in an attempt to elevate the lid. This brow action can raise a drooping lid an additional 3 to 5 mm.

Conversely, if a peripheral facial nerve palsy develops, the frontalis on the homolateral side will lose its normal tone and sag to a lower position. Therefore, with a third nerve palsy the brow on the affected side will be higher than normal, and with a peripheral seventh nerve palsy the brow on the affected side will be lower.

ACKNOWLEDGMENT

This study was supported in part by a grant from the French Hospital Foundation for Medical Research and Education, San Francisco, California.

REFERENCES

1. Warwick R: *Eugene Wolff's Anatomy of the Eye and Orbit*. E07, Philadelphia, W.B. Saunders, 1976.
2. Clemente CD: *Gray's Anatomy*. Philadelphia, Lea & Febiger, 1985.
3. Jones LT, Wobig JL: *Surgery of the Eyelids and Lacrimal System*. Birmingham, Aesculapius, 1976.
4. Anderson RL, Beard C: The levator aponeurosis. Attachments and their clinical significance. *Arch Ophthalmol* 95: 1437, 1977.
5. Doxanas MT, Anderson RL: Oriental Eyelids. An anatomic study. *Arch Ophthalmol* 102: 1232, 1984.
6. Doxanas MT, Anderson RL: *Clinical Orbital Anatomy*. Baltimore, Williams & Wilkins, 1984.
7. Beard C, Quickert M: *Anatomy of the Orbit*. Birmingham, Aesculapius, 1977.
8. Kuwabara TK, Cogan DG, Johnson GC: Structure of the muscles of the upper eyelid. *Arch Ophthalmol* 93: 1189, 1975.
9. Anderson RL: Medial canthal tendon branches out. *Arch Ophthalmol* 100: 981, 1982.
10. Lemke BN, Stasior OG: The anatomy of eyebrow ptosis. *Arch Ophthalmol* 100: 981, 1982.
11. Hawes MJ, Dortzbach RK: The microscopic anatomy of the lower eyelid retractors. *Arch Ophthalmol* 57: 943, 1964.
12. Putterman AM, Urist MJ: Surgical anatomy of the orbital septum. *Ann Ophthalmol* 8: 319, 1974.
13. Jones LT: The anatomy of the upper eyelid and its relation to ptosis surgery. *Am J Ophthalmol* 57: 943, 1964.
14. Anderson RL, Dixon RS: The role of Whitnall's ligament in ptosis surgery. *Arch Ophthalmol* 97: 705, 1979.
15. Colin JRO, Beard C, Wood I: Experimental and clinical data on the insertion of the levator palpebrae superioris muscle. *Am J Ophthalmol* 85: 792, 1978.
16. Beard C: *Ptosis*. St. Louis, CV Mosby, 1976.
17. Beard C: Muller's superior tarsal muscle: anatomy, physiology and clinical significance. *Ann Plast Surg* 14: 324, 1985.
18. Isaksson J: Studies on congenital genuine blepharoptosis. *ACTA Ophthalmol* T2 (Suppl): 18, 1962.
19. Berke RN, Wadsworth JAC: Histology of levator muscle in congenital and acquired ptosis. *Arch Ophthalmol* 53: 413, 1955.

20. Wesley RE, McCord CD, Jones NA: Height of the tarsus of the lower eyelid. *Am J Ophthalmol* 90: 102, 1980.
21. Milder B, Weil BA: *The Lacrimal System.* Norwalk, Connecticut, Appleton-Century-Crofts, 1983.
22. Tse DT, Anderson RL, Fratkins JD: Aponeurosis disinsertion in congenital entropion. *Arch Ophthalmol* 101: 436, 1983.
23. Collin JRO, Rathbun JE: Involuntional entropion. *Arch Ophthalmol* 96: 1058, 1978.
24. Dryden RM, Leibsohn J: Levator aponeurosis in blepharoplasty. *Ophthalmology* 85: 718, 1978.
25. Putterman AM: Ectropion of the lower eyelid secondary to Muller muscle-capsulopalpebral fascia detachment. *Am J Ophthalmol* 85: 814, 1978.
26. Dryden RM, Leibsohn J, Wobig J: Senile entropion. *Arch Ophthalmol* 96: 1883, 1978.
27. Jones LT: Anatomy of the lower eyelid. *Am J Ophthalmol* 49: 29, 1960.
28. Roy FH: *Ocular Differential Diagnosis*, ed 2. Philadelphia, Lea & Febiger.
29. Records RE: Eyebrows and eyelids. In Duane TD, Jaeger EA: *Biomedical Foundations of Ophthalmology*. Philadelphia, Harper & Row, 1982, vol 2.
30. Hornblass A, Adachi M, Wolintz A, Smith B: Clinical and ultrastructural correlation in congenital and acquired ptosis. *Ophthal Surg* 7: 69–78, 1976.

CHAPTER 2

Physiology and Neurology of the Eyelid

CARL J. HANIG, M.D.
ALBERT HORNBLASS, M.D., F.A.C.S.

The primary function of the eyelids and eyebrows is to synchronously protect the globe from external injury, while preventing the cornea from drying out. Another function of the eyelids is to regulate the amount of light entering the eye. Also, the eyelids and eyebrows play a major role in facial expressions (1). This chapter will discuss the function of the eyelids in relation to their anatomic design, as well as the neuroophthalmic mechanisms that make these functions possible. The physiology of the eyebrow is discussed elsewhere in this text.

SKIN AND APPENDAGES

The skin of the eyelids is one of the thinnest in the body. Its elasticity and loose attachment to underlying structures (except at the brow and lid margin) are important to its function as the covering layer to eyelid structures; these features also provide a potential space for inflammatory exudation and infection. Loss of elasticity later in life may result in excess eyelid skin obstructing the visual field (*hooding*) (2). This skin is covered by vellus hair follicles with adjacent sebaceous glands. Eyelid skin and follicles are abundantly supplied with a network of nerve endings (3).

The eyelid skin includes several creases: an upper eyelid crease, a lower eyelid crease, a malar crease, and a nasojugal crease (Fig. 2.1). The upper crease is formed by the insertion of levator aponeurosis fibers into the subcutaneous layer. This crease is lower and more poorly developed in the Oriental eyelid, in which the orbital septum fuses with the levator below the superior tarsal border, and the inferior extension of preaponeurotic fat produces an upper lid fullness. The lower eyelid crease is formed analogously by the insertion of the capsulopalpebral fascia fibers. The higher fusion of this structure with the orbital septum in orientals may produce a fuller lower lid, or epiblepharon (4). The malar and nasojugal creases demarcate the inferior border of eyelid skin. They are fixed to bone and limit the spread of fluids between the eyelids and lower face.

The cilia (eyelashes) protect the eye from foreign material. They are arranged in five to six rows in the upper lid, and three to four rows in the lower lid. The uneven arrangement of the rows allows for the loss of cilia without leaving gaps in the protective barrier they provide. The cilia lack arrector pili muscles, but the follicles are surrounded by the garlands of cholinesterase reactive nerve fibers (as are the glands of Zeiss and Moll), suggesting their importance in the protective blink reflex (3).

SENSORY INNERVATION

The upper eyelid is supplied by the ophthalmic division of the trigeminal nerve. This purely sensory nerve arises from the trigeminal (Gasserian) ganglion and enters the cavernous sinus where, after giving proprioceptive branches to the oculomotor, trochlear, and abducens nerves, as well as dural and tentorial branches, it divides

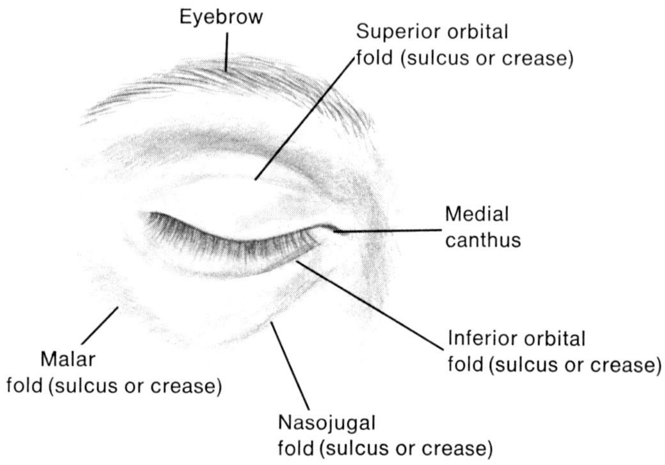

Figure 2.1. Surface anatomy of the eyelids. (From Hornblass A: *Tumors of the Ocular Adnexa and Orbit.* St. Louis, CV Mosby, 1979.)

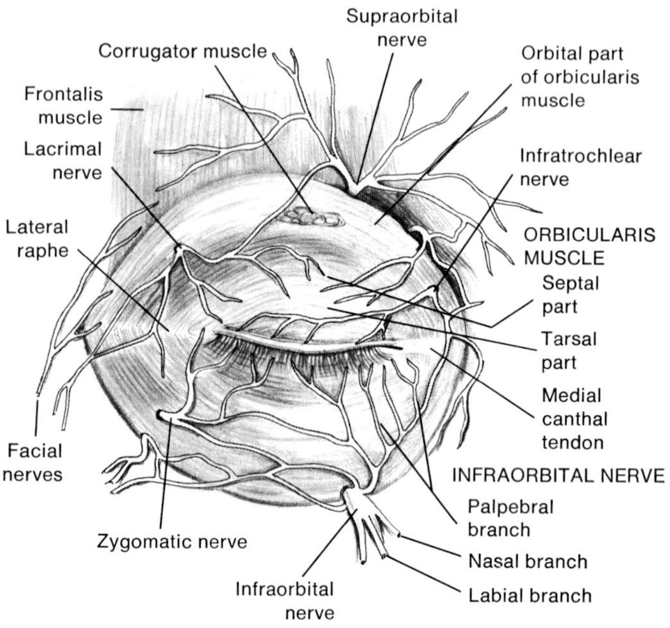

Figure 2.2. Sensory nerves of the eyelids (From Hornblass A: *Tumors of the Ocular Adnexa and Orbit.* St. Louis, CV Mosby, 1979.)

into the frontal, lacrimal, and nasociliary nerves. These enter the orbit via the superior orbital fissure.

The *lacrimal nerve* divides, with the upper division supplying upper lid skin and conjunctiva, and the lower anastomosing with a branch of the maxillary division. The *frontal nerve*, after giving off the supratrochlear nerve to the forehead, becomes the *supraorbital nerve*, and exits through the supraorbital notch, innervating the upper lid, forehead, and frontal sinus. The *nasociliary nerve* supplies the ciliary ganglion and long ciliary nerves to the globe; the infratrochlear nerve to the medial canthus, upper lid skin and conjunctiva, and lower lid; and nasal fibers to the anterior septum and lateral nasal walls, middle and inferior turbinates, and skin of the tip of the nose.

The lower eyelid is supplied primarily by the maxillary division of the trigeminal nerve. This purely sensory nerve passes from the trigeminal ganglion, through the middle cranial fossa (where it is embedded in dura lateral to the cavernous sinus), through the foramen rotundum into the pterygopalatine fossa. Here it gives off the sphenopalatine, posterior superior alveolar (supplies maxillary sinus, upper molars, and gums), and zygomatic nerves before passing through the inferior orbital fissure to become the *infraorbital nerve.*

The infraorbital nerve passes through the infraorbital groove, exiting through the infraorbital foramen to supply the lower lid, side of the nose, and upper lip. The *zygomatic nerve* also traverses the infraorbital fissure into the orbit, where it divides into the *zygomaticofacial nerve* (supplying the skin over the zygoma), and the zygomaticotemporal, which anastomoses with the lacrimal nerve, carrying with it parasympathetic fibers. Additional alveolar branches from the infraorbital nerve, arising in the infraorbital groove, supply the premolar upper teeth and gums (Fig. 2.2–2.4).

ASCENDING PATHWAYS

The sensory divisions of the trigeminal nerve enter the brainstem on the anterior aspect of the pons, together with the smaller motor division. Most sensory fibers descend in the *spinal trigeminal tract* to reach the nucleus of the spinal tract. This nucleus mediates primarily the perception of pain and temperature. The more rostral *main sensory nucleus* also receives sensory fibers and mediates the sense of touch. Fibers from both nuclei cross the midline and then project to connections in the thalamus. A third sensory nucleus, the *mesencephalic nucleus*, receives projections primarily from the muscles of mastication and oral cavity and is felt to be involved in proprioceptive mechanisms (5).

THE PALPEBRAL FISSURE

The palpebral fissure is a critical consideration in ophthalmic plastic surgery. Fox (6) studied the palpebral fissure in a group of 1732 patients. The most frequent adult length was 28 mm, with 83% of patients between 25 and 30 mm. Most growth occurred in the first 10 years of life (from a length between 18 and 21 mm in infants under 1 year of age). The average fissure width was between 8 and 11 mm (93.7%), with minimal growth after the first few weeks of life.

Movement of the palpebral fissure is closely related to movement of the globe. In upgaze and downgaze, action by the extraocular muscles and shifts in the distribution of the orbital contents result in a rotation of the plane of the palpebral fissure to remain perpendicular to the visual axis. Analogous rotations in position of the canthi on medial and lateral gaze are noted. Retraction of the globe, as in Duane's syndrome, results in a retraction and narrowing of the palpebral fissure. The involvement of the palpebral fissure in the lacrimal tear pump and its secretory function are discussed elsewhere in this text (7).

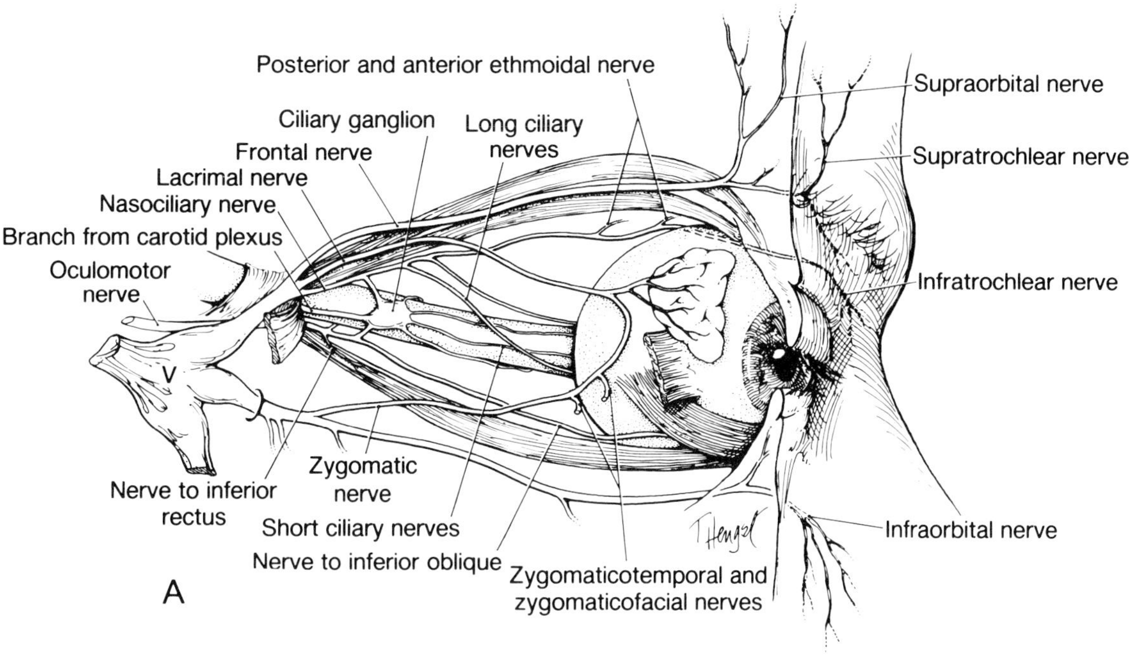

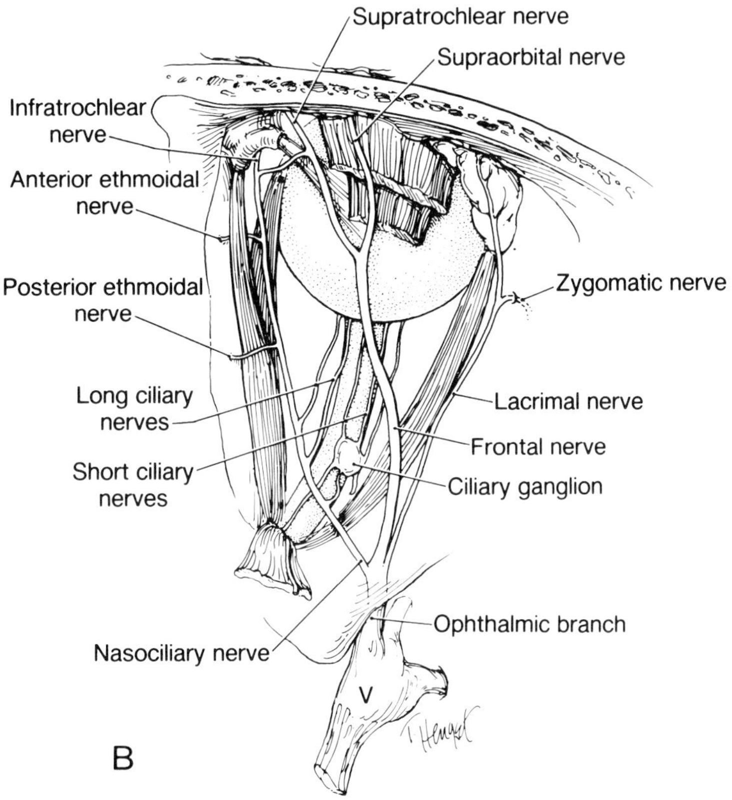

Figure 2.3. Branches of the ophthalmic division of the trigeminal nerve. *A*, From laterally. *B*, From above. (From Miller RN: In Walsh, Hoyt (eds): *Clinical Neuro-ophthalmology*, ed 4. Baltimore, Williams & Wilkins, 1985, vol 2.)

EYELID MOTILITY

The upper and lower eyelids form a complex system of movements, which can be thought of as two opposing motor systems, one for opening and one for closing the palpebral fissures. These systems involve both voluntary and involuntary controls, via the oculomotor and facial nerves, as well as the sympathetic nervous system. The

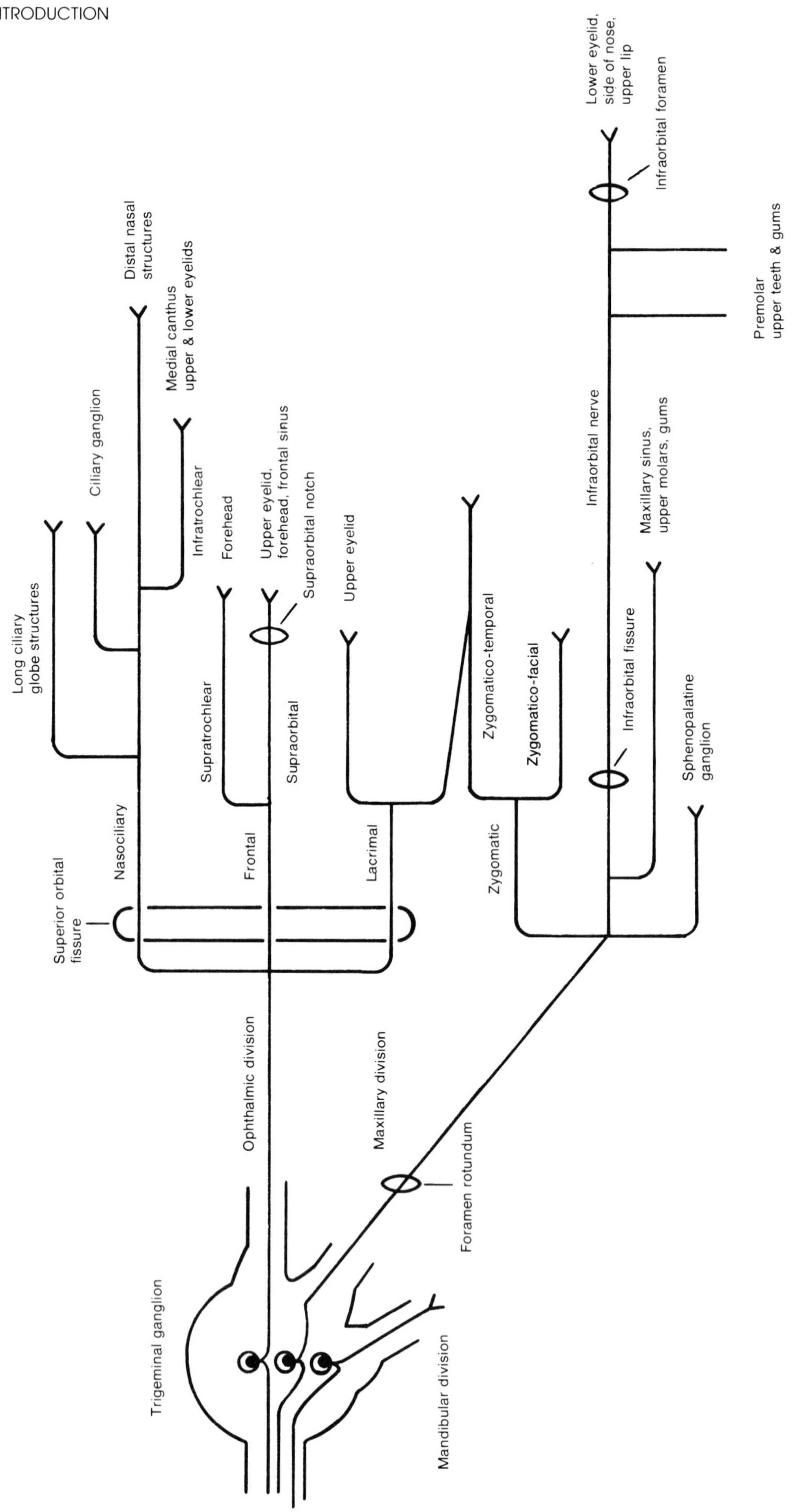

Figure 2.4. Schema of trigeminal nerve.

opening and closing mechanisms will be considered separately, but in actuality these mechanisms act in coordination with each other.

OPENING MOVEMENTS

The Upper Eyelid

The action of elevation of the upper eyelid is accomplished primarily via the *levator palpebrae*. This voluntary skeletal muscle is innervated by the superior branch of the oculomotor nerve. *Mueller's muscle* (superior palpebral muscle) originates from the underside of the levator. This involuntary smooth muscle receives its sympathetic innervation via the oculomotor nerve, which picks up sympathetic fibers from the carotid artery in the cavernous sinus (5). The levator is responsible for raising the upper lid, while Müller's muscle aids the levator in maintaining this position. Müller's muscle also reflects changes in the state of arousal and the activity of the sympathetic nervous system (e.g., drooping in states of drowsiness and fatigue or retraction in fright and anger). The action of this muscle may be demonstrated by topical agents, i.e., adrenergic agents will increase lid retraction, while guanethidine will decrease it (8).

The upper lid follows the visual axis closely on vertical movements. This movement has been shown to be solely a function of the levator, with progressively increasing electrical activity within the levator as gaze moves progressively higher. No orbicularis activity is noted in this action, as shown by electromyographic studies (9). This following movement has also been found to be independent of gravity. Control of this following movement is cortical and is related to the control of vertical shifts of the visual axis in the occipital cortex (8).

The levator muscles of both upper eyelids are bilaterally and equally innervated. This extension of *Hering's law*, which was originally applied to pairs of extraocular yoke muscles, is frequently demonstrated in patients presenting with a unilateral ptosis. In an attempt to elevate the ptotic eyelid, excess innervation is supplied to that lid's levator muscle and, by Hering's law of equal innervation to agonist muscles, to the contralateral levator muscle as well. The result is a contralateral upper lid *retraction*, which will resolve with correction of the opposite lid's ptosis (10, 11). In considering this phenomenon, one must recall that both levator muscles receive their innervation from a single midline nucleus at the caudal end of the oculomotor nucleus (Fig. 2.4).

The eyelid muscles also obey *Sherrington's law* of reciprocal innervation. Electromyographic studies show complete absence of orbicularis activity in different positions of gaze, including extreme downgaze, and a corresponding inhibition of the levator on voluntary eye closure. Changes from extreme upward to downward gaze are produced by variations in the innervation supplied to the levator muscle, with no involvement of the orbicularis.

Levator function. Adequate evaluation of levator function is critical in ptosis surgery and will be considered in greater detail elsewhere in this volume. For the purpose of this discussion several key points will be mentioned briefly. First, evaluation of the levator muscle must be isolated from the action of the frontalis muscle, which may add up to 5 mm of lid elevation. In Beard's classification, over 8 mm of levator excursion constitutes good levator function, with 15 mm of excursion considered normal. Two millimeters of excursion is attributed to transmitted movement from the superior rectus muscle. Because of its origination from the levator muscle, Müller's muscle will not give any lid elevation in the absence of levator function (1).

One must consider the role of Whitnall's ligament in lid elevation. This condensation of fibrous tissue in the superior orbit directs the elevating action of the levator muscle, whose fibers generate a primarily posteriorly directed force of contraction. The importance of preserving this structure in ptosis surgery is stressed (12).

The Lower Eyelid

Unlike the upper eyelid, the lower eyelid lacks a voluntary muscle for opening movements. The lower lid retractors are the *capsulopalpebral fascia* and *inferior palpebral muscle*. The capsulopalpebral head originates from the inferior rectus muscle (thus the corresponding movement of the lower lid in downgaze) and divides into two portions in order to fuse with the capsule of the inferior oblique muscle (the location of the inferior oblique makes it susceptible to injury during surgery of the lower lid retractors). These two portions then join anterior to the inferior oblique muscle to form *Lockwood's ligament*, which then continued anteriorly as the capsulopalpebral fascia to insert into the lower tarsal border.

The inferior palpebral muscle is analogous to Müller's muscle of the upper lid and is under sympathetic control. It originates from the capsulopalpebral head of the inferior rectus muscle and is concentrated in the region of the inferior fornix. Studies have indicated that the inferior palpebral muscle does not insert into the tarsal border. The theory of capsulopalpebral disinsertion in entropion and ectropion was not upheld in one recent study, although the termination of the inferior palpebral muscle was further from the tarsal border in these cases than in controls (13, 14)

Supranuclear Control

The corticobulbar and extrapyramidal systems both contribute to the levator nucleus, and levator tonus is related to the level of arousal. Levator action is linked to and parallels that of the superior rectus muscle in all positions of gaze. The notable exception is during forced lid closure, where the levator is inhibited while the superior rectus is activated (*Bell's phenomenon*).

Synkinesis between the levator and trigeminal nuclei is sometimes observed and may be either a normal occurrence, as in a child who simultaneously opens the mouth and eyes widely, or an abnormal one, as in the *Marcus Gunn phenomenon* [discussed elsewhere in this text (15)]. Supranuclear abnormalities of levator innervation may result in ptosis (although this is much more frequently secondary to a sympathetic deficiency, as in Horner's syndrome) or in lid retraction [as is seen in mesencephalic lesions (5)].

EYELID CLOSURE

Voluntary and involuntary closure of the eyelids is produced by the action of the orbicularis muscle. In discussing the action of this muscle in lid closure, it is necessary to consider the three functional components: the pretarsal, preseptal, and orbital divisions. Each of these units has specific functions attributed to it (Fig. 2.5).

Blinking

A blink is a brief closing of the palpebral apertures and refers to a bilateral action. The *blink fibers* of the pretarsal orbicularis are the principal units involved in this contraction. The closing phase may vary from 50 to 120 ms and is divided into three phases: a slow phase (during which the levator is inhibited), followed by a fast, and then another slow phase. There is also medial movement of the lids during blinking, especially in the lower lid—this is probably due to the relative laxity of the lateral lid attachments. The *mixed blink and volition fibers* of the preseptal region are involved in blinking to a lesser extent. The *volitional fibers* of the preseptal and orbital orbicularis muscle are discussed later (Fig. 2.6) (16, 17).

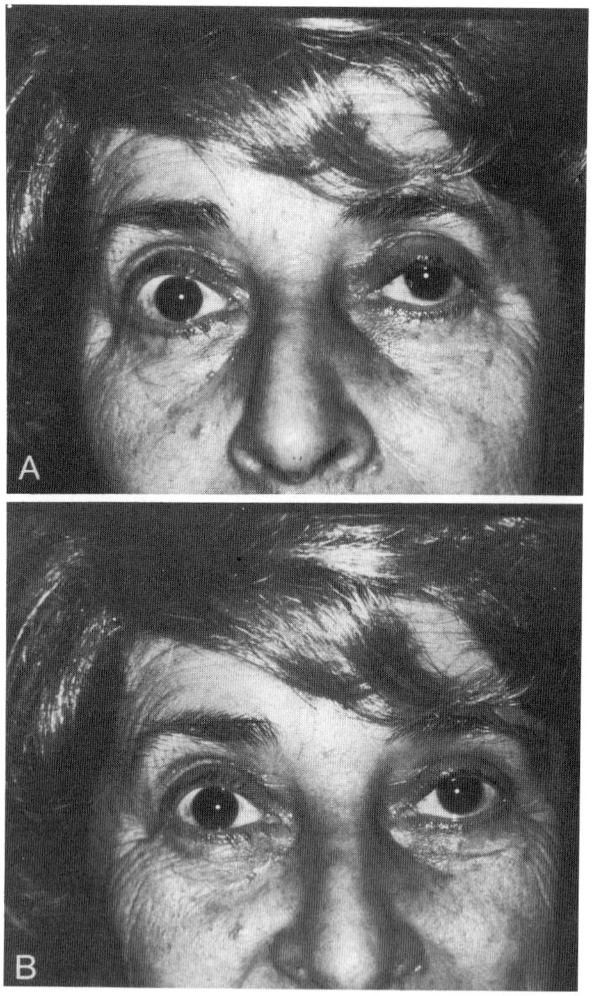

Figure 2.5. Demonstration of Hering's law as applied to the levator muscles. *A*, Ptosis of upper eyelid with retraction of opposite upper lid. *B*, After instillation of neosynephrine into the ptotic eye with subsequent decrease in ptosis; a small decrease in the retraction of the opposite upper lid is noted.

Blinking may be either periodic, voluntary, or reflex. *Reflex blinking* is mediated through the brainstem. The *orbicularis reflex* may be elicited by either tapping the orbicularis muscle (Wartenberg; a monosynaptic proprioceptive reflex) or another part of the face (e.g., glabellar tap; monosynaptic and polysynaptic components). The *corneal blink reflex*, which is elicited by touching the cornea, is a polysynaptic reflex mediated by the trigeminal afferent pathway. Auditory stimulation may also produce a blink (cochleopalpebral, auropalpebral reflexes), as will palatal stimulation (palatopalpebral reflex). The *reflex blink to a flash of light* has a longer latency than the other reflexes discussed and may have a cortical component as may the *menace* reflex (16).

Periodic blinking refers to the involuntary eye closure that occurs throughout the day. This closure is infrequent in infants (1 or 2 blinks/min), averages 15 to 16 blinks/min in adults, and frequently occurs at moments of relaxation or preceding changes in direction of gaze. The rate is influenced by emotion (which increases the rate) and level of alertness (which decreases the rate). The rate of periodic blinking is thought to be mediated by the basal ganglia and/or reticular formation. This is supported by the decreased blink rate in patients with Parkinson's disease and progressive supranuclear palsy (18).

Voluntary eyelid closure is mediated by the pyramidal system, via the corticobulbar tract. *Winking* is a unilateral

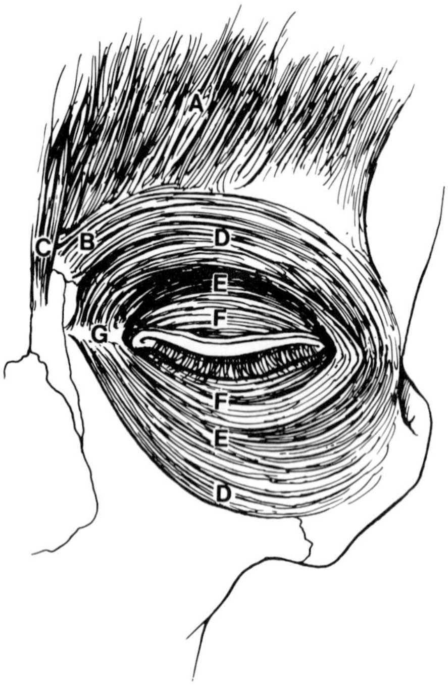

Figure 2.6. Musculature of the brow and eyelids. *A*, Frontalis muscle. *B*, Corrugator superciliaris. *C*, Procerus. *D*, Orbital orbicularis. *E*, Preseptal orbicularis. *F*, Pretarsal orbicularis. *G*, Medial canthal tendon. (From Doxanas MT, Anderson RL: *Clinical Orbital Anatomy*. Baltimore, Williams & Wilkins, 1984.)

form of voluntary lid closure, in which the orbicularis and levator contract simultaneously. Voluntary closure involves the *volitional fibers* of the preseptal and orbital orbicularis. With maximal closure, the skin of the upper and lower lids overrides the tarsi, as is seen in ocular blepharospasm (19).

Disorders of insufficiency of lid closure may be supranuclear, brainstem or facial nerve (e.g., Bell's palsy) related, or neuromuscular. Disorders of excessive eyelid closure may also be either central (e.g., essential blepharospasm) or peripheral (e.g., hemifacial spasm, myotonic dystrophy).

REFERENCES

1. Beard C: *Ptosis*, ed 3. St. Louis, CV Mosby, 1981, pp 26–31, p 81.
2. Hornblass A: *Tumors of the Ocular Adnexa and Orbit*. St. Louis, CV Mosby, 1979, pp 17–41.
3. Montagna W, Ford DM: Histology and cytochemistry of human skin, *Arch Derm* 100: 328–335, 1969.
4. Doxanas MT, Anderson RL: Oriental eyelids. *Arch Ophthalmol* 102: 1232–1235, 1984.
5. Miller NR: In Walsh, Hoyt (eds): *Clinical Neuro-Ophthalmology*, ed 4. Baltimore, Williams & Wilkins, 1985, pp 932–988, 1004–1040.
6. Fox SA: The palpebral fissure. *Am J Ophthalmol* 62: 73–78, 1966.
7. Doane MG: Interaction of eyelids and tears in corneal wetting and the dynamics of the normal human eyeblink. *Am J Ophthalmol* 89: 507–516, 1980.
8. Records RE: *Physiology of the Human Eye and Visual System*. New York, Harper & Row, 1979, pp 1–24.
9. Bjork A: Electromyographic studies on the coordination of antagonistic muscles in cases of abducens and facial palsy. *Br J Ophthalmol* 38: 605–615, 1954.
10. Gay AJ, Salmon ML, Windsor CE: Hering's law, the levators, and their relationship in disease states. *Arch Ophthalmol* 77: 157–160, 1967.
11. Schechter RJ: Ptosis with contralateral lid retraction due to excessive innervation of the levator palpebrae superiorus. *Ann Ophthalmol* 10: 1324–1328, 1978.
12. Anderson RL, Dixon RS: The role of Whitnall's ligament in ptosis surgery. *Arch Ophthalmol* 97: 705–707, 1979.
13. Doxanas MT, Anderson RL: *Clinical Orbital Anatomy*. Baltimore, Williams & Wilkins, 1984, pp 80–82.
14. Hawes MJ, Dortzbach RK: Microscopic anatomy of the lower eyelid retractors. *Arch Ophthalmol* 100: 1313–1318, 1982.
15. Lubkin V: The inverse Marcus Gunn phenomenon. *Neurology* 35: 249, 1978.
16. Hoyt WF, Loeffler JD: Neurology of the orbicularis oculi. In Smith JL (ed): *Neuro-ophthalmology*. St. Louis, CV Mosby, vol 2, 1965, pp 167–205.
17. Gordon G: Observations upon the movements of the eyelids. *Br J Ophthalmol* 35: 339–351, 1951.
18. Loeffler JD, Slatt B, Hoyt WF: Abnormalities of the eyelids in Parkinson's disease. *Arch Ophthalmol* 76: 178–185, 1966.
19. Moses RA: The eyelids. In Adler (ed): *Physiology of the Eye*, ed. 7. St. Louis, CV Mosby, 1981, pp 1–15.

CHAPTER 3

General Principles and Considerations

RAYMOND REICH, M.D.

THE OCULOPLASTIC SURGEON

Ophthalmic plastic and reconstructive surgery, while ancient in many of its applications, has only in recent decades come into its own as a distinct surgical subspecialty, with its own discipline, principles, and highly skilled practitioners. The explosion of technological and surgical advances in recent years has been phenomenal in all branches of medicine and in ophthalmology in particular. Oculoplastic surgery has burgeoned, with its own literature, meetings, and ever-increasing innovations. The practitioner of oculoplastic surgery, whether the subspecialist or the general ophthalmologist, must keep up with these advances but must also subscribe to other, more traditional, considerations.

Surgeons must be aware of their own limitations. Detailed knowledge of periocular anatomy, a sense of the nature and behavior of periocular tissue, and the capacity to make and alter surgical decisions on the spot, can only be provided by adequate training and experience. The question of whom to operate upon and whom to refer must be carefully weighed by all surgeons.

While our fund of information has increased over the past 5000 years, our intelligence remains about the same. It is well known that bright, innovative thinkers, with much less accrued information to draw upon than we now have, have left their mark on medicine since time immemorial.

BRIEF HISTORY OF OCULOPLASTIC SURGERY

Fox, Duke-Elder, Arrington, Rogers, and others—and more recently Katzen—have documented fascinating histories of oculoplastic surgery.

Plastic and periocular plastic procedures are among the oldest documented operations. Susruta, a Hindu physician of the 6th or 7th century BCE, describes his techniques for facial plastic reconstructions, especially in the region of the nose (the amputation of which was a popular form of punishment in his time). Some of the ancient Indian techniques applicable for skin grafting resurfaced in early 19th century European literature.

Naturally, over the years, things that bothered people the most were the most likely to be addressed by physicians. Thus dacryocystitis and its treatment by cauterization—and later fistulization—appear in the 1st and 2nd century CE Roman literature of Celsus and Archigenes.

Cicatricial entropion secondary to trachoma—an old and widespread disease—drove patients and surgeons to great lengths to relieve the unrelenting trichiasis. Some of the early procedures of Celsus and Paul of Aegina were as intelligent and innovative as they were horrible and disfiguring. They displayed an understanding of the anatomic lamellae of the eyelid.

Avicenna, Ibn Rashid, Maimonides, and others of the 10th–13th century Arabic-speaking world described their diagnosis and treatment of oculoplastic disorders.

Some practitioners, such as the Tagliocozzis of medieval Italy, kept some of the secrets of their art restricted to their own families. Tagliocozzi did publish, in Venice, in 1597, a plastic surgery textbook, *De Curtorum Chirurgia per Institionem*.

It was in the 19th century that much of what we would recognize today as reasonable oculoplastic procedures was developed. Pedicle flaps, lid-shortening procedures, levator resection, dacryocystectomy, lacrimal probing, conjunctival surgery, and free skin grafting appeared in relatively primitive but basically modern form.

An interesting chapter in the history of skin grafting concerns the heterograft, or "zoograft" from rats, rabbits, pigs, and fowl. John Davis, in a 1919 text on plastic surgery, describes the early apparent take of these grafts; the initial healing phase; and then their inevitable, abrupt, and at that time, inexplicable demise.

Aseptic technique, the success of "pinch" grafts on granulating surfaces, and then enhanced experience with larger split and full-thickness grafts in the late 19th century revolutionized the concept of skin grafting and opened new possibilities for oculoplastic reconstruction.

THE OCULOPLASTIC PATIENT

Like the eye itself, the ocular adnexae subjected to surgical manipulation must maintain their functional as well as their physical integrity. The eyes occupy such a central position in a patient's overall appearance and self image that great care must be taken to satisfy cosmetic considerations in the essentially noncosmetic patient, as well as functional considerations in the cosmetic patient.

Perhaps the most important consideration in the initial process of patient-doctor selection is that the two understand each other. Listen to the patients. Establish a good relationship. Be certain, as the doctor, that you know precisely what patients want and expect. Make certain, as well, that patients understand exactly what is involved in the surgery, what risks there are, what the likely benefits are, what the preoperative and postoperative routines will be, and what is expected of them. Discuss fee arrangements in advance. Document the visual acuity.

Does the patient have a reasonable attitude toward the surgeon and the proposed surgery? Is it being done because the patient wants it, or to please someone else? Does the patient truly understand the nature of the disorder? Does the patient with the basal cell tumor know that he or she indeed has cancer? Has this patient previously sued another physician over a related matter? Can this patient be satisfied? (See the chapter by Hornblass for a more extensive discussion on this subject.)

These questions must be carefully considered at the time of the first interview. A second interview, just prior to the procedure, may be helpful in cementing the doctor-patient relationship and in clearing up any unanswered questions on either side. It was during such a second interview that this author discovered that the attractive young woman sitting across the desk from him who indeed has a slight ptosis of the temporal aspects of her brows, wanted her brows lifted so that "the teenagers in the street will stop making animal noises" at her.

In cosmetic cases in particular, the psychological status of the patient is of critical concern. Olley and Thompson, in the psychiatric literature, have compiled a six-point profile of patients who should not be considered for cosmetic surgery (also see the chapter by Gurfein):

1. Tentative patients whose chief motivation for the surgery is the instigation of friends or relatives;
2. Patients with unrealistic expectations who expect magical results and wish to improve acceptance of themselves by others without having to actively modify their behavior or personality;
3. Patients who can only vaguely describe their problem or what they desire;
4. Paranoid patients who exhibit exaggerated, bizarre, or overly sexualized descriptions of the deformity;
5. Depressed or hypochondriacal patients;
6. Insatiable cosmetic surgery patients.

In addition to the chief complaint that brought the patient to the doctor, the surgeon must also consider other oculoplastic factors in the patient's face and point these out to the patient. The patient's general health must be taken into account, both from the standpoint of surgical and anesthetic risks, as well as possible underlying factors in the pathogenesis of the presenting problem. It is better to find out beforehand what medications a patient takes. It is late, in the operating room, to discover that the bleeding patient is on anticoagulants.

In this litigious era, the need for adequate preoperative documentation is obvious. Photographs are essential, serving not only to document the preoperative situation but to remind patients later, if necessary, what they looked like before. Contemporary technology permits easily and inexpensive videotaping of patients' preoperative condition as well as their informed consent.

These considerations, skillful surgery, and general good sense and good will help ensure a mutually gratifying experience for doctor and patient.

OCULOPLASTIC TISSUE

Periocular tissue is special. Its surgery, in turn, requires a special discipline. Perhaps nowhere else in the body are form, function, and appearance so intimately bound together.

Lid skin is the thinnest and finest in the body, lending itself extremely well to reconstructive manipulation but also rendering it hard to match with autologous tissue. It is delicate, and in turn, must be handled with great delicacy.

Flaps may be tiny and easily spoiled by rough handling or improper instrumentation. Fine forceps, such as a 0.3 mm or occasionally a 0.12 mm, small skin hooks, fine, sharp scissors and knives, and proper needles and needle holders are necessary. Great care must be taken in dissection, tissue manipulation, hemostasis, tissue orientation and suture placement in order to achieve satisfactory results.

Eyelid anatomy is extremely complex, and an intimate knowledge of this anatomy is mandatory for the oculoplastic surgeon. A sense of aesthetics and an appreciation of symmetry are well developed in the superior surgeon.

NEEDLES, SUTURES, INSTRUMENTS

The most capable craftsman requires the proper tools to allow full expression of his abilities. The oculoplastic surgeon, similarly, in order to take full advantage of the array of instruments, needles, and sutures available, must be familiar with them and their various applications.

Before addressing a wound, the surgeon must decide which instruments to use to manipulate that wound and which suture and needle to use (see chapter by Eliasoph).

NEEDLES

There are four principal configurations in needles used in ophthalmic plastic surgery (Fig. 3.1): The *cutting needle* has a triangular-shaped cross section and a sharp cutting edge along the inner diameter of the circle (usually 3/8 circle) that lends itself to deeply placed sutures.

The *reversed cutting needle* is also triangular in cross section but has a cutting edge along the outer diameter of the circle that aids in penetrating hard tissue. Either of these two needles work well in skin.

The *spatula needle* is flatter, with sharp sides. It can penetrate superficially yet securely and is therefore particularly useful for anchoring sutures in tari or sclera.

Taper needles have a round cross section and a sharp tip. These needles work well in loose connective tissue, but they may be difficult to use in tissue with more "drag" resistance.

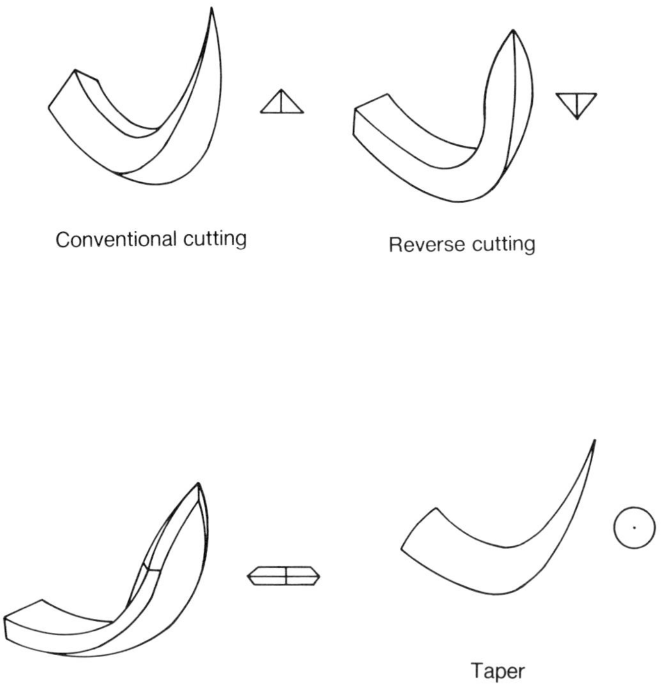

Figure 3.1. The four most commonly used needle configurations in ophthalmic plastic surgery.

SUTURES

Nonabsorbable sutures most commonly used in oculoplastic surgery are silk, nylon or Prolene, Supramid, and Mersilene or Dacron.

The most commonly used suture is probably 6-0 silk. It handles very well, is soft and pliable, and produces "just the right amount" of tissue reaction. In most cases, nylon can be substituted for silk. Smooth and less reactive than silk, nylon is the classical suture for subcuticular closures.

Supramid is a permanent suture used for deeply placed support, such as anchoring to periosteum. Mersilene and Dacron may be similarly used for deep, long-lasting fixation. Their tendency to produce somewhat more of a tissue reaction may be an advantage in producing a solid bond.

The advantage of absorbable sutures is that they are indeed absorbed when their work is done. While the rate of absorption varies, plain gut generally lasts 4–7 days, while chromic gut lasts 7–14 days. These are produced from sheep intestines. The synthetic absorbables in common use, considered less reactive than gut, are Dexon and Vicryl. For deep closures 4-0 and 5-0 sutures are usually used, while 6-0 and 7-0 are used for tarsus, mucosal surfaces, and skin closures in small children.

NEEDLE HOLDERS

The Castroviejo ophthalmic needle holder, in its many variations, is the most useful all-purpose needle holder in oculoplastic surgery. It is comfortable to use with needles accompanying 4-0 to 7-0 sutures and leaves the surgeon in good control of needle and suture flow. A smaller ("micro") needle holder, of similar construction, is best suited for finer needles bearing 8-0 to 10-0 sutures.

Some surgeons are accustomed to the Kalt needle holder, which is still in common use and is designed for intermediate gauge sutures. Some find the tendency for the suture length to become entangled in the thumb-activated lock quite annoying. A classic plastic (Webster) needle holder is also suitable for intermediate (4-0 to 6-0) sutures.

FORCEPS

There is a wide variety of preferences in forceps among surgeons. Essentially, the choices are "smooth" or "toothed" and "gross," "fine," or "extra fine." The fine-toothed Bishop-Harmon forcep is the author's preference for handling lid skin. The full-thickness lid may be held with Graefe or Adson forceps. The proper forcep feels comfortable in the surgeon's hand, handles tissue delicately yet effectively, and affords the surgeon total control of the tissue.

SCISSORS

The proper choice of a scissor is of great importance in facilitating the work to be done. Straight and curved, sharp tipped and round tipped, Stevens scissors or iris scissors are good general purpose instruments. Westcott scissors are excellent for finer tissues, while small Metzenbaum scissors should be used for heavier tissues.

TRAY

A general purpose oculoplastic instrument tray need not be cluttered with a great many instruments but should contain an adequate variety to permit the surgeon to address, with delicacy and purpose, each aspect of periocular tissue in the manner most suited for it. A simple tray might include:

Castroviejo needle holder;
Micro needle holder;
Straight, sharp iris scissor;
Straight Stevens scissor;
Curved Stevens scissor;
Westcott scissor;
Small Metzenbaum scissor;
Adson forceps;
Graefe forceps;
Fine-tooth forceps;
Smooth tissue forceps;
Skin hooks;
Desmarres retractor;
Fine rake retractors;
Measuring device;
Bard-Parker handle;
No. 15 blade;
No. 11 blade;
Special instruments as required:
Fascia needle stripper, drill, periosteal elevator, etc.

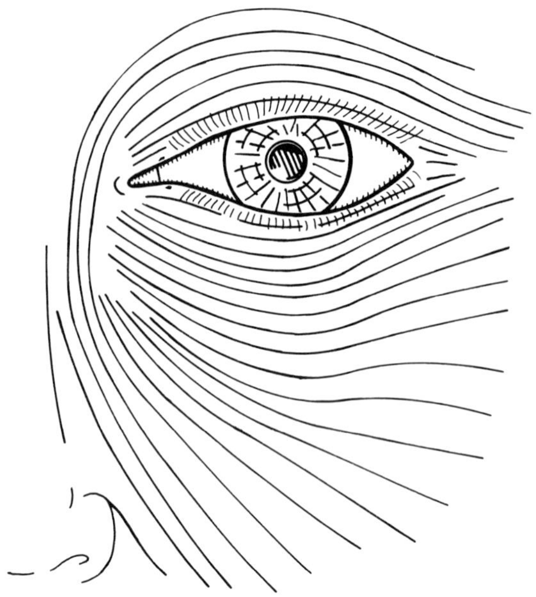

Figure 3.2. The lines of Langer. These represent the natural skin cleavage lines in the periorbital region.

INCISIONS

A well-made incision is the first step in a well-done operation. Wounds should be cleanly and sharply incised along planned and premarked lines. Unless a bevel is specifically indicated, the cut should be perpendicular and aided by good lighting, exposure, and traction as needed. The natural crease lines of the face and the lines of Langer serve as guides for well-oriented incisions which may heal with little or no discernible scarring (Fig. 3.2).

Even where general anesthesia is employed, it is frequently useful, to define tissue planes and to provide homostasis, to infiltrate the operative site with a solution of epinephrine–containing local anesthetic mixed with hyaluronidase. The latter agent may be particularly helpful when operating on scarred tissue.

CLOSURE

Architects frequently comment that no matter how well-done or how solidly built a construction job is, it is usually judged by its surface finishing. Careful attention to suturing technique is most likely to provide satisfactory "surface finishing" in periocular surgery. Careless or improper suturing may result in unsightly scarring. Scars are generated by closure that is too tight or too loose, improper edge orientation, infection, blood clots, and retained foreign matter. Ragged edges or necrotic tissue must be cut away.

Tissue layers must be carefully identified and closed accordingly. Deep closure, where indicated, eliminates dead space and its potential for infection and provides strength for the wound. The skin edges should just lie together under no tension. Tension in the skin closure tends to widen the resulting scar. Subcutaneous sutures should be placed with their knots facing internally to avoid their presenting through the wound.

The skin edges, when properly apposed, are left slightly everted. In the healing process, contraction tends to occur in an anteroposterior direction, so that slight eversion at the time of closure helps prevent a depressed scar.

Careful spacing and orientation of the needle passages is necessary to achieve the desired result. Directing the needle passage so that slightly more deep tissue than superficial tissue is included in the bite will help effect proper edge orientation and avoid inversion. Entry and exit points should be equidistant from the wound. Fortunately, lid skin is quite "forgiving" and may mask some degree of technical inadequacy in suturing.

Small bites of skin and removal of sutures at the proper

time also contribute to satisfactory results. There are numerous suture techniques that may be applied, as indicated, to the various aspects of periocular tissue:

Thin lid skin responds equally well to *running* or *interrupted sutures*. A running technique is particularly useful for the rapid and effective closure of long, tension-free incisions. Suturing skin against tension will usually result in ectropion, "hooding," or unnatural folds (Figs. 3.3–3.5).

Horizontal mattress sutures are useful in providing broad areas of support and may be quickly placed. A typical site for this type of suture is the skin graft donor area behind the ear.

Vertical mattress sutures provide both deep and superficial support in the same area, and are useful in closure against tension. The so-called near-far/far-near suture and its variations provide similar advantages (Fig. 3.6).

Subcuticular closure is an aesthetically pleasing approach that is especially useful in the brow area or in thicker eyelid skin. It is technically difficult to perform in the thinnest skin. Typically a 5-0 nylon suture is used, with the ends anchored or left free in "pull out" fashion. Each needle entry site is precisely opposite the preceding exit site, at approximately 3-mm intervals. Because it provides very little strength to the skin closure itself but serves mainly to finely appose skin edges, an adequate tension-free subcutaneous closure must be provided first (Fig. 3.7).

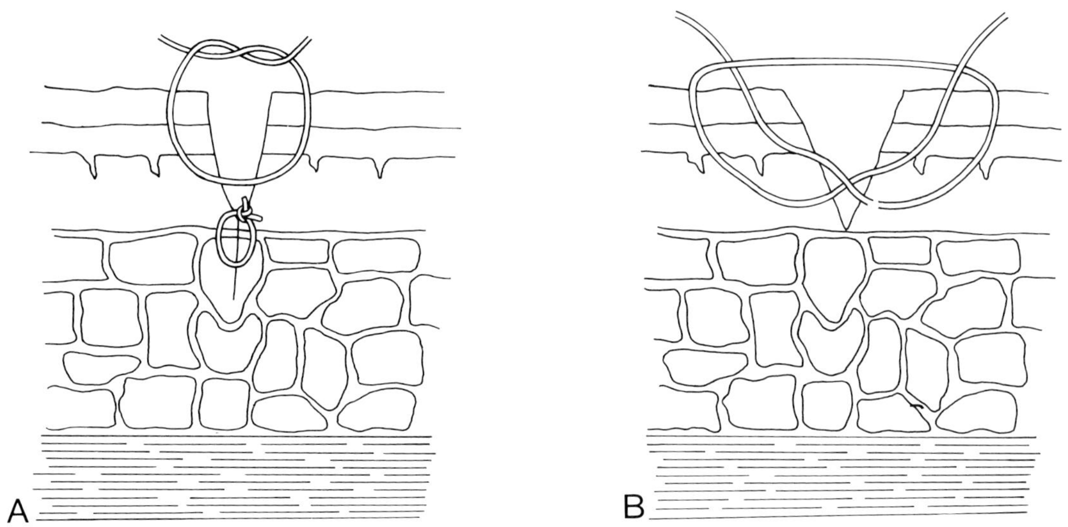

Figure 3.3. *A,* Layered closure eliminates dead space and adds strength. *B,* Near-far/far-near suture.

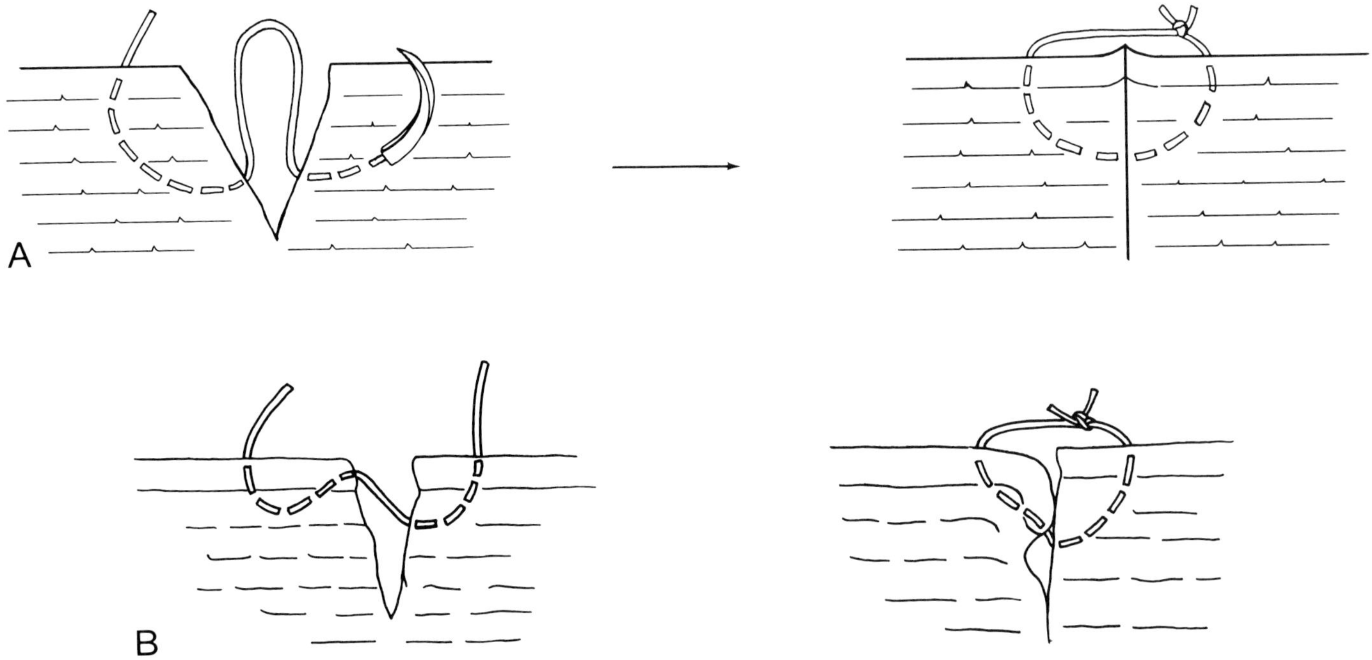

Figure 3.4. *A,* A well-placed suture is carefully spaced and oriented. *B,* A poorly executed suture will result in a misaligned wound and an unsightly scar.

Delicate skin tips at the juncture of three suture lines may be damaged by direct handling or may not fall together well enough with direct closure. Here the *half-buried horizontal mattress suture* serves to bring the tips together without actually involving them in the suture bite. In this technique the needle is passed through the skin near one tip, subcutaneously beneath the second and third tips, and then out through the skin of the first tip adjacent to its entry site to complete the circle (Fig. 3.8).

Knots are tied with "just the right amount" of tension—a sense borne of experience. The novice surgeon tends to tie too tightly.

The appropriate time for suture removal varies with location and choice of suture material. Leaving sutures in too long may result in epithelialized suture tracts, which must later be opened individually and predispose to scarring.

The most commonly used periocular material, 6-0 or 7-0 silk, can usually be removed by the third or fourth day. Prolene and nylon, as less reactive materials, may require another day's healing before removal. In most cases the wound should still be supported after early suture removal with sterile tape strips. Once properly applied to a dry surface, these strips may hold the wound together for another few days. Antibiotic ointment may still be used; it diffuses through the tape to the skin without loss of adhesion.

A common and annoying problem a surgeon may encounter when approaching the end of a sutured incision is the "dog ear." A dog ear is likely to result, especially in elliptical incisions, if the long diameter is less than 2–3 times the short diameter. Several corrective approaches are available. The dog ear may be excised as a second ellipse, thus elongating the wound, which in turn is closed directly. Alternately, an M-Y plasty may be performed, in

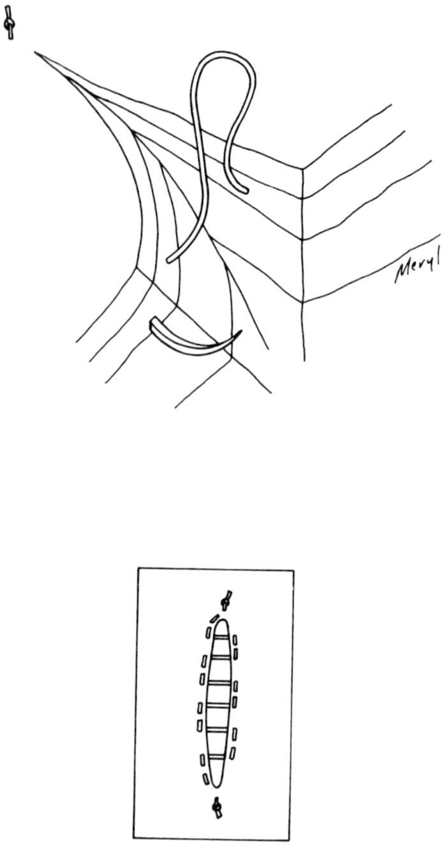

Figure 3.7. Subcuticular sutures run just below the surface of the skin, with entry and exit sites carefully aligned.

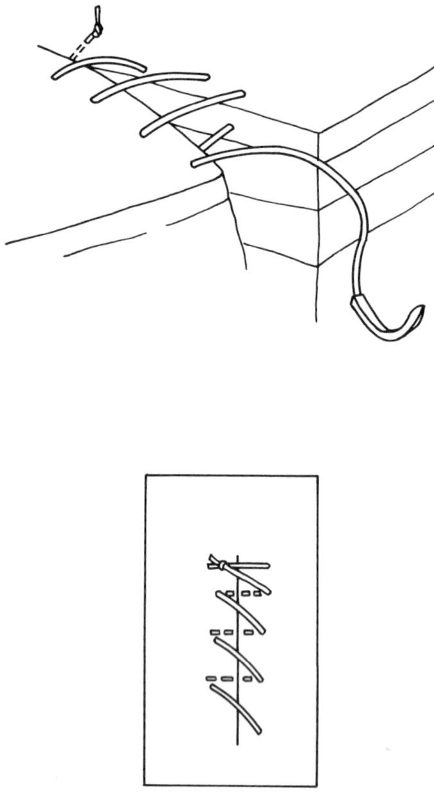

Figure 3.5. A simple, running closure.

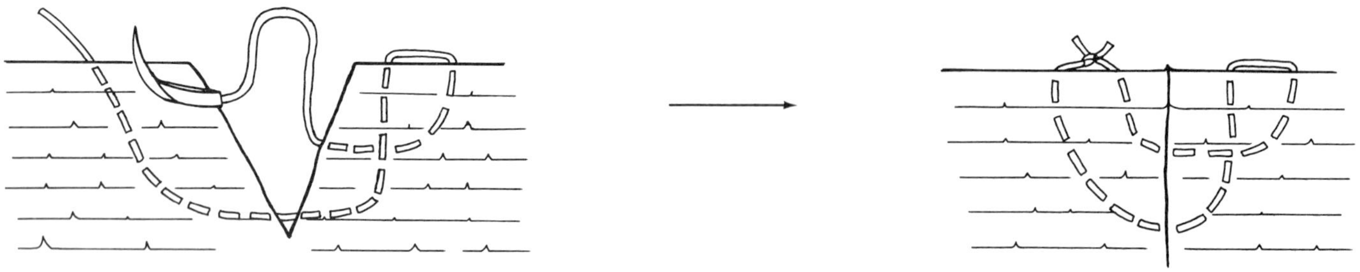

Figure 3.6. The vertical mattress suture, like the near-far/far-near suture, affords strength and depth to the wound closure.

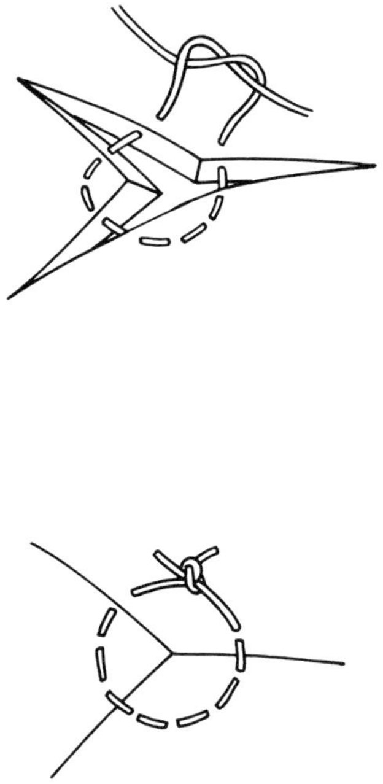

Figure 3.8. The half-buried horizontal mattress suture.

which the excision of two small triangles debulks the dog ear from the sides with the tip neatly laid down at the end of the linear incision (Fig. 3.9).

HEMOSTASIS

A good operation can be spoiled by a postoperative hemorrhage, which can deform a wound and ruin a graft. Therefore, good hemostasis should be achieved (see chapter by Wertenheill).

Patients on anticoagulants should discontinue these drugs preoperatively if medically permissible. Patients will often not realize that aspirin is indeed an anticoagulant and may deny taking such medication when in fact platelet function may be severely reduced. They should be asked specifically about aspirin and coumadin.

Preoperative infiltration with epinephrine-containing solutions, as previously mentioned, can be extremely helpful in minimizing bleeding. Of course, careful consideration must be given to the patient's medical status and the compatibility of epinephrine with the general anesthetic agent used.

The epinephrine in most local anesthetic preparations comes in a concentration of 1:100,000. This can be diluted down several times to increase the safety factor, while still remaining an efficacious hemostatic agent. Epinephrine-related compounds may also be used intraoperatively in the form of soaked pledgets placed on bleeding sites and held with pressure. This is particularly useful for bleeding mucosal surfaces in lacrimal surgery.

Infiltration with epinephrine does not work instantaneously. To derive the greatest benefit, the surgeon should administer the injection at least 10 minutes prior to making the incision.

During surgery, a slow, general ooze of blood is sometimes best handled with pressure and patience. Pinpoint electrocautery, either unipolar (Bovie) or bipolar (Wetfield), is the mainstay of intraoperative hemostasis. Larger blood vessels may be clamped and electrocoagulated. In all cases, care must be taken not to burn adjacent tissue excessively.

Thrombogenic agents can be extremely useful in cases of persistent oozing. Gelfoam induces the release of thromboplastin, which in turn initiates coagulation. Thrombin mediates the transformation of soluble fibrin to insoluble, clot-forming fibrin. Avitene powder, microfibrillar collagen, also stimulates and supports the clotting mechanism.

Postoperatively, ice packs may reduce the likelihood of bleeding as well as edema. Moderate-pressure dressings may be helpful in some cases, while light dressings, which permit inspection of the eye or operative site, may be indicated in others. In anophthalmic surgery, of course, greater pressure may be safely applied.

Hypertrophic scars may be avoided by gentle tissue handling and precise, tension-free closures. Wounds kept clean, free of crusts, and annointed with a daily dose of antibiotic ointment are likely to heal well. Scars that do develop may be reduced and softened by steroid injection and by a massage with steroid ointment and cocoa butter.

WOUND HEALING

In the clean surgical wound, with tissue apposition provided by sutures, initial sealing occurs within hours. On the surface, epithelial cells begin to bridge the gap and provide a barrier to infection. Within the wound, a clot forms which seals the defect. The inflammatory phase of the healing process is thus initiated, with the appearance of leukocytes and phagocytes to cleanse the wound of microbes and necrotic tissue and prepare the way for healing.

Fibrocytes and fibroblasts in the margin of the wound are transformed into metabolically active cells migrating across the wound, through, and supported by, the clot, at a rate of approximately 0.2 mm/day. As the fibroblasts from each side of the wound meet, by the 2nd or 3rd day, resorption of the inflammatory material begins.

Solid cords of endothelial cells from the cut ends of capillaries similarly migrate along the fibrin meshwork, canalize, and anastomose with those from the other side. The lymphatics undergo a similar process as well.

The clot has now, by the 3rd to 4th day, become "organized," and consists of a highly vascularized, active connective tissue with residual inflammation. This is granulation tissue, which is present in minimal amounts in a clean wound healing by primary union and which figures more prominently in less well-apposed wounds healing secondarily.

Collagen, which is laid down by the 4th or 5th day, strengthens the repair. It is believed that vitamin C is needed to mediate the precipitation of soluble procollagen

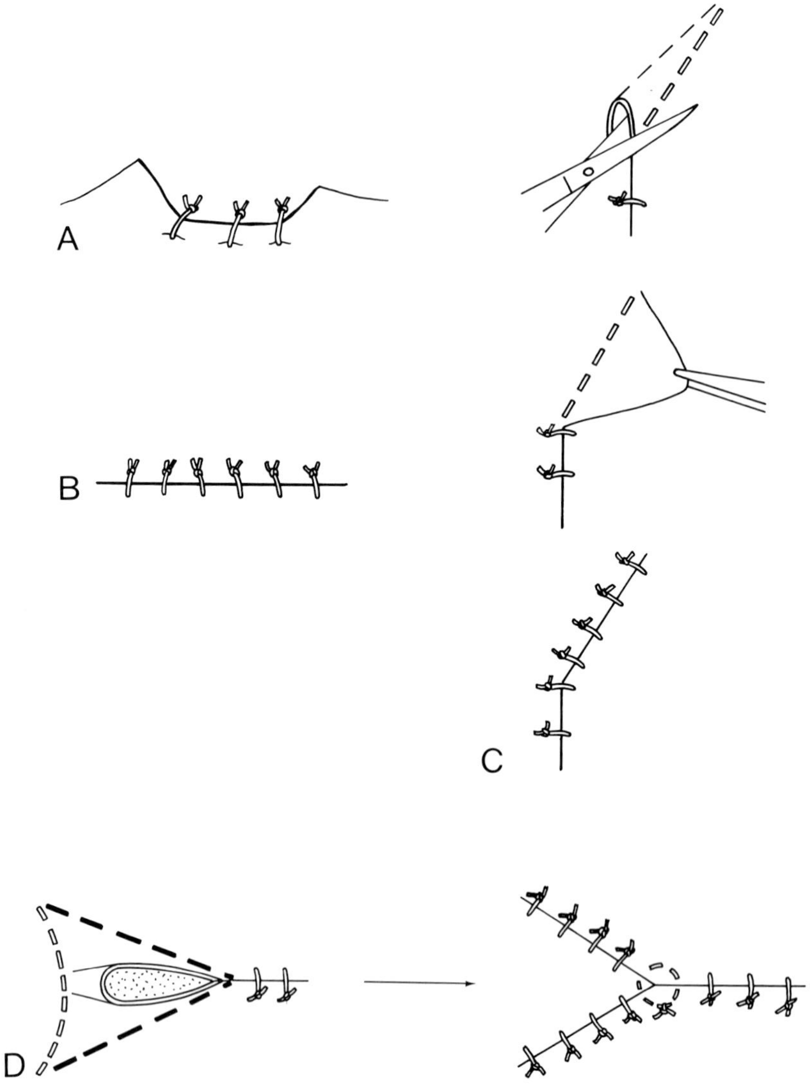

Figure 3.9. The dog-ear dilemma. *A,* The problem. *B,* The ideal solution, upon elongation of the ellipse. *C,* Elongation and resection of a triangle, as dictated by facial lines. *D,* M-Y plasty, with a half-buried horizontal mattress suture to preserve the tips.

into insoluble collagen fibers. The epidermis, meanwhile, has largely healed by epithelial proliferation.

As the scar matures, vascularization is diminished, the collagen shrinks and some is resorbed, and fibroblasts disappear. The scar begins to contract. Maximum strength is achieved by about the 10th week, although most of the strength is present already by the 14th day.

SKIN FLAPS

Ophthalmic plastic surgery frequently involves the transposition of tissue from its original position to fill or correct a defect. When it is completely removed from its donor site, a *free graft* has been performed. When its base and blood supply are left intact, it is called a *flap.*

Some flaps, especially thicker ones, tend to scar more than free grafts, but they do carry their own blood supply and may thus be useful in scarred areas where the inherent blood supply may not suffice to support a free graft. The thickness possible in such a flap may also serve to fill a deep defect that would be inadequately filled by a thin free graft. Infection and pigment changes are also less likely than with a free graft. As with any plastic maneuver, careful planning before creating the flap is critical:

A *sliding flap* may be nothing more than the undermining of skin to allow a tension-free primary closure. There is no change in the direction of the skin (Fig. 3.10).

An *advancement flap* is a freed-up tongue of tissue brought in to close a gap, such as in a Cutler-Beard lid sharing procedure. In essence, a three-sided flap is advanced from an area of abundant tissue. This maneuver is easier in older patients with loose skin. Another example is a flap brought in from the temple to close a lower eyelid defect (Fig. 3.11).

A *rotational flap* involves the rotation of skin and subcutaneous tissue into a surgical defect. The direction of the skin is changed as the flap is rotated about a pivot point. A semicircular rotational flap from the temple to repair large defects of the lower lid, as described by Tenzel, is an example. The radius of the arc through which the flap is rotated is the line of greatest tension. Relief for this tension line, if needed, is provided by a backcut from the pivot point along the base of the flap (Fig. 3.12).

Transposition flaps are usually long and resorted to when much tissue is needed in a nonadjacent area. An example is the midline forehead flap, which is sometimes used to replace lost eyelids (Fig. 3.13).

A *hammock flap* retains its insertion at both ends for better blood supply. Under conditions unconducive to free skin grafting, a hammock from the upper lid may be used to fill a defect across the lower lid.

The *Z plasty* is a classic flap maneuver and, because of its great importance and usefulness, will be described in some detail: Its principal use is to revise contracted scars, adding up to 30% of available tissue along the lines of tension. The change in direction of the lines of stress that produces the lengthening also has its own inherent benefit. Thus, the gain in length relieves contractures, and the change in direction minimizes facial scars.

Whereas straight lines may contract, the broken-up lines of the Z plasty distribute the contractile forces in different directions. The Z plasty breaks up linear scars, lengthens the line of contracture, and prevents its recurrence by redirecting the scar along the lines of minimal tension (Fig. 3.14).

The "Z" consists of two opposing triangles that are transposed. Typically, the arms are of equal length and the angles are set at 60°. Increase in length, which is the desired result, is proportional to the length of the arms. Thus, the angle controls the percent of increase, while limb length controls the actual increase (Fig. 3.15).

Choice of angle and limb length are not strictly arbitrary. The larger the angle, the greater the gain. But the larger the angle, the more difficult it is to transpose the triangles. Smaller angles are easier to work with but produce fragile flaps with little effect. Thus, while angles of 30–90° are possible, 60° is the largest angle that permits ready trans-

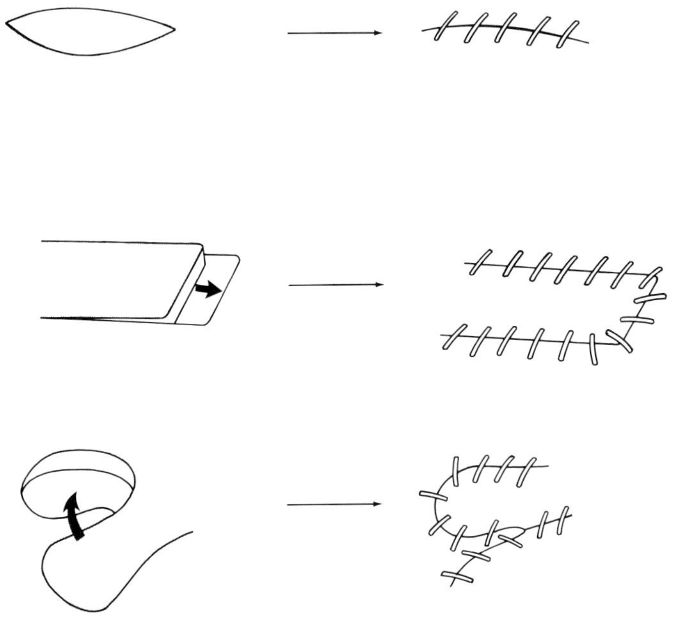

Figure 3.10. Examples of flaps. *Shaded areas* represent the undermining necessary to move the flap into place.

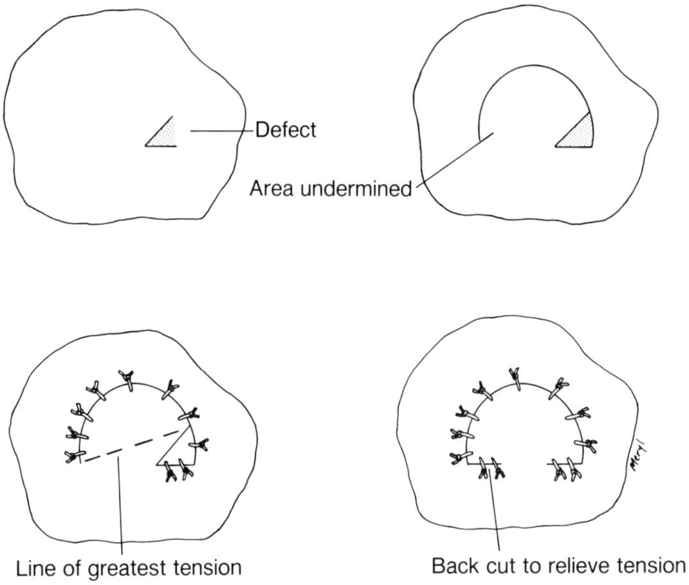

Figure 3.12. A rotational flap, depicting a back-cut to relieve tension.

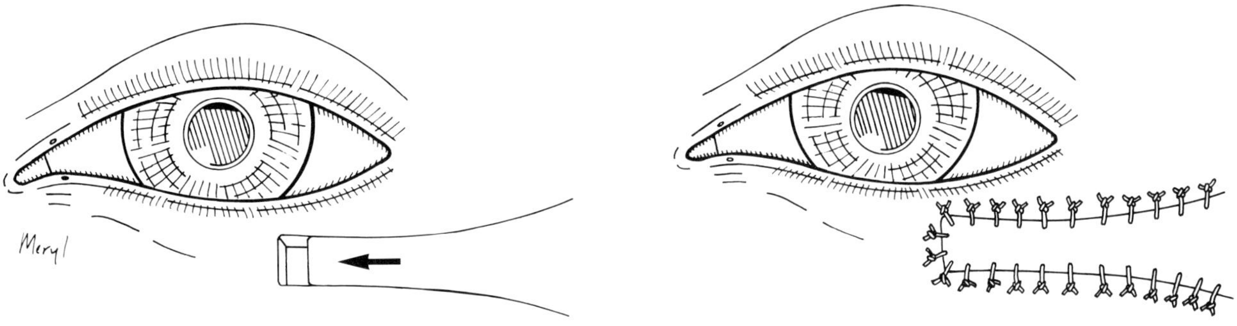

Figure 3.11. A schematic depiction of an advancement flap in the periocular region.

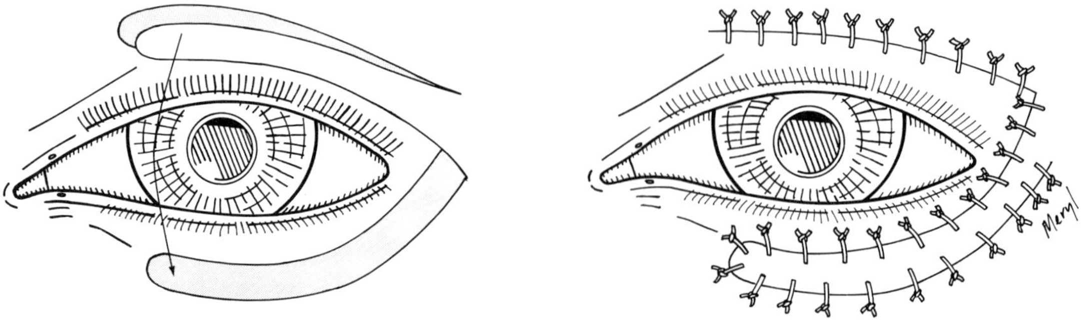

Figure 3.13. This transitional flap provides the tissue benefits of a full-thickness graft while maintaining the advantage of an attached base for nutritional support.

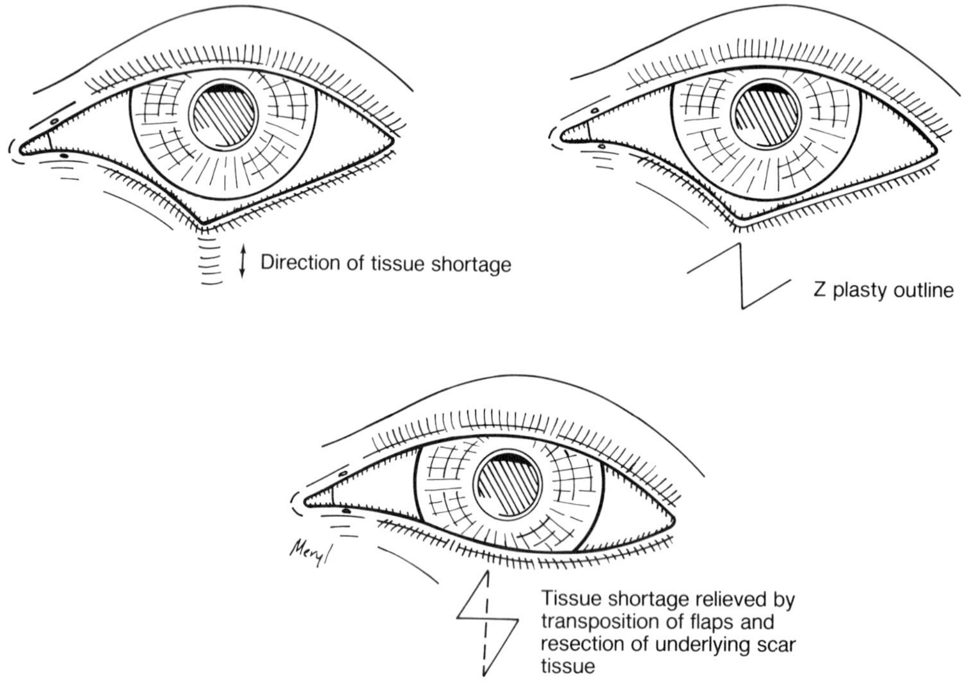

Figure 3.14. A contracted scar, deforming the lower eye- lid, is relieved by a Z plasty.

position of the triangles while producing the greatest increase in length along the central arm (Fig. 3.16).

Elaborate charts that predict the theoretical percentage gain in length for each angle chosen have been worked out. These values are not strictly true but theoretical: the biomechanical properties of tissue vary from the strictly mathematical predictions. Simply put, if the skin is not loose enough, the transposition will be less effective.

The length of the limbs of the "Z" similarly has its theoretical and practical considerations. The limbs are constructed equal in length to the central segment. The greater the length of the central segment, the greater the length gained. Long-limbed Z's tend to produce scars and may be difficult to achieve, because they are limited by the amount of tissue available for transposition. A series of small Z's to break up a long scar generally works much better, although some lengthening is sacrificed. A single, long scar is thus avoided.

Depressed and hypertrophic scars respond well to Z plasty. Postsurgical epicanthal folds and lid contour deformities are common indications in the periocular region. The central line of the initial "Z" is drawn along the scar line, or the line of greatest tension. The central line of the completed "Z" should conform, if possible, to the natural lines of the face, such as the lines of Langer or the nasolabial fold.

When the flaps are finely dissected and elevated, the cicatricial tissue must be completely resected to allow the rotation to take place. The triangles are transposed and carefully sutured into place. Tips, as always, must be handled gently, and, particularly in the case of a multiple Z plasty, care must be taken not to lose track of the transpositions and inadvertently suture a triangle back into its original position (Fig. 3.17).

A *V-to-Y plasty* is an alternate procedure for lengthening skin along lines of tension. It may sometimes be used in correcting minor cicatricial ectropion. A "V" is drawn, the skin is undermined, and then closed as a "Y." Skin is thus drawn from the sides of the base of the Y to fill the

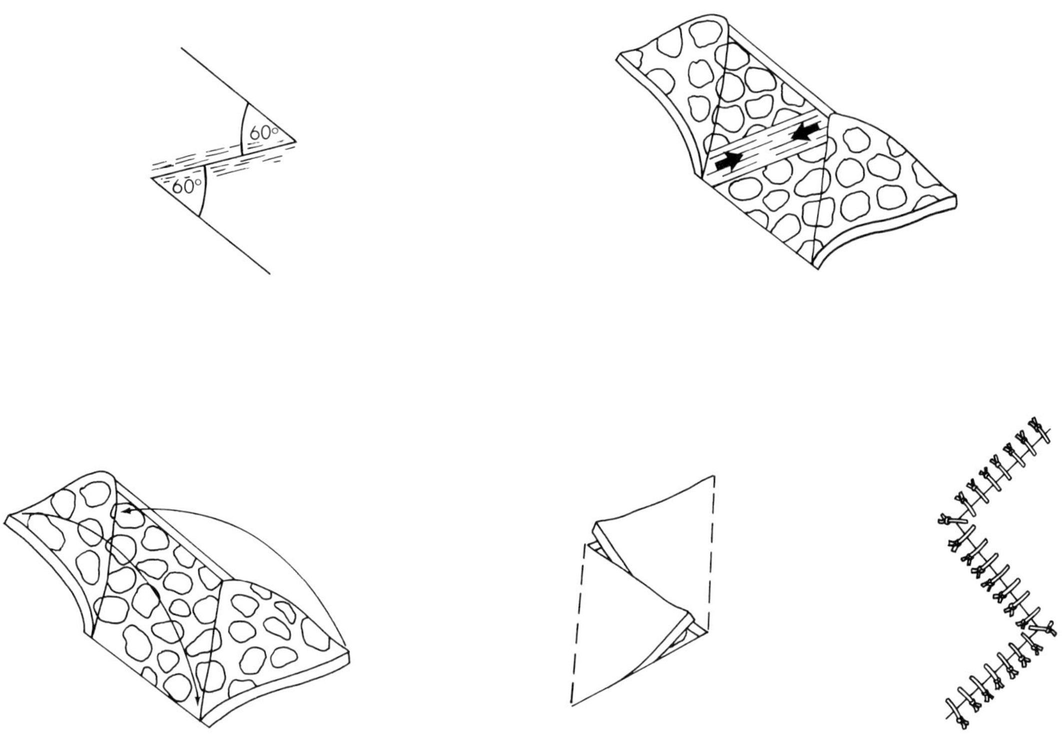

Figure 3.15. A Z plasty set at 60° angle. The central line is along the scar. Cicatricial tissue is removed and the flaps are transposed.

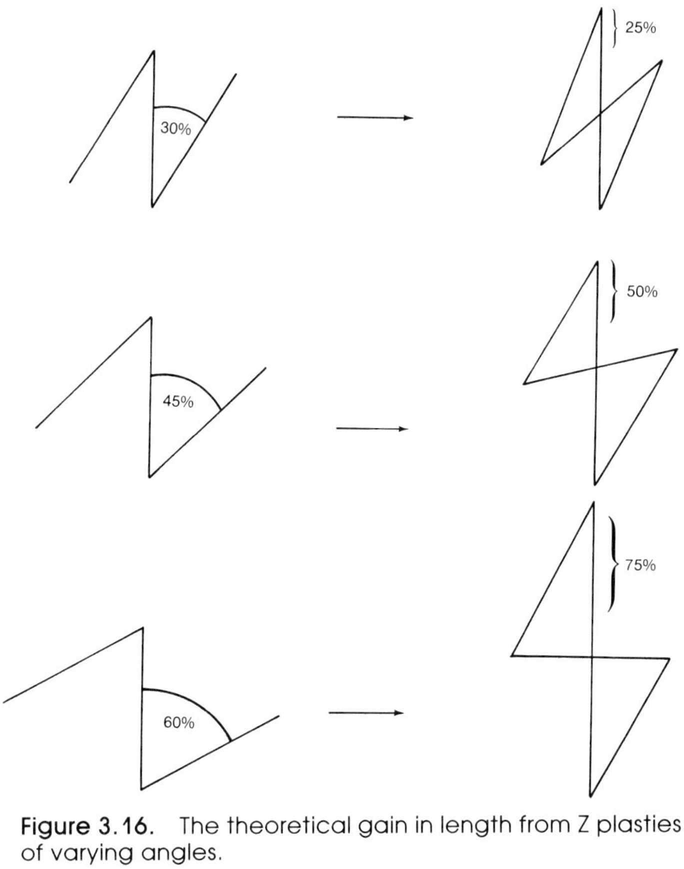

Figure 3.16. The theoretical gain in length from Z plasties of varying angles.

gap, tightening perpendicular to the base and lengthening parallel to it (Fig. 3.18*A*).

In a *Y-to-V plasty*, which may be used to repair an abnormal epicanthal fold, a "Y" is incised and undermined, and closed as a "V". Tissue is added perpendicular to the base of the Y, and shortened parallel to it (Fig. 3.18*B*).

A *rhomboid flap* closed a rhomboid-shaped defect with a triangular flap of smaller size rotated into place. Adequate undermining is necessary to free up the tissue sufficiently to close the donor site as well as to rotate the flap freely. This technique may be useful in the temporal region or over the brow. It was described by Limberg in a Russian monograph on plastic surgery in 1947 and later adapted for oculoplastic use (Fig. 3.19).

The *W plasty* breaks up a long, linear scar perpendicular to the crease lines of the face into a series of interdigitating triangles. This results in a series of small, more-or-less horizontal lines, some of which will now lie within the creases or at least parallel to them. The forehead is a typical location for this type of procedure.

While the incision may be carefully marked off freehand, a W plasty knife, or W plasty incision guides, are available for precise work. The scar is resected, and the triangles, with arms 3–5 mm long, are mobilized and sutured into place. (Fig. 3.20*A*). The first lobe of a bilobed flap is rotated into a round defect. The second, a smaller lobe, fills the space vacated by the first lobe, and its defect, in turn, is closed linearly. In this way, tissue may be borrowed from an area with relatively lax skin that permits mobilization and advancement to close a defect in an area that does not (Fig. 3.20*B*).

The *0-to-Z plasty* converts a round defect into a Z-shaped linear one. Sufficient skin must be present to permit adequate mobilization for this technique, which may be useful in the temple or in closing the donor site for a dermis-fat graft to the socket (Fig. 3.21).

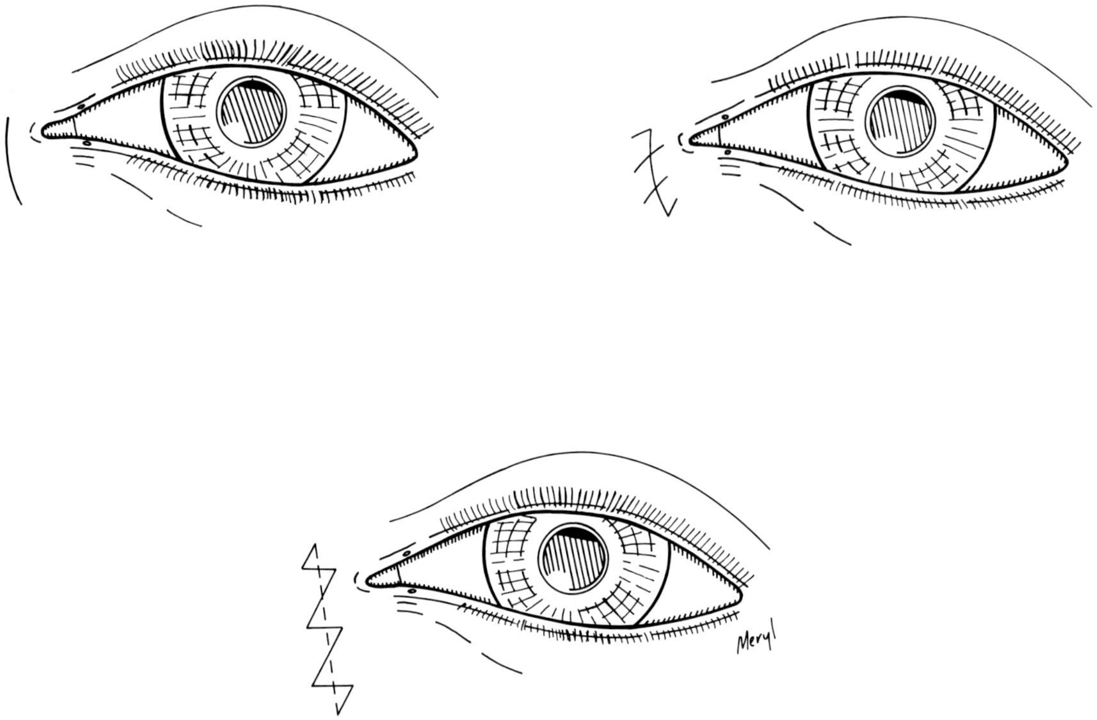

Figure 3.17. A multiple Z plasty to correct a pericanthal fold.

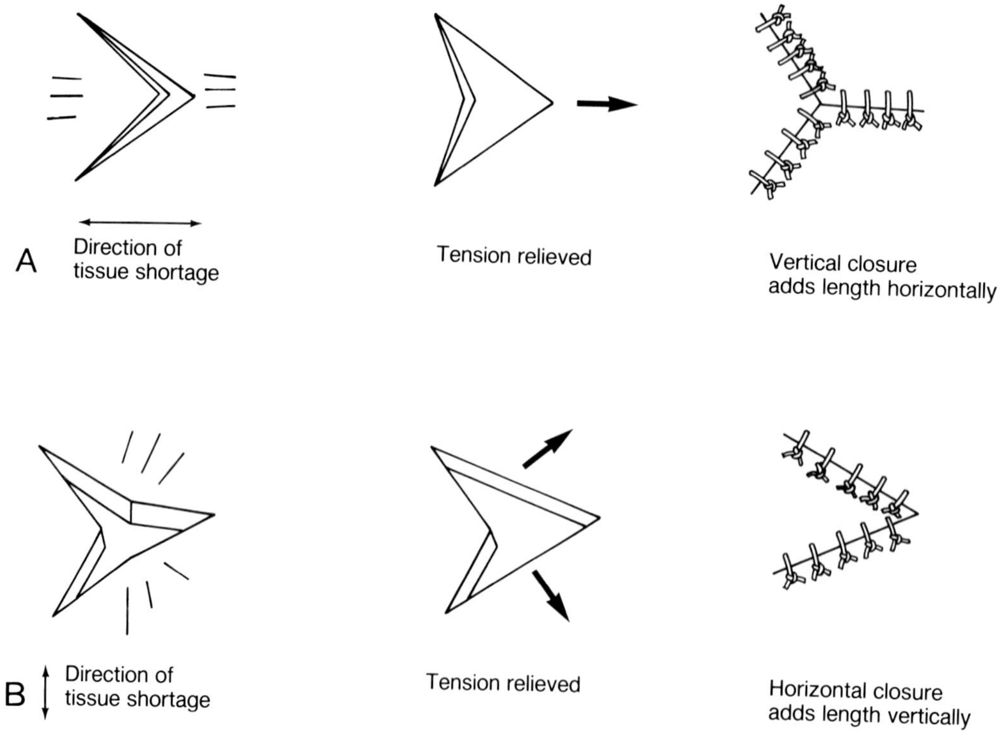

Figure 3.18. *A,* V-to-Y plasty. *B,* Y-to-V plasty.

SKIN GRAFTS

Whereas flaps are rotated, advanced, or transposed into a defect, a true, free graft is entirely transplanted from another location.

Several terms should be defined first to facilitate this discussion: An *autograft* originates in the patient's own body. A *homograft* is derived from another individual of the same species. A *heterograft* comes from another species; *zoograft* is a historical term for animal-derived grafts

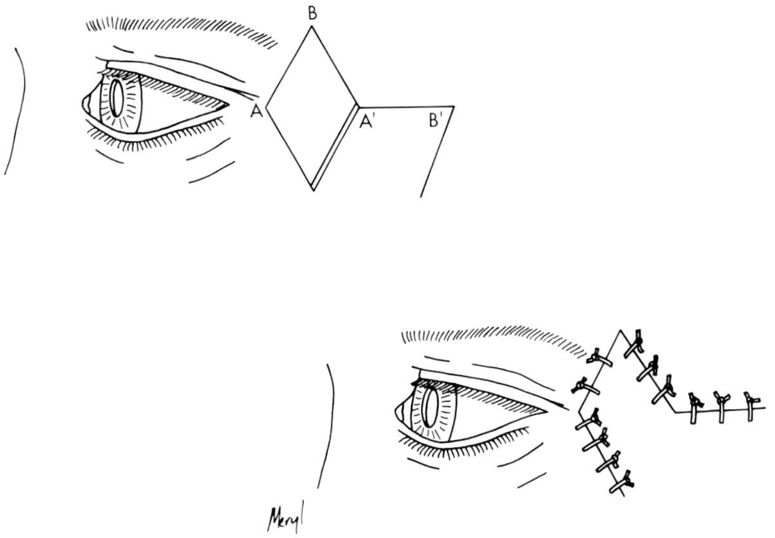

Figure 3.19. A rhomboid flap to correct a defect at the temple.

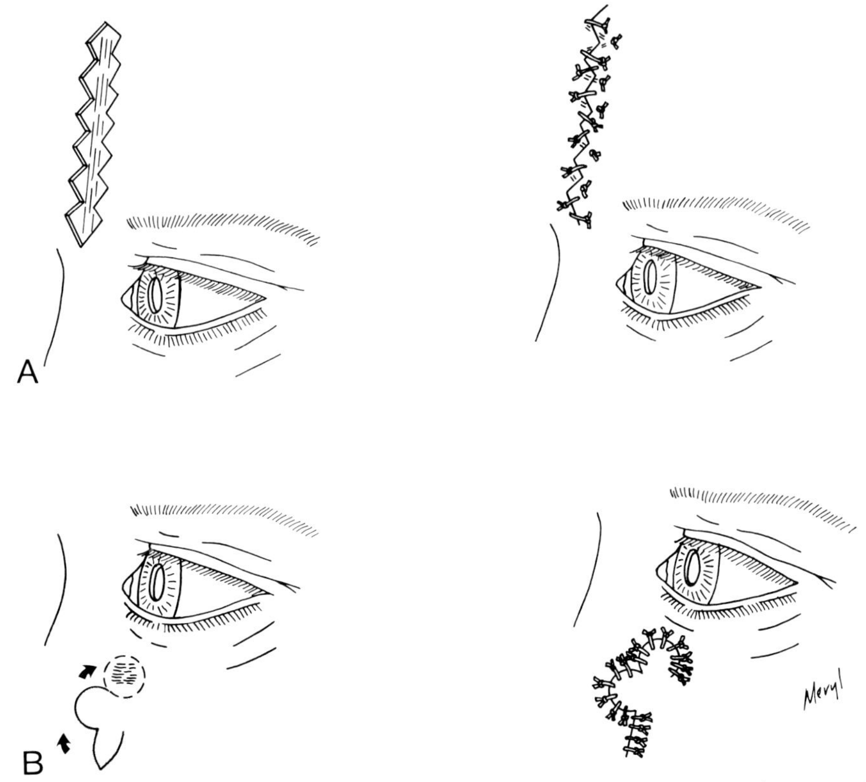

Figure 3.20. *A*, A long W plasty to close a forehead defect. *B*, A classical bilobed flap to correct a defect in the lower lid near the nose.

to humans. A *free graft* is totally uprooted from its source and transplanted. A *flap* or *pedicle graft*, as noted above, retains part of its original attachment.

A *full-thickness* skin graft includes the dermis as well as epidermis and carries with it a normal complement of sweat glands, sebaceous glands, and hair follicles. A *split-thickness* skin graft includes the epidermis but only part of the dermis, and may be thin (0.015 inch), intermediate, or thick (0.10 inch). Thin and intermediate split-thickness grafts contain few sweat glands, sebaceous glands, or hair follicles (Fig. 3.22).

There are relative advantages and disadvantages to each technique. By and large, the best functional and cosmetic results are obtained with full-thickness skin grafts. Color and texture are good, and contraction is less than with split-thickness grafts.

The full-thickness graft, however, is limited by the availability of donor material. The donor sites, of course,

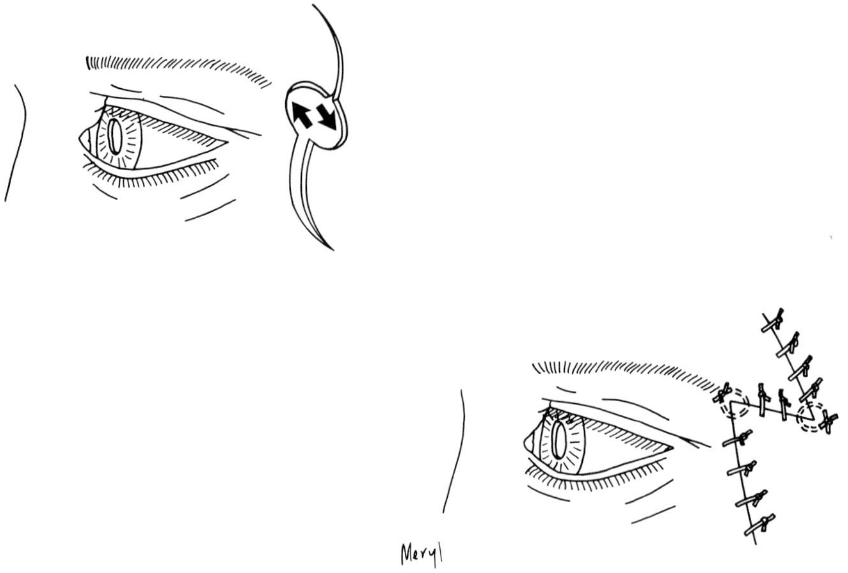

Figure 3.21. An O-to-Z plasty.

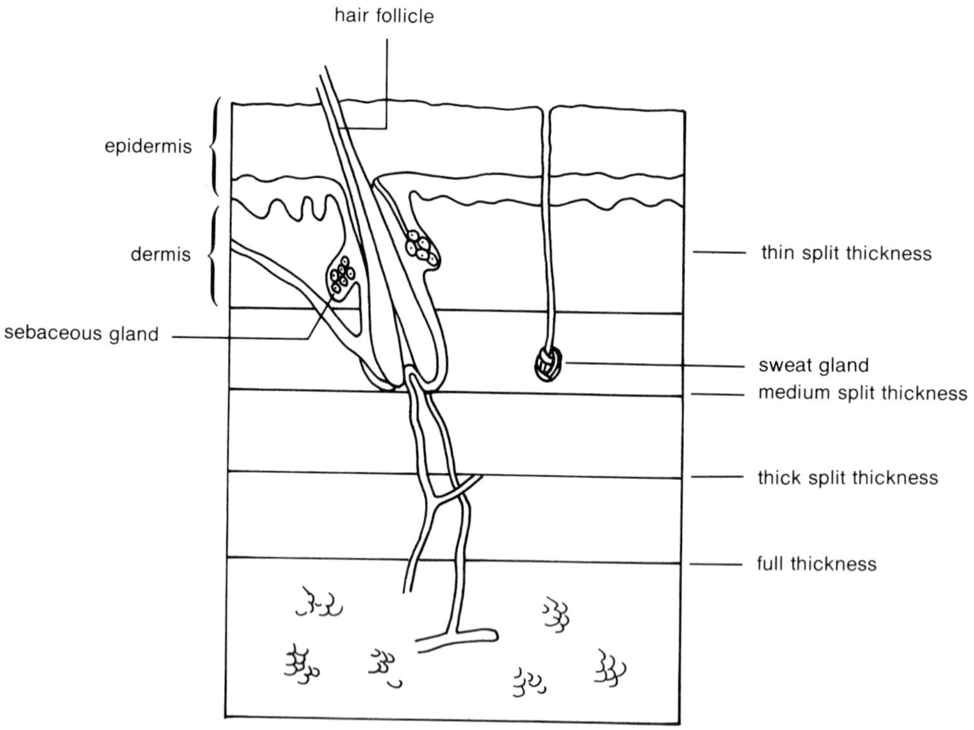

Figure 3.22. A schematic cross section of skin and the cutting levels of various graft thicknesses.

require additional surgery for closure. Also, the challenge of viability is greater in a graft that is thicker. Because vascularization of the graft proceeds more slowly, the chances of failure are greater and the optimal conditions are somewhat more demanding than with a split-thickness graft.

Split-thickness skin can be harvested in much greater quantity, is pliable, viable, and its donor site, which is generally on the thigh or upper, inner arm, requires no closure. It is well-suited for application to granulation tissue, which will not support a full-thickness graft. It can be applied directly to periosteum-free orbital bone and will take somewhat more readily on capillary-poor irradiated tissue. Split-thickness grafts, however, are more prone to change with time, resulting in color and texture variation and tissue contraction. The latter is a particular problem with split-thickness grafts, although stretching may mitigate this process as the scar matures.

DONOR SITES

The best source and the best color match for a full-thickness graft to the eyelids is the thin, pliable skin of the upper eyelid, from which a graft of up to 4 cm may be obtained in suitable patients. The next most desirable site is the skin behind the ears. A fairly large graft can be taken (two similar donor sites are available), and the color and texture match is reasonably good. The donor defect can be closed primarily, or if deemed necessary, with a split-thickness graft from another area. For larger pieces of full-thickness skin, the supraclavicular area and the upper inner arm are possible donor sites. Nonlid skin tends to shrink more than lid skin does, and larger grafts should be taken to compensate for this (Fig. 3.23).

Split-thickness donor sites suitable for the periocular region include the supraclavicular area, the upper inner arm, and the retroauricular area. Some surgeons prefer split-thickness skin from one of these sites for grafting to the upper eyelid as its thinness aids in the motility needed for an upper eyelid. The abdomen and thigh provide large donor areas of good split-thickness skin, but this is not very suitable for the face. It is, however, useful for lining a socket.

SKIN GRAFT SURVIVAL

While a skin graft ultimately requires vascularization and integration into its recipient bed, its immediate metabolic needs must somehow be met before these processes can possibly take place. Without a nutritive supply and an outlet for waste products, the graft cannot survive the immediate postoperative period.

Studies have shown that this function is served by a serum-like fluid derived from the host bed, a process called "imbibition." Fibrin initially anchors the graft in place, although this is, of course, a rather tenuous attachment. The fibrin clot is ultimately organized into a fibrous attachment, typically by the 10th day.

The graft dermis is invaded by capillary sprouts from the host; anastomoses between the host and graft vasculatures take place and host erythrocytes find their way into the graft. Circulation into the graft has been documented by 48 hours postoperatively. Where this vascularization is slow or delayed, a blue or "cyanotic" graft results. As circulation into the graft improves, a healthy pink color develops.

Because of its thinness, a split-thickness graft is considered more viable than a full-thickness graft for several reasons: serum imbibition alone may be sufficient to support it for a longer period of time; revascularization may occur more quickly because of the shorter distance anastomosing vessels must travel; and indeed the richest capillary bed is found in the more superficial layers of the skin.

To succeed, a graft must have a well-vascularized bed that is capable of producing serum imbibition for its early metabolic support and capillary buds for subsequent revascularization. Immobilization of the graft on its recipient bed is critical to assure nutrient exchange and allow for capillary ingrowth.

By the 3rd month, subcutaneous fat can be found, and, if not too much scarring is present in the graft bed, the graft will become reinnervated as host nerve fibers penetrate it. With time, sensation in the graft will approximate that of the surrounding skin.

Proper technique in obtaining, preparing, and laying-in a graft is essential in maximizing the chances for a take. Infection will kill a graft; therefore, scrupulous asepsis must be observed. Many surgeons routinely use prophylactic parenteral antibiotics postoperatively. The graft itself may be soaked in an antibiotic solution prior to its being sutured into place.

The recipient bed must be adequately prepared. Scar tissue should be excised. To receive a split-thickness graft, granulation tissue should be thinned and smoothed out to prevent shrinkage. Full-thickness grafts are not placed over granulation tissue.

The blood supply of the recipient area should be assessed. Will it support a free graft? Will it perhaps support a split-thickness but not a full-thickness graft? When in doubt, it might be safer to consider a pedicle flap graft, which brings with it its own inherent blood supply.

Because a free graft depends upon the absorption of nutrients from its host bed, the presence of blood pooling under the graft may be fatal to it. Hemostasis must be very good—but overcautization can be a fatal flaw as well. Some surgeons elect to puncture a graft to allow for the egress of blood. Any pooled fluid under a graft must be drained if the graft is to succeed.

The graft itself, from a carefully chosen and preferably hairless site, must be meticulously harvested, prepared, and, of course, gently handled.

FULL-THICKNESS SKIN GRAFT

A full-thickness graft, typically spindle-shaped, is planned, marked, outlined by knife incision, and excised thinly with scissors. A template of the recipient bed may be useful in determining the size and shape of the graft.

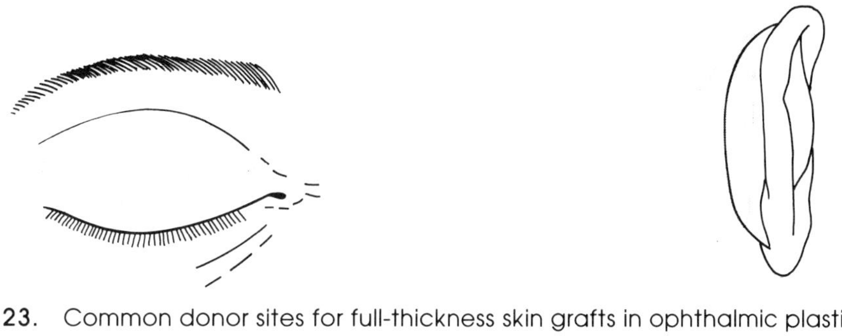

Figure 3.23. Common donor sites for full-thickness skin grafts in ophthalmic plastic surgery.

The skin is first ballooned away from the underlying tissue with an injection of epinephrine-containing local anesthetic. The graft is then laid over the surgeon's finger and carefully defatted and thinned out with delicate scissors. In inadequately defatted, in addition to potential problems with viability, the graft may also end up thick or lumpy. The donor site is sutured closed.

The graft is cut to shape, leaving it slightly oversized to allow for shrinkage. Too large a full-thickness graft will be too thick as it heals. It is anchored into place with 5-0 or 6-0 silk sutures, and then definitively sutured with running or interrupted 6-0 or 7-0 silk. The anchor sutures may be left long to tie a pressure stent into place. Small pieces of Telfa, soaked in antibiotic and then wrung out, are placed over the graft and covered with another piece of Telfa cut to the size and shape of the graft. This stent, held in place by the anchor sutures, serves to provide diffuse, even pressure over the entire graft (Fig. 3.24).

Some surgeons prefer a removable dressing, so that blood collecting under the graft can be detected and evacuated. The graft should be minimally manipulated until it is well integrated and the sutures removed.

SPLIT-THICKNESS SKIN GRAFT

While it is possible to obtain a split-thickness skin graft freehand, this requires a great deal of skill, and, in this technological age this technique is probably a lost art.

The Humby knife was developed in the 1920s and consists of a roller attached to a knife. The thickness of the graft is determined by setting the knife-roller distance with a calibration device.

Drum dermatomes, such as the Padgett-Hood device and its later refinement by Reese, allow for greater accuracy (Fig. 3.25). An adhesive material is applied to the donor site, and, in the Reese unit, a tape is attached to the drum so that the graft will ultimately adhere to the tape. The thickness is set (0.2 to 0.8 mm), and as the drum is rolled over the skin, the blade is brought into play. The tape and graft are then easily removed from the drum, and the thin skin can be readily laid into recipient bed, with or without the tape. Primary contraction, discussed below, will not occur with the tape in place.

The electric dermatome, developed by Brown in the 1940s, permits the rapid removal of large strips of split-thickness skin. The donor skin is lubricated with sterile mineral oil to permit the smooth flow of the instrument. The area is kept taut by the assistant, and as the dermatome is advanced, the emerging graft is drawn up and supported by the assistant. A calibrated dial sets the thickness. Width guides allow the surgeon to determine the width of the graft, which may be up to 3 inches (Fig. 3.26).

Air-driven dermatomes, such as the Stryker or Hall units, operate much like the Brown device but require no electricity. The Davol dermatome, developed in 1965 and recently improved, is battery powered with a disposable cutting head (Fig. 3.27).

The Castroviejo electric dermatome-mucotome is discussed under "Mucous Membrane Grafts." The donor site is covered with Telfa or Zeroform gauze and bandaged. Thin graft donor sites heal within 10 days, with little

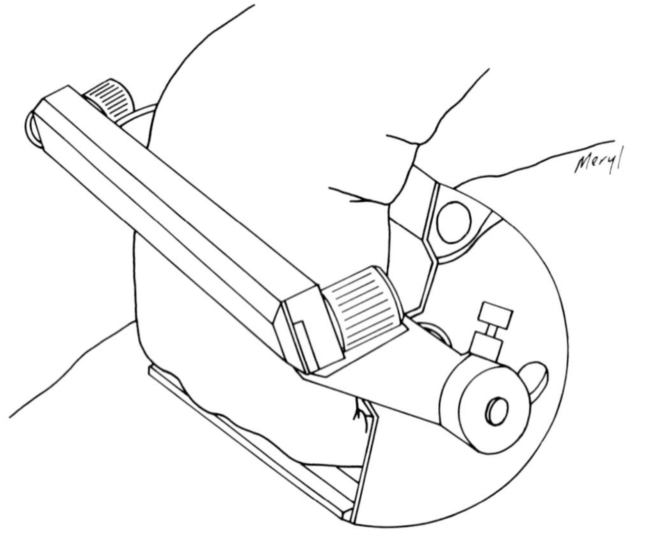

Figure 3.25. A drum-type dermatome for split-thickness skin grafts.

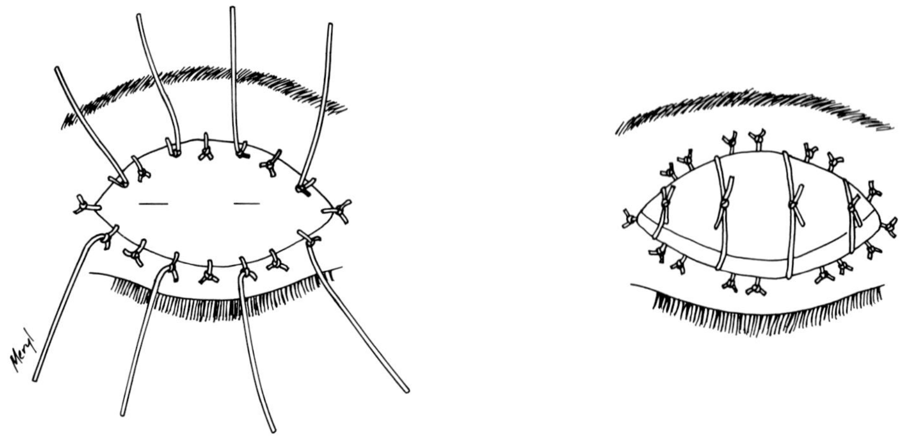

Figure 3.24. A skin graft sutured into place, with perforations to allow for the egress of blood. A stent is tied over the graft with sutures left long for this purpose.

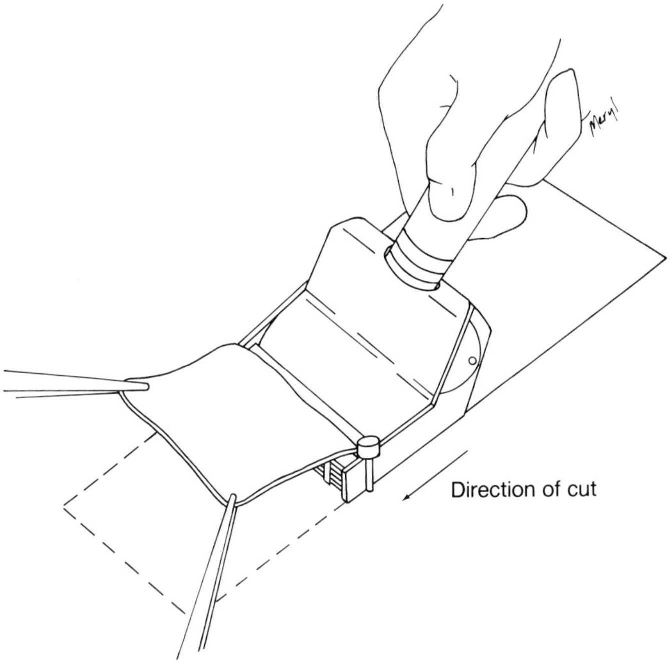

Figure 3.26. An electric dermatome raising a split-thickness skin graft.

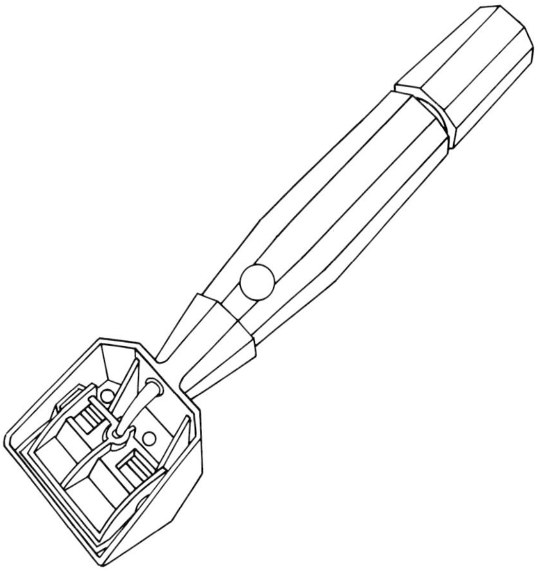

Figure 3.27. A cordless electric dermatome with a disposable cutting head.

residual sequelae. Thicker graft donor sites (70–90% of the dermis) heal in 3–8 weeks but often leave permanent scars. Epidermal regeneration is usually good; dermal regeneration, however, may be poor, with replacement of lost dermis by scar tissue. Loss of elasticity is likely.

CONTRACTION

Graft contraction is described as "primary" or "secondary." Primary contracture results from the inherent elastic properties of the skin and occurs immediately upon harvesting the graft. Because the elastic fibers are found principally in the dermis, full-thickness grafts tend to contract more at this stage than split-thickness grafts and thicker, dermis-bearing, split-thickness grafts will contract more than thinner ones.

Shortly after the removal of a graft, the apparent difference in size between the graft and the donor site from which it was just removed can be amazing and indeed frightening. This kind of contracture is readily reversed by stretching as the graft is sutured into place.

Secondary contracture is a more serious matter. It is a postoperative process that begins on about the 10th day and may continue for up to 6 months. It is at least partly related to factors at the recipient site, such as mobility. A rigid recipient bed is less likely to produce a contracting graft than a more mobile one, such as an eyelid. Thicker grafts contract secondarily less than thinner grafts. A complete take contracts less than a graft in which there is a partial loss, as the lost area heals by contraction and epithelialization from surrounding skin.

When an eyelid is being grafted, leaving the lid on a slight stretch for several days will help minimize contraction of the graft. Massage, with or without steroids, is also helpful in maintaining the size and smoothness of the graft.

MUCOUS MEMBRANE GRAFTS

Mucosal grafts, either split or full-thickness, may be required in oculoplastic reconstructions. Loss of fornices, as may occur in the anophthalmic socket, contracted socket, symblepharon, recurrent pterygium, and cicatricial entropion with trichiasis, are among the more common indications for bulbar or palpebral conjunctival grafts.

The donor sites usually chosen for such grafts are the conjunctiva of the fellow eye (bulbar or fornix-derived) or the oral mucosa (lower lip, cheek, and upper lip). Nasal mucosa, usually as a composite chondromucosal graft, may be used in special circumstances. Vaginal mucosa is rarely used in oculoplastic procedures.

The lower lip is an excellent site for obtaining mucous membrane grafts, as it provides a relatively large area and heals very well with virtually no scarring. It serves well for large socket or cul-de-sac grafts. Because it retains its pink color, buccal mucosa can be unsightly in a visible location. Here a thin, split-thickness mucous membrane graft obtained with an electric mucotome will be less obvious.

In addition to the lower lip, the cheeks provide additional mucous membrane. The tissue here is somewhat thicker and more difficult to obtain. Care must be taken not to harm the parotid duct outlet in the process.

The recipient area is prepared first, and good hemostasis is achieved. The donor site is ballooned up with an injection of epinephrine-containing anesthetic solution. A full-thickness graft is taken freehand, and, as in a full-thickness skin graft, it is turned over and thinned out to excise submucosal fatty and glandular tissue (Fig. 3.28).

Split-thickness mucosal grafts are harvested with a Castroviejo mucotome or a Davol dermatome. They range in thickness from 0.1 to 0.6 mm. For replacing bulbar conjunctiva, the graft should be no thicker than 0.3 to 0.4 mm. Socket linings may be 0.5 to 0.6 mm. The submucosal injection allows the tissue to be cut taut and flat, so that a smooth, even graft is obtained. The gauge is set, and the head of the instrument is applied at a 45° angle and pressed firmly as it advances. An assistant lifts and supports the graft as it emerges in a strip 10–15 mm wide (Fig. 3.29). It is important to keep the proper orientation to avoid confusion later as to which side of this ultrathin membrane is up. The graft should also be larger than the

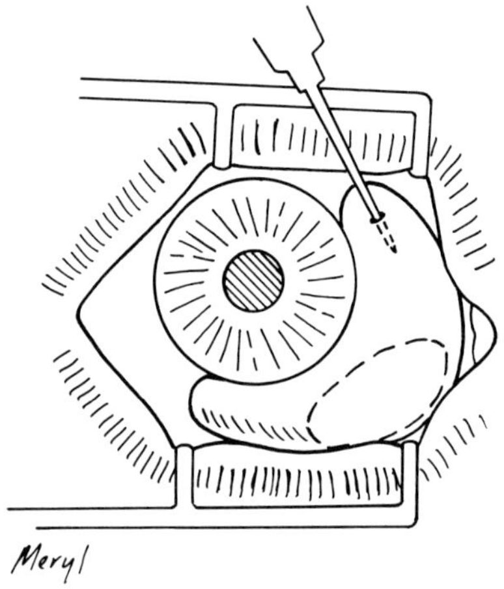

Figure 3.28. A conjunctival graft harvested from the superior bulbar conjunctiva, after first ballooning with epinephrine-containing anesthetic.

recipient area, as substantial shrinkage is anticipated (30–50%). The donor site is left to heal spontaneously, and usually does heal quite nicely in about 2–3 weeks. An antiseptic mouthwash is recommended during the healing process. In addition to sutures, immobilization of the graft should be assured with the use of conformers or stents.

The best cover for the sclera is autogenous conjunctiva, which may be obtained from the fellow eye. Available amounts are limited, however. Bulbar conjunctiva is probably superior to forniceal conjunctiva for replacing visible bulbar conjunctiva defects, as it is thinner and highly transparent.

The conjunctiva is ballooned up with epinephrine with xylocaine. Assessment of the size of the graft should be made before this injection, as the conjunctiva expands greatly and may look deceptively large. The graft is carefully dissected with Westcott scissors. Here too it is critical not to lose track of which side is up when the graft is free. It should be immediately anchored to the recipient site with fine absorbable sutures and stented into place as indicated.

The lateral upper fornix should be avoided so as not to damage the lacrimal gland ducts. The donor site does not normally require closure, although a few fine sutures, if desired, will keep it from spreading.

Other materials, natural and alloplastic, are finding increasing use in oculoplastic reconstructions. Cartilage, to replace tarsus, may be obtained from the nose together with mucous membrane. An alternate site is the ear. Some surgeons use rib cartilage. Bone, tarsus, fascia lata (autogenous or homogenous), dermis with fat, and bank sclera have their uses in reconstructive procedures. Silastic (in ready-made sheets or quick-curing liquid form), Supramid, and Teflon add to the surgical armamentarium. The applications of these materials will be discussed in the appropriate chapters on reconstructive techniques.

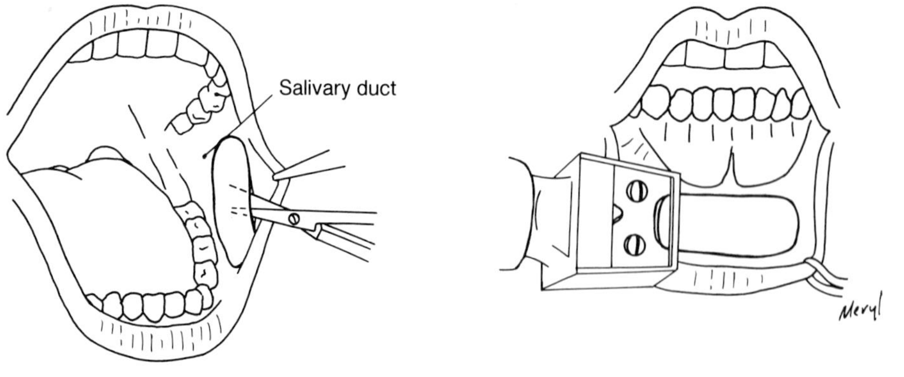

Figure 3.29. Preparation of thick and thin mucous membrane grafts from the oral cavity.

CONCLUSION

Mankind has learned that despite its many shortcomings, its capacity to grow and to achieve cannot be fathomed. Some view this in a secular context. Others see it as God's mandate to continue and complete acts of Creation. As far as we have come from the first, primitive attempts to heal and, in a sense, recreate the human body, we cannot conceive what tomorrow's developments may bring. And so, we will continue to learn, to build, to strive, to perfect. It is in our nature to do so. Our particular subject of interest, ophthalmic plastic and reconstructive surgery, is an ideal model for this striving, and a most appropriate vehicle for its expression.

SUGGESTED READINGS

Arrington GE: *A History of Ophthalmology*. New York, MD Publications, 1959.

Beyer CK, Albert DM: The use and fate of fascia lata in ophthalmic plastic and reconstructive surgery. *Ophthalmology* 88: 869–886, 1981.

Borges AF: *Elective Incisions and Scar Revision*. Boston, Little, Brown & Co., 1973.

Bullock JD, Koss N, Flagg SV: Rhomboid flap in ophthalmic plastic surgery. *Arch Ophthalmol* 90: 203, 1973.

Callahan MA, Callahan A: *Ophthalmic Plastic and Orbital Surgery*. Birmingham, Aesculapius, 1979.

Converse JM: *Reconstructive Plastic Surgery*. Philadelphia, WB Saunders, 1977, vol 1.

Dineen P: *The Surgical Wound*. Philadelphia, Lea & Febiger, 1981.

Dupuis C, Rees TD: Historical notes in blepharoplasty. *Plast Reconstr Surg* 47: 246–251.

Duke-Elder S, MacFaul P: The ocular adnexa. *System of Ophthalmology*. London, Kimpton, 1974, vol 13.

Fox SA: *Ophthalmic Plastic Surgery*, ed 5. New York, Grune & Stratton, 1976.

Fox SA: Basic techniques in lid surgery: their origins and their apocrypha. *Am J Ophthalmol* 50: 384, 1960.

Grabb WC, Smith JW (eds): *Plastic Surgery*. Boston, Little, Brown & Co., 1973.

Iliff CE, Iliff WJ, Iliff NT: *Oculoplastic Surgery*. Philadelphia, WB Saunders, 1979.

Katzen LB: History of cosmetic oculoplastic surgery. In Putterman A (ed): *Cosmetic Oculoplastic Surgery*. New York, Grune & Stratton, 1982.

Lubkin V: Psychologic Aspects of Ophthalmic Plastic Surgery. In Silver B (ed): *Ophthalmic Plastic Surgery*. American Academy of Ophthalmology and Otolaryngology, Rochester, MN 1977, pp 43–45.

McGregor IA: *Fundamental Techniques of Plastic Surgery and Their Surgical Applications*. Baltimore, Williams & Wilkins, 1972.

Milani MR, Kornfeld DS: Psychiatry and surgery. In Kaplan HI, Freedman AM, Seddock BJ (eds): *Comprehensive Textbook of Psychiatry*. Baltimore, Williams & Wilkins, 1980, vol 3, pp 2056–2069.

Mustarde JC: *Repair and Reconstruction in the Orbital Region*. Baltimore, Williams & Wilkins, 1966.

Putterman A (ed): *Cosmetic Oculoplastic Surgery*. New York, Grune & Stratton, 1982.

Rees TD: *Aesthetic Plastic Surgery*. Philadelphia, WB Saunders, 1980.

Robbins SL: *Pathology*. Philadelphia, WB Saunders, 1968.

Rogers BO: History of skin transplantation. In Troutman RC et al (eds): *Plastic and Reconstructive Surgery of the Eye and Adnexa*. Washington, Butterworth, 1962.

Soll DB: *Management of Complications in Ophthalmic Plastic Surgery*. Birmingham, Aesculapius, 1976.

Tenzel RR: Reconstruction of the central one-half of an eyelid. *Arch Ophthalmol* 93: 125, 1975.

Wilkins RB, Kulwin DR: Skin and Tissue Techniques. In McCord CW (ed): *Oculoplastic Surgery*. New York, Raven Press, 1981.

CHAPTER 4

Anesthesia in Ophthalmic Plastic Surgery

GIL A. EPSTEIN, M.D.

The choice of anesthesia is an integral part of ophthalmic plastic surgery. The surgeon must assess the age, physical condition, and psychological status of the patient along with proposed surgical procedure. An understanding of the various modalities will enable the surgeon to provide maximum comfort with as little possible risk.

As a rule, children are best operated on under general anesthesia. Some adult procedures (orbital, lacrimal, enucleation) are best suited for general anesthesia. For eyelid procedures, either local or regional anesthesia may be used to achieve optimal cosmetic results.

PRESURGICAL EVALUATION

A complete medical history should be available to the surgeon. Working with the patient's family practitioner, internist, or pediatrician is helpful to the surgeon and often comforts the patient. The surgeon should be aware of medications the patient takes, presence of allergies, social habits, and previous surgical experiences. This is the time to decide which medications should be taken and which should be discontinued. The present trend is to allow patients their oral cardiac and antihypertensives with 30 cc of water. If an anesthesiologist is to be present, he or she should evaluate the patient. A compassionate interview will instill confidence and security in the patient.

PREANESTHETIC MEDICATION

A wide variety of sedatives, tranquilizers, and pain medications are available for preanesthesia. For the patient undergoing general anesthesia, the premedication can be ordered by the anesthesiologist and often includes an anticholinergic to reduce secretions. For those patients having local anesthesia, the premedication should be tailored to the individual patient as well as the surgical procedure and technique. Although many preanesthetic medications are available, the following discussion includes the four categories of drugs most frequently used: (*a*) Hypnotic-sedative, (*b*) tranquilizers, (*c*) narcotics-analgesics, and (*d*) anticholinergics.

HYPNOTIC-SEDATIVES

The hypnotic-sedatives are general central nervous system (CNS) depressants that are frequently used to calm and relieve apprehension. Barbiturates are the oldest group of hypnotic-sedatives, and secobarbital (Seconal) and pentobarbital (Nembutal) are the most often prescribed. The usual hypnotic dose is 100 mg orally, 90 minutes prior to surgery. For children 3–4 mg/kg is used. Consideration should be given to the respiratory depressive action. If sleep is undesirable during an ophthalmic plastic procedure (levator surgery, blepharoplasty) barbiturates should be avoided.

Chloral hydrate is a nonbarbiturate hypnotic-sedative whose main action is sleep. It has worked well in the author's experience as a premedication for nitrous oxide-oxygen conscious sedation in reducing nausea. The usual dose in adults is 500–1000 mg, 30–60 minutes prior to surgery.

TRANQUILIZERS

This group of medication primarily relieves anxiety. Amnesia may be produced as well as some sedation. The benzodiazepines are the most widely used tranquilizers, of which diazepam (Valium) is most frequently prescribed. There is questionable potentiation of narcotic effect by diazepam as well as antiemetic effect. The usual dosage is 5–10 mg in adults administered orally or intramuscularly 1 hour prior to surgery. Caution should be used in elderly patients because of potential disorientation. Tolerance of diazepam is often seen. Diazepam has anticonvulsive properties and may help reduce CNS toxicity from local anesthetics. If diazepam is given intravenously, it should be given slowly in 1- to 2.5-mg increments.

Phenothiazine derivatives are often used to potentiate the effect of narcotics. Promethazine (Phenergan) is most widely used; the usual dosage is 25–50 mg intramuscularly 30–60 minutes before surgery. Hydroxyazine pomate (Vistaril) is a similar drug but is not truly in the phenothiazine group. Hydroxyzine pomate similarly potentiates the action of narcotics as well as provides antiemetic, sedative, and tranquilizing effects. The usual dosage in adults is 12.5–75 mg intramuscularly 30–60 minutes preoperatively.

NARCOTIC ANALGESICS

The primary use for preanesthetic narcotics is pain relief. Anticipated painful local anesthetic injections as well as reduction in pain associated with lying for prolonged time are important considerations. Secondary functions of narcotics are euphoria or sedation. Narcotics produce respiratory depression that may last 2–3 hours; these should be used cautiously in patients with pulmonary diseases. Postural hypotension is occasionally encountered and should be considered in the ambulatory patient. Nausea and vomiting are common side effect of narcotics but may be reduced when combined with phenothiazine-like compounds. Morphine sulfate and meperidine (Demerol) are the most likely used narcotic analgesic preanesthetic medications. Dosage for morphine sulfate is 2–10 mg intramuscularly 1 hour preoperatively. Meperidine is usually prescribed 12.5–100 mg intramuscularly 1 hour preoperatively. Sublimase (Fentanyl) is a synthetic narcotic analgesic with similar properties to morphine and meperidine. It is given intravenously in doses of 0.25 mg–1 mg and has onset of action within 5 minutes. It can cause occasional muscular rigidity. Ultra-short-acting synthetic narcotics (Sufentonil and Alfentanil) are presently being introduced which may be of great use in out-patient surgery that is increasing in popularity.

Naloxone hydrochloride (Narcan) is the most widely used narcotic antagonist to reverse confusion or excess sedation produced by narcotics. The usual dosage is 0.1–0.4 mg and is administered intravenously.

ANTICHOLINERGICS

The primary use of anticholinergics is for its antisialagogue effect; they also prevent vagal reflexes encountered with general anesthesia. Atropine sulfate and scopolamine are the most commonly used. The usual adult dose of atropine is 0.4 mg intramuscularly 30–60 minutes prior to surgery, or intravenously just prior to induction of general anesthesia. Although scopolamine is a better antisialagogue, it has less antivagal effect. Caution is advised with geriatric patients as they can occasionally become restless and disoriented. The usual dose of scopolamine is 0.4–0.6 mg intramuscularly.

Glycopyrolate (Robinol) is rapidly becoming the most frequently used anticholinergic because (*a*) it has an increased anticholinergic potency, (*b*) it produces little sedation, and (*c*) it does not have tachycardia as a side effect. The usual adult dose is 0.2 mg intramuscularly.

GENERAL ANESTHESIA

The definition of general anesthesia is reversible unconsciousness with loss of sensation of pain. Indications for general anesthesia in patients undergoing ophthalmic plastic surgical procedures are (*a*) infants and children; (*b*) patient preference, unless the procedure necessitates patient cooperation; (*c*) extensive and prolonged procedure; (*d*) patients with mental disorders or uncooperative patients; (*e*) patients unable to lie still because of muscular-skeletal disorders.

An anesthesiologist usually administers and monitors the general anesthesia. A proper history and physical examination by the anesthesiologist will determine the optimal general anesthetic that should be given. The ophthalmic plastic surgeon should be familiar with the commonly used agents. General anesthetic agents may be administered parenterally, by inhalation, orally, or rectally.

Thiopental (Pentothal) and methoxatal (Brevitol) are members of the barbiturate family and are usually administered intravenously. They act rapidly and are primarily used as inducing agents prior to the use of inhalation general anesthesia. These agents also may be used to relieve the fear or discomfort from local injection. One half to one third the usual induction dose is used under these circumstances.

Dissociation anesthesia is produced by ketamine, which rapidly produces analgesia, anesthesia, and dissociation from the surroundings. Ketamine is indicated in pediatric patients undergoing short procedures that do not necessitate endotracheal anesthesia. Hypertension, tachycardia, increased intraocular pressure, and nystagmus are frequent side effects. Hallucinations, confusion and fright are occasionally seen in the postrecovery period. Because of the multitude and frequency of side effects, the long recovery time, and the lack of antagonist, I do not advocate its use in ophthalmic plastic surgery.

Halothane is perhaps the most widely used general inhalation anesthetic; it is especially used in children. It is a nonexplosive agent that produces little nausea. Heptatoxicity has been reported with halothane, especially with repeated administrations. Halothane sensitizes the myocardium to catecholamines, so care must be taken to avoid excessive epinephrine injections for the purpose of hemostasis.

Nitrous oxide is a less potent analgesic than halothane; however, it is frequently combined with other agents to potentiate action. Nitrous oxide in combination with oxygen is a safe method for sedations and is discussed in detail in the second half of this chapter. Enflurane (Ethraine) and isoflurane (Forane) are now the most widely used inhalation agents for adults in the United States. Enphraine (Ethraine) is a nonflammable agent with the advantage of less myocardial sensitivity to catecholamines. A seizure pattern is seen on electroencephalogram in 2% of patients. Renal toxicity is also suspected. Forane is an isomer of Ethraine and does not have the CNS or renal toxic effects of Ethraine.

LOCAL ANESTHESIA

Local anesthetics are agents that produce loss of sensation in a circumscribed area. There are two general types: topical and injectable. These agents work by inhibiting excitation at nerve endings or blocking conduction in peripheral nerves. Local anesthetics are classified into esters or amides based on the chemical linkage between two of their components, the lipophilic aromatic and the hydrophilic amide. Cocaine, procaine, and tetracaine are esters; while lidocaine, mepivicaine, bupivocaine, and etidocaine are amides. Allergic reactions are most commonly seen with the ester group. Cocaine blocks nerve reuptake of norepinephrine, whereas all others prevent nerve depolarization by preventing entrance of sodium ions that are essential for nerve conduction. Chemical properties of local anesthetics account for their increased tissue penetration in higher-alkaline solutions. The onset and duration of action of these agents depend on the length of time the drug is protein bound. Esters are eliminated in the plasma by pseudocholinesterone, while amides are degraded in the liver. Toxic reactions are due to blood absorbability and occur infrequently in ophthalmic plastic surgery. This is because small volumes are necessary for surgery. Central nervous system stimulation (excitement, apprehension, nausea) or depression (drowsiness, respiratory failure, and cardiovascular collapse) may occur. Since all local anesthetics, with the exception of cocaine, are vasodilators, tachycardia, hypotension, and syncope may be seen as toxic effects.

Epinephrine is often mixed with local anesthetics, thereby causing vasoconstriction. This prolongs the duration of action and decreases toxicity from blood absorption. However, side effects from epinephrine (tachycardia, hypertension, CNS stimulation) should be considered in predisposed patients.

TOPICAL AGENTS

Cocaine Hydrochloride

Cocaine was discovered by Koller in 1884 and derives from the erylthroxylin coca bush. It was the first anesthetic used topically in ophthalmology. Its mechanism of action is by blocking reuptake of nonepinephrine at the nerve terminal. It has vasoconstrictive aspect and should not be used with epinephrine. Cocaine has an additional sympathomimetic effect and is often used to diagnose Horner's syndrome. Cocaine toxicity makes its use rare today. However, it is useful in lacrimal surgery to vasoconstrict mucous membranes; gauze strips soaked in 5% cocaine solution are packed into the nasal cavity.

Tetracaine Hydrochloride (Pontocaine Hydrochloride)

This widely used drug has rapid onset (under 30 seconds), with a duration of action of 15 to 20 minutes. It is available in 0.5–2% solution. Like cocaine, tetracaine is toxic to the cornea, usually manifesting as superficial punctuate keratopathy. Many patients complain of burning until the anesthetic effect is reached. Sterile vials are available for intraoperative use.

Proparocaine Hydrochloride (Ophthaine, Ak-Taine, Alcaine)

Proparocaine has similar actions as tetracaine. Although there is less toxicity to the cornea and less discomfort, there is a higher incidence of allergic reaction (conjunctival injection, lid swelling, superficial punctate keratopathy). It is available in a 0.5% solution but is not available for intraoperative use.

INJECTABLE AGENTS

Various injectable local anesthetics are available. The differences are mainly speed of onset and duration of action. Table 4.1 lists the most widely available commercial products. Epinephrine hydrochloride is frequently added to local agents to cause vasoconstriction, which decreases systemic absorption and prolongs the anesthetic effect thereby decreasing toxicity. Another advantage is

Table 4.1
Local Anesthetic Agents for Injection

Agent	Onset	Duration	Maximum Dose
Procaine (Novocaine)	<5 min	30–60 min	10–14 mg/kg
Lidocaine (Xylocaine)	<5 min	2–3 h	4–7 mg/kg
Mepivicaine (Carbocaine)	5 min	2 h	4.5 mg/kg
Bupivicaine (Marcaine)	10 min	>6 h	3–5 mg/kg
Etidocaine (Duranest)	3–5 min	>6 h	4–5 mg/kg

the increased hemostasis at the operative site. Systemic effects of epinephrine are tachycardia, palpitations, tremor, apprehension, pallor and hypertension. Epinephrine should be used cautiously in patients with significant heart disease, hypertension and thyrotoxicosis.

Hyaluronidase (Wydase) is frequently added to local anesthetics to increase tissue permeability, which shortens the onset of anesthetic effect. The increased tissue spread from hyaluronidase enables the surgeon to use less anesthetic; however, the duration of anesthetic effect is decreased.

Procaine Hydrochloride (Novocaine)

Procaine, one of the first local anesthetics available for injection, was first synthesized in 1905. It has an onset of action within minutes and lasts 30 to 60 minutes. Procaine is most commonly used in 1 to 2% solutions. Toxic effects include nausea, convulsion, and cardiovascular collapse when dosages exceed those recommended. It is therefore rarely used today.

Lidocaine Hydrochloride (Xylocaine)

Lidocaine is perhaps the most widely used local infiltrative anesthetic. Its action is similar to procaine but has a quicker onset of action, better tissue diffusion, and longer duration of action. Lidocaine is most commonly available in 1% or 2% solution. Some feel that 2% solution gives a more potent and longer duration of action. Others feel that there is no difference in its action and 2% solution is more toxic. Systemic toxicity is manifested by nausea, vomiting, drowsiness, personality change, hypotension, and convulsions. Care must be taken when soaking sponges or gauze in solution of lidocaine because systemic absorption may occur. Maximum amounts of lidocaine recommended are 3 mg/kg without epinephrine, 5 mg/kg with epinephrine, and no more than 500 mg under any circumstance. Lidocaine is available for topical use in a 4% solution.

Mepivicaine Hydrochloride (Carbocaine)

Mepivicane is similar to lidocaine in terms of dosages, duration of action, and toxicity. It is used when the patient has allergy to other local anesthetics.

Bupivicaine Hydrochloride (Marcaine)

Bupivicaine is one of the longest-acting local anesthetics and is useful in long ophthalmic plastic procedures. Because of its long onset of action, bupivicaine is often mixed with lidocaine to combine short onset with long duration. It is most commonly available in 0.5% and 0.75% solutions. Bupivicaine has similar toxicity as lidocaine, but cardiotoxic reactions (asystole) and respiratory arrest have been reported with the use of 0.75%. The maximum dose of bupivicaine recommended is 250 mg.

Etidocaine Hydrochloride (Duranest)

The agent is gaining popularity because of the short onset of action and the prolonged anesthetic effect. The chemical properties are similar to Lidocaine. It is most commonly available in 0.5–2% solutions, with 250 mg as the maximum safe dose.

METHODS OF LOCAL INJECTION OF ANESTHETIC AGENTS

INFILTRATIVE ANESTHESIA

Injecting local anesthetic directly into the area to be operated on is the most widely used method to produce anesthesia. For best control, a 25- to 30-gauge needle is an optimal size. Periodic aspiration of the syringe is useful in preventing direct intravenous administration. The surgeon may try to limit the amount of agent delivered when seeking sensory anesthesia without motor akinesia. This is most applicable to levator surgery when lid levels are assessed intraoperatively.

Infiltrative anesthesia is frequently uncomfortable; this can be minimized by a slower rate of injection and the comfort and assuredness of another person's hand (nurse, anesthetist, anesthesiologist). Often a short-acting sedative (pentobarbitol) or nitrous oxide–oxygen can be given to prevent discomfort and induce amnesia. The discomfort from infiltrative anesthesia is due more to the activity of the anesthetic solution (particularly containing epinephrine) than from needle penetration.

REGIONAL ANESTHESIA

Injection of anesthetic agents into nerve bundles requires knowledge of the anatomy of the orbit and eyelids. Regional or nerve block anesthesia avoids tissue distortion as opposed to infiltrative anesthesia and requires less agent to produce a similar anesthetic effect. Separation of motor and sensory anesthesia can be achieved with regional anesthesia. Refer to the chapter on anatomy for a detailed description of the nerve supply to the orbit and lids. A synopsis of the practical anatomy is given in Figure 4.1.

Frontal Nerve Block

The frontal and lacrimal nerves supply the majority of sensation in the upper lids. These nerves enter the orbit through the superior orbital fissure and follow the roof of the orbit between periosteum and intermuscular membrane. The entrance of these nerves is approximately 4 cm posterior to the superior orbital margin. The technique of frontal nerve sensory anesthesia, which was advocated by Hildreth and Silver, has gained popularity.

A retrobulbar (4 cm) needle (22 or 23 gauge) is placed in the center of the superior orbital rim and the needle is directed posteriorly so that it hugs the roof of the orbit (Fig. 4.2). An index finger placed over the supraorbital notch can aid in needle placement and care must be taken to not deviate from a central line to avoid perforating supraorbital vessels. When the needle is fully inserted, the syringe is aspirated to ensure no direct placement in vessel. One half to 0.75 ml is all that is usually necessary to achieve sensory anesthesia (Fig. 4.3). Caution is advised not to inject in the periosteum or the anesthesia will be ineffective. If the anesthetic is placed within the intermuscular membrane, levator akinesia may ensue (Fig. 4.3).

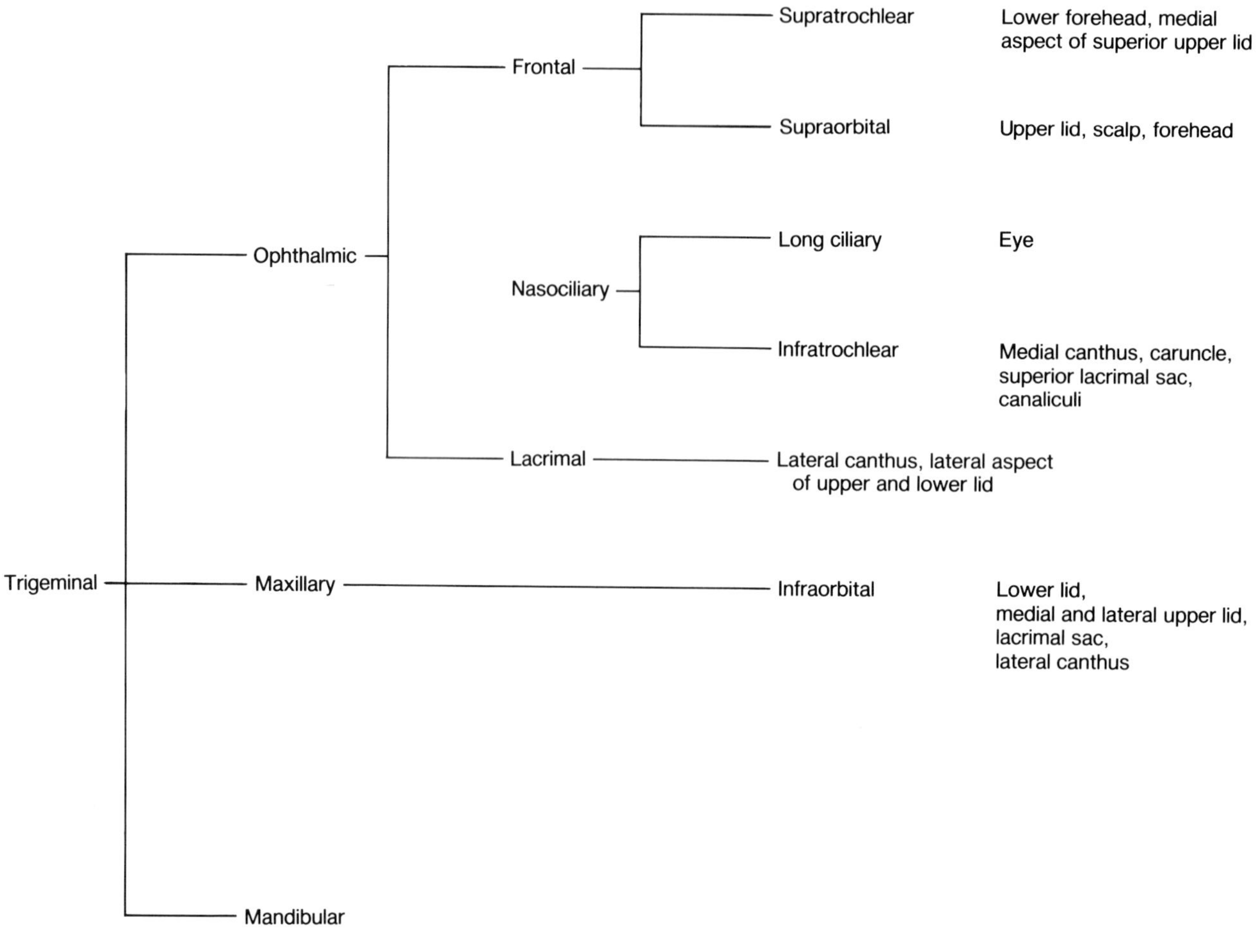

Figure 4.1. Sensory innervations of the eyelids and orbit.

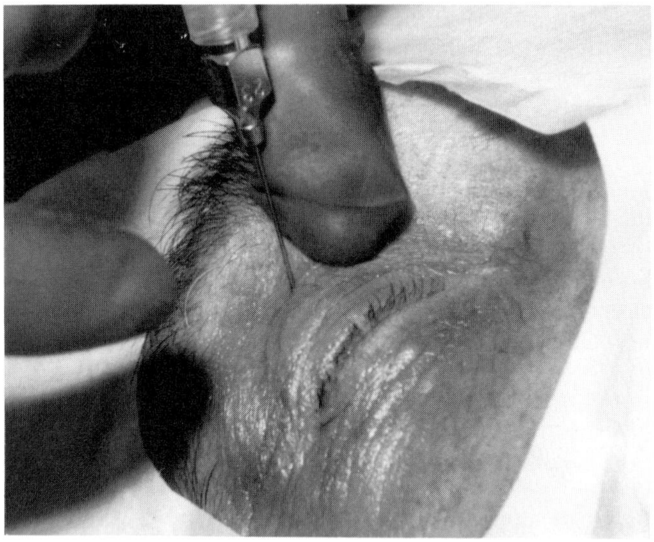

Figure 4.2. Frontal nerve block—retrobulbar needle hugs the superior orbital roof.

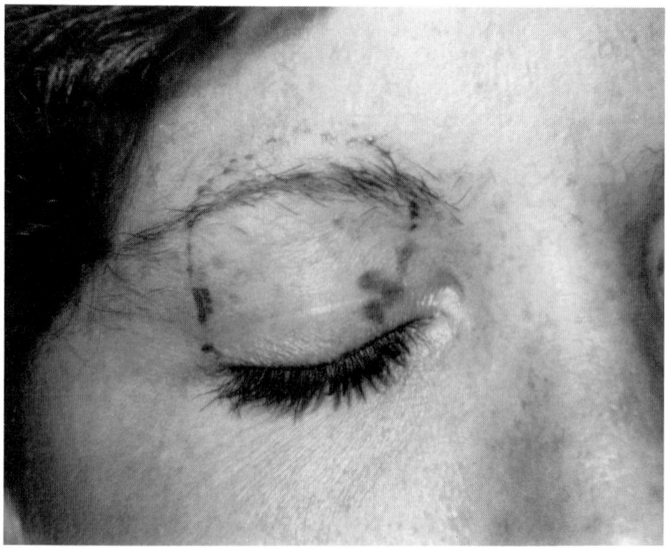

Figure 4.3. Area of anesthesia from frontal nerve block.

The supratrochlear and the supraorbital nerves are branches of the frontal nerve, and the infratrochlear nerve bundles are branches from the nasociliary nerve. Each may be selectively blocked. Infratrochlear and supratrochlear regional blocks are useful in lacrimal surgery (Fig. 4.4). These nerves lie just below the palpable trochlea, and

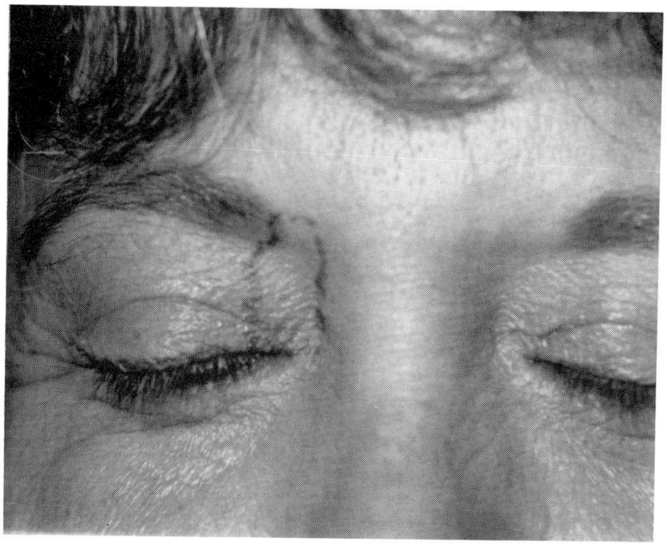

Figure 4.4. Area blocked by supratrochlear block.

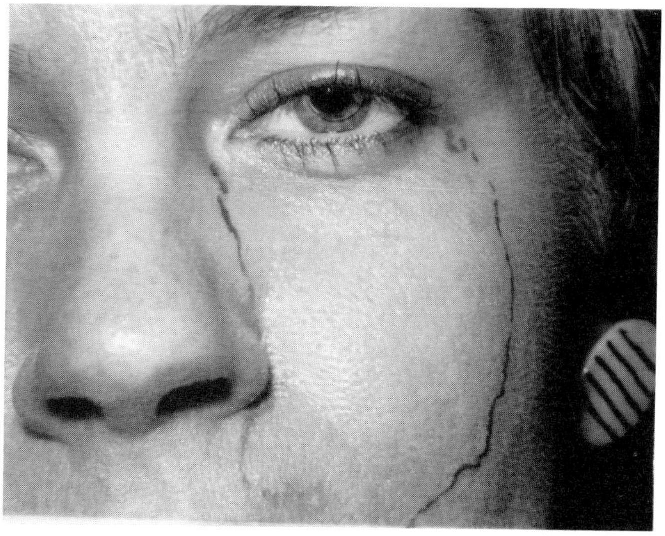

Figure 4.5. Area anesthetized from infraorbital regional block.

a retrobulbar needle is placed posteriorly 1.5–2.5 cm hugging the medial orbit. A supraorbital block is not advocated due to the close proximity of the supraorbital vessels.

The infraorbital nerve is a branch of the maxillary nerve which is the second branch of the trigeminal. The infraorbital nerve courses through the infraorbital canal and emerges from the infraorbital foramen, which is approximately 1.5 cm below the inferior orbital rim and is in line with the supraorbital notch and pupil. The needle should be placed into the foramen and into the canal; this will anesthetize the lower lid, inferior lacrimal sac, upper lid and upper central teeth (Fig. 4.5).

The lacrimal nerve is a division of the ophthalmic nerve that innervates the lateral canthus, lateral aspect of the upper and lower lids, and lacrimal gland. The needle penetrates the superior-most aspect of the lateral orbital wall and traverses posteriorly 2.5 cm to achieve selective anesthesia of the nerve.

NITROUS OXIDE–OXYGEN CONSCIOUS SEDATION

Conscious sedation is a valuable adjunct to local anesthesia in ophthalmic plastic surgery. Nitrous oxide-Oxygen when used in combination is the most popular inhalation technique and is widely used in the dental community. The ophthalmic plastic surgery community is most likely uninformed about N_2O due to its association in producing general anesthesia. With increasing numbers of patients undergoing cosmetic surgical procedures attention must be directed at making the surgical experience pleasant and the patient comfortable. Safety is also a significant consideration in view of increasing outpatient surgery. Subanesthetic effects of N_2O-O_2 provide a safe, effective, and controllable tool in providing patient comfort.

HISTORICAL PERSPECTIVES

Joseph Priestly first synthesized N_2O in 1772. Twenty years later, Sir Humphrey Davy commented on its properties. In 1799, Davy constructed a gas delivery machine. Horace Wells, who is credited as the discoverer of general anesthesia, had a tooth extracted in 1844 under the influence of N_2O. In 1868, Edmund Andrews commented on asphyxia caused by 100% N_2O and advocated combination with O_2. Since the 1940s the dental community has begun to establish the technique of conscious sedation using subanesthetic doses of N_2O-O_2 and has developed much of modern-day delivery systems.

CHEMISTRY

Nitrous oxide is an inorganic inhalation agent that is colorless and is without significant odor or taste. Nitrous oxide is prepared in equilibrium between its liquid and gaseous phases. It is marketed in blue steel cylinders as opposed to oxygen, which comes in pure gaseous form and is sold in green tanks. Nitrous oxide supports combustion similar to O_2. The blood-gas solubility is low, which accounts for its rapid onset and recovery.

PHARMACOLOGY

Nitrous oxide primarily affects the central nervous system. It is the weakest of all general anesthetics. The pharmacologic effects of N_2O vary with the concentration and are thus dose related. The subjective reaction to N_2O applicable in conscious sedation are those in Table 4.2 and correspond to the stages of anesthesia. Cardiovascular effects correlate to inhaling 100% O_2 and include a minimal rise in mean arterial pressure due to increased peripheral vascular resistance. There is insignificant reduction in cardiac output. There are no significant effects on the respiratory system. Nitrous oxide is primarily excreted by the pulmonary system, with a small amount excreted by skin. The major side effect is nausea and is dose related. Some authors feel nausea is more likely in a patient with

Table 4.2
Subjective Symptoms of Nitrous Oxide-Oxygen Conscious Sedation

- Stage I Anesthesia
  - Level 1
    - Feeling of relaxation
    - Tingling sensation in fingers, lips, or tongue
    - Feeling of warmth
  - Level 2
    - Humming, droning, buzzing sounds
    - Lethargy
    - Drowsiness
    - Euphoria
    - Analgesia
  - Level 3
    - Hallucination
    - Dreams
    - Fears (falling, dying)
    - Nausea
- Stages II–IV Anesthesia—Unconscious

Table 4.3
Objective Signs of Nitrous Oxide-Oxygen Conscious Sedation

- Stage I Anesthesia
  - Level I
    - Normal relaxed, fully conscious. Follows directions
  - Level 2
    - Relaxed, euphoric, less aware of surrounding. Follows directions but is slower
  - Level 3
    - Brow perspiration, body stiffening, claw hand, less aware of surroundings—usually does not follow directions
- Stage II Anesthesia-rigid, active, unpredictable movements

an empty stomach as opposed to an individual who has had a light meal.

Table 4.3 details the objective signs of N_2O-O_2 sedation analgesia that correspond to the level and stage of anesthesia. Particular attention should be paid to those signs of stage I level 3 as this is too deep a stage to safely utilize N_2O-O_2. When using a nasal cannula, however, this level is virtually never reached.

INHALATION SEDATION EQUIPMENT

A gas source machine is available either as a portable or central system. Although more costly, a portable system is most flexible for ophthalmic plastic surgery (Fig. 4.6). Nitrous oxide is commercially available in blue colored steel cylinders, while oxygen comes in green cylinders. A portable system contains "E" size tanks. Two N_2O and two O_2 cylinders can be connected to the analgesic portable machine. The E size tanks contain approximately 1600 liters of N_2O and 650 liters of O_2. To eliminate the possible inadvertent connection of wrong gases, there is a pin index safety device universally recognized and utilized (Fig. 4.7). An advantage to the portable system is readily visible volume gauges.

Although the initial cost of a central system is greater,

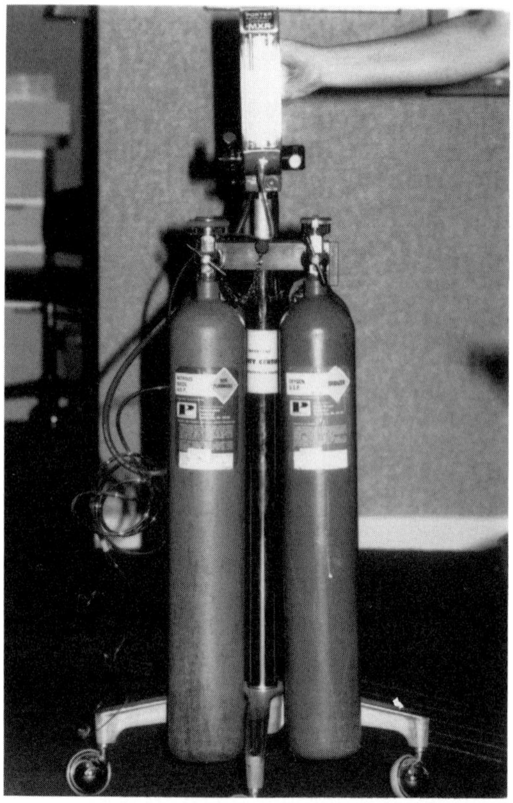

Figure 4.6. A standard portable analgesic gas machine.

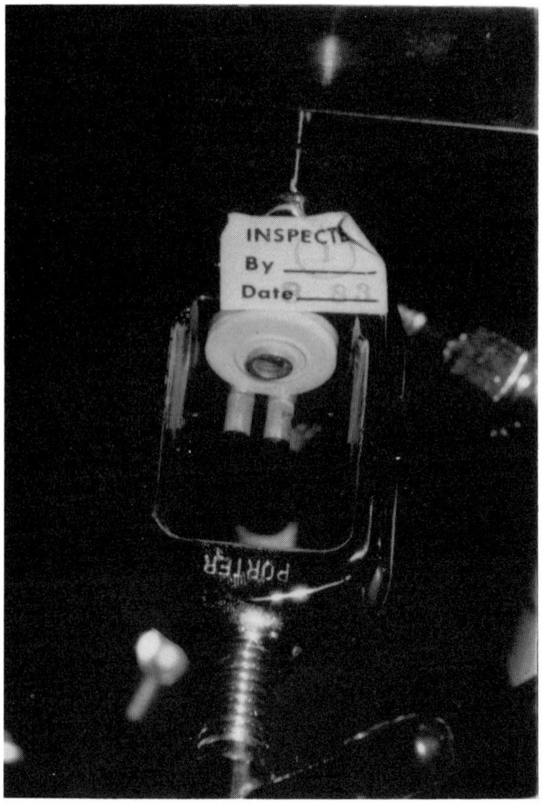

Figure 4.7. Pin safety index that prevents inadvertent improper tank connection.

it is cheaper to operate than a portable one. More than one room can be serviced. Larger tanks containing up to 10 times as much gas may be used. The tanks are usually stored in a separate storage area where the volume gauges are located. A manifold system can add a second tank of gas without interrupting the bulky refill or tank exchange process. If a central system is desired, it should be installed by a reputable dealer in accordance with accepted fire protection and compressed gas standards.

The analgesia machine is a gas delivery system specifically for administering conscious sedation, as opposed to an anesthetic machine which can deliver general anesthesia. These are the safety factors present in analgesia machines:

1. *Minimum oxygen flow:* A preset minimum flow of O_2 is given to the patient. This may be specified as a certain percentage of O_2 (customarily above 20%) or as a minimum flow of O_2 (customarily 3 to 5 liters/min).
2. *Automatic shutoff:* In the event that O_2 is depleted, an analgesia machine has a fail-safe mechanism of shutting off and eliminating further flow of N_2O.
3. *Maximum N_2O concentration:* Analgesia machines will deliver a specified maximum concentration of N_2O (usually 70–80%).
4. *A nonrebreathing circuit:* If a mask is employed, all exhaled gases cannot be rebreathed.
5. *Flush valve:* The ability to fill the system with 100% O_2.

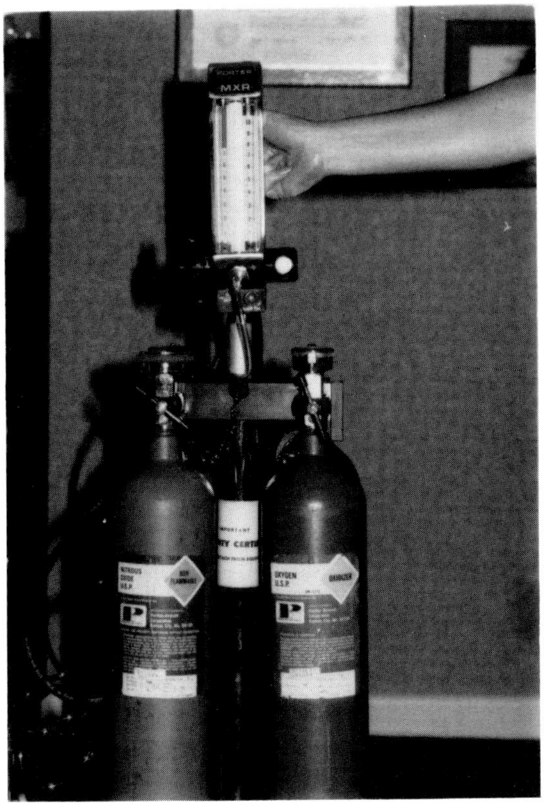

Figure 4.8. Flow meters that measure gas nitrous oxide and oxygen mixture, which is expressed in liters per minute.

Flow meters indicate in liters per minute the amount of N_2O and O_2 delivered (Fig. 4.8). Many systems also calculate the percentage of each gas delivered. For ophthalmic plastic surgical procedures, I advocate use of a standard nasal cannula (Fig. 4.9). It is easily connected directly to the gas machine and is less cumbersome than conventional nasal masks. The cannula allows the surgeon conventional preparation and draping so as to maintain sterility (Fig. 4.10). This cannot be achieved with standard nasal masks. In addition, the cannula will not distort the lower lid. Because the nasal cannula does not fit snugly with the nares, a diffusion effect is created between room air and N_2O-O_2. Thus higher flows of gas are necessary to obtain sufficient concentrations of N_2O. With a nasal cannula concentrations of greater than 25% N_2O are rarely if ever achieved.

There has been concern regarding the possible toxic effects of trace N_2O levels on operating room personnel. Of particular attention is the issue of spontaneous abortion in pregnant women. Corbett showed an increase in fetal death in rats exposed to 1% N_2O. Repeat studies did not confirm this. Two other studies found no toxicity to rat fetuses exposed to room concentrations of N_2O up to 50%. There is no evidence of change in male fertility or muta-

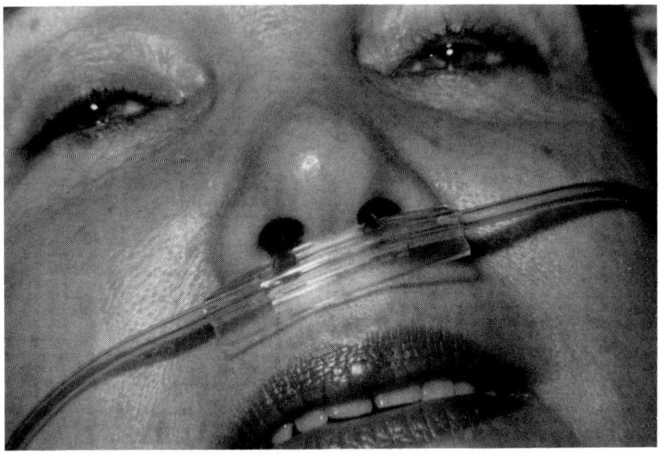

Figure 4.9. A nasal cannula in place.

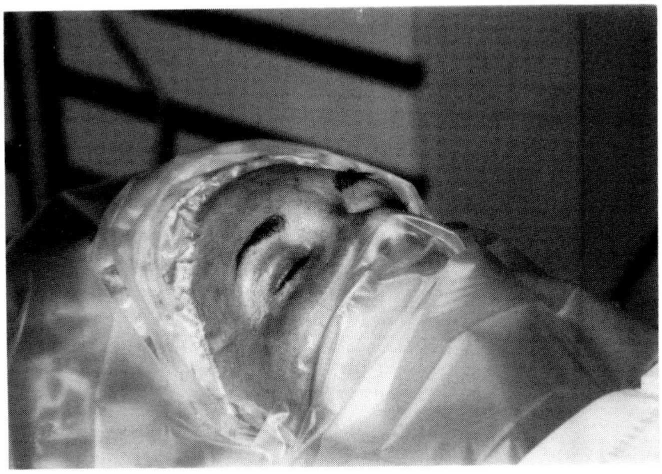

Figure 4.10. With the use of nasal cannula, the patient can be prepared and draped in the customary fashion.

Table 4.4
Indications for Nitrous Oxide-Oxygen Conscious Sedation

1. *Elimination of fear:* Especially useful in those patients who fear eye or eyelid manipulations. Commonly thyroid patients and children are more fearful.
2. *Cardiac patients:* N_2O-O_2 conscious sedation eliminates stress which may cause unnecessary outpouring of endogenous epinephrine. Discussion with the cardiac patient's general practitioner is advised.
3. *Mentally retarded patient:* Although general anesthesia is preferred, patients with mild retardation are good candidates.
4. *Hypertension:* Stress and anxiety are reduced greatly and often a more stable blood pressure is achieved.
5. *Mild asthma:* Anxiety and stress, which often precipitate asthmatic attacks, are reduced. N_2O is not a respiratory irritant and is not likely to precipitate an asthmatic attack. Additionally, allergy to N_2O is virtually unknown.
6. *Children*

genesis. There is no substantiated evidence of birth defect, however, office personnel should be properly advised. Adequate ventilation rapidly eliminates trace amount of N_2O. Some operating rooms utilize scavenger systems that collect and dispose of leaked gases. These systems are costly and probably unnecessary unless nearly continuous utilization and poor ventilation are present.

INDICATIONS FOR CONSCIOUS SEDATION IN OPHTHALMIC PLASTIC SURGERY

It is the goal of all ophthalmic plastic surgeons to make the surgical experience pleasant for the patient. The use of N_2O-O_2 technique alters the patient's mood as to reduce fear, apprehension and pain threshold. Many ophthalmic plastic surgery procedures necessitate consciousness and cooperation in obtaining the optimal results. The N_2O-O_2 technique eliminates the need for parenteral hypnotic, sedative, or analgesic medications that may have undesired prolonged effects. The advantage of N_2O-O_2 is the rapid induction and rapid recovery that can thereby be pulsed. If a lid measurement is important to the success of ptosis surgery, the N_2O may be shut off and the patients may be evaluated as if no medication is affecting them. The N_2O-O_2 technique allows for reduced recovery room time.

The avoidance of parenteral hypnotics, sedatives, and analgesics is most beneficial when dealing with office-based outpatient surgery. This is particularly useful when operating on an elderly patient. Examples of medications avoided when using conscious sedation include meperidine, morphine sulfate, diazepam, hydroxyzine pomeate, and barbiturates. Inhalation conscious sedation allows continuous verbal contact with the patient. The physician is thus able to alter the dosage of analgesia. Although most dentists employ N_2O-O_2 without monitoring the patient, a nurse periodically evaluates the vital signs of the patient. An updated emergency chart is available at all times. The need for an anesthetist, recovery room personnel, and equipment are eliminated when parenteral medications are avoided.

TECHNIQUES OF ADMINISTRATION

The nasal cannula is taped to the cheek, and the patient can then be prepared and draped. When the analgesia machine is turned on, 100% O_2 is delivered at approximately 6 liters/min. When N_2O is added, the O_2 is lowered to 2 to 3 liters/min. A 50% concentration of N_2O (2 to 3 liters/min) is begun. The patient is asked to breathe in through the nose and out through the mouth. After a minute or two, the patient is asked: "Do you feel fine?" "Do you feel tingling around your mouth?" "Are you feeling high?" This is usually accomplished in a matter of minutes, but in some patients it may be necessary to increase the flow of N_2O to 60 or even 70% concentration until the desired affect is achieved. While the N_2O is being initiated, the patient is asked not to talk so as to eliminate further dilution of gas. A portable stereo with lightweight headphones is useful in distracting the patient from talking with the surgeon. When a state of relaxation and euphoria is achieved, local anesthesia may be administered. To stop N_2O, one shuts off the flow meter knob and raises the O_2 to 6 to 8 liters/min. It is felt that by giving large-flow O_2, the effects of N_2O can be more rapidly eliminated.

Table 4.5
Contraindications of Nitrous Oxide-Oxygen Conscious Sedation

Nasal obstruction
Acute rhinitis
Nasal tumor
Nasal deformity
Acute respiratory disease
Pneumonia
Tuberculosis
Bronchitis, chronic obstructive lung disease
Severe asthma
Psychiatric patients
Severe cardiac disease
Congestive heart failure, pulmonary edema
Severe angina
Pregnancy
Teratogenic effects with N_2O shown in rat embryo. No documentation in humans. No known effect on long-term exposure to N_2O during pregnancy.

PATIENT INDICATIONS AND CONTRAINDICATIONS

Ideally, one should obtain a "medical clearance" prior to doing lid surgery, especially in patients with cardiovascular and pulmonary diseases. Table 4.4 is a guideline of the indications for N_2O-O_2 conscious sedation technique. Table 4.5 outlines the contraindications of the technique.

ADJUNCT MEDICATIONS

It is well recognized that parenteral medications described previously can work synergistically with N_2O-O_2.

However, safer medications can be employed to potentiate the effect of N_2O as well as reduce nausea. These medications are preferred:

1. Chloral hydrate 500-1000 mg orally ½ hour prior to surgery;
2. Diazepam 2 to 7.5 mg orally ½ hour prior to surgery.

SUMMARY

Nitrous oxide-oxygen conscious sedation is an effective technique that has little risk of complications. Rapid induction and recovery make it especially useful in ophthalmic plastic surgery, where lid measurements and suture placement are crucial in achieving optimal results. Nitrous oxide-oxygen is particularly useful in office-based outpatient surgery, usually allowing the surgeon to eliminate more potent parenteral hypnotics, sedatives, and analgesics, which may have significant side effects. The pleasurable experience of the patient along with excellent physician control make the inhalation sedation N_2O-O_2 technique an invaluable adjunct in ophthalmic plastic surgery.

SUGGESTED READINGS

Allen GD: *Dental Anesthesia And Analgesia.* Baltimore, Williams & Wilkins, 1972.

Atkinson WS: *Anesthesia in Ophthalmology*, ed 2 Springfield, Illinois, GC Thomas, 1965.

Bennett CR: *Conscious Sedation In Dental Procedure.* St. Louis, CV Mosby, 1974.

Bron AJ, McKenzie PJ: Ocular anesthesia. In Rice TA, Micheals RG: *Ophthalmic Surgery*, ed 4. St. Louis, CV Mosby, 1984.

Bruce RA, McColdrick KE, Oppenheimer P: *Anesthesia for Ophthalmology.* Birmingham, Alabama, Aesculapius, 1982.

Callahan A: *Surgery of the Eyelids and Ocular Adnexa.* Birmingham, Alabama, Aesculapius, 1966.

Corbett TH, Cornell RG, Endres JD, Millard RI: Effects of low concentrations of nitrous oxide in rat pregnancy. *Anesthesiology* 39: 299–301, 1973.

Dorch JA, Dorch SE: *Understanding Anesthesia Equipment.* Baltimore, William & Wilkins, 1984.

Duane D (ed): *Clinical Ophthalmology.* Hagerstown, Maryland. Harper & Row, 1976.

Felts JA, Silver B: Anesthesia. In Stewart WB: *Ophthalmic Plastic and reconstructive Surgery.* Rochester, Minnesota, American Academy of Ophthalmology, 19??.

Ferstandig LL: Trace concentration of anesthetic gases: a critical review of the disease potential. *Anesth Analg* 57: 328–345, 1978.

Goodman LS, Gillman A: *The Pharmacological Basis of Therapeutics*, ed. 6. New York, 1980.

Gruen G: Inhalation Analgesia And Sedation. In Clark JW (ed): *Clinical Dentistry.* Hagerstown, MD, Harper & Row, 1979.

Hildreth HR, Silver B: Sensory block of the upper eyelid. *Arch Ophthalmol* 77: 230, 1967.

Journal of the American Medical Association: Standards and guidelines for cardiopulmonary resuscitation and emergency cardiac care. *JAMA* 244: 453–509, 1980.

Katzen LB, Karvelis JJ: Anesthesia, analgesia, and amnesia. In Putterman AM: *Cosmetic Oculoplastic Surgery.* New York, Grune & Stratton, 1982.

Leopold I: Advances in anesthesia in ophthalmic surgery. *Ophthal Surg* 5–13, 1974.

Mazze RI, Wilson AI, Rice SA, Baden JA: Effects of nitrous oxide on fetal development and male fertility in mice. *Anesthesiology* 55: A188, 1981.

Myers, EJ. In Krupin T, Waltman SR (eds): *Complications in Ophthalmic Surgery.* Philadelphia, Lippincott, 1983.

Shane SME: *Conscious Sedation For Ambulatory Surgery.* Baltimore, University Park Press, 1983.

Snow JC: *Anesthesia in Otolaryngology and Ophthalmology.* New York, Appleton-Century-Crofts, 1982.

CHAPTER 5

Anesthetic Considerations for Oculoplastic Surgical Procedures

IRVING BERLIN, M.D.

The choice of anesthesia, whether local or general, is made primarily by the surgeon and patient and secondarily by the anesthesiologist. This selection should be based on several considerations:

1. The age, physical, and mental status of the patient (very few children younger than their middle teens are candidates for local anesthesia);
2. The presence of concurrent diseases and the type of surgery to be performed;
3. The emotional preparedness of a surgeon to cope with an awake patient;
4. The skill and ability of the anesthesiologist.

Some possible complications of local anesthesia are briefly presented next:

1. Reactions to injected drugs are not common because of the small amounts used for oculoplastic procedures, but drug sensitivity is sometimes encountered.
2. Inadvertent intravascular injection may cause mild excitement, tachycardia, neurocirculatory collapse, and respiratory or circulatory arrest.
3. If a retrobulbar injection is required, hemorrhage may occur, which can warrant postponement of the surgery.

At our institution, 70–80% of all ocular surgery is performed under general anesthesia.

The outcome of an oculoplastic procedure may well be determined by the competence of the anesthesiologist. Increased bleeding due to the anesthetic technique used can jeopardize the surgical repair. Therefore, sound anesthetic measures should be practiced, and these begin with the preoperative visit. The anesthesiologist should review the chart to evaluate the physical status of the patient, check the laboratory data, and discover what medications are regularly being taken, which may determine what premedication and what anesthetic agents to use.

During the preoperative visit the nature of the surgical procedures is noted and the individual requirements of the patient are assessed in order to avoid confusion in the operating room. Decisions such as proper placement of the intravenous infusion, use of an orotracheal or nasotracheal tube, and location of the anesthetic equipment can be made during this visit to eliminate any delay in starting the procedure and to allow maximum freedom around the surgical field (Figs. 5.1–5.3).

While assessing these requirements, the patients fears and anxieties are also explored. Gaining the patients confidence with an explanation of what is going to take place in the operating room may engender remarkable cooperation even in children (Fig. 5.4).

Premedication should not be routine and should be tailored for each patient. A drowsy, hopefully amnesic but cooperative patient is the goal. For children we use pentobarbital (Nembutal) suppositories 2 hours preoperatively followed by intramuscular atropine or scopolamine 1 hour preoperatively. Children often fall asleep from the suppository and are not even aware of the intramuscular injection. Adults receive a tranquilizer followed by a narcotic and atropine or glycopyrrolate (Robinul). The antiemetic effect of the tranquilizer is desirable because it allows a quite smooth awakening in the recovery room. The belladonna alkaloids are not only important in drying secretions of the respiratory tract but they also diminish the reflex activity of the pharynx, larynx, and heart. Atropine causes less delirium in the recovery period than

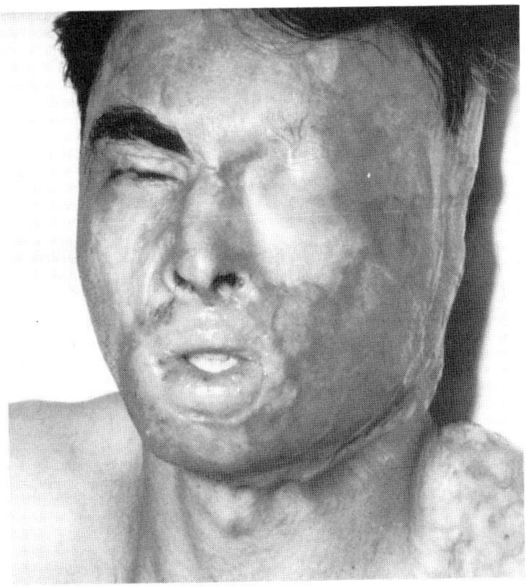

Figure 5.1. Problem: Burn patient for surgery with inability to open mouth.

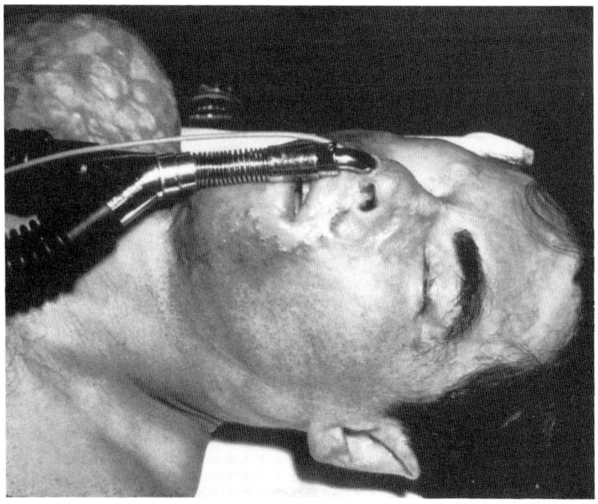

Figure 5.2. Solution to problem: Nasal intubation.

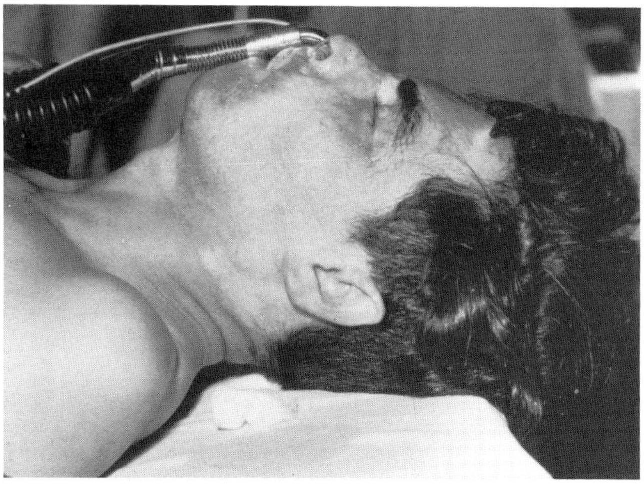

Figure 5.3. Burn patient prior to draping.

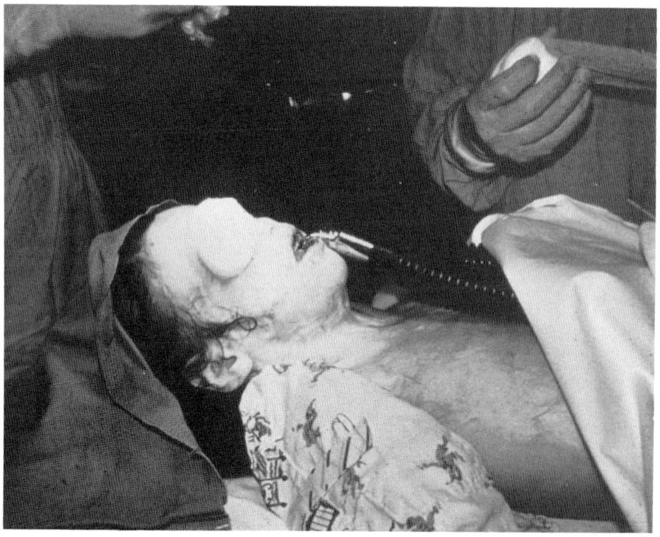

Figure 5.4. Seriously burned child anesthetized for many surgical procedures.

scopolamine, especially in children, and is my personal preference.

After the appropriate monitoring equipment is placed, induction of anesthesia is begun. Precordial stethescope, pulse monitor, electrocardiogram, temperature probe in children, and pulse oximeter are utilized and applied at appropriate times during the induction.

Children are induced with a mixture of nitrous oxide and oxygen (N_2O-O_2), and halothane is slowly introduced followed by intubation. Maintenance is achieved with this mixture via nonrebreathing or semiclosed systems in relatively deep planes.

Adults are induced with thiopental sodium (Pentothal). Intubation is facilitated by using a short-acting muscle relaxant (succinycholine). Prior to intubation, we spray the epiglottis, larynx, and trachea with 6–10 ml of 2% lidocaine. The topical anesthetic is important in bridging the gap between the waning effect of the thiopental and muscle relaxant before an adequate depth of anesthesia is reached with the inhalation agent. This can prevent straining or bucking of the endotracheal tube. Lidocaine is rapidly absorbed from the mucosal surfaces and may also have a systemic effect, thereby preventing annoying arythmias.

Enflurane or isoflurane combined with N_2O-O_2, with the patient breathing spontaneously, is our method of choice. Neuroleptanalgesia is another technique that may be used. Combinations of meperidine (Demerol) and diazepam (Valium), morphine and diazepam, droperidol and sublimase (Fentanyl) now Versed (Midazolam) are all useful techniques when inhalation agents are contraindicated; however, this method normally has a longer recovery period.

Oral or nasal intubation is essential for operations performed around the head and neck because it provides complete access to the operative site. The anesthetic equipment must not be cumbersome and should be practically inconspicuous. In patients with suspected difficult intubation problems, the use of blind nasal intubation or a fiberoptic endoscope may be considered (Fig. 5.5).

Anesthetic equipment must be tailored for oculoplastic procedures. The anesthetic machine should be equipped with rebreathing hoses (6–8 inches) longer than conventional hoses to allow full access for surgeon and assistants and any equipment that may be required (Fig. 5.6).

I do not use long-acting muscle relaxants for several reasons. Muscle relaxation is not necessary for oculoplastic procedures and in some cases may preclude the surgeon's ability to identify branches of the facial nerve with a nerve stimulator. Due to the necessary rapid turnover of our procedures, reversing the effects of long-acting muscle relaxants and straining on the endotracheal tube prior to complete reversal is avoided.

Intraoperative bleeding or oozing can be a major obstacle to reconstruction in oculoplastic procedures. This may be due to several reasons; light anesthesia with straining on the endotracheal tube may be one of these reasons. The converse is also true: deep anesthesia with depressed, unassisted respirations may build up CO_2 with vasodilation, thereby causing troublesome oozing. The surgeon's changing of a patient's head position may kink or partially kink an endotracheal tube and cause partial obstruction. Increased bleeding for no apparent medical or surgical reason should alert the anesthesiologist to check the circuit.

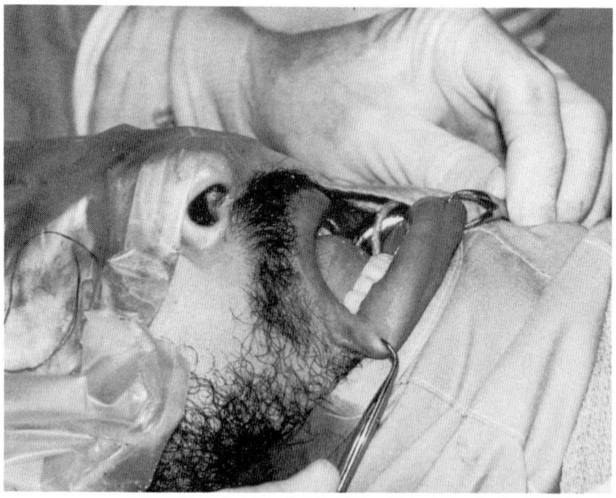

Figure 5.5. Surgeon preparing to take a mucous membrane graft.

Proper positioning of the operating table can be an advantage in reducing bleeding during surgery. The head should be elevated 15–20° to facilitate venous drainage; especially in obese patients, this position decreases pressure of the abdominal contents on the diaphragm thereby minimizing expiratory resistance that may contribute to oozing.

Our technique of using high concentration of anesthetic gases coupled with a head-up tilt of the operating table and injection of local anesthetic by the surgeon can produce relative hypotension with much less intraoperative bleeding.

There are few indications for inducing profound hypotension in oculoplastic surgery. However, if this is indicated and if the patient's physical condition allows this technique, hypotensive agents are available. Ganglion blocking drugs may be used. Trimetaphan by intermittent drip or sodium nitroprusside are most commonly used. The use of propranolol will both lower the dose requirements of these agents and avoid undesirable reflex tachycardia. There are serious risks associated with the use of these agents, including cerebral thrombosis, myocardial problems, central retinal artery thrombosis, and oliguria. Patients must be carefully screened. Drug-induced hypotension should be reserved for those operations where the benefits outweigh the risks.

Careful management in the recovery room is critical. A soft nasal airway is more readily tolerated by the reacting patient. No airway obstruction should be tolerated. Nausea and/or vomiting should be controlled expeditiously. Prochlorperazine and droperiodol are very effective anti-

Figure 5.6. Position of anesthesiologist and anesthesia machine at level of patient's knees.

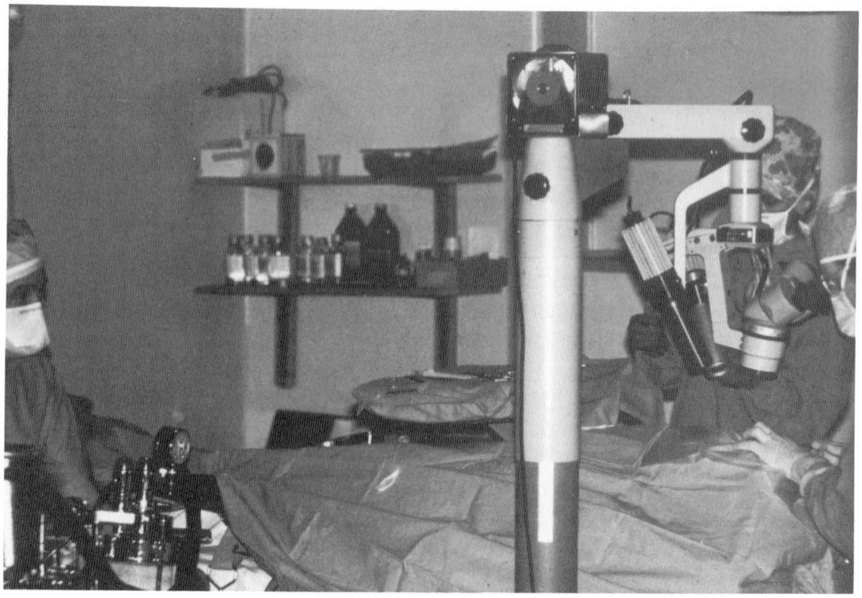

emetics. Hypertension should be treated by first determining the possible cause and then instituting the appropriate therapy.

Many oculoplastic procedures except in children may be performed under local analgesia. However, those patients who do not wish to be awake during surgery may preclude local analgesia; patients with a language problem and who may not be cooperative; and operative procedures where infiltration may distort and hinder the reconstruction. Well-conducted and well-managed general anesthesia can at least approximate and even surpass operative conditions of local analgesia.

CHAPTER 6

Wound Healing

ROBERT B. WILKINS, M.D.
STEVEN J. LAUKAITIS, M.D.

This chapter will consider two aspects of wound healing applicable to the oculoplastic surgeon. The first is the physiology of wound healing in four phases. The second is a practical approach towards wound healing. It emphasizes concepts related to wound healing and scar formation.

PHYSIOLOGY OF WOUND HEALING

Wound healing may be divided into four phases that are based on specific proceedings within a wound. These phases are *inflammatory phase*, *fibroblastic phase*, *wound contraction*, and *scar maturation*.

INFLAMMATORY PHASE

Immediately following any traumatic or surgical wounding, the response is the commencement of the inflammatory phase. It is characterized by a vascular response with hemostasis, which progresses to a cellular and tissue response (Table 6.1).

Initially, the vascular response is the vasoconstriction of affected blood vessels. It is accompanied by the formation of hemostatic plugs from accumulating clotting products, which include platelets, fibrin, and thrombin. After vasoconstriction, vasodilatation occurs. The vasodilatation promotes stasis of blood flow and exudation of chemotactic factors within plasma protein. These factors increase the number of polymorphonuclear neutrophils in the affected area. This cellular response increases over the next 12–48 hours. The neutrophils undergo cell lysis and release granules containing lysozymes. Extracellular debris, fibrin, and bacteria (which also have accumulated in the area) are enzymatically degraded by the lysozymes. Simultaneously, monocytes and macrophages phagocytize this digested material.

During this phase, the groundwork for further wound healing occurs. New vascular buds appear from preexisting capillaries along the wound edge. Later, fibroblasts appear in the perivascular connective tissue, setting the stage for the fibroblastic phase of wound healing.

FIBROBLASTIC PHASE

About 4 to 5 days after injury, the fibroblast phase prevails (Table 6.2). Characteristic is a proliferative rather than an exudative response to injury. This proliferation includes heightened vascular and fibroblastic activity and lasts 2–4 weeks. The new capillary buds formed previously acquire muscle coats and differentiate into arterioles and venules, with continual migration into the wound edge.

The activity of the fibroblasts peaks during the fibroblastic phase. The migration of fibroblasts occurs into the wound edge, and, with mitosis, the fibroblast population multiplies. Also, activated macrophages produce a substance that stimulates fibroblastic growth.

Wound reconstruction is the principal role of the fibroblast. Along with its migration and multiplication, the fibroblast also secretes extracellular substances necessary for wound matrix. Collagen, glycoproteins, and mucopolysaccharides are deposited in the spaces created by the loss of tissue.

Collagen production by the fibroblast is substantial during the fibroblastic phase and exceeds collagenolysis. A temporary, hypertrophic scar may occur during these 2–4

Table 6.1
Inflammatory Phase

- Vascular Response
  - Vasoconstriction
  - Vasodilatation
  - Hemostasis
  - Chemotaxis
- Cellular Response
  - Polymorphonuclear neutrophils
  - Monocytes
  - Macrophages
- Tissue Response
  - Capillary buds
  - Fibroblasts

Table 6.2
Fibroblastic Phase

- Capillary Buds
  - Arteriole formation
  - Venule formation
- Fibroblasts
  - Migration
  - Mitosis
  - Synthesis of extracellular substances
- Collagen
- Mucopolysaccharides
- Tensile Strength

weeks. These hypertrophic scars regress spontaneously with scar maturation.

The morphology of the wound changes during collagen synthesis. Wounds examined microscopically at 10 days exhibit a haphazard orientation of collagen fibrils. Over the next 3 months, these fibrils coalesce to form irregular masses of collagen bundles that reorient to the prevailing skin tension. Concomitantly, intramolecular and intermolecular collagen bonding by covalent cross-linking adds rigidity to the structural collagen. Ground substances consisting of mucopolysaccharides and glycoproteins add an amorphous matrix between cells and fibers. These ground substances are also secreted by the fibroblast.

The collagen in a wound is responsible for the tensile strength of the wound. Tensile strength is defined as "the ability of the wound to resist rupture." Initially, a wound exhibits poor tensile strength but, with the maturation of collagen, the tensile strength increases rapidly. Three phases of collagen maturation have been identified. In the first phase, the early tensile strength is directly related to the concentration of collagen. With collagen cross-linking, the tensile strength increases exponentially. Orientation of the cross-linked fibrils maintains the tensile strength.

The direction of the skin tension determines the intensity of wound healing. Generally, the skin tension is parallel to the underlying muscle fibers and skeletal system. Consequently, incisions perpendicular to the lines of skin tension create maximal wound contractures. This stimulates excessive collagen deposition and poor orientation of the scar.

WOUND CONTRACTION AND GRANULATION

Wound contraction occurs concurrently with the fibroblastic phase and continues for several months. It is the process by which the area of the open wound diminishes by centripetal movement of the surrounding skin and the wound edge. It involves movement of the dermis and the overlying epithelium. Initially, the contraction involves only movement of existing tissue. This contraction creates stress on the surrounding tissues with thinning, stretching, and increasing tension. To compensate, intussusceptive growth occurs by which the overlying epithelial cells multiply to cover the increased surface area and to decrease the tension. The dermal elements (hair follicles and glands) become more widely separated with the addition of collagen. These processes preserve the original thickness of the surrounding tissue and return the taut skin to a more normal tension.

If contraction of a wound is incomplete, granulation tissue is formed. Granulation tissue consists of collagen, blood vessels, and specialized fibroblasts called "myofibroblasts." These cells contain elements similar to smooth muscle cells, including contractile properties from inherent myofibrils. These fibrils appear to generate the contractile force necessary to unite gaping wound edges. As these edges are being apposed, collagen synthesis remains constant or decreases. Beneath the advancing edge, collagenolysis predominates and helps to remodel the scar.

SCAR MATURATION

The maturation process continues for years, but the scar reaches maximum strength at 10–12 weeks. Most healed wounds are weaker than the tissue surrounding them. The point of greatest weakness is the interwoven junction between scar collagen and normal collagen. Usually, a scar will never be as strong as the tissue it replaces. Even after a year, wounds of skin and fascia will be 15–20% weaker than the normal surrounding tissue.

Regeneration of hair follicles and sebaceous glands begins about 4–6 weeks after injury. At this time, the migrated epidermal tissue differentiates with downward projections into the dermis, maturing as hair follicles. The sebaceous glands originate as outpouchings from these projections, rapidly maturing into active sebaceous glands at the same time.

During scar maturation, some absorption and remodeling of the scar occurs. About 6–12 months after wounding, there is a continuation of intramolecular and intermolecular collagen cross-linking; this may be longer in fibrous tissue such as fascia. Facial tissue heals slowly in comparison to other tissue and may not gain its ultimate strength until a year or more.

Intermittent changes in skin tension during the first 6 months may cause a reactivation and proliferation of scar tissue. This is well illustrated by a scar that is perpendicular to the transverse crease lines of the lower lid. A linear scar perpendicular to the longitudinal pull of the orbicularis muscles is alternately stretched and relaxed as the muscle contracts. This stimulates a proliferative process by the fibroblasts, causing scar hypertrophy. In contrast, a scar parallel to the skin crease lines will remain linear and appear cosmetically acceptable.

CLINICAL ASPECTS ASSOCIATED WITH EXCESS SCAR FORMATION

Excess scar formation, hypertrophic scars, and keloids are the bane of the cosmetic surgeon. In most people, widening of a normally thin scar may be prevented if certain inciting factors related to wound healing are kept in mind. All may exacerbate excessive collagen deposition and scar formation. The factors, which are discussed next, are outlined in Table 6.3.

Inflammation is necessary for wound healing. However, excess inflammation adds to the production of collagen. Wound areas fraught with debris, necrotic tissue, or bacteria promote excess inflammation. Failure to remove dirt from a traumatized wound may result in tatooing and scar hypertrophy. This can impede wound healing, extending the proliferative phase, causing a poor cosmetic result. Cleansing of the wound with irrigation, gentle manipulation of wounded tissue, and judicious cautery keep iatrogenic inflammation to a minimum and help to promote rapid wound healing (Fig. 6.1).

All wounds are contaminated with bacteria. What stimulates the prolongation of the inflammatory phase in perceivably sterile wounds is uncertain. In the presence of bacteria, there is a greater stimulus for macrophage activation. This leads to the production of an activating factor that stimulates fibroblast multiplication and secretion of collagen, which may promote excess scar formation.

Table 6.3
Factors Related to Excess Scar Formation

Inflammation
Infection
Suture Materials
Skin Tension
Hematoma
Age
Surgical Technique

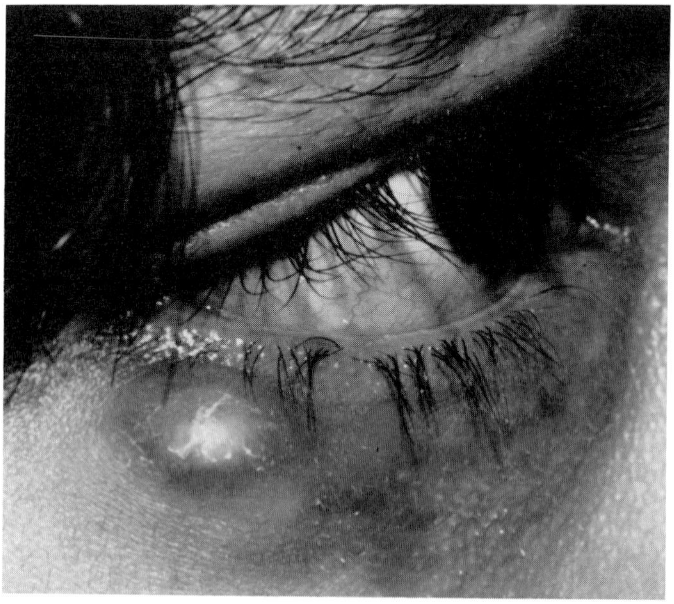

Figure 6.1. Suture granuloma: This patient exhibits chronic inflammation from a retained suture following lower lid blepharoplasty. Note the excess granulation tissue from an extended phase of wound healing.

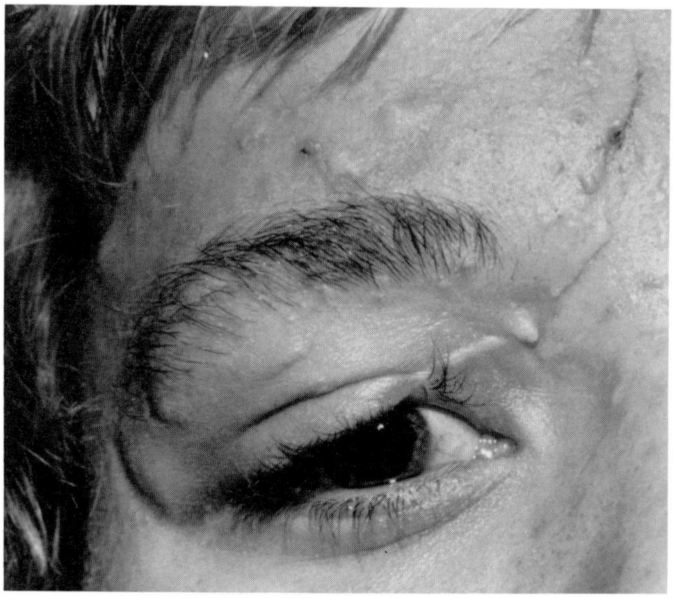

Figure 6.2. Hypertrophic scar: These scars are elevated and remain within a normal skin incision.

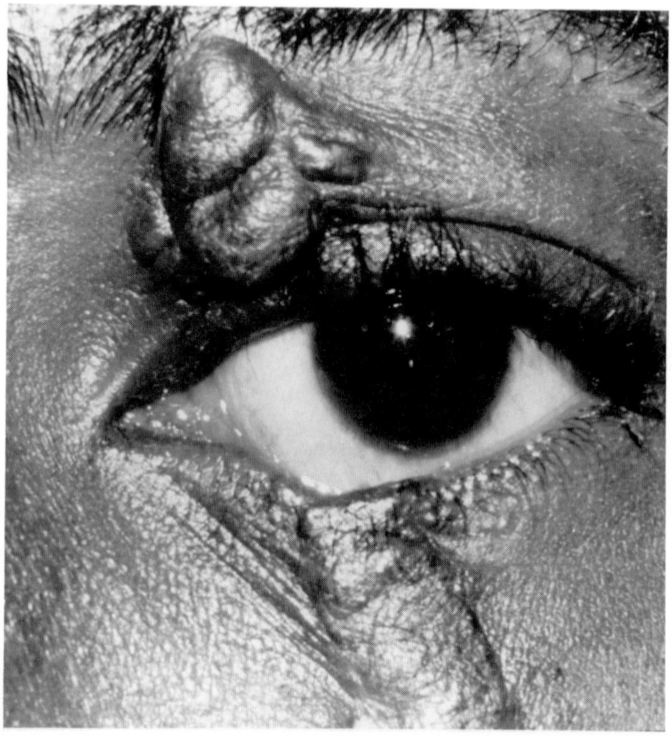

Figure 6.3. Keloid formation: Keloids extend beyond the normal skin incision and invade the surrounding normal tissue.

Suture material is a foreign body and may produce a lag in wound healing. Absorbable sutures have been noted to form a haven for bacterial growth, which may create an infected wound with delayed healing.

All tight skin sutures normally induce a small area of ischemia with focal necrosis. However, those skin sutures that are knotted with excessive tension eventually exhibit vascular proliferation of the wound and a propensity towards excess scar production. By the judicious placement of subcutaneous sutures, less tension is necessary for skin closure.

Skin tension influences the physical properties inherent to wound healing. Maximal contraction of wounds results in a scar influenced by skin tension lines. Skin tension is discussed in a later section.

Hematomas act as foreign bodies. They inevitably become organized (if not evacuated), leading to excess fibroplasia and unsightly scar conformation. Hematomas also promote bacterial growth since they are an excellent medium. Hematomas are prevented by fastidious hemostasis utilizing blunt pressure, careful cautery, and thrombin packs.

Children exhibit a greater tendency toward excessive scar production. This is probably related to the physiologic status of the skin. The greater elasticity of children's skin may be the inciting factor for a faster and excessive healing response. In contrast, adults with loss of skin elasticity hide scars more readily among wrinkles.

Poor surgical technique induces poor wound healing. Instrument-induced trauma inflicted by forceps without teeth, excessive cautery, and sponge rubbing rather than blotting create unnecessary inflammation that can impede wound healing. Poor wound apposition creates unsightly scars. It goes without saying that proper closure of wounds in layers generally leads to a fine, linear scar.

KELOIDS AND HYPERTROPHIC SCARS

Keloids and hypertrophic scars are related in that both exhibit collagen hyperproduction exceeding collagenolysis. Although both have decreased collagenase production, their clinical characteristics are different. Hypertrophic scars are elevated, remain within a normal skin incision, and improve spontaneously with time (Fig. 6.2). Conversely, keloids extend beyond the normal skin incision; they invade the surrounding tissue and eventually recur after surgical excision (Fig. 6.3). The factors responsible for keloid formation are not fully understood.

LINES OF MINIMAL TENSION

The clinical significance of the lines of minimal tension applies to scar conformation. Surgical incisions parallel to these lines have minimal contraction and fine linear scars. In contrast, wound incisions traversing these lines exhibit scar hypertrophy.

The lines of minimal tension are associated with the underlying muscle fiber direction, such that these lines are parallel to muscle fibers. With muscle contraction, *a minimal tension is exerted on the overlying skin parallel to the force of muscle contraction.* Consequently, with a scar parallel to this force, minimal tension will be exerted on the healing wound.

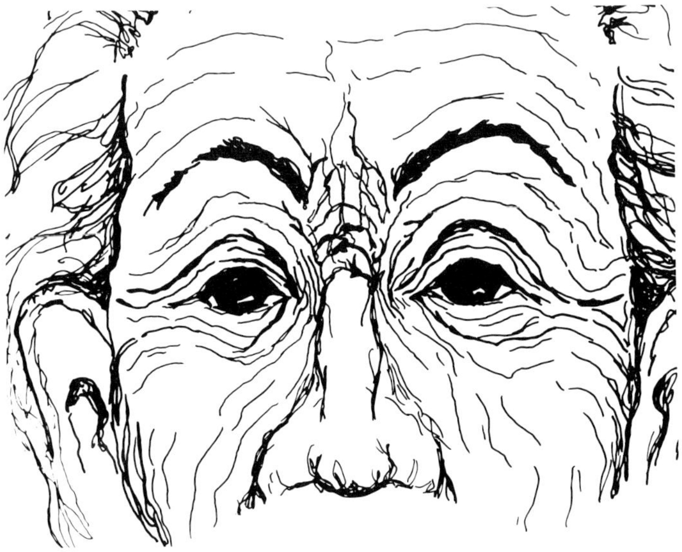

Figure 6.4. Lines of minimal tension and skin wrinkles: Surgical incisions parallel to these lines have minimal contraction that result in fine linear scars.

Skin wrinkles generally follow the lines of minimal tension. Anatomically, they may represent the dermal attachment of an underlying muscle fiber or aponeurosis. Examples include the orbicularis oculi in the lower lid and the terminations of the levator aponeurosis that create the upper lid crease. Between these wrinkles are skin folds, which are loosely connected to the underlying tissue.

It is important to realize that skin wrinkles are not lines of minimal tension. A number of muscles contracting in unison create skin wrinkles that may not follow the lines of minimal tension of individual muscle fibers. For example, the glabella region exhibits vertical wrinkle lines that are accentuated by the simultaneous contractions of the procerus, corrugator supercilii, and the orbicularis oculi. The lateral crow's foot angulating across the zygoma is formed by the muscular contractions of the orbicularis oculi and the zygomaticus muscle.

The lines of minimal tension and skin wrinkles are ideal guidelines for the direction of elective incisions and are useful concepts to the cosmetic surgeon. When the incision is placed in these positions, a better-quality scar is obtained. Incisions traversing these lines will exhibit scar hypertrophy, regardless of meticulous wound closure (Fig. 6.4).

SUGGESTED READINGS

Converse JM: *Reconstructive Plastic Surgery.* Philadelphia, WB Saunders, 1977.

Dineen P: *The Surgical Wound.* Philadelphia, Lee & Febiger, 1981.

CHAPTER 7

Instrumentation for Ophthalmic Plastic and Reconstructive Surgery

IRA ELIASOPH, M.D., F.A.C.S.

Instrumentation for surgery must be planned prior to any actual operation. Surgeons should be able, when necessary, to improvise and use the tools at hand when unexpected situations arise. We must have the flexibility to revise the preoperative surgical plan as circumstances dictate, especially in trauma and tumor cases. We must have a proper grounding in anatomy, physiology, and pathology to select surgical methods wisely. We must also increase our understanding of surgical mechanics in regard to how our hands work and how our instruments aid as accessories to our fingers.

This discussion is not designed to be an instrument catalog. References to any specific instrument are intended to advise the novice and suggest some review or rethinking for the experienced surgeon. Good surgery proceeds in orderly fashion without apparent haste and with proper preparation and planning, gentle handling of tissues, careful dissection, use of appropriate materials, and meticulous closures. We should try to find instruments that are the best design for their particular purpose. If we have selected properly, we can do much of our work with fewer tools and fewer changes. Be aware of the need for instruments to be in proper condition; therefore, use them for their intended purpose and have them repaired or adjusted if they are even slightly "off." Use of a delicate forceps or a needle holder on something heavier than that for which it was designed soon makes it unusable. A primary tool is the combination of preoperative photographs and measurements, which should be in the operating room and visible to the surgeon as appropriate, prior to and during surgery. Photography is a subject of its own, but it is part of the instrumentation we require. Get good, consistent photographs. At the end of this chapter are some suggested instrument lists (Fig. 7.1, Appendix 1).

Local anesthesia should be administered, with rare exceptions, by the operating surgeon, to verify the solution administered and the specific area of anesthesia desired. This avoids use of epinephrine when possible and when not possible, permits minimal injected volume of the agent. It also will allow for adequate surface anesthesia with akinesia in doing a procedure such as an external levator aponeurosis repair or tuck. The needles used should be shorter, rather than longer, and of very fine caliber when injecting into the thin eyelid skin. Injecting first at the least sensitive area and working from that spot is useful. Injecting slowly is much more comfortable for the patient, and introducing the needle for the next segment through the margin of tissue already anesthetized is also helpful. When possible, inject through tissue to be removed in a blepharoplasty or direct brow lift, but *avoid* injecting into an area of tumor of inflammation. Direct the point of the needle so that movement by the patient (or the surgeon) will not be toward the globe or other structures to be avoided.

Markings on the skin are often needed, and these should be done prior to distorting the tissue by injection and without pull on the tissues by the head drapes. If possible, the patient should be sitting up for the marking and for the intraoperative assessment in instances where gravity changes the upright from the supine tissue relationships. In all cases, the head and upper body should be elevated enough to relieve the pressure of the abdominal content into the thorax and to lower venous and arterial pressure to the head. Even with a marker that makes a broad line, the edge of its mark will place an incision accurately.

General anesthesia eliminates the need for injection in the surgical area and makes possible surgery on children and some geriatric patients who otherwise would not be

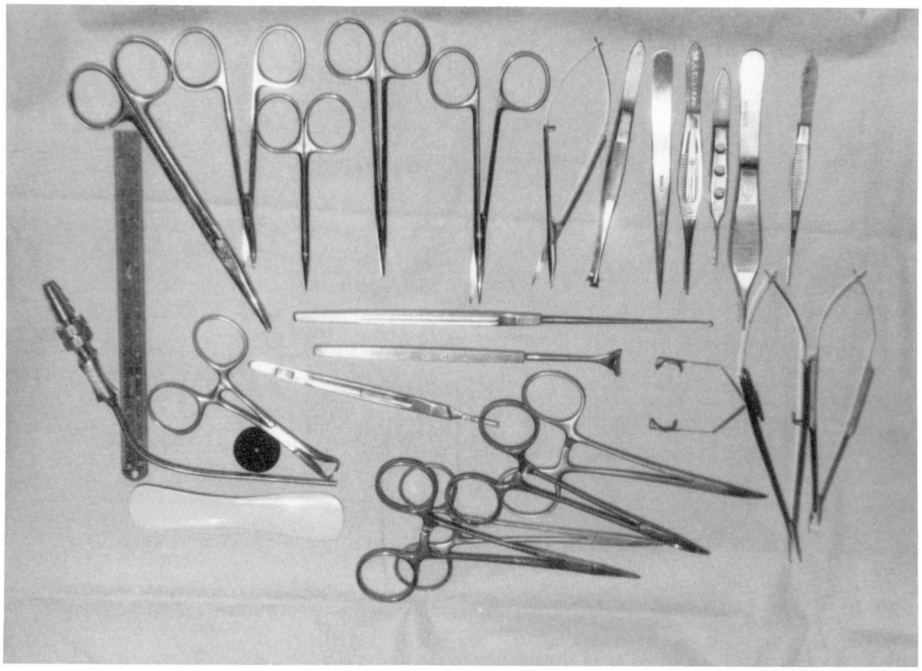

Figure 7.1. Primary lid tray.

able to cooperate for the procedure. General anesthesia is preferred for surgery involving bone in most instances. On entering the operating room, the surgeon should speak to the patient and help the patient to be as relaxed as possible in the operating environment. The patient data, photos, and measurements should be posted in an accessible place. Emergency resuscitation equipment should be regularly checked. Special instruments should be checked with nurse or technician, suture needs reviewed, and local anesthetic solutions checked. For certain procedures, standing gives the surgeon much better positioning and flexibility. After scrubbing, see that the patient is properly draped to block out areas outside the surgical field, to allow for repositioning of the head as needed (even to sitting up for some situations), and, in cosmetic procedures and ptosis corrections, to assure that the draping does not push or pull at the face. Check that wiring or tubing for cautery, suction, drill, or your headlight are not too short to allow proper ease of movement. You should not have to delay surgery significantly for accomplishing the photography, nor should you have to have any but the briefest communication with the photographer.

It would be hoped that you can review videotapes of at least some of your operations. Set aside time and look at that pair of hands working as though they were not yours. Use of many instruments should be like gesturing in a speech: the hand approaches, makes the stroke, and returns to a rest position. A curved scissors is almost impossible to utilize for a straight cut, a short suture needle will not go through both edges of an incision, omission of a skin hook giving traction makes the wound closure uneven. The classical scalpel blade shape works very well for most skin incisions and must be held and used in the proper manner. The "belly" of the blade should be drawn along the incision line and the tissue incised vertically. Exceptions, of course, exist, such as the bevel needed in doing a direct brow lift to avoid incising the hair follicles. A pointed blade is useful when the incision to be made is a stab wound of limited length. In doing a median type of tarsorrhaphy, as an example, splitting the lid at the gray line and removing a few millimeters of conjunctiva can be neatly done with a pointed blade. An angulated blade such as a keratome blade is useful when reaching around a corner is necessary to incise the nasal mucosa, as in dacryocystorhinostomy or in dissection in the orbit.

Knives and dermatomes for obtaining grafts must be particularly chosen and meticulously maintained. A graft is taken with a cutting system that will provide donor tissue of proper uniform thickness and size slightly larger than the defect to be filled. Cutting with the CO_2 laser is becoming an accepted method of dissecting and cauterizing for highly vascular tumors and in patients with bleeding disorders.

Scissors are not only for cutting but are tools for surgical dissection. The finger loops allow controlled spreading of the blades to separate tissues and then to cut where indicated. Blunt-pointed scissors (straight Stevens scissors 4½ inches or 11.4 cm) are the most useful in extending incisions and defining anatomical planes. In doing the dissection for lower lid blepharoplasty skin-muscle flap, a curved Metzenbaum scissor (5¾ inches or 14.6 cm length) is suitable. In doing a coronal incision for forehead lift, a longer scissor of 9 inches or 22.9 cm is needed and may be useful in the temporal approach to a depressed fracture of the zygoma. In trimming small skin flaps, a fine-pointed scissor of standard or spring-back (Westcott) type is very good, particularly with serration on one blade to keep the tissue from sliding away. Finger loops (rather than spring-opening) scissors must be used for spreading, keeping in mind that a long-handled and short-bladed scissor gives very little separation at its tips.

The Graefe fixation forceps is useful for grasping the lid

margin by sliding one blade inside at the canthus and shifting to the desired location on the lid before tightening and raising it.

A toothed Adson forceps will hold heavier tissues effectively that fine forceps will not. Brow skin or scalp and the tarsal plate are examples of tissues for which this instrument is well suited. For many surgical procedures, a fine-toothed forceps of the Bishop Harmon or Lester design is excellent. The forceps design of Ramon Castroviejo for use on the globe for cornea or sclera is of little use in oculoplastic work, because the teeth were not designed for skin and fascia and will often slip. A bayonet shaping with either serrated tips or teeth is frequently superior to a straight design when working in the orbit, as in drawing orbital tissue from a floor fracture.

A curved or angulated forceps may help in certain tight corners to allow tissue to be grasped perpendicularly along its cut edge.

Tying forceps are often inadequate because they are out of alignment or are designed to hold only at the very tip. A smooth-surfaced suture thread, moist with irrigating solution or with a touch of fatty tissue, cannot be reliably grasped with many of the forceps available.

Hemostatic forceps that are fine and light (mosquito clamps) usually suffice in ophthalmic work, and frequently hemostasis is accomplished by means of a cautery device. The small disposable battery-operated hot-wire cauteries are fair. Most ophthalmic plastic surgeons favor the wet-field bipolar forceps cautery, which coagulates the tissue between the forceps tips. The heavy-duty electric cauteries with a second electrode plate elsewhere against the patient's skin may allow current to pass along blood vessels or through tissue from the surgical field toward the second electrode. In doing a lateral orbitotomy (Kronlein), the bleeding from the cut edges of the bone can be stopped effectively with firm application of bone wax.

Last, we must see clearly what we do, and working in a bloody pool is potentially disastrous. Gauze squares and cotton-tipped applicators must be put in your field of vision and separated to be picked up easily.

Retractors, whether smoothly curved, such as a Desmarres or Arruga, or a simple sharp hook or rake, can hold something out of the way or in a particular position. Lid specula and retractors that can be attached to the drapes are fine, but the self-retaining retractors I have seen seem to be of little help. The malleable ribbon retractor in different widths can be shaped for specific orbital exploration.

Take particular pains to set the position of a drill or chisel so that its cutting point or edge has free access without contacting soft tissue. A drill should be run for several seconds and started and stopped two or three times before being turned toward the patient to determine that the bit is in place properly and for you to be aware of whatever torque the drill has in your hands.

Needle holders used in most ophthalmic surgery are light, fine instruments for the placement of extremely fine-diameter suture material with swaged-on needles that are precisely sharpened segments of fine wire.

In a deep location a small half-curve needle can be properly guided with a straight needle holder on its long axis, but a curved needle holder holds at an angle and cannot direct the needle around in a proper arc through the tissue.

Choose needles that are long enough to traverse the tissue you require. Straight needles are of little use in ophthalmic work, but the curve is an improvement only if the surgeon follows the curve. Generally, needles designated "3/8 curve" are provided. The "1/2 curve" needle is good in a confined space, as in suturing the flaps of a dacryocystorhinostomy.

On completion of the actual surgery, apply dressings to protect wounds from contamination, mechanical stresses, or pressures that cause the patient discomfort. Often, no dressings are indicated. For many incisions, cover can be provided with adhesive of porous material that is available in a variety of widths (Steri-strips), and a nonadherent pad (Telfa) can be cut to shape and secured by hypoallergenic paper tape. Cold compresses to decrease swelling are used in the immediate postoperative period after such procedures as blepharoplasty.

Instrumentation is a whole scheme for accomplishing a procedure. Learn about instruments used in other fields; they suggest ways of dealing with some of our surgical problems.

Suggested Instrument Lists

GENERAL OFFICE CHECKLIST

Examination and measurements specific to the problem
General eye examination, Schirmer test, facial asymmetry, exophthalmometry, transillumination
General medical status, allergies, bleeding status, written clearance from internist
Psychological evaluation, psychiatric consultation as appropriate
Photographs and drawings
Informed consent (Why does this problem require this type of surgery? What this operation will *not* do!)
Scheduling: Office, hospital ambulatory, in-patient
Duration of operation
Anesthesia: general, local, standby
OR contacted for special needs: (e.g., fascia lata, cryoprobe, bone screws, headlight)

GENERAL OPERATING ROOM CHECKLIST

Photographs, measurements, drawings
Anesthetic solutions
Sutures and implants
Special instruments, check function of electrical devices
Monitoring equipment
Emergency equipment for resuscitation
Visual check of instrument tray
Review of operative sequence with assistant, nurse, OR technician, and photographer

POSTOPERATIVE ADJUNCTS

Ointments and massage
Cosmetics, artificial lashes, tattooing
Contact lenses, spectacles (prisms, convex or concave, tinting)
Ocularist
Eyelash curler, suction bulb, muscle hook
Further surgery and/or dermabrasion, skin peel, hair transplant

PRIMARY LID TRAY

Plain forceps, fine
Adson forceps, toothed
Bishop-Harmon forceps
Eliasoph tying forceps
Jeweler's forceps
Graefe fixation forceps
Westcott scissors
Stevens scissors, curved and straight
Double-pointed scissors, fine
Fine scissors with no-slip serration
Metzenbaum scissors, medium
Single skin hooks
Desmarres retractors
Barraquer lid speculum
Protective contact lenses
Jaeger lid plate
Knife handles, No. 9
Skin marker
Ruler
Mosquito clamps, curved and straight
Towel clips
Castroviejo needle holders, curved and straight
Frazier suction tip
Syringes, 3 ml and 10 ml
Needles, 25 gauge ⅝ inch
Irrigation
Cotton-tipped applicators
Gauze squares
Sutures
Steri-strips
Bipolar cautery
Scalpel blades, No. 15
Anesthetic drops
Anesthetic for injection

ANCILLARY TRAYS

LACRIMAL IRRIGATION

Bowman probes
Punctum dilators
Stainless safety pin
Cannulas (smooth blunted 23 gauge needle)

Syringe, 3cc
Cotton-tipped applicators
Irrigation fluid (balanced salt solution, antibiotic eye drops, dilute methylene blue, fluorescein, boiled milk, saccharine anesthesia eye drops, anesthetic for injection)

NASAL PACKING

Bayonet forceps
Nasal specula, adult and child sizes
Ribbon gauze packing
Cocaine, 4% solution

CANALICULUS REPAIR

Primary lid tray
Lacrimal irrigation tray
Crawford intubation set with hook (Jedmed)
Veirs rods
Bonn forceps or other very fine-toothed forceps
Nylon sutures, 10-0
Operating microscope

ORBITAL

Primary lid tray and dacryocystorhinostomy tray
Right angle retractor
Ribbon retractors
Shovel retractor
Heavy scissors (for implants)
Heavy scalpel (for implants)
Bristow elevator
Gillies elevator
Periosteal elevators, Freer and McKenty
Stainless steel wire
Wire cutters
Hemostats
Floor implants
Supramid sheets
Teflon sheets
Stryker saw and blades
Headlight (fiberoptic)
Cryoprobe

DACRYOCYSTORHINOSTOMY

Lacrimal irrigation tray and nasal packing tray
Small osteotomes and chisel set
Mallet
Rongeurs, end- and side-cutting, two each
Kerrison punches, two
Hall air drill
Hand lacrimal trephine (preferred by some surgeons)
Stryker saw and trephines (preferred by some surgeons)

GRAFTING

Small surgical set (for dermis-fat graft and others)
Covered petri dish (for graft tissue)
Fascia stripper
Dermatome or mucotome
Lip clamps

ENUCLEATION

Primary tray
Muscle hooks
Enucleation scissors
Berens tampon speculum (or testtube)
Enucleation snare
Implants
Ball introducer

PTOSIS

Primary tray
Optional addition of ptosis clamps, Erhardt clamps, muscle hooks, graft set with fascia stripper

CORONAL INCISION

Metzenbaum scissors, long
Bayonet forceps, long
Bayonet forceps long on bipolar cautery
Suction tip, long
Codman stapler

BLEPHAROSPASM

Nerve stimulator

SUTURES

Listings are Ethicon, unless specified	
Black silk, double-armed	
4-0 micropoint cutting G3	783G
6-0 G1 or TG-140-8	1732G
7-0	7733G
10-0	
Gut, chromic	
3-0 cutting CP-2 needle	886H
4-0 micropoint cutting G3	793G
4-0 one-half circle spatula S2	1798G
6-0 TG 140-8	1735G
Gut, plain	
Dacron, doubly armed, cutting needles	
4-0, 5-0	(Davis and Geck)
Mersilene	
4-0 green RD-1 needle or white spatula S-4	
5-0 white spatula S-14	
Prolene	
5-0 blue monofilament, one-half circle	
Spatula OPS-%	8625G
Nylon black monofilament cutting	
P-1 or P-3	697G
Polydek silky II, Teflon-coated	
4-0 one-half circle	(Deknatel)
Supramid	
3-0	(S. Jackson Co.)
Surgical steel	
5-0 cutting P-3 one-half-circle spatula, doubly armed	

MISCELLANEOUS

Crawford lacrimal intubation set 28-0185 with "crochet hook" (Jedmed, 1430 Hanley Industrial Court, St. Louis, Missouri 63144)
Jones Pyrex tubes, sets, and replacements (Gunther Weiss, 14380 NW Science Park Dr., Portland, OR)
Hornblass or Smith Shields, Smith symblepharon shields (Mager and Gougelman, 120 East 56 St., New York, NY 10022)
Shannon orbital implants (John J. Kelley, 1930 Chestnut St., Philadelphia, PA 19103)

CHAPTER 8

Oculoplastic and Strabismus Series Photography

WILLIAM SHIELDS, B.A., C.R.A.

Oculoplastic photography serves a variety of medical, educational, and legal purposes; however, irrespective of the intended use, the biomedical photographer's primary objective is to produce an accurate representation of the patient's condition. This is not quite as easy or simple as it might seem. Variations in perspective, lighting, and makeup can create the same photographic impressions as plastic surgery. The selection of materials and processing techniques are important factors in determining the contrast, gray scale, and resolution of the photograph. Portrait photographers spend years developing techniques to minimize minor defects and to enhance or obscure contours of the client's face. The biomedical photographer utilizes these same techniques but not with the purpose of enhancing or obscuring a patient's facial characteristics, but rather with the purpose of producing an accurate representation of the patient's condition.

The oculoplastic photograph must not only document the patient's condition; it must also be comparable, that is, all the photographic variables must remain constant for the preoperative and postoperative study—the change in the patient's condition must be the only variable. In order to ensure that the change in the patient's condition is the sole variable, a photographic protocol must be prepared for each study. The process of designing and writing this protocol is called *photographic standardization.* This process is the most important aspect of the photographic procedure; the photographs are only valuable if they are an accurate representation of the patient's condition and if the postoperative series can be reliably compared with the preoperative series without considering distortions introduced by the photographic technique.

Oculoplastic photography standardization can be divided into two categories: *studio considerations* and *processing and handling considerations.* Studio considerations include perspective and distortion, color, exposure, lighting, fields of view, magnification, patient positioning, and camera and studio equipment. Processing and handling considerations include the film processing and printing protocols and the clerical procedures, that is, billing, recordkeeping, and the filing of the photographs. Although this chapter will stress the technical procedures, the clerical procedures are important—the photographic studies are worthless if you cannot find them.

Standardization not only enhances the quality and reliability of the photographs but also increases the photographer's efficiency. If all the routine technical procedures and problems are resolved in advance, the photographer can concentrate on relaxing the patient and eliciting the patient's cooperation.

In addition to oculoplastic photography, this chapter will discuss the techniques and equipment used in surgical photography.

STUDIO CONSIDERATIONS

PERSPECTIVE AND DISTORTION

Perhaps the most difficult variable to understand and control in studio patient photography is the distortion introduced by photographing the patient from an incorrect perspective. Perspective is the representation of a three-dimensional subject on a two-dimensional plane. The normal, or "true perspective," is defined as "the two-dimensional representation of a subject as the three-dimensional subject would normally be viewed." Any perspective other than the true perspective would be said to be distorted. In order for a photograph to be a valid representation of the patient and thus of clinical value it must be as free as possible of distortion.

There are three primary factors than can cause distortion: lens design, camera viewpoint, and film-to-subject distance. Modern lens design has all but eliminated the distortion at one time inherent in lens design. Camera viewpoint and film-to-subject distance are of a more immediate concern to the biomedical photographer since they can be controlled in the studio.

Camera viewpoint is defined as "the angle at which the optical axis transects the vertical and horizontal plane of the subject." If the optical axis is any any angle other than 90° to the horizontal and vertical axis, the photograph will have an abnormal perspective as a result of distortion (Fig. 8.1). Camera viewpoint distortion results from either poor patient positioning or incorrect camera alignment; that is, the horizontal and vertical plane of the subject must be parallel to the film plane and the principle lens plane. The camera alignment can be easily standardized by the use of a monopod (or tripod) and a small level. Patient head position is a more difficult problem since it depends on the cooperation of the patient. A headrest attached to the posing chair is helpful, but it must be comfortable and unobtrusive. For many patients it is extremely difficult to maintain the correct position for more than a few minutes; therefore, speed is essential.

Film-to-subject distance distortion is a more subtle form of abnormal perspective and can be easily overlooked by the photographer unless special care is taken with the design of the photographic procedure. As we said before, true perspective is defined by the way we perceive others in daily interaction. That is, socially and professionally, we interact with other people face to face at a distance of from 40 to 60 inches; therefore, a photograph taken of a person's face from a distance between 40 and 60 inches would have a normal perspective (Fig. 8.2). If that same subject was photographed from a distance of less than 40 inches, it would appear distorted, as it would if it was photographed at a distance greater than 60 inches. For the sake of standardization, 56 inches has become the accepted distance.

Since this type of distortion is a result of the film-to-subject distance, a lens must be selected that will give adequate magnification at the film plane from the proper distance. When you select a lens, keep in mind that head size varies and, therefore, you should not select a lens that fills the negative area with the average subject. Lens selection and magnification will be discussed in more detail later in the chapter.

The point of focus is also a critical factor in film-to-subject distance distortion. It cannot be assumed that if the focus is set at 56 inches, the same film-to-subject distance will be maintained, unless the point of focus is also the same. In serial photography over a 3- to 4-month period, the photograph will not have the same perspective unless you standardize the focus on a particular anatomical landmark. The eyelashes or the lid margin are the most common landmarks for the frontal views. The lateral views present a somewhat more difficult problem, there being no obvious anatomical landmarks at the point of interest; the anterior pole of the cornea, although not ideal, seems to provide the only adequate point of focus (Fig. 8.3).

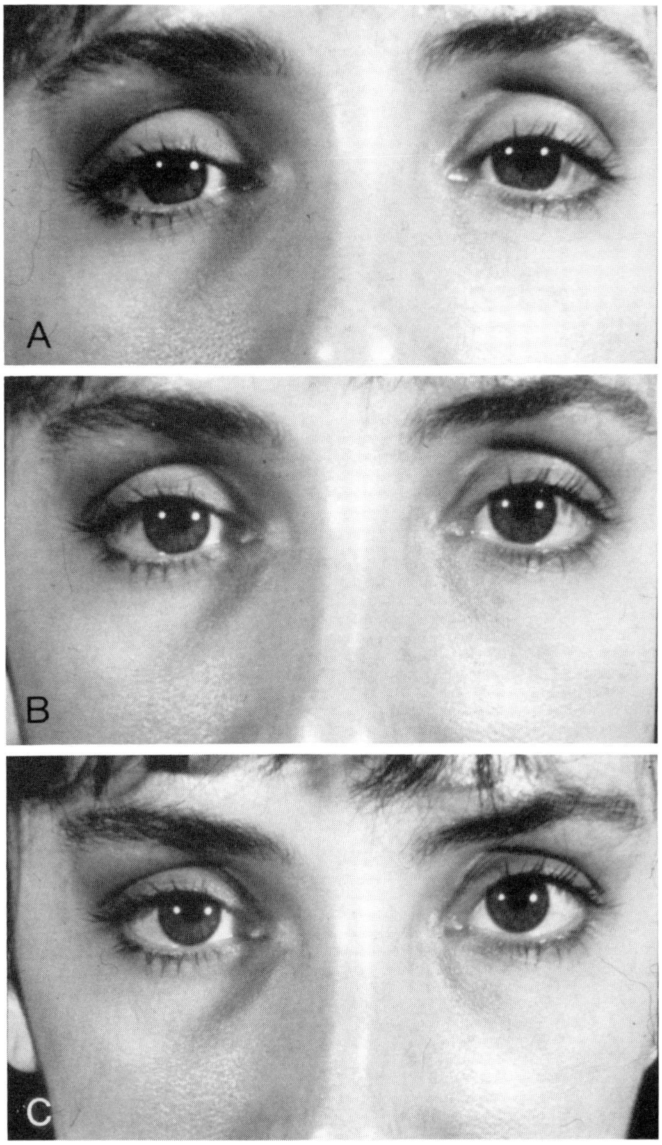

Figure 8.1. Camera viewpoint distortion. *A*, Distortion introduced when the camera is slightly lower than, and tilted up toward, the patient. *B*, Normal perspective. *C*, Distortion introduced when the camera is slightly higher than, and tilted down toward, the patient. Compare the shape of the nose and the orbital section of the lid.

LIGHT AND EXPOSURE

The second area to be addressed for the standardization process is lighting and exposure. Light is the very essence of photography; all of our visual understanding of the world is determined by the interaction of light and the physical world. Exposure is the relationship between light and the photographic emulsion; however, before discussing exposure, we must first understand the elementary characteristics of light. Once we have reviewed these char-

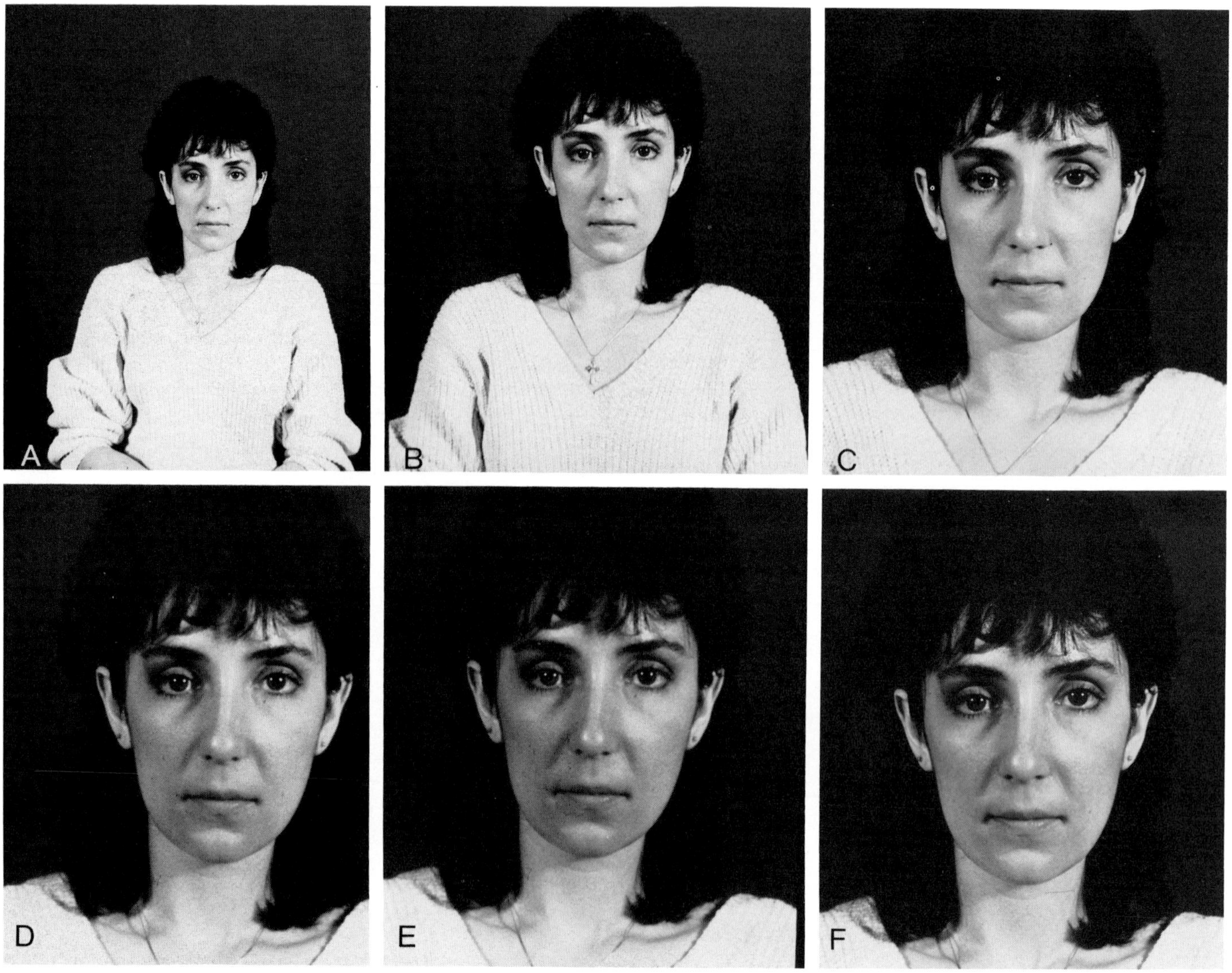

Figure 8.2. Irrespective of the focal length lenses used, the perspective will be identical if the film-to-subject distance is the same. *A*, 35-mm lenses at 56 inches. *B*, 50-mm lenses at 56 inches. *C*, 70-mm lenses at 56 inches. *D*, Enlargement of *panel A*. *E*, Enlargement of *panel B*. *F*, Enlargement of *panel C*. The perspective of *panels D*, *E*, and *F* is identical.

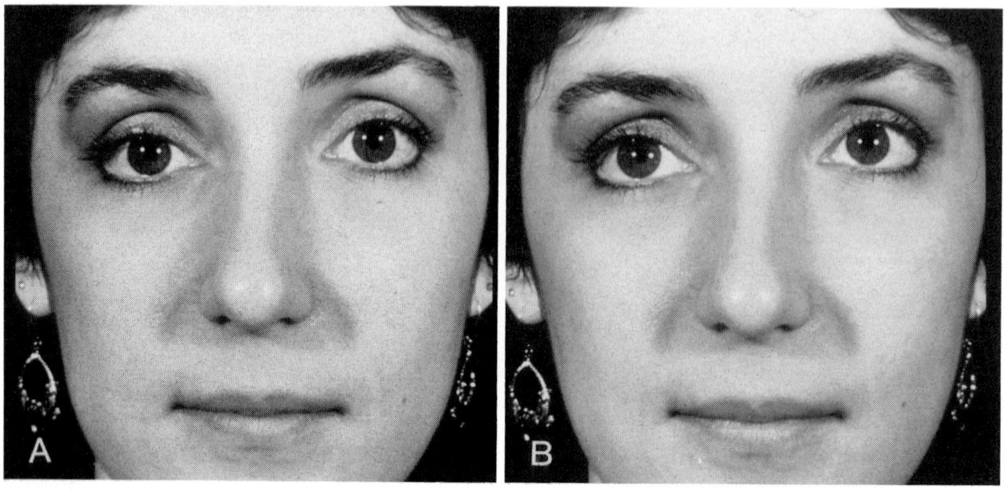

Figure 8.3. Instruct the patient to look directly at the lens. If the patient is daydreaming, the eyes will appear out of focus. *A*, Eyes focused. *B*, Daydreaming.

acteristics and the basic principle of exposure, we will discuss various light sources and lighting techniques for the oculoplastic patient.

The three characteristics of light that concern the biomedical photographer are the quality of the light, the color temperature of the light, and the intensity of the light. The quality of the light is the "directional or nondirectional characteristic" of the light. If the source of the light is small and intense, the shadows cast by the light will be sharp and deep; the sun on a cloudless day is a good example of a strong directional light source. Conversely, if the source of the light is large and diffuse, that is, nondirectional, there will be weak or indistinct shadows as you would experience on an overcast day. Since our visual perception of shape is determined by shadows, the biomedical photographer needs a directional light to distinguish the topography of the face and a nondirectional light to lighten the shadows without creating new and contradictory shadows. The directional light is generally called the "main or key light" and the nondirectional light is called the "fill light."

The second consideration is the color temperature of light. White light is made up of various combinations of wavelengths of the visible spectrum. The mix of the wavelengths emitted by a light source is determined by the physics of the source and the amount of energy consumed by the source. The light from each source is compared with the light emitted by a heated theoretical "blackbody" and is thereby designated with a color temperature. Color temperature is measured in degrees Kelvin; the scale is similar to the centigrade scale except it is based on absolute zero (−270°C) instead of the melting point of ice. Unlike the human eye, which accommodates for various color temperatures, color photographic film is sensitive to these variations and must be properly matched with the light source. If color film is used under the wrong lighting conditions, the color balance of the film will shift, resulting in a color cast. For instance, if daylight color film is used indoors with tungsten illumination, the photograph will have an orange cast; conversely, if tungsten film is used outside in the daylight, the photograph will have a blue cast.

The third characteristic, the intensity of light, is the quantity or strength of the light and is one of the factors that determines film exposure. Exposure is the product of the intensity of the light at the film plane and the time during which the light acts on the photographic emulsion. In the camera the aperture controls the intensity of the light, and the shutter controls the duration of the exposure. Most modern 35-mm cameras are equipped with a light meter positioned close to the film plane to help calculate the correct exposure. If the source is an electronic flash, the duration of the light is too short to register on the camera's internal light meter. Special light meters designed to measure the intensity of the electronic flash are available, but they are prohibitively expensive. An alternative method for calculating the intensity of the electronic flash is to use the guide numbers provided by the manufacturer. Most flash units have a chart or a wheel calculator on the back of the unit to calculate the exposure from the flash to subject distance, the guide number, and the film speed. The latest electronic meters have provided an even simpler method of calculating flash intensity by incorporating a light-sensitive cell, generally a "thyristor circuit," into the flash unit, which measures and controls the output of the flash.

Flash calculators as well as light meters are calibrated to determine the exposure for a subject with a reflectivity of 18%—a green lawn has a reflectivity of 18%. Since most oculoplastic patients do not have a reflectivity of 18% (Caucasians and blacks have approximate reflectivities of 92% and 10%, respectively), the calculated or metered exposure reading is not necessarily the correct exposure. Most of the variables in oculoplastic photography can be controlled; therefore, in the beginning it is probably easiest to determine the correct exposure by bracketing a set of exposures around the metered reading. For example, if the metered reading is *f*11 at 1/60 of a second, photograph the patient using the following *f*-stops at 1/60 of a second, *f*16, *f*16 plus 1/2 stops, *f*11, *f*11 plus 1/2 stops, and *f*8. Bracketing in the preceding manner ensures that the correct exposure will be used. Be sure to take thorough notes so that the correct exposure can be correlated with the patient's skin tone.

LIGHTING EQUIPMENT

Lighting equipment is manufactured in many shapes, types, outputs, and sizes; it is almost as varied as the types of cameras and lenses manufactured. Despite this variety, we can reduce all of this equipment into two categories for producing artificial light: incandescent lamps, or continuous sources, and electronic discharge lamps, or stroboscopic sources. Incandescent sources, which were once pervasive, have taken a backseat to electronic flash sources over the last 15 years; however, a weak incandescent source is still used with most professional electronic flash sources to serve as a "focusing" or "modeling light."

Incandescent sources are hot, which is uncomfortable for both the photographer and the patient and potentially dangerous. They also consume a great deal of energy, and their color temperature is not as stable as electronic flash sources.

For all these reasons, the electronic flash is preferred over the incandescent sources. As I said before, electronic flashes are available as either manual or automatic units. Although the automatic units are excellent for the amateur photographer, the manual units are preferred by the professional photographer because of the consistency of the light output. If you already own an automatic unit, it probably has a manual mode of operation.

For location photography in your office, electronic flash units are light, small, and extremely portable. The smaller units are generally powered by batteries, rather than the AC power required by the incandescent sources. In close-up photography, it is important for the light source to be as close as possible to the camera lens; incandescent sources of sufficient power are much too large and hot for such close work.

Two types of electronic flashes are used for close-up work: ring lights and small point sources. A ring light is a circular electronic flash tube that is attached to the front end of the camera lens. This type of source provides a flat shadowless illumination designed primarily for cavity work. Except when photographing such cases as the socket after an enucleation, most external eye photography requires a small diffuse point source that produces a directional illumination, permitting the ophthalmologist to appreciate the effect of the subject's topography and the depth relationship.

As a side note, the depth relationships are also influenced by the depth of field, which is a factor of the size of the lens' aperture: as the diameter of the aperture decreases, the depth of field increases; conversely, as the diameter of the aperture increases, the depth of field decreases. Since the aperture is an exposure determinant, the aperture cannot be closed down unless the strength of the light is sufficient to compensate for the light lost to the smaller aperture opening. Electronic flash units, even the very small portable ones, are sufficiently powerful to permit a small aperture.

Flash units for close-up work are manufactured with either a ring light or a point source, and one manufacturer has designed a unit that combines both the ring light and the point source. The only disadvantage to these units is that they can be a little unmanageable; you might wonder if they were designed for someone with three hands. Despite the "Rube Goldberg appearance," these units can be very effective if used properly and with patience.

LIGHTING TECHNIQUE

The next step in the standardization process is patient lighting. Since our usual understanding of the subject is primarily dependent upon the interaction of light and the subject, a great deal of care must be taken to ensure that the lighting techniques we use to document the oculoplastic patient do not minimize or maximize the patient's condition. The lighting technique must be consistent so that the preoperative and postoperative photography are comparable, that is, the lighting technique must be identical throughout the life of the series.

In addition to neutrality and consistency, the lighting technique must also consider "standard conditions," which means that the lighting must be similar to the lighting conditions under which the subject is generally seen. Since our lighting orientation is the sun, we consider a normally lit subject one that is softly illuminated from above. Although this consideration is purely psychological, if we do not incorporate it into our overall lighting, the unnatural quality of the light will be distracting. Because the patient will be viewed most often under normal lighting conditions, the objective of the photographic study therefore is to document patients preoperatively and postoperatively as they would be seen under normal conditions.

The first rule to keep in mind when designing a lighting technique for a particular condition is to keep it simple. Going back to our psychological condition in terms of what we perceive as normally lit subjects: First, we are accustomed to a light from above, and second, we are accustomed to only one main light. The more complicated the lighting technique becomes, the greater the danger of violating one of these principles. That is not to say that no more than one light can be used, but when four and five lights are used, it becomes extremely difficult to maintain the integrity of the lighting design. In oculoplastic photography, as with most types of photography, there should be only one dominant light; any secondary lights must be subordinate and subservient to the main light. One of the dangers in patient photography is forgetting the patient: the more complicated the techniques and equipment used by the photographer, the less attention and time the photographer can give to the patient.

In this chapter, we will limit our lighting design to two lights so that the photographer will not inadvertently violate one of the basic principles and so that an inordinate amount of time to adjust lights can be avoided. As such, we have eliminated the two least important lights in a general setup: the hair light and the background light.

The *main light*, as its name implies, is the most important light and the one for which placement is most critical. Most commonly, the main light is a diffuse directional light from above that casts soft shadows. The main light should cause "catch lights" in the eyes; if it is too high, you will not be able to see the catch lights and must therefore lower it. A patient with deep eye sockets will require a much lower main light than a patient with a normal socket; otherwise, the socket will be hidden by the shadows cast by the main light. The second light that we use is the *fill light*. The purpose of this light, which is always subservient and subordinate to the main light, is to lighten the shadows cast by the main light. The fill light is an on-camera axis light and as such illuminates everything that the camera sees, including the area illuminated by the main light. The main light, on the other hand, is an off-camera axis light and provides the dimensional quality to the photograph. Although the positioning of the fill light is considerably easier than the main light, it can also be tricky. If possible, avoid causing a second catch light in the eye; if it cannot be avoided, it is permissible to retouch the second catch light in a black-and-white photograph. Unfortunately, color slides cannot be readily retouched. It should be noted that this is the only instance where retouching is permissible in oculoplastic photography.

The next consideration in lighting design after the placement of the lights is the *lighting ratio*. The lighting ratio refers to the relative intensity of the main light to the fill light in terms of the total effect. For instance, a typical lighting ratio is 3:1, which means that the main light is three times as strong as the fill light when considered together. In oculoplastic photography 3:1 is a good lighting ratio for both color and black-and-white photographs. There are two simple methods of establishing a 3:1 lighting ratio. The first is through the use of the aperture scale as a distance scale. For example, if the main light is 8 feet from the subject, the fill light should be 11 feet from the subject; if the main light is 11 feet from the subject, then the fill light should be 16 feet from the subject. The second method is through the use of an *incident light meter*. An incident light meter reads the light of the source from the patient position. When taking a reading of the main light, you should place the incident light meter at a position that is illuminated by the main light. When taking a reading of the fill light, place the incident light meter at the position illuminated by the fill light. These readings must be taken when both the main and the fill light are one.

The use of electronic flash units makes the process of establishing lighting ratio more difficult; however, the same methods can be used if you have an incident electronic flash meter or if the modeling light on the electronic flash units are in a known proportion to the output of the flash tube.

Unlike perspective, exposure, and color temperature, lighting ratios are subjective (i.e., there is no right or wrong ratio). The lighting ratio is completely dependent on the preference of the ophthalmologist. The only hard and fast rule is consistency between the preoperative and the postoperative views.

Once one is familiar with the general principles of lighting, it is relatively easy to apply these principles to the particular photographic study required. In this section, we will examine two external eye photographic studies, the *strabismus series* and the *eye plastic series*, that are very dissimilar in purpose and will therefore require two entirely different lighting approaches.

In the strabismus series (Fig. 8.4), the ophthalmologist is interested in the range of motion of the eye, whereas in the eye plastic series, the ophthalmologist is interested in the lids, orbits, and tissue surrounding and covering the eye. Since in the strabismus series, we are not interested in the topographical characteristic of the eye or orbital region, but in the range and coordination of motion of the eyes, this study uses a very flat, almost shadowless light. Although theoretically this should be done with a main light raised slightly above the camera position, it is much more convenient to use two lights evenly balanced and positioned 45° to either side of the medium place of the subject and slightly above the camera axis. These lights act as one main light and produce a very soft and even illumination.

In the eye plastic series (Fig. 8.5), the ophthalmologist is not so much interested in studying the eye itself but rather the architecture of the skin that surrounds and covers the eye. Since the subject of the photographic study is the topography of the orbital region, a highly directional lighting design that will illustrate the texture and quality of the orbital tissue is required. The study should include (*a*) an overall photograph of the patient's face, (*b*) medium close-up photographs of both eyes open and closed and both eyes looking up and down, and (*c*) close-up photographs of anteroposterior (frontal) and lateral views of each eye. This series requires two basic lighting setups: one for the anteroposterior and one for the lateral views.

For the frontal view the two lights should be balanced and positioned 45° to either side of the median plane of the subject and approximately 45° above the camera. This setup will provide even illumination and have the directional characteristics necessary to illustrate the topography. For patients with deep-set eyes, it may be necessary to lower the lights slightly to avoid the shadows cast by the brows—only lower the lights if the eye is not picking up the catch light.

The lateral views require a main light and a fill light. The key light is positioned such that the edge of the light highlights the bridge of the nose and skin across the lower lid. The fill light is positioned slightly above the camera position and balanced for a ratio of 3:1 with the main light. This light is used to fill in the deep shadows cast by the key light (Fig. 8.6).

MATERIALS, EQUIPMENT AND SPACE

The materials and equipment used for this type of work vary greatly, depending on the financial and technical limitations placed on the photographer. Most professional photographic equipment is of comparable quality, and so the particular system you select is only of minor importance.

For black-and-white work, I have found that the 120-film format provides the resolution and grain structure necessary to document the fine details of the cutaneous aspects of the orbit. I have found that Plus-X film developed in stock solution of DK-50 at 68°F for 6 minutes will provide an excellent tonal range with adequate negative density. There are many combinations of film developer that can be used for this type of work; however, one rule should be kept in mind: achieve the desired contrast through lighting, not through film development. I have found that printing the negatives on Polycontrast Rapid II RC paper and developing them in a 1:2 solution of Dektol produces excellent results.

In addition to the black and white 5 × 7 prints, 35-mm color transparencies are made for all patients. For the color transparency series, I recommend Kodachrome 64 slide film. Although the resolution and color balance of the Kodachrome film is excellent, the 3- to 4-day processing time available in most of the country may make it necessary to use one of the Ektachrome transparency films available that can be processed in-house—unless you are as fortunate as I am to have arranged an overnight Kodachrome service that enables us to provide a fast turnover time.

Because of the 3- to 4-day turnover time required for the black-and-white prints and the color transparencies, we have a Polaroid camera available for emergencies, which we use with Polaroid Type 667 coatless black-and-white Land film.

One of the annoying problems that can crop up and ruin a photographic study is film spoiled by improper handling and storage. Even though the proliferation of air conditioners and centrally controlled humidifiers has minimized this problem, care should be taken to ensure that proper storage and handling conditions are met. Film, whether unprocessed or processed, must be protected from x-rays, harmful gases, high relative humidities, and high temperatures; unprocessed film stored for more than 4 weeks should be kept frozen.

In addition to the storage condition, it is important to process exposed film as soon as possible. Exposed color film is particularly sensitive to color balance fluctuation between the time it is exposed and processed. For processed film it is important to minimize the film exposure to light; this is particularly critical for color transparencies, which should not be projected for longer than 1 minute.

Because of its excellent optics compactness and reliability, we have chosen the Hasseblad system for our black-

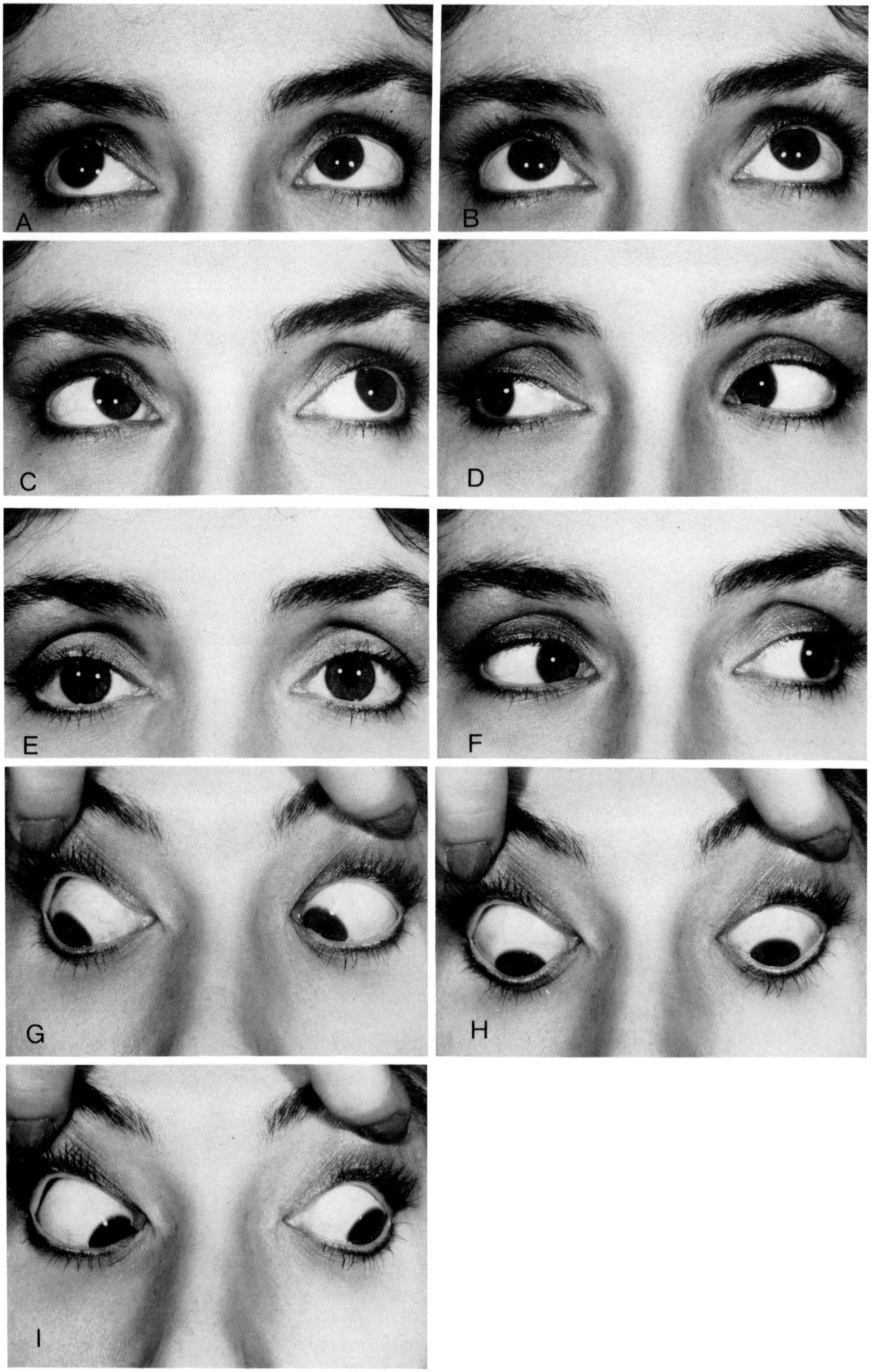

Figure 8.4. The strabismus series; the nine cardinal gazes.

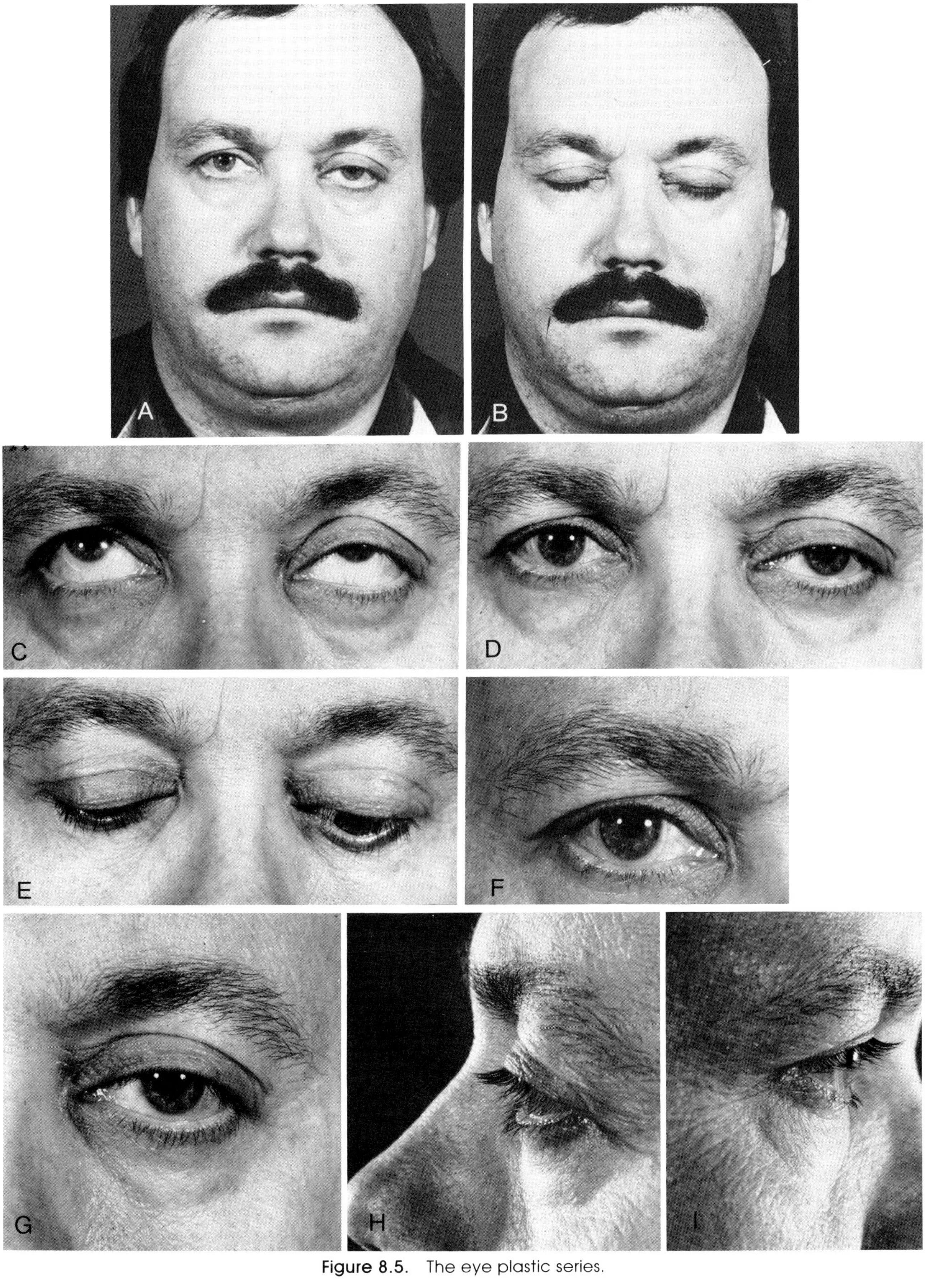

Figure 8.5. The eye plastic series.

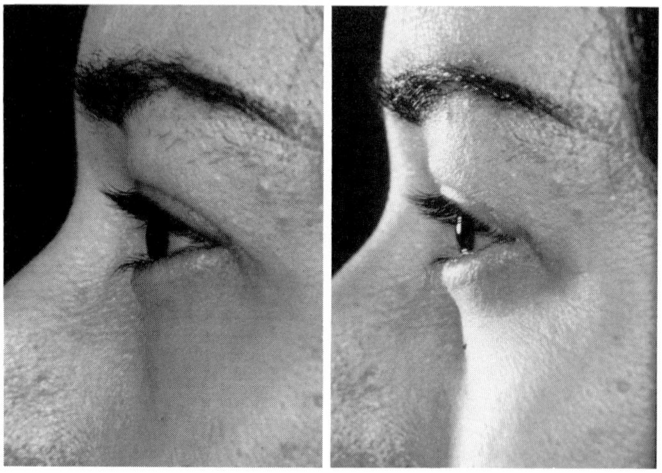

Figure 8.6. Comparison of lighting techniques to illustrate orbital region. The photograph on the left is a relatively flat light design compared with the photograph on the right, which utilizes a lighting technique designed to highlight the topographic characteristics of the orbital region.

and-white work. Our Hasseblad 500 C/M body is equipped with a magnifying hood and a 12-frame film magazine. We use a 150-mm sonar lens with a Hasseblad 21 extension tube; for closer views, we use a Proxor F-1m close-up lens. For the color transparencies, we have selected the Nikon F2 body and a Micro-Nikon 105-mm lens. With these systems, we are able to provide the surgeon with identical views in both color and black and white.

This type of work requires a studio or at least a dedicated area. The area need not be large, but in order to work comfortably, it should not be any smaller than 15 × 10 feet. An area should be provided for patients to remove makeup and arrange their hair such that it does not obscure any details of the face. A minimum of two lights are required; either electronic flash or floodlights is acceptable. However, as I stated previously, floodlights are hot and can become very uncomfortable. The heat radiating from the lights will quickly cause the patient to perspire, which must be avoided. For these reasons the electronic flash system is preferable. The studio should be equipped with a sturdy chair with an extension to position the head. In order to avoid accidents, the chair should not be on wheels.

A monopod is also very helpful for this type of work because it enables you to level the camera before shooting; remember the dramatic effects that a slight camera tilt can have on perspective. The background need not be large; 40 × 40 inches is sufficient. Colored backgrounds should be avoided since they tend to confuse the interpretation of the patient's skin pigmentation in the color transparency. A black or white background is much too stark, and the 18% gray is slightly too dark. As a rule of thumb, we look for a background with a reflectivity of approximately 30%.

PHOTOGRAPHY IN THE OPERATING ROOM

Documentation of surgical procedures presents some unique problems for the ophthalmic surgeon. Most general surgical procedures do not require special equipment; however, the ophthalmic surgeon's operating site is so small that special equipment is required. Let us first consider surgical procedures done with an operating microscope. Unfortunately, the microsurgical procedure cannot be adequately documented with a hand-held camera or the traditional video camera. Since I am familiar with the Zeiss operating microscope, and it is one of the most common, I will confine this discussion to equipment designed for this particular instrument. Although the optical design of the other operating microscopes are different, the general principles discussed in this section are applicable to all the various operating microscopes.

In order to obtain the same view and adequate magnification, the camera must utilize the microscope in order to document the procedure. The optics of the microscope serve as the camera lens, and therefore the camera body must be conjugated with the optics of the microscope such that the point of focus is the same for the film plane as it is for the surgeon.

In order to divert or split the light traveling through the microscope to the surgeon's oculars, a beam splitter is inserted just before the binocular head. This beam splitter has two ports: one for assisting the surgeon and a second one for documentation. Zeiss manufactures two beam splitters, the Beam Splitter 50 and the Beam Splitter 70. The Beam Splitter 50 sends 50% of the light to the surgeon and 50% of the light to the camera. The Beam Splitter 70 sends seven times the amount of light to the camera as it does to the surgeon. Almost every photographer in the field will prefer the Beam Splitter 70 over the Beam Splitter 50 because we always need the additional light, but then we are not the ones who are performing the surgery. Unless you can purchase both beam splitters, the Beam Splitter 50 is the most versatile and will adequately serve most of the needs of the photographer.

Photoadapters are generally classified by their *focal length.* Simply stated, the focal length of a lens is a measure of the light-bending power of a lens or lens system when we take into account the refractive index and shape. Focal length is important in photography because it decides the magnification of the image (i.e., the longer the focal length, the larger the image). Ophthalmologists are more familiar with the term "diopter" to express the power of a lens. A diopter is the reciprocal of the focal length in meters. When the power of a lens is stated in diopters (d), its focal length is given by 100/d in centimeters. In photography only supplementary close-up lenses are expressed in diopters.

The focal length of a lens or photoadapter is generally engraved on the mount: f = 90 mm. This should not be confused with the *f*-number, which is designated as "*f*8" or "*f*/8" and also engraved on the lens mount.

The *f*-number is a numerical expression of the relative

aperture of a lens at its different stops. The *f*-number is equal to the focal length divided by the effective diameter of the lens opening. In still photography it is used in conjunction with the shutter speed and the film speed to determine the exposure. The lens or adapter will generally have a series of *f*-numbers that correspond to different aperture settings and are engraved on a ring on the lens. This means that the higher the *f*-stop number, the smaller the opening and therefore the less light transmitted. However, the lens or adapter will be catalogued by its largest aperture (and correspondingly its smallest *f*-number).

The first adapter introduced on the market for the Zeiss operating microscope was the single camera adapter (Fig. 8.7); one was designed to accept video/cine, another was designed to accept still photography. Even though the beam splitter had two ports, one was reserved for the assisting surgeon, so in order to videotape a procedure and photograph it at the same time, the microscope would have to be moved, the adapters changed and then redraped before the surgery continued, which was too time consuming to be practical. As the need for documentation increased, many surgeons wanted to be able to videotape and photograph a procedure. Video was also needed so the surgery could be viewed by the nurses and technicians assisting with the operation.

The first company to design a dual adapter for the Zeiss operating microscope was a specialty optical house called Designs for Vision. The success of the Designs for Vision adapter, the Telestill Photo Adapter (Fig. 8.8), spurred

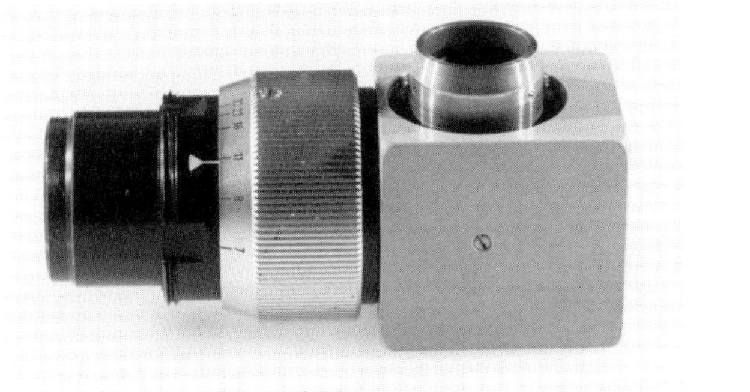

Figure 8.7. Single camera adapter with built-in aperture.

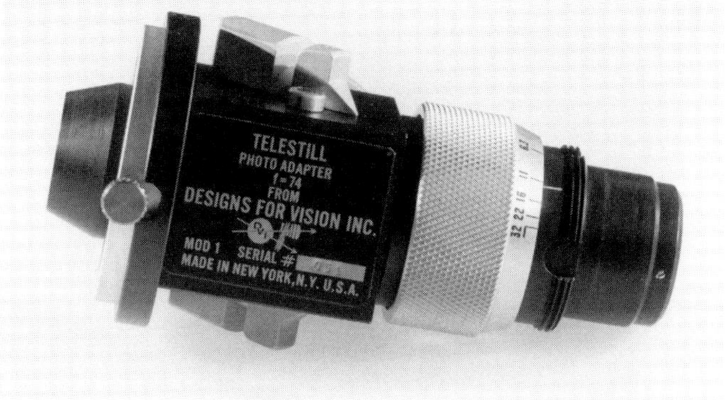

Figure 8.8. Telestill photoadapter: focal length, 74 mm.

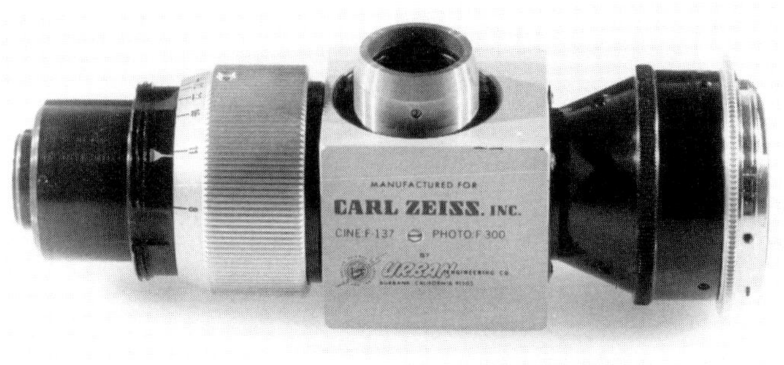

Figure 8.9. Zeiss Urban Dual Camera Adapter: focal length, 137 mm.

Zeiss to introduce their own dual adapter called the Zeiss Urban Dual Camera Adapter (Fig. 8.9).

The Telestill Photo Adapter is a front surface mirror adapter with a lever to alternate between the video/cine port and the still port. This adapter is manufactured in three different focal lengths and sells for approximately $1200.

The Zeiss Urban Dual Camera Adapter is also manufactured in three focal lengths. The Zeiss adapter uses a beam splitter instead of the front surface mirror design of the Telestill Photo Adapter so that it is not necessary to alternate between the video/cine port and the still photography port; video/cine and still photography can be done simultaneously. In order to eliminate the switching lever of the Telestill Photo Adapter, Zeiss had to split the light beam once again which decreased the illumination at the two documentation ports by about 25%. For the majority of ophthalmic surgery, the illumination system of the microscope is adequate, and this does not present a problem; in posterior segment surgery the maximum amount of light is necessary and therefore the Telestill Photo Adapter is preferable.

In microsurgical procedures the camera body is only of minimal importance; with the proper adapters almost any quality 35 mm camera can be used for this type of work.

The next problem encountered is releasing the shutter. Since the surgeon's are scrubbed and the microscope is often draped, it is difficult to reach the camera shutter release without contaminating the surgical field. This problem can be overcome with an infrared transmitter and receiver designed to release the shutter from a distance. The Contax Infrared Controller S Set is designed for use in the operating room and had a range of approximately ten unobstructed feet, but it should be tested in your particular setting.

SUGGESTED READINGS

Abrahamson Jr, IA: An ophthalmologist's approach to anterior segment photography. *J Ophthal Photogr* 4: 1981.

Christopher KW: "External Eye Photography: Equipment and Technique," *J Ophthal Photogr* 4: 1981.

Dickason WL, et al.: Pitfalls of comparative photography in plastic and reconstructive surgery. *Plast Reconstr Surg* 58: 1976.

Eastman Kodak Co: *Clinical Photography*. Eastman Kodak Co., 1972.

Eastman Kodak Co: *Electronic Flash: The Kodak Workshop Series*. Rochester, NY, Eastman Kodak Co., 1981.

Eastman Kodak Co: *Kodak Color Films*, ed 8. Rochester, NY, Eastman Kodak Co., 1980.
Eastman Kodak Co: *Kodak Professional Black and White Films*. Rochester, NY, Eastman Kodak Co., 1984.
Eastman Kodak Co: *Kodak Professional Photoguide*, ed 1. Eastman Kodak Co., 1981.
Eastman Kodak Co: *Photography with Large Format Cameras*. Rochester, NY, Eastman Kodak Co., 1973.
Eastman Kodak Co: *Professional Photographic Illustration Techniques*. Rochester, NY, Eastman Kodak Co., 1978.
Eastman Kodak Co: *Professional Portrait Techniques*. Rochester, NY, Eastman Kodak Co., June 1980.
Engel CE: *Photography for the Scientist*. London, Academic Press, 1968.
Foldes J: *Large Format Camera Practice*. New York, Amphoto, 1969.
Gray DE: Developing standards and measuring performance in biomedic production. *J Biol Photogr Assoc* 47: 1979.
Hoerenz P: The operating microscope IV. Documentation. *J Microsurg* December: 1980.
Krugman ME, et al.: Facial series of photographs as viewed by the plastic surgeon with special emphasis on the nose. *J Biol Photogr Assoc* 47: 1979.
Langford MJ: *Advanced Photography*. London, Focal Press, 1974.
Langford MJ: *Basic Photography*. London, Focal Press, 1974.
Neldette CB: *Neldette's Handbook of Photography and Reprography*.
Sherwin RB: *Legal Aspects of Photography*. New York, Amphoto, 1973.
Shields WJ: Clarification of some terms used often by videographers. *Ophthalmol Times* April 15: 1984.
Shields WJ: Describe types of photoadapters used in documentary microsurgery. *Ophthalmol Times*. June 15: 1984.
Shields WJ: External eye photography reported to require standardized technique. *Ophthalmol Times*. Feb 15: 1984.
Shields WJ: Guidelines offered to assist in external eye photography. *Ophthalmol Times*. Jan 15: 1984.
Shields WJ, et al.: Strabismus and eye plastic photography. *J Ophthal Photogr* 5: 29–35, 1982.
Utz P: *Video User's Handbook*. Englewood Cliffs, NJ, Prentice-Hall, 1980.
Zarem HA: Standards of photography. *Plast Reconstr Surg* July, 1984.

CHAPTER 9

Psychological Implications of Ophthalmic Plastic Surgery

HADASSAH NEIMAN GURFEIN, PH.D.

Of all the human characteristics, physical beauty is one of the most prized and coveted by all members of society. Attractive people receive warmer reactions and are generally more highly regarded than homely people. It is not surprising, therefore, that physical attractiveness is integral to the mental health, emotional well-being, and positive self-image of the average person.

> If we lived in a world in which the way we look made no difference in the responses we get, there would be no demand for aesthetic plastic surgery. However, such is not the case. We live in a social world in which the face of a person is perceived as an index of the person himself. Influenced as we are by stereotypes of facial configuration, features, and expressions that are presumed to indicate such qualities as personality, intelligence, character traits, and temperament, not to mention what has become (particularly in the United States) an obsessive concern with looking young and beautiful, the person whose face deviates from the norm not only receives differential treatment but becomes the helpless victim of negative judgments, prejudice and discrimination (1).

Despite the benefits of plastic surgery, it also has its own set of psychological reactions because it involves the act of surgery, which is in itself a traumatic invasion of body space, and because it tampers with body image (2). These related concepts of body space and body image are keys to understanding surgery's potential for psychological trauma. Surgical patients are asked to undergo a suspension of ego functions through anesthesia and an invasion of the boundaries of the body ego.

Additional stress is created by the anxieties related to any change in body shape. Such anxieties have been expressed over the centuries in legends, myths, and stories of gigantism, dwarfism, and other transformations. Patients may experience surgically produced bodily changes, whether positive or negative, as stressful.

"Body image is the perception of one's own body at a given point in time. Body image distortion is the discrepancy between the actual body and the body as reflected in one's mental representation" (3). Some degree of body image distortion is probably close to universal. All of us experience some part of ourselves as bigger, smaller, fatter, thinner, more beautiful, or uglier than is actually the case. We never see ourselves exactly as others see us. It is all a matter of degree.

Body image distortions may be minimal or pathological. An anorectic woman who sees herself in the mirror as overweight confronts a body image that does not coincide with the way she is perceived by everyone around her. Similar confusion about one's appearance may result in a great deal of anxiety after cosmetic surgery, even when the surgery itself is entirely successful.

Such confusion is not merely caused by the change in appearance but also by the significance the change has to an individual. Confusion is heightened by the fact that when a person looks different, the world starts reacting to him or her differently, although inside that person feels the same (3).

Surgery for aesthetic purposes is becoming accepted by our society as an endeavor as legitimate as any other in the medical profession. But the stigma associated with undergoing surgery for the improvement of one's appearance still has not entirely disappeared. The reluctance to accept aesthetic surgery may be traced to our biblical heritage, which decrys the concept of vanity. The Book of Proverbs instructs that "charm is deceptive, and beauty is vain (5)." Goldwyn points out the interesting paradox of our culture, which admires wealth gained through work more than it admires inherited wealth but inverts that value when the wealth consists of physical beauty (6). The irony is that the very culture which once devalued plastic surgery and viewed it as capricious may in fact be responsible for maintaining the values which will result in its proliferation.

Bearing in mind our culture's ambivalence on this subject, it is easy to understand why patients undergoing plastic surgery may experience psychological conflicts over and above those normally experienced by other surgical patients. Guilt and fear of punishment may accompany elective plastic surgery, particularly if complications ensue.

The ophthalmological surgeon should also consider the special significance of the eye as a person's window to the world and its role as a communication device, object of beauty, and conveyor of sexuality. The eye is valued by both its owner and beholder as the vehicle of perception and is therefore a key to one's success in all human interaction and functioning.

The rest of this chapter attempts to clarify the psychological aspects of successfully performing ophthalmic plastic surgery. It addresses stated reasons for seeking surgery as well as motives and expectations. The importance of the doctor-patient relationship will be discussed, including some of the surgeon's own motivations in performing surgery. A description of candidate selection is followed by assessment techniques. The conclusion deals with postoperative care.

REASONS FOR SEEKING SURGERY

The reasons for ophthalmological plastic surgery fall into two major categories: (*a*) functional problems that include malformations that are congenital or acquired through trauma (pain) or pathological processes and (*b*) cosmetic improvement of malformations that are congenital or acquired. Each condition carries with it a different set of psychological considerations.

FUNCTIONAL PROBLEMS

When vision or life are in danger, the reasons for seeking surgery are straightforward and decision-making is usually relatively easy. However, it should not be taken for granted that there are no psychological difficulties in patients undergoing noncosmetic ophthalmic plastic surgery.

Congenital Malformation

A congenital deformity of one dating from early childhood can adversely affect the personality of children, influencing their character structure and concept of body image. The defect becomes incorporated into their personality through the integration of their own awareness of the defect, and their perception of how others react to them (7). The attitude of the parents and siblings is the single most important factor in determining how children view themselves and function in the world. For example, the process of separation and individuation from mother, which occurs approximately between ages 18 to 24 months, is influenced by the way others, and the mother in particular, react to the child (7a). Separation will be discouraged if the environment is either hostile or overprotective. The child will then perceive the world as a cold, threatening, or frightening place and will not successfully negotiate this crucial developmental stage. If the deformity is very conspicuous, the rejection or overprotectiveness from both the family and/or the outside world may cause serious psychological damage to the child. It is crucial that the parents accept the child with the deformity without guilt or anxiety. Thus, early correction through plastic surgery can be helpful in preventing serious emotional problems. Surgery is particularly indicated for conditions that cannot be outgrown and cause impairment of vision and unattractiveness.

Acquired Malformation

Malformations acquired later in life by accident or disease are less often associated with psychological complications, since the formed personality is less vulnerable. Of course, the basic (premorbid) personality structure of patients will influence their reaction to this stress.

A condition requiring radical surgery, such as enucleation, is an exception since the physical alteration and emotional impact resulting from this operation are of a tremendous magnitude and may require a major life adjustment.

COSMETIC SURGERY

Cosmetic surgery, and especially blepharoplasty, is becoming increasingly popular as a valid reason for plastic surgery. Some elect it to improve on nature's endowment and some want to restore what has deteriorated with age. Striving to look younger is now common and acceptable among both sexes; it is a legitimate reason for plastic surgery and a realistic goal.

While cosmetic surgery has become an ordinary luxury for the affluent, it has always been a practical necessity for professional performers and entertainers, who are continually in the public eye and rely on their looks for employment.

PATIENT MOTIVATION AND EXPECTATION

Motivation and expectation differ among patients seeking plastic surgery. Inappropriate motives are usually related to unrealistic expectations. Timing is an important factor to consider, as it may be related to motivation. It is necessary to determine who is motivated for the surgery: the patient or other family members. The wish for surgery should come from the patient and should not be suggested by family members or the surgeon. Patients who are not self-motivated may blame the surgeon for any disappointment they may experience.

FUNCTIONAL PROBLEMS

Motivation for nonelective plastic surgery is self-evident and includes saving the sight and/or life of the patient.

Congenital and Acquired Malformations

Congenital and acquired malformations or growths are valid and obvious motives for plastic surgery. The aim is to repair and restore proper functioning and/or appearance to the eye. The patient should be informed of realistic expectations, especially if perfection cannot be achieved.

Requests for surgical correction of longstanding deformities should be regarded with suspicion unless there is indication of longstanding dissatisfaction. If the deformity is longstanding, it is advisable to find out why patients waited until the present in view of their previous knowledge of the availability of corrective surgery. Such patients may have minimized the appearance of the deformity in their mind via the coping mechanisms of denial and minimization, which helped them to face the world. It is important to ascertain whether the relief of present emotional or psychological stress is the reason that surgery is now being sought. Psychological evaluation is often necessary in such cases (7).

The surgeon should be cautious when the patient's concern about the malformation is disproportionate to the seriousness of the condition. Patients who desire plastic surgery for minor malformations are those who view these malformations as more obvious than they are. These patients are usually very demanding. The more insignificant the malformation that concerns the patient, the more the likelihood of postoperative dissatisfaction (8). Although the stated reason is sometimes valid, one must prove to uncover underlying motives. Frequently these patients have emotional problems unrelated to the deformity. The importance that preconscious and unconscious factors play in a patient's motivation for surgery was pointed out by Meyer and associates (9), who studied rhinoplasty patients and found that interpretation may center around the following conflicts: sexual identification, ambivalence in identification with parents, the sexual symbolism of the nose, the wish for surgery, and concepts of body image. Ophthalmic surgery patients may be motivated by similar conflicts.

COSMETIC SURGERY

The most immediate and common motive for blepharoplasty is the removal of sagging skin and wrinkles in order to look younger, less tired and more attractive (10). That is why the majority of blepharoplasty patients are middle-aged women who are experiencing any number of bodily changes, such as menopause and general physical deterioration. Such motivation is appropriate. However, reasonable and attainable motives for plastic surgery are often accompanied by less legitimate and unrealistic underlying motives. Sometimes these are openly expressed by the patient, but oftentimes, they reveal themselves only after some probing. For example, a patient may hope to become less shy, more confident, less inhibited. Surgery may be sought to realize a desire to feel rejuvenated or to recapture a sense of vigor, youth, and self-confidence. This may mean finding a better job, getting promoted, saving a marriage, or finding a spouse. There may be a wish to compete romantically and professionally with younger people at a time when individuals are reckoning with their position in life, unrealized ambitions, and failures. Another common unconscious motivation is the restoration of a loss caused by divorce, job loss, child leaving the house, or death. Patients may not be aware of these unconscious motives until they fail to be achieved after surgery.

Patients such as these, with unrealistic expectations, will undoubtedly be dissatisfied with the surgical results of blepharoplasties, which cannot possibly cure all of life's ills. It is therefore crucial that the surgeon ascertain the patients' motives before surgery in order to determine their suitability for the operation and whether surgery will help them to achieve their goal. The soundness of the motivation will indicate the likelihood of satisfaction with the surgical results.

Occasionally the motivation for plastic surgery is a change in ethnic identity. Oriental people often choose to have plastic surgery performed on their eyes in order to assume a more Western look. Since ethnic appearance plays an integral part in the formation of body image, it is likely that discomfort with one's ethnic appearance will manifest itself during adolescence. This is a good age for such an operation since changes are relatively rapidly incorporated into the body image (3). On the other hand, when performing a routine blepharoplasty on an Oriental patient, the surgeon should be especially careful to preserve the Oriental configuration of the eyelids unless the patient indicates otherwise. Disturbance of this superficial manifestation of ethnic identity could be traumatic.

These precautions should not keep the surgeon from performing blepharoplasty when the request is legitimate, because as long as patients are emotionally stable, even those whose expectations are somewhat unrealistic will be able to adjust to reality after the operation.

PATIENT SELECTION

The factors that determine a patient's suitability for plastic surgery vary with each category, and there are different implications before, during, and after surgery. The most important factors in patient selection should be appropriate motivation and realistic expectation.

PORTRAIT OF THE IDEAL PATIENT

If we were to describe the perfect candidate for ophthalmological plastic surgery, our imaginary patient would possess the following characteristics: A female baby with a gross congenital deformity whose parents are stable, supportive, and understanding of their child and have a firm sense of the realistic expectations of the corrective surgery; or a middle-aged or older woman with sagging eyelids leading a stable personal and professional life and desiring a blepharoplasty. Her motive would be to achieve a younger and realistically more attractive appearance. Her motive would be even more credible if the blepharoplasty were something that she had been thinking about for quite a while or, if she were having it performed again, 10 years later, after having been satisfied with the previous results. The best prognosis is found among patients who have an actual disfigurement, whose appearance is important for their career, who are aging and want to look younger, or who have wanted surgery for a long time (11).

AGE AS A SELECTION FACTOR IN PATIENTS WITH CONGENITAL DEFORMITIES

Congenital deformities should be operated on as early in life as possible—preferably before the age of 10 months (12). Well-meaning parents often delay surgery until a child is older, by which time the psychological damage is already done (1). Goin and Goin (3) suggest that when operating on an infant, it is important for the parents to have seen the deformity so they can appreciate the contrast before and after the surgery. If delay is necessary, surgery should be deferred until the children are capable of understanding what is going to happen and can express their fears and worries. Surgery should be performed before the child enters school and easily becomes an object of curiosity and social rejection. The most ideal age would be 3–4 years. Ages to avoid are approximately 12–24 months, because of increased separation anxiety, and age 5 in boys, because of anxiety about body mutilation at this age.

DANGER SIGNALS

Surgeons can greatly reduce, or even eliminate the risk of dissatisfied patients and malpractice suits by selecting patients wisely. Awareness of, and alertness to, the characteristics of the potentially troublesome patient contribute to a successful selection process. The literature is replete with cautions and descriptions of problematic patients (3, 6, 10, 13–15).

Bizarre behavior, delusions, hallucinations, marked deterioration in functioning, illogical thinking, flat affect, social withdrawal, and isolation are causes for concern. Avoidance of eye contact, inappropriate smiles, and blank stares may accompany these symptoms. They suggest the presence of a psychotic condition. Further investigation of such patients should include a detailed social history. Patients whose contact with reality is weak can become acutely psychotic from the surgery (10). Severely psychotic patients will most likely not be rational enough to cooperate with the surgeon. However, as long as the patient's motivations, understanding, and expectations are consonant with reality surgery can be performed. Clarkson and Stafford-Clark (16) rightly point out that the presence of psychosis accompanied by delusions about the body part to be operated on is the only absolute contraindication to cosmetic surgery. Severe forms of psychopathology do not necessarily contraindicate surgery (7).

Intense mood distortion. Intense mood distortion may indicate an affective disorder. Sadness, loss of interest or pleasure in usual activities, a feeling of hopelessness or worthlessness, loss of appetite, insomnia, somatic complaints and diminished ability to concentrate may indicate a depressive disorder. Depressed patients may hope to lift their depression through plastic surgery. Such temporary relief is likely to be followed by a recurrence of the depression and regret over the surgery.

Exaggerated exuberance, over-optimism, incessant talking or activity. Flight of ideas, grandiosity, and an inability to stick to one subject may indicate mania. Such a patient may make unreasonable and impulsive demands. Failure to comply with the medical regimen is likely. Surgeons should be especially wary of the manic patient who is often an affable person capable of charming them into agreeing to the surgery before they perceive the manic's disturbance.

Secretiveness, suspiciousness, distrustful, and brittle behavior. Persecutory ideation, extreme sensitivity, blaming others, silence and evasiveness when confronted with sensitive subjects may indicate the presence of a paranoid condition. Because of the lucid and clear manner in which the paranoid discusses many subjects, this condition may be difficult to detect. An extreme paranoid condition in which the patient is not in touch with reality should serve as a warning not to operate. Patients who exhibit mild suspiciousness yet retain a firm hold on reality may be appropriate candidates for surgery provided they receive the reassurance they are seeking and a full explanation of the procedures.

Of course, not all excessive displays of emotion reflect mental illness. Nevertheless, the presence of unusual behavior is a signal that some disturbance may exist necessitating further investigation. This may indicate a personality disorder that will be manifested in problematic behavior that will interfere with a smooth surgical course.

The following are some behavioral clues that do not necessarily indicate psychosis but that may indicate psychopathology and necessitate further inquiry:

Obsessive, detailed, and repetitive questioning. Overly lengthy complex reasons for surgery betray intense anxiety and are often characteristic of one of the following: (*a*) depressed individuals seeking reassurance but actually disclosing their pessimism; (*b*) obsessive-compulsive individuals whose thoughts are dominated by certain upsetting and repetitious themes, who carry out certain unpleasurable ritualistic routines in order to relieve anxiety—they will demand to know all the details of the procedure and set perfectionistic standards; (*c*) hypochondriacal individuals who describe their expectations in great detail and continually inquire into the pathologic meaning of minor events or normal postoperative events—these patients may be critical of the surgery no matter how successful it is (10).

Excessively fastidious appearance. This may indicate an exaggerated concern with keeping oneself intact and maintaining a perfect image. This concern may be applied to the plastic surgery in such a way that insignificant details are blown out of proportion. This behavior belies considerable insecurity and is often exhibited by the paranoid or obsessive-compulsive person.

Inappropriate, hostile, or critical remarks. Irritability, anger, identity disturbance (e.g., "I do not know who I am"), intolerance of being alone, emptiness, boredom, a history of intense and unstable interpersonal relationships, and impulsivity, (e.g., sexual promiscuity, substance abuse, and self-damaging acts) reflect a borderline personality disorder. Such patients can be operated on provided they have realistic expectations. Hostility is often expressed through nonpayment of bills. These patients are consumed with envy and fantasies of revenge. Surgeons should not allow themselves to be provoked by their anger. It is best to point out that their anger has nothing to do with the reality of the present situation. Clear, firm limits should help avoid difficulties.

Grandiose sense of self-importance or uniqueness. Self-involvement; fantasies of success, brilliance, beauty, and love; exhibitionism; seeking admiration; indifference, rage; humiliation; or emptiness in response to criticism or failure characterize many of the patients who come to the plastic surgeon. These characteristics reflect a narcisstic character disorder. Such patients often expect special favors and are surprised when they are treated like others without entitlement. Functioning is characterized by exploitiveness, inability to appreciate how others feel, and relationships that alternate between overidealization and devaluation. Setting limits is very important. Such people do not appreciate special favors but view them as their entitlement. Their demands will increase. They should be treated as other patients. They often will not be pleased no matter how successful the result.

Overly dramatic, reactive, or intense behavior. Exaggerated, or excited behavior to attract attention is characteristic of a histrionic personality disorder. While often superficially charming, such people are egocentric, demanding, dependent, helpless, constantly seeking reassurance, and manipulative. Such individuals are very trusting of others, suggestible, and initially respond positively to an authority figure they think can magically solve their problems. They are easily influenced by others. The surgeon should be aware of their attempt to control the opposite sex or enter into a dependent relationship.

Vague and evasive answers. If a patient provides excessive confusing details, indicates confusion of reasons and goal for surgery, or fails to make eye contact while answering your questions, it may indicate the presence of the following conditions: schizophrenia, depression, mania, or insufficient exploration into the reasons for surgery.

Rudeness, pushiness, or messiness. Treating the surgeon's office as his or her home may indicate a patient's lack of regard for following doctor's orders and for convention, such as paying bills.

History of dissatisfaction with previous surgeries. Patients who relate numerous unsatisfactory consultations or surgery addicts who have previously undergone plastic surgery for the same purpose are candidates for future disappointment. Multisurgery patients usually have gross psychopathology with strong masochistic tendencies (17). Their aims are seldom achieved by yet another operation. Patients who alternate concern from one body part to another, who have real or imagined deformities, and who change from one surgeon to another may never find satisfaction. The surgeon should not be flattered into accepting such patients just because they are critical of past doctors but praise him or her. This pattern of dissatisfaction is more than likely to continue and may end in litigation (4).

Cursory answers and an off-hand attitude. This type of behavior may reflect an impulsive decision, lack of a strong desire for the operation, or underlying hostility. Impulsive behavior, such as a demand for an immediate operation, may reflect a general impulsive character style. Such patients are more likely to regret having had the operation.

In general, it is a good idea for surgeons to follow their intuition. If the patient arouses a sense of discomfort and uneasiness, surgeons should follow their trained instincts and either obtain more detailed background information or refer the patient for a psychological consultation. A poor prognosis is suggested if any of the following are present: a history of dissatisfaction with previous surgery, a history of psychiatric hospitalization, unreasonable motivation, inappropriate expectations, impulsive decisions, or a possibility of litigation (8, 11). The surgeon should be able to reject a request for surgery either because of the patient's psychological instability or inappropriate motivation.

PATIENT ASSESSMENT

The purpose of the assessment interview is to determine whether plastic surgery is appropriate for a particular patient at this particular time. While it is not possible to delve into the psyche of all patients, the motives, expectations, and personality of the patient should be assessed by means of observation and a casual open-ended dialogue or a structured interview. Surgeons can become adept at assessing a patient's potential for successful plastic surgery by employing a technique that utilizes their training as symptomotologists. It is worthwhile to carefully scrutinize a prospective patient with the goal of avoiding future misunderstandings, malpractice suits, or disappointments either on the part of the patient or the surgeon.

Before the initial interview, perhaps while in the waiting room, patients should be presented with an information pamphlet on plastic surgery procedures. The pamphlet should outline realistic expectations, preoperational and postoperational procedures, and possible side effects. Alerting patients to possible postoperative depression and disappointment will help many to traverse this difficult period. This provides the first step in ensuring realistic expectations and in dispeling any illusions or misapprehensions the patient might have about the operation.

When the assessment indicates that surgery is contraindicated, surgeons should explain to the patient the reasons for their decision. If the surgeons recognize that the patient is attempting to solve a psychological problem via surgery, they should tactfully and sensitively suggest that psychotherapy might be a more effective way of dealing with the problem. Patients are often appreciative of a doctor's sensitivity and awareness of their emotional needs.

Ideally, the surgeon should take time to conduct the

assessment interview before going on to discuss the more technical aspects of the surgery. Surgeons should use their first meeting with the patient as an opportunity to gather as much information as possible. Because of time pressures it may be necessary for a busy plastic surgeon to employ a psychologist, social worker, or nurse practitioner who is trained to conduct the initial interview. The interview should include the following questions:

1. Why do you want surgery?
2. Why did you choose this particular time to have the surgery?
3. Whose idea was it?
4. How long have you been considering the surgery?
5. What do you hope to achieve from this operation?
6. How do you think your life will be different after plastic surgery?
7. Have you had any previous consultations with plastic surgeons? Tell me about them.
8. Have you ever had an operation? Tell me about your experience.

The interview should answer the following questions:

1. Are patient's and surgeon's goal in accordance?
2. Can surgery satisfy the patient's aim and fantasies?
3. Can the patient accept a result that is less than perfect?
4. Will the patient regret the surgery and be angry with the surgeon and initiate litigation?
5. Will the patient's ego strength allow him or her to withstand the operation without decompensation?

Since direct questions do not always reveal the true motives of a patient, open-ended inquiries about job and marriage should be included in the interview. Remarks such as "I like to get to know may patients, tell me about yourself" encourage self-disclosure. The doctor or the designated interviewer should encourage the patient to expand upon answers that indicate cause for concern. General observations of facial expressions, body language, and patient's style of responding may be revealing.

If, after the initial interview, it is still unclear whether an operation is advisable because of psychological considerations, an outside psychological or psychiatric consultation should be sought.

When the patient is a child, careful preparation with adequate explanation is imperative. Ideally, psychological counseling would be routinely offered to help children deal with preoperative, operative, and postoperative procedures. For very young children, dramatizing the surgical procedure with dolls is very helpful. The surgical and hospital experience may be responded to with isolation, depression, or acting out. Behavior such as temper tantrums, crying, nightmares, and bedwetting are common. Supportive parents are essential for helping a child successfully negotiate the continued trauma of hospitalization and surgery.

Do not underestimate or shortcut the interview procedure. The time you spend in assessment and establishing a positive relationship will pay off and eliminate time spent dealing with problems that could have been avoided. Do not hesitate to recommend preoperative counseling; this is beneficial for both patient and surgeon.

DOCTOR-PATIENT RELATIONSHIP

The quality of the doctor-patient relationship is second in importance only to the technical expertise of the surgeon. In order to completely abdicate responsibility for their body and accept the gift of beauty and healing, patients must have absolute trust in the surgeon (7). Trust increases the likelihood of mutual satisfaction between doctor and patient. The relationship is particularly important to patients who are obliged to relinquish control of their body and appearance to the surgeon during the operative procedure.

Patients are in such awe of a surgeon's powers that they view him or her as omnipotent and feel beholden to the surgeon. Surgeons, therefore, have serious responsibility for their patient's emotional well-being. This respect and often idealization can help surgeons maintain their authority in the eyes of their patients, but it should be borne with a sense of humility and not used to intimidate the patient.

It is the surgeon's responsibility to promote trust by showing genuine concern and empathy and by being communicative, approachable, and serious about the patient's concerns. Patients can detect a physician's insincerity, lack of caring, and indifference. Such behavior makes patients feel as if they are imposing on the surgeon. It strips them of their dignity and does not reflect well on the physician.

Establishing a good preoperative relationship with the patient will give the surgeon something to fall back on should there be any reason for dissatisfaction with the results of the surgery. Patients will more easily accept a result that fell short of their expectations if a good patient-doctor rapport existed from the start. A good doctor-patient relationship is more effective for gaining trust than intimidation or flaunting one's reputation.

In each case, surgeons should examine their own motives for surgery. A keen awareness of their own goals and needs may enable surgeons to select candidates wisely and help surgeons choose appropriate courses of surgery. Physicians must be aware of their own needs and not use them as a reason for operating. It will prevent confusing their own needs with those of the patient's.

It is advisable for the surgeon to exercise caution when suggesting surgery, even to a patient who exhibits a severe defect resulting from trauma or previous surgery (7). Although some patients who desire surgery are reluctant to ask for it and are waiting for the doctor to suggest it, they will often blame the doctor if they are not entirely pleased with the outcome.

Some surgeons feel a slight imperfection is enough to warrant aesthetic improvement in order to create some beautiful ideal. That is not necessarily in the patient's best interests.

Lubkin (7) offers some useful insights into situations that trigger misguided motives on the part of surgeons for operating: (*a*) being manipulated by the patient for the patient's own ends; (*b*) being unable to resist appeals; (*c*) being tempted beyond their professional capacity by the social status of the patient; (*d*) wishing to add a particular type of case to their roster; (*e*) being unsure that they can control this particular patient; (*f*) performing the operation more for their own needs than those of the patient.

If the patient is a young child, the above issues require even closer attention, particularly the development of trust, since the operation could be even more traumatic. The parents' relationship with the doctor determines the child's view of the doctor, and the doctor can be viewed either as aloof, intimidating, and mercenary or as benevolent and trustworthy. The importance of the doctor-patient relationship should not be underestimated.

POSTOPERATIVE RESULTS

PATIENT SATISFACTION

The aim of reconstructive surgery is not only physical improvement but an improvement in the self-image and psychological well-being of the patient. If the patient is happy, the operation has been a success. Patients are more easily satisfied with plastic surgery results than are their surgeons. When patients are satisfied, disappointed surgeons who have not met their own criterion of success are advised not to express their discontent.

It is of paramount importance to establish a mutually respectful and trusting preoperative doctor-patient relationship. Some patients will be unhappy even if the surgery is successful. This initial good feeling will dispose the patient to give the doctor the benefit of the doubt.

Although complications are rare, patients should be warned about them during the initial interview and in a pamphlet. Such warning will make the patient less angry with the surgeon and more accepting of an unsatisfactory result.

When Surgeon and Patient Agree

If patients find the results of their operation unsatisfactory, surgeons should wait for patients to express their disappointment and should then tell the patient whether they agree. If the complaint is valid, it will probably not vanish and may come back to haunt the surgeon. Agreement with the patient will gain the surgeons respect and trust and protect their integrity. If surgeons agree with their patients in a nondefensive way, the surgeons will be protecting their integrity, gaining the respect and trust of the patient, and possibly even improving their reputation for the future.

The next step is to offer a remedy if possible. One possibility is to suggest a remedial operation, at no charge, or at least at a greatly reduced cost. It is extremely important to continue to be attentive to these patients. This does not necessarily mean giving more time, just making the time spent more meaningful to patients by focusing on their concerns. If nothing can be done surgically, the surgeon should not be tempted to try. Patients should be provided with sufficient psychological support to enable them to accept the result by maintaining a close relationship.

In some of these instances the fault lies in the screening process, which should have lead to the rejection of candidates for whom surgery could not achieve the desired goal.

When Surgeon and Patient Disagree

The greatest dilemma exists when the surgeon is pleased with the results and the patient is not. As the surgeon gains experience, he or she will become adept at screening out patients who are bound to be disappointed. In the meantime, the surgeon should not show anger. Anger will alienate patients and cause them to be hostile and vindictive. It is important for surgeons to be honest and express their disagreement. But they should show patients the respect of listening and trying to understand what they are saying. The specific complaints should be addressed. Surgeons should show concern and empathy and, taking the complaints into account, explain why they believe the operation was a success. Offering the name of a colleague for a second opinion often reassures the patient that the surgeon is confident that the result was indeed successful.

Patient's temporary disappointment. Most aesthetic operations are followed by some degree of psychological alteration or disturbance (6). Even when patients consider the surgery a success and are happy with their improved appearance, they may still experience a sense of loss and require a period of emotional adjustment. Such disappointment could be the product of postsurgical depression, guilt, remorse or anxiety and will probably ebb. The surgeon should be reassuring, calm, kindly, and resist the temptation not to see this patient frequently. The patient may merely need help in weathering a brief storm.

Depression immediately following cosmetic surgery is most often seen in particularly fastidious and meticulous people because of their reaction to the swelling, bruising, dirty bandages, and oily hair. They need to be reminded that these are only temporary effects.

Some patients pay great attention to detail at a later stage rather than immediately following surgery. They point out small imperfections or irregularities. Often they are simply trying to show how observant they are in an attempt to regain some measure of control over their own bodies. This should not necessarily be taken as displeasure with the operation.

An operation resulting from trauma caused by an accident is always a shock and accompanied by depression. To facilitate adjustment, psychological counseling for the patient and family members is always indicated. Concerns of the patient include appearance, social acceptability, and continued ability to work. The higher the level of preoperative psychological adjustment, the easier it will be for the patient to adapt after the operation.

GENERAL GUIDELINES FOR POSTOPERATIVE PSYCHOLOGICAL CARE

Surgeons should communicate with their patients immediately following surgery, since this is a particularly vulnerable time. An unsightly appearance, inability to attend to personal hygiene, loss of control, general feeling of physical weakness, and fear of mutilation heighten the patient's anxiety and dependency needs. Since patients often do not know what to expect, they turn to the doctor for an interpretation of the results. The surgeon should explain in some detail what took place during the operation. This helps the patient feel more in control, less mystified and part of the process. If the operation has been successful, it is important that the surgeon tell this to the patient. Do not assume that the patient knows it or shares that opinion. Silence on the part of the surgeon is often mistaken for disappointment. Surgeons should ask patients how they feel about the operation. Preoperative and postoperative pictures are useful especially when the patient or family and friends "see no difference." Open communication between doctor and patient will result in a confirmation that the expenditure of time and money plus the physical and psychological risks were well worth it.

Enucleation and Extenteration

Postoperative psychology is quite naturally somewhat different for removal of the eye because of the more serious medical and psychological implications. Lubkin (7) advises that "the removal of a blind eye, even an unsightly blind eye, should not be lightly proposed." For the patient whose life it saves, it may not be as distressing. Nevertheless, eye removal, even when prompted by a serious or life-threatening condition, often causes severe postoperative depression, isolation, and withdrawal (7).

Intensive psychological counseling should be strongly and routinely suggested to avert emotional problems that may result. Patients should undergo in-depth preoperative counseling regarding the consequences of the operation. Dealing with normal anticipatory grief reactions helps postoperative adjustment. Counseling should address (*a*) loss of vision, castration anxiety, and annihilation anxiety; (*b*) life-and-death issues that may have arisen; (*c*) altered self-image; (*d*) public reaction; (*e*) phantom-limb syndrome, in which the patient imagines the eye to still be in place, either with or without its attendent preoperative pain; and (*f*) whether use of an eye patch or a facial prosthesis is recommended.

SUMMARY

Facial malformation, whether congenital or acquired, has a significant impact on the reactions of others and on one's self-esteem. Despite beneficial effects of plastic surgery there is potential for psychological distress. Expectations should be realistic and should not be based on promises that cannot be fulfilled. Frequently, the idea of undergoing plastic surgery results from emotional problems unrelated to the deformity, and surgery will probably not solve the problem. Surgeons can greatly reduce the risk of dissatisfied patients and malpractice suits through careful patient selection.

Mutual agreement between patient and physician, with respect to the objectives of surgery, should help ensure mutual satisfaction with the outcome.

Evaluation of the psychological as well as the medical state of the patient should make it more likely that all needs are addressed. Patient selection should take into account age, basic personality structure, social environment, expectations, and motivations. Assessment of candidates should include a preoperative interview and possibly a questionnaire.

Some characteristics of potentially troublesome patients are depression, paranoia, obsessions, compulsions, narcissism, bizarre behavior, emotional lability, excessive anger, erratic life history, and a history of multisurgery. If serious questions about the psychological state of the patient arise, a psychological consultation should be arranged.

A good doctor-patient relationship that promotes trust, confidence, and concern facilitates a smooth surgical and postoperative course. Good medical care includes attending to the patient's emotional, as well as medical needs during the weeks and months following the operation.

Plastic surgery shares some of its objectives with psychotherapy. Plastic surgeons and psychotherapists both aim to enhance a person's self-image and self-confidence. Ophthalmic plastic surgeons should therefore have an especially high level of psychological awareness and, as much as any other physician, should see in each of their patients a whole and distinct person.

REFERENCES

1. Macgregor FC: The place of the patient in society. *Aesthet Plast Surg* 5: 19–26, 1981.
2. Milani MR, Kornfeld DS: Psychiatry and surgery. In Kaplin HI, Freedman AM, Saddock BJ (eds): *Comprehensive Textbook of Psychiatry, III.* Baltimore, Williams & Wilkins, 1980, pp 2056–2069.
3. Goin JM, Goin MK: *Changing the Body: Psychological Effects of Plastic Surgery.* Baltimore, Williams & Williams, 1981, pp 39–138.
4. Macgregor FC: Patient dissatisfaction with results of technically satisfactory surgery. *Aesthet Plast Surg* 5: 27–32, 1981.
5. Proverbs 31 verse 30.
6. Goldwyn RM: *The Patient and the Plastic Surgeon.* Boston, Little, Brown & Co., 1981, pp 34–46.
7. Lubkin V: Psychological and legal considerations in opthalmic plastic surgery. In Soll DB: *Management of Complications in Opthalmic Plastic Surgery.* Birmingham, Alabama, Aesculapius, 1976, pp 359–365.

7a. Mailer M, Pine F, Bergman A: *Psychological Birth of Human Infant Symbiosis and Individuation.* New York, Basic Books, 1975.

8. Macgregor FC: Social and psychological considerations in an aesthetic plastic surgery. In Rees TD (ed): *Aesthetic Plastic Surgery.* W. B. Saunders, Philadelphia, 1980, pp 27–38.
9. Meyer E, Jacobson WE, Edgerton MT, Canter A: Motivational patterns in patients seeking elective plastic surgery. I. Women who seek rhinoplasty. *Psychosomat Med* 22: 193–201, 1960.
10. Shulman BH: Psychiatric issues in cosmetic blepharoplasty. In Putterman A (ed): *Cosmetic Oculoplastic Surgery.* New York, Grune & Stratton, 1981, pp 46–51.
11. Shulman BH: Psychiatric assessment of the candidate for cosmetic surgery. *Otolaryngol Clin North Am* 13: 383–389, 1980.

12. Macgregor FC, Abel TM, Bryt A, Lauer E, Weissmann S: *Facial Deformities and Plastic Surgery: A Psychosocial Study.* Springfield, Illinois, Charles C Thomas, 1953.
13. Hornblass A: Patient selection for cosmetic oculoplastic surgery. In Putterman A (ed): *Cosmetic Oculoplastic Surgery.* New York, Grune & Stratton, 1982, pp 28–31.
14. Apton AA: *Your Mind and Appearance: A Psychological Approach to Plastic Surgery.* New York, Citadel Press, 1951, pp 167–179.
15. Rees TD: Selection of patients. In Rees TD, Wood-Smith D (eds): *Cosmetic Facial Surgery.* Philadelphia, WB Saunders, 1973, pp 17–26.
16. Clarkson P, Stafford-Clark D: Role of the plastic surgeon and psychiatrist in the surgery of appearance. *Br Med J* 15: 1768–1771, 1960.
17. Lubkin V: Psychological aspects of ophthalmic plastic surgery. In Silver B (ed): *Ophthalmic Plastic Surgery*, ed 3. Rochester, Minnesota, American Academy of Ophthalmology and Otolaryngology, 1977, pp 43–45.

CHAPTER 10

Medical Legal Aspects

PHILIP A. SHELTON, M.D., J.D., F.A.C.S., F.C.L.M.

Most ophthalmologists are increasingly and uncomfortably aware of the impact of federal and state law on their medical practices. The law, in its broad generic sense, has always been present as the set of rules by which groups of people live. As our society has become more complex and more rights and responsibilities have been added, these rules or laws have become more numerous and intrusive due to the increasing diversity of interests between individuals.

While some honest attempts have been made to simplify paperwork requirements, codify laws using plain language, reduce court back-log, and find alternate means of resolving disputes such as arbitration and mediation panels, little headway has been made against the tidal forces of increasing civil litigation and governmental regulation.

This chapter will attempt, in a small way, to give the ophthalmologist some understanding of the current "hot spots" in the law along with a broad overview of the major areas of interface between the law and our medical practices.

The area of malpractice litigation is probably of most interest to individual ophthalmologists although the broader questions of governmental and administrative regulation are of more long-term importance to the profession in general. This chapter will consider only the issues of medical malpractice. Most of the cases cited will be ophthalmic, but significant plastic surgical and noneye cases may be used for illustration of trends.

MALPRACTICE LITIGATION

The ultimate dispute mechanism in our civilized society is the adversary proceedings, or court trial. Historically, its roots may be in the selection of individual or tribal champions who fought in mortal combat for the idea, land, principle, etc. in contention. It has since become highly stylized and more complex but still consists of a referee (judge), two or more adversaries (parties), their champions (attorneys), and a jury or finder of facts. The rationale for this system is the conviction that it is the best way to discover the truth.

Unfortunately, the abrasive aspects of the adversary system often evoke angry, confused, and indignant responses from the physician who is not trained in its rules or familiar with its mechanisms. These responses are uniformly counterproductive. Our medical training will support us well if we remember to maintain a posture of equanimity when confronted by the unexpected or unfamiliar.

In order for a plaintiff to prevail in a malpractice suit, he/she must prove *each* of four elements:

1. The physician had a duty to the patient.
2. The physician breached the applicable standard of care (negligence).
3. The negligent act of omission was the *cause* of damage.
4. There was in fact damage.

Failure to prove *each* of these elements should result in a nonsuit or verdict for the physician.

DUTY TO THE PATIENT

This is usually not a problem area once the doctor-patient relationship has been established. The questions that sometimes arise have to do with the degree of contact necessary to establish or dissolve the relationship. This duty arises from the acceptance by physicians *or their office staff* of an appointment to see a patient with a specific medical problem. If after accepting such an appointment the physician decides not to see the patient, he should timely notify the patient in writing (registered, return receipt requested) to seek other medical aid and offer valid suggestions on where such aid can be found. In *Maltempo v. Cuthbert* (1) the most recent extension of the physician's duty occurred when a physician covering for Mr. Maltempo's family doctor was called by the patient's wife. Dr. Cuthbert was told that Mr. Maltempo, a diabetic, was very ill and in jail, and the family was concerned that he was not getting proper care from the medical personnel in prison. Dr. Cuthbert assured the family that he would check the situation and call them if any problems arose. He called the jail and was told that Mr. Maltempo was being treated by the jail physician, Dr. Freeman. Dr. Cuthbert never called Dr. Freeman, never visited the jail, and never called the Maltempo family again. Mr. Maltempo died by aspiration of vomitus shortly thereafter, and Dr. Cuthbert was found liable for breach of his duty to communicate with the Maltempo *family*—since he undertook a duty to a person not even his own patient.

The Virginia case of *Lyons v. Graether* (1977) (2) seems to outline the barest minimum contact necessary to establish the duty or doctor-patient relationship. A new patient made an appointment to see the doctor with a specific complaint (vaginal infection). When the patient arrived at the physician's office, he refused to see her because she was accompanied by her seeing-eye dog. He made no effort to recommend another physician for her. She delayed finding another gynecologist and suffered harm thereby. The court stated that the physician, by his employee, had accepted an appointment at a specific time for a specific problem and that at the least he was duty bound to refer her elsewhere for care which he had not provided.

Thus, your staff can make you liable without your ever having seen or even spoken to the patient.

Other areas where your staff may cause the physician liability by extension of agency law principles (i.e., vicarious liability) are not hard to find. In *Rosenblum v. Bloom* (3) a dermatologist's newly employed technician put 100% trichloracetic acid on a patient's face instead of the 5% solution ordered by the physician. On the trial court level, the physician was found to be liable for failing to exercise the duty of control and supervision over his employee. On appeal, the judgment for the plaintiff and adequacy of the award were affirmed.

In *McBride v. Saylin,* (4) an early 1936 case, the vicarious liability of the general practitioner owner of an "industrial emergency hospital" was affirmed when his contractural employee, a general practice resident, failed to diagnose a perforated cornea with an intraocular foreign body that ultimately led to the loss of the eye. The standard of care of a general practitioner was held to include the use of x-rays and suspicion of a corneal perforation in the presence of a history of a nail head injury with "air bubbles and rust in the cornea."

In those cases where a physician speaks directly to a patient or even to another physician about the patient (e.g., emergency room physician) and either makes a diagnosis, suggests therapy, or makes a follow-up appointment, the duty to the patient is even more evident.

In a recent case (5) of cataract extraction with subsequent complications, an attempt was made by the patient to suppress the opinion of the second treating ophthalmologist, who failed to find that the defendant ophthalmologist's actions were the cause of the plaintiff's loss of vision. The patient claimed that since the second doctor had treated the patient, admission of his statement would breach the physician-patient privilege. The appeals court found the trial courts' disallowance of this testimony to be in error, reversed the finding for the plaintiff and remanded for a new trial on the grounds (*a*) that there was no longer an ongoing doctor-patient relationship and (*b*) that courts normally find a waiver of physician-patient privilege on health and medical history which the patient/plaintiff has put into issue.

BREACH OF THE STANDARD OF CARE

Establishment of the Standard of Care

The standard typically quoted is, "That degree of skill and learning ordinarily used under the same or similar circumstances by members of the profession." For ophthalmology all jurisdictions use at least a statewide, and most now use a national, standard. In *McCormack v. Linberg* (6) and in *Logan v. Greenwich Hospital Association* (7) the court specifically held that the standard of care for a specialist is national, not local, and a specialist must be held to the same standard of care as other specialists in the field. It generally requires expert testimony to establish a breach of this standard as such matters are beyond the competence of the lay jury. The major exception is called *res ipsa loquitor* or "the thing speaks for itself." This doctrine, if applicable, will allow the case to go to the jury without expert medical testimony to support it. The general rule is, that the circumstances must be of such a character where a layman is able to say, as a matter of common knowledge and observation, that the consequences of professional treatment were not such as ordinarily would have followed if due care had been exercised. Thus the res ipsa doctrine generally applies to sponges left in operative sites. Res ipsa has specifically been ruled *inapplicable* in ophthalmology cases where a viral corneal infection occurred postthyroidectomy [*Merritt v. Deaconess Hospital et al.* (8)], where endophthalmitis occurred following cataract surgery [*Adams v. EENT Hospital et al.* (9) and *Schofield v. Idaho Falls Latter Day Saints Hospital* (10)], and where a retinal detachment followed a cataract extraction with vitreous loss [*Stundon v. Stadnick* (11)].

In the area of ophthalmic plastic and reconstructive surgery res ipsa has also been ruled inapplicable in cases of infection following scar excision [*Pink v. Slater* (12)], corneal scarring due to lagophthalmos following rhizotomy [*Wagner v. Olmedo* (13)], and ptosis following lid block anesthesia for pterygium excision [*Charlton v. Montefiore* (14)].

In *Miller v. Scholl* (15), the court ruled that failure to use phacoemulsification as an alternate procedure in 1973 did not constitute negligence since:

> Mere evidence that the conduct of the surgeon did not measure up to the standards of a single member of the profession as opposed to the standards of the profession *as a whole* (emphasis ours) does not support a submission of negligence in a malpractice action, for the basic and fundamental reason that the standards of a single member of the profession may be higher or lower than the standards of the profession as a whole.

In the matter of timely referral to subspecialists, the Supreme Court of Wyoming in the 1981 case of *Siebert v. Fowler* (16) found for the defendant ophthalmologist in the absence of specific expert testimony that one with the requisite skill, diligence, and knowledge would have referred the diabetic patient to a retinal specialist for laser treatment at an earlier time.

In a most interesting 1983 case [*Sikorski v. Bell* (17)], the Court of Appeals of Georgia stated that unnecessary surgery may not be malpractice if a patient is fully informed and the surgery is performed adequately. In this case of a patient with advanced glaucoma, a surgical procedure was done with resultant suprachoroidal hemorrhage and a total loss of vision. The plaintiff's expert suggested that alternate nonsurgical procedures could have been utilized, but he did not adequately contradict the defendant ophthalmologist's proof as to his compliance with the applicable standard of care.

By far the most significant change in the standard of care is represented in the trilogy of Washington State cases: *Helling v. Carey* [1974 (18)], *Gates v. Jensen* [1979 (19)], and *Harris v. Groth* [1983 (20)].

The Helling court concluded that failure to test for glaucoma in patients under 40 was negligent in spite of uncontradicted expert testimony that this was not the standard of care. The court invoked a judicially determined standard of care based on the 1932 decision of the T. J. Hooper (21), in which a tugboat had damaged its barges in tow in stormy seas because of failure to have a radio receiver which would have given an updated weather report. Tugs did not usually carry radio receivers, but Judge Learned Hand said in the opinion: "Courts must in the end say what is required; there are precautions so imperative that even their universal disregard will not excuse their omission."

Following the Helling case, the Washington State legislature redefined the standard of care to the exercising of that degree of skill, care, and learning *possessed* by other persons in the same profession. The court in *Gates v. Jensen* held that this is a much broader standard than exercising the degree of skilled care and learning *practiced* by other persons in the same profession. This reasonable prudence test may therefore require a standard of practice that is higher than that exercised by the medical profession. Thus, the court found for the plaintiff where the defendant ophthalmologist failed to do visual fields and a dilated fundus exam in a patient whose tension was in the glaucoma suspect range and who subsequently suffered damage to her optic nerves.

The most recent case in this trilogy (*Harris v. Groth* 1983) was won by the ophthalmologist because the jury instruction requested by the plaintiff was overly broad and did not correctly state the law. It is questionable at best if the angle closure glaucoma in this case could have been court reiterated its view that a "reasonable prudence" standard is applicable in the state of Washington rather than an "average practitioner" standard.

No other state has yet followed this "reasonable prudence" or court-imposed standard, but the trend seems to be in that direction.

In summary, there seems to be a tendency to extend the required standard of care beyond that ordinarily *used* by members of the profession locally to that level of skill, care and learning *possessed* by other professionals often on a national level. In making this decision the court will balance ability, impact, and cost. This tends to accelerate the speed by which the standard of care approaches the state of the art (22).

Informed Consent

In early malpractice cases the touching of someone's body without their consent was a "battery." The modern view is that the standard of care requires the physician to inform the patient of the nature of the proposed treatment, alternate therapies including none, and the risks and reasonably expected benefits of each one and only then secure their consent. A growing minority of states has ruled that the disclosure should be such that a reasonable patient could make an intelligent choice based on its contents. This standard does *not* require expert witness testimony as to the usual actions of the physicians in the specialty.

In the majority of states however, the standard of disclosure required is "measured by those communications a reasonable medical practitioner in the same branch of medicine would make under the same or similar circumstances" (23). In addition these states require expert medical evidence to establish this standard.

The recent case of *Welch v. Whitaker* (24) concurred in the directed verdict in favor of the ophthalmologist who alledgedly failed to warn the patient of the possibility of corneal scarring subsequent to the removal of a corneal foreign body and rust ring. No expert medical evidence was presented by the patient-plaintiff on the issues of the standard of disclosure, the standard of care of removal of the foreign body, and the proximate cause of the corneal scarring.

In the vast majority of states the patient-plaintiff must then prove that a reasonable patient as well as the individual plaintiff would not have given consent had they been informed of the risk or outcome that actually transpired.

There are exceptions to the informed consent doctrine that relieve the physician from the duty to fully disclose. Medical emergencies and patient incompetency (which may require guardian consent) are clear examples. Voluntary waiver, where patient knowingly and intelligently decline to be informed in order to reduce their anxiety upon disclosure, is a rarely used but available exception. The most controversial is the therapeutic exception, where it is *clearly* poor medical practice and potentially harmful to the patient's health to fully disclose the risks. The problem with the therapeutic exception is to balance the individual patient's right to make informed decisions against society's policy, which encourages procedures needed to maintain a health populace.

On a trial court level, the Massachusetts Superior court

in *Precourt v. Frederick* (25) allowed a jury verdict to stand against the defendant ophthalmologist who was found negligent by failing to inform his patient with recurrent uveitis, that use of systemic steroids might cause aseptic necrosis of bones and joints. There was no expert evidence that this was usual practice, but Massachusetts joins a growing number of states following reasonable patient standard of required disclosure. This case was reversed on appeal. The majority of the court held that the risk of aseptic necrosis was "so remote as to be negligible" and therefore Dr. Frederick did not have a duty to disclose this risk. The dissenting judge concurred in the result but only on the grounds that since the critical dose and time relationship for the causation of aseptic necrosis by systemic steroids is unknown, the plaintiff's statement of his potential unwillingness to proceed with only the second of two courses of prednisone had the risk of aseptic necrosis been disclosed was insufficient evidence on causation to allow submission to the jury.

Contrasting the Precourt case is the 1979 North Dakota case of *Winkjer v. Herr* (26). Here the defendant ophthalmologist did not notify the patient that the use of Phospholine iodide could cause cataracts. The court found for the defendant and stated, ". . . information does not indicate at what levels and over what length of time the drug has been shown to possibly cause cataracts. There can be no liability for a physician to disclose a risk that was unknown in the manner in which a particular drug or treatment was prescribed."

An interesting case of apparent invalidation of a signed consent form was found in the New Mexico case of *Toppino v. Herhohn* (27). In this case, involving plastic reconstruction of a woman's breast, the surgeon's statements "we'll get this right" and "this will be right" were held to be an express warranty of results in spite of a signed consent form which said" . . . though good results are expected they cannot be and are not guaranteed." The court held that since the defendant did not raise the defense based on the alleged conclusiveness of the signed surgical consent at trial, he could not raise it on appeal.

In the North Carolina case of *Estrada v. Jaques* (28) the appeals court reversed the summary judgment of the lower court in favor of the defendant, based on the presumed validity of a signed consent form. The appeals court held that a signed consent form is not given conclusive weight. Rather it is only *some evidence* of valid consent and is not sufficient to grant automatic summary judgment under a North Carolina statute governing signed consent forms. Knowledge of procedures is not a broad enough disclosure. Patients must be informed of their usual and most frequent risks and hazards. Since the procedure in question was experimental (embolization technique) the patient must be told additionally of the experimental nature of the procedure, any uncertainty regarding risks of the procedure, and the known or projected most-likely risks.

Georgia, on the other hand in *Butler v. Brown* (29), has held that its state's medical consent statute merely requires disclosure of the general terms of treatment and not of the accompanying risks. Such written consent is "conclusively presumed to be a valid consent in the absence of fraudulent misrepresentation of material facts in obtaining the same."

In *Moore v. Fragatos* (30), however, a waiver of the right to a jury trial by signing a preadmission arbitration agreement was deemed to be an invalid waiver of a constitutional right since the patient was not given all necessary "material" information such as the composition of the malpractice arbitration panel and therefore the waiver could not be deemed "intelligent". Also, the fact that the agreement was signed when the patient was in pain and about to enter the hospital for surgery, when his state of mind was not fully clear, would have been enough to make the waiver of rights "involuntary" and therefore invalid.

Although *Moore v. Fragatos* is not an informed consent case, the principles enunciated by its holding certainly seem to allow a patient to challenge the presumption that a signed consent form means that valid consent has in fact been obtained.

Of interest is the judgement of an actionable assault against an ophthalmologist [*Shulman v. Lerner* (31)] who removed a chalazion surgically rather than just having it "merely punctured" as had been done by the doctor's associate in the past. In addition, the defendant removed a freckle from the eyelid adjacent to the chalazion without getting the patient's permission. The patient-plaintiff, although a dentist, was held not to have consented to surgery on his eyelid although he did not object upon viewing preparation of the syringe and draping of the eye.

In the case of *Dondashi v. Fine* (32), the plaintiff was found to be entitled to a new trial on the issue of informed consent even though he had signed a consent form. The Florida statute creates a conclusive presumption that a signed consent is valid *only if* certain presumptions are met. The patient had orbital floor fracture repaired and had lost light perception thereafter. The patient and his expert witness denied the preoperative presence of diplopia and enophthalmos.

The court held that "under the circumstances" the patient, who had a language problem and undeniably tore up the first consent form, did not fulfill the required presumptions since he did not have knowledge that the second form was a consent form nor did he have a general understanding of the procedure, risks and hazards, and medically acceptable alternatives.

In *Lacy v. Laird* (33) the minor plaintiff (over age 18 when the age of majority was 21) was entitled to only nominal damages for technical "assault" for performance of a nasal plastic procedure. The procedure was carried out nonnegligently and the only issue was the absence of consent of the patient's parents or guardian. The court agreed that the consent of the minor 18 year old was sufficient but the real question was that the right of consent rests with the parents or guardian whose liability for support and maintenance of their child may be greatly increased by an unfavorable result from the operational procedures upon the part of the surgeon.

Lest you think that all of the informed consent decisions have gone to the plaintiffs, *Yates v. Harms* (34) held that the physician need not apprise the patient of each infinitesimal, imaginative, or speculative element that would go into the making of the risks of the procedure. Thus the possibility of endophthalmitis following cataract extraction did not have to be disclosed.

In addition, *Valenci v. Beamen* (35) held that the physician's testimony as to his habit and custom of warning approximately 250 patients that previous year of the potential hazards of eye surgery, could not be impeached by a specific witness if the physician never stated that he told *every* patient or *that specific* patient. The testimony of the plaintiff's witness, who wished to testify that she had never received any warnings, was not permitted in the absence of evidence that the witness was among the approximately 250 patients that the defendant claimed to have warned.

Another very important informed consent decision, although not an ophthalmological case, was *Logan v. Greenwich Hospital Association.* In 1983, the Supreme Court of Connecticut held in this case that *all* alternative modes of treatment, including those that might be more hazardous, had to be disclosed to the patient. In addition, the court stated that medical care in Connecticut was henceforth to be judged against a national standard rather than a local statewide standard.

Thus the trend seems to be toward the reasonable patient standard of disclosure, with physicians having almost no relief from the requirement of an exhaustive recitation of all possible alternatives and complications, even those they may never have encountered. This pendulum has swung to the extreme, and some counterforce is hopefully due and may be apparent in *Hook v. Rothstein.* In this case the court pointed out that the physician should be concerned with the patient's best interests and not what a lay jury, untrained in medicine and employing perfect hindsight, might later conclude he or she should have disclosed. [Referral to dissent in *Scaria v. St. Paul Fire and Marine Insurance Company*, 227 NW2d 647,659 (1975).] However, if a state-of-the-art alternative is safe, effective, and of reasonable cost and availability it should be disclosed, even if not recommended (36).

CAUSATION

Once plaintiffs have demonstrated a breach (negligence) in the applicable standard of care, they must connect the negligent act or omission with the damage suffered. The standard for proving causation is generally "reasonable medical probability," not simply possibility. In almost all cases proof of causation requires expert testimony.

In most jurisdictions the defendant-physician may be called up by the plaintiff as a fact witness. There is variability, however, between jurisdictions as to whether the defendant-doctor may be used as a medical expert by the plaintiff. In most states defendants are subject only to questions as to facts but are not required to give their expert medical opinion. Local legal guidance on this point is essential. (*Mcdermott v. Manhattan Eye and Ear Hospital.*

In *Hall v. Bacon* (38) the plaintiff was not entitled to recover against his physicians even if they were negligent in failing to diagnose and notify the patient of his injury. There was no expert evidence offered that the 36-day delay in diagnosis of the fractured orbit caused the fat atrophy and enophthalmos. In fact, the plaintiff's expert said that a delay in surgery was indicated in the presence of excessive facial swelling as was present in this case. In addition, the prolongation of pain and suffering was not actionable in the absence of expert testimony that the cause of the pain and suffering was due to the failure to timely diagnose the orbital fracture.

In *Lazenby v. Beisel* (39), the patient became blind following a retrobulbar hemorrhage. The defendant's expert suggested that failure to do a lateral canthotomy and give intravenous doses of Diamox or mannitol decreased the patient's chance to maintain his sight, which was lost due to increased intraocular pressure. The appeals court held that the trial court erred in instructing the jury that negligence is a legal cause of injury if it lessens a person's chance of complete recovery. No evidence was given that using a lateral canthotomy and giving intravenous doses of Diamox or mannitol would probably have salvaged the patient's vision.

In *Edwards v. the United States* (40), the plaintiff failed to prove that a flat anterior chamber following cataract extraction in his right eye, which spontaneously reformed within 5 days, was the cause of the patient's subsequent glaucoma, which was controlled on medication. The court stated: "The decision to delay surgery was a judgment decision and the evidence is not persuasive that the judgment exercised was in error." Also, ". . . since plaintiff's left eye has greater pressure than his right, it is illogical to ascribe the pressure in the right eye to the cataract surgery or treatment of the right eye . . . ."

There are some cases, chiefly those involving wrongful death, where the standard of causation is altered to "if there was any substantial possibility of survival and defendant has destroyed it, he is answerable" [*Hicks v. United States* (41)]. There does not seem to be a tendency for the courts to apply this doctrine of "best last chance" to eye cases, but the possibility always exists that in a truly desperate situation it may be invoked.

DAMAGES

Damages are usually clearly evident and measurable by loss of visual acuity or field, diplopia, cosmetic defects, lost wages, etc. Pain and suffering, while subjective, can be objectively valued by the jury upon persuasive evidence.

An interesting eye case held that a patient does *not* have a duty to submit to cataract surgery in order to reduce the damages caused by malpractice. In a 1979 case [*Frisnegger v. Gibson* (42)], the patient sustained a cataract subsequent to the perforation of his eye by the defendant ophthalmologist, who was injecting the eyelid preparatory to chalazion removal. The patient suffered severe depression and refused to have the cataract removed, which had incapacitated him. This trial court properly approved a reasonable person test for the jury to determine if damages should be reduced rather than the mandatory test requested by the defendant.

OTHER LEGAL CONSIDERATIONS

Statute of Limitations

This is the time limit following the alledged malpractice event during which the court will hear the case at all. This is totally a matter of state statute and varies widely between jurisdictions. Of interest are two cases in which fraudulent reassurance tolled or delayed the running of the statute of limitations.

In *Hundley v. Martinez* (43) an ophthalmologist continually reassured the patient from August 1, 1962 until May 22, 1963 with statements that the eye "was all right" and "getting along fine". The court found that these reassurances were positive acts of fraud and tolled the statute of limitations so that the suit entered on May 5, 1965 fit within its 2-year limit.

In *Smile v. Lawson* (44), silence itself was held to be fraudulent concealment and tolled the statute of limitations. The court based this decision on the fiduciary or trust relationship that a physician has with the patient and therefore places on the physician a greater duty of disclosure than merely not to commit *active* fraud or misrepresentation. The real issue in this case was whether the physician was *aware* of cutting both recurrent laryngeal nerves during thyroidectomy and was therefore fraudulently concealing this fact when he reassured the plaintiff that her voice problems would get better spontaneously, without telling her of the specific problem. The court held that there was sufficient evidence to allow this question to get to trial and therefore tolled the statute of limitations on the above reasoning.

Subsequent Tortfeasors

In a case [*DeNike v. Mowery* (45)] where an auto accident resulted in orbital and facial injuries, the plaintiff settled with the original tortfeasor upon the reliance of his plastic surgeon that he would have "a socially acceptable face, satisfying to his security and business activities". He later sued the physician for malpractice. The physician's entire defense was based on the general rule that when an original tortfeasor causes injury, he or she is responsible for complications (including malpractice) of the subsequent treating physician. The physician did not deny the allegations of malpractice.

There are many variations on these rules based on the jurisdiction involved, but the DeNike court held that since neither the plaintiff nor the original tortfeasor was aware or could have been aware of the malpractice at the time of their settlement and therefore could not and did not contemplate this additional damage, the original release could not operate to release the physician who is not a true joint tortfeasor but rather an independent successive wrongdoer.

Conspiracy to Discourage Expert Witness

In *Clancy v. Gooding* (45) the plaintiff, who had filed a medical malpractice suit based on eyelid surgery, attempted to ammend the complaint alleging that the insurance company (Physicians Mutual) had engaged in a conspiracy to prevent the patient from obtaining expert medical testimony by pursuing a policy "which discourages a member physician from testifying against another member physician." The court held that these were two independent actions and could not be joined because it would be "confusing to the jury." The court held that the statute of limitations on the malpractice suit would not prevent the conspiracy suit from being filed as a separate lawsuit.

SUMMARY

It is often a traumatic and frightening experience for an ophthalmologist to be involved as a defendant in a medical malpractice suit. The initial shock should not precipitate irrational or angry behavior that is counterproductive to the physician's interests. Cooperation with one's attorney is essential to secure the best possible defense. While even a careful opthalmologist may be sued for nonmeritorious claims, avoidance of malpractice litigation is enhanced by following a few simple rules:

1. Be kind to your patient: Nothing breeds litigation like hostility.
2. Keep good records: They are essential to your defense and unparalleled as the best available evidence.
3. Inform your patients of all the possibilities: Only the physician can ask, "Do you understand what you have been told or read? If not, what are your questions?"
4. Do not be afraid of second opinions: They increase your stature in the patient's view (47).
5. Write lots of letters: Document your records with return-receipt-requested letters discharging patients, following up on significant no-shows, explaining complex points to patients, etc.
6. Be careful what you say about others: Careless words may entrap another physician in a needless malpractice suit. If your remark was malicious ("that butcher", "quack"), you may be sued for slander. Be wary of violating patient privacy and confidentiality by remarks over the phone while within another person's range of hearing.
7. Train and control your employees: They are your agents when acting within the scope of their employment. Document job descriptions and the protocols they must follow for all phases of their work. From telephone manners and questions to the technical aspects of fundus photography or other procedures, your staff's negligence will usually be viewed as your negligence (48).

NOTES

1. U.S. Court of Appeals 5th Cir., Nov. 21, 1974.
2. 239 S.E. 2d 103, Va., 1977.
3. 492 S.W. 2d 321, Texas, 1973.
4. 56 P. 2d 941, Calif., 1936.
5. Trujillo v. Puro 683 P.2d 1963, 101 N.M. 408, 1984.
6. McCormack v. Linberg 352 N.W.2d 30 Minn. App., 1984.
7. Logan v. Greenwich Hospital Association, 465 A.2d 294, Conn., 1983.
8. 357 N.E. 2d 65, O., 1975.
9. La App., 346 So. 2d 327, La, 1977.
10. 409 P. 2d 107, Idaho, 1965.
11. 469 P. 2d 16, Wyo., 1970.
12. 281 P.2d 272, Calif., 1955.
13. 365 A.2d 643, Del., 1976.
14. 45 Misc. Rep. 2d 153, Sup. Ct. Queens, N.Y., 1/15/65.

15. 594 S. W. 2d 324, Mo., 1980.
16. 637 P. 2d 255, Wyo., 1981.
17. 307 S. E. 2d 701, GA. App., 1983.
18. 519 P. 2d 981, Wash., 1974.
19. 595 P. 2d 919, Wash., 1979.
20. 663 P. 2d 113, Wash., 1983.
21. 60 F. 2d 737, 2nd Cir., 1932.
22. State of the Art v. The Standard of Care: Shelton, P.A. *Int. J. of Cataract Surgery* 1:7, Sept. 1984.
23. Hook v. Rothstein, 316 S.E. 2d 690, S.C. App., 1984.
24. Welch v. Whitaker, 317 S.E. 2d 758, S.C. App., 1984.
25. Precourt v. Fredericks, S.J.C. Mass. S-3457 8/19/85, Dockett #41128 Oct., 1983.
26. 277 N.W. 2d 579, N.D., 1979.
27. 673 P.2d 1318, 1983.
28. Estrada v. Jones, 321 S.E. 2d 240, N.C. App., 1984.
29. 290 S.E. 2d 293, GA. App., 1982.
30. 321 N.W. 2d 781, Mich. App., 1982.
31. 141 N.W. 2d 348, Mich., 1966.
32. 397 So. 2d 442, Fla. App., 1981.
33. 139 N.E. 2d 25, Ohio, 1956.
34. 393 P. 2d 982, Kan., 1964.
35. 509 P. 2d 274, N.M. App., 1973.
36. Shelton PA: State of the art v. the standard of care. *Int J Cataract Surg* 1:7, Sept. 1984.
37. 16 App. Div. Rep. 2d 374, N.Y., 1962.
38. 453 P.2d 816, Idaho, 1969.
39. 425 So. 2d 84, Fla., 1983.
40. 497 F. Supp. 379, Ala., 1980.
41. 368 F. 2d 626, 4th Cir., 1966.
42. 598 P. 2d 574, Mont., 1979.
43. 158 S.E. 2d 159, W.V., 1967.
44. 435 S.W. 2d 325, Mo., 1968.
45. 418 P.2d 1010, Wash., 1966.
46. 647 P.2d 885, N.M., 1982.
47. Shelton PA: Second opinions—A guide to the perplexed. *Int J Cataract Surg* 2:3, Feb. 1985.
48. Shelton PA: Vicarious liability and the employer/employee relationship. *Int J Cataract Surg* 1:2, Jan. 1984.

SECTION II

CONGENITAL AND DEVELOPMENTAL ANOMALIES

CHAPTER 11

Congenital Eyelid Coloboma

RICHARD P. CARROLL, M.D., F.A.C.S.

A coloboma is an embryologic cleft of uncertain etiology. Eyelid colobomas are unilateral or bilateral full-thickness defects that may involve the upper or lower lids, and may be associated with colobomas or other anomalies of the globe. Upper lid colobomas are usually isolated findings, whereas lower lid colobomas are frequently associated with facial clefts, lacrimal anomalies, dermoids, or dental defects.

Colobomas are most often found at the junction of the inner and middle thirds of the upper lid and at the junction of the middle and outer thirds of the lower lid. There is usually an absence of all lid structures except the myocutaneous junction in the upper lid defects, whereas in the lower lid, structures will be poorly formed but usually identifiable. The defects range in size from tiny triangular notches in the lower eyelid to large rectangular defects in the upper eyelid. Associated trichiasis or ridges of skin from the coloboma to the cornea may complicate management.

EMBRYOLOGY

Mesoblastic folds fuse from the inner to the outer canthus between the 32- and 37-mm stages of development. During this period, the meibomian glands, cilia, orbicularis muscle, and tarsal plates differentiate. The fused structures then divide, so that in the 50-mm embryo the upper and lower eyelids can be identified (1).

ETIOLOGY

While the etiology of eyelid colobomas is uncertain, theories have included pressure necrosis from amniotic bands, localized failure of mesoblastic folds to fuse, viral infections in utero, vitamin imbalance, and poor placental circulation. Heredity seems to play a minor role except in the Treacher Collins' syndrome, which is an autosomal dominant trait of varying penetrance and expressivity. Lower lid colobomas are a feature of this mandibulofacial dysostosis.

TREATMENT

Medical treatment of lid colobomas includes ocular lubricants, moist chambers, and bandage contact lenses. Eyelid colobomas can be repaired electively unless the globe is threatened by exposure. If surgical correction of a large upper lid defect is delayed in an infant, an examination under anesthesia should be performed to assess the status of the globe, and all concerned should be instructed to notify the managing ophthalmologist immediately should signs of exposure develop. In fact, even large defects are often remarkably well tolerated if the extraocular motility is intact. Cosmetic considerations, psychological trauma to the patient or parents, and the treatment of associated defects are other relative indications for surgical correction.

The horizontal pull of the canthal tendons will often make colobomas appear larger clinically. Therefore, before making a final decision on how to correct the defect, while the patient is under anesthesia, the edges of the coloboma should be grasped and pulled together with toothed forceps or skin hooks to determine the true size of the defect. While satisfactory repair can almost always be accomplished with one procedure, the possibility of needing additional procedures should be discussed preoperatively. For example, tethering of the levator complex during the repair of a large upper lid defect may result in a postoperative ptosis that will need secondary repair.

The most appropriate procedure to use in the repair of an eyelid coloboma will depend on the size, configuration, and location of the defect as well as the presenting symptoms and signs. Small notches in the outer thirds of the lower eyelids such as those seen in the Treacher Collins' syndrome often require no specific treatment and may become less noticeable as other features of the syndrome are corrected. On the other hand, small defects in the nasal portion of the lower eyelid associated with lacrimal anomalies, as seen in Figure 11.1, may require attention to satisfactorily repair the lacrimal drainage apparatus. Other factors such as the quality of the surrounding tissues, associated anomalies, and the visual status of the globe must be considered. The latter is particularly important if a lid-sharing technique is being considered in a young patient in whom occlusion amblyopia is a postoperative possibility.

PENTAGONAL REPAIR WITH OR WITHOUT CANTHOLYSIS

Many eyelid colobomas can be surgically repaired by converting the coloboma into a pentagonal defect and repairing it as one would repair a lid margin laceration. After freshening the edges of the coloboma, the surgeon places the sutures through the raw edges into firm tissue such as tarsus or periosteum. A technique for repair of full-thickness pentagonal defects is described in detail in the chapter on "Management of Eyelid Trauma." As in all eyelid margin repairs, precise alignment of the margin with correct suture placement and suture tension is necessary to avoid postoperative notching (Fig. 11.2). This complication can occur as a result of pressure necrosis from tying the margin sutures too tightly or from wound separation because sutures have been tied too loosely.

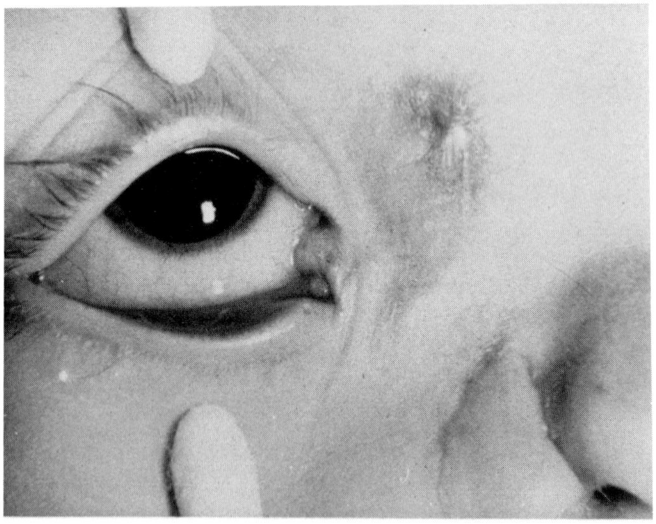

Figure 11.1. Small nasal lower lid coloboma associated with lacrimal anomalies and a facial cleft.

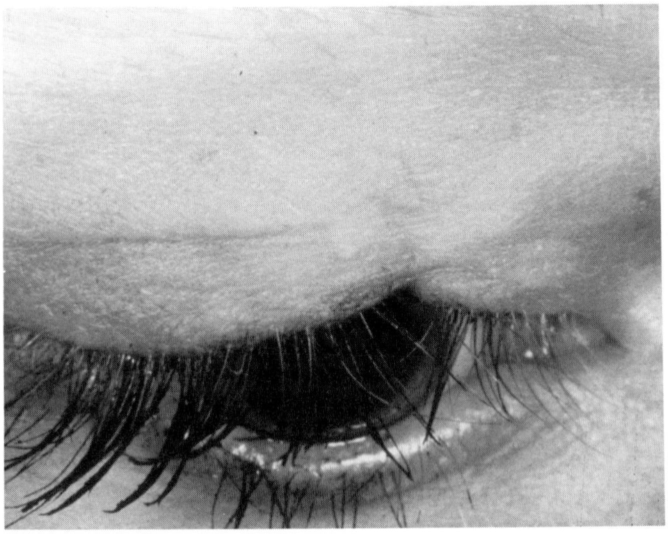

Figure 11.2. Eyelid margin notch following repair of an upper lid coloboma.

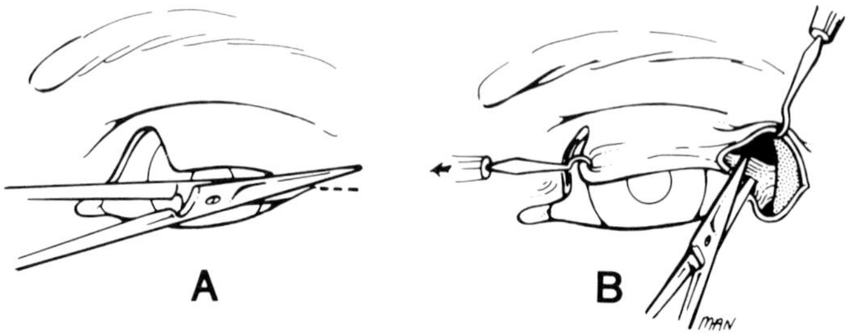

Figure 11.3. *A*, Canthotomy. *B*, Cantholysis of the upper limb of the lateral canthal tendon.

While there should be no undue tension on the eyelid margin closure, tension-relieving sutures are no longer recommended because of the additional inflammatory reaction they cause in the repaired tissue. An additional 2 to 3 mm of relaxation may be obtained by a cantholysis of the appropriate limb of the lateral canthal tendon (Fig. 11.3). The canthal incision requires no suturing. Almost all colobomas of lower eyelids can be repaired by primary repair of a pentagonal defect with or without cantholysis. Upper lid colobomas that cannot be repaired with this technique can usually be reconstructed using the versatile semicircular skin muscle flap described by Tenzel (2). This technique when properly performed can be used to repair defects that involve up to 50–60% of the lid. For the rare patient in which more than 50% of the eyelid is involved, the Tenzel technique can be used in combination with other reconstructive techniques. Lid-sharing techniques, while frequently recommended in the past, are virtually coloboma and should be avoided in young patients because of the possibility of postoperative occlusion amblyopia.

TENZEL MYOCUTANEOUS FLAP

The technique for reconstruction of colobomas using the Tenzel flap is shown in Figure 11.4. The myocutaneous flap is designed away from the eyelid to be reconstructed with the size of the semicircular flap determined by the size of the coloboma. An outline of the flap is drawn with a marking pencil, after which 0.5 ml of 1% Xylocaine with epinephrine is injected beneath the proposed flap for hemostasis. A perpendicular incision is made through skin and orbicularis with a razor blade knife, taking care not to bevel the edges of the flap. The skin muscle flap is then elevated with curved blunt scissors.

A small canthotomy is next performed. The size of this incision should be only large enough to admit a tiny, straight scissor to perform a lateral cantholysis of the lid to be reconstructed. Following cantholysis, the remaining portion of the eyelid as well the semicircular flap can be elevated. This maneuver, however, will not allow for advancement of the flap into the defect, which requires aggressive undermining and incision of deeper eyelid attachments. These attachments include the attachments of the eyelid retractors and the orbital septum to the periosteum overlying the lateral orbital rim. In reconstruction of the upper eyelid, care must be taken not to injure the lacrimal gland or its ductiles during this part of the procedure. Once adequate mobilization of the eyelid and semicircular flap has been achieved, it is advanced into the defect. As in primary closure of the coloboma, the edges of the defect should be freshened to create a pentagonal configuration. An eyelid margin closure is then carried out.

Finally, attention is directed to the lateral canthal angle, which is reconstructed subcutaneously with absorbable sutures. These sutures are placed through the undersurface of the semicircular flap into the periosteum overlying the lateral orbital rim. It is essential that these periosteal sutures be placed to prevent postoperative nasal migration of the lateral canthal angle or laxity in the reconstructed eyelid. A 6-0 silk suture is then used to reconstruct the angle, and multiple 6-0 silk sutures are then used to complete the closure in the lateral canthal area. The patient is instructed to use a Fox shield at bedtime and to keep the sutures meticulously clean. Superficial sutures are removed in 4–5 days. Eyelid margin and lateral canthal angle sutures are removed in 7–10 days.

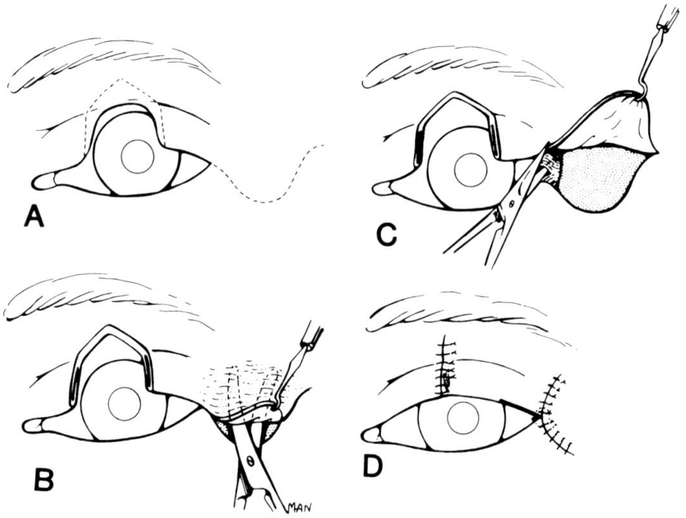

Figure 11.4. Semicircular myocutaneous flap. *A*, Marking of incisions. *B*, Undermining of semicircular flap. *C*, Cantholysis of upper limb of lateral canthal tendon. *D*, Closure.

SUMMARY

Definitive reconstruction of a congenital eyelid coloboma can usually be performed on an elective basis. Primary closure after freshening the edges of the defect, sometimes combined with cantholysis or reconstruction with Tenzel's semicircular myocutaneous flap alone or in combination with other techniques, will accomplish the reconstruction. Lid-sharing techniques such as the Cutler-Beard flap should be avoided in the pediatric patient.

REFERENCES

1. Mann IC: *Developmental Abnormalities of the Eye.* Philadelphia, JB Lippincott Co, 1957.
2. Kidwell EDR, Tenzel RR: Repair of congenital colobomas of the lids. *Arch Ophthalmol* 97: 1931–1932, 1979.

CHAPTER 12

Congenital Euryblepharon

STEPHEN L. BOSNIAK, M.D.

Euryblepharon is a primary symmetric enlargement of the horizontal palpebral apertures. This entity does not include secondary enlargement of the palpebral apertures from buphthalmos, staphylomata, or proptosis. Although rare, it has been described in the ophthalmic literature on several occasions (1–27). Desmarres (2) coined the term *euryblepharon* in 1854 from the Greek work "eury" meaning "broad."

There may be a familial tendency for this lid deformity to occur. Waardenburg (12) described a woman with 31-mm horizontal palpebral apertures. Her three sons had palpebral apertures of 35 mm, 29 mm, and 31 mm. Byron Smith has performed surgery on a father and daughter with congenital euryblepharon (Fig. 12.1). J. R. Woltz (15) also described this condition in two members of the same family. Shannon and Flanagan (28) described it as an autosomal dominant trait that may be seen in several members of the same family in its milder forms.

CLINICAL PRESENTATION

The horizontal palpebral aperture normally averages 28–30 mm in length (21, 22). It increases from 18.35 mm at birth to 29.68 mm at 24 to 26 years; one-half of this increase occurs in the first 4 years of life (16). It is slightly less in females. Some variations in the size and shape of the palpebral apertures are obviously racial, but extreme variations are abnormal. Most of these patients have elongated lid margins, a shortage of lid skin, and a downward and lateral displacement of the outer canthi. The increased lid margins are particularly evident in relation to the globe and the orbit. There may be a prominent ectropion and a gutter between the globe and the lateral canthal angle. Eyelid closure will accentuate the lid margin eversion. As a rule all four lids are usually involved, but involvement of only the upper (17–19) or the lower lids (13, 14) or unilateral involvement (24) have been described. Mild forms of euryblepharon may become less apparent with body growth (22).

Patients with congenital euryblepharon may present with an entire spectrum of deformities. They may have a slight lengthening of their lid margins and palpebral apertures (Fig. 12.2) or more pronounced defects that have associated lagophthalmos with conjunctival and corneal exposure (Fig. 12.3). These severe defects, the S-shaped palpebral aperture, (25) seem to bridge the gap between the congenital ectropion–euryblepharon syndrome and the Treacher Collins'–Franceschetti's syndromes. Even though the lid margin remains intact, the shortage of skin and the canthal deviation resemble colobomas and hypoplasia of the infraorbital rim (26).

Associated anomalies have been described: ptosis (7, 23–25) telecanthus without epicanthal folds (24, 25), a double row of meibomian glands (24), lateral displacement of the inferior punctum (24), latent nystagmus (20), and esotropia (2, 23).

ETIOLOGY

The etiology of congenital euryblepharon is unknown. Several theories have been advanced. Abnormal skin tension, pull of the platysma and defective separation of the lids may result in localized displacement of the lateral

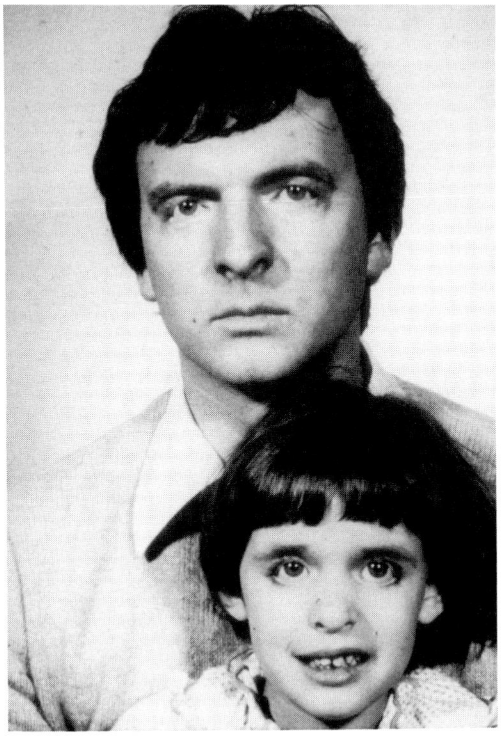

Figure 12.1. The father is pictured 20 years after correction of congenital euryblepharon with free skin grafts to both lower lids. The 5-year old daughter is pictured preoperatively. Dr. Byron C. Smith operated on both the father and the daughter.

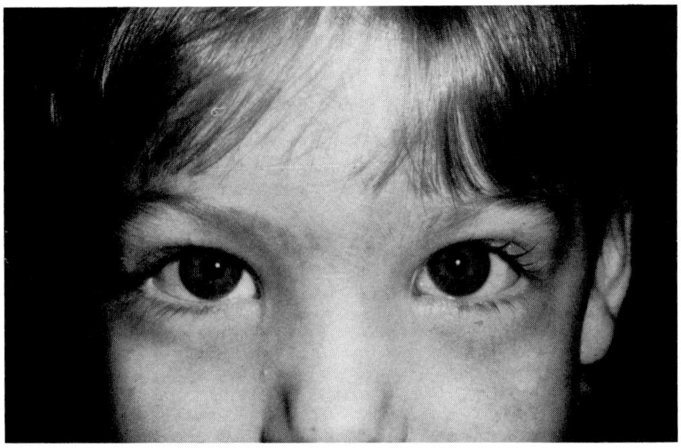

Figure 12.2. A 3-year old girl with mild euryblepharon and a slight lateral gutter between the globe and the lateral canthal angle.

canthi and an abnormal enlargement of the palpebral aperture (3). Congenital hypoplasia or absence of the orbicularis oculi could explain many of the features of this syndrome (18). It seems obvious that the shortage of eyelid skin, perhaps secondary to a defect in lid disjunction, is responsible at least in part for the deformity of the palpebral aperture.

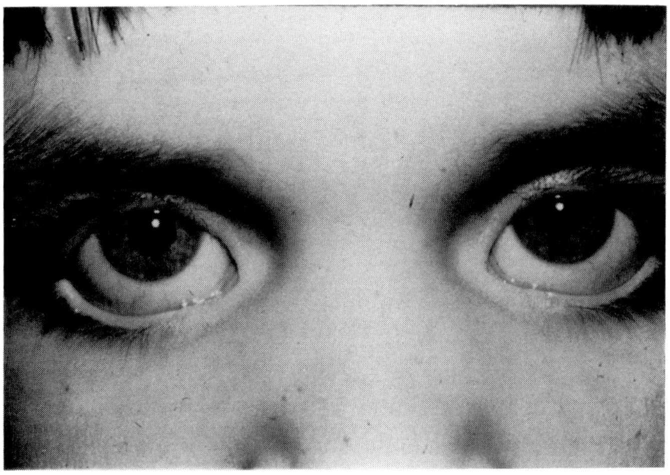

Figure 12.3. Prominent lagophthalmos with a markedly elongated lid margin and shortage of eyelid skin.

SURGICAL CORRECTION

For mild, generalized enlargement of the palpebral apertures lateral tarsorrhaphies will adequately correct the euryblepharon (16).

When the downward and lateral displacement of the outer canthus is more prominent, a lateral canthoplasty may be necessary to correct the deformity (24). The redundant lower lid margin is resected (Fig. 12.4), the inferior arm of the lateral canthal tendon is detached and refixated to bone posterior to the lateral orbital rim. Two holes are drilled through the lateral orbital rim, and the lateral canthal tendon is secured in to the proper position with 5-0 stainless steel wire (Fig. 12.5). The lateral canthal angle and lid margin are reapproximated with 6-0 black silk sutures.

If there is restriction of lid closure secondary to shortage of eyelid skin, retroauricular skin grafts will lengthen the anterior lamella of the lid (1, 7, 24–26) (Fig. 12.6). The lid is put on stretch with a 4-0 black silk suture in the lid margin. A paraciliary incision is made and extended beyond the canthus. The full extent of the skin deficit is demonstrated by gap between the edges of the incision, with the lid on stretch and the orbicularis and orbital septum released. A free retroauricular skin graft is fashioned with its maximum width 10% greater than the maximum height of the lid defect. The graft is sutured into position with nonabsorbable sutures and covered with a pressure patch after the lid has been immobilized with a traction suture. As the lower lid deformity is usually more prominent, the lower lids should be corrected first. If corneal exposure is not a problem, then upper lids may be corrected 6 months later. Skin grafting can be combined with lateral canthoplasties.

For the severest of deformities the reconstruction may be accomplished in stages. First, a free tarsal graft and a

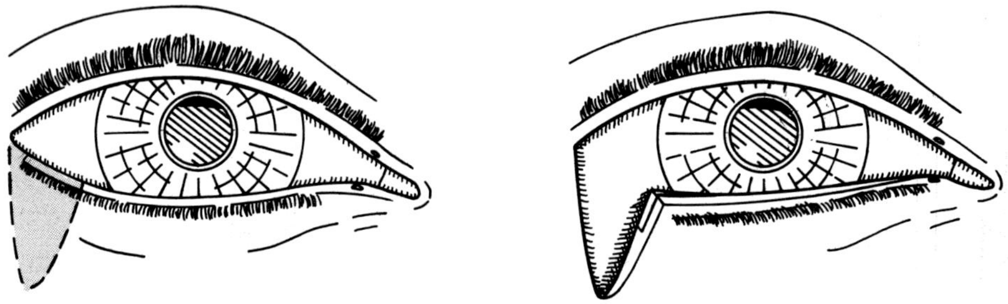

Figure 12.4. Resection of redundant lower lid margin.

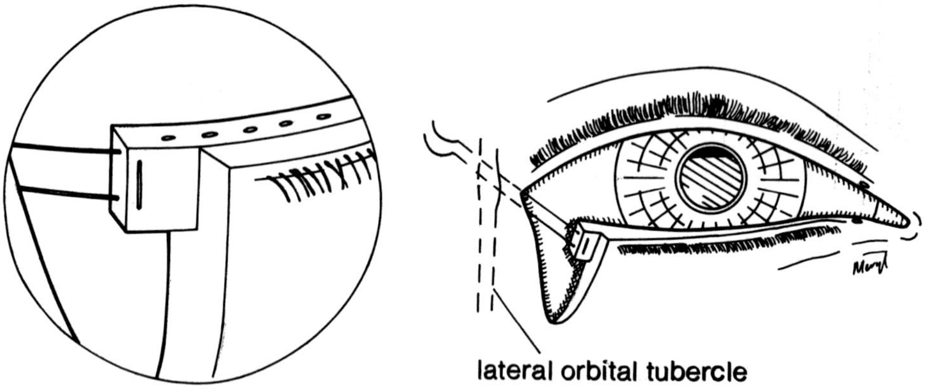

Figure 12.5. The lateral canthal angle may be reconstructed by detaching the lateral canthal tendon and refixating it to the lateral orbital wall posterior to the rim.

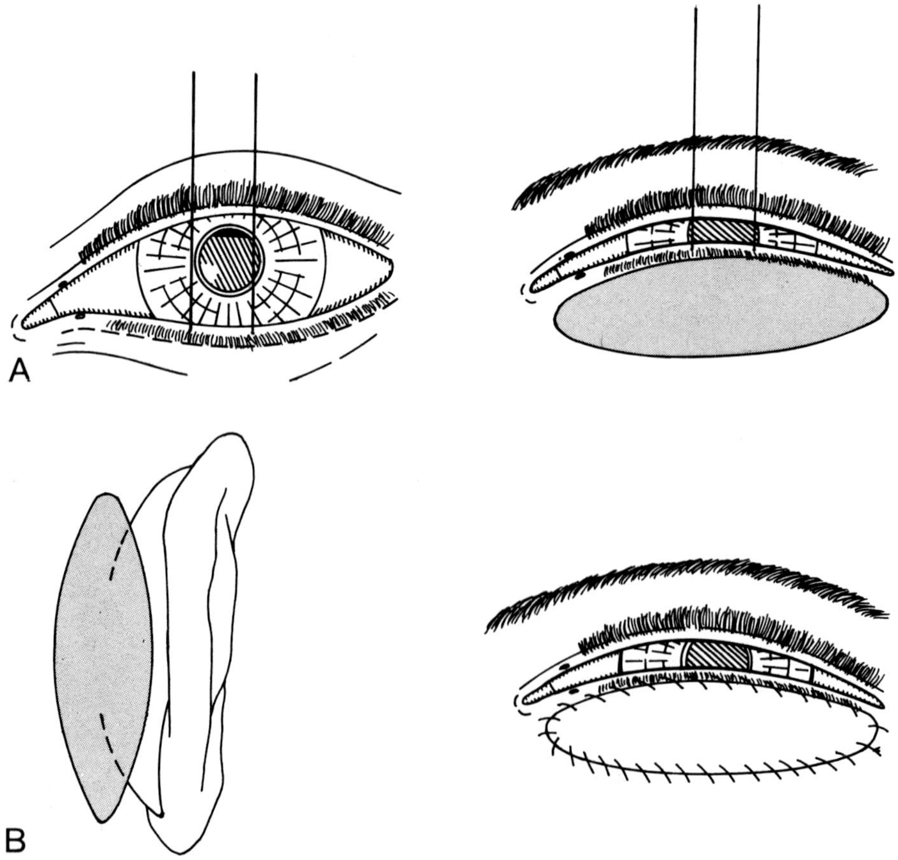

Figure 12.6. When there is marked shortage of eyelid skin, free retroauricular skin grafts will be necessary to lengthen the anterior lamella.

lateral canthoplasty may be used to reestablish a lateral canthal angle. Second, a free retroauricular skin graft can be used to vertically lengthen the anterior lamella of the lid.

REFERENCES

1. Harley RD: *Pediatric Ophthalmology.* Philadelphia, WB Saunders Co., 1975, p 241.
2. Desmarres E: Trait theorique et. practique des maladies des yeus. *Paris* 1: 468, 1854.
3. Schreiber L: *Graefe-Saemisch Handbush des gesammte Augenheilkunde*, ed 3. Leipzig, 1924, p 571.
4. Lindberg JG, *Klin Mbl Augenheilk* 81: 665, 1928.
5. Seefelder R: *Kurzes Handbuch der Ophthalmologie.* Berlin, 1930, vol 1, p 604.
6. Weve H, Ned T: *Geneesk.* 80: 1213, 1936.
7. Gordon S, Cragg BH: Congenital ectropion associated with bilateral ptosis. *Br J Ophthalmol* 28: 520, 1944.
8. Leffertstra, quoted in Duke-Elder: *Oostel Ooghelk gez.* 1958.
9. Ostriker PJ, Lasky MA: Congenital eversion of the upper eyelids. *Am J Ophthalmol* 37: 779, 1954.
10. Mazahar, M: Congenital eversion of the upper eyelids. *Br J Ophthalmol* 39: 702, 1955.
11. Hopen JM: Congenital eversion of the upper eyelids. *Arch Ophthalmol* 53: 118, 1955.
12. Waardenberg PJ, Franceschetti A, Klein D: *Genetics and Ophthalmology.* London, Oxford University Press, 1961, p 235.
13. Gupta JS, Kumar K: Euryblepharon with ectropion. *Am J Ophthalmol* 66: 554, 1968.
14. Gupta AK, Ramanurthy S, Shukan KM: Euryblepharon. A case report. *J Pediatr Ophthalmol* 9: 173, 1972.
15. Wolter JR: Familial euryblepharon. *Pediatr Ophthalmol* 9: 175, 1972.
16. Keipert JA: Euryblepharon. *Br J Ophthalmol* 59: 57, 1975.
17. Steiner L: Familiar Abnorm Weite Lidspalte Infolge Hypoplasie des Tarsus. *Klin Monatsbl Augenheilkd* 153: 708, 1968.
18. LaRocca V: Plastic repair of a congenital deformity of the external canthus. *Am J Ophthalmol* 31: 1469, 1948.
19. Ismail AM: Abnormalities of the configuration of the palpebral aperture. *Bull Ophthalmol Soc Egypt* 62: 219, 1969.
20. Davis GV, Lauring L: Familial euryblepharon associated with latent nystagmus alternating sursumduction and esotropia. *J Pediatr Ophthalmol* 11: 86, 1974.
21. Duke-Elder S, Cook C: *System of Ophthalmology.* London, Kimpton, 1963, vol 3, part 1, p 310.
22. Duke-Elder S: *System of Ophthalmology.* London, Kimpton, 1964, vol 3, pt 2, p 841.
23. Gupta AK, Saxera P: Euryblepharon with associated ocular anomalies. *J Pediatr Ophthalmol* 13: 163, 1976.
24. McCord, CD, Chappell J, Pollard ZF: Congenital euryblepharon. *Ann Ophthalmol* 11: 1217, 1979.
25. Mustarde JC: *Repair and Reconstruction in the Orbital Region, A Practical Guide.* New York, Churchill-Livingston, 1980, p 351.
26. Tessier P: *Plastic Surgery of the Orbit and Eyelids.* New York, Masson, 1981, p 148.
27. Feldman E, Bower SF, Morgan SS: Euryblepharon: a case report with photographs documenting the condition from infancy to adulthood. *J Pediatr Ophthalmol* 17: 307, 1980.
28. Shannon GM, Flanagan J: Disorders of the lids. In Harley RD (ed): *Pediatric Ophthalmology.* Philadelphia, WB Saunders, 1975, p 241.

CHAPTER 13

Congenital Anomalies of the Eyelid and Socket

ROGER KOHN, M.D.

Included within this chapter is a detailed chronicle of the principle congenital and developmental anomalies of the eyelids and socket. These varied disorders represent tissue deficiencies, structural abnormalities, and tumors. Due to their relative infrequency, complications arising from surgical correction have not been documented in the literature. Uncomplicated congenital ptosis and congenital lacrimal dysfunction will be discussed elsewhere within this volume.

CONGENITAL EYELID COLOBOMAS

Congenital eyelid colobomas typically manifest as full-thickness deletion defects in a triangular configuration (Fig. 13.1). They may occasionally assume a quadrilateral, W, or irregular shape, while partial-thickness colobomas may occur in the lower eyelid. These partial-thickness defects may retain orbicularis oculi muscle, tarsal elements, cilia, or glandular structures. Such retained tissues are usually malformed and malpositioned. The coloboma edge is rounded and covered with conjunctiva. Defect size may range from a small indentation at the eyelid margin to absence of almost the entire eyelid, suggesting ablepharon.

Colobomas are most frequently encountered at the medial aspect of the upper eyelid or at the lateral aspect of the lower eyelid. Typically unilateral, colobomas may also be bilateral and on occasion have involved all four eyelids. Symmetrical defects are not uncommon, and multiple colobomas may occur on one eyelid.

Since their initial description by Jacques Guillemeau in 1585, eyelid colobomas have been associated with a myriad of ocular, periorbital, and facial defects. Associations have included microphthalmos, corneal opacification (from exposure), corectopia, coloboma of the iris or choroid, anterior polar cataract, lens subluxation, epibulbar dermoid, caruncle malformation, symblepharon, nasolacrimal obstruction, eyebrow malformation, orbital dermoids, Treacher Collins' syndrome (Fig. 13.2), Goldenhar's syndrome, and cleft lip and palate.

The pathogenesis of congenital eyelid colobomas results from delayed or incomplete union of mesodermal sheets of the frontonasal and maxillary processes. Although rarely hereditary, occasionally a dominant pedigree is observed.

Timing of surgery should be a manifestation of the degree by which the cornea is threatened by desiccation (see the chapter by Carroll). Upper eyelid colobomas are more prone to exposure, while lower eyelid colobomas frequently cause trichiasis. Exposure becomes a significant factor when more than one third of either eyelid is missing. The clinically apparent size of a coloboma may be misleading. The disrupted orbicularis oculi muscle causes the surrounding normal eyelid elements to horizontally retract away from the defect in a manner similar to cutting a stretched rubberband. This artifactually expands the coloboma. The true extent of the defect may be determined simply by approximating the defect's edges.

Most colobomas are small, allowing surgery to proceed electively during the first 4 years of life if Bell's phenomenon is intact. During this interval, medical management is essential to avoid exposure. In mild cases, lubricating ointment and drops given frequently may prove sufficient. In more severe cases a moisture chamber or bandage soft contact lens may also be required. Surgery becomes urgent if significant corneal exposure ensues despite these measures.

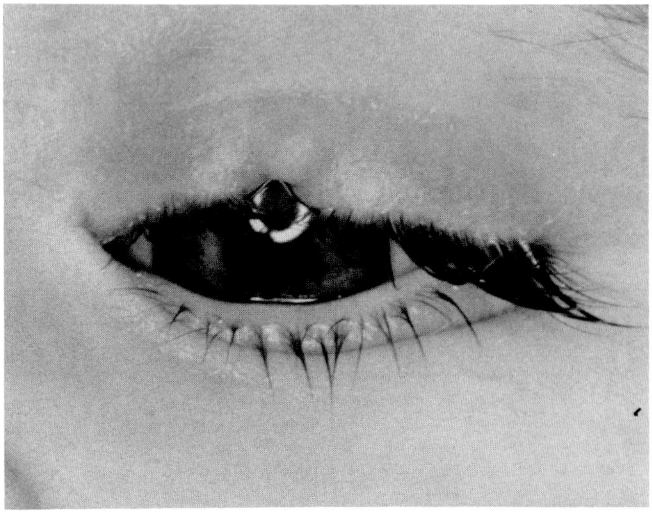

Figure 13.1. Typical coloboma, full thickness and of triangular configuration.

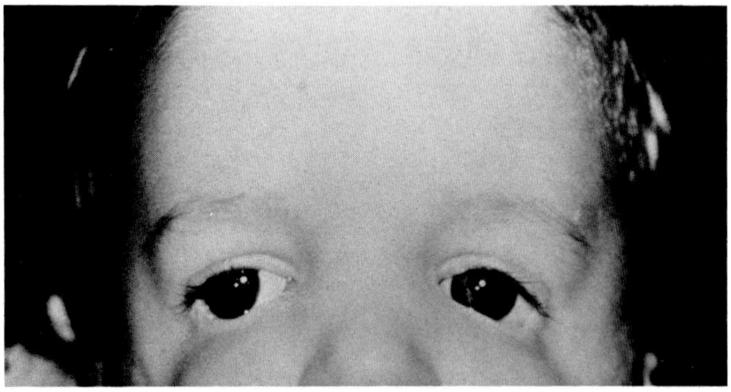

Figure 13.2. Coloboma of the lateral aspect of the lower eyelid in Treacher-Collins' syndrome.

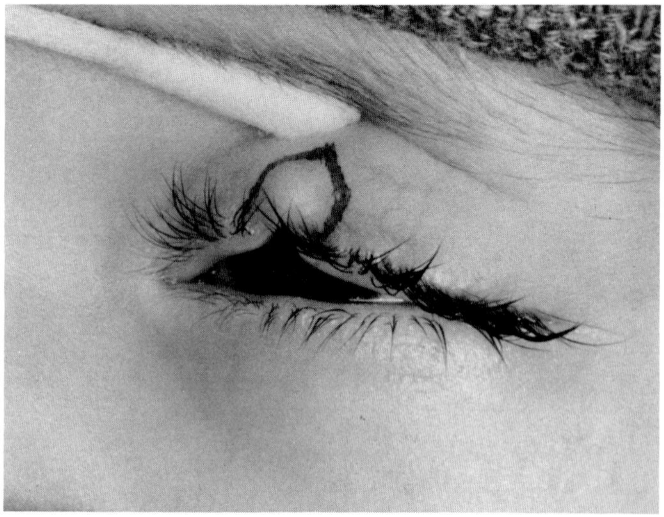

Figure 13.3. Pentagonal demarcation around coloboma.

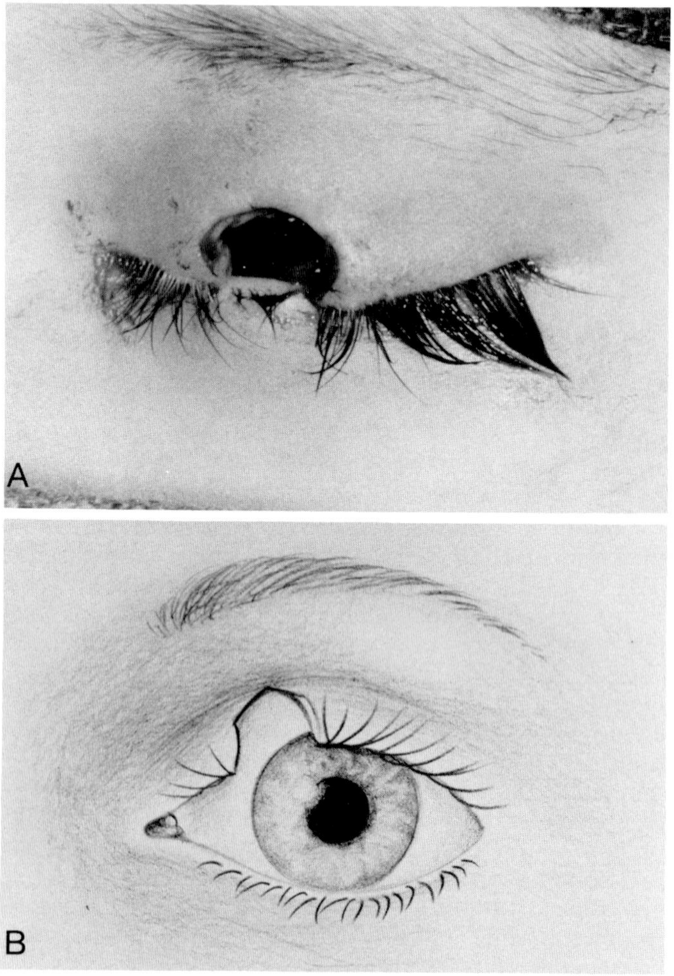

Figure 13.4. *A, B,* Coloboma margins surgically freshened.

Most colobomas involve less than 30% of the eyelid, allowing reconstruction by simply freshening the margin of the defect, converting it to a pentagonal configuration, (Figs. 13.3 and 13.4) and closing by direct approximation. All normal eyelid tissue should be preserved to minimize the scope of reconstruction.

Eyelid reconstruction is structured around reformation of the eyelid margin. Although three margin sutures would be ideal for this purpose, the small anatomy in these young children often allows placement of only two such sutures (Fig. 13.5). An anterior eyelid margin suture of 7-0 silk (or chromic) is inserted just anterior to the gray line, engaging each side of the defect. Immediately posterior to the gray line a similar 7-0 silk (or chromic) suture is placed, engaging both sides of the defect. Each suture should penetrate 2 mm deep into the tarsus and emerge 2 mm from each cut edge of the eyelid margin (Fig. 13.6). Placement of the anterior suture should carefully avoid damage to the nearby eyelash follicles. As each of these sutures is placed, it should be temporarily tied with a slip knot to determine the accuracy of apposition. Any suture that does not achieve optimal approximation should be replaced. The posterior suture should be tied first and then tunneled anteriorly underneath the anterior suture, which is tied last (Fig. 13.7). This minimizes corneal epithelial disruption by the eyelid margin suture line. These sutures should be left long and secured to the opposing cheek or

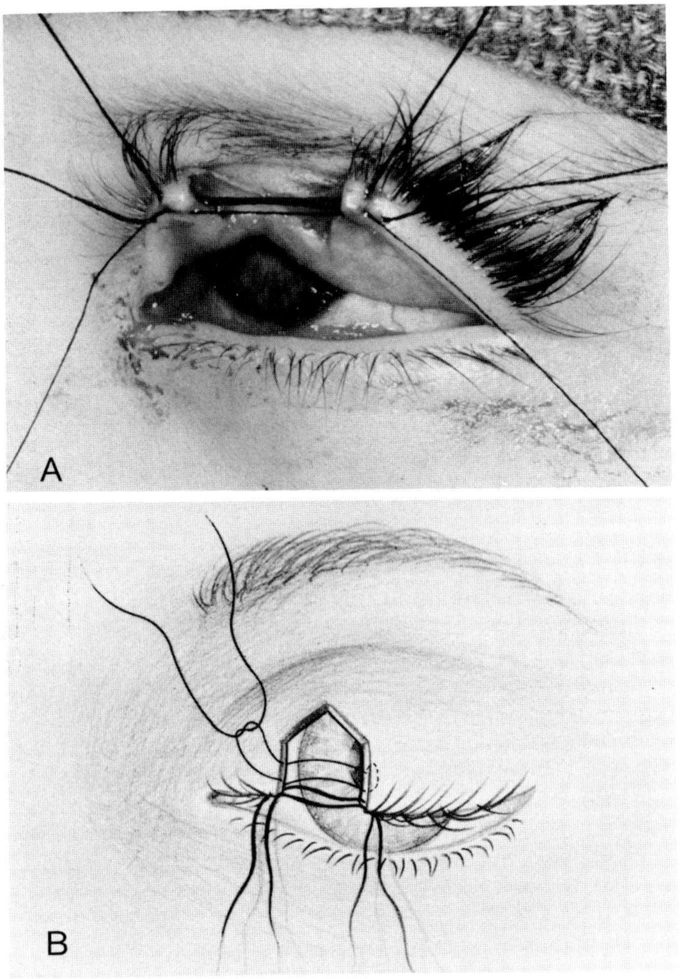

Figure 13.5. *A, B,* Anterior and posterior eyelid suture placement.

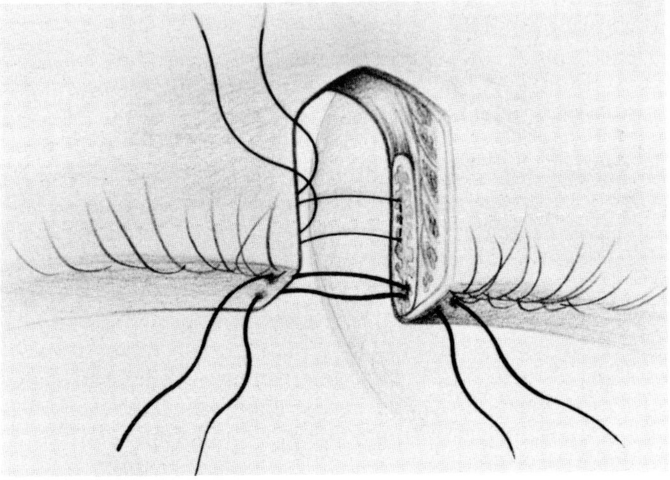

Figure 13.6. Placement of eyelid margin sutures depicted in cross section.

brow respectively to minimize any postoperative notching tendency (Fig. 13.8). The tarsus is then approximated with a 7-0 vicryl mattress suture, followed by skin closure with 7-0 silk (or chromic). The skin sutures may be removed 6

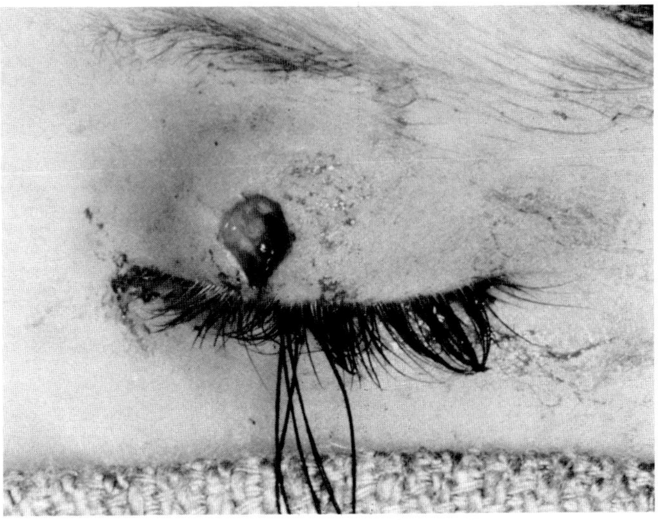

Figure 13.7. Eyelid margin sutures tied.

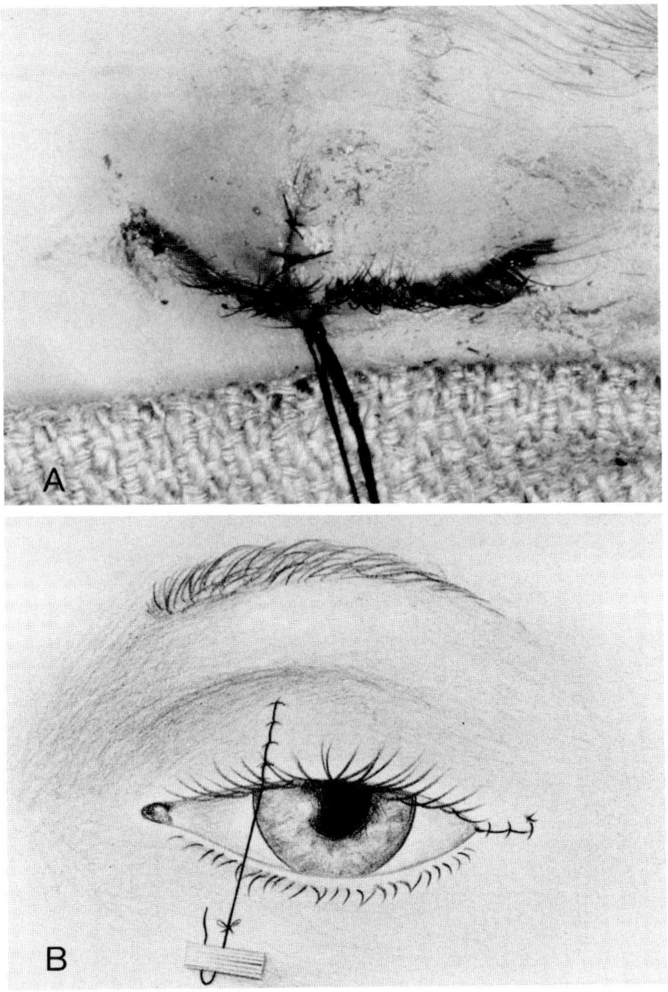

Figure 13.8. *A, B,* Eyelid margin sutures secured to cheek to minimize postoperative notching.

days postoperatively, while the eyelid margin sutures should remain under mild traction for 10 days.

Colobomas involving 30–50% of the eyelid will addi-

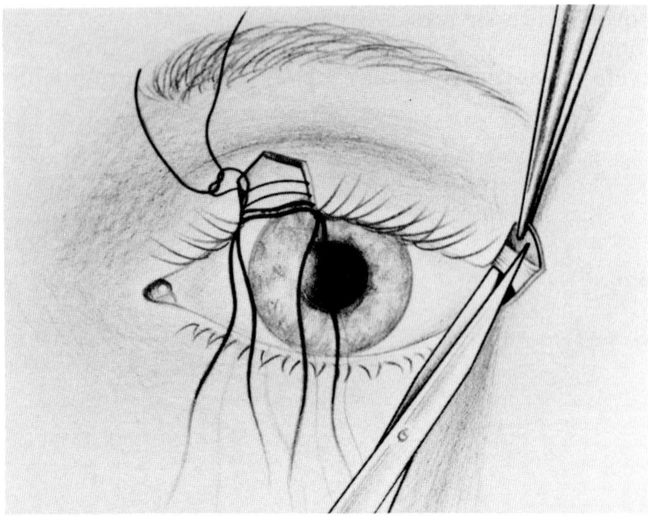

Figure 13.9. Lateral cantholysis to enhance coloboma closure.

tionally require a lateral canthotomy with lysis of the appropriate crus of the lateral canthal tendon (Fig. 13.9). Defects greater than 50% are rare, but can be preferentially reconstructed with Mustarde or Tenzel rotational flaps, which are described elsewhere in this volume. Hughes or Cutler-Beard eyelid sharing flaps are not recommended as they would cover the globe for 3 months and may predispose to deprivation amblyopia in these young children.

MICROBLEPHARON AND ABLEPHARON

Microblepharon is an extremely rare vertical forshortening of full-thickness eyelid tissue first described by Fuchs in 1885. Either eyelid can be affected, although the upper eyelid is more commonly involved. Lagophthalmos and corneal desiccation are often mild when Bell's phenomenon is intact. Marked degrees of microblepharon may approach ablepharon, with rudimentary cutaneous nodules in place of the eyelid. The globe may vary from normal to vestigial. Microblepharon has been additionally associated with absent eyelashes and eyebrows, and auricular, oral, and genital abnormalities (see the chapter by Hornblass and Reifler).

Speculation on the pathogenesis of microblepharon suggests four possible causes: (*a*) primary growth failure of eyelid tissue, (*b*) normal initial formation with subsequent destruction and absorption of eyelid tissue, (*c*) temporary fusion of the eyelids during fetal development, or (*d*) a widespread coloboma.

Management should be based upon the specific tissue deficiencies of each case and the functional integrity of the globe. Cheek rotation flaps, eyelid-sharing advancement flaps, pedicle rotation flaps, and full-thickness retroauricular skin grafts, alone or in partial combination, may prove useful.

EURYBLEPHARON

Euryblepharon, as first reported by Desmarres in 1854, depicts an anomalous bilateral symmetrical enlargement of the palpebral aperture that is associated with enlarged eyelids. Horizontal palpebral fissure length may be 35 mm in this condition, compared with 25–30 mm in normal individuals. Although euryblepharon is stable, the extreme flaccidity of the eyelids may in time result in lateral ectropion of the lower eyelids, decreased blink response, and lagophthalmos.

The etiology is unknown, although speculation has centered around a hypoplasia of the orbicularis oculi muscle. Hereditary associations documented in euryblepharon have not fallen into clear autosomal or sex-linked categories. It may occasionally present as a manifestation of Down's syndrome.

These patients may surgically benefit from horizontally shortening the lateral aspect of the upper and lower eyelid. The wound closure should incorporate a lateral canthoplasty to further shorten the palpebral fissure.

CRYPTOPHTHALMOS

Cryptophthalmos was first reported by Zehender and Manz in 1872 and depicts a very rare failure of eyelid fold formation (from mesodermal and ectodermal nondifferentiation), resulting in failure of eyelid formation. This is subdivided into three groups: (*a*) Typical (complete) cryptophthalmos is the most common form whereby skin replaces the eyelids, passing smoothly from the forehead to the cheek and completely covering and attaching to the subjacent globe. Eyebrow hair and lashes are absent in this form. (*b*) Partial (incomplete) cryptophthalmos occurs when facial skin fuses with the medial aspect of the globe, replacing the eyelid in that region. The lateral eyelid is normal in this form. (*c*) Congenital (abortive) symblepharon depicts the fusion of the upper eyelid to the upper aspect of the globe, while the cornea is covered by keratinized stratified squamous epithelium. The superior punctum is absent and xerosis of the globe may result.

This disorder is typically bilateral and symmetrical, although unilateral and asymmetrical cases have been reported. Its occurrence is sporadic, with occasional autosomal recessive or dominant pedigrees elicited.

Associated ophthalmic features may include microphthalmos, small or absent anterior chamber, absent trabecular meshwork and Schlemm's canal, subluxated lens, either absence or adherence of iris and lens to corneal endothelium, atrophic ciliary body, variable choroidal colobomatous cysts, dermoids, supernumerary brow, absent hair follicles, and absent lacrimal and accessory lacrimal glands. These associated findings often render the visual prognosis poor.

Associated nonophthalmic features may include dyscephaly (including meningomyelocele), mental retardation, otolaryngologic malformations (inner, middle, and outer ear anomalies; deafness; preauricular tags; nasal clefts; abnormal nares; cleft lip and palate; and laryngeal atresia), genitourinary malformations (hypospadius, undescended testes, clitoral hypertrophy, renal agenesis), cardiac malformations, syndactyly, umbilical hernia, anal atresia, frontal and temporal bone flattening, and abnormal hair distribution.

Histopathologic examinations in cryptophthalmos have demonstrated metaplastic changes from the corneal epithelium to skin. The orbicularis oculi muscle and levator palpebrae superiorus muscle are well represented, while the tarsal plate and conjunctiva are rudimentary or absent.

Treatment is directed toward functional and cosmetic eyelid reconstruction. The palpebral aperture must be promptly parted in the neonate to allow any potential for formed vision. In parting the eyelids, the subjacent globe must be carefully protected and preserved. The opening should be made at the point of eyelid fusion. If this landmark is indistinct, the incision should run along the horizontal axis as defined by the angles of the medial and lateral orbital rims (see the chapter by Katowitz).

SYNDROME OF BLEPHAROPTOSIS, BLEPHAROPHIMOSIS, EPICANTHUS INVERSUS, AND TELECANTHUS (KOHN-ROMANO SYNDROME)

Although reports of the various elements of this condition date to the 1920s, this disorder was first completely collated into a distinct syndrome by Kohn and Romano in 1971. It is thereby recognized as the tetrad of blepharoptosis, blepharophimosis, epicanthus inversus, and telecanthus based upon clinical and hereditary characteristics (see the chapter by Beard).

The ptosis is usually severe, demonstrating a levator palpebrae superiorus that is hypoactive and fibrotic (Fig. 13.10). One case with dehiscence of the levator aponeurosis has also been noted (Fig. 13.11). These patients have hypoplasia of the tarsal plate with absence of the eyelid fold and smooth overlying skin that correlates with the very poor levator function commonly found. Vertical brow width is increased from constant utilization of the frontalis muscle for lid lifting. To compensate for the severe ptosis, the head may assume a backward tilt while the chin arches upward (Fig. 13.10).

Blepharophimosis denotes a diminution of horizontal palpebral fissure length from a normal 25–30 mm to 18–22 mm in this condition (Fig. 13.10).

Epicanthus inversus folds originate in the lower eyelid and sweep superiorly and medially over the inner canthus (Fig. 13.10). This may diminish the normal canthal depression. The caruncle and plica semilunaris are hypoplastic and secluded beneath the epicanthus inversus fold.

Telecanthus as defined by Mustarde denotes increased distance between the internal canthi (Fig. 13.10). This is subdivided into primary and secondary forms based upon radiologic evidence of hypertelorism. In this syndrome the length of the medial canthal tendon is increased from a normal 8–9 mm to 13 mm.

Additional eyelid features include the upper eyelid margin's characteristic S-shape and the lower eyelid margin's downward concavity, particularly laterally, which may

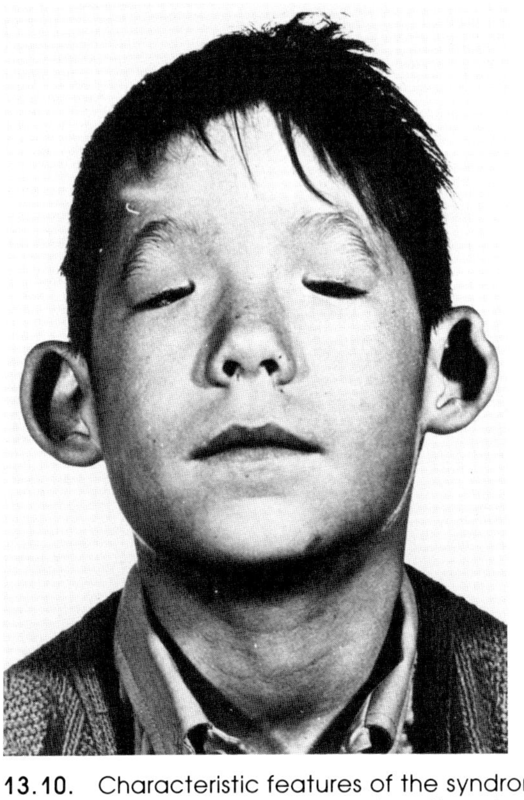

Figure 13.10. Characteristic features of the syndrome of blepharoptosis, blepharophimosis, epicanthus inversus, and telecanthus (Kohn-Romano syndrome).

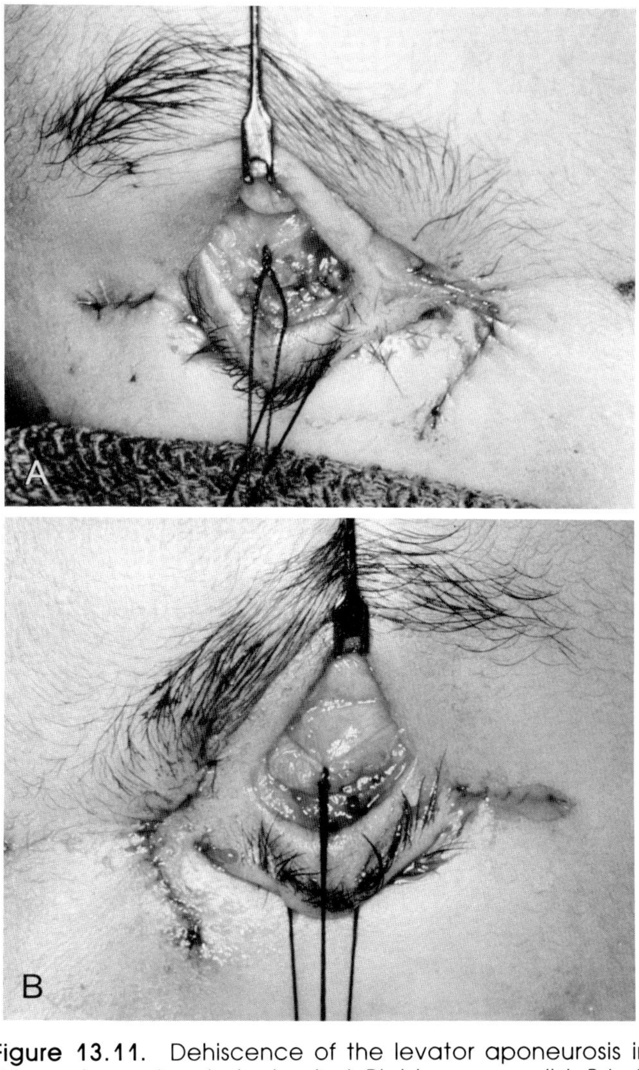

Figure 13.11. Dehiscence of the levator aponeurosis in this syndrome (central suture). *A*, Right upper eyelid. *B*, Left upper eyelid.

result in ectropion. Trichiasis was additionally present in several reports. The lacrimal system is often affected. The lower punctum is uniformly laterally displaced, while the upper punctum is medially displaced. Posterior ectopia of the lower punctum and aplasia of the upper punctum were recently described (Fig. 13.12). Other variations may include stenosis of all canaliculi, elongation of the horizontal canaliculi, and punctal reduplication.

Additional ophthalmic features include microphthalmos, exotropia, esotropia, underaction of the superior rectus muscle with limitation of upgaze, underaction of the inferior rectus muscle with limitation of downgaze, nystagmus, and optic disc colobomas.

Additional facial features include a broad and flat nasal bridge with a bony deficiency at the supraorbital rim and brow. The palate may be high arched (Fig. 13.13), and the ears may be low set and cupped with an overhanging helix (Fig. 13.10). Despite the patient's appearance, mental status is normal, although some patients have developed secondary psychological problems from their cosmetic handicap. This condition is quite stable over time (Fig. 13.14).

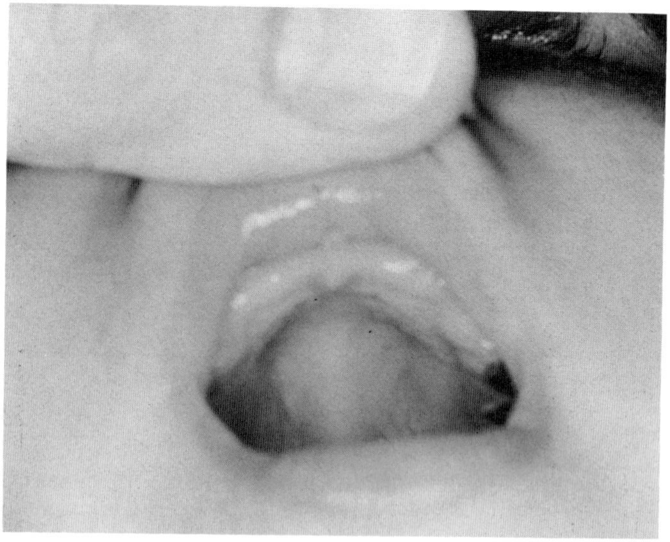

Figure 13.13. High-arched palate is variably present in this syndrome.

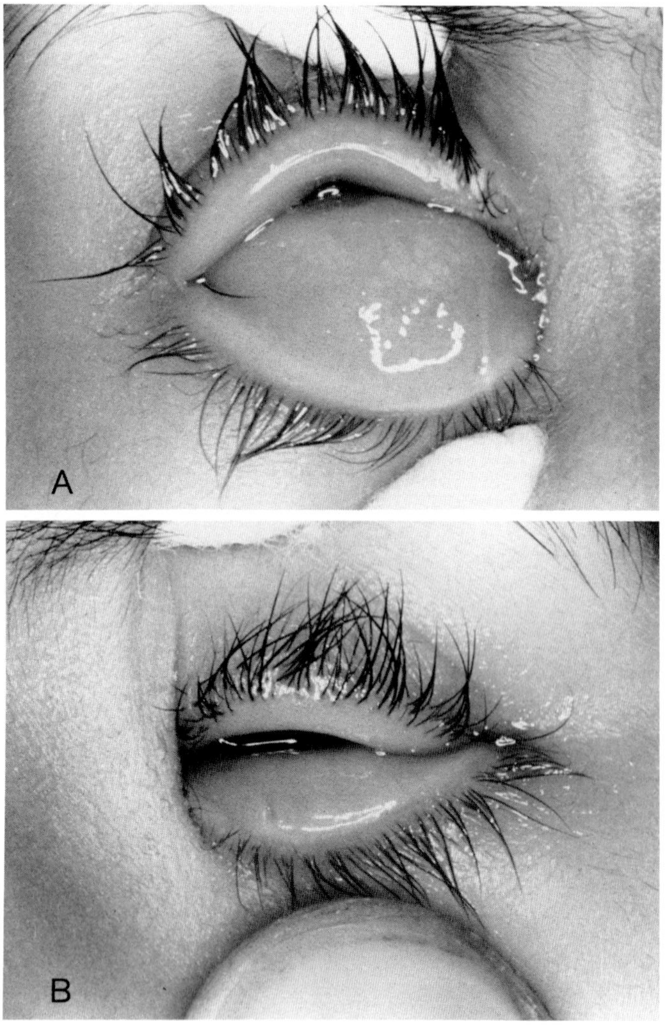

Figure 13.12. Posterior and lateral ectopia of the lower punctae. *A*, Right lower punctum. *B*, Left lower punctum.

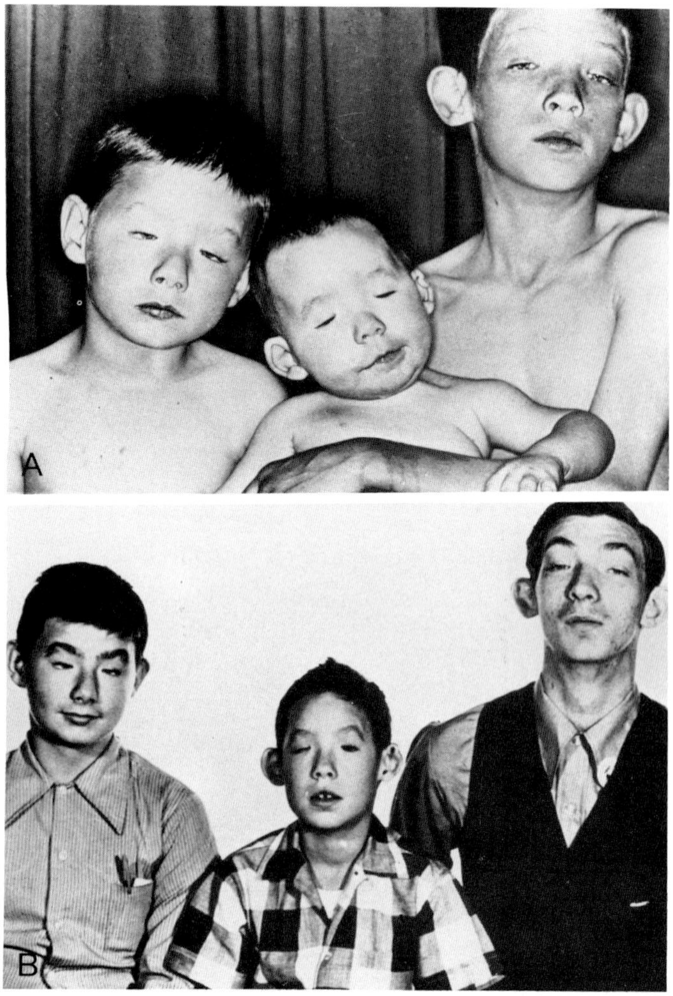

Figure 13.14. The stability of this condition is demonstrated by the 7-year interval between photographs of these siblings.

The syndrome is associated with an increased incidence of amenorrhea. This correlates with the autosomal dominant hereditary pattern with essentially 100% penetrance, occuring more commonly in males and expressed more commonly through male lineage (Fig. 13.15). Sporadic cases are occasionally found. All chromosomal studies have proven normal.

Management is often deferred until the preschool years when the anatomy becomes larger and easier to work with. The surgery is based upon a medial canthoplasty, which eliminates the epicanthus inversus and telecanthus while reducing the blepharophimosis.

Traditional approaches to the medial canthoplasty have included Y-V plasty and Mustarde's quadrilateral flaps. The latter is simply a Y-V plasty with a superimposed double Z-plasty. The double-Z component does not contribute to reduction of the epicanthus inversus fold but does accentuate the resultant scar as considerable suture material is placed in a small region (Fig. 13.16). For this reason quadrilateral flaps have proven less efficacious than Y-V plasty.

The Y-V plasty also has several notable disadvantages. In this technique the leading edge of the "V" is maximally advanced, while the remainder of this flap is advanced progressively less. A second disadvantage results from the prominent V-shaped scar which does not conform well to Langer's lines (Fig. 13.17).

In either technique the superficial head of the medial canthal tendon is shortened. Most cases require transnasal wiring, although occasional mild cases have benefitted from simply resecting the medial canthal tendon and securing it to periosteum or bone at the anterior lacrimal crest.

I have recently made two modifications in the surgical technique for this disorder. A C-U plasty is used rather than Y-V plasty. This provides appreciable advancement of the entire flap, not just the apex, and conforms to Langer's lines. Additionally, severance of the insertion of the antagonist lateral canthal tendon results in more effective advancement of the medial canthal tendon in transnasal wiring. This is comparable to the augmentative effect of recession and resection in strabismus surgery.

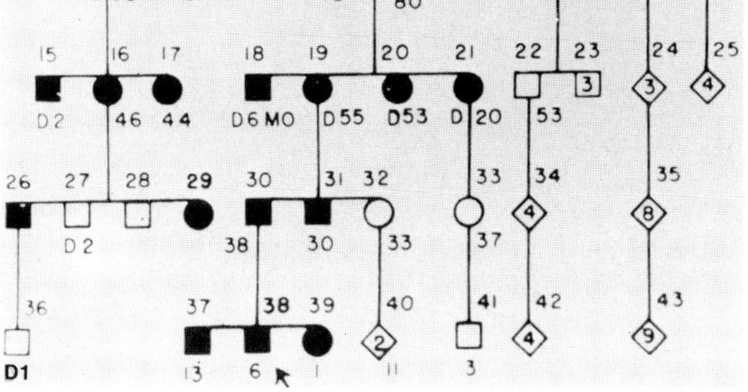

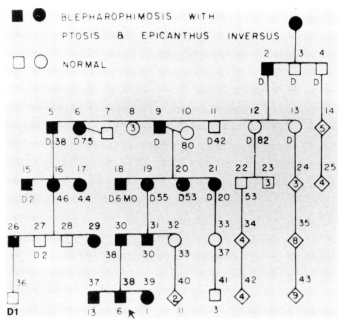

Figure 13.15. Pedigree demonstrating autosomal dominance, strong penetrance, and disproportionate expression through male lineage.

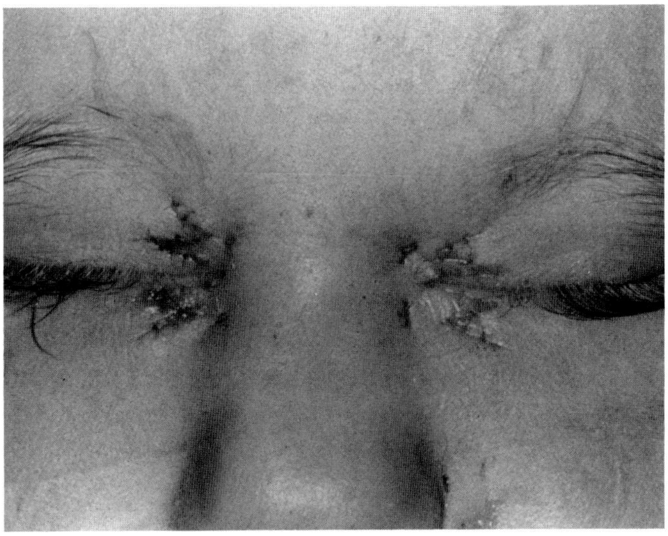

Figure 13.16. Quadrilateral flaps demonstrating considerable suture material placed within small anatomic region.

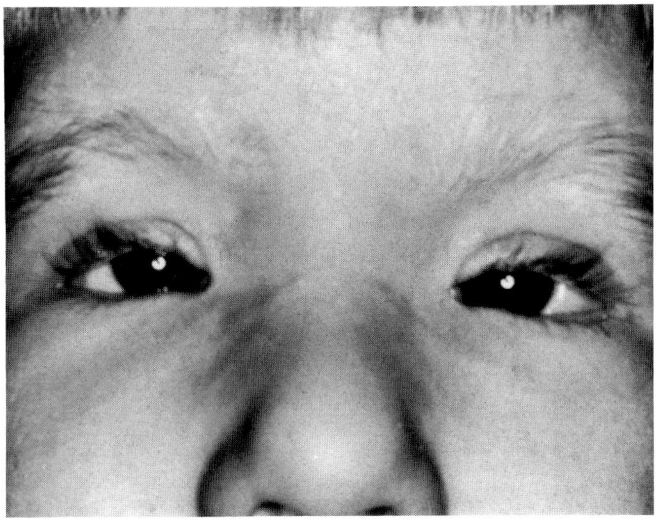

Figure 13.17. Y-V plasty 1 year postoperatively demonstrating prominent scar and limited medial mobilization.

Author's Technique

The inner canthus incision site should be marked bilaterally with methylene blue. This should assume a C-shaped crescentic configuration with approximately 7 mm of tissue incorporated within the defined skin muscle excision site (Fig. 13.18). The size can be modified somewhat to accentuate or lessen the excision from one case to

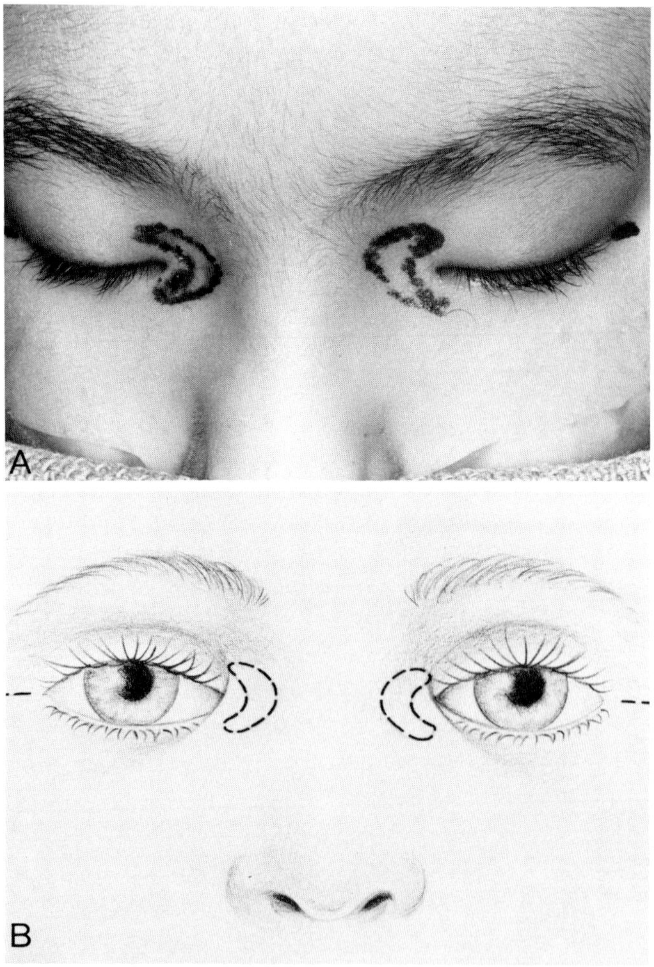

Figure 13.18. C-shaped crescentic configuration of the inner canthus excision site.

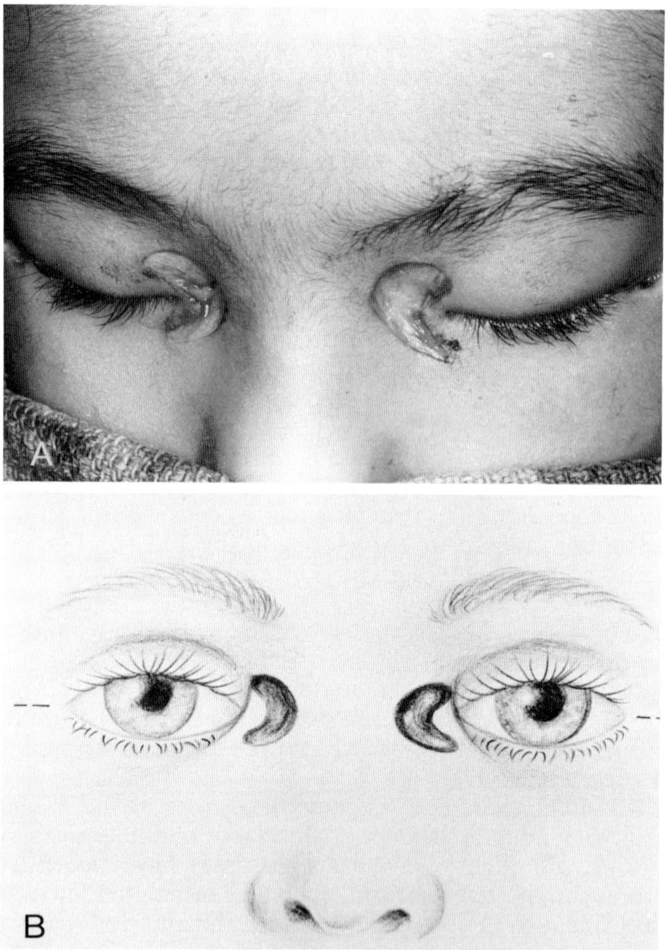

Figure 13.19. Appearance following skin muscle excision.

another. The "C" should be placed approximately 5 mm medial to the inner canthus and should not approach the nearby canalicular system. Skin and muscle should be excised according to these lines (Fig. 13.19). The incision is carried to the anterior lacrimal crest where the superficial head of the medial canthal tendon is isolated and resected with one side secured with either a 27-gauge wire or a 2-0 Supramid suture (Fig. 13.20).

A 3-mm horizontal incision is made just lateral to the outer canthus overlying the lateral orbital rim. Through this incision the lateral canthal tendon is isolated at the lateral orbital tubercle and completely disinserted (Fig. 13.21). Skin is closed with running 7-0 silk (or chromic). The medial mobility of the medial canthal tendon will now be appreciably enhanced.

In mild cases the resected superficial head of the medial canthal tendon may be secured to periosteum or bone at the anterior lacrimal crest. Most cases, however, require transnasal wiring.

In wiring, a bony window is fashioned in the posterior lacrimal and anterior ethmoidal areas. The lacrimal sac should be displaced somewhat laterally to avoid damage. Sufficient bone should be removed to accommodate a Wright needle for wire or suture passage. The Wright needle enters the bony window on the side without suture

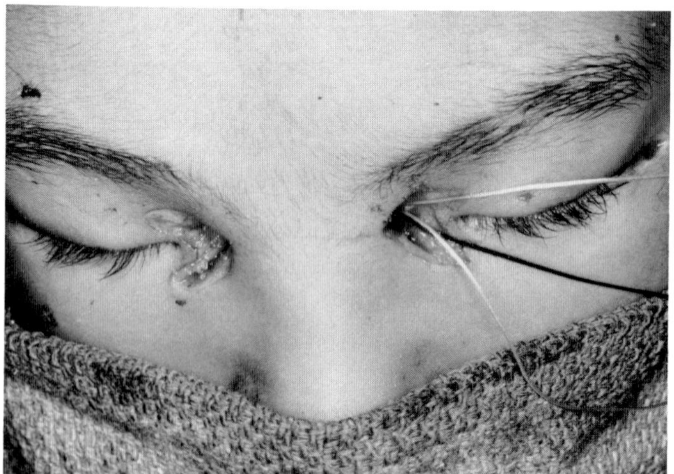

Figure 13.20. Superficial head of medial canthal tendon resected and secured with 2-0 Supramid suture.

or wire. It is then passed through the nasal septum emerging through the opposite bony window (Fig. 13.21). Some pressure is required to penetrate the septum. Careful attention must be focused to prevent momentum from carrying the needle immediately through the second window, as the medial globe is in close approximation. The

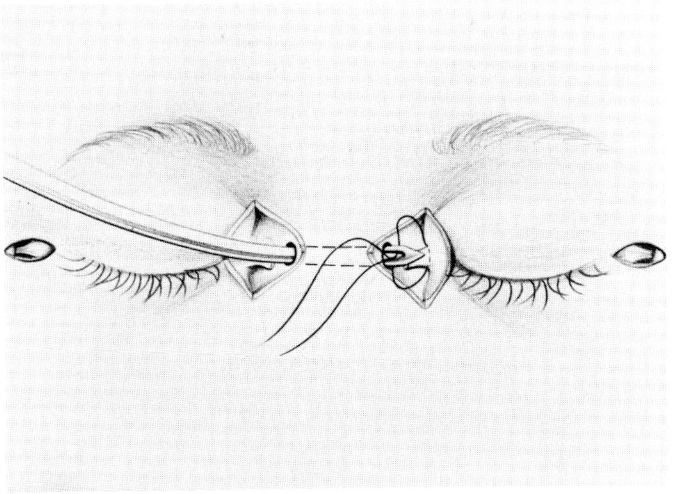

Figure 13.21. Transnasal passage of Wright needle through the bony windows and nasal septum to receive the Supramid suture. The lateral canthal tendon has been disinserted from the lateral orbital tubercle.

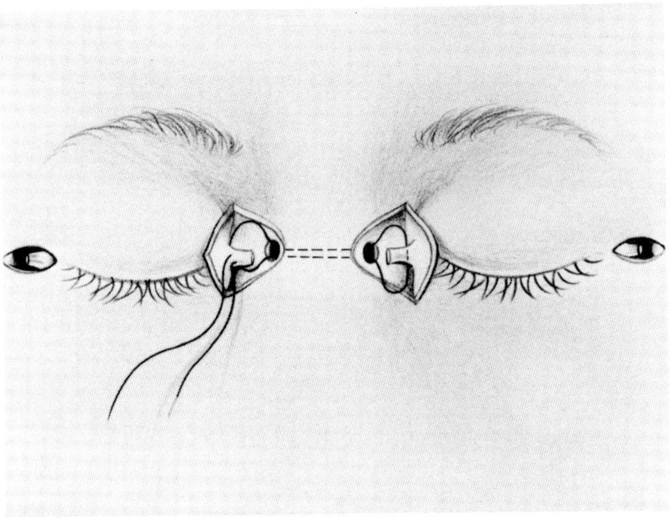

Figure 13.22. Supramid suture secured to superficial heads of both medial canthal tendons through bony windows.

Supramid suture or wire should be placed through the eyelet opening in the Wright needle, and this material becomes properly positioned as the Wright needle is withdrawn. The Supramid or wire is then secured to the second medial canthal tendon to provide maximal advancement of the medial canthal structures (Fig. 13.22). Tightening should be snug and secure but not so tight that tendon necrosis and suture disengagement ensues. The suture material gains some stability from its passage through the nasal septum. Medial advancement is enhanced by the previous lysis of the lateral canthal tendons.

The C-shaped skin muscle flap is mobilized medially and may be further tailored to reduce the epicanthal fold and telecanthus. This is secured with three interrupted 5-0 Vicryl horizontal mattress sutures to hold the advancing flap in position. The skin is closed with running 7-0 silk (or chromic) to maximize cosmesis. The resultant inner canthus suture line assumes a somewhat U-shaped configuration (Fig. 13.23).

This procedure affords additional medial mobilization beyond that achieved by Y-V plasty and results in a less visable scar, owing to its conformity to Langer's lines (Fig. 13.24).

Ptosis is corrected as the final stage of the first procedure or at a second operation. Usually frontalis suspension is required due to the very poor levator function present in these cases. In selected patients, though, with less ptosis and demonstrable levator function, a maximum levator resection may prove adequate. The one case with bilateral levator aponeurosis dehiscence was corrected by dehiscence repair alone.

Rare cases with severe blepharophimosis may be helped by an enhanced lateral canthoplasty with conjunctival reattachment to hold the outer canthus in a more open configuration. Cases with lower eyelid ectropion are quite amenable to retroauricular full-thickness skin grafting.

ANKYLOBLEPHARON

Ankyloblepharon, as first described by von Ammon in 1841, is a partial fusion of the eyelids over a portion of

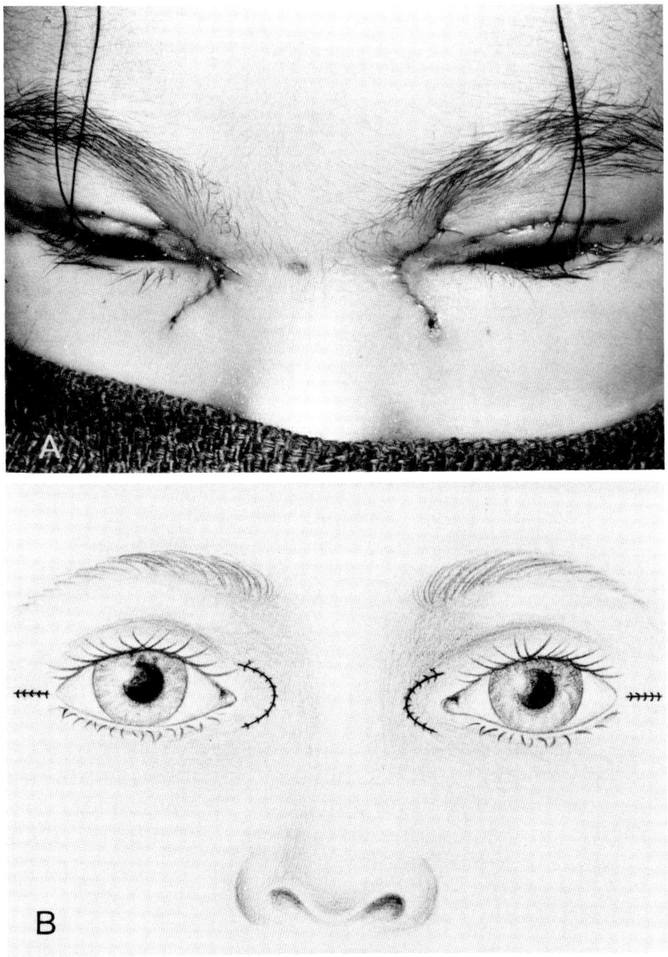

Figure 13.23. *A, B,* Resultant U-shaped suture line at inner canthus and small suture line at outer canthus.

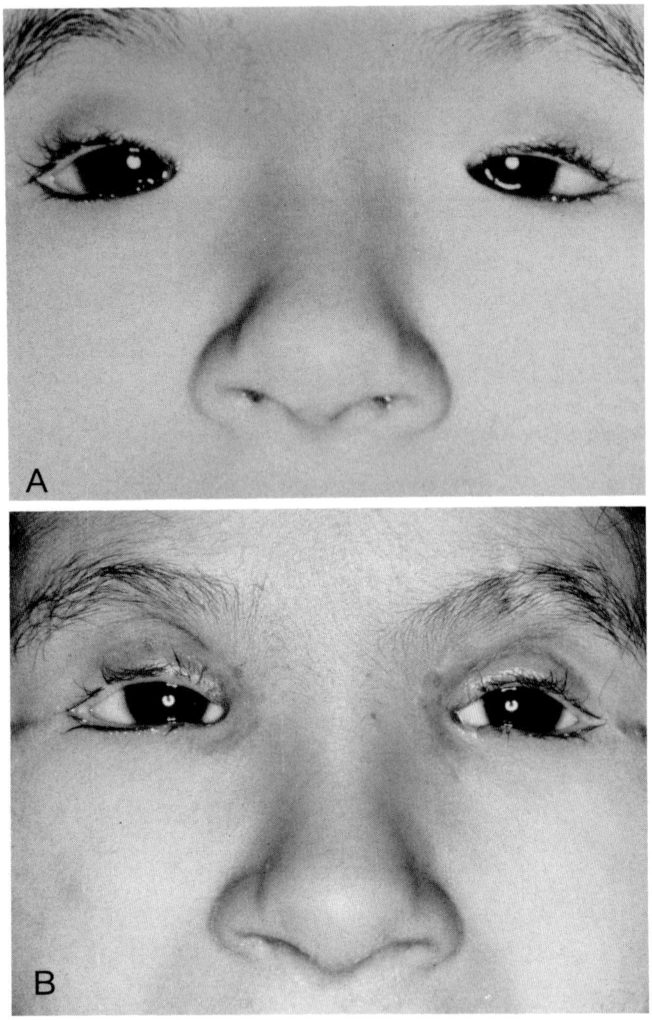

Figure 13.24. C-U plasty. *A*, Preoperative appearance. *B*, Postoperative appearance demonstrating limited scar conforming to Langer's lines and significant improvement of this condition.

their length that produces horizontal forshortening of the palpebral aperture. This fusion occurs most commonly at the outer canthus, erroneously suggesting exotropia (pseudoexotropia). Occasionally an inner canthal ankyloblepharon is noted that may result in pseudoesotropia. Ankyloblepharon may be associated with other anomalies including anophthalmos, microphthalmos, and congenital phthysis bulbi.

The pathogenesis has been attributed to developmental arrest resulting in growth aberration at either canthus. Many cases have a hereditary component, usually dominant, although sporadic cases are seen.

The treatment of this condition involves incising the fused portion of the eyelid margin. The appropriate conjunctival and cutaneous surfaces are then joined to reapproximate normal anatomy.

ANKYLOBLEPHARON FILIFORME ADNATUM

Ankyloblepharon filiforme adnatum is a rare disorder first described by von Hasner in 1881. It consists of fine attachments of extensile tissue fusing various portions of the upper and lower eyelids together. This reduces the vertical palpebral fissure width and appreciably interferes with eyelid movement. The bands may be unilateral or bilateral, single or multiple, symmetrical or asymmetrical. These attachments arise at the gray line, posterior to the cilia and anterior to the meibomian gland orifices. They are composed of a central vascularized connective tissue core surrounded by stratified squamous epithelium. Associated findings occasionally may include cleft lip, cleft palate, adherent pinna, intraoral anomalies, ventricular septal defect, patent ductus arteriosis, syndactyly, hydrocephalus, meningomyelocele, imperforate anus, and the popliteal-pterygium syndrome.

The etiology of ankyloblepharon filiforme adnatum has been attributed to an interplay between a temporary arrest of epithelium and a rapid proliferation of mesenchyme, allowing the union of mesenchymal tissue along various points of the upper and lower eyelid margin. Subsequent eyelid movement stretches these attachments into formed bands. Although usually sporadic, autosomal dominant and recessive patterns have been reported.

Treatment involves simply severing the attachments. The resultant epithelial tags will subsequently rapidly involute.

CONGENITAL ENTROPION AND EPIBLEPHARON

Congenital entropion of the lower eyelid is an uncommon, usually asymptomatic disorder first reported by Frontmuller in 1847. This condition is manifested by an inward rolling of the eyelid margin causing the cilia to point inward toward the globe (Fig. 13.25). Confusion may result with the more common condition, epiblepharon, in which a horizontal redundant medial skin fold induces a vertical orientation of the cilia (Fig. 13.26). Both conditions may at times coexist and disproportionately occur in Orientals.

Improper development of the distal lower eyelid retrac-

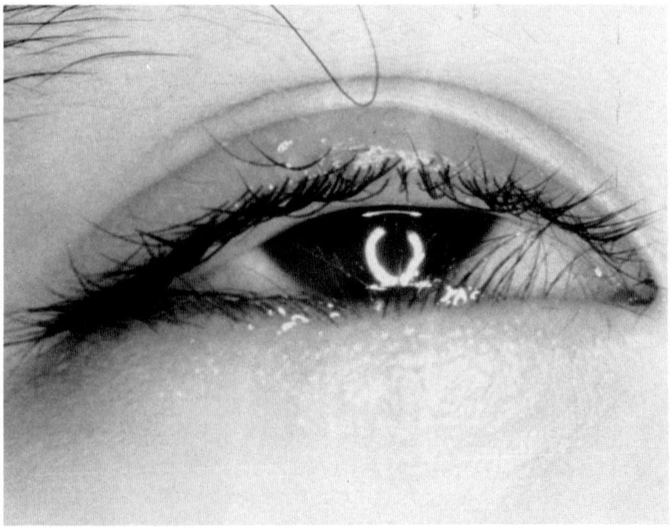

Figure 13.25. Congenital entropion with inward rolling of eyelid margin, and cilia pointing inward toward the globe.

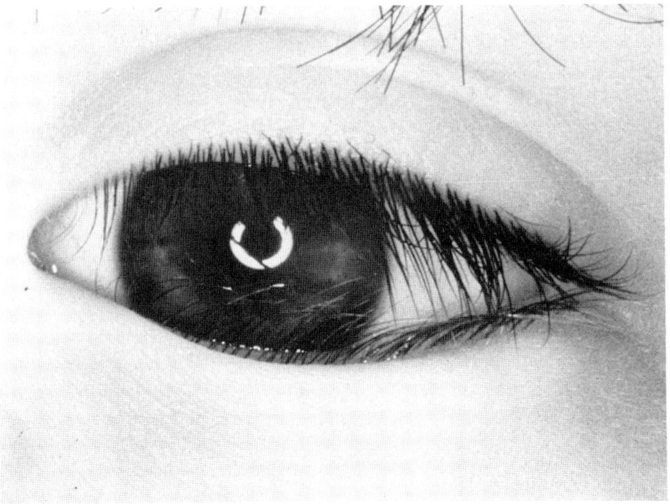

Figure 13.26. Epiblepharon with redundant medial skin fold causing vertical orientation of the cilia.

tor with attenuation or dehiscence near the tarsal plate appears to be a common etiologic denominator in congenital lower eyelid entropion and epiblepharon. Secondary forms of congenital entropion can result from epicanthal folds, microphthalmos, and anophthalmos. These cases are caused by mechanical factors.

The clinical course of congenital entropion is often asymptomatic with spontaneous resolution. Therefore, surgery should be reserved for those cases that persist and threaten the cornea. When surgery is indicated, the recommended procedure is the tuck of the inferior aponeurosis as described by Jones and Reeh.

In this procedure a horizontal incision is made 3 mm below the lower eyelid margin, traversing the central 80% of the eyelid. The incision is carried to the lower tarsal border excising preseptal orbicularis oculi muscle encountered in the process. Five interrupted 5-0 silk (or chromic) sutures close the wound. Each suture should be passed in a backhand manner that engages skin and tarsus above, then penetrates the orbital septum and engages the inferior aponeurosis below, and finally emerges through skin at the lower limb of the incision. Tying these sutures with imbrication achieves the tuck and imparts outward rotation to the eyelid. The backhand suture placement minimizes the risk of penetrating the inferior sclera, which is in close proximity to the inferior aponeurosis of these young children.

Epiblepharon also improves and often resolves by age 3 as eyelid skin stretches. During this period conservative treatment with lubricating ointment will help spare the cornea. Surgery should be reserved for rare persistent cases. These may be corrected by either excising the skin and orbicularis oculi muscle comprising the redundant fold or by placing Quickert-Rathbun eyelid crease sutures.

Congenital entropion of the upper eyelid results from either congenital horizontal tarsal kink, as reported by Callahan, or cicatrization from inflammatory or infectious factors. Kink occurs from an anomalous fixed-inward rotation of the distal tarsal margin that causes the cilia to abrade the cornea. This may be corrected by resecting that portion of tarsus involved in the kink process. Congenital cicatricial entropion may be repaired by a Wies tarsal splitting procedure as modified by Ballen.

CONGENITAL ECTROPION

Primary congenital ectropion of the lower eyelid is an extraordinarily rare condition with occasional familial associations. Instead, congenital ectropion is more commonly seen as a disorder secondary to microphthalmos, buphthalmos, euryblepharon, tumors of the eyelid, or as part of the syndrome of blepharoptosis, blepharophimosis, epicanthus inversus, and telecanthus (Kohn-Romano syndrome) (Fig. 13.27). In the latter condition ectropion results from vertical skin deficiency. Such cases are corrected utilizing retroauricular full-thickness skin grafting to the lower eyelid. Rare cases of congenital ectropion due to excessive horizontal eyelid length are managed by horizontal eyelid shortening such as the Bick procedure.

Congenital ectropion of the upper eyelid presents as a total eversion as first described by Adams in 1896. This is postulated to arise from birth trauma interfering with venous drainage. The resultant chemosis everts the eyelid and triggers orbicularis oculi muscle spasm. Orbicularis oculi muscle hypotonia has also been suggested as an etiology. Conservative management involving lubricating ointments, a moisture chamber, and traction sutures placed at the eyelid margin often prove adequate. Persistent cases may additionally require excision of prolapsed conjunctiva.

MEDIAL CANTHAL TENDON ECTOPIA

Medial canthal tendon ectopia is a rare disorder in which the tendon and attached canthal structures are vertically displaced, particularly inferiorly (Fig. 13.28). Here, the medial canthal tendon inserts at the junction of the medial orbital wall and the infraorbital rim with the inferiorly displaced lacrimal sac subjacent. Nasal cleft deformities have been associated with this condition. The etiology is considered to be a developmental arrest during the second month of embryonic life. Treatment consists of a medial canthal Z-plasty with supraplacement of the medial canthal tendon. Any concurrent lacrimal obstruction should also be corrected.

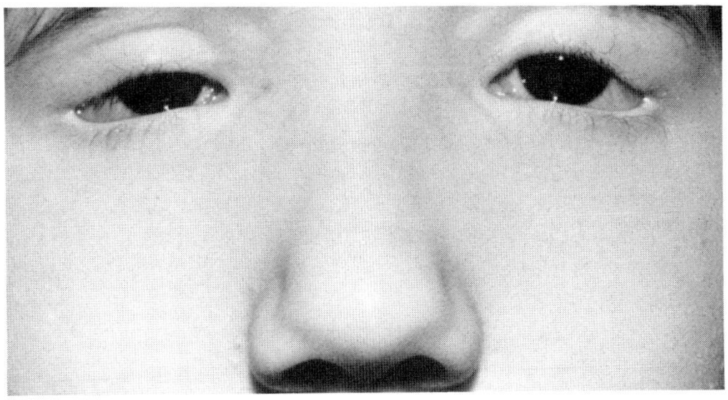

Figure 13.27. Congenital ectropion of the lateral portion of both lower eyelids in the syndrome of blepharoptosis, blepharophimosis, epicanthus inversus and telecanthus (Kohn-Romano syndrome).

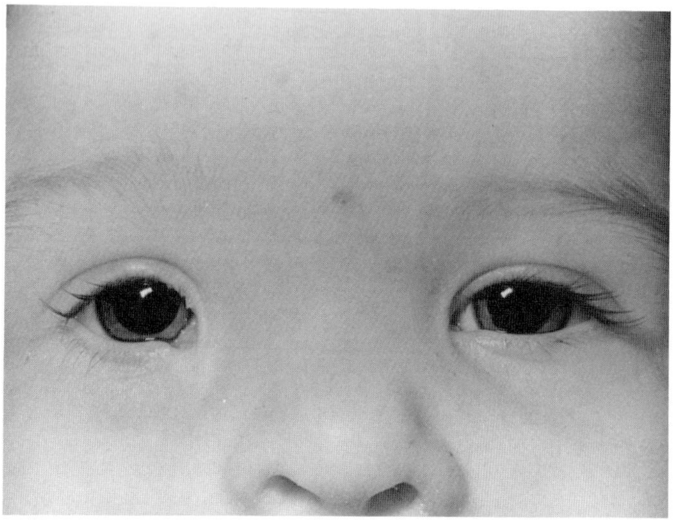

Figure 13.28. Medial canthal tendon vertical ectopia in a newborn.

CONGENITAL CLINICAL ANOPHTHALMOS

True anophthalmos is an exceptionally rare disorder manifested by failure in the outgrowth of the primary optic vesicle. This results in total nonrepresentation of essential ocular structures derived from neuroectoderm. Microphthalmos is more commonly seen, whereby these tissues are variably represented. Clinical distinction between anophthalmos and microphthalmos is often indistinct and may be discernible only upon subsequent postmortem examination of serial sections of the orbit. Hence, the term "congenital clinical anophthalmos" is appropriate to describe both entities.

Anophthalmos was first noted by Lycosthenes in 1557, with the first complete clinical description by Bartholin in 1657. It has been embryologically subdivided into three categories.

Primary anophthalmos results from suppression of the optic vesicle during differentiation of the optic plate, following formation of the rudimentary forebrain. This results in absence of the optic nerve and neuroectoderm derivatives. Clinically, orbital and palpebral tissues are present, albeit underdeveloped, as they are not dependent upon the optic vesicle for differentiation.

Secondary (complete) anophthalmos results from an intrauterine insult during pregnancy, which suppresses development of the entire forebrain. This causes numerous major abnormalities not compatible with life.

Degenerative anophthalmos results from absorption of the optic vesicle after its initial formation. The bony orbit, eyelids, lacrimal system, conjunctiva, extraocular muscles, cornea and sclera are not dependent on the optic vesicle for development. Therefore, they may be present with some degree of differentiation.

Congenital clinical anophthalmos most commonly presents as a small amorphous nodular mass near the orbital apex. The surrounding orbit is formed but is shallow, with overlying small and sunken eyelids (Fig. 13.29). Commensurately, the palpebral aperture is horizontally forshortened (Fig. 13.30). Cilia, meibomian glands, punctae, lacrimal tissue, and extraocular muscles are variably present. The optic nerve is usually absent, which reduces optic foramina size.

Anophthalmos may be associated with eyelid colobomas, clefting disorders, polydactyly, cardiac malformations, mental retardation, craniofacial anomalies, and central nervous system defects. Most primary cases are sporadic, although dominant, recessive, and sex-linked cases have all been reported.

Surgery is best deferred until maximum benefit has been derived from mechanically stretching the fornices with progressively larger conformers beginning within the first several weeks of life. Conformers should be changed at 1- to 2-week intervals. Initially, even the smallest conformer may not fit or self retain. At this stage soft malleable conformers may have to be trimmed to size and secured with 4-0 silk mattress sutures. These sutures are placed at

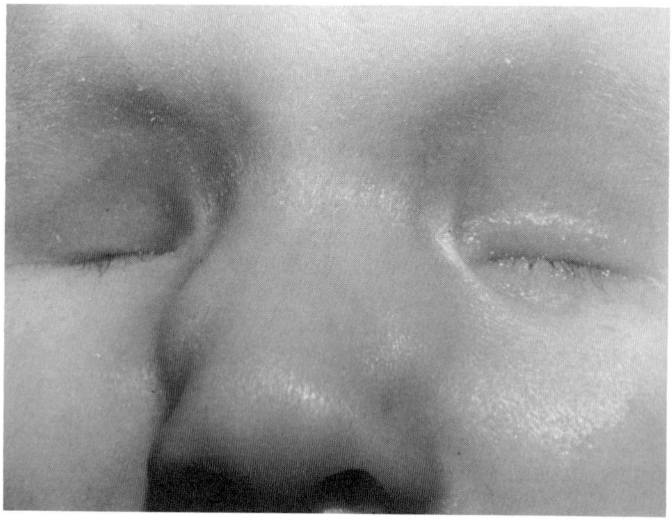

Figure 13.29. Bilateral congenital clinical anophthalmos with small and sunken eyelids.

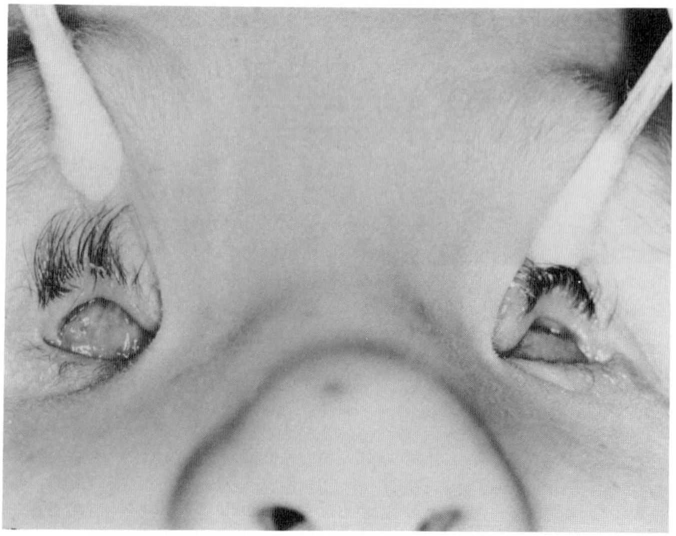

Figure 13.30. Bilateral congenital clinical anophthalmos with palpebral fissures horizontally foreshortened.

the superior and inferior aspect of the conformer, penetrating the respective conjunctival fornix, engaging periosteum at the orbital rims, and emerging through the skin where they are tied over rubber bolsters to avoid skin excoriation (Fig. 13.31). After a short time retention sutures will not be required. Pressure conformers may also prove useful in socket enlargement. In either system vertical expansion exceeds horizontal expansion.

Eyelid and socket surgery rarely proves necessary for this condition. Early surgery promotes scar tissue formation, which significantly impedes any potential mechanical socket expansion. Therefore, all surgery should be delayed until this process has been completed.

Orbital volume may be reduced 50–60% in these cases. The ocular vestige should be left as this provides a better stimulus to orbital growth than would an enucleation sphere.

Should the fornices remain insufficient, they may be augmented by mucous membrane grafting. These grafts are harvested from the lower lip internal to the vermillion border. A Castroviejo mucotome set at 0.3 mm thickness is optimal for this purpose. Thinner grafts may shred, while thicker grafts will penetrate the fat layer of the lip and scar. These grafts are sutured with 7-0 chromic into a "bed" surgically opened in the fornices. They may be further supported by a stent or conformer (Fig. 13.32).

The palpebral fissue can be horizontally lengthened by a lateral canthotomy and canthoplasty. Major eyelid reconstruction is rarely indicated. Should this be required, Tenzel and Mustarde flaps are preferable to Hughes or Cutler-Beard flaps as they are not dependent on the underdeveloped eyelids for donor tissue.

DERMOID CYSTS

Dermoid cysts are benign choristomas. During development ectoderm and periosteum are in close apposition to bony suture lines. Pieces of ectoderm may become pinched off when suture lines close. As the skin develops so will this ectodermal tissue, but the tissue will develop in an ectopic location and form dermoid cysts (Fig. 13.33).

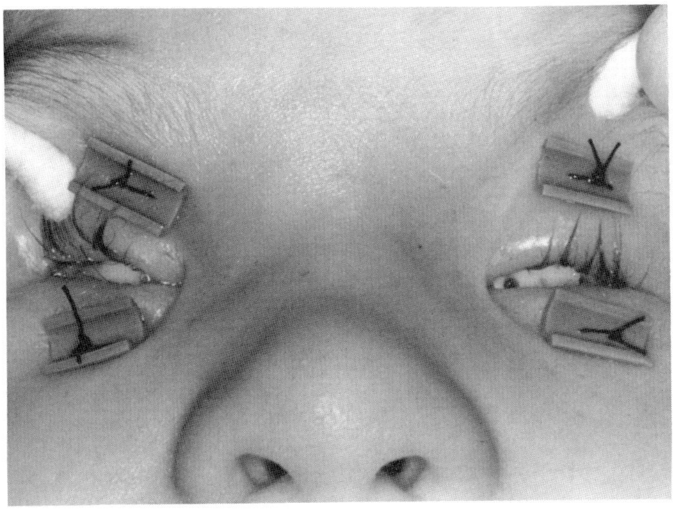

Figure 13.31. Soft, malleable conformer secured with 4-0 silk mattress sutures that have been tied over bolsters.

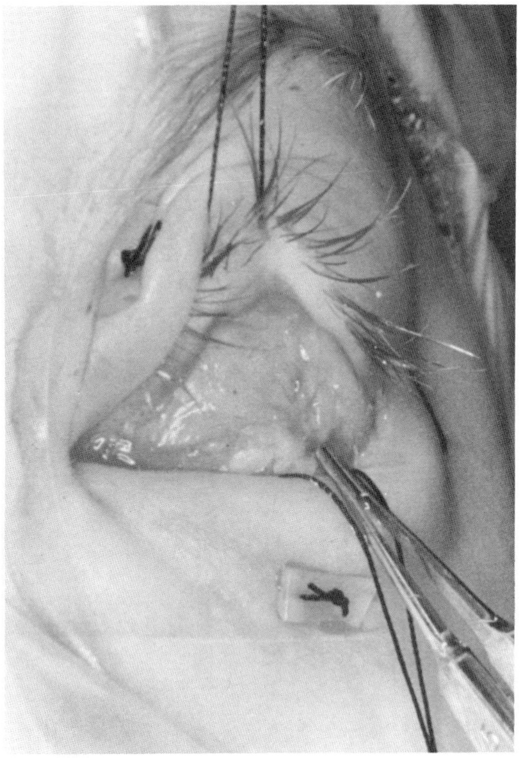

Figure 13.32. Mucous membrane grafts sutured into fornices with 7-0 chromic sutures.

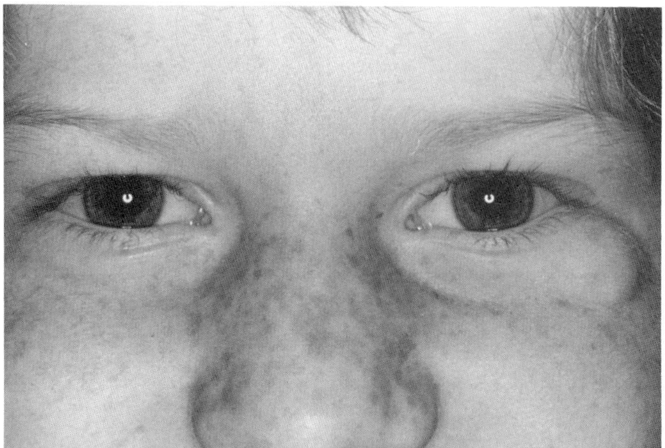

Figure 13.33. Dermoid cyst in atypical location.

They most commonly occur at the anterior aspect of the superior temporal orbit fixed to periosteum near the zygomaticofrontal suture (Fig. 13.34). They are less commonly seen in the deeper orbit in proximity to the sphenoid bone.

The peak incidence of orbital dermoids is from three to ten years of age, while fewer may manifest in the third or fourth decades. In childhood, dermoids typically present as a painless subcutaneous mass lesion of irregular configuration. They are firm and minimally mobile, although not usually attached to the overlying skin.

Superficial dermoids rarely present with radiologic evidence of bone erosion, while their deeper counterparts

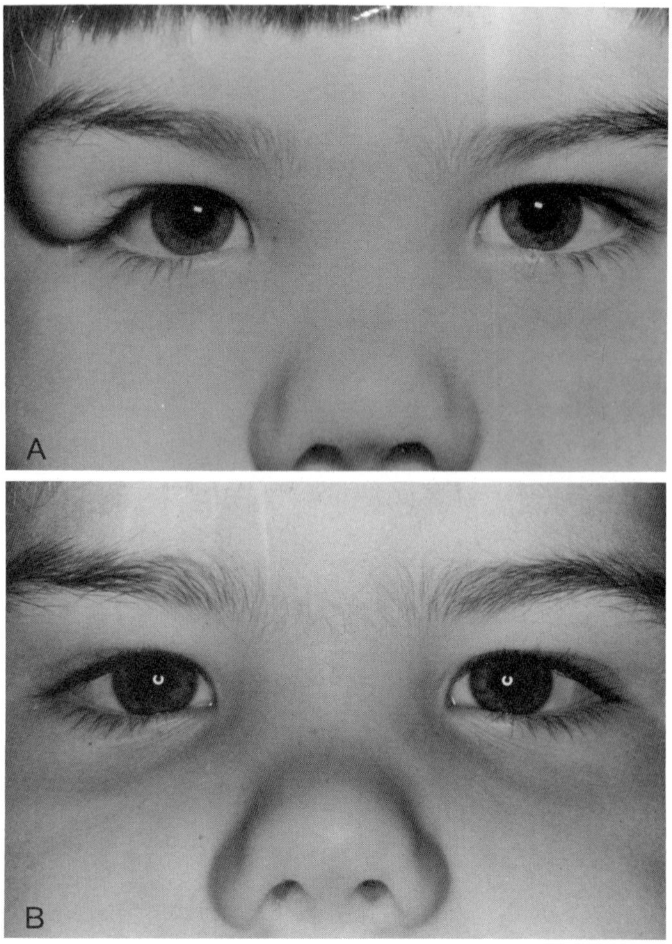

Figure 13.34. *A*, Dermoid cyst in characteristic location. *B*, Appearance following surgical removal.

may demonstrate moderate fossa formation or erosion through orbital bone. Ultrasonographically, dermoids have smooth, well defined contours with good sound transmission. They demonstrate variable amplitude internal echos due to the variable internal contents of these lesions. The degree of posterior extension can often be defined on B-scan ultrasonography. Computed axial tomography (CAT) scans may further demarcate these lesions, which may be highlighted by increased density of the surrounding bone.

Histopathologically, orbital dermoids are composed of epidermal tissue mixed with one or more dermal adnexal structures or skin appendages such as hair follicles, sebaceous glands, and sweat glands. Microscopically, they have a prominent cystic structure lined by keratinizing epidermis that may contain keratin, hair, or fat.

Superficial orbital dermoids can be readily removed through a skin incision directly over the cyst. The dissection must carefully avoid disrupting the capsular lining since the sebaceous material, if released into the orbit, will set up a moderate granulomatous inflammatory reaction. Diverticula, if present, should also be excised as they may provide a source of recurrence.

Deep orbital dermoids often necessitate a Kronlein lateral orbitotomy for removal. Should they extend through the sphenoid bone toward the intracranial space, they are best removed in conjunction with a neurosurgical approach.

Some orbital dermoids present subconjunctivally (Fig. 13.35). The indications for surgical removal of such lesions are somewhat conservative as blepharoptosis, motility disturbances, and lacrimal gland obstruction may be encountered as postoperative sequelae. Indications for removal of subconjunctival dermoids include: direct obstruction of the visual axis, anisometropic amblyopia secondary to pressure-induced astigmatic changes, and significant cosmetic disfigurement (see the chapter by Reifler and Hornblass).

ORBITAL TERATOMA

Orbital teratomas are exceedingly rare, with fewer than 60 cases in the literature. They present in the newborn as a unilateral progressively expanding polycystic tumor. Although usually confined to the orbit, bony erosion with intracranial extension can occur. Teratomas form mucin, which collects within and expands the cysts to enormous proportions. Marked enlargement of the eyelids and orbit may result (Fig. 13.36). The globe is normally developed, although the cornea and optic nerve may become compromised from marked proptosis. Clinical examination demonstrates a cystic nonreducible mass that readily transilluminates. Some solid elements may also be present.

The evaluation of a suspected teratoma should include plain radiographs of the orbit and skull, CAT scans of the orbit and anterior cranial areas, and ultrasonography. This should demonstrate a circumscribed cystic mass with calcifications variably present. The surrounding orbit may be considerably enlarged. These studies should characterize and localize the tumor to facilitate surgical planning.

The differential diagnosis of congenital orbital teratoma in a neonate should also include rhabdomyosarcoma, undifferentiated sarcoma, lymphoma, lymphangioma, hemangioma, hematoma, neuroblastoma, neurofibroma, meningocele, encephalocele, inflammatory pseudotumor,

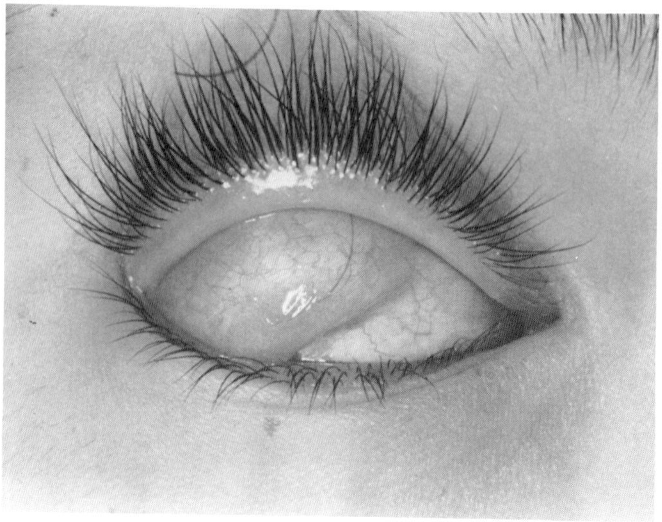

Figure 13.35. Dermoid cyst with subconjunctival presentation and hair emerging through the surface.

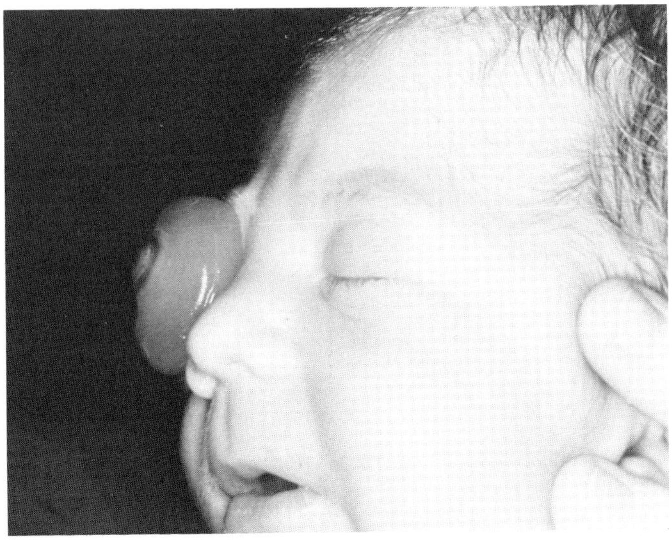

Figure 13.36. Orbital teratoma with marked proptosis and enlargement of the eyelids (Courtesy of Arthur Grove, M.D.).

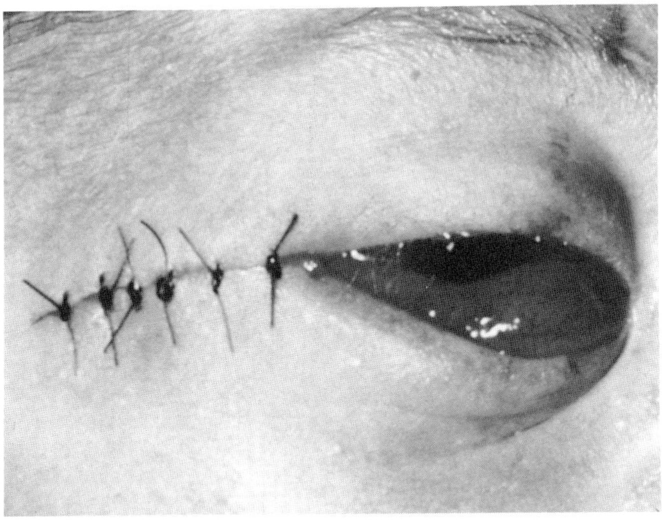

Figure 13.37. Appearance immediately following surgical removal of orbital teratoma depicted in Figure 13.36 (Courtesy of Arthur Grove, M.D.).

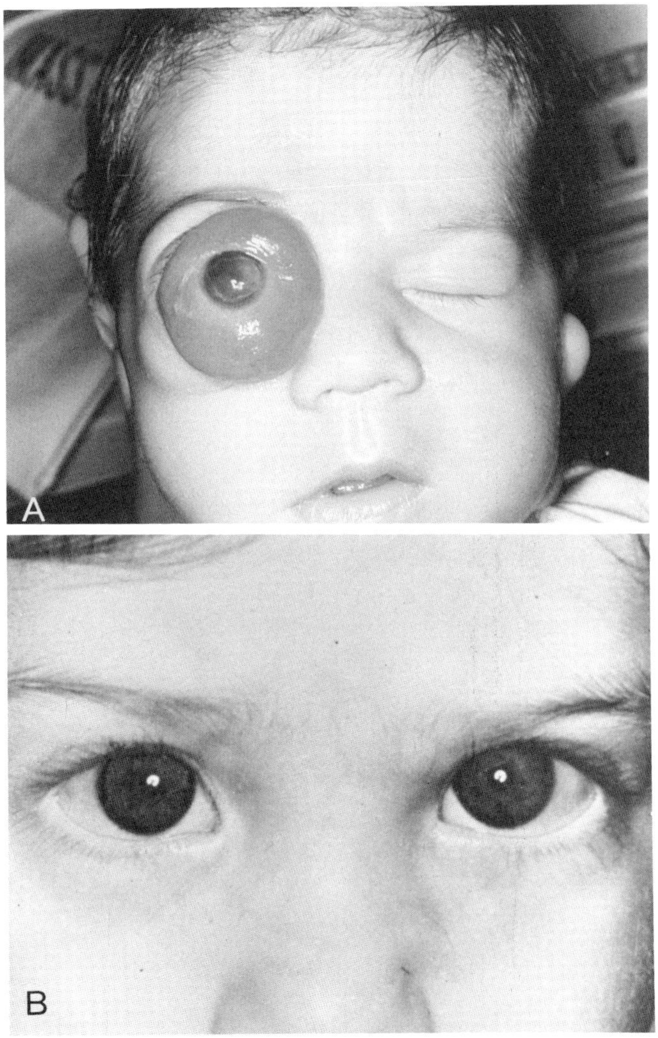

Figure 13.38. Preoperative (*A*) and postoperative (*B*) appearance of child with orbital teratoma. Vision was restored to 20/40 in this eye (Courtesy of Arthur Grove, M.D.).

dermoid cyst, microphthalmos with cyst, congenital cystic eyeball, and congenital glaucoma with buphthalmos.

Histopathologically, teratomas are composed of tissues representative of two or three germinal layers. Although principally composed of ectoderm, endodermal and mesodermal components are also represented. Differentiation may vary from an amorphous mass to complete fetal architecture. Malignant degeneration rarely occurs. The extensive fluid accumulation within these encapsulated cysts causes teratomas to be clinically destructive beyond their benign histologic structure.

The globe must be continuously protected during the preoperative assessment period. Prompt surgical removal of these tumors is essential, preserving the globe for vision or cosmesis if at all possible (Fig. 13.37). Surgery usually requires a lateral or anterolateral orbitotomy. Teratoma removal can sometimes be facilitated by coexistent needle aspiration of the fluid-filled encapsulated cysts to reduce tumor size. Although exenteration has been used in the past, many teratomas can be removed while retaining the globe with useful vision resulting in some cases (Fig. 13.38).

SUMMARY

Congenital anomalies of the eyelids and socket comprise a variety of tissue deficiencies (congenital eyelid colobomas, microblepharon/ablepharon, cryptophthalmos, congenital clinical anophthalmos), structural abnormalities (euryblepharon; the syndrome of blepharoptosis, blepharophimosis, epicanthus inversus, and telecanthus; ankyloblepharon; ankyloblepharon filiforme adnatum; congenital entropion/epiblepharon; congenital ectropion; medial canthal tendon ectopia) and tumors (dermoid cysts, orbital teratoma). The known clinical characteristics, history, pathogenesis, genetic transmission and treatment of these uncommon disorders are completely presented.

SUGGESTED READINGS

Barber J, Barber L, Guerry D, Geeraets W: Congenital orbital teratoma. *Arch Ophthalmol* 91: 45, 1974.

Baylis H, Bartlett R, Cies W: Reconstruction of the lower lid in congenital microphthalmos and anophthalmos. *Ophthalm Surg* 6: 36, 1975.

Biglan A, Buerger G: Congenital horizontal tarsal kink. *Am J Ophthalmol* 89: 522, 1980.

Butler M, Eisen J, Henry J: Cryptophthalmos with an orbital cyst and profound mental and motor retardation. *J Pediatr Ophthalmol Strab* 15: 233, 1978.

Callahan M, Callahan A: *Ophthalmic Plastic and Orbital Surgery.* Aesculapius, Birmingham, 1979.

Carroll R, Wilkins R, Fredricks S, Small R: Congenital medial canthal tendon malposition. *Ann Ophthalmol* 10: 665, 1978.

Chang D, Dallow R, Walton D: Congenital orbital teratoma: report of a case with visual preservation. *J Pediatr Ophthalmol Strab* 17: 88, 1980.

Codere F, Brownstein S, Chen M: Cryptophthalmos syndrome with bilateral renal agenesis. *Am J Ophthalmol* 91: 737, 1981.

Cullen J: Orbital diploic dermoids. *Brit J Ophthalmol* 58: 105, 1974.

Feldman E, Bowen S, Morgan S: Euryblepharon: A case report with photographs documenting the condition from infancy to adulthood. *J Pediatr Ophthalmol Strab* 17: 307, 1980.

Geeraets W: Ocular syndromes (Kohn-Romano Syndrome). Lea and Febiger, Philadelphia, 1976.

Gilbert H, Smith R, Barlow M, Mohr D: Congenital upper eyelid eversion and Down's syndrome. *Am J Ophthalmol* 75: 469, 1973.

Golden S, Perman K: Bilateral clinical anophthalmia. *Southern Medical Journal* 73: 1404, 1980.

Gupta J, Kumar K: Euryblepharon with ectropion. *Am J Ophthalmol* 66: 554, 1968.

Ide C, Davis W, Black S: Orbital teratoma. *Arch Ophthalmol* 96: 2093, 1978.

Johnson C: Epicanthus and epiblepharon. *Arch Ophthalmol* 96: 1030, 1978.

Johnson C: Epiblepharon. *Am J Ophthalmol* 66: 1172, 1968.

Kazarian E, Goldstein P: Ankyloblepharon filiforme adnatum with hydrocephalus, meningomyelocele, and imperforate anus. *Am J Ophthalmol* 84: 355, 1977.

Keipert J: Euryblepharon. *Brit J Ophthalmol* 59: 57, 1975.

Kennedy R: Growth retardation and volume determination of the anophthalmic orbit. *Am J Ophthalmol* 76: 294, 1973.

Kidwell E, Tenzel R: Repair of congenital colobomas of the lids. *Arch Ophthalmol* 97: 1931, 1979.

Kohn R, Romano P: Blepharoptosis, blepharophimosis, epicanthus inversus, and telecanthus—A syndrome with no name. *Am J Ophthalmol* 72: 625, 1971.

Kohn R: Additional lacrimal findings in the syndrome of blepharoptosis, blepharophimosis, epicanthus inversus, and telecanthus. *J Pediatr Ophthalmol Strab* 20: 98, 1983.

Kohn R: Correction of telecanthus utilizing C-U plasty, medial canthal tendon shortening and lysis of the lateral canthal tendon. Presented at the American Society of Ophthalmic Plastic and Reconstructive Surgery, San Francisco, October, 1985.

Lemke B, Stasior O: Epiblepharon. *Clin Pediatr* 20: 661, 1981.

McCarthy G, West C: Ablepharon macrostomia syndrome. *Dev Med Child Neurol* 19: 659, 1977.

Patipa M, Wilkins R, Guelzow K: Surgical management of congenital eyelid coloboma. *Ophthalm Surg* 13: 212, 1982.

Pollard Z, Calhoun J: Deep orbital dermoid with draining sinus. *Am J Ophthalmol* 79: 310, 1975.

Quickert M, Wilkes D, Dryden R: Nonincisional correction of epiblepharon and congenital entropion. *Arch Ophthalmol* 101: 778, 1983.

Reeh M, Beyer C, Shannon G: *Practical Ophthalmic Plastic and Reconstructive Surgery.* Lea & Febiger, Philadelphia, 1976.

Rodrigue D: Congenital ectropion. *Can J Ophthalmol* 11: 355, 1976.

Rosenman Y, Ronen S, Eidelman A, Schimmel M: Ankyloblepharon filiforme adnatum. *Am J Dis Child* 134: 751, 1980.

Sassani J, Yanoff M: Anophthalmos in an infant with multiple congenital anomalies. *Am J Ophthalmol* 83: 43, 1977.

Soll D: *Management of Complications in Ophthalmic Plastic Surgery.* Aesculapius, Birmingham, 1976.

Stern E, Campbell C, Faulkner H: Conservative management of congenital eversion of the eyelids. *Am J Ophthalmol* 75: 319, 1973.

Sugar H: The cryptophthalmos-syndactyly syndrome. *Am J Ophthalmol* 66: 897, 1968.

Waring G, Shields J: Partial unilateral cryptophthalmos with syndactyly, brachycephaly, and renal anomalies. *Am J Ophthalmol* 79: 437, 1975.

CHAPTER 14

Congenital Ptosis

CROWELL BEARD, M.D.

Congenital ptosis is discussed here as that ptosis with which a patient may be born, but it is limited to the type caused by a developmental lack of striated fibers in the levator muscle. This type comprises the majority of ptosis patients seen. Other types of ptosis with which a patient may be born are discussed elsewhere in this volume.

A brief review of the history of the treatment of congenital ptosis is given. The pathophysiology of congenital ptosis is considered from the standpoint of light and electron microscopic studies correlated with clinical signs of the condition. The details of an adequate preoperative examination for the determination of effective surgical treatment are outlined. A quantitative approach to the surgical treatment of the various degrees of congenital ptosis is given as well as the details of six operations that the author has found to be effective in treating almost any of the cases of congenital ptosis that might present. Some typical results from the author's practice are depicted. Since complications are a part of ptosis surgery, the usual ones and their treatment are considered.

By reviewing the material considered here, surgeons who wish to include the treatment of ptosis in their practice should find the answers to most of the questions they will have in the treatment of what I will call "true congenital ptosis."

HISTORY

The surgical treatment of ptosis was probably limited to the excision of upper eyelid skin until the 19th century. Scarpa (1), in *Diseases of the Eye* (published in 1806) speaks of the excision of "integuments at the upper part of the relaxed eye-lid in the vicinity and direction of the superior arch of the orbit." In a few instances, this is still an acceptable operation.

During the 1800s, when some progress was being made in many types of surgery, the surgery for ptosis became more sophisticated. The first-known levator resection, performed by Bowman (2), was reported in 1857. It was done by the conjunctival approach to the levator aponeurosis. In 1883, Eversbusch (3) reported the first skin approach levator shortening, an aponeurosis tuck. Brow suspension by sutures was done in 1880 by Dransart (4), and in 1893 by Hess (5). Brow suspension by buried skin strips was done by Panas (6) in 1886 and by Tansley (7) in 1895. The Motais (8) operation and the Parinaud (9) procedure for ptosis repair by suspension from the superior rectus muscle were both reported in 1897.

Since the turn of the century, the levator muscle, the frontalis muscle, and the superior rectus muscle have continued to be used as power sources for elevation of a ptotic eyelid. The procedures for their usage and the indications for the use of each have changed greatly.

Lapersonne (10), Blaskovics (11), Agatston (12), Iliff (13), Fox (14), Leahey (15), Johnson (16), Berke (17) and Jones (18) offered improved techniques for levator shortening. Some form of one of their procedures is the favorite of most of the current ptosis surgeons.

Brow suspension ptosis repair has been improved by the use of better suspension materials, the best being autogenous fascia lata as recommended by Wright (19) in 1922. Many types of nonabsorbable suture material have been used. The favorites have been Supramid and silicone rubber.

Superior rectus eyelid suspension has been done by forming an adhesion between the tarsus and the superior rectus muscle at or near the muscle's insertion. Various methods of producing this adhesion have been used. These operations have been (or should have been) abandoned because of motility and corneal problems that followed the surgery in most instances. Singh and Singh (20) recently devised a procedure that separates the superior rectus muscle from the globe and attaches it totally to the lid. This allows independent action between the lid and the globe and causes less danger of keratitis.

The operation of Fasanella and Servat (21), which is a vertical shortening of the tarsus and Müller's muscle, was introduced in 1961. It has limited use in congenital ptosis, as it is only useful in mild cases with good levator function. It is a good operation for some cases of acquired ptosis, particularly in elderly patients.

Recent attempts have been made to utilize the lid-elevating power of Müller's muscle in the treatment of congenital ptosis. Jones (18), Mustardé (22, 23), Collin and Beard (24), and Sisler (25) have attempted to retain this muscle's function. Sufficient experience with these procedures to allow for conclusions to be drawn is currently lacking.

PATHOPHYSIOLOGY

The term *congenital ptosis* is a poor one. The word "congenital" implies "existing at or before birth." the condition that is being discussed here fits this definition. But, other types of ptosis existing since birth such as jaw-winking ptosis, congenital fibrosis of the extraocular muscles, congenital oculomotor nerve palsy, congenital misdirected third nerve, the traumatic ptosis of birth injury, the ptosis of the blepharophimosis syndrome, and perhaps other types, also are included in the term "congenital." They are different entities from "true congenital ptosis", have separate causes, and are treated differently.

The type of ptosis being discussed here comprises well over half of the ptosis population. It deserves a descriptive name in the ptosis classification to separate it from the other types of ptosis previously mentioned. Since it is not my purpose to try to change the classification that has become common through usage (even though I do not like it), I will, for this chapter, usurp the term "congenital ptosis" to signify this common entity and leave the other types of ptosis with which a person might be born to others. To emphasize the importance and independence of this syndrome, I will call it "true congenital ptosis."

In 1955, Berke and Wadsworth (26) demonstrated by light microscopy that there was a deficiency of striated muscle fibers in the levator muscle in true congenital ptosis. The degree of this deficiency is directly proportional to the severity of the ptosis and to the diminution of levator function (the millimeter excursion of the upper lid margin when the patient changes gaze from eyes-down to eyes-up). Their histologic findings were later given confirmation by the electron microscopic studies of Hornblass, Adachi, Wolintz, and Smith (27).

This deficiency of striated muscle fibers in the levator muscle in true congenital ptosis is present at birth and remains stationary throughout life. It is considered to be a localized developmental dystrophy of unknown cause. Most of the cases seen are sporadic, but some present with a positive family history of blepharoptosis.

A levator muscle with a deficiency of striated muscle fibers will not only be unable to hold its eyelid at a proper level but will be unable to contract adequately to raise the lid on upgaze and to relax adequately to allow the lid to depress on downgaze. The slight-to-moderate lid lag on downgaze is usually diagnostic of true congenital ptosis.

The dystrophy is unilateral in about 75% of the cases. In a small number of cases (about 5%) there is a weakness of elevation of the ipsilateral eye, perhaps due to a superior rectus muscle weakness. Biopsy studies of these superior rectus muscles have not been reported, and the pathologic nature of the elevation weakness has not been established. It is reasonable to postulate that since the levator muscle and the superior rectus muscle originate from the same embryologic bud, the superior rectus might in some instances be involved with the same developmental dystrophy as the levator muscle. Indeed, it seems odd that it does not happen more often. In some cases, the limited globe elevation appears more like a double-elevator palsy. This would not be so simple to rationalize, and I know of no plausible explanation.

DIAGNOSTIC EXAMINATION

The preoperative examination of ptosis patients is the most important step in their care. The condition must be accurately classified as to type and degree in order that appropriate treatment may be planned.

HISTORY

The surgeon should question about the family history of ptosis and other ocular abnormalities such as visual deficiency and strabismus. The birth history, including term, type of delivery, birth injury, and birth weight should be noted. The time that the parent or the physician first noted the ptosis is of importance. The parent should be asked whether the ptosis has remained stationary, improved, or worsened. Early photographs, if available, may be helpful.

It is well to question the parent as to whether or not the child sleeps with the ptotic eye partially open. Little has been said of this phenomenon. It is caused by the inability of the dystrophic levator muscle to fully relax and is comparable to the slight lid lag on downgaze that true congenital ptosis patients have.

Unfavorable response to previous anesthesia, particularly malignant hyperthermia, by either the patient or close relatives should be noted. If the history suggests this, a creatine phosphokinase (CPK) determination should be made. If it is high, the operation should be postponed until appropriate prophylactic treatment (Dantrolene) can be given.

The child's development, both physical and mental, are often of importance with reference to the ptosis and its treatment. The child's postoperative cooperation, or lack of it, may affect the final result.

EXAMINATION

If the child is old enough, the visual acuity should be determined. While some idea of the refractive state of the eyes should be determined, I do not feel that a cycloplegic refraction adds much to the record, although I would not argue with those who would include it for completeness of the examination and the record. A manifest retinoscopy or a neutralization of the glasses worn should suffice. An examination of the extraocular movements and a cover test should be done. About 1 ptosis patient in 5 or 6 will have some type of motility problem, with or without amblyopia. The patient should be checked for the presence of Bell's phenomenon.

Attention should now be directed to the ptotic eyelid. Inspection of the patient with the head straight and with the patient looking at the examiner will indicate whether or not significant ptosis exists. If it does, the degree of drooping can be rather accurately estimated by comparing the lid margin's level on the cornea with that on the normal side. In bilateral ptosis the levels can be compared to the average level, which is about 2 mm below the upper limbus. Good landmarks are the limbus and the upper pupillary border, which are about 4 mm apart when the pupil is not noticeably dilated or constricted. A lid with its margin at the pupillary border is about 2 mm ptotic, which is "mild." If it covers the pupil slightly, it is 3 mm ptotic, which is "moderate." If it bisects the pupil, it is 4 mm ptotic, which is "severe." In true congenital ptosis the drooping is very rarely more than 4 mm, although I have seen it as much as 6 mm. It is well to check the estimates obtained above by millimeter ruler measurements. It is difficult to measure some children's lid slits with a ruler, as they may shy away from this instrument when it is held as close as is necessary. The estimates are usually quite accurate.

Some ptosis surgeons measure the lid slits with the patient looking up and down as well as in the primary position. Some of us do not have enough gymnastic ability to take these measurements, and many children fail to cooperate sufficiently for the measurements to be significantly accurate. I do not attempt it. It stands to reason that the relative degree of ptosis will increase on upgaze because the involved levator will not elevate the lid. It also stands to reason that the lid slit will increase in size on downgaze if there is a lid lag. If the ptotic lid is lower than its fellow on downgaze, we are *not* dealing with true congenital ptosis. An estimate or measurement of the amount of ptosis combined with a note as to the relative position of the eyelid on downgaze are all that are needed at this stage of the examination.

The most important part of the preoperative examination is the measurement of the levator function, the millimeter excursion of the upper lid margin when the patient looks from far down to far up. When this measurement is being taken, it is well to apply thumb pressure on the brow to prevent the frontalis from raising the brow and adding slightly to the excursion. The measurement should be taken several times until a consistent reading is obtained. Normal readings will vary from 12 to 16 mm. The excursion in true congenital ptosis will vary from 2 mm to about 12 mm. A measurement of 8 mm or more is considered "good." One of 5 mm to 7 mm is "fair," while 4 mm or less is "poor." It is probable that when a consistent measurement of only 2 mm is obtained, the levator muscle is not active, and the excursion is transmitted from the superior rectus muscle.

The pupils should be checked for equality and for reactions. In true congenital ptosis they should be normal. The media and fundi should be examined and abnormalities noted. One should look for evidence of neurological disease that might have ptosis as a symptom. Tumor, inflammation, and hereditary and degenerative diseases would be the principal suspects. Signs of one or another of them are occasionally found during a ptosis examination.

Preoperative and postoperative photographs are an important part of the ptosis patient's record. They are routinely taken with the patient looking straight ahead, up, and down.

From the above routine steps the ptosis can be classified as to type and degree. If it turns out that they are dealing with true congenital ptosis, surgeons can now plan an approach for effective treatment. If the ptosis proves to be acquired, or one of the other types of "congenital" ptosis with which the patient might have been born, the treatment can best be planned after further study, and sometimes after consultation with other specialists.

TREATMENT

WHEN TO OPERATE

The treatment of almost all cases of true congenital ptosis is surgical. The first decision to be made is when to operate. I often hear it said that surgery should be postponed until the ages of 4 or 5. This is true in some cases, but the age of the patient is not the critical factor. Technically, levator resection or brow suspension can be done at any age. The small size of the parts to be altered should not bother the ophthalmologist or the plastic surgeon. A more important factor is the accuracy of the preoperative examination. With a few conceptions, as soon as one knows what procedure to do and can figure how much to do, the patient is operable.

The emotional status of a small child must be taken into account. Reactions to previous surgery or illness will be helpful in determining whether or not they are ready for surgery. A child's reactions to examination will also help surgeons in their decision. If, at a younger age than 4, the patient seems mature enough to reason with, surgery can be planned at any convenient time.

If the levator function is poor enough to make brow suspension essential and if the surgeon feels (as I do) that autogenous fascia lata is the suspension material of choice, he or she must be sure that the leg is long enough to make it possible to obtain fascia of adequate length. This would be a minimum of 7 to 8 cm. Shorter pieces can be spliced, but the graft is not as secure. We are usually thinking of a minimal age of 3 years, but I have seen children at the age of 1 year who could be treated by autogenous fascia lata brow suspension. One can ask, "Why not use preserved fascia?" The best reason that I can think of is that it is not as good. Reactions are more severe, and there is a definite tendency for it to lose its effectiveness after a period of time. Since this operation is meant to last a lifetime, a material should be used that has the greatest potential for fulfilling this requirement. I believe that homogenous fascia should be used only when autogenous material is unobtainable.

The question of whether early surgery is harmful or helpful has not been settled. Merriam and associates feel that early surgery can lead to high astigmatic refractive errors (28). Hoyt and associates feel that postponing the surgery can lead to high myopia (29). None of Hoyt's cases had true congenital ptosis. I have no opinion as to which concept is the best one to believe in. I have not seen either complication in the patients that I have been able to follow for long periods.

I have not seen amblyopia result from true congenital ptosis although it has been feared and has been reported. When I have seen a ptotic lid and an amblyopic eye, there has *always* been strabismus, anisometropia, or a high astigmatic error to account for the uncorrectable vision.

The psychological aspect of blepharoptosis should be taken into account. I have noticed that children usually do not become aware of the deformity until they start kindergarten. Preschool playmates make little note of it, but a strange new group of classmates tends to ask questions and to give nicknames. These tend to make impressions on some sensitive psyches. Therefore, the ideal time for surgery precedes this step toward maturity.

The proper time to plan ptosis surgery is (*a*) when the surgeon has been able to examine the patient satisfactorily enough to allow classification of the ptosis as to type and degree, (*b*) when the patient has matured enough to make a good operative and postoperative patient, (*c*) when the leg is long enough to furnish adequate fascia lata if brow suspension is indicated, and (*d*) preferably before the child is ready to start school.

CHOICE OF OPERATION

It is without question that the best power source with which to elevate the ptotic eyelid is the levator muscle. This muscle is ideally positioned and innervated. The only good excuse for not using it would be when it is obviously incapable of adequately performing this lid-elevating function. In general, poor levator function (4 mm or less of excursion) signifies this state.

When levator resection is to be done, the surgeon must have some plan regarding the amount of levator complex to resect. Some prefer to set the lid margin at a predetermined level on the cornea at the operating table. I do not like this method because it involves some variables that are difficult to control. The depth of the anesthesia, determination of the position of the globe while the patient is under general anesthesia and draped, and the tension made on the levator during the placement of the fixing sutures all make a difference in the amount of resection that will be necessary to place the lid margin at the desired level. I consider it more accurate to resect a predetermined amount of levator tissue.

There are no infallible rules or formulas for the amount of levator resection that will always lead to a perfect result. Experience in treating a large number of cases has led to the approximations that will be outlined in the following paragraphs. It must be emphasized that these figures must only be used for true congenital ptosis. They are a useful guideline that will lead to good results in most cases. Experienced operators will alter them in accordance with their own techniques and results.

In mild (2 mm) true congenital ptosis, the levator function is always good (8 mm or more). Either a Fasanella-Servat operation or a levator resection of 12 or 13 mm by either the conjunctival or the skin approach will raise the lid adequately. One wonders why such large resections are necessary. I believe that it is because all of the standard levator resection operations include the total excision of Müller's muscle, or otherwise make it ineffective, and thereby create the effect of increasing the ptosis by 2.5 mm. The Fasanella-Servat procedure only shortens Müller's muscle by about one third of its length, and it continues to exert a lifting power on the lid. Therefore, its smaller resection seems to be equally as effective as a larger levator resection.

Moderate (3 mm) true congenital ptosis has a levator function of either good (8 mm or more) or fair (5–7 mm) in almost all cases. If the levator function is good, a resection of 14 to 17 mm will suffice. If the function is fair, a resection of 18 to 22 mm will be required. Again, either approach is acceptable, the decision being determined by the surgeon's preference.

Severe (4 mm or more) true congenital ptosis never has a levator function of more than 7 mm. If the function is in the 5- to 7-mm range, a resection of 23- to 27-mm should be done by the skin approach. When this approach is used, the shortened levator can be advanced on the tarsus, and a little more lid elevation can be obtained. Also, maximum resections are easier to obtain when skin approach procedures are used. If the levator function is only 3 or 4 mm, a "supermaximum" levator resection (up to 30 mm) is an option, but usually not a very good one. Ordinarily, brow suspension becomes a necessity.

There are times, however, when the levator function is borderline and when a trial of levator shortening is indicated. This is particularly true when the ptosis is bilateral. Here, a symmetrical slight undercorrection might be preferable to full correction by "unnatural" brow suspension. If levator resection is tried and proves unsuccessful, brow suspension can be done as a secondary procedure.

In those cases with less than 4 mm of levator function the primary procedure should be brow suspension. Since a patient who has had severe unilateral true congenital ptosis with poor levator function treated by unilateral brow suspension presents a bizarre asymmetry in life that is not cosmetically appealing, we have been excising the terminal part of the levator muscle and its aponeurosis on the normal side to convert the unilateral ptosis into a bilateral one. Then, we have been elevating both lids symmetrically with bilateral fascia lata brow suspension (30). The appearance in life of two lids elevated by frontalis action is much more pleasing than that of the elevation of one lid by a normal levator and one by brow suspension. Some have performed the same bilateral brow suspension but have omitted the levator excision on the normal side. I have done this variation on occasion, but I do not feel that the overall appearance is as good, particularly in upgaze. Here, the intact levator overrides the brow suspension leading to asymmetry. It is fortunate that most cases of severe true congenital ptosis with less than 4 mm of levator function are bilateral. Here, there is no question as to the proper procedure. Bilateral brow suspension (preferably with autogenous fascia lata) is the operation of choice.

The true congenital ptosis with weakness of elevation of the ipsilateral eye requires a slightly different approach. If the eyes are level in the primary position, it is best to ignore the hypotropia and treat the ptosis by the rules previously given. However, if levator resection is the operation to be done for the particular ptosis, the amount of resection should be increased by 3 or 4 mm. If there is hypotropia when the eyes are in the primary position, the vertical strabismus should first be corrected by surgery, which is outside of the scope of this chapter. The ptosis should then be reevaluated. The correction of the strabismus will often increase the ptosis measurably.

SURGICAL TECHNIQUES

In the previous section, reference was made to six operations, one for weakening of the normal levator in patients with severe unilateral ptosis with poor levator function, one for obtaining fascia lata, and four for the correction of blepharoptosis. There are many other operations that may be useful to the ptosis surgeon, but by the use of these six procedures almost all cases of true congenital ptosis can be successfully treated. These are the operations that I have used most frequently in my ptosis surgery:

Levator Excision

As previously discussed, it is occasionally good treatment to create a ptosis of the normal eyelid for the sake of symmetry. Excision of the terminal levator muscle, its aponeurosis and attached Müller's muscle is shown in Figure 14.1. This operation is an easy and an effective one for this purpose. It is also useful in the treatment of jaw-winking ptosis, to nullify the synkinetic eyelid movements preparatory to brow suspension.

Fasanella-Servat Operation

This procedure was reported as a "levator resection procedure." It is really a shortening of Müller's muscle and the upper third of the tarsus. When the lid is everted preparatory to applying the curved hemostats shown, the levator aponeurosis retracts upward and out of the operative field. As performed for many years, a combination of continuous mattress and running sutures was used without complication. This was made possible by the availability of a fine 6-0 plain gut suture that was gas sterilized and rapidly softened in the conjunctival sac. It did not irritate the cornea. This suture material is no longer available; and *substitutes should NOT be used with this suture placement as keratitis will almost surely result.* The suturing technique that I now use is shown in Figure 14.2. A single running 6-0 plain gut suture is placed subconjunctivally to avoid its contacting the cornea. A temporary "pullout" suture holds the tissues in position while the subconjunctival suture is being placed.

Levator Resection by the Conjunctival Approach

The procedure shown in Figure 14.3 has been modified from the operation of Agatston (12). The levator aponeurosis is easy to identify, as it is the first layer encountered when an incision is made through the tarsus close to its upper border. The operation is easily and quickly done. The recovery period is more rapid than that following skin approach levator resection. I prefer it for mild or moderate true congenital ptosis and for levator resection following undercorrection (see "Complications").

Levator Resection by the Skin Approach

This operation (Fig. 14.4) has been modified slightly from the procedure of Johnson (16) and that of Berke (17). Identification of the levator aponeurosis is made easy by carrying the dissection through the full thickness of the lid and then identifying it from its posterior aspect. In this way and at this level there are few confusing layers.

Obtaining Fascia Lata and Brow Suspension Using Autogenous Fascia Lata

The "harvesting" of fascia lata is not a difficult procedure. Ophthalmologists can learn it easily. There are several methods described using different instruments. I am including one using the Masson stripper. The Crawford and the Mustardé strippers are both good, as are others.

There are several techniques for the placement of fascia lata in the eyelid. The technique of Crawford (31) is one of the better ones. It allows good control of the contour of the lid margin by having two areas of suspension.

Fascia lata removal is shown in Figure 14.5, and its placement by the Crawford method is shown in Figure 14.6.

RESULTS

The results of the treatment of true congenital ptosis by the methods outlined have been quite good (Figs. 14.7–14.12). By "good," it is meant that the final result was very close to what had been predicted preoperatively. The result depends largely upon the preoperative levator function. When it is 8 mm or more, the lid can usually be

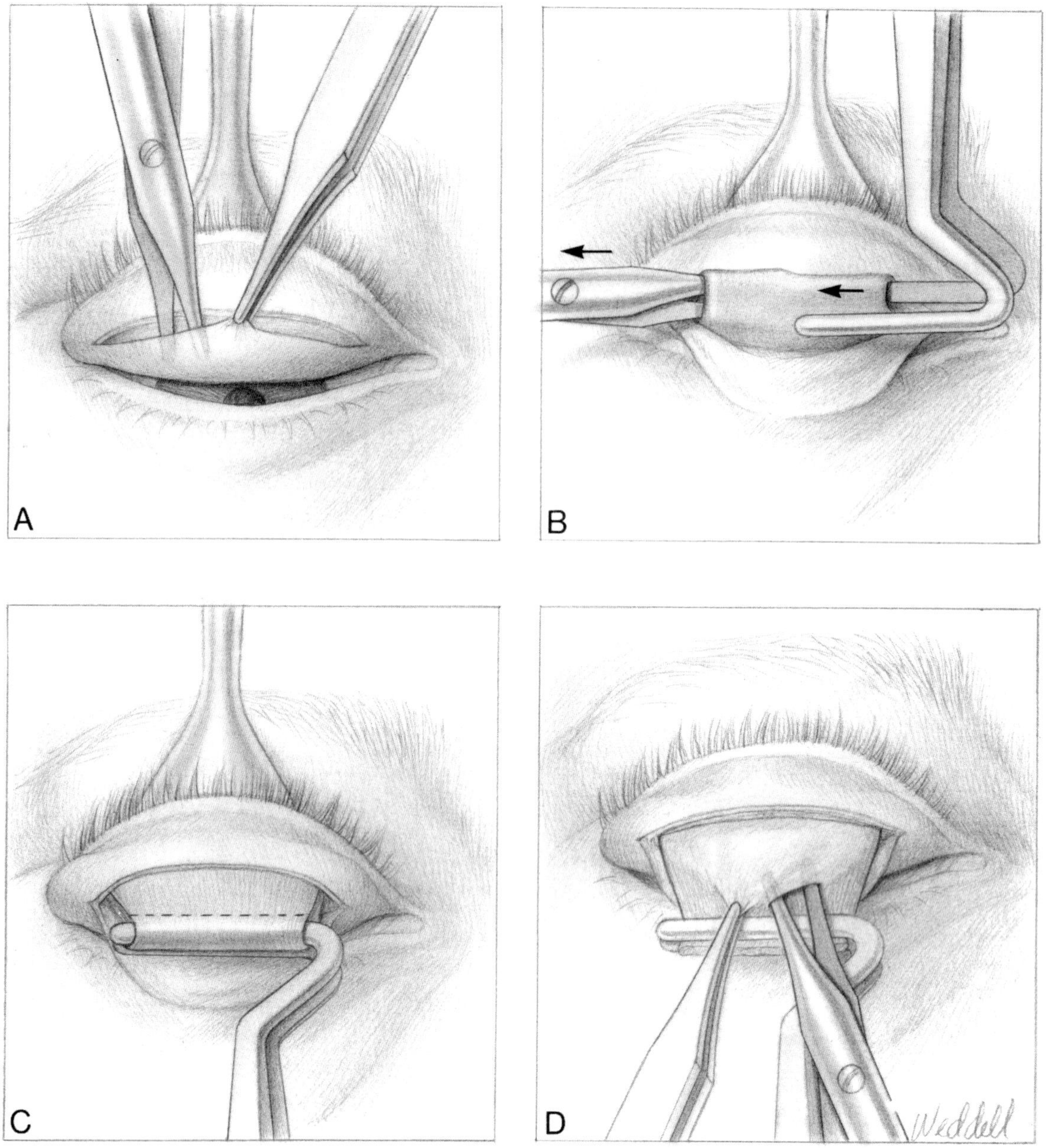

Figure 14.1. Excision of levator muscle. *A*, The lid is everted over a lid retractor. A shallow incision is made through the conjunctiva at the upper border of the tarsus. The conjunctiva is undermined from Muller's muscle. *B*, The levator aponeurosis and Muller's muscle are undermined with scissors. A ptosis clamp is inserted as the scissors is withdrawn. *C*, The clamp is rotated downward, and the tissues held in it are separated from their terminal attachments. *D*, The orbital septum is elevated from the levator aponeurosis. *E*, The horns of the levator aponeurosis are cut with small snips in direct view until the levator tissue can be delivered into the wound. *F*, The levator muscle is clamped about 15 to 20 mm above the ptosis clamp and divided in the crush mark. When bleeding has been controlled, by cautery if necessary, the levator muscle is allowed to retract into the orbit. *G*, The conjunctival wound is closed with a subconjunctival 6-0 plain catgut suture. (Adapted from Beard C: *Ptosis*, ed 3. St. Louis, CV Mosby, 1981.)

placed within a millimeter of the desired height, often exactly at it. The lid excursion will still be deficient but not sufficiently so to be noticeable. The postoperative lid lag will be slightly increased over its preoperative state. The patient may sleep with the operated eye open by a small amount, but this does not seem to cause keratitis. Both parent and patient are usually satisfied with the result obtained.

When the levator function has been only fair, the lid height is also usually satisfactory. The lid lag is apt to be

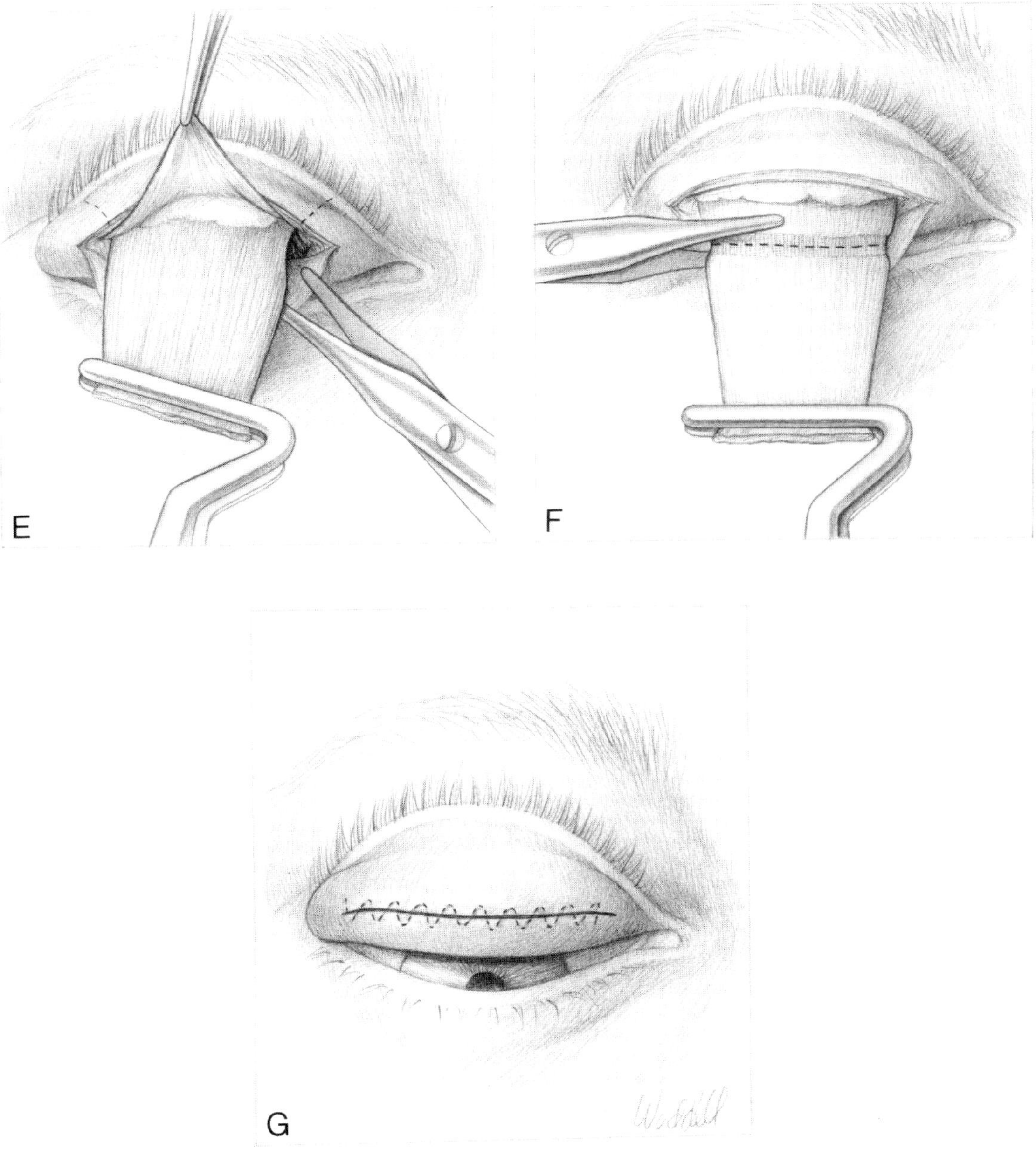

Figure 14.1. *E–G.*

noticeable and the blink is asymmetric. The patient takes an excellent picture, which looks impressive when compared with the preoperative photo. The patient and family can usually be convinced that the result is good. But, "touch up" operations are often useful in making both doctor and patient happier. The final result is often better when the ptosis was bilateral. Symmetrical lid lag and deficient blink are cosmetically acceptable.

When the levator function has been poor, the result is never as good as one would want. Since this can be anticipated, the patient and/or family should be forewarned. The lid lag from brow suspension is not preventable. While the eyes should open well, they will not close as well. Fortunately, the eyes being somewhat open at night does not seem to bother the patient. The corneas of young patients seem to adjust quickly to exposure. Lubricants at bedtime may be needed, but usually not for over a few weeks.

If maximum or supermaximum levator resection has been done for a case with poor levator function, the lid lag is almost as bad as that following brow suspension, but it is a little less noticeable. The principal disadvantage of this type of treatment is that the result is often not permanent. In a matter of several months, or even years, many of the lids that seemed to be adequately elevated have tended to redevelop some degree of ptosis, sometimes as bad as the preoperative state. Secondary operations are then indicated. If repeated levator shortening is done, the postoperative lid excursion is apt to be reduced. Usually brow suspension is needed.

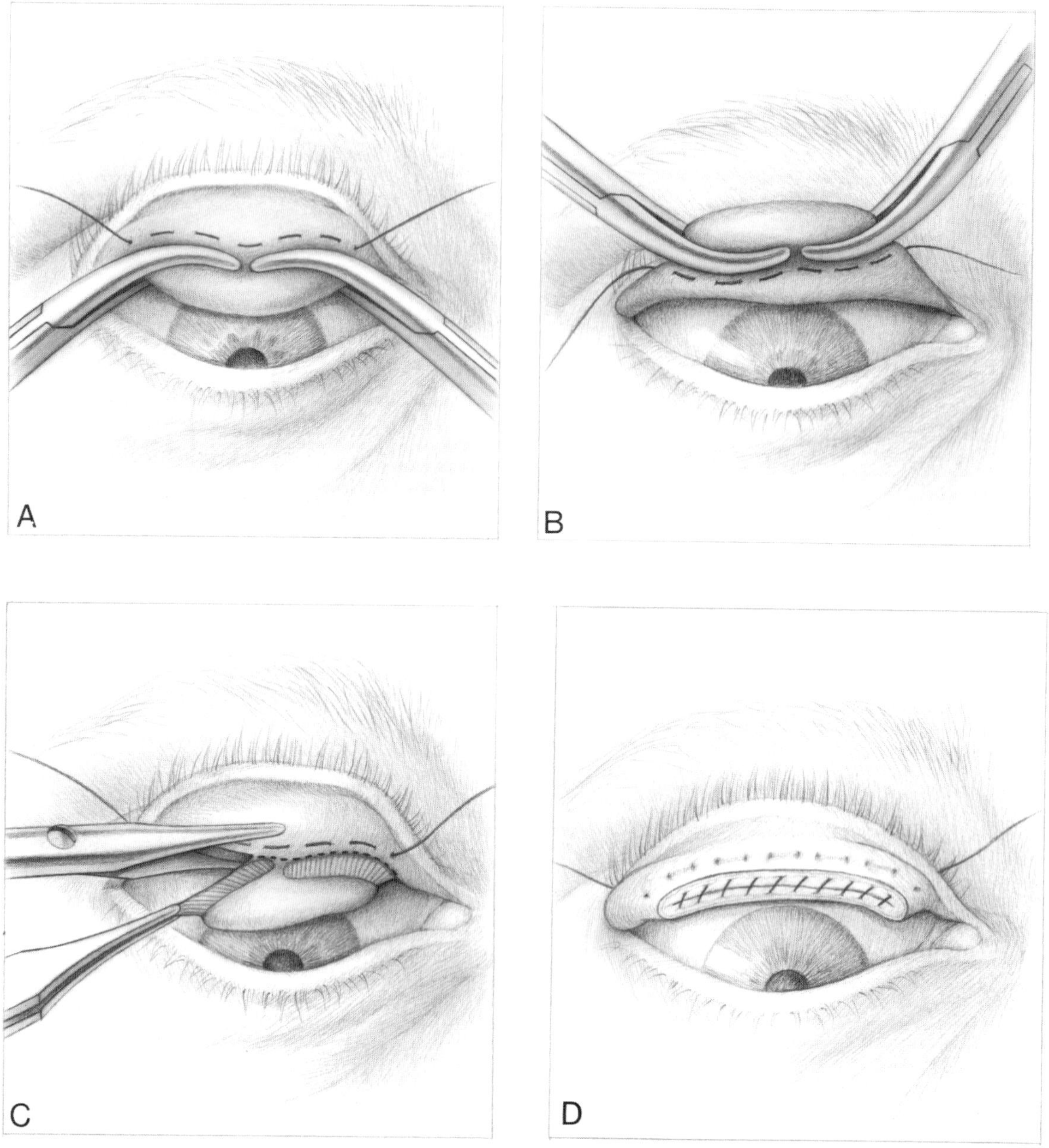

Figure 14.2. Fasanella-Servat operation (modified). *A*, The eyelid is everted. A lid retractor is not used as it would force the levator aponeurosis down into the operative level. Two hemostats are placed as shown. The bases are forced toward the lid margin, and the tips are forced toward the top of the tarsus. This prevents postoperative "peaking". A temporary monofilament suture is placed in running mattress fashion above the clamps. *B*, The clamps are turned upward to show the underside of the monofilament suture placement. *C*, The clamps are removed. The tissues included (tarso-conjunctiva, upper third of the tarsus, lower third of Muller's muscle and a small amount of palpebral conjunctiva) are excised along the crush marks. *D*, A double-armed 6-0 plain catgut suture placed subconjunctivally joins Muller's muscle to the top of the tarsus. The two ends of this suture are brought out through the full thickness of the lid where they can be locked to the skin or their ends loosely tied together. The monofilament suture is now withdrawn. By this suture placement no suture material will touch and irritate the cornea. (Adapted from Beard C: *Ptosis*, ed 3. St. Louis, CV Mosby, 1981.)

COMPLICATIONS

A complication should be considered as something that is present postoperatively that will need further treatment or something that might have been prevented. Ptosis repair has its share of complications. Ptosis repair is a type of surgery in which every result cannot be expected to be perfect. Disappointment by patient and/or surgeon should not necessarily be considered a complication. Indeed, if the possible outcomes of the surgery are considered and

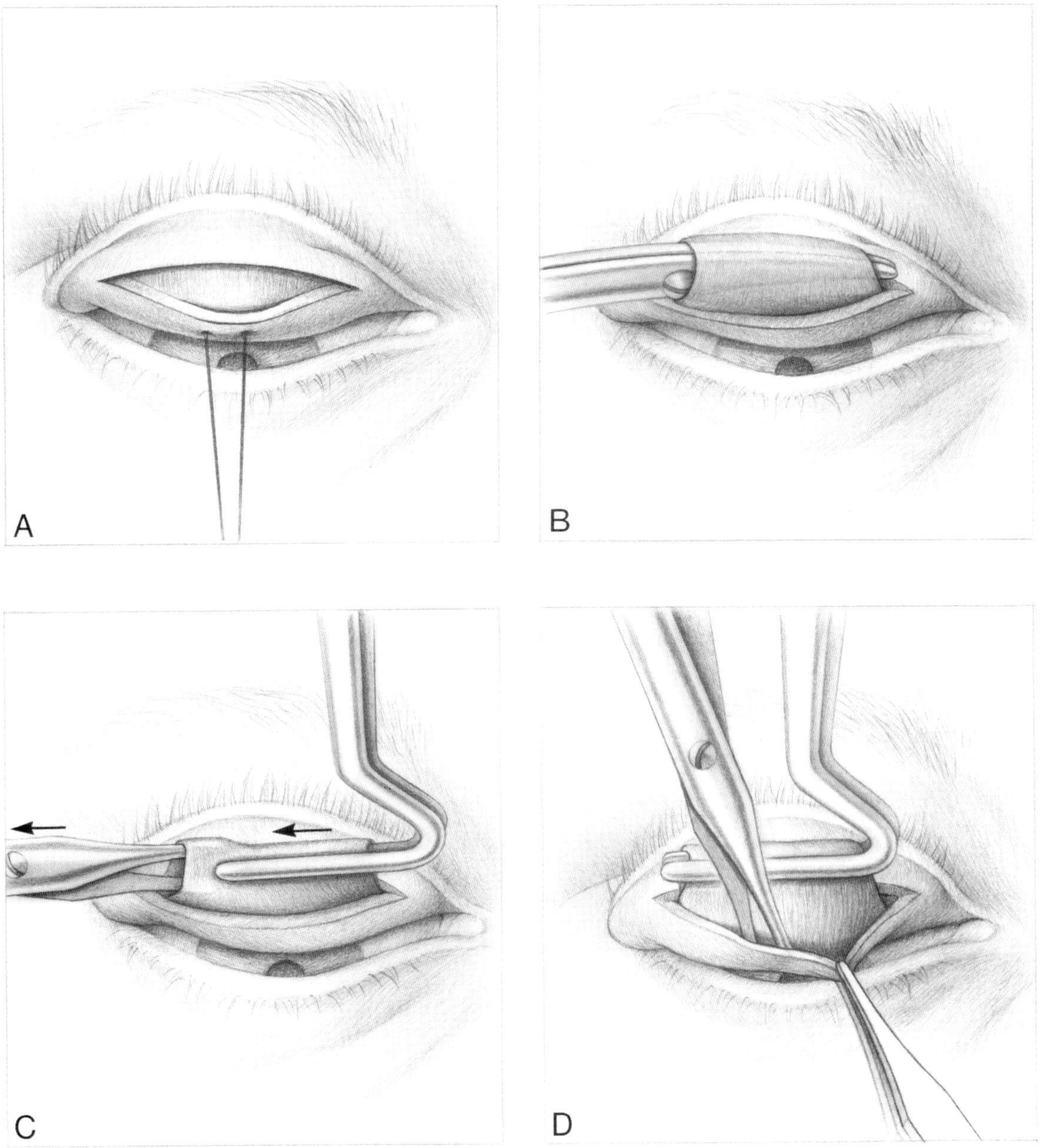

Figure 14.3. Levator resection by the conjunctival approach. *A*, The upper lid is everted. The upper border of the tarsus can be fixed with a suture or held by the assistant with a forcep. A scratch incision is made through the tarsus and into the pretarsal space from 1 to 3 mm below its upper border. *B*, The levator aponeurosis, which is the next layer, is undermined with scissors. *C*, A Berke ptosis clamp is made to follow as the scissors is withdrawn. It is well to place the clamp as shown with the handle up. *D*, The tarsal remnant is used for traction. The attachment of Müller's muscle is severed from the upper tarsal border, and the conjunctiva is undermined to the height of the superior fornix. *E*, The tarsal remnant is excised. *F*, The handle of the Berke ptosis clamp is rotated downward and the levator aponeurosis is divided from its terminal attachments. *G*, Traction is made on the ptosis clamp. The orbital septum is identified and is elevated from the levator aponeurosis. Preaponeurotic fat can usually be identified at this stage of the dissection. *H*, Traction is made on the ptosis clamp. The levator muscle is here prevented from delivery into the wound by the intact levator horns. These can be palpated. Snipping them under direct view is done until the amount of levator tissue desired can be brought into the operative field. *I*, Three double-armed sutures (5-0 chromic catgut is good) are placed in the levator muscle at a predetermined height above the clamp. *J*, The sutures are made to engage the edge of the fornix conjunctiva. The excess levator is excised. *K*, The needles are brought through the tarsus at its upper edge and are carried through the full thickness of the lid, to emerge at the desired site of the lid crease. *L*, A cross section shows the suture path through the levator, fornix conjunctiva, upper edge of the tarsus, through the full thickness of the lid and through a bolster. The levator is shortened, the continuity of the conjunctiva is reestablished, and the lid crease is formed by this suture placement. A Frost suture is placed in the lower lid and taped to the brow for corneal protection. (From Beard C: *Ptosis*, ed 3. St. Louis, CV Mosby, 1981.)

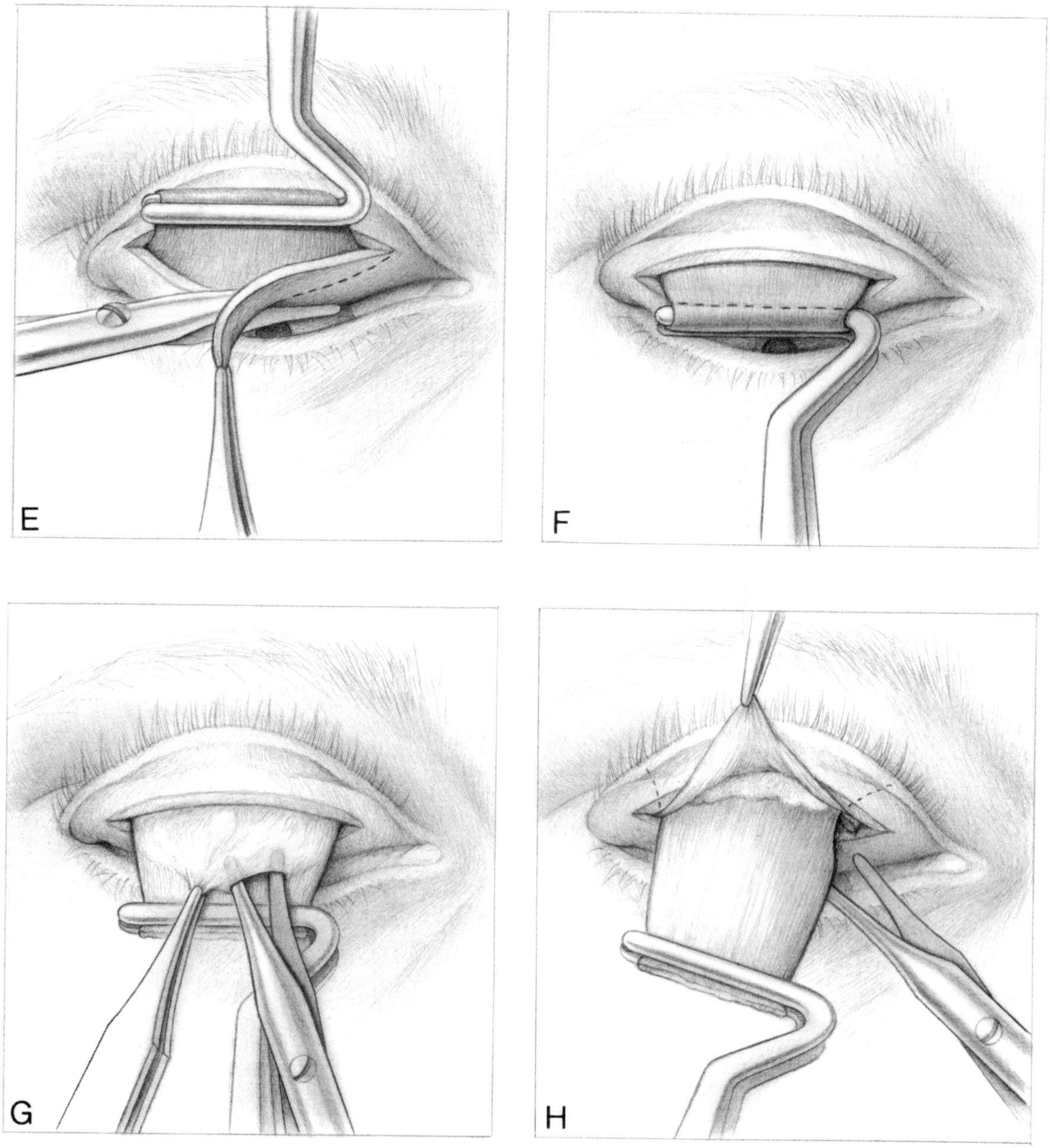

Figure 14.3. *E–H.*

explained preoperatively, postoperative dissatisfaction should not be the significant factor that it is.

By far, the most frequent complication of true congenital ptosis surgery is undercorrection. Overcorrection is occasionally seen. Usually it follows reoperation. These and the other complications that are seen from time to time and their treatment will be discussed.

UNDERCORRECTION

Undercorrection is the result of the resection of too little of the levator muscle and/or its aponeurosis or of using levator resection when brow suspension was indicated. When the levator function has been good, the lid tends to rise over a period of up to 2 months after the surgery. When the levator function has been fair, it may also rise, but to a lesser degree. When the levator function has been poor, the lid tends to remain at the same level or to drop slightly in the weeks after the operation. It may drop considerably over the years to come. For these reasons, it is well to postpone evaluation and decision as to further surgery for at least 2 months.

Undercorrection can be reduced in frequency by taking good preoperative measurements and by resecting the full indicated amount of tissue at surgery. It may be better to take a millimeter or so more than planned because of the tendency toward undercorrection at the first operation for true congenital ptosis. Suture slippage should not be a problem if the sutures are firmly tied. There is little room for careless surgery.

In unacceptable undercorrection still exists after a pe-

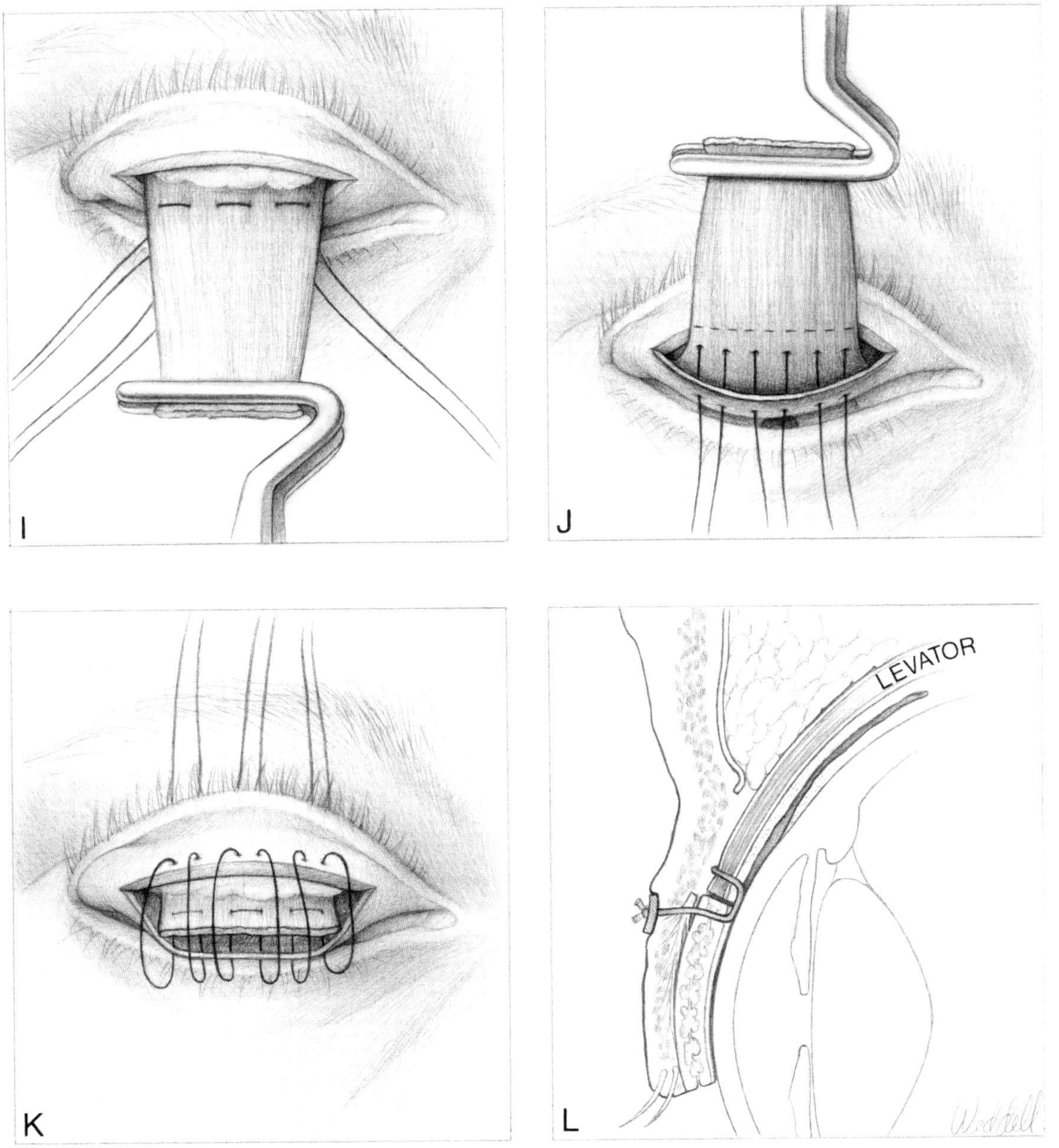

Figure 14.3. *I–L.*

riod of 2 months or more, additional surgery is indicated. The ptosis should then be evaluated as to degree and severity as was done originally. The amount of resection to be done is determined as before. However, there is a tendency to resect too much the second time, and for this reason it well to resect a millimeter or so less than planned. Also, because of the overcorrection danger, I usually use the conjunctival approach in which I tie the sutures externally. This makes them available for early removal in case of overcorrection.

If the undercorrection is only 2 mm or less, a vertical resection of about 4 mm of posterior lamellar lid tissue above the upper tarsal border may give the lid the needed extra lift. This can also be done by a Fasanella-Servat type of posterior resection if the tarsus has not been previously shortened. A full-thickness supramarginal lid resection as recommended by McCord (32) is another way of "touching up" a mild undercorrection.

If the levator function is less than 5 mm and the residual ptosis is more than 3 mm, brow suspension is probably the best secondary procedure. If the ptosis is unilateral, I am of the opinion that the terminal part of the normal levator should be excised and that for the sake of symmetry both lids should be suspended from the brows with fascia lata.

OVERCORRECTION

While overcorrection of true congenital ptosis is rare, it is distressing to the patient and embarrassing to the surgeon. Fortunately, it is fairly easy to treat successfully.

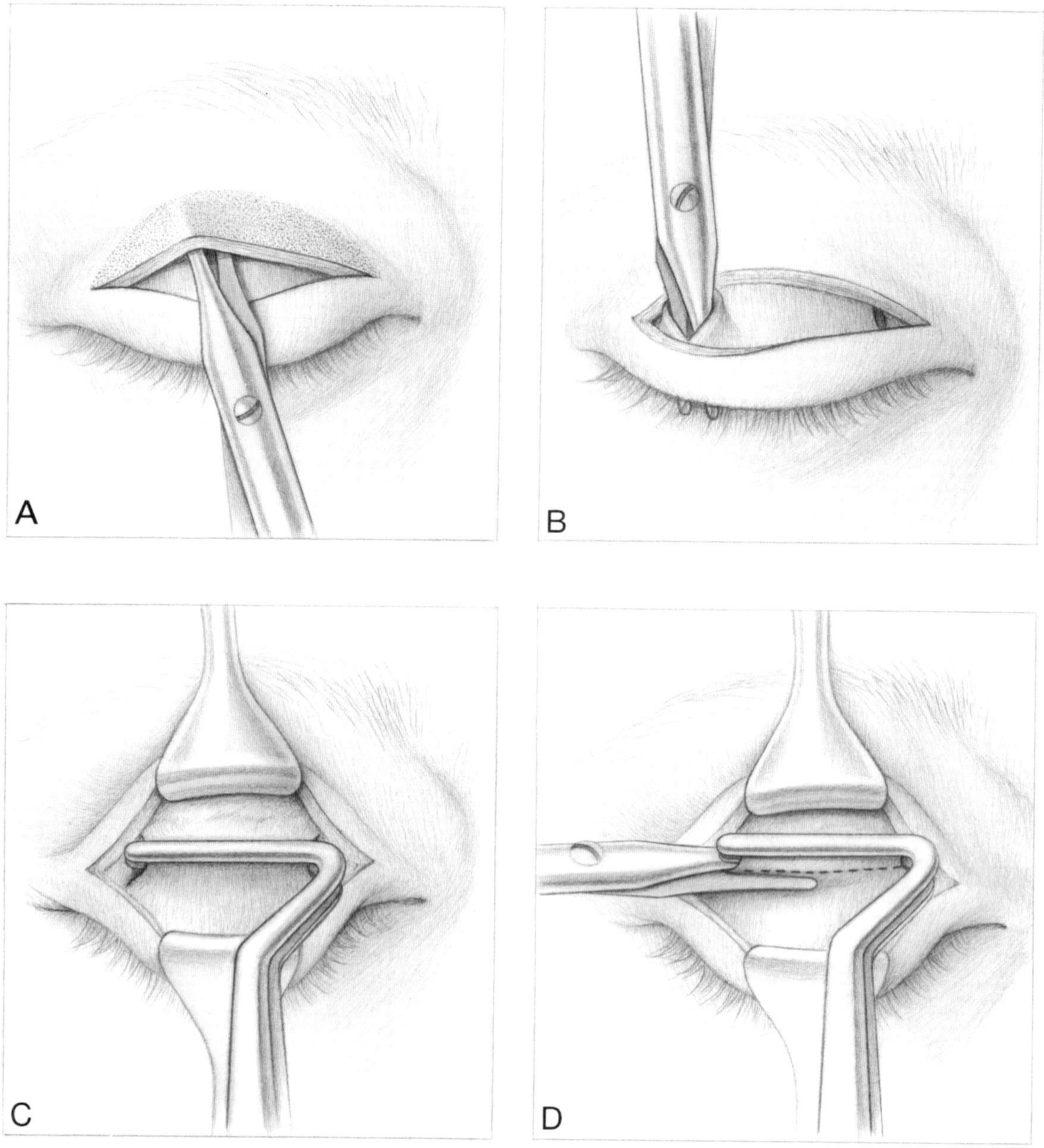

Figure 14.4. Levator resection by the skin approach. *A*, A skin incision is made at the desired lid crease level. The skin and preseptal orbicularis muscle are undermined superiorly for a distance of 6 or 7 mm. *B*, Incisions are made with scissors at the two ends of the skin incision. They are made through the full thickness of the lid, into the superior fornix. *C*, A Berke ptosis clamp is placed between the two incisions, the deep blade lies upon the conjunctiva at the upper tarsal border. *D*, The tissues included in the ptosis clamp are divided from their attachments at the upper tarsal level. *E*, The clamp is rotated upward, exposing the palpebral conjunctiva. This is undermined and freed from the ptosis clamp. *F*, The conjunctiva is brought downward to its original position. *G*, The conjunctiva is resutured to the upper tarsal border using 6-0 plain catgut. Müller's muscle and the levator aponeurosis are now easily identified. *H*, The ptosis clamp is now lowered, and the orbital septum is elevated from the levator aponeurosis exposing the preaponeurotic fat pad. *I*, Traction is made on the ptosis clamp, and the medial and lateral horns of the levator aponeurosis is severed by small snips made under direct view. Some 20 mm of levator can now be delivered into the wound. If a larger resection is planned, it may be necessary to cut the superior transverse ligament on the two sides of the muscle. *J*, The planned amount of levator tissue resection is measured. Three 5-0 chromic catgut sutures are placed in the levator at this level and tied with double knots. *K*, The excess levator tissue is excised below the sutures. *L*, The three sutures are fixed to the anterior surface of the tarsus and tied with single knots. *M*, If the contour is satisfactory, triple knots are tied. If not, the sutures can be removed and replaced in the tarsus until they are felt to be at the proper levels. If the resection has been large, a crescent of skin is removed above the original incision. *N*, Three skin sutures of 6-0 plain catgut are placed. They are fixed to the levator muscle to assure the postoperative presence of the lid crease. *O*, Additional skin sutures are placed as needed. The fornix conjunctiva is checked for prolapse (see "Complications"). A Frost suture is placed in the lower lid and taped to the brow for corneal protection. (From Beard C: *Ptosis*, ed 3. St. Louis, CV Mosby, 1981.)

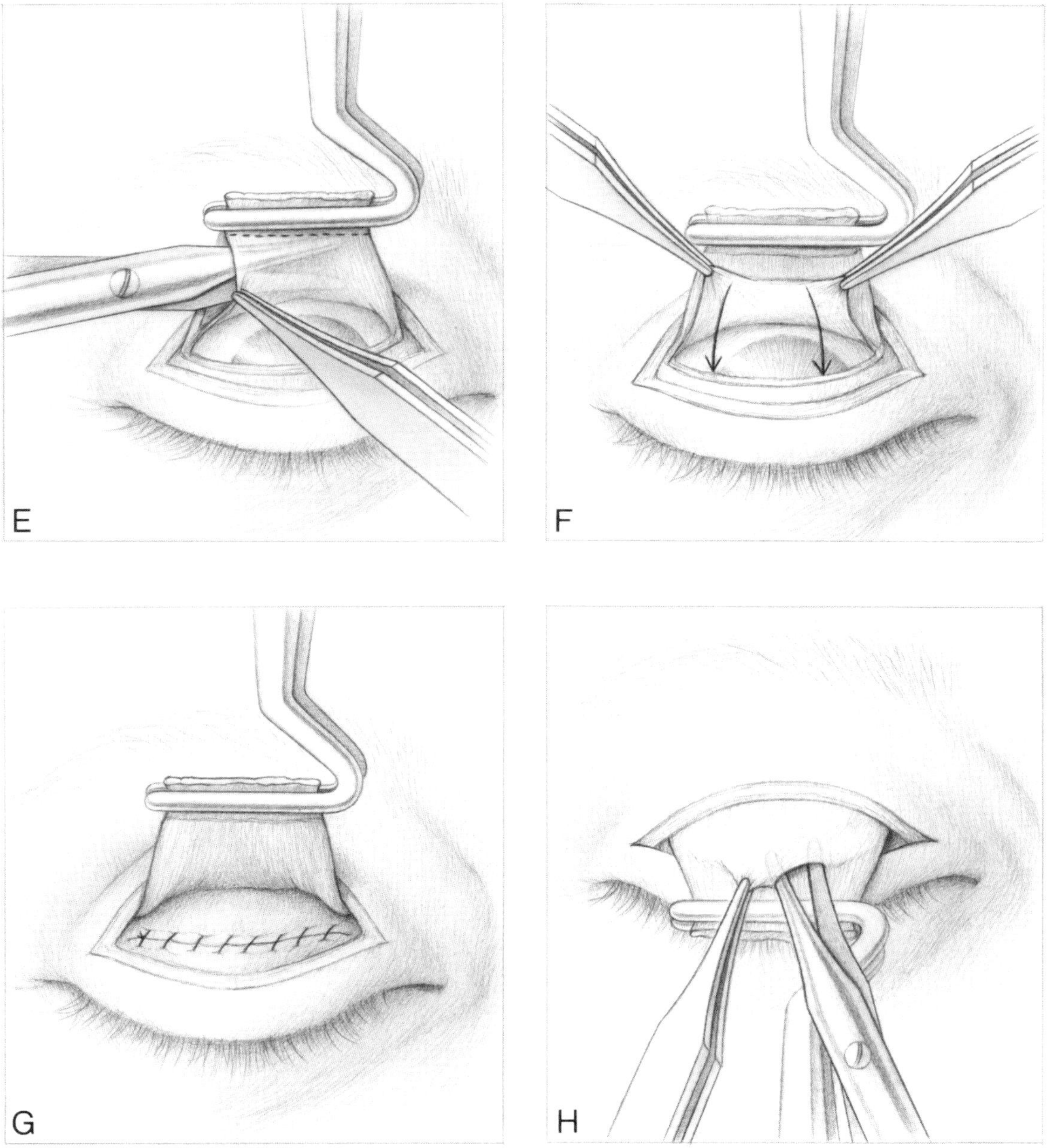

Figure 14.4. *E–H.*

If overcorrection is noted at the first dressing and if the operation has been done by the conjunctival approach, the center suture should be removed. If the lid is still high on the following day, the medial and lateral sutures are removed. Usually, enough adhesion has formed by this time that the lid does not fall completely. The level is checked daily. If the lid remains high after a day or two, "squeezing" exercises are started. If there is still overcorrection, massage is started with the patient looking down. The massage is given in a downward direction, and is performed for 5 or 10 minutes two or three times a day.

During the 2nd week more drastic steps should be taken if the overcorrection persists. The lid can be doubly everted on a Desmarres retractor and traction made on the lid. This requires general anesthesia in children but can be done under local anesthesia in cooperative adults. This maneuver can be repeated if necessary, and if the process does not become a problem from the anesthesia standpoint.

If the above regime has not been successful in lowering the eyelid, it is best to allow the tissues to heal and to plan on corrective surgery at a later period. The length of the waiting period should be about 2 or more months. During this period, I usually have the patient continue massage. Sometimes I have thought that it helped a little. If there is lagophthalmos, corneal lubrication must be kept in mind. Burning, tearing, and corneal staining are symptoms and signs that active treatment is essential. A moisture shield

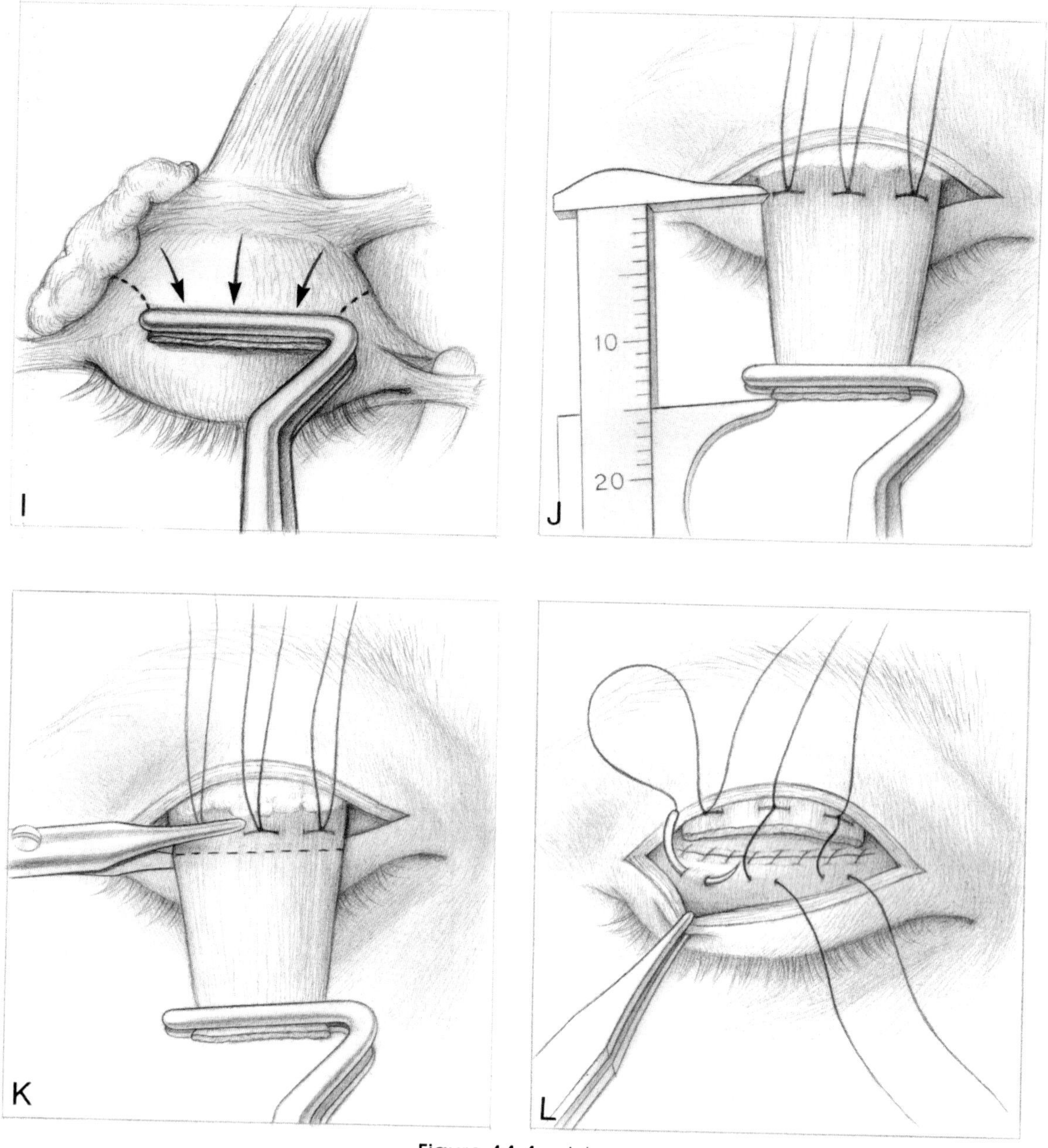

Figure 14.4. *I–L.*

may be necessary, but usually taping of the lids at night, along with the use of artificial tears and ointments, will suffice.

When the lid appears "quiet," the amount of overcorrection is assessed. The amount of excess elevation is measured.

An overcorrection of 1 mm or slightly more can be relieved by a levator tenotomy. The lid is anesthetized and everted on a Desmarres retractor. A scratch incision is made through the tarsus about 1 mm below and parallel to its upper border. The incision is carried deeper until the wound edges spread by about twice the amount of desired effect (33). A reverse-Frost suture is then placed in the upper lid and is taped to the cheek to hold the lid on downward traction.

An overcorrection in the region of 2 or 2.5 mm can be relieved by Berke's recession of the levator with suture fixation (33). This can be effectively done by starting with the tenotomy described above. When the levator tissue has been divided, the dissection is carried superiorly along the anterior surface of this muscle until it can retract. A running 6-0 plain catgut suture is used to fix the cut edge of the levator and the tarsoconjunctiva to the preseptal muscle fibers. The suture is placed in such a way that it will hold the conjunctival edges apart by about twice the amount of the desired lowering of the lid. The denuded area left open covers with conjunctival epithelium within a matter of 4 or 5 days. A reverse Frost suture holding the lid with downward traction enhances the effect of the procedure.

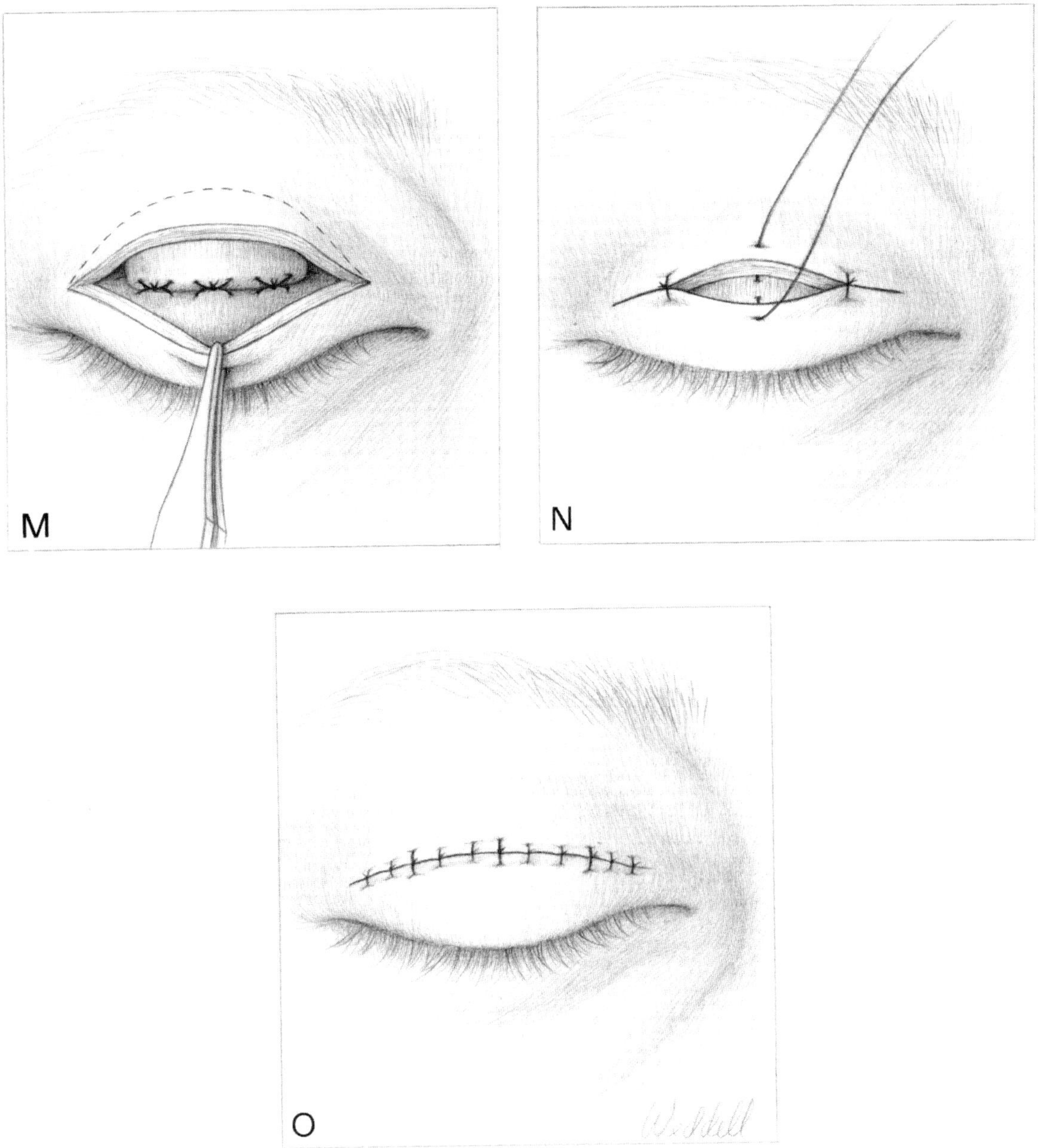

Figure 14.4. *M–O.*

If the overcorrection amounts to 3 mm or more, the above procedures will help but will usually result in insufficient lowering of the lid. In these instances I prefer to recess the levator with a spacer to separate it from the tarsus. Various materials have been used. An excellent one is banked human sclera that has been cleaned of uveal and Tenon's capsular remnants and preserved in 70% isopropyl alcohol. I have found it practical to separate the tissues with a spacer of preserved sclera that has been leached with water or saline for 8 to 10 hours and placed in Neosporin solution for an hour or so before use. It should be about twice the width of the desired eyelid lengthening. I prefer to cover the sclera with a flap of conjunctiva, but some feel that this is not necessary. Again, a reverse Frost suture to hold the lid on downward tension should be used.

LID LAG, LAGOPHTHALMOS AND KERATITIS

Some degrees of lid lag follows the correction of most cases of true congenital ptosis. This can hardly be considered a complication unless it results in corneal irritation caused by exposure. The patients often sleep with the eye slightly (or moderately) open but without drying or irritation of the cornea. Examination may show a minimal corneal stain, but the eye usually remains white and comfortable. In those cases where there are mild symptoms, the use of artificial tears in the daytime and a bland ointment at night will usually result in cessation of symp-

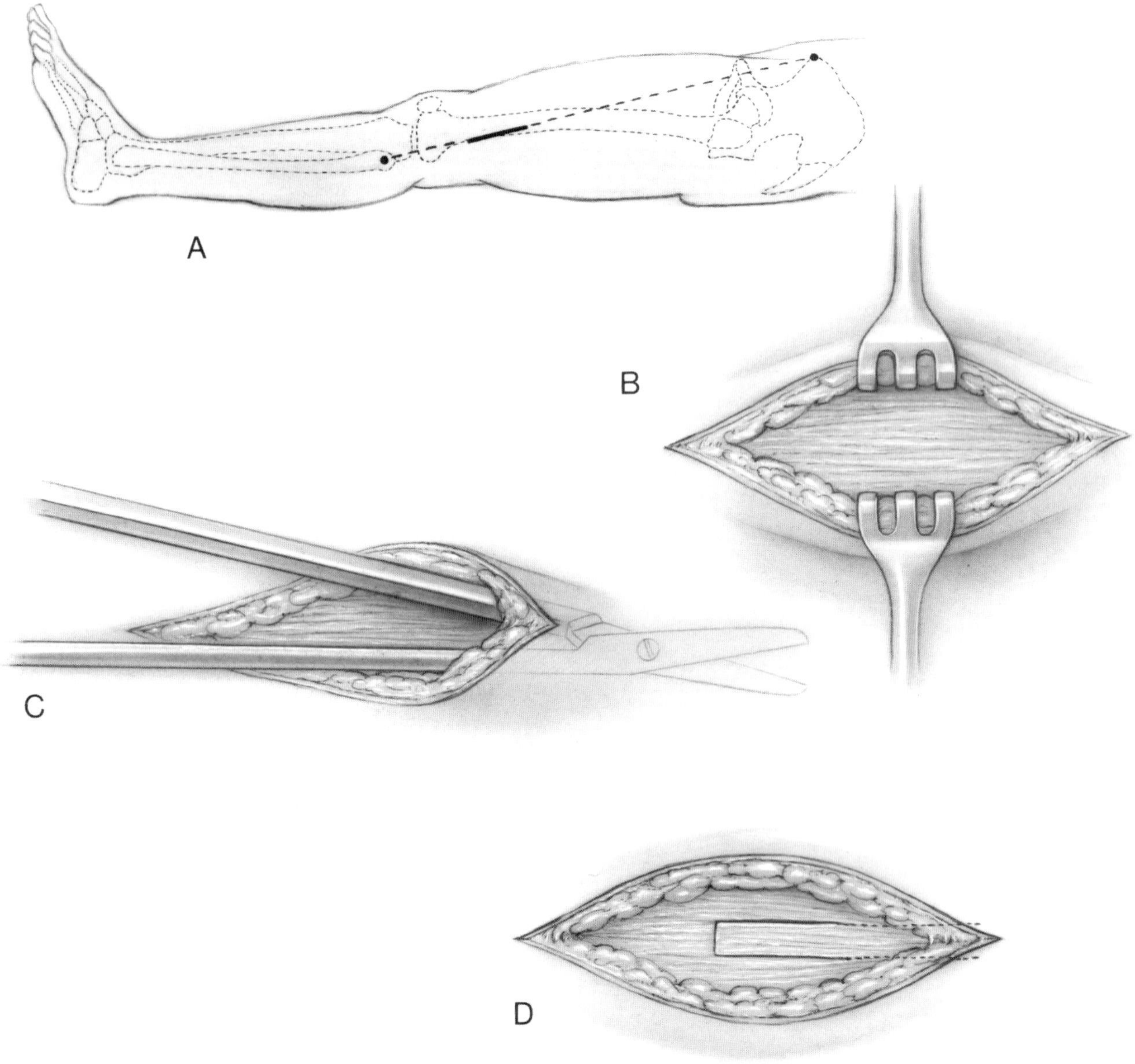

Figure 14.5. Obtaining fascia lata. *A*, The leg incision site is marked before the leg is draped. It is along a line joining the head of the fibula and the anterior superior iliac spine. It starts 5 or 6 cm above the knee joint and is 7 or 8 cm in length. *B*, The incision is carried through the skin and subcutaneous fat until the white and glistening fascia lata is exposed. *C*, The fat is elevated from the fascia lata for 8 or 10 cm by blunt dissection. *D*, Two linear incisions are made in the fascia, about 5 or 6 mm apart. From these two incisions the fascia is opened upward for a few centimeters by scissors stripping with the blades held open about 10° or by some other instrument such as the handle of a groove director. The two linear incisions are then joined by a cut between them at their lower ends. *E*, A fascia stripper is used to engage the tongue of fascia lata previously prepared. The Masson stripper is shown. *F*, The tongue of fascia is held firmly with a clamp, and the stripper is forced upward until it meets firm resistance. The strip is cut with the mechanism on the stripper being used. For bilateral surgery a second strip is taken. Each of them can now be divided lengthwise into two strips 2 or 3 mm wide and 8 to 10 cm long. *G*, The fascia is not sutured. The fat layer is closed with interrupted 4-0 plain catgut. The skin is closed with 4-0 silk. Alternate sutures can be of the vertical mattress type. (From Beard C: *Ptosis*, ed 3. St. Louis, CV Mosby, 1981.)

toms. The frequency of application can then be reduced. Usually in a few weeks the medication can be discontinued.

If the lid lag is so severe that it takes a conscious effort for the patient to close the eye, lagophthalmos exists. In this instance, keratitis of a more severe nature will result. This is extremely rare in the treatment of true congenital ptosis. The use of upper lid massage, combined with moisture shields or taping of the lids, may be necessary. If the condition fails to respond favorably to these measures, a bandage lens may be tried. If this is not practical and rapidly successful in at least stabilizing the process, one

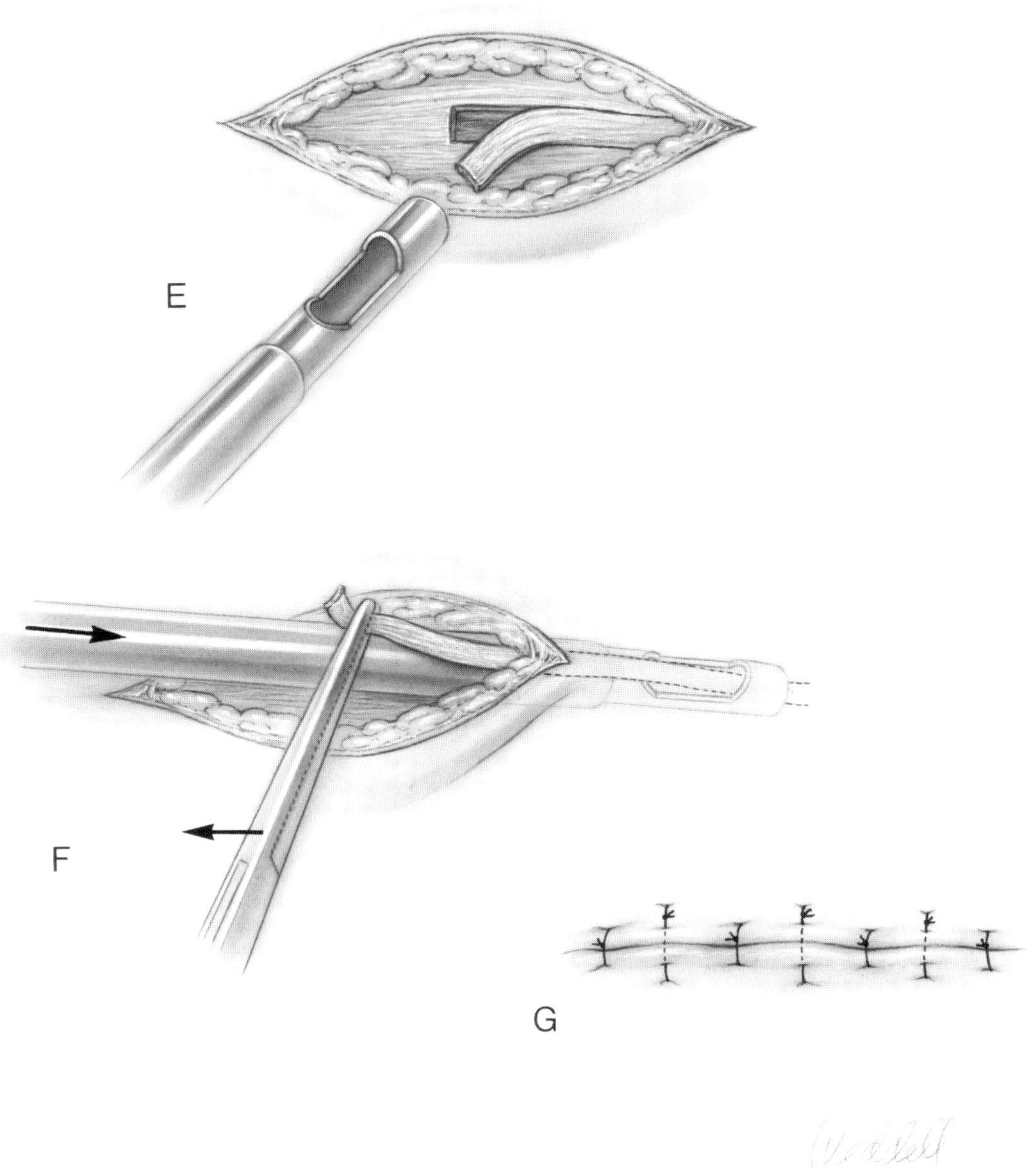

Figure 14.5. *E–G.*

must consider the surgical lowering of the lid as discussed in "Overcorrection."

ENTROPION AND ECTROPION

These complications are occasionally seen. Undue tensions on either the anterior or posterior lamellae of the lid may cause the lid margin and the lash line to be directed in an abnormal postoperative position. It may become less marked with massage, which may be tried for a period of observation unless the cornea is endangered. It is usually necessary to surgically rearrange the pretarsal tissues in order to relieve the abnormality. They may be adjusted upward or downward on the tarsus and fixed to it with three or four mattress sutures. This may be combined with excision of a preseptal crescent of skin if this tissue is redundant.

LID CREASE AND LID FOLD ABNORMALITIES

A lid crease that is too high or too low results from a skin incision that has been too high or too low if the skin approach has been used or from sutures that have been brought out at an improper level if the conjunctival approach has been used. The crease can be lowered by excising skin and underlying scar between the desired level and the existing level. Raising a crease that has been placed too low may be done by suture fixation of the skin to the underlying tissues at the desired level. Unfortunately, this is apt to expose the scar of the misplaced crease. This may or may not be of significance.

The fold of skin that normally overlies the lid crease may be redundant if the levator resection has been large and excess skin has not been excised. This is a complication that is somewhat disfiguring but which is easily rem-

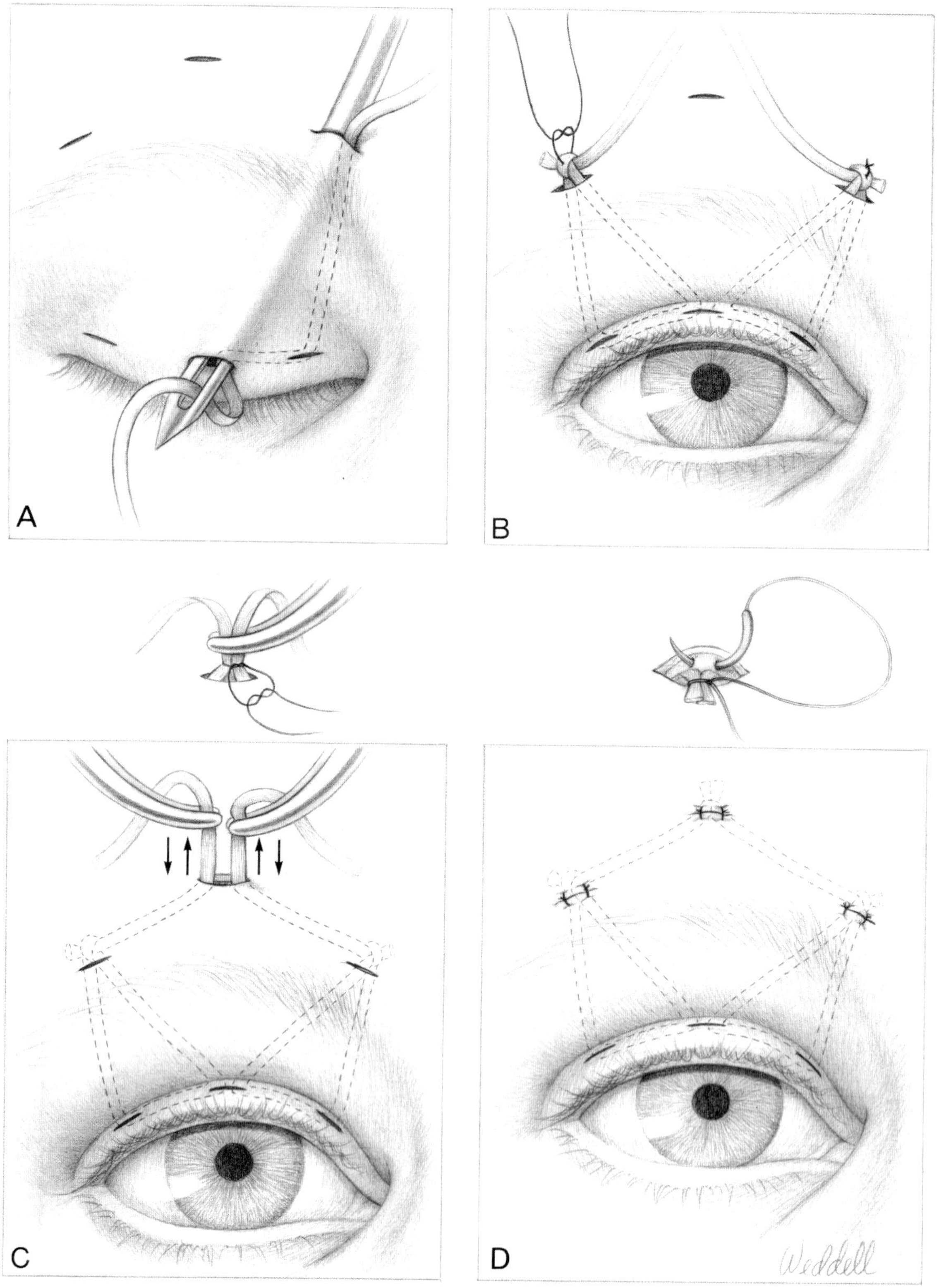

Figure 14.6. Brow suspension with fascia lata (Crawford). *A,* A total of six stab incisions are made as shown. Three are made about 2 or 3 mm above the lash line and penetrate to the tarsus. Three are made above the brow and penetrate to the periosteum of the frontal bone. Bleeding from the latter incisions may be brisk but subsides with time and pressure. With the use of a Wright needle or other similar instrument one of the fascia strips is placed in triangular fashion as shown. The fascia lies so that it is firmly fixed to the tarsus by the fibers of the levator aponeurosis attaching here. The vertical fascia is placed deep to the preseptal muscle fibers but superficial to the orbital septum. *B,* The second strip of fascia is similarly placed. The ends of each triangle of fascia are tied together with double knots, which are then reinforced with 5-0 chromic catgut ties. The knots retract into the medial and lateral

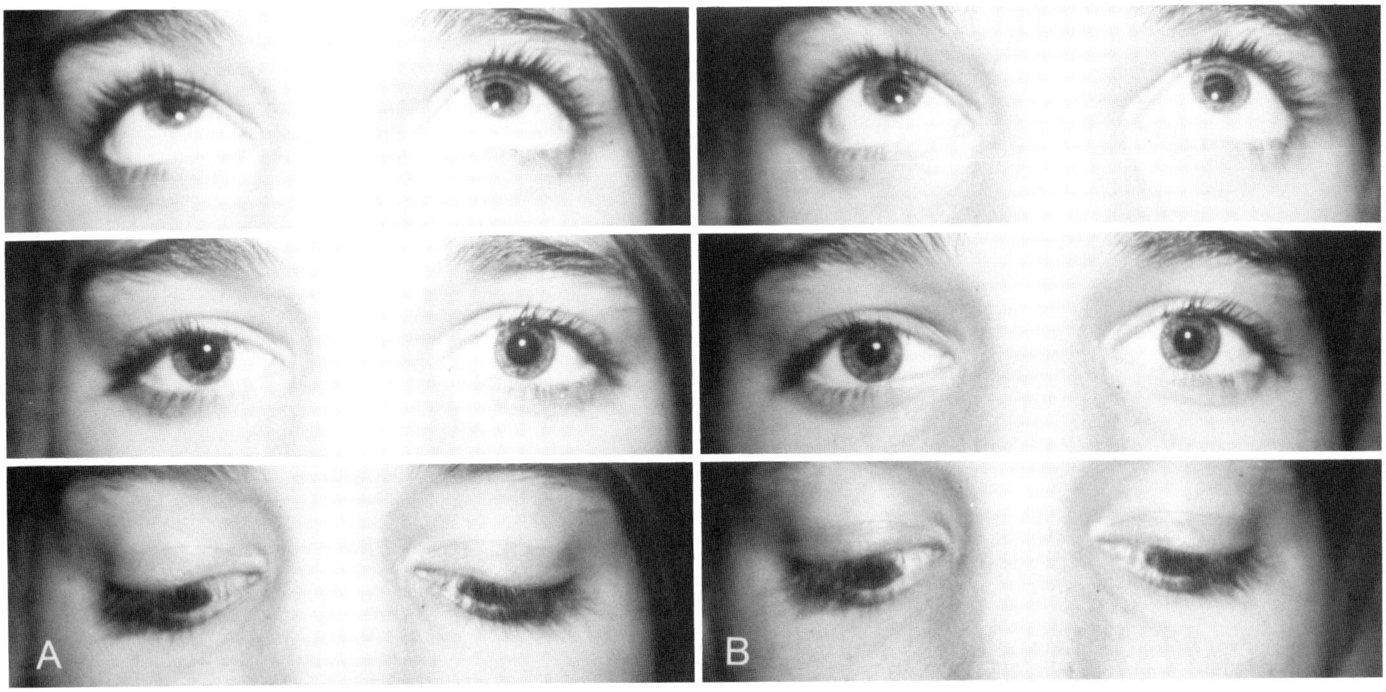

Figure 14.7. Mild (1.5 mm) "true congenital ptosis" with good (12 mm) levator function before (*A*) and after (*B*) Fasanella-Servat operation.

edied by the excision of a crescent of skin above the lid crease.

LOSS OF EYELASHES

This complication is easier to prevent than to relieve. If, during the lid dissection, the lash follicles come into view, it is best to back up and dissect no further at this level. If the follicles are damaged, the lashes will come out and most often will not regrow. Lash transplants of brow hair are technically not difficult, but they are seldom satisfactory in appearance. They require more grooming and trimming than the average child or male adult is willing to do. Older female patients can create a better appearance with artificial lashes.

CONJUNCTIVAL PROLAPSE

Prolapse of the conjunctiva of the upper fornix into the palpebral aperture sometimes follows large levator resections. If the conjunctiva prolapses at the conclusion of surgery and cannot be readily and easily replaced, two or three loosely tied mattress sutures between fornix and skin will serve to prevent later prolapse.

If the prolapse is not discovered until the first dressing, it may recede spontaneously. Steroid drops or ointment may hasten the process. If after a period of a few weeks prolapse still persists, the exposed roll of conjunctiva can be excised with minimal anesthesia. I have done this on young children by combining topical anesthesia with vocal encouragement.

HEMORRHAGE

The abundant blood supply of the eyelids creates a nuisance at surgery, but one that is usually easily overcome. There are a few larger type vessels that require cautery but usually none that require ties. Pressure and a little time will stop the oozing. The field must be dry before closure is done. Suturing of the skin in skin approach procedures often leads to brisk surface bleeding. This stops without treatment in most cases. If it does not, light cautery will suffice.

It is late bleeding that leads to concern. This may result from spontaneous breakdown of the clot at a bleeding point or it may result from minor or major trauma. The bleeding that finds its way to the outside is startling, particularly if it presents as spurting or dripping from the wound. However, as long as it is not backing up into the

brow incisions. *C*, The free ends of fascia from each triangle are passed beneath the skin to the center brow incision where each is fixed with a clamp. They are individually tightened and loosened until the lid contour seems correct. The two strips are then grasped with a single clamp at skin level. The strips are tightened until the lid margin begins to shelve away from the cornea. They are then loosened until lid contact with the cornea is barely made. A 5-0 chromic catgut ligature is placed around both strips, as shown in the *inset*, and tied tightly. *D*, The excess fascia is excised. One end of the ligature suture is then fixed to the subcutaneous tissue at the upper edge of the central brow incision, as shown in the *inset*. The frontalis fibers lie in this layer. The brow incisions are closed with 6-0 plain catgut sutures. The skin incisions near the lash line need not be sutured. A Frost suture is placed in the lower lid and taped to the brow for corneal protection. (From Beard C: *Ptosis*, ed 3. St. Louis, CV Mosby, 1981.)

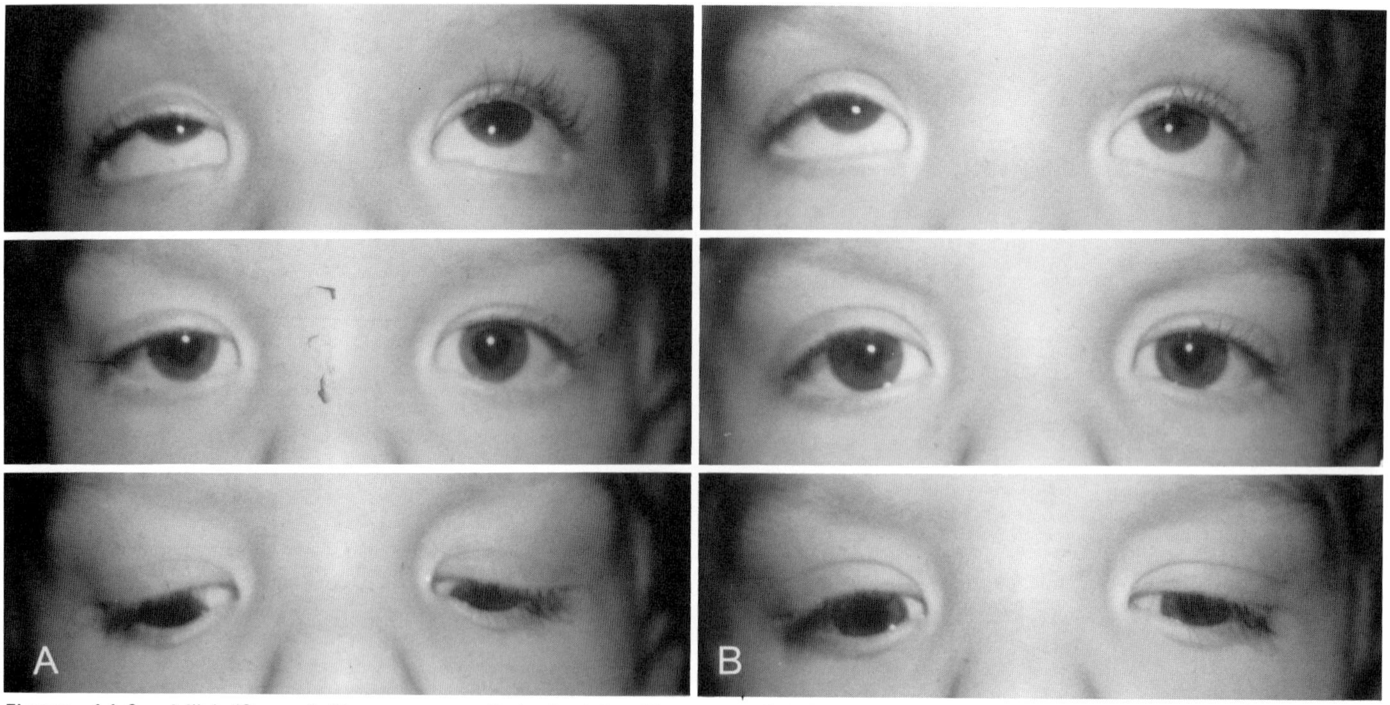

Figure 14.8. Mild (2 mm) "true congenital ptosis" with good (9 mm) levator function before (*A*) and after (*B*) small (13 mm) levator resection by the conjunctival approach.

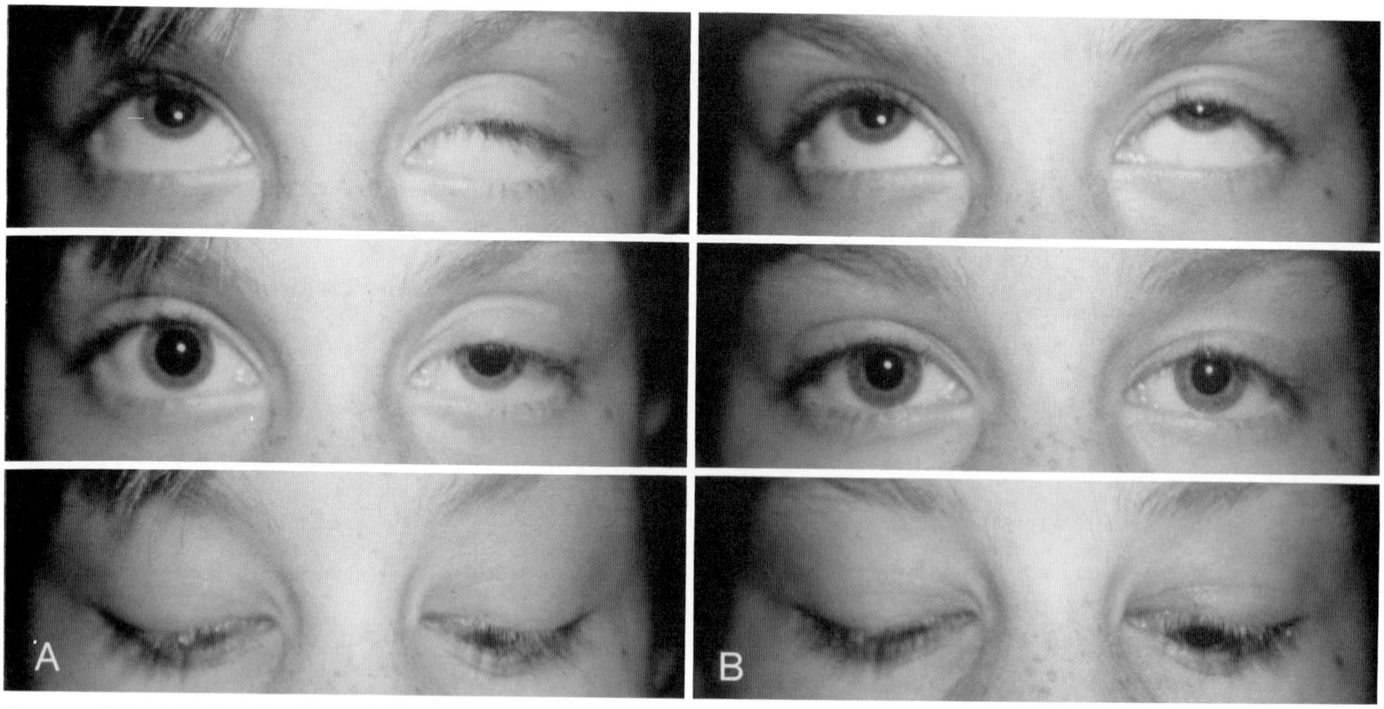

Figure 14.9. Moderate (3 mm) "true congenital ptosis" with good (8 mm) levator function before (*A*) and after (*B*) moderate (17 mm) levator resection by the conjunctival approach.

operative area and causing a hematoma, it will not jeopardize the final result. The bleeding may stop with time and pressure, in which case a pressure dressing should be applied and left in place for 2 or 3 days.

If generalized pressure does not stop the bleeding, finger pressure applied to a point above the medial or lateral canthus may be effective in stopping it. In this case, a suture can be blindly placed through the skin at this point to attempt to surround and ligate the feeding vessel central to the bleeding point. Only if the above efforts fail should the wound be opened and the bleeding vessel located and cauterized or tied.

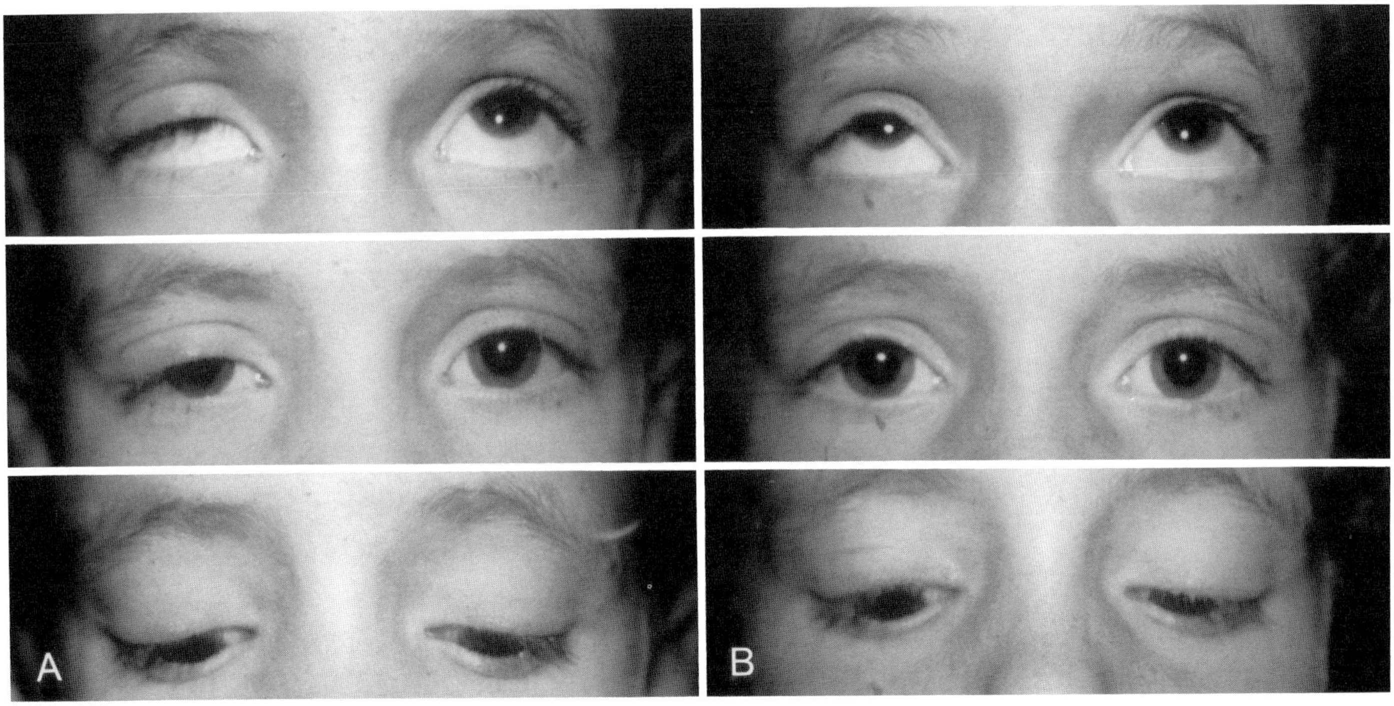

Figure 14.10. Severe (4 mm) "true congenital ptosis" with fair (6 mm) levator function before (*A*) and after (*B*) maximum (25 mm) levator resection by the skin approach.

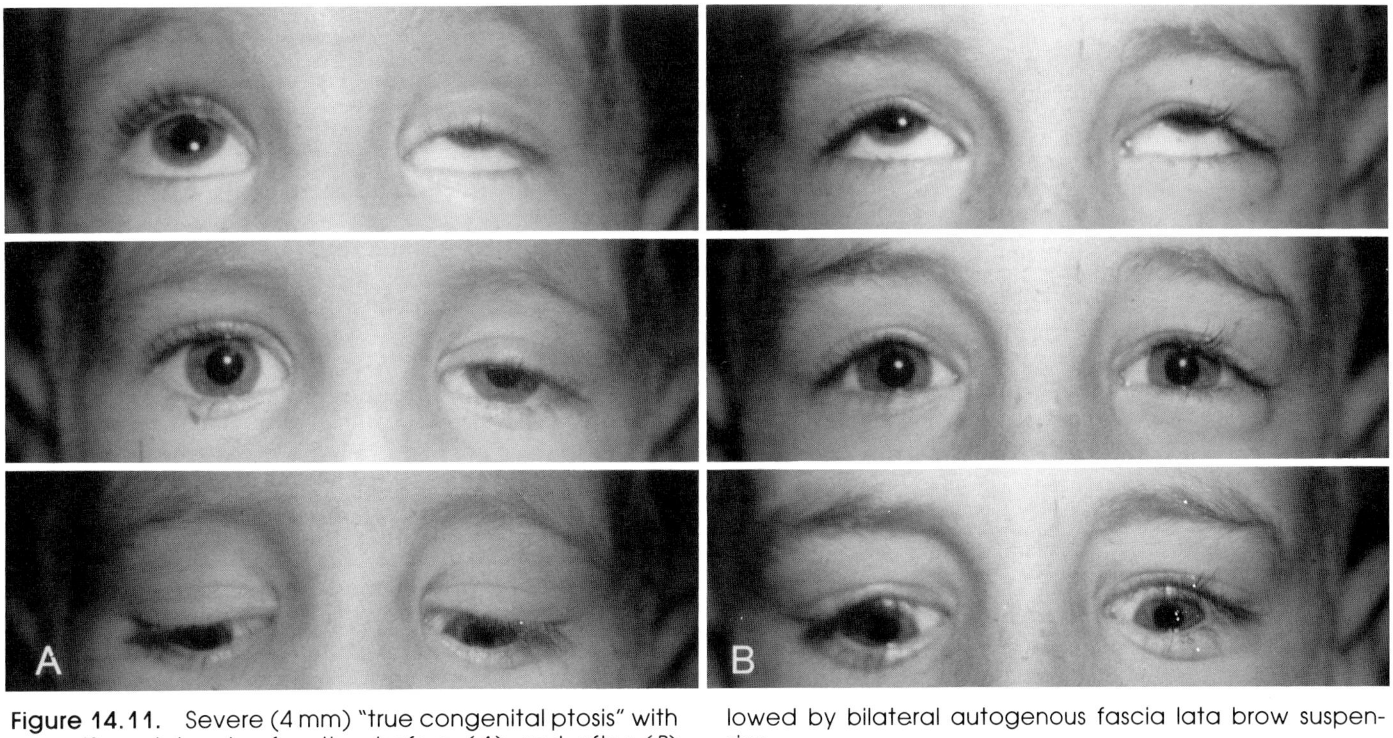

Figure 14.11. Severe (4 mm) "true congenital ptosis" with poor (3 mm) levator function before (*A*) and after (*B*) excision of levator aponeurosis and terminal muscle followed by bilateral autogenous fascia lata brow suspension.

If there is hematoma function without current bleeding, it may be possible to aspirate or otherwise evacuate it. In all likelihood the result will have been compromised and reoperation at a later date will be necessary.

INFECTION

The eyelid's abundant blood supply may be an annoyance at surgery, but it makes the area resistant to infection. Pyogenic infection is quite rare in ptosis repair. When it

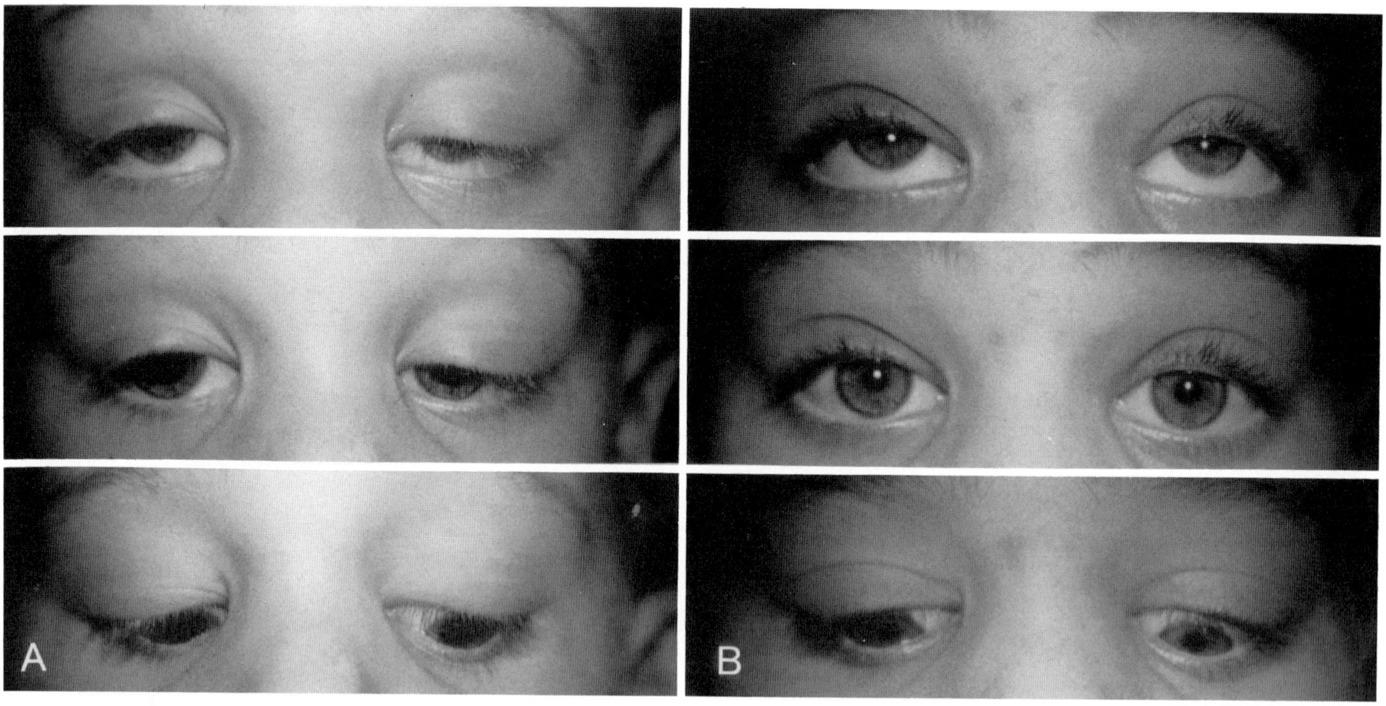

Figure 14.12. Severe (right, 4 mm; left, 5 mm) "true congenital ptosis" with poor (right, 3 mm; left, 2 mm) levator function before (*A*) and 5 years after (*B*) bilateral autogenous fascia lata brow suspension.

does occur, it will usually respond to antibiotic treatment without permanent effect on the result.

Delayed chronic infection is quite common after the use of nonabsorbable suture in brow suspension surgery. It can only be relieved by removal of the suture. It is my belief that the use of these sutures in the treatment of true congenital ptosis is almost never indicated, and this complication should almost never occur.

EXTRAOCULAR MUSCLE IMBALANCE

A temporary vertical muscle imbalance will occasionally follow supermaximum levator resection. This is probably the result of traction on the superior rectus muscle through the fibrous connections that exist between its sheath and the sheath of the levator muscle. It should be short-lived as the connective tissues will stretch. Only rarely should vertical muscle surgery be needed, and it should be delayed for several months until the imbalance is stationary.

Injury to the reflected tendon of the superior oblique muscle can follow blind cutting of the horns of the levator aponeurosis. If traction is made upon the ptosis clamp while the cuts are being made, and if the cutting is restricted to small snips in direct view until the muscle can be delivered into the wound, the oblique muscle's tendon will not be damaged. If the tendon should be inadvertently severed, it would be extremely difficult and probably ineffective to try to repair it. Minimal imbalance seems to result if a compensatory myomectomy of the ipsilateral inferior oblique muscle is done.

CONCLUSIONS

Congenital ptosis, which is called "true congenital ptosis" in this chapter, comprises the majority of ptosis patients. It is due to a developmental dystrophy of the levator muscle, usually isolated but sometimes associated with a weakness of elevation of the ipsilateral eye. The functional capacity of the dystrophic levator muscle varies with the relative number of striated muscle fibers it contains. This capacity can be fairly accurately estimated by evaluating the degree of ptosis and the amount of eyelid excursion as the patient shifts gaze from eyes down to eyes up.

When the condition is severe enough to warrant treatment, surgery is the only logical choice. The ptotic eyelid can be raised by a vertical shortening of its posterior lamella (the Fasanella-Servat operation), by shortening the levator muscle or by suspending the lid from the brow with some type of material. Of the materials currently being used, autogenous fascia lata is by far the best. The surgical results are best when the levator function is good and vertical lid shortening or levator resection is indicated and performed. When brow suspension is used, the result can never be as good. When this operation is necessary, the best results will follow if bilateral surgery is done. For the sake of symmetry, it is sometimes wise to create and treat a bilateral condition in dealing with unilateral ptosis. This is done by excising part of the levator complex on the normal side followed by bilateral autogenous fascia lata brow suspension.

The surgery of ptosis is not difficult, but a thorough

knowledge of eyelid anatomy is essential. A well-planned and well-executed procedure should result in a highly satisfactory result in the vast majority of cases.

REFERENCES

1. Scarpa A: *Practical Observations on the Principal Diseases of the Eyes.* London, Cadell and Davies, 1806, p 130.
2. Bowman WP (cited by Bader D): Report of the chief operations performed at the Royal London Ophthalmic Hospital, for the quarter ending September, 1857. II. Eyelids, 51 operations. *R Lond Ophthalmol Hosp Rep* 1: 34, 1857–1859.
3. Eversbusch O: Zur operation der congenitalen blepharoptosis. *Klin Monastbl Augenheilkd* 21: 100, 1883.
4. Dransart HN: Un cas de blepharoptose opere par un procede special a l'auteur. *Ann Oculist* 84: 88, 1880.
5. Hess C: Eine operationsmethode gegen ptosis. *Arch Augenheilkd* 28: 22, 1893.
6. Panas P: D'un noveau procede operatoire applicable au ptosis congenital et au ptosis paralitique. *Arch Ophtal (Paris)* 6: 1, 1886.
7. Tansley JO: A congenitao ptosis case and operation. *Trans Am Ophthalmol Soc* 7: 427, 1895.
8. Motais M: Operation du ptosis par la greffe tarsienne d'une languette du tendon du muscle droit superieur. *Ann Oculist* 118: 5, 1897.
9. Parinaud H: Noveau procede operatoire du ptosis. *Ann Oculist* 118: 13, 1897.
10. Lapersonne F: Sur quelques modifications dans les operations du ptosis. *Arch Opht* 1: 497, 1903.
11. Blaskovics L: A new operation for ptosis with shortening of the levator and tarsus. *Arch Ophthalmol* 52: 563, 1923.
12. Agatston SA: Resection of the levator palpebrae muscle by the conjunctival route for ptosis. *Arch Ophthalmol* 27: 994, 1942.
13. Iliff CE: A simplified ptosis operation. *Am J Ophthalmol* 37: 529, 1954.
14. Fox SA: *Ophthalmic Plastic Surgery.* New York, Grune & Stratton, 1952.
15. Leahey BD: Simplified ptosis surgery: resection of the levator palpebrae by the external route. *Arch Ophthalmol* 50: 588, 1953.
16. Johnson CC: Blepharoptosis: a general consideration of surgical methods with results in 162 operations. *Am J Ophthalmol* 38: 129, 1954.
17. Berke RN: Results of resection of the levator muscle through a skin incision in congenital ptosis. *Arch Ophthalmol* 61: 177, 1959.
18. Jones LT: The anatomy of the upper eyelid and its relation to ptosis surgery. *Am J Ophthalmol* 57: 943, 1964.
19. Wright WW: The use of living sutures in the treatment of ptosis. *Arch Ophthalmol* 51: 99, 1922.
20. Singh D, Singh M: Total transplantation of the superior rectus muscle for ptosis. *Trans Ophthalmol Soc (UK)* 98: 71, 1978.
21. Fasanella RM, Servat J: Levator resection for minimal ptosis: another simplified operation. *Arch Ophthalmol* 65: 493, 1961.
22. Mustardé JC: Experiences in ptosis correction. *Trans Am Acad Ophthalmol Otolaryngol* 72: 173, 1968.
23. Mustardé JC: Problems and possibilities in ptosis surgery. *Plast Reconstr Surg* 56: 381, 1975.
24. Collin JRO, Beard C (cited by Beard C): *Ptosis*, ed 3. St. Louis, CV Mosby, 1981, p 191.
25. Sisler HA: Preserving and maximizing the effect of Müller's superior tarsal muscle in levator surgery for blepharoptosis. *Orbit* 1: 113, 1982.
26. Berke RN, Wadsworth JAC: Histology of levator muscle in congenital and acquired ptosis. *Arch Ophthalmol* 53: 413, 1955.
27. Hornblass A, Adachi M, Wolintz A, Smith B: Clinical and ultrastructural correlation in congenital and acquired ptosis. *Ophthalmic Surg* 7: 69, 1976.
28. Merriam WW, Ellis FD, Helveston EM: Congenital blepharoptosis, anisometropia, and amblyopia. *Am J Ophthalmol* 89: 401, 1980.
29. Hoyt CS, Stone RD, Fromer C, Billson FA: Monocular axial myopia associated with neonatal eyelid closure in human infants. *Am J Ophthalmol* 91: 197, 1981.
30. Beard C: A new treatment for severe unilateral ptosis and for ptosis with jaw-winking. *Am J Ophthalmol* 59: 252, 1965.
31. Crawford JS: Repair of ptosis using frontalis muscle and fascia lata. *Trans Am Acad Ophthalmol Otolaryngol* 60: 672, 1956.
32. McCord CD Jr: An external minimal ptosis procedure—external tarso-aponeurectomy. *Trans Am Acad Ophthalmol Otolaryngol* 79: 683, 1975.
33. Berke RN (cited by Beard C): *Ptosis*, ed 3. St. Louis, CV Mosby, 1981, pp 235–240.

CHAPTER 15

Dermoid and Epidermoid Cysts of the Eyelid

DAVID M. REIFLER, M.D.
ALBERT HORNBLASS, M.D.

Dermoid and epidermoid cysts are developmental lesions that frequently occur in and around the orbital and periorbital region. These cysts are classified as *choristomas* (1–3). A choristoma is a congenital lesion composed of essentially normal tissue that is not normally found at the involved site. The basic nature of dermoid and epidermoid cysts has long been recognized. We have no better explanation for the etiology of these cysts than that proposed in 1853 by Verneuil; that is, the inclusion and sequestration of a pouch of skin in deeper tissues during fetal development (4). As discussed below, the cyst walls are typically composed of a keratinizing stratified squamous epithelium (1–5) although the epithelium may fail to demonstrate keratinization (6, 7). Dermal appendages are present in the walls of the dermoid cyst, whereas in epidermoid cysts these structures are absent (1–5). The content of the cysts therefore may vary from predominately desquamated epithelium to a more oily mixture of debris and sebaceous secretions. Since dermoid and epidermoid cysts have a similar clinical presentation and presumably similar etiology, they will be discussed together, although the pathologic and clinical distinctions will also be noted.

Dermoid and epidermoid cysts most commonly occur in the more anterior orbital and periorbital regions (Table 15.1) (2–5). Although these cysts may occur in the orbital roof and deeper within the orbit, the discussion in this chapter will be concerned primarily with the much more common anterior lesions.

INCIDENCE

Approximately 50% of dermoid and epidermoid cysts occur in the head and neck region, and of these, about 60% are situated in the lid and brow (4). Dermoid cysts tend to involve contiguous, anterior orbital and eyelid structures (8, 9). This has led to a variability in the tabulation of the incidence of these cysts by location (9). Some authors characterize dermoid and epidermoid cysts as usually being primary tumors of the orbit that involve the lid secondarily (2), whereas others have excluded anterior dermoids from their series of orbital tumors (10). Despite the differences in reporting statistics, it is well accepted that anteriorly located cysts are relatively common, particularly in children, while deep orbital dermoid and epidermoid cysts are much more rare.

Over 50% of anterior dermoid cysts are located in the superotemporal quadrant (4, 5). In the lid, the next most common location is superonasal, followed by inferonasal and, last, inferotemporal (4, 5).

CLINICAL PRESENTATION

When dermoid cysts present as a lid mass, they are generally well circumscribed and nontender. In the superotemporal quadrant, they may be confined anteriorly within the brow and lid (Fig. 15.1) or extend posteriorly in the area of the lacrimal gland fossa (Fig. 15.2) or deeper within the temporal orbit (Fig. 15.3). When the cyst extends posteriorly, it may be less freely moveable and this

Table 15.1
Location of Orbital Dermoid Cysts[a]

Location	Percentage
Upper temporal quadrant	62
Upper nasal quadrant	19
Lower nasal quadrant	4
Lower temporal quadrant	0
Deep within the orbit	3
Unspecified	12

[a] From Iliff C, Green WR: *Orbital tumors in children.* In Jakobiec FA (ed): *Ocular and Adnexal Tumors.* Birmingham, AL, Aesculapius, 1978, p 673.

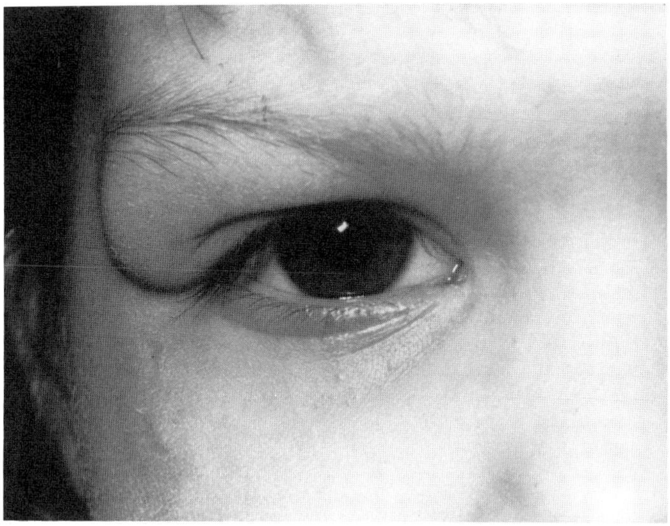

Figure 15.1. Dermoid cyst of the temporal portion of the right upper lid and brow. The cyst was attached to the periosteum of the superior orbital rim without having a posterior orbital extension.

posterior component may produce smooth pressure erosion of the bony orbital wall (so-called fossa formation). Some authors have described the location of the cysts as deep to both muscle and periosteum (11), but a clearly defined periosteal covering may not be found and the tumor may be entirely confined to preseptal tissues. A greater portion of the circumference of the cyst can be palpated when the lesion is entirely within the lid and brow. The anterior tissues of the lid overlying the cyst are distorted and the protuberant swelling may have the appearance of being suspended from the temporal-most aspect of the orbital rim (Figs. 15.1 and 15.2). Typically, the skin is otherwise normal and may be moved freely over the tumor (3, 5, 11). These characteristic clinical findings are in contrast to the more diffuse benign eyelid tumors of childhood such as plexiform neurofibroma (Fig. 15.4) or hemangioma (Fig. 15.5).

Compared with the typical presentation of temporally located dermoid and epidermoid cysts, medially located cysts have certain distinguishing clinical characteristics. Typically, there is a unilateral appearance of fullness in the medial canthal area that results in an asymmetric broadening of the base of the nose and involves only the most medial aspect of the lid (Figs. 15.6 and 15.7). Although the deformity may be noticed early in infancy, the slow growth of the tumor may delay further consultation until later in childhood. The mass, which is usually quite firm to palpation, tends to be intimately connected to the underlying periosteum. The fixation to the surrounding tissues may be broadly based and extend superiorly to the peritrochlear tissues and inferiorly to the medial canthal tendon (Fig. 15.8). In contrast with the loosely arranged tissues in the temporal eyelid, the tightly apposed structures of the medial canthus limit movement of the lesion upon clinical palpation.

Unless there is a significant extension of the tumor posterior to the equator of the globe, proptosis will not occur. However, larger cysts, both medially and temporally, may cause displacement of the globe with resulting diplopia and restricted motility (5).

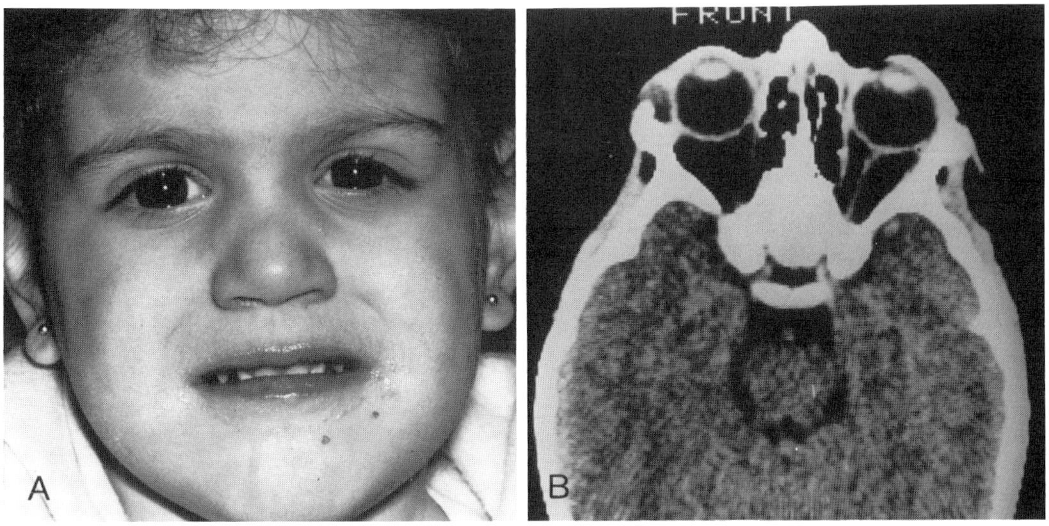

Figure 15.2. *A,* Dermoid cyst of the left upper lid and superotemporal orbit. *B,* Computed tomogram showing the cystic nature of the lesion and its posterior extent in the lacrimal gland fossa.

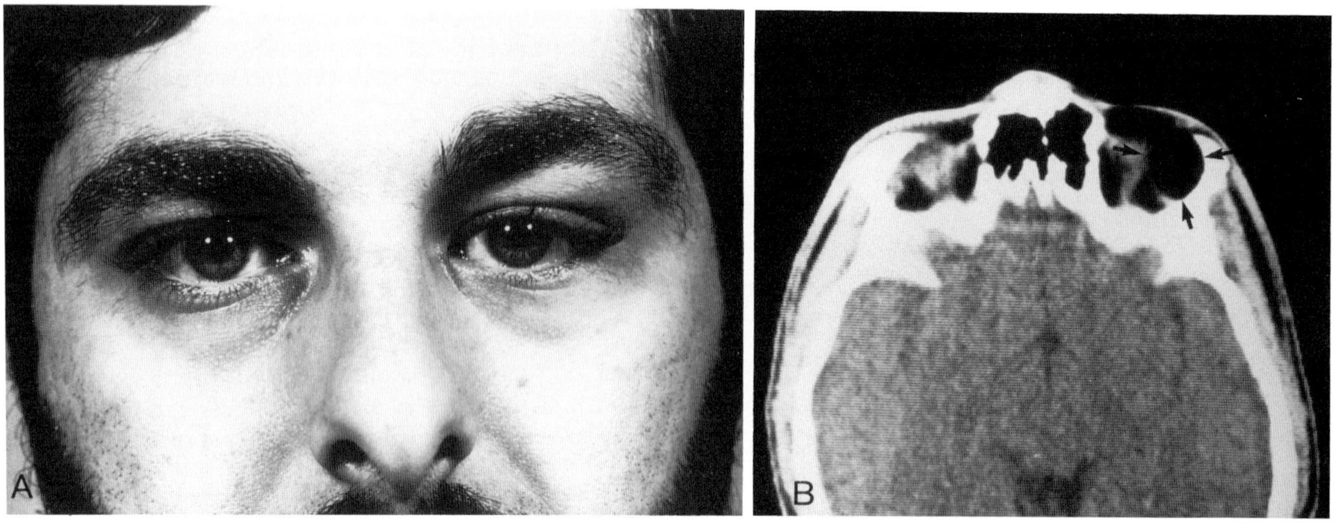

Figure 15.3. *A,* Dermoid cyst of the left orbit in an adult. *B,* Computed tomogram shows the cystic nature and deep orbital extent of the lesion.

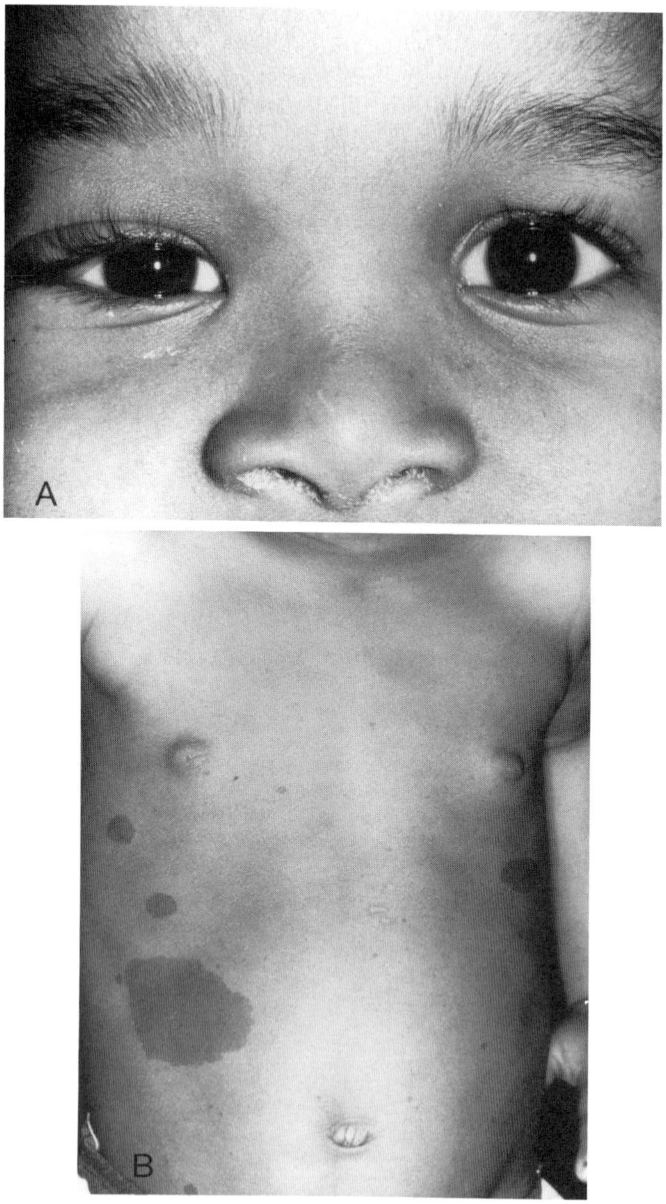

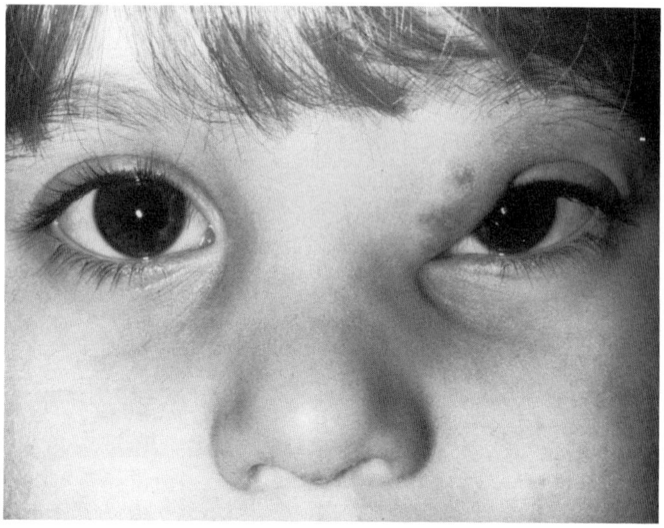

Figure 15.5. Capillary hemangioma of the left upper lid. Unlike dermoid cysts of the medial canthus, the tumor was not adherent to the periosteum and was rather soft to palpation. Involvement of the skin with the capillary vessels was pathognomonic.

Anterior dermoid cysts are generally well circumscribed and have a spherical or oval shape. When anterior dermoid cysts are excised, they are usually smaller than 1.0 cm to 1.5 cm in size (5). Rarely, a fistulous tract may extend across the lid or toward the tip of the nose (12). Rupture with accompanying inflammation may result from accidental trauma or as a complication of surgery. This may lead to a larger, multilobulated, or less discrete lesion (3, 11). If the nature of the lesion is not appreciated, the surgeon may mistakenly perform an incision and drainage

Figure 15.4. Plexiform neurofibroma of right upper lid in a patient with neurofibromatosis. In contrast to a dermoid cyst, the lesion was diffuse rather than localized (*A*), and the patient was found to have numerous cafe au lait spots (*B*), which confirmed the diagnosis.

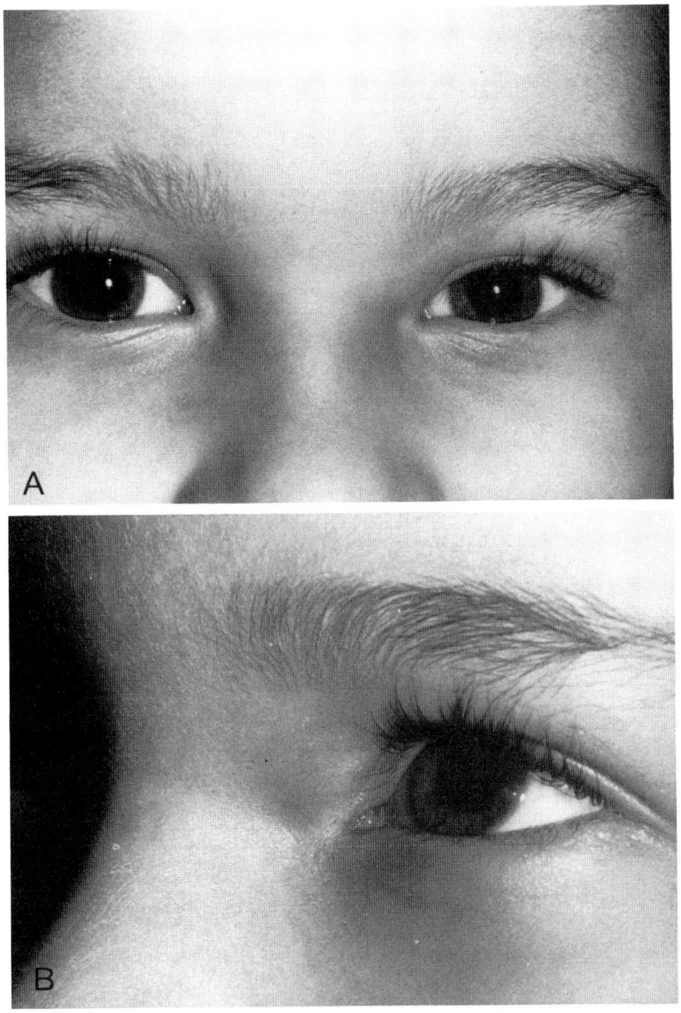

Figure 15.6. Dermoid cyst of the left medial canthus. *A,* The gradually progressive asymmetry eventually was noticed by the patient's parents. *B,* The lesion was firmly adherent to the underlying bone and the medial canthal tendon.

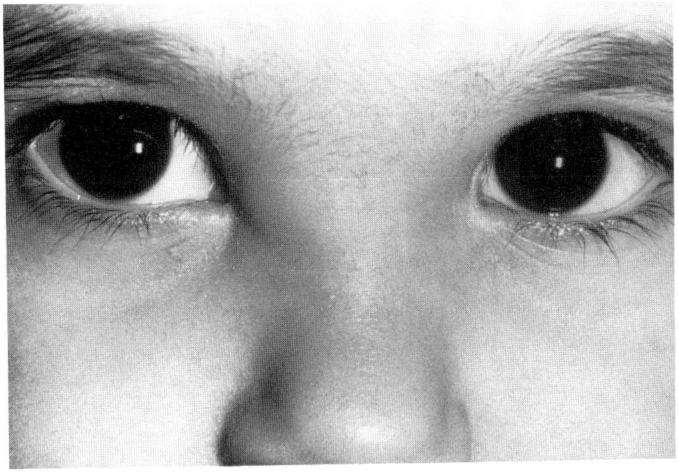

Figure 15.7. Epidermoid cyst of the right medial canthus. The asymmetric broadening at the base to the nose became quite obvious.

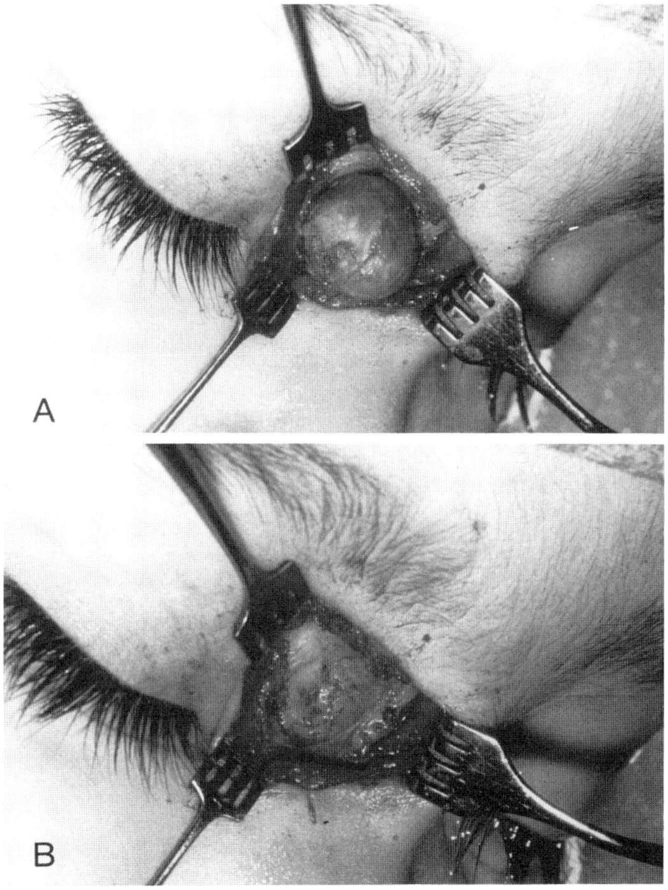

Figure 15.8. Intraoperative photographs of patient shown in Figure 7. *A,* The epidermoid cyst extends from the trochlea to the medial canthal tendon. *B,* After removal of the tumor and adherent periosteum, the "fossa formation" can be demonstrated.

of the cyst, which will only lead to further inflammation rather than a cure.

An attachment of dermoid cysts to bone or periosteum is present in about 20% of cases (5). Cysts with fossa formation in the medial or temporal quadrants particularly tend to have some degree of fusion with the periosteum. When growth extends mainly anteriorly into the temporal aspect of the upper lid, there is frequently an attachment to the bone by a fibrous band (2). This may cause some degree of restriction in the passive movement of the cyst on palpation. We have recently had one case of a superotemporal dermoid cyst associated with cyst formation in the adjacent palpebral lobe of the lacrimal gland (dacryops). In this case, the dacryops may have been due to mechanical blockage or a combination of hypersecretion and weakening of the duct walls (14).

Although deeply situated dermoids that arise within the diploe or suture lines produce characteristic radiographic findings (15), more anteriorly located cysts usually do not show any abnormalities when conventional roentgenograms are used. Plain roentgenograms are useful in distinguishing dermoid cysts from sinoorbital mucocele, meningocele, or encephalocele. In these latter conditions, polytomography or computed tomography can further define a communication with the sinuses or cranial cavity.

Some authors feel that special x-ray studies are probably not indicated in cases of typical superotemporal dermoid cyst (5). However, the composition and posterior extent of the lesion may be demonstrated by computed tomography, and therefore, this particular study may be of great value. The cystic nature of this lesion is well appreciated using computed tomography (Figs. 15.2 and 15.3). The contents of a dermoid cyst may show a radiologic density equivalent to or less than that of water, depending upon the proportion of fatty sebaceous secretions (16).

Compared with typical dermoid and epidermoid cysts, conjunctival cysts and cystic conjunctival dermoids show certain deviant clinical features. They are more apt to occur in a superomedial or medial location than typical dermoid or epidermoid cysts (7). Cysts that are possibly conjunctival in origin may also occur superotemporally in the palpebral lobe of the lacrimal gland (dacryops, lacrimal gland duct cysts) (14, 17, 18). A congenital sequestration of conjunctiva may be the origin of lacrimal gland duct cysts in some cases (17), although most of these lesions are acquired and probably arise from an enclosed and dilated lacrimal gland duct (14, 18). Dacryops is distinguished from dermoid and epidermoid cysts by its localization of symptoms and clinical findings to the palpebral lobe of the lacrimal gland. Still, the computed tomographic appearance of dacryops in the superotemporal quadrant of the orbit (17) may be reminiscent of dermoid cysts. However, as in the case of conjunctival dermoid (7), dacryops is characteristically not associated with an osseous defect (18).

PATHOPHYSIOLOGY

Periorbital dermoid cysts develop along lines of closure of a fetal fissure. Presumably, an infolding of the ectoderm results in a sequestration of epithelial structures (3, 4, 11, 13). Attachment of the periosteum is sometimes seen, particularly in proximity to a cranial bony suture. Dermoid and epidermoid cysts are almost entirely composed of dermal elements. The dermoid cyst is distinguished from the teratoma, which contains all three germ layers and less than 90% is composed of dermal elements (11).

The presence of a keratinizing squamous epithelium and dermal appendages such as pilosebaceous apparati or sweat glands characterize the dermoid cyst (Fig. 15.9; Refs. 1–5). Hair shafts, if present, are usually found plastered against the inside of the cyst wall, presumably displaced by keratinaceous and sebaceous debris. The hair shafts sometimes may be observed through the cyst wall at the time of surgery (Fig. 15.10). Dermal appendages may be numerous or few, and the term *epidermoid cyst* is applied when these appendages are absent. However, extensive histologic sectioning to completely rule out the presence of dermal adnexal structures is generally impractical, since this information is of little clinical importance.

Other types of related cysts may show a nonkeratinizing epithelium except at the points at which hair shafts enter the cyst. Jakobiec (7) has referred to this latter type as "conjunctival dermoid," noting that the epithelium frequently contains scattered mucus-secreting goblet cells and other features of conjunctiva. Simple conjunctival cysts may be congenital or acquired and are structurally analogous to epidermoid cysts since appendageal structures are absent. The classification of epithelial lined cysts, as summarized in Table 15.2, follows that proposed by Jakobiec.

In contrast to a solid, epibulbar dermoid tumor, the epithelium of the dermoid cyst is invaginated (3). Dermoid cysts contain desquamated epithelium, cholesterol, fat, hair and sebaceous secretions. Depending on which constituent predominates, the contents may be keratinaceous (epithelium) or more oily and fluid (sebaceous) (3–5). In the lids, the epithelial debris and secretions of dermoid cysts are generally a creamy white color and have a consistency that has been likened to that of toothpaste (19). In epidermoid cysts, desquamated epithelial products may be arranged in homogeneous, concentric layers containing numerous cholesterol crystals, which gave rise to the older designation of *cholesteatoma* or *pseudocholesteatoma* (4). In dermoid cysts, the oily, sebaceous secretions may turn a dark brown color due to hemorrhage and secondary hemosiderin production (3). These descriptions of cholesteatomas and oil cysts were classically applied to deeper orbital lesions. The contents of dermoid cysts frequently cause a chronic inflammatory response of variable intensity (Fig. 15.11). Histopathologically, inflammatory cells may be seen in the dermoid capsule, and there is frequently an associated thickening of the cyst wall. Microperforations in the cyst wall that allow even a small egress of the toxic contents may be responsible for inciting this inflammatory process. Epidermoid cysts, which lack sebaceous material, tend to have cyst walls that are thinner and less inflamed. Rupture of a dermoid cyst, either spontaneously or through accidental or surgical trauma, may give rise to a more dramatic response that subsequently develops into a smoldering granulomatous inflammation (3–5).

As previously mentioned, epithelial-lined cysts in the periorbital region show a variable composition that includes variations in keratinization (6, 7) and the degree of inclusion of appendageal structures. Although the dysembryogenetic basis for this phenomenon is unknown, it seems likely that the final composition of these cysts depends upon the nature and developmental potentialities of the incorporated elements (7).

TREATMENT

The potential for gradual enlargement, spontaneous or traumatic rupture, or even posterior orbital growth and its attendant complications justifies definitive surgical excision of dermoid cysts in most cases. The excision of an

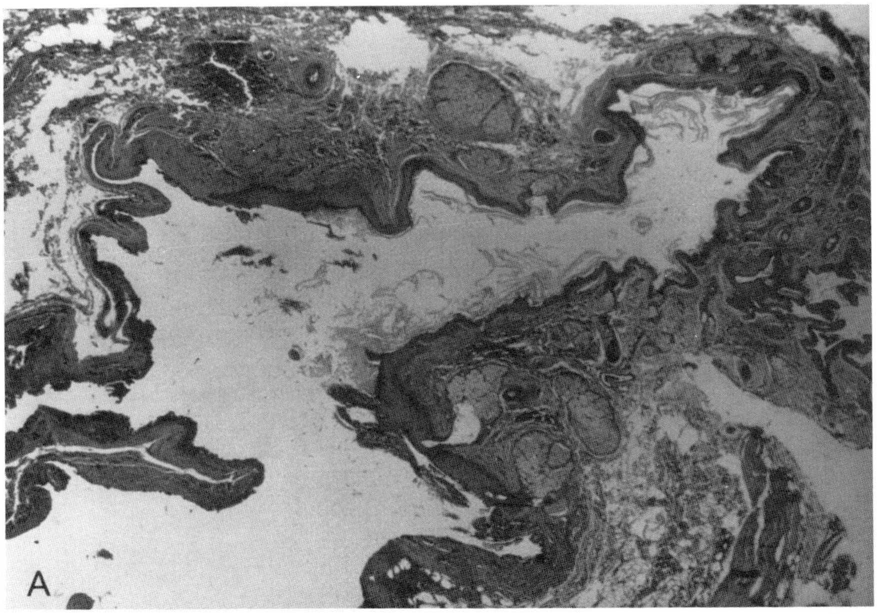

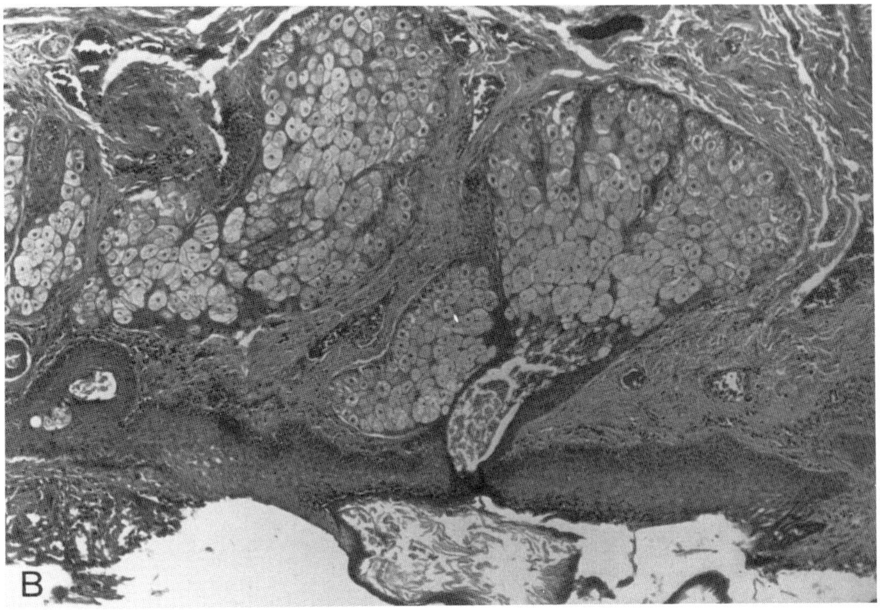

Figure 15.9. Dermoid cyst. Histopathology reveals a keratinizing squamous epithelium (*A*) with pilosebaceous apparati embedded in the dermis-like wall of the cyst (*B*). (Hematoxylin and eosin.)

anterior dermoid cyst is a relatively simple matter. However, care must be exercised to remove the tumor in toto without rupturing the capsule (12). In the event of spillage into the surrounding tissues, the contents of a dermoid cyst can produce an intense inflammatory reaction (3). A direct surgical approach with good exposure will minimize undue manipulation and pressure upon the cyst (Fig. 15.12). Following a suitably placed skin and muscle-splitting incision, further blunt dissection of the orbicularis muscle and surrounding soft tissue is performed. Meticulous dissection will decrease the chances of cyst rupture and trauma to important adjacent structures.

When the wound margins are retracted apart and in a posterior direction, a greater portion of the cyst is exposed. Tightly wound cotton applicators can further expose the more posterior aspect of the cyst. A cryoprobe may be used to apply traction to the cyst wall, although this technique is quite optional. Dissection with the use of sharp scissors then completes the excision of the cyst, and care is exercised to avoid perforation of the cyst wall during dissection. When the cyst is adherent to the bone, the overlying periosteum is removed with the tumor. In the presence of previous rupture of the cyst, all fibrous or loculated extensions of the cyst should be removed. Meticulous hemostasis will reduce postoperative ecchymosis.

After the subcutaneous tissues are closed in a layered fashion with absorbable sutures, the skin should be closed with interrupted or subcuticular sutures. In young children, the use of interrupted absorbable sutures of 6-0 polyglactin or 6-0 mild chromic gut avoids the adverse emotional and physical trauma of suture removal. The exposed ends of these absorbable sutures eventually fall

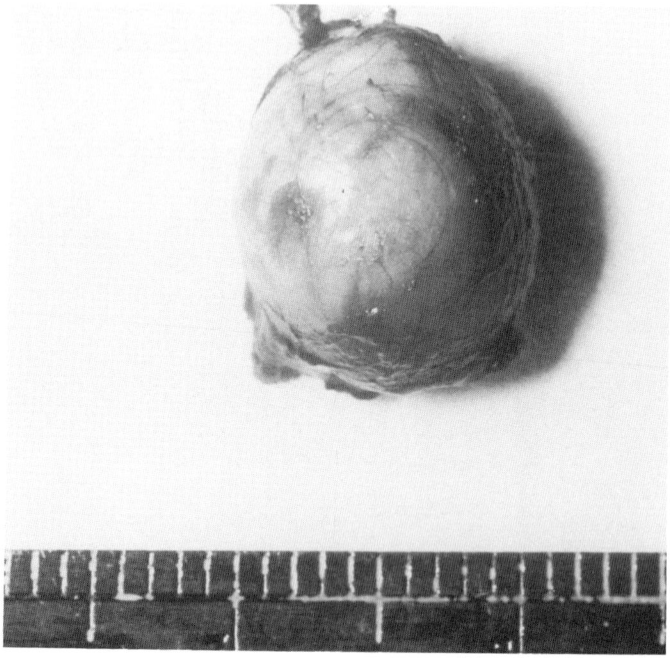

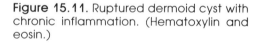

Figure 15.10. Excised dermoid cyst. A smooth capsule surrounded this oval shaped cyst. Hairs could be observed within the cyst at the time of removal.

Table 15.2
Classification of Ocular Adnexal Epithelial-Lined Cysts[a]

	Dermal Appendages	
	present	absent
Keratinizing epithelium	Dermoid cyst	Epidermoid cyst
Nonkeratinizing epithelium	Conjunctival dermoid	Conjunctival cyst

[a] From Jakobiec FA, Bonanno PA, Sigleman J: Conjunctival adnexal cysts and dermoids. *Arch Ophthalmol* 96: 1404–1409, 1978.

off and yield good cosmetic results, particularly if the incision was properly chosen to camouflage the scar (Fig. 15.13).

In the temporal aspect of the upper lid, the surgical incision can be placed just below and parallel to the eyebrow (Fig. 15.12) or in the upper lid crease. If the cyst is small and readily accessible through the conjunctival fornix, a transconjunctival surgical approach may be used (Fig. 15.14). However, visibility of a cyst through the conjunctiva may be associated with a posterior orbital extension (Fig. 15.2), and surgical exposure and total removal of the cyst may therefore be easier via a skin approach. With a properly planned incision and adequate exposure, complications such as cyst rupture or lacrimal dysfunction can usually be avoided.

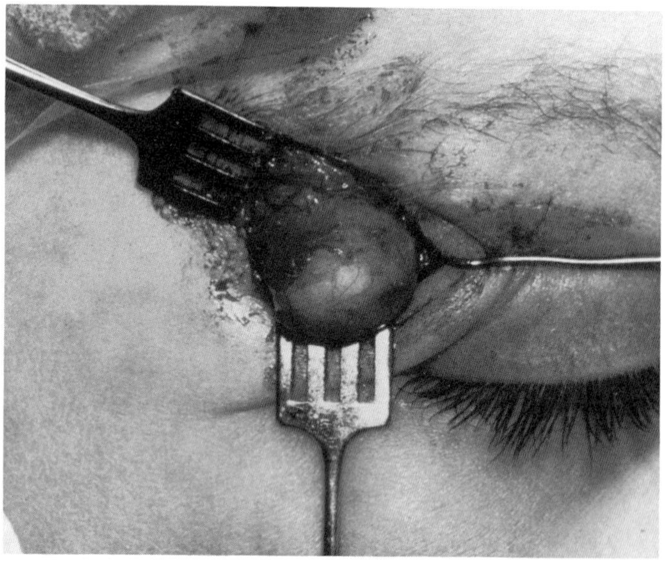

Figure 15.12. An infrabrow skin incision was used to expose the dermoid cyst. Figure 15.1 shows the preoperative appearance.

Figure 15.11. Ruptured dermoid cyst with chronic inflammation. (Hematoxylin and eosin.)

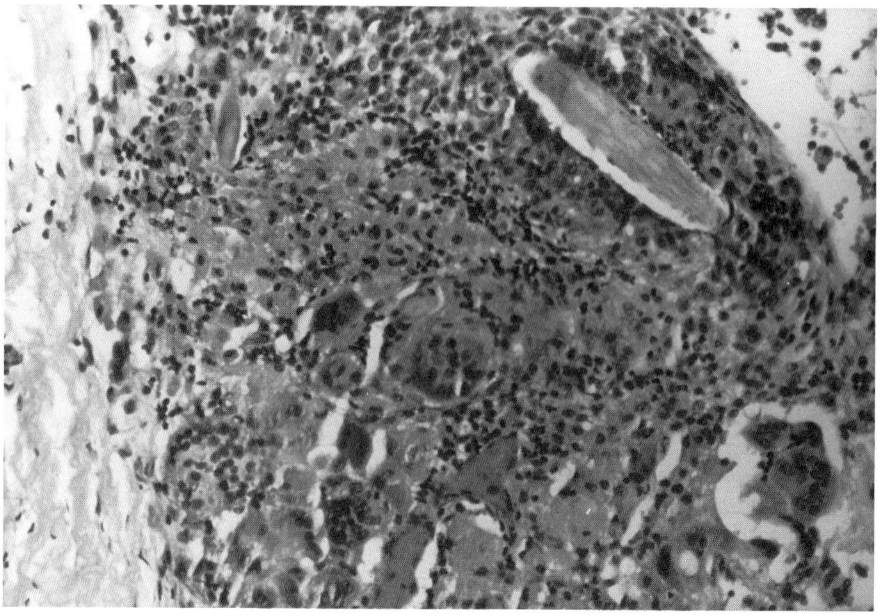

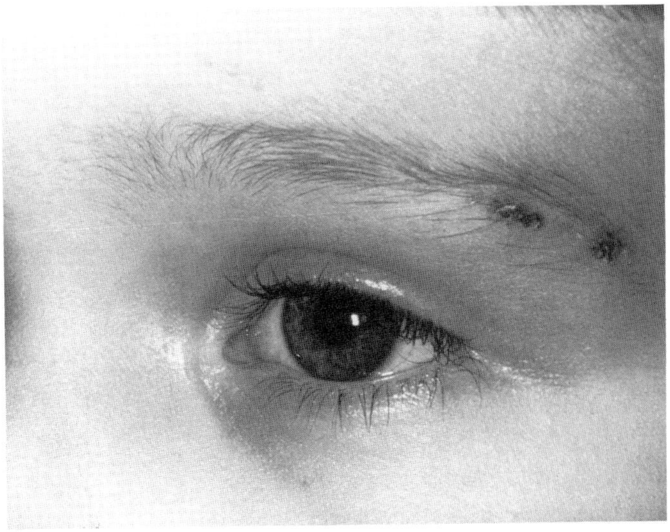

Figure 15.13. Three weeks after removal of a dermoid cyst. Some of the 6-0 polygalactin (Vicryl) sutures have already fallen out.

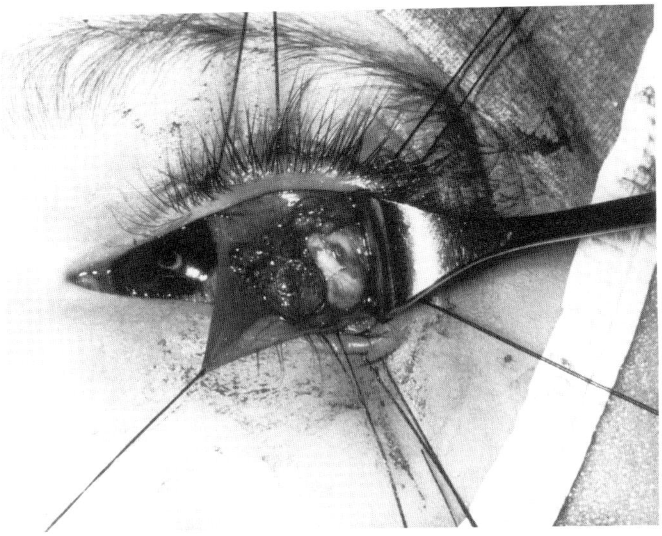

Figure 15.14. A transconjunctival surgical approach was used in the removal of this dermoid cyst, which had a small extension beneath the orbital rim.

COMPLICATIONS

Rupture of the cyst wall may produce considerable inflammation caused by the toxic sebaceous secretions. If this complication is noted intraoperatively, copious irrigation of the wound should follow removal of all identifiable portions of the cyst (2). Recurrence of a cyst may occur when a portion of the cyst wall is left behind. These complications are avoided when an unruptured cyst is completely excised. In cases of previous rupture and inflammation, care should be taken also to completely remove scar tissue that may harbor trapped islands of viable epithelial cells (11).

Unsightly scars are rarely a problem. In the medial canthus, a web-like scar may develop, but this may be amenable to digital massage and resolve in time without further treatment.

In the superotemporal quadrant, the potential for a disturbance of lacrimal gland secretion has already been mentioned. The potential for this complication probably only exists when there is a significant posterior orbital component that requires surgical dissection in this region. Similarly, dissection in the region of the trochlea could conceivably cause a disturbance of ocular motility. The possibility of injury to the temporal branch of the facial nerve when deeper orbital surgery is required has also been mentioned (11).

SUMMARY

Dermoid cysts of the lid are classified as "choristomas" and show a variety of adnexal structures including pilosebaceous apparati. Epidermoid cysts lack adnexal structures. Many of these eyelid dermoids are contiguous with an anterior orbital portion. This is of clinical importance but has led to a variation in reporting the actual incidence of eyelid versus orbital lesions. Both anterior orbital and eyelid dermoid cysts occur most commonly in the superotemporal quadrant. Posterior orbital dermoid and epidermoid cysts are much more rare. These congenital cysts show gradual enlargement but may increase more rapidly in size when the cyst wall is ruptured. The treatment of choice is complete surgical excision of the cyst without rupture of the cyst wall.

REFERENCES

1. Yanoff M, Fine BS: *Ocular Pathology. A Text and Atlas.* Hagerstown, MD, Harper & Row, 1975, p 526.
2. Nicholson DH, Green WR: Tumors of the eye, lids and orbit in children. In Harley RD (ed): *Pediatric Ophthalmology.* Philadelphia, WB Saunders Co, 1975, p 923.
3. Reese AB: *Tumors of the Eye,* ed 3. Hagerstown, Harper & Row, 1976, p 41.
4. Duke-Elder S: Normal and abnormal development. In Duke-Elder S (ed): *System of Ophthalmology.* St. Louis, CV Mosby, 1964, vol 3, pt 2, p 956.
5. Iliff C, Green WR: Orbital tumors in children. In Jakobiec FA (ed): *Ocular and Adnexal Tumors.* Birmingham, AL, Aesculapius, 1978, p 673.
6. Moffatt PM: An orbital dermoid (lined by skin and modified conjunctiva). *Br J Ophthalmol* 25: 428–430, 1941.
7. Jakobiec FA, Bonanno PA, Sigelman J: Conjunctival adnexal cysts and dermoids. *Arch Ophthalmol* 96: 1404–1409, 1978.
8. Harley RD: Disorders of the lids. *Pediatr Clin North Am* 30: 1145–1158, 1983.
9. Shields JA, Bakewell B, Augsburger JJ, et al: Classification and incidence of space-occupying lesions of the orbit. A survey of 645 biopsies. *Arch Ophthalmol* 102: 1606–1611, 1984.
10. Henderson WJ: *Orbital Tumors,* ed 2. New York, Grune & Stratton, 1980, p 75.
11. Wang MKH, Macomber WB: Tumors of the eyelids and orbit. In

Converse JM (ed): *Reconstructive Plastic Surgery*, ed 2. Philadelphia, WB Saunders Co, 1977, vol 2, p 874.
12. Dayal Y, Hameed S: Periorbital dermoid. *Am J Ophthalmol* 53: 1013–1016, 1962.
13. Iliff CE, Ossofsky HJ: *Tumors of the Eye and Adnexa in Infancy and Childhood.* Springfield, IL, CC Thomas, 1962, p 95.
14. Duke-Elder S, MacFaul PA: The ocular adnexa. In Duke-Elder S (ed): *System of Ophthalmology.* St. Louis, CV Mosby, 1974, vol 13, pt 2, p 638.
15. Pfeiffer RL, Nicholl RJ: Dermoids and epidermoids of the orbit. *Trans Am Ophthalmol Soc* 46: 218–243, 1948.
16. Blei L, Chambers JT, Liotta LA, DiChiro G: Orbital dermoid diagnosed by computed tomographic scanning. *Am J Ophthalmol* 85: 58–61, 1978.
17. Brownstein S, Belin MW, Krohel GB, et al: Orbital dacryops. *Ophthalmology* 91: 1424–1428, 1984.
18. Hornblass A, Herschorn B: Lacrimal gland duct cysts. *Ophthal Surg* 16: 301–306, 1985.
19. Ophthalmologic Staff of the Hospital of Sick Children, Toronto: *The Eye in Childhood.* Chicago, Year Book Medical Publishers, 1967, p 94.

CHAPTER 16

Tarsal Kink Syndrome

STEPHEN L. BOSNIAK, M.D.

The tarsal kink syndrome is a rare severe form of congenital entropion of the upper lid. In this entity there is a prominent posterior angulation of the midportion of the tarsal plate. There is a true inversion of the upper lid margin and trichiasis with corneal ulceration. This form of congenital entropion is more severe than the mild rotation of the upper lid lashes that occurs secondary to epiblepharon (1, 2).

CLINICAL PRESENTATION

Kettesy described an entropion "caused by folding of the tarsus" in 1948. Callahan coined the term *tarsal kink syndrome* in 1966 (4) and presented one case. Since then only three additional case reports have been published (5–7). The clinical presentations were very similar in each of these five cases. The children were born with corneal ulcers, upper lid edema, blepharospasm, and upper lid trichiasis (Figs. 16.1 and 16.2). In all cases a horizontal ridge transversing the horizontal expanse of the upper lid could be palpated. After lid eversion a corresponding tarsal-conjunctival groove could be identified (Fig. 16.3). There was concurrent ptosis in two cases (6, 7). Eyelid creases were lacking in three cases. In three of the published cases, before the lid deformity was recognized, a postpartum corneal ulcer progressed despite apparently adequate medical therapy. Three of the cases involved the right upper lid, one case involved the left upper lid, and one case was bilateral. In one case there was associated birth trauma (7).

Because of the rarity of this condition, there is often a delay in its recognition. Once the diagnosis has been established, the surgeon must choose from the various surgical alterations and then immediately begin amblyopia therapy.

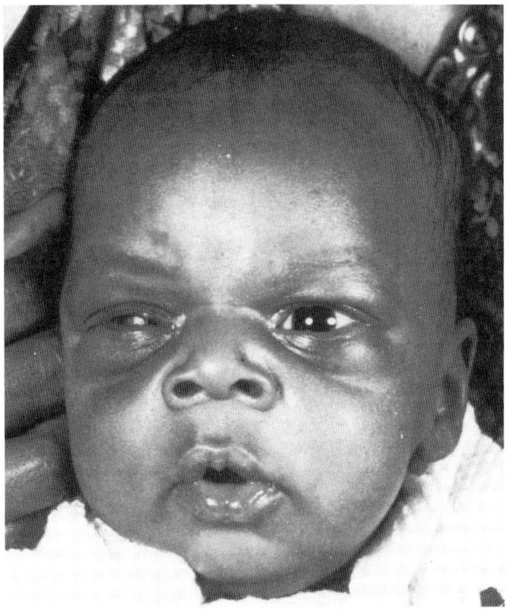

Figure 16.1. A 2-month old child with a tarsal kink of his right upper lid. (From Bosniak SL, Hornblass A, Smith B: Reexamining the tarsal kink syndrome. *Ophth Surg* 16: 437–440, 1985.)

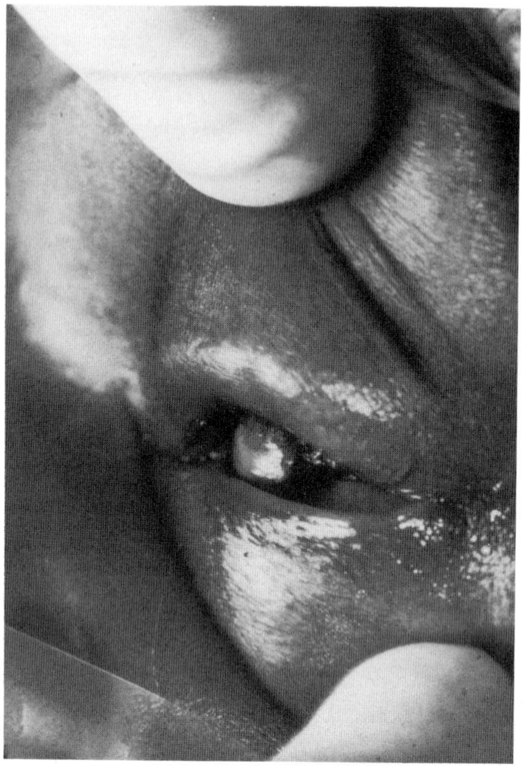

Figure 16.2. Trichiasis and corneal ulceration secondary to the tarsal kink. (From Bosniak SL, Hornblass A, Smith B: Reexamining the tarsal kink syndrome. *Ophth Surg* 16: 437–440, 1985.)

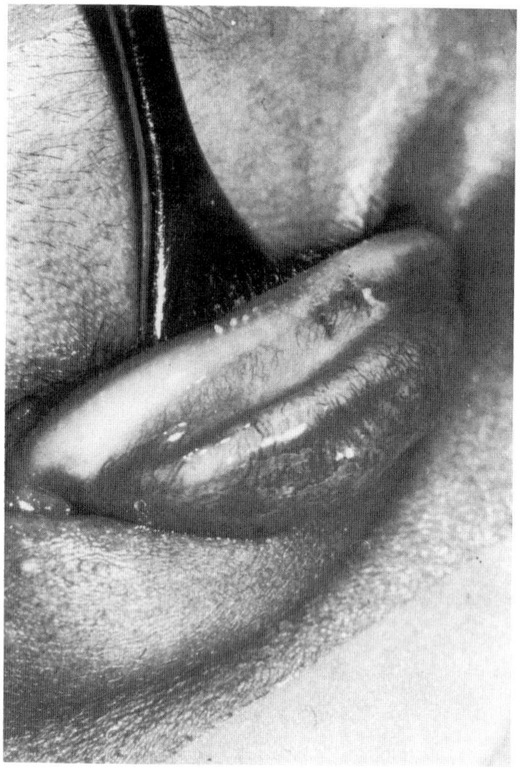

Figure 16.3. There is an obvious tarsal-conjunctival groove evident on lid eversion. (From Bosniak SL, Hornblass A, Smith B: Reexamining the tarsal kink syndrome. *Ophth Surg* 16: 437–440, 1985).

ETIOLOGY

Several hypotheses have been offered as to the etiology of this entity. Kettesy (3) postulated that severe conjunctival inflammation and secondary edema of the upper fornix with bulging and drooping of the conjunctiva initiates a chain of events that leads to the formation of a tarsal kink. He further theorized that a temporary paralysis of the levator allowed the heavy superior fornix to bend the maleable tarsal plate. After levator function returned, the tarsal fold persisted and the lid margin was drawn toward the cornea. Bosniak, Hornblass and Smith (7) postulated in utero positional stress on an immature tarsus as a cause of the tarsal kink. They also suggested corneal ulceration as an initiating event, secondary blepharopasm, and tertiary permanent distortion of a still-malleable tarsus. It is unlikely that this lid deformity is caused by a defect in lid disjunction (which normally occurs between the 5th and 6th month in utero) as there are no associated lid margin abnormalities (8). Because of the rarity of this entity there is no apparent genetic predisposition.

SURGICAL CORRECTION

LID STABILIZATION

Kettesy (3) described stabilizing the lid by "smoothing out" the tarsus over a gauze roll and fixating it with mattress sutures (Fig. 16.4).

Bosniak, Hornblass, and Smith (7) stabilized the lid with a series of mattress sutures and a lateral suture tarsorraphy. Three 4-0 black silk mattress sutures were placed from the palpebral conjunctiva inferior to the tarsal angulation, exited from the skin above the kink, and tied over bolsters (Fig. 16.5). A 4-0 black silk mattress was used for the lateral tarsorraphy, passed from the inferior pretarsal skin, through the anterior tarsus, out the grey line, into the superior grey line, through the anterior superior tarsus, out the skin, and tied over a bolster (Fig. 16.5).

TARSAL FRACTURING AND MARGINAL ROTATION

The upper lid is everted over a Desmarres retractor. A no. 15 Bard Parker is used to incise the palpebral con-

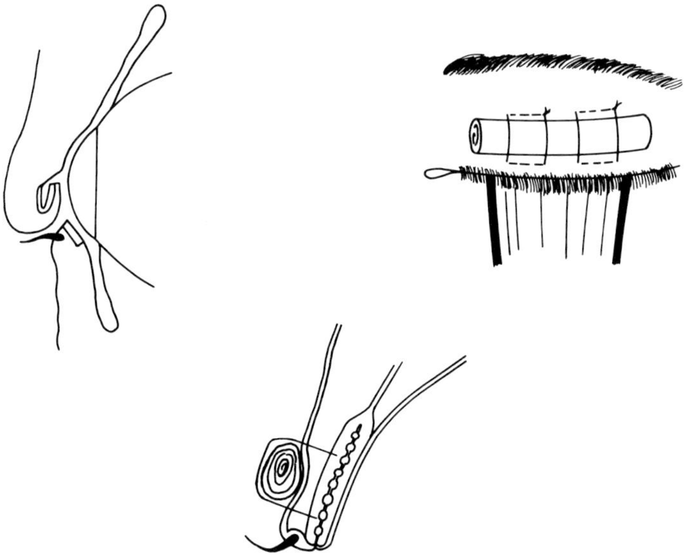

Figure 16.4. Kettesy lid stabilization. The lid is smoothed out by fixating a gauze or Telfa roll over mattress sutures.

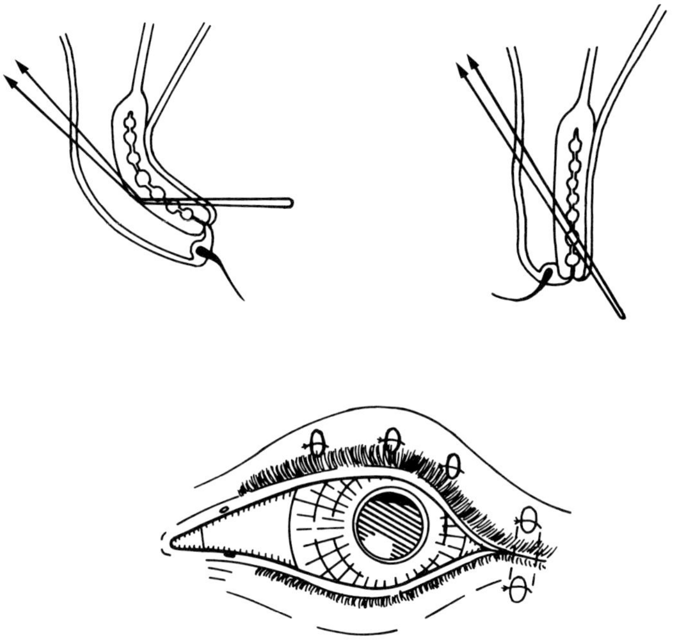

Figure 16.5. The lid may be stabilized by placing a series of mattress sutures from the inferior angulated tarsus through the skin and preseptal orbicularis and tying them over bolsters. A lateral suture tarsorraphy prevents further in-turning of the lid margin.

junctiva and overlying the tarsal groove. The incision is deepened through the tarsus. The lid margin is rotated with three 4-0 black silk mattress sutures placed from the palpebral conjunctival surface at superior edge of the tarsal incision, through the posterior aspect of the superior tarsus, through the inferior pretarsal orbicularis muscle and pretarsal skin, and tied over bolsters (Fig. 16.6).

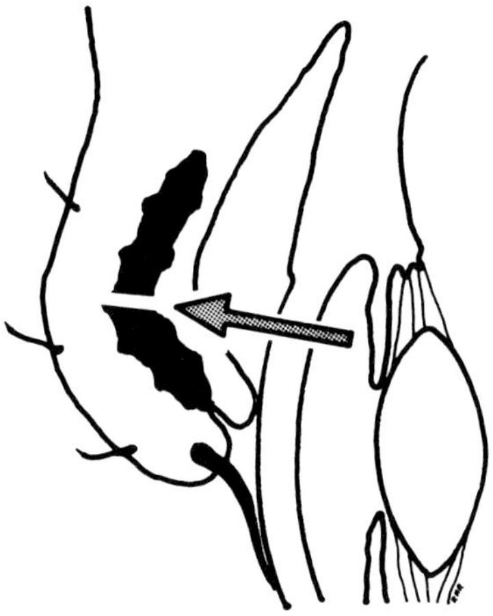

Figure 16.6. Tarsal fracturing and marginal rotation with lid eversion sutures (suture placement as in Fig. 16.7).

The tarsal fracturing and marginal rotation may also be accomplished with a complete transverse blepharotomy and marginal rotation (Fig. 16.7) (11, 12).

TARSAL RESECTION AND REPAIR WITH SCLERAL GRAFT

Callahan (4) resected the angulated tarsus via an anterior approach, then reapproximated the levator aponeurosis and Müller's muscle to the tarsal remnant. Theoretically this could result in a vertical shortening of the upper lid.

Posterior tarsal conjunctival resection of the kinked tarsus and replacement with sclera would not result in a vertical shortening of the posterior lamella. Tenzel (13) combined this procedure with marginal rotation.

The lid is everted. Horizontal tarsoconjunctival incisions are made inferior and superior to the kink. The rectangular segment of tarsus and conjunctiva is resected. A free scleral graft of dimensions matching the defect in the posterior lamella of the upper lid is fashioned. The graft is secured to the remaining tarsus with buried interrupted sutures of 5-0 chromic. It is stabilized with 4-0 black silk mattress sutures, brought through the skin, and tied over bolsters (Fig. 16.8).

LAMELLAR TARSOPLASTY

McCarthy (6) described an anterior lamellar tarsal resection. The anterior tarsal surface is exposed via a lid crease incision. A one-half thickness lamellar dissection is performed from 1 mm below the superior tarsal margin to just above the cilia follicles. The excised tarsus is then reversed, repositioned into the tarsal bed, and fixed with absorbable sutures (Fig. 16.9). The skin is closed, and a lid crease formed.

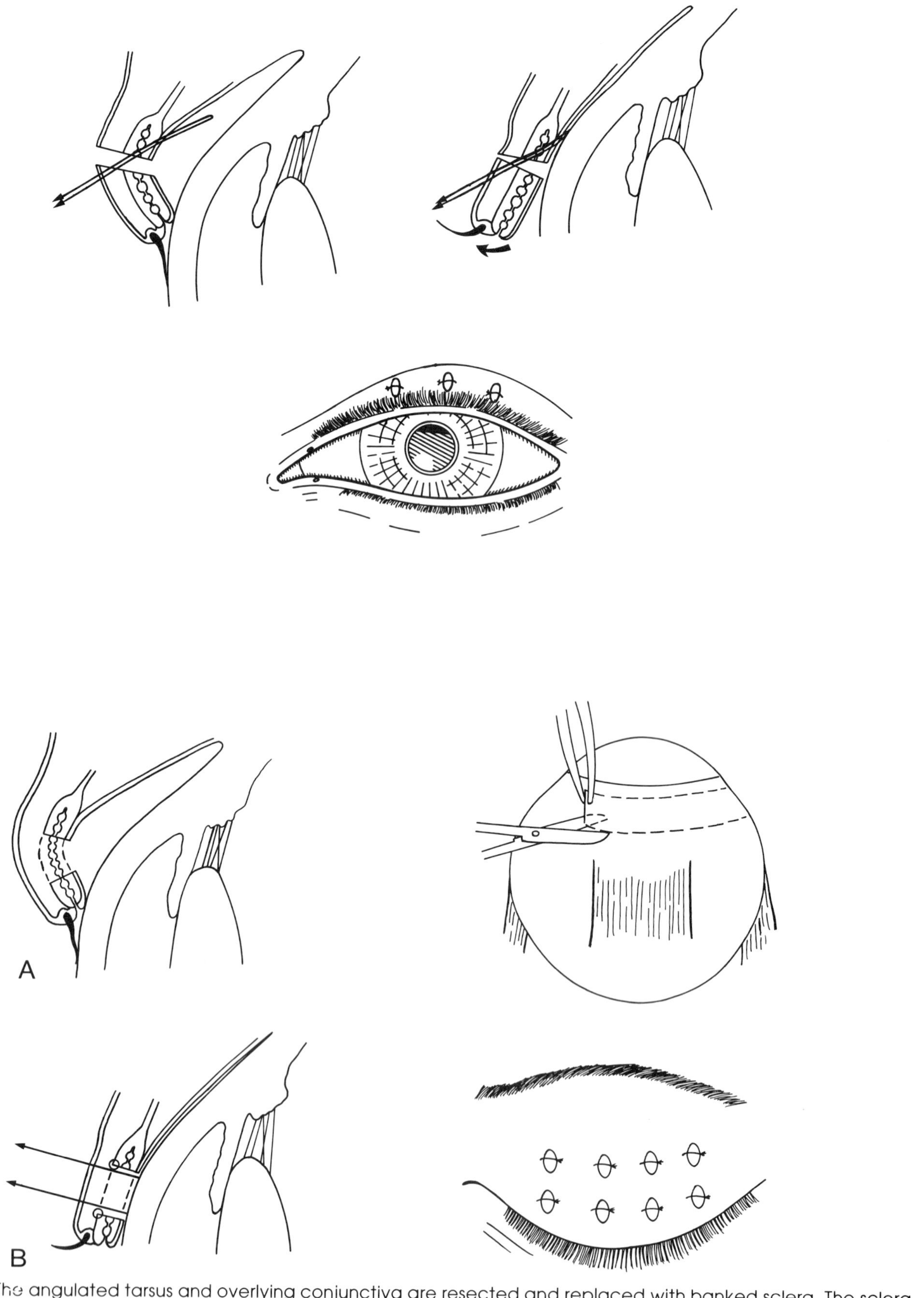

Figure 16.8. The angulated tarsus and overlying conjunctiva are resected and replaced with banked sclera. The sclera is sutured to the remaining tarsus with absorbable sutures and fixed to the lid with 4-0 black silk sutures tied over bolsters.

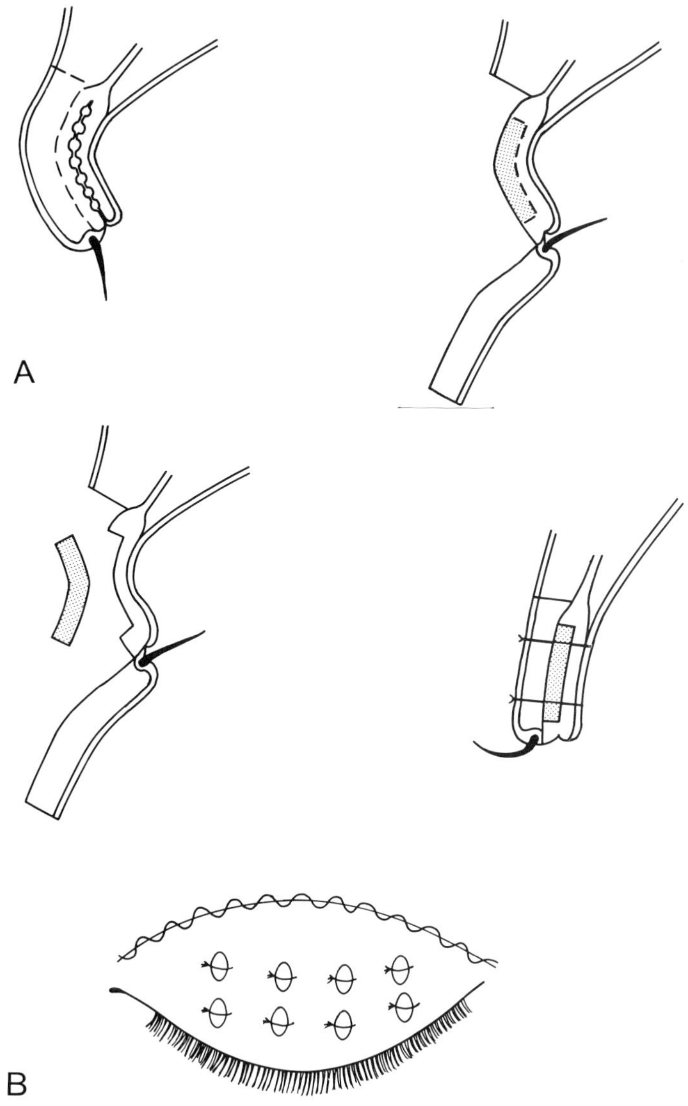

Figure 16.9. Lamellar tarsoplasty. The anterior one half of the tarsal plate is resected, reversed, and resutured to the tarsal bed.

REFERENCES

1. Hiles DA, Wilder LW: Congenital entropion of the upper lids. *J Pediatr Ophthalmol* 6: 157, 1969.
2. Firat T, Ozkan S: Bilateral congenital entropion of the upper eye lids. *Br J Ophthalmol* 57: 753, 1973.
3. Kettesy A: Entropion in infancy caused by folding of the tarsus. *Arch Ophthalmol Bd* 39: 640, 1948.
4. Callahan A: Congenital entropion. In Callahan A (ed): *Reconstructive Surgery of the Eyelids and Ocular Adnexa.* Birmingham, Alabama, Aesculapius, 1966, pp 37–40.
5. Biglan AW, Buerger G: Congenital horizontal tarsal kink. *Am J Ophthalmol* 89: 522, 1980.
6. McCarthy RW: Lamellar tarsoplasty—A new technique for correction of Horizontal tarsal kink. *Ophth Surg* 15: 859, 1984.
7. Bosniak SL, Hornblass A, Smith B: Re-examining the tarsal kink syndrome. *Ophthal Surg* 16 (7): 437–440, 1985.
8. Ozanics V, Jakobiec FA: Prenatal development of the eye and its adnexa. In Jakobiec FA (ed): *Ocular Anatomy, Embryology and Teratology.* Philadelphia, Harper & Row, 1982, pp 84, 85.
9. Fuchs HE: Stellway-Snellen suture. In Duane A (trans): *Textbook of Ophthalmology.* Philadelphia, JB Lippincott, 1923, p 882.
10. Feldstein M: A method of correction of entropion in aged persons. *Eye, Ear, Nose and Throat Monthly* 39: 730–731, 1983.
11. Wies FS: Cicatrical entropion. *Trans Am Acad Ophthalmol Otolaryngol* 59: 503, 1955.
12. Ballen PH: A simple procedure for the relief of trichiasis and entropion of the upper lid. *Arch Ophthalmol* 72: 239, 1964.
13. Tenzel RR, Miller GR, Rubenzik R: Cicatrical upper lid entropion. Treated with banked scleral graft. *Arch Ophthalmol* 93: 999, 1975.

CHAPTER 17

Xeroderma Pigmentosum

ALAN D. ANDREWS, M.D.
KENNETH H. KRAEMER, M.D.

The rare, hereditary syndrome, xeroderma pigmentosum (XP), is principally characterized by a markedly increased susceptibility to sunlight-induced cutaneous and ocular damage. Clinical manifestations include acute sun sensitivity (i.e., easy "sunburning"), photophobia, freckling and other pigmentary abnormalities, atrophy of the skin, and both benign and malignant cutaneous or mucosal tumors. Some persons with XP also manifest a progressive central nervous system degeneration.

The biochemical hallmark of XP is a reduced capacity to repair the DNA damage that occurs when cells are exposed to ultraviolet (UV) light. Ten different genetic subtypes of XP have been identified thus far, each apparently having a distinct DNA repair defect different from the others.

Age of onset, severity, and rate of progression of the clinical abnormalities vary greatly among XP patients. This variability is a function of the numerous different XP genotypes, the difference in cumulative sunlight exposure among affected individuals, and probably other, as yet undetermined, genetic and environmental differences among the patients. Since early diagnosis and the institution of strict sun-avoidance measures can make a tremendous positive difference in the life of persons with XP, it is important to suspect this diagnosis even when manifestations are few and relatively minor.

EPIDEMIOLOGY

Xeroderma pigmentosum has been reported in all races and virtually all regions of the world. Estimates of the prevalance of XP vary widely, however. For instance, in the United States and Europe, XP has been estimated to occur in 1 of 250,000 persons (1), while in Japan, estimates are 1 of 40,000 persons (2). Males and females are equally affected (1); the rate of parental consanguinity in families with affected individuals is high (3, 4); and the parents of persons with XP do not, as a rule, exhibit any of the clinical manifestations of XP. It thus appears that most cases of XP are inherited in an autosomal recessive fashion. There is, however, one report of a family that may carry a dominantly inherited form of XP (5), and it is possible that one or more of the less common genetic forms of XP, i.e., forms for which only one or two affected individuals have been identified, could be inherited in a manner different from that of the more common genetic subgroups.

CUTANEOUS ABNORMALITIES

Some but not all XP patients experience an acute sunburn-like erythema of the skin after only mild to moderate sun exposure. When present, this clinical manifestation is usually the earliest sign of XP, and is often noted following the child's first significant exposure to sun. The reaction is confined to those skin surfaces actually exposed to sunlight; thus, it is most often seen on the face and arms. In severe reactions blisters and subsequent desquamation of the skin may occur. Clinical studies (6) and patient histories indicate that XP patients may have a delayed peak erythema response, i.e., the time between exposure to ultraviolet light and the attainment of the most intense erythema may be longer in XP patients than that of sunburn reactions in normal individuals. Also, the erythema may last much longer than usual, e.g., up to several weeks or more. Other studies suggest that a history of marked acute sun sensitivity in an XP patient may be associated with a poorer prognosis than that for an XP patient with no such history (7).

Almost all persons with XP, whether or not they experience acute sun-sensitivity reactions, do eventually develop chronic skin changes in those areas that are repeatedly exposed to sunlight. These chronic changes occur and progress gradually over a period of years; they most often begin to appear within the first few years of life, but in some patients these changes do not first become clinically apparent until the second or third decade of life.

Usually the first change to be noted is a pattern of unusual freckling, i.e., early and abnormally numerous pigmented macules, most of which are clinically indistinguishable from normal freckles (ephelides). But with time, patients develop many larger, darker, and more irregular lesions, resembling, both clinically and histopathologically, lentigo simplex, lentigo senilis and, sometimes, lentigo maligna. Achromic (white) macular spots also develop, interspersed with the pigmented lesions, often giving a "salt and pepper" appearance to sun-exposed areas of skin (Figs. 17.1–17.4).

Soon after the appearance of abnormal pigmentation most patients also begin to develop telangiectasia of the most highly sun-exposed skin. The telangiectatic lesions may be single, venous dilatations of various lengths or tangled masses of small vessels. Atrophy and dryness of the skin also begin to appear at this time and may progress to produce large areas of tightened, atrophic, and usually depigmented skin, especially on the central face. In severe cases, the mouth may appear "pinched" and patients may be unable to fully open their mouth. *Poikiloderma* is a term often used to describe the combination of irregularly increased and decreased pigmentation, atrophy, and telan-

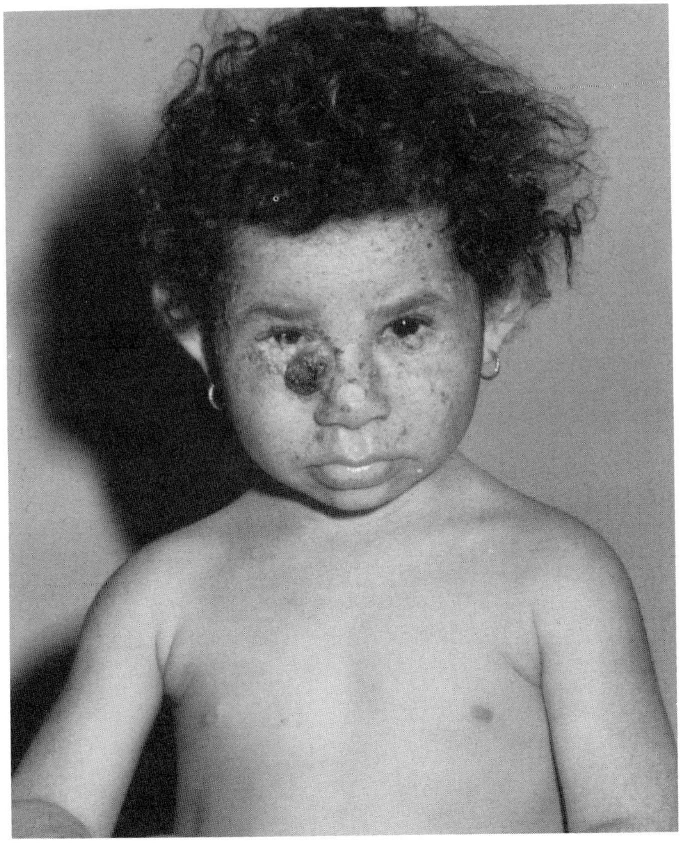

Figure 17.1. Palestinian Arab girl, age 3, with marked freckling of the face and sparing of the chest. Crusted squamous cell carcinomas beneath right eye and on both lower eyelids. Corneal cloudiness in right eye. (From Kraemer KH, Slor H: Xeroderma pigmentosum. *Clin Dermatol* 3: 33–69, 1985.

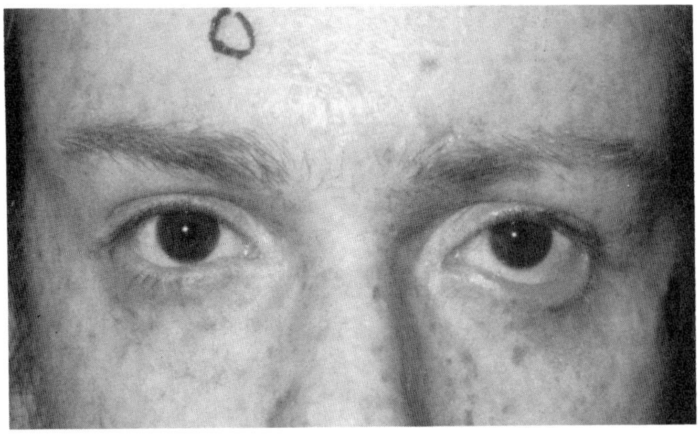

Figure 17.2. Boy, age 17, with xeroderma pigmentosum showing typical pigmentary changes of skin, plus conjunctival inflammation, and ectropion of left lower lid.

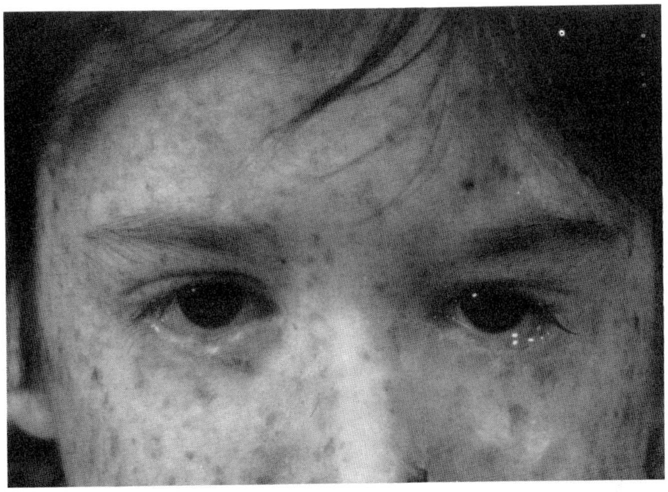

Figure 17.3. Boy, age 10, with xeroderma pigmentosum showing typical pigmentary changes (irregular freckles), scarring from surgery on left cheek, and crusted actinic keratosis of left nares. He has ectropion, loss of lashes, and basal cell and squamous cell carcinomas of the lower lids.

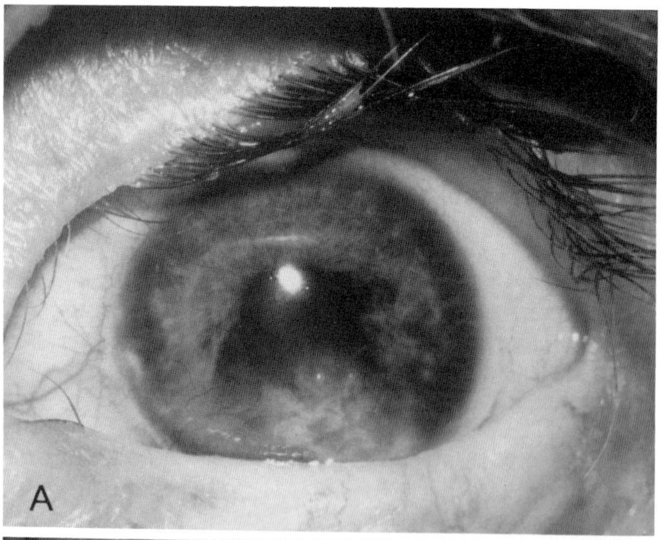

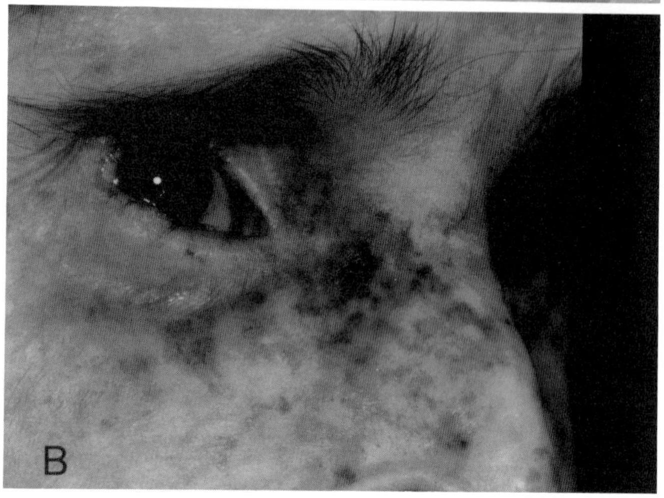

Figure 17.4. *A,* Corneal clouding, conjunctival telangiectasia with vascularization of a portion of the cornea, and atrophy, telangiectasia, and loss of lashes of the lower lid of a 28-year-old patient with xeroderma pigmentosum and Cockayne's syndrome. *B,* Same patient with xeroderma pigmentosum and Cockayne's syndrome. The freckling, achromic areas and atrophy are typical of xeroderma pigmentosum. The beak-like nose, sunken eyes, and loss of subcutaneous tissue are similar to those manifestations in patients with Cockayne's syndrome. (From Kraemer KH, Slor H: Xeroderma pigmentosum. *Clin Dermatol* 3: 33–69, 1985.)

giectasias of the skin. This same pattern can be seen on the sun-exposed skin of much older persons without XP who spend many years in the sun, such as farmers or other outdoor workers; it can be seen also in persons suffering chronic radiodermatitis from radiation therapy.

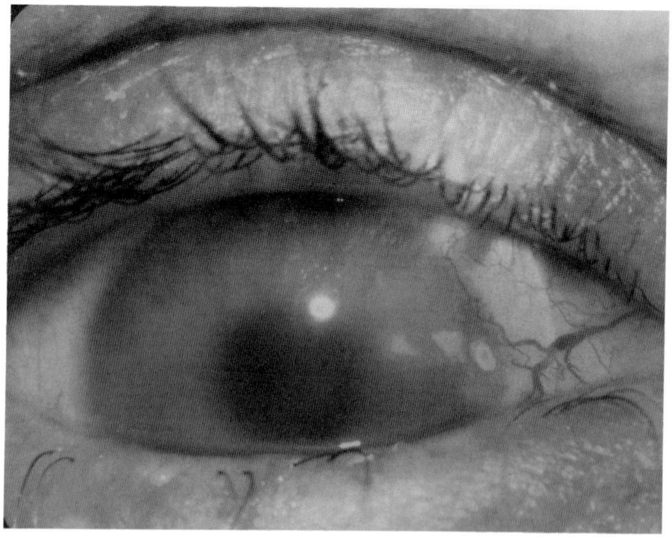

Figure 17.5. Corneal clouding, conjunctival telangiectasia with vascularization of a portion of the cornea, and telangiectasia and loss of lashes of the lower lid in a 28-year-old patient with xeroderma pigmentosum. She is wearing a soft contact lens for protection of the cornea. She subsequently had a partially successful corneal transplantation. (From Kraemer KH: Xeroderma pigmentosum. In Demis DJ, Dobson RL, McGuire J: *Clinical Dermatology.* Hagerstown, MD, Harper & Row, 1980, vol 4, pp 1–33.)

Finally, XP patients begin to develop skin neoplasms, the first such growths appearing anywhere from age 2 or 3 to as late as the 3rd or 4th decade of life. Most often the earliest lesions consist of benign keratoses, warty papillomas, angiomas, and premalignant actinic keratoses. Occasionally fibromas, angiofibromas, and neurofibromas have been reported. Keratoacanthomas also may develop.

Malignant skin tumors may appear at a very early age. In a recent study of the XP literature by Kraemer and associates (8) the median age of XP patients at the time of their first-reported skin cancer was 8 years, and the overall frequency of basal and squamous cell carcinomas in XP patients was estimated to be almost 5000-fold greater by age 20 than that for the general population in the United States. Basal and squamous cell carcinomas of the skin are by far the most common malignancies reported in XP patients, but the incidence of malignant melanoma is greatly increased in XP also, as much as 2000-fold the expected incidence by age 20 (8). A high frequency of malignant neoplasms, mostly squamous cell carcinomas, of the anterior tip of the tongue have been reported in XP patients, especially in those of African and Middle Eastern ancestry (9, 10).

Sarcomas of the skin have been reported in XP patients but are not common (11).

OCULAR ABNORMALITIES

Most XP patients develop photophobia and conjunctivitis at an early age, often at the time of or even before the earliest cutaneous signs of XP. However, a few patients from Israel have been reported who developed significant

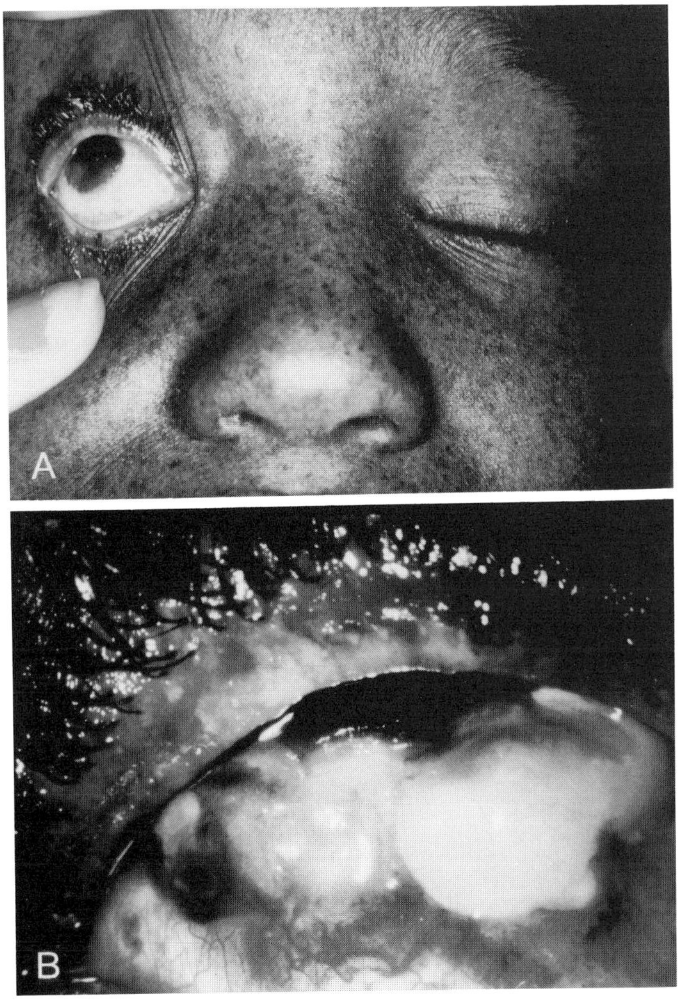

Figure 17.6. *A,* Black American girl, age 7, with xeroderma pigmentosum. She had freckling of her face with severe photophobia. Conjuctival injection and corneal cloudiness is seen in her right eye. *B,* Two years later a protruding squamous cell carcinoma was removed from her right eye.

cutaneous changes of XP on the face without any appreciable conjunctivitis (10). In some cases acute blepharitis, iritis, and keratitis may also occur.

Changes of the lids and conjunctivae usually parallel those of the ultraviolet-damaged skin on the rest of the

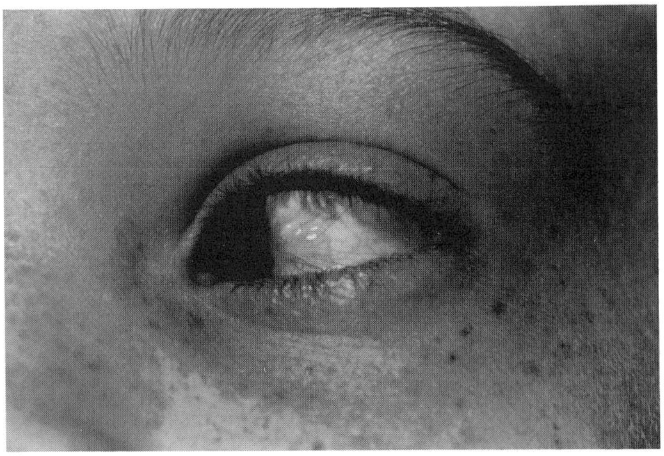

Figure 17.7. Squamous cell carcinoma of conjunctiva near corneoscleral limbus in an 8-year-old patient with xeroderma pigmentosum. (From Kraemer KH: Xeroderma pigmentosum. In Demis DJ, Dobson RL, McGuire J: *Clinical Dermatology.* Hagerstown, MD, Harper & Row, 1980, vol 4, pp 1–33.)

face, including the development of pigmentary abnormalities, telangiectasia, and atrophy. Atrophy of the lids is a major source of subsequent ocular problems, including ectropion and madarosis, and resultant exposure keratitis. Corneal opacification may result from such keratitis, and synechiae or atrophy of the iris can result from iritis. Conjunctival inflammation may occasionally lead to vascularization of the cornea (Figs. 17.2–17.6).

A variety of benign inflammatory growths of the conjunctivae and cornea have been reported, including pingueculae, pterygiums, symblepharons, pigmented phlyctenule-like lesions, and staphylomas of the cornea (12).

Benign and malignant tumors of the lids occur with similar frequency and histologic type to tumors of the sun-exposed skin elsewhere (Figs. 17.1 and 17.3). In addition, intraepithelial epitheliomas and squamous cell carcinomas of the conjunctivae may arise, especially at the corneal-scleral limbus (Figs. 17.6 and 17.7). Primary tumors of the cornea have included epitheliomas, squamous cell carcinomas, sarcomas, and melanomas (12). Benign fibromas and papillomas of the iris have been reported also. However, the funds of the eye is unaffected in XP, presumably because it is effectively shielded from ultraviolet light by the anterior structure of the eye.

NEUROLOGIC ABNORMALITIES

Xeroderma pigmentosum associated with severe neurological and somatic abnormalities is sometimes referred to as the "DeSanctis-Cacchione syndrome" after two Italians, DeSanctis and Cacchione, who in 1932 (13) reported three brothers with such a clinical picture. The list of possible neurologic or somatic abnormalities associated with XP includes microcephaly with progressive mental deterioration (sometimes beginning in the first or second year of life), low intelligence, hypoflexia or areflexia, progressive sensorineural deafness, choreoathetosis, ataxia, spasticity, retarded growth, and retarded sexual development. Only a few patients have been reported with all of these abnormalities. More often, patients with XP have only one or a few of these abnormalities, and the majority of reported cases of XP have none of these associated neurological or somatic abnormalities (1, 12).

Pathologically, patients with XP and associated neurologic abnormalities have a simple loss of neurons, especially from the cerebral cortex and cerebellum, without evidence of an abnormal storage process, inflammatory changes, or gliosis (1, 13, 14). Affected patients may suffer a progressive lower motor neuron degeneration, which is probably responsible for the often reported hypoflexia or areflexia (1, 13).

OTHER ABNORMALITIES

Deficient growth and sexual development have been reported primarily in those XP patients with the early onset and rapid progression of severe neurologic abnormalities. No consistent pattern of abnormalities in clinical laboratory tests has been identified among such patients (12).

Neoplasms of internal organs have been reported in XP, and the recent study by Kraemer and associates (8) has found evidence to suggest that the incidence of certain relatively uncommon internal malignancies, such as brain cancers, and nonglossal oral cavity cancers is greatly increased among patients with XP. Whether the incidence of other internal malignancies, especially those more common among the general population, is increased in XP remains an open question at this time.

XP WITH COCKAYNE'S SYNDROME

Interestingly, two individuals have been reported, each of whom suffered from both XP and another, very rare, autosomal recessive disorder known as Cockayne's syndrome (1, 15). The features of Cockayne's syndrome include cachectic dwarfism, sunsensitivity, deafness, mental retardation, normal pressure hydrocephalus, a "wizened" facial appearance, decreased nerve conduction velocities, optic nerve atrophy, and a "salt and pepper" pigmentary retinal degeneration. The increased reflexes and fundus changes served to differentiate these two patients from patients with the DeSanctis-Cacchione syndrome. The cutaneous changes in these two patients were typical of those found in XP, and unlike those in other reported cases of Cockayne's syndrome, in which pigmentary abnormalities and skin cancers are not found. Each of these individuals, as it turns out, has a unique DNA repair defect, different from that of all other XP patients so far studied, and different from each other as well (15). Nevertheless, the coincidence of these two patients, each having both XP and Cockayne's syndrome strongly suggests that, as in XP, defective DNA repair also may play a role in the pathology of Cockayne's syndrome (Fig. 17.4).

DNA REPAIR DEFECTS

Extensive research into the biochemistry of human DNA repair mechanisms and their role in a variety of biologic phenomena, including cancer cause and prevention, has been performed in vitro with cells derived from patients with xeroderma pigmentosum. Detailed reviews of this research are available (1, 10, 12, 16), and we will herein briefly summarize only certain findings pertaining specifically to XP. The first report showing that cells from XP patients were defective in DNA repair capacity was that of Cleaver, in 1968 (17). He showed that the so-called nucleotide excision repair pathway was defective in XP cells. This repair pathway is composed of a series of enzymes that act in sequence to remove certain aberrant chemical "lesions" from DNA.

The chemical "lesion" most studied is the pyrimidine dimer, a covalent linkage between two adjacent pyrimidine bases on one strand of the double-stranded DNA molecule. This lesion, readily caused by UV radiation, distorts the DNA helix and interferes with normal translation and replication of the DNA. Other lesions of DNA, caused by any of a variety of chemical mutagens and carcinogens, also interfere with DNA function, and are also repaired by the nucleotide excision repair pathway. Most XP cells, it turns out, are apparently defective in an early step in this repair pathway. The consequences of such defects are that cells from XP patients are killed more readily by UV radiation (and by many chemical mutagens); XP cells show increased levels of UV-induced chromosome breakage, of UV-induced sister-chromated exchanges, and of UV- and chemical-induced mutations (7, 10, 12). Some or all of these cellular phenomena may of course be relevant to the increased incidence of sunlight-induced skin cancers in XP patients.

In 1972, researchers in the Netherlands showed that fusion of cells from certain XP patients could result in multinucleated cells in which DNA excision repair levels were restored to normal; this phenomenon is termed *complementation.* These investigators identified three different "complementation groups," i.e., different genetic forms of XP, each having a repair defect unique from the others (18). Subsequent work by Kraemer and associates (19) and others has expanded the number of complementation groups to eight (15, 20, 21). Hence, at least eight different genetic defects in the DNA excision repair pathway can result in the XP phenotype.

Furthermore, another group of XP patients, first identified by Burk and co-workers (22), have normal DNA excision repair. The cells from these patients, who are designated "XP variants" have been found to be defective in a separate DNA repair process known as "postreplication repair." In normal cells, this process, by as yet undetermined molecular mechanisms, apparently allows DNA to replicate in the presence of some unrepaired pyrimidine dimers or other chemical lesions in the template DNA. While most patients with the variant form of XP have had all the classical clinical manifestations of XP, there is a subgroup of XP variants, formerly referred to as having "pigmented xerodermoid" in whom the classical pigmentary and neoplastic abnormalities are quite delayed in onset, e.g., into the fourth decade or later (10).

TREATMENT

Early diagnosis, close medical monitoring for detection of neoplasms, and complete protection from UV radiation exposure are the most important aspects of management in XP. The latter, when begun at an early age, has been shown to result in a marked reduction of the serious cutaneous and ocular changes of XP. Unfortunately, there is no known treatment for the neurological abnormalities of XP.

Protection from UV radiation involves many considerations. Sunlight is the principal source of UV light in our environment, but patients must also avoid exposure to UV light from artificial sources, such as germicidal lamps, sunlamps, and even the common cool white fluorescent lamp, if unfiltered, as this source, too, emits small amounts of potentially harmful UV radiation. Incandescent lamps appear to be safe for XP patients, as does exposure to sunlight or other UV sources filtered through window glass. Patients should adopt a life-style that minimizes potential UV exposure (e.g., indoor and/or night jobs); children should only play outdoors if they can be provided with a shelter that totally blocks direct UV exposure. Clothing should cover as much of the skin surface as possible. Outdoor activity should be limited to early mornings and late afternoons. Wide-brimmed hats and long hair styles should be encouraged. Sunglasses that are completely opaque to UV light should be worn whenever the patient is outdoors. The glasses should be equipped with side shields to protect eyelids and periorbital skin. In the car, windows should always be closed. Any areas of skin not fully covered by clothing should be covered with opaque sun blocking agents (zinc oxide or titanium dioxide), thick makeup, or at the very least, with chemical sunscreens having a sun-protection factor rating of 15 or more.

The detection of neoplasms involves frequent medical examinations, preferably at least every 3 months, and instruction of the patient and/or patient's family in the recognition of skin cancers. Examinations should always include the eyes (including conjunctival areas normally covered by the lids), the nares, the mouth (especially the tongue), and the scalp.

Premalignant actinic keratoses can be treated by liquid nitrogen cryotherapy or by topical 5-fluorouracil. Large areas containing many keratoses can be treated effectively with dermatome shaving, dermabrasion, or split-thickness skin grafts (12).

Malignant lesions in XP patients are treated by the standard modalities utilized for such malignancies in patients without XP, e.g., electrodessication and curettage, cryosurgery, surgical excision, and chemosurgery. X-radiation therapy is tolerated without unusual reactions by most XP patients. One must keep in mind that conservation of tissue is even more important in XP than in normal patients, due to the increased likelihood that further surgery in the same vicinity may be required in the future. This is especially important around the eyes (Fig. 7.8).

Artificial tears or soft contact lenses may help keep the cornea moist and protect it against trauma when the patient has developed lid deformities. Corneal transplants have been used to restore vision after severe keratitis and corneal opacification, but corneal vascularization may increase the chances of transplant rejection (12).

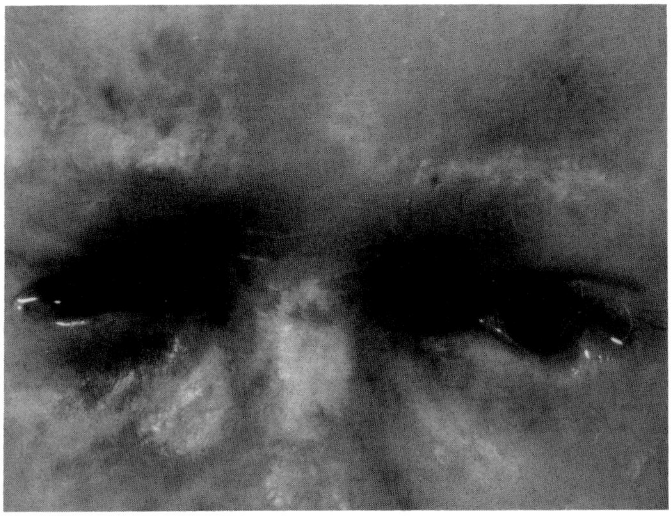

Figure 17.8. Patient, age 27, had marked photophobia since early childhood. She had multiple basal cell and squamous cell carcinomas of the face and eyelids with numerous skin grafts. She has an unusual "inverse" pattern of pigmentation with marked freckling of the abdomen and chest and diminished pigment on the face. (From Kraemer KH, Slor H: Xeroderma pigmentosum. *Clin Dermatol* 3: 33–69, 1985.)

REFERENCES

1. Robbins JH, Kraemer KH, Lutzner MA, et al: Xeroderma pigmentosum: An inherited disease with sun sensitivity, multiple cutaneous neoplasms, and abnormal DNA repair. *Ann Intern Med* 80: 221–248, 1974.
2. Neel JV, Kodai M, Brewer R, Anderson RC: The incidence of consanguineous matings in Japan; With remarks on the estimation of comparative gene frequencies and the expected rate of appearance of induced recessive mutations. *Am J Hum Genet* 1: 156–178, 1949.
3. El-Hefnawi H, Rasheed A: Xeroderma pigmentosum: A further clinical study of 12 Egyptian cases. *J Egypt Med Assoc* 45: 106–141, 1962.
4. Takebe H, Miki Y, Kozuka T, et al: DNA repair characteristics and skin cancers of xeroderma pigmentosum patients in Japan. *Cancer Res* 37: 490–495, 1977.
5. Anderson T, Begg M: Xeroderma pigmentosum of mild type. *Br J Dermatol* 62: 402–407, 1950.
6. Pawsey SA, Magnus IA, Ramsay CA, et al: Clinical, genetic and DNA repair studies on a consecutive series of patients with xeroderma pigmentosum. *Q J Med* 48: 179–210, 1979.
7. Andrews AD, Barrett SF, Robbins JH: Xeroderma pigmentosum neurological abnormalities correlate with colony-forming ability after ultraviolet radiation. *Proc Natl Acad Sci USA* 75: 1984–1988, 1978.
8. Kraemer KH, Lee MM, Scotto J: DNA repair protects against cutaneous and internal neoplasms: Evidence from xeroderma pigmentosum. *Carcinogenesis* 5: 511–514, 1984.
9. Plotnick H: Xeroderma pigmentosum and mucocutaneous malignancies in three black siblings. *Cutis* 25: 311–313, 1980.
10. Kraemer KH, Slor H: Xeroderma pigmentosum. *Clin Dermatol* 3: 33–69, 1985.
11. Hadida E, Marill FG, Sayag J: Xeroderma pigmentosum (A propos

de 48 observations personelles). *Ann Dermatol Syphiligr* 90: 467–496, 1963.
12. Kraemer KH: Xeroderma pigmentosum. In Demis DJ, Dobson RL, McGuire J: *Clinical Dermatology*. Hagerstown, Md., Harper & Row, 1980, vol 4, pp 1–33.
13. DeSanctis C, Cacchione A: L'idiozia xerodermica. *Riv Sper Freniatr* 56: 269–292, 1932.
14. Yano K: Xeroderma pigmentosum with changes in the C.N.S.: A histological study. *Folia Psychiatr Jpn* 4: 143, 1950.
15. Moshell AN, Ganges MB, Lutzner MA, et al: A new patient with both xeroderma pigmentosum and Cochayne syndrome establishes the new xeroderma pigmentosum complementation group H. In Friedberg E, Bridges B (eds): *Cellular Responses to DNA Damage.* New York, Alan R Liss, 1983, pp 209–213.
16. Cleaver JE: DNA repair deficiencies. In Fleischmajen R (ed): *Progress in Diseases of the Skin.* Grune & Stratton, New York, 1984, vol 2.
17. Cleaver JE: Defective repair replications of DNA in xeroderma pigmentosum. *Nature* 218: 652–656, 1968.
18. DeWeerd-Kastelein EA, Keijzer W, Bootsma D: Genetic heterogeneity of xeroderma pigmentosum demonstrated by somatic cell hybridization. *Nature* 238: 80–83, 1972.
19. Kraemer KH, DeWeerd-Kastelein EA, Robbins JH: Five complementation groups in xeroderma pigmentosum. *Mutation Res* 33: 327–340, 1975.
20. Arase S, Kozuka T, Tanaka K, et al: A sixth complementation group in xeroderma pigmentosum. *Mutation Res* 59: 143–146, 1979.
21. Keijzer W, Jaspers NG, Abrahams PJ, et al: A seventh complementation group in excision-deficient xeroderma pigmentosum. *Mutation REs* 62: 183–190, 1979.
22. Burk PG, Lutzner MA, Clarke DD, et al: Ultraviolet-stimulated thymidine incorporation in xeroderma pigmentosum lymphocytes. *J Lab Clin Med* 77: 759–767, 1971.

CHAPTER 18

Ablepharon, Microblepharon, and Cryptophthalmos

DAVID M. REIFLER, M.D.
ALBERT HORNBLASS, M.D.

Ablepharon may be defined as a congenital anomaly in which there is total absence of both the upper and lower eyelids. At birth, there may be severe corneal exposure or cryptophthalamos may be present, in which case the cornea and eyelid folds are replaced by skin that passes smoothly over the orbital margin (1). Both ablepharon with cryptophthalmos and ablepharon without cryptophthalmos have occurred in siblings and in children with bilaterally asymmetric findings (2–4). When ablepharon with cryptophthalmos is unilateral, the opposite side may be entirely normal (5) or show various anomalies including eyelid colobomata (6), severe microblepharon with symblepharon formation (3), or ablepharon without cryptophthalamos (2–7).

Microblepharon, a less severe form of eyelid involvement, is defined as a vertically shortened eyelid, usually with normal eyelid structures (8). Mild degrees of microblepharon are rarely associated with widespread congenital anomalies. However, in the more severe forms of approaching ablepharon, associated anomalies are frequently found (8). The association of congenital eyelid deformities with other congenital anomalies has been recognized since the first report of cryptophthalmos by Zehender (9) in 1872. These anomalies include meningoencephalocele (9), abnormal hairline (3), deformities of the ear and nose (2, 10, 11), cleft lip and palate (12), irregular dentition (7, 11), ankyloglossia (10), laryngeal atresia (13), syndactyly (3, 12, 14, 15), ventral hernia (7, 10), and genitourinary abnormalities (2, 10, 14). The term "cryptophthalmos syndrome" has been applied to the broad spectrum of these associated findings (16).

A classification of congenital eyelid fold abnormalities is shown in Table 18.1. Ablepharon, microblepharon, and cryptophthalmos are the least common of these abnormalities and probably comprise a continuous spectrum of related conditions (17). Eyelid coloboma is also an uncommon condition, although not quite so rarely seen (discussed elsewhere in this volume). Contralateral eyelid coloboma is occasionally seen in cases of ablepharon (6), which suggests common pathogenetic factors. Eyelid colobomas have also been grouped within a broader system of classification for facial and craniofacial clefts (18, 19), but a clear relationship between ablepharon/microblepharon and the various types of facial clefts has not been established. The most common forms of congenital eyelid fold abnormalities involve the various types of congenital ptosis. These are discussed elsewhere in this volume.

The ablepharon-macrostomia syndrome has a distinctive set of anomalies that include either ablepharon or microblepharon, an enlarged fish-like mouth, and the absence of lanugo (Fig. 18.1; Refs. 7, 17). This syndrome shares several features in common with other cryptophthalmos syndromes, particularly the abnormally shaped ears and nose, ventral hernia, and genitourinary anomalies.

The evidence linking the rare conditions of ablepharon, microblepharon, and cryptophthalmos may be summarized as follows. First, an asymmetric concurrence of these different conditions is sometimes seen in fellow eyes of the same individual where anomalies are bilateral. Second, different formes frustes of these anomalies may be present within different members of a single family. Third, ablepharon, microblepharon, and cryptophthalmos have been described in association with similar patterns of multiple organ system anomalies (16, 17).

PATHOPHYSIOLOGY

PATHOGENESIS

A review of eyelid development is helpful in understanding congenital eyelid abnormalities. The upper and lower eyelid anlage appear early in the second month (16–20 mm) of fetal development (8, 20). The eyelid folds elongate and contact each other at about 10 weeks (32–45 mm). The eyelids normally separate at about 6 months (180–200 mm). This separation has been attributed to keratinization and holocrine secretion of lipid at the eyelid margin (21). Migrations of neural crest cells are also now known to contribute to the eyelids and corneal stroma (22).

The mechanisms involved in the formation of ablepharon may vary between cases. Ablepharon may result from either a primary failure of eyelid development, as first suggested by Zehender (9). Alternatively, a destruction and subsequent absorption of the eyelids may account for the anomaly in other cases (10). The presence or absence of lashes in cryptophthalmos has been interpreted by some authors as giving some insight into the pathogenesis of this condition (21). This finding does not distinguish between the possible mechanisms, i.e., primary failure of

Table 18.1
Classification of Congenital Eyelid Fold Abnormalities[a]

Cryptophthalmos (ablepharon)
Microblepharon
Coloboma
Epicanthus, ptosis and abnormalities of the levator palpebrae superioris

[a] From Mann I: *Developmental Abnormalities of the Eye.* London, Cambridge University Press, 1937, p 395.

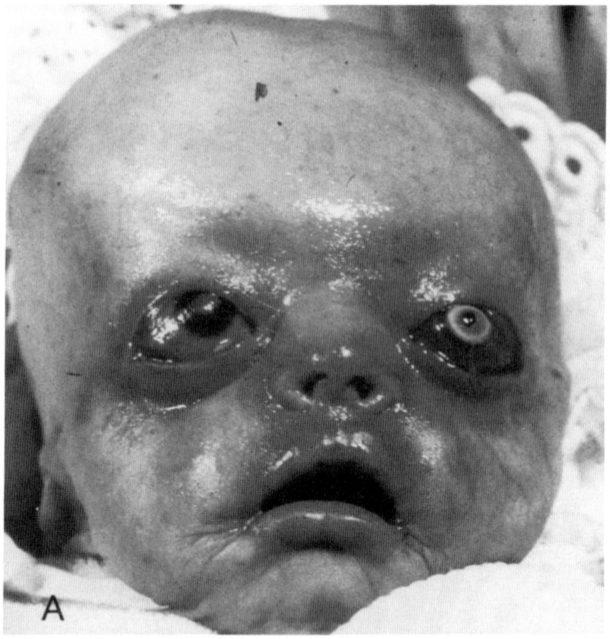

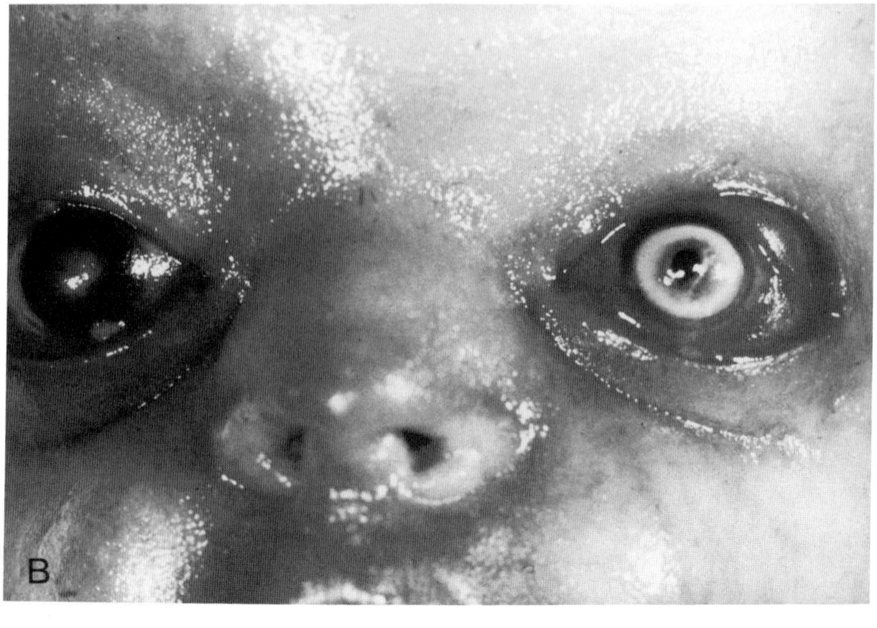

Figure 18.1. A case of ablepharon-macrostomia in a 10-day-old infant. *A,* Abnormal findings included an absence of eyebrows, vertically shortened eyelids, right corneal opacity, left corneal perforation, anomalous pinnae and macrostomia. *B,* Severe, bilateral corneal exposure with corneal opacity in the right eye and corneal perforation in the left eye. (From Hornblass A, Reifler DM: Ablepharon macrostromia syndrome. *Am J Ophthalmol* 99: 552–556, 1985.)

Table 18.2
Syndromes Associated with Ablepharon and/or Cryptophthalmos

Microblepharon
Mild degree: usually no syndromic associations
Severe forms approaching ablepharon: associated anomalies likely (6)[a]
Ablepharon without cryptophthalmos
Ablepharon macrostomia syndrome (8) (see text)
Cryptophthalmos
Cryptophthalmos syndrome (16) (see text)
Malformative syndrome with cryptophthalmos (14)
Cryptophthalmos
Dyscephaly (including meningocele, anomalies of ear, nose, lip and palate)
Syndactyly
Genital malformations
Cryptophthalmos-syndactyly syndrome (3)
Cryptophthalmos
Syndactyly
Presence or absence of additional anomalies
Fraser syndrome (2)
Cryptophthalmos
Auricular defects
Abnormal genitalia

[a] References are in parentheses.

eyelid fold development, failure of lid separation, or secondary destruction. However, theories of a local inflammatory or destructive process (10), or mechanical interference of eyelid development by amniotic bands (6), seem inconsistent with the frequent syndromic presentations of ablepharon that include a variety of visceral anomalies. A summary of the various syndromes associated with ablepharon and/or cryptophthalmos is shown in Table 18.2.

The two different forms of ablepharon, i.e., with and without cryptophthalmos, probably represent a genetically determined autosomal recessive disorder with a wide range of expression. Parental consanguinity is present in 15% of cases (3), and many familial cases of two or three siblings have been reported (2, 4, 9, 10, 14). Azevedo, Biondi, and Ramalho (4) reported a pair of monozygotic twins with differing expressions of ablepharon. One of the twins was born with bilateral cryptophthalmos and one with ablepharon on the right and cryptophthalmos on the left.

HISTOPATHOLOGY

Duke-Elder (6) interpreted the skin over the globe in cryptophthalmos as representing a keratinized transformation of the corneal epithelium into true integument. The keratinizing epithelium is many cell layers thick and may show irregular ingrowths of rete peg-like formations into the deeper layers. The outer surface includes well-formed sweat and sebaceous glands (10). Although the orbicularis and levator may be present in cases of cryptophthalmos, the tarsal plate and meibomian glands are generally absent (6). The basal cell layer contains melanin.

In microblepharon, all of the eyelid structures are represented, but the lids are vertically shortened. The corneal epithelium may be normal initially or show dermoid patches, as in cases of eyelid colobomas. Secondary changes in the cornea may also occur, including ulceration, perforation, and scar formation.

TREATMENT, RESULTS, AND COMPLICATIONS

The treatment of severe microblepharon or ablepharon represents a formidable challenge, due to the problem of severe corneal exposure and the extensive reconstructive surgery that may be required (17, 23). In cryptophthalmos, the smooth keratinized tissue that covers the globe, which is perhaps metaplastic cornea and conjunctiva (12), is not amenable to surgery since an incision through this tissue may enter directly into the inside of the eye (1). The prognosis for vision in such cases of cryptophthalmos is virtually hopeless. However, reconstruction of the eyelids may afford some cosmetic improvement, particularly when there is partial cryptophthalmos (2–3). The visual prognosis is somewhat better, although still guarded, in the situation of ablepharon without cryptophthalmos. Despite the grotesque appearance of these children, early surgical management must be directed primarily toward correcting functional defects and only secondarily toward correcting cosmetic deformities. The use of vestigial lid structures is particularly advantageous in reconstruction (17).

Total reconstruction of an eyelid in microblepharon and ablepharon differs in many respects from that frequently encountered in large eyelid reconstructions following traumatic loss or tumor excision since both the upper and lower eyelids are usually involved simultaneously. The principles utilized in two-stage, lid-sharing procedures such as the Hughes procedure (24) or the Cutler-Beard bridge flap method (25, 26) may have to be modified or abandoned in favor of alternate methods. Even in the presence of sufficient donor lower lid tissue for a bridge flap procedure, nearly all of the tarsal plate is left to maintain the integrity of the bridge of the lower lid margin (27). The implantation of material such as eyebank sclera within the advanced bridge flap, may give an added measure of stability to the reconstructed eyelid and prevent inward rotation. This modification has been used in an infant with extensive bilateral upper eyelid colobomas (27). The temporary blepharorrhaphy inherent in lid-sharing reconstructive techniques serves a dual purpose of providing corneal protection and mobilization of tissue for reconstruction. Unfortunately, ipsilateral lid-sharing procedures are not possible when there is a lack of sufficient donor tissue. In unilateral cases a viable composite eyelid graft taken from the contralateral side may at least partially furnish the tissue required for reconstruction (28). Nourishment of such composite grafts is best assured by an overlying skin flap and mobilization of the underlying conjunctiva.

Sole reliance on free skin grafts placed directly over mobilized conjunctiva may lead to failure since viability of the graft depends entirely on conjunctival flaps (29). In some cases, as in the ablepharon-macrostomia syndrome

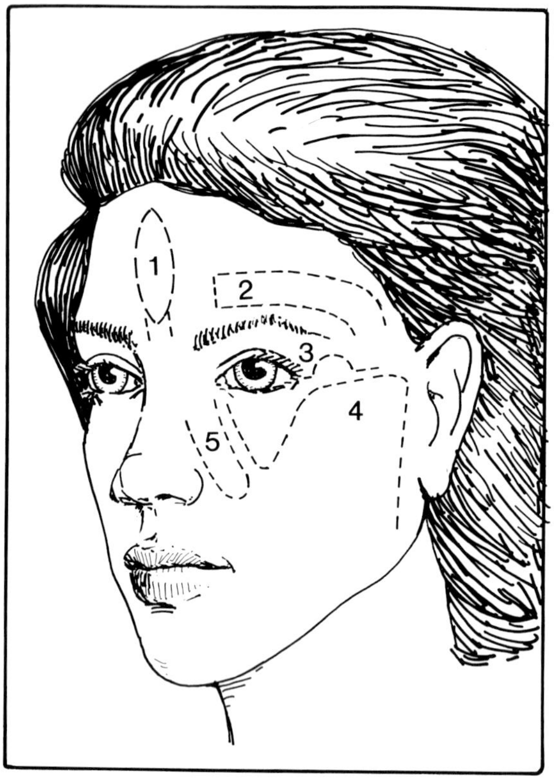

Figure 18.2. Diagram of local periorbital skin flaps. Local flaps available for eyelid reconstruction include (*1*) median forehead, (*2*) supraorbital, (*3*) temporal semicircular, (*4*) cheek, and (*5*) nasolabial flaps.

(17), there may be a great deal of redundant posterior auricular and cervical skin. When used in combination with other techniques, this excess tissue may be an excellent source for free skin grafts. Although there may be an absence of lanugo at birth, this skin can become hair bearing with time.

Local, periorbital skin flaps may be used to reconstruct the anterior eyelid lamellae in cases of severe congenital eyelid defects. Local flaps available for eyelid reconstruction include median forehead, supraorbital, temporal, cheek, and nasolabial flaps (Fig. 18.2; Refs. 30, 31). Preparation of skin flaps for the treatment of ablepharon and allied conditions requires a posterior lining of mucous membrane. Mobilization of the residual conjunctival from the fornices may be possible in these cases, unless there is extensive ankyloblepharon and symblepharon formation. Even though they are much thicker than eyelid skin, local skin flaps have a high rate of long-term viability. The use of combinations of techniques, such as the advancement of a semicircular skin flap over a composite eyelid graft (31), may contribute to the overall reconstruction effort.

The factors influencing visual prognosis in cases of ablepharon, microblepharon, and cryptophthalmos include the severity of primary and secondary corneal abnormalities, the presence of associated ocular pathology, and the healing responses to plastic and reconstructive surgery.

REFERENCES

1. Yanoff M, Fine B: *Ocular Pathology. A Text and Atlas*, ed 2. Philadelphia, Harper & Row, 1982, p 215.
2. Fraser GR: Our genetical load. A review of some aspects of genetical variation. *Ann Hum Genet* 25: 387–415, 1962.
3. Sugar HS: The cryptophthalmos-syndactyly syndrome. *Am J Ophthalmol* 66: 897–899, 1968.
4. Azevedo ES, Biondo J, Ramalho LM: The cryptophthalmos in two families from Bahia, Brazil. *J Med Genet* 10: 389–392, 1973.
5. Howard RO, Fineman RM, Anderson B, Moseley N, Gilman M, Rothman S: Unilateral cryptophthalmos. *Am J Ophthalmol* 87: 556–560, 1979.
6. Duke-Elder S: *System of Ophthalmology*. St. Louis, CV Mosby, 1964, vol 3 pt 2, p 829.
7. McCarthy GT, West CM: Ablepharon macrostomia. *Develop Med Child Neurol* 19: 659–672, 1977.
8. Mann I: *Developmental Abnormalities of the Eye*. London, Cambridge University Press, 1937, p 395.
9. Zehender W: Eine Missgeburt mit hautuberwachsenen Augen oder Kryptophthalmos. *Klin Monatsblat Augen* 10: 225–249, 1872.
10. Gupta SP, Saxena RC: Cryptophthalmos. *Br J Ophthalmol* 46: 629–632, 1962.
11. Ide CH, Wollschlaeger PB: Multiple congenital abnormalities associated with cryptophthalmia. *Arch Ophthalmol* 81: 638–644, 1969.
12. Zinn S: Cryptophthalmia. *Am. J. Ophthalmol* 40: 219–223, 1955.
13. Chiari H: Congenitales Ankylo-et Symblepharon und congenitale Atresia Laryngis bei einem Kinde mit mehrfachen anderweitigen Bildungsanomalen. *Prager Zeit Heil* 4: 143–154, 1883.
14. Francois J: Malformative syndrome with cryptophthalmia. *Int Ophthalmol Clin* 8: 817–837, 1968.
15. Dinno ND, Edwards WE, Weiskopf B: The cryptophthalmos-syndactyly syndrome. *Clin Pediatr* 13: 219–224, 1974.
16. Goodman RM, Gorlin RJ: *Atlas of the Face in Genetic Disorders*, ed 2. St. Louis, CV Mosby, 1977, p 262.
17. Hornblass A, Reifler DM: Ablepharon macrostromia syndrome. *Am J Ophthalmol* 99: 552–556, 1985.
18. Tessier P: Anatomical classification of facial, craniofacial and laterofacial clefts. In Tessier P et al (eds): *Symposium on Plastic Surgery in the Orbital Region*. CV Mosby, St. Louis, 1974, p 189.
19. Tessier P: Anatomical classification of facial, craniofacial and laterofacial clefts. *J Maxillofac Surg* 4: 69–74, 1976.
20. Ozanics V, Jakobiec FA: Prenatal development of the eye and its adnexa. In Duane TD, Jaeger EA (eds): *Biomedical Foundations of Ophthalmology*. Philadelphia, Harper & Row, 1982, vol 1, ch 3, p 14.
21. Anderson H, Ehlers N, Matthiessen ME: Histochemistry and development of the human eyelids. *Acta Ophthalmol* 43: 642–668, 1965.
22. Noden DM: Periocular mesenchyme Neural crest and medodermal interactions. In Duane TD, Jaeger EA (eds): *Biomedical Foundations of Ophthalmology*. Philadelphia, Harper & Row, 1982, vol 1, ch 13, p 14.
23. Waring GO, Shields JA: Partial unilateral cryptophthalmos with syndactyly brachycephaly and renal anomalies. *Am J Ophthalmol* 79: 437–449, 1975.
24. Hughes WL: A new method for rebuilding a lower lid. *Arch Ophthalmol* 17: 1008–1017, 1937.
25. Culter NL, Beard C: A method for partial and total upper lid reconstruction. *Am J Ophthalmol* 39: 1–7, 1955.
26. Smith B, Obear M: Bridge flap technique for large upper lid defects. *Plast Reconstr Surg* 38: 45–48, 1966.
27. Wesley RE, McCord CD: Transplantation of eye bank sclera in the Culter-Beard method of upper eyelid reconstruction. *Ophthalmology* 87: 1022–1028, 1980.
28. Putterman AM: Viable composite grafting in eyelid reconstruction. *Am J Ophthalmol* 85: 237–241, 1978.
29. Smith BC, Nesi FA: Upper lid loss due to formalin injection: Surgical reconstruction. *Ophthalmology* 86: 1951–1953, 1979.
30. Achauer BM, Menick FJ: Salvage of seeing eyes after avulsion of upper and lower lids. *Plast Reconstr Surg* 75: 11–15, 1985.
31. Putterman AM: Combined viable composite graft and temporal semicircular skin flap procedure. *Am J Ophthalmol* 98: 348–354, 1984.

SECTION III

DISEASES OF THE EYELIDS

CHAPTER 19

Regional Contact Dermatitis of the Periorbital Area

ALEXANDER A. FISHER, M.D.

An important factor influencing the development and type of contact dermatitis is the area that is exposed to the contact allergen. The eyelids are one of the most sensitive areas. Any substance used on the scalp, face, or hands may produce allergic eczematous contact dermatitis of the eyelids, while those primary sites remain unaltered. Airborne pollen and dust and all types of volatile agents may affect the eyelids first and exclusively. Eyelash curlers may produce eyelid dermatitis because of sensitivity to the rubber edge of the nickel-plated portion of the appliance. Marked edema of the eyelids is often a feature of poison ivy and hair dye dermatitis.

Contact dermatitis is the most common eruption of the eyelid. The skin of the area is very susceptible to irritants and allergens. This may be because of its thinness (0.55 mm as compared with the thickness of the integument of the face, which measures about 2.0 mm) or because of rubbing with the hands and fingers, which become exposed to many substances.

COSMETICS

Contact dermatitis of the lids and periorbital area is more often caused by cosmetics applied to the hair, face, or fingernails than by cosmetics applied to the eye area. It is important to bear in mind that the sites to which some of these cosmetics are applied may not be affected.

This is particularly true for hair dye and nail polish. Allergic and irritant reactions to face creams, makeup (foundation lotions and bases), and blushers may likewise be limited to the eyelids (1).

Two principal forms of contact dermatitis attributable to eye-area cosmetics are recognized: *allergic contact dermatitis* and *irritant (toxic) contact dermatitis* (2). The morphologic features of these two forms are not always readily distinguishable. The degree of inflammation may be of the same order (usually mild to moderate), and the interval may be the same between the initial exposure and the onset of the dermatitis. Furthermore, potential irritants in eye area cosmetics and in cosmetics in general are usually weak; repeated exposures are often required to induce a reaction. Nor do all exposed individuals react, as they generally do with strong irritants (3).

PATCH TEST RESPONSE

The patch test response to allergens and irritants may likewise be indistinguishable. Erythema and/or edema at the patch test site may be elicited by either of these. An eczematous vesicular reaction diagnostic of delayed allergic hypersensitivity in response to potential allergens in eye makeup is by no means the rule. Consequently, interpretation of patch test results may be difficult, and the likelihood of irritant false-positive reactions needs to be borne in mind.

The cause of contact dermatitis of the eyelid is not always readily ascertainable. The following approach is recommended, especially when more than one cosmetic is suspect:

Step 1. Take a detailed history of exposure; this should include inquiry as to agents other than eye-area cosmetics that are known to elicit localized contact dermatitis of the eyelids, the introduction of a new product, and the renewal or refill of a previously used product. Modification and revision of formulations without a change in nomenclature or packaging is not an uncommon practice in the cosmetic industry. The method used to remove eye makeup also merits attention. Eye-area cosmetics may be removed by face creams, wet (chemically treated) facial tissues, or eye makeup removers.

Step 2. When the history is not sufficiently revealing of when more than one cosmetic appears to be involved, the *use test* is often helpful in pinpointing the causative agent. In my experience the use test is often more rewarding than an open or closed patch test with the product because of the high incidence of false-positive and false-negative reactions in response to patch testing. To carry out the use test, the product is generally applied 2 or 3 times a day for at least 4 or 5 days to the back of the ear or to a selected site on the flexor aspect of the forearm. Although a positive test (i.e., reproduction of the dermatitis) is significant, a negative response does not necessarily exclude the test substance as causative.

Step 3. *Patch tests* with the components (open or closed, depending on the chemical nature of the ingredient) of the product(s) incriminated by the history and use test are carried out in an attempt to identify causative allergen(s). Most cosmetic companies are ready to comply with a physician's request for such materials (see Appendix).

Appropriate interrogation and the use test will eliminate a good deal of unnecessary patch testing. Patch tests and photopatch tests should be used as confirmatory tools, not as the first line of investigation. The need for experience with the patch test technique despite its seeming simplicity and with the pitfalls of reading and interpretation cannot be overemphasized. As yet, there is no diagnostic test for irritant (toxic) contact dermatitis.

EYELID IRRITATION AND CONJUNCTIVAL REACTIONS

Stinging and burning of the eyes and lids on application of an eye-area cosmetic appear to be the most common complaints. These subjective symptoms are usually transitory and unaccompanied by objective signs of irritation. Evaporation of volatile components, such as mineral spirits, isoparaffins, and alcohol, and the presence of potential irritants such as propylene glycol and soap emulsifiers in the eye-area formulations are among the principal causes. In some instances tolerance increases with subsequent applications so that the offending product does not have to be discarded.

Conjunctivitis may be elicited by physical irritants (e.g., mascara flakes, eyeshadow dust, particles of eyeliner, and mascara extenders such as nylon or rayon fibers), chemical irritants (e.g., solvents and soap emulsifiers), and potential allergens (e.g., preservatives and fragrances).

Irritation Due to Mascara

Water-based mascara may contain a number of soap emulsifiers such as sodium borate and ammonium stearate, which are formed by interaction of stearic acid with ammonium hydroxide; these agents may be irritating to certain individuals with better tolerance for an anhydrous waterproof mascara. Conversely, an individual who does not tolerate waterproof mascara or waterproof eyeliner may tolerate their water-based counterparts. In the event that neither type of mascara or eyeliner is tolerable, a cake mascara or a cake eyeliner may be tried. Maybelline Cake Mascara, Lumilane Cake Mascara (Orlane), and Maybelline Ultra Liner Cake Eyeliner have only half the number of chemicals currently found in water-based and waterproof formulations. The potential for irritation is thus considerably reduced. This is not true for Channel's Compact Mascara, which is highly complex. Similarly, individuals who cannot use cream eyeshadow may tolerate pressed powder eyeshadow and vice versa.

Conjunctival Pigmentation Due to Eyeliner

Conjunctival pigmentation caused by eyeliner is a consequence of applying eyeliner to the conjunctival side of the lid instead of the exterior lid adjacent to the lashes. Unless the upper lid is everted to bring the aggregates of pigment deposited along the upper margin of the tarsal conjunctiva into view, this complication may be missed. Twelve cases were reported by Zuckerman (4) and another was reported by Jervey in 1969 (5). Although some patients complain of discomfort, tearing and itching, most are asymptomatic and do not require treatment.

Sensitivity to Eye Cosmetic Preservatives

Parabens. Parabens, with few exceptions, are common to all eye-area products. These esters of parahydroxybenzoic acid frequently are combined with at least one other antimicrobial such as phenylmercuric acetate, imidazolidinyl urea (Germall 115) or quaternium 15 (Dowicil 200) to ensure adequate protection against yeasts, molds, and pseudomonads, which are widely distributed in nature. Clinique's Resistant Eyeliner and Basic Eye Emphasizer are paraben-free; they contain sorbic acid as a preservative. Paraben-sensitive individuals however, do not necessarily have to avoid paraben-containing cosmetics. According to Fisher (6), patients sensitized to parabens may nevertheless tolerate paraben-containing cosmetics even on the thin skin of the eyelids provided the product is applied to normal skin that was not subjected to a dermatitis in the past. This is the so-called *paraben paradox*.

Other additives. Diisopropanolamine used in cosmetic gloss formulations to "set up" the gel has produced allergic contact dermatitis from an eyeshadow and a "blushing" gel (7). Ditertiarybutyl hydroquinone, an antioxidant in eyeshadow, produced an eyelid dermatitis (8).

Formaldehyde donors. Quaternium-15, imidazolidinyl urea, and DMDM hydantoin are formaldehyde donors. The latter is used less frequently than the other two compounds. Quaternium-15 has been shown to be a more active formaldehyde releaser than imidazolidinyl urea (9). Allergic reactions may be elicited by the compound per se or by the released formaldehyde. Fisher (10) maintains imidazolidinyl urea is a much safer preservative than quaternium 15 for formaldehyde-sensitive individuals. Potassium sorbate is also used as a preservative in eye-area products. Sensitization to this agent is reported (11).

Sensitivity to Eye Cosmetic Aids

Artificial Eyelash Adhesives. False eyelashes consist of synthetic or natural fibers, including human hair, mounted on a thin fabric strip. The adhesive is a mixture of rubber latex, cellulose gums, casein solubilized with a very mild alkali or other resins and water. The adhesive is formulated to be nonirritating and to permit easy removal of the lashes by simply peeling them off. This rubber latex rarely irritates the eyelids. I have encountered no instances of allergic reactions to it.

Eyelash Curlers. Nickel-sensitive patients may acquire eyelid dermatitis from nickel-plated eyelash curlers and tweezers. Such curlers and tweezers should be replaced by the stainless steel variety. Formerly, rubber-tipped eyelash curlers produced eyelid dermatitis in rubber-sensitive patients.

REACTIONS TO OTHER COSMETICS

Nail Polish Dermatitis

Nail polish dermatitis is an "ectopic" dermatitis since sensitized individuals do not acquire dermatitis of the nails or paronychial area but elsewhere such as the eyelids and neck (Fig.19.1). The dry nail polish becomes polymerized and is not a sensitizer (12). The sensitizing toluenesulfonamide formaldehyde resin in ordinary nail polish may be replaced by a "hypoallergenic" polyester resin (Clinique).

Sensitivity to Hair Cosmetics

Hair dyes, bleaching agents containing ammonium persulphate, perfumed hair sprays, hair-setting lotions, and shampoos containing formaldehyde may affect the eyelids without producing scalp or forehead dermatitis. Paraphenylenediamine sensitivity, and ammonium persulphate in particular, may produce marked edema of the eyelids (Figs. 19.2 and 19.3).

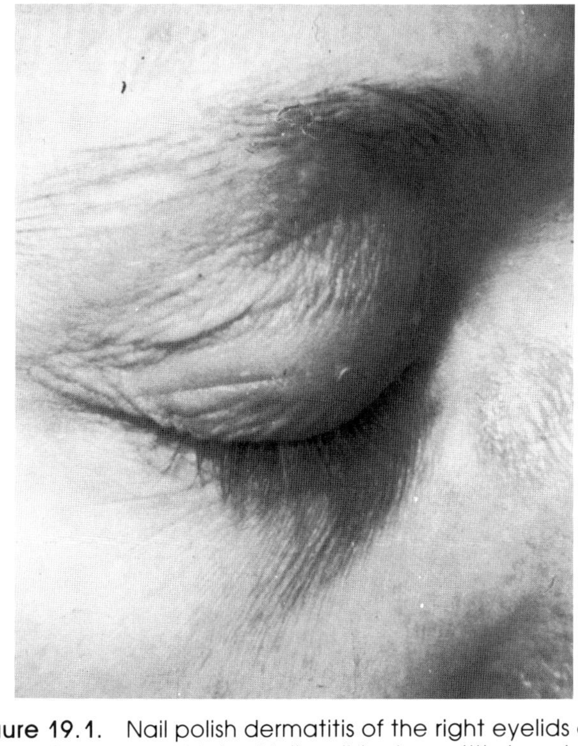

Figure 19.1. Nail polish dermatitis of the right eyelids and sides of the nose. Note: Nail polish dermatitis is ectopic and does not affect the paronychial area.

EYESHADOW MIMICKING ORBITAL CALCIFICATION ON X-RAY

A single case of bilateral curvilinear supraorbital shadows was found on x-ray examination of the skull of a patient complaining of increasing headaches that were

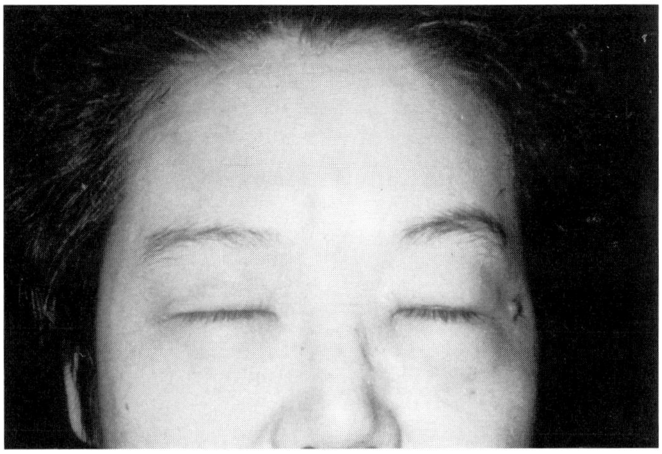

Figure 19.2. Edema and dermatitis of the eyelids and periorbital area due to hair dye sensitivity from allergic reaction to paraphenylenediamine, the most common hair dye.

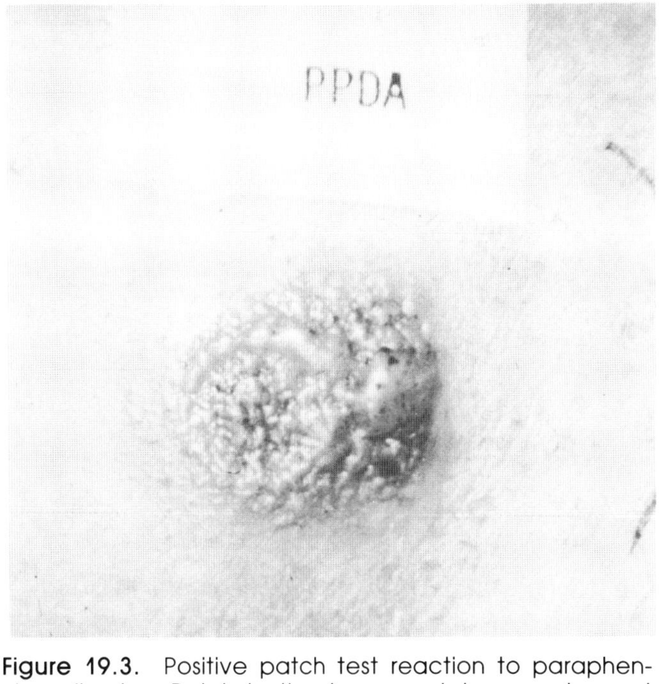

Figure 19.3. Positive patch test reaction to paraphenylenediamine. Patch testing is a mandatory requirement before dying the hair with this compound. This is often not done, as was the case in Figure 19.2.

initially interpreted as calcification. It was noted that the patient wore a large amount of eye makeup, which suggested the possibility of an artifact. The curvilinear shadows disappeared after the eye shadow was removed. Incidentally, a subsequent survey of 25 types of eye shadow showed that many were radiopaque because of bismuth, magnesium silicate, and iron oxides within the formulations (13).

OPHTHALMIC PREPARATIONS

The following preservatives may produce not only conjunctivitis but also eyelid dermatitis in sensitized individuals (14): benzalkonium chloride, an antiseptic which is one of the most widely used ophthalmic preservatives (Table 19.1, Fig. 19.4); thimerosal (merthiolate), another compound widely employed as an ophthalmic medication preservative (Table 19.2); and chlorbutanol, a very rare sensitizer whose preparations (Table 19.3) may be used when allergic reactions are present to thimerosal and benzalkonium chloride.

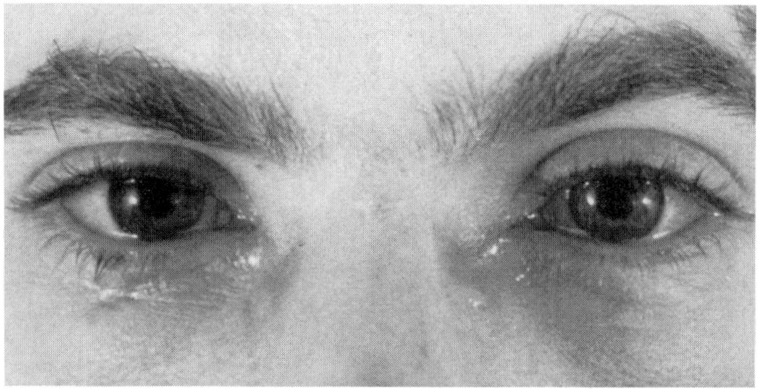

Figure 19.4. Conjunctivitis and dermatitis of the eyelids, due to allergic reactions to benzalkonium chloride in eye drops.

Table 19.1
Commonly Used Preservative in Ophthalmic Preparations

Benzalkonium chloride–containing
Atropsiol
Clear Eyes
Dacriose
Epifrin
FML Liquifilm
Humorsol 0.125% ophthalmic solution
Humorosol 0.25% ophthalmic solution
Inflamase
Inflamase Forte
Isopto Carbachol
Isopto Carbachol
Metimyd Ophthalmic Suspension
Metreton Ophthalmic Suspension
Murine For Your Eyes
Optimyd Ophthalmic Solution
P.V. Carbachol Liquifilm
Sodium Sulamyd Ophthalmic Ointment
Tear-Efrin
Tearisol
Visine Eye Drops
Benzalkonium chloride–free
Soaclens (Alcon)
Vasocon (Cooper)

Table 19.2
Ophthalmic Products Containing Thimerosal (Merthiolate)

Adapta (Alcon BP)[a]
Soaclens (Alcon BP)
Allerest (Pharmacraft)
Collyrium Drops (Wyeth)
Murine (Abbott)
Prefrin Z (Allergan)

[a] Some ophthalmologists are prescribing this product as an artificial tear substitute.

Table 19.3
Ophthalmic Products Containing Chlorobutanol

Lacril Artificial Tears (Allergan)
Liquifilm Tears (Allergan)

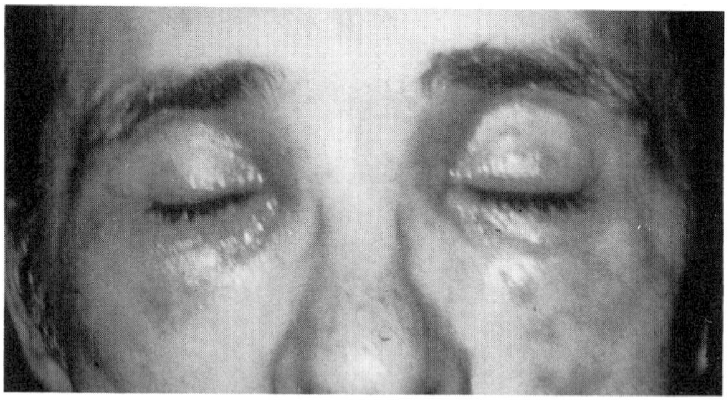

Figure 19.5. Contact dermatitis due to neomycin in an ophthalmic preparation.

Table 19.4
Patch Test Series: Topical Ophthalmic Preparations Including Contact Lens Solutions

Paraben mix 15% (3% each: ethyl, methyl, butyl, benzyl, propyl) (PET)
Phenylmercuric acetate 0.05% PET
Phenylmercuric nitrate 0.05% PET
Thimerosal 0.1% PET
Propylene glycol 10% AQ
Sorbic acid, 5% PET
Benzalkonium chloride, 0.01% PET
Benzethonium chloride, 0.1% AQ
Chlorohexidine, 1% AQ
Chlorobutyanol, 1% AQ
Epinephrine chloride 0.1% AQ
Pilocarpine chloride 0.1% AQ
Isopto carbachol 1%
Acetozolamide 0.1%
Mannitol 2% in alcohol
Epifrin 1%

PET = petrolatum
AQ = aqueous

The antimicrobial neomycin may produce a contact dermatitis when used in ophthalmic preparations (Fig. 19.5). A patch test series of ophthalmic preparations is outlined in Table 19.4.

Phenylmercuric Nitrate and Acetate. These chemicals are used occasionally in ophthalmic products. Table 19.4 lists a "patch test series" for testing for preservatives in ophthalmic solutions including contact lens solutions.

OTHER IRRITANTS

Paper. Facial tissues containing perfume, formaldehyde or benzalkonium chloride may produce dermatitis in sensitized individuals. Newsprint, carbon paper, etc. will produce eyelid dermatitis, particularly in certain individuals who are sensitized to formaldehyde.

Plants. The Rhus family of plants, in particular, may produce marked swelling of the eyelids with minimum dermatitis of the face.

Airborne Contactants. Household sprays, insecticides, animal hairs, and occupational volatile chemicals can produce eyelid dermatitis.

Eyelid Dermatitis Due to Fruits. The oil of lemon peel and the dyes of Florida orange skin can cause eyelid dermatitis.

Match Dermatitis. The phosphorous sesquisulfide in "strike anywhere" matches may produce marked eyelid dermatitis (15). Such patients should use "safety" matches or cigarette lighters. Match dermatitis usually affects the eyelids and face, particularly the left side. The dermatitis may also affect the thighs and hands. Contact urticaria of the eyelids may occur.

Even nonsmokers who do not use matches may acquire the dermatitis if they are near individuals who use matches, since apparently the allergen may become airborne (16). Contact urticaria of the eyelids was ascribed to the use of "strike anywhere" matches (17).

Quinazoline Yellow (D&C Yellow 11) Eyelid Dermatitis. Calnan (17) reported that Yellow D&C #11 dye produced an eyelid dermatitis due to the presence of this dye in an eye cream.

Other compounds producing dermatitis of the eyelids include lanolin (Fig. 19.6) and vitamin E preparations (Fig. 19.7).

TREATMENT

Contact dermatitis in the periorbital region may be treated with the application of cold milk compresses. I usually have the patient put whole or skim milk into a small basin and add ice cubes. The patient then applies the compresses to the involved area, for intervals of 10 minutes. This is then followed by application of 1% hydrocortisone ointment.

If there is any secondary infection apparent, Ilotycin (erythromycin) ophthalmic ointment is prescribed. Diphenhydramine capsules (25 to 50 mg) on retiring may be helpful in acute cases. In extremely severe cases, a 4-day course of prednisone (40–60 mg) may be required.

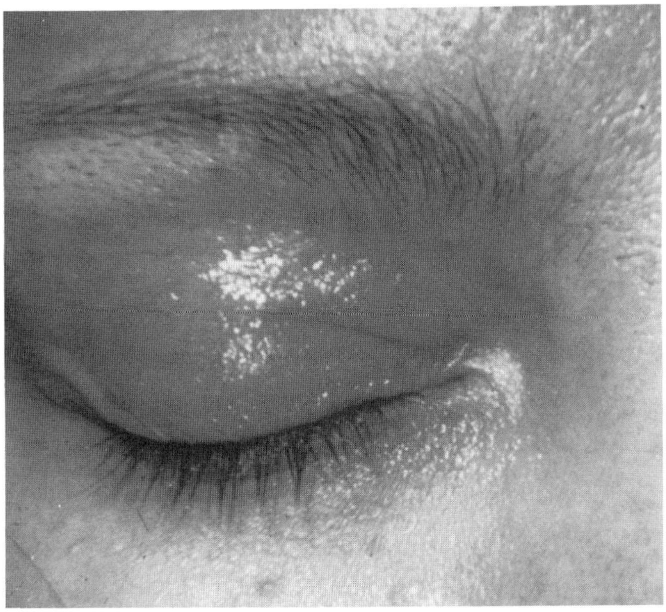

Figure 19.6. Dermatitis of the eyelid due to lanolin.

EDITOR'S COMMENT

Dr. Alexander A. Fisher, an outstanding dermatologist, has had a lot of experience in contact dermatitis. Dr. Fisher outlines the causative factors in contact dermatitis in the periorbital area. He stresses that contact dermatitis is the most common eruption of the skin in the periorbital area. Since the skin is very thin, it is extremely susceptible to irritants and allergens. It is also an area where patients frequently rub their eyes and therefore will bring various contaminants to the area. The list of cosmetics and the various other agents that cause contact dermatitis are enumerated in this chapter. Fortunately most of these are transient and do not leave a permanent residuant.

The use of thio-tepa has been used in the treatment of recurrent pterygium. It should be pointed out that this has been reported to cause vitiligo in patients with pigmentation, and it would be another drug to avoid in the periorbital area.

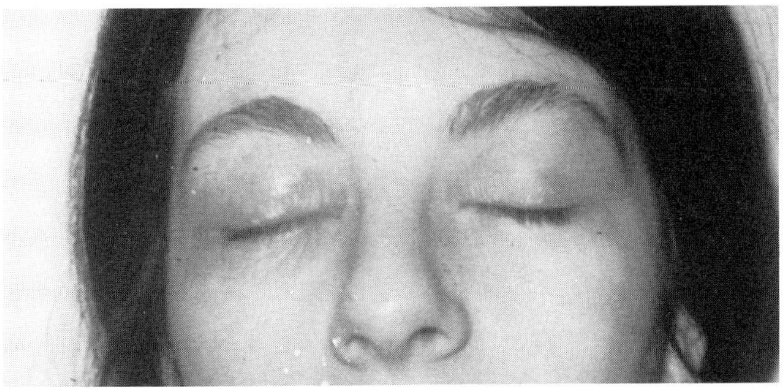

Figure 19.7. Dermatitis of the eyelids due to vitamin E in a cream.

REFERENCES

1. Pascher F: Adverse reactions to eye area cosmetics and their management. *J Soc Cosmet Chem* 33: 249, 1982.
2. Mathias TCG, Maibach HI: Cutaneous irritation: factors influencing the response to irritants. *Clin Toxicol* 13: 333, 1978.
3. Mohajerin AH: Common cutaneous disorders of the eyelids. *Cutis* 10: 279, 1972.
4. Zuckerman BD: Conjunctival pigmentation due to cosmetics. *Am J Ophthalmol* 62: 672, 1966.
5. Jervey JH: Mascara pigmentation of the conjunctiva. *Arch Ophthalmol* 81: 124, 1969.
6. Fisher AA: The paraben paradoxes. *Cutis* 12: 830, 1973.
7. Cronin E: Di-isopropanolamine in an eyeshadow. *Cont Derm Newsl* 13: 364, 1973.
8. Calnan CD: Ditertiarybutylhydroquinone in eyeshadow. *Cont Derm Newsl* 13: 368, 1973.
9. Jordan Jr, WP, Sherman WT, King SE: Threshold responses in formaldehyde-sensitive subjects. *J Amer Acad Derm* 1: 44, 1979.
10. Fisher AA: Allergic contact dermatitis from germall-115; a new cosmetic preservative. *Cont Derm* 1: 126, 1975.
11. Fisher AA: Cutaneous reactions to sorbic acid and potassium sorbate. *Cutis* 25: 350, 1980.
12. Fisher AA: Allergen replacements in allergic dermatitis. *Int J Derm.* 16: 319, 1977.
13. Forman WG, McDowell RV, Shivers JA, Steele JR: Cosmetic eye shadow mimicking orbital calcification (letter to the editor). *JAMA* 235: 2695, 1977.
14. van Ketel WG, Melzer-van Riemskijk FA: Conjunctivitis due to soft lens solutions. *Cont Derm* 6: 321, 1980.
15. Steele MC, Ive FA: Recurrent facial eczema in females due to 'strike anywhere' matches. *Br J Derm* 106: 477, 1982.
16. Ive FA: Studies in Contact Dermatitis XXI. Matches. *Trans St. John's Hosp Derm Soc* 53: 135, 1967.
17. Calnan CD: Quinazoline Yellow SS in cosmetics. *Cont Der* 2: 160, 1976.

Patch Test Kit Instructions[a]

The purpose of this system is to deliver an allergen in the various vehicles from a single standardized bottle. When you receive the patch test kit, all of the plastic bottles will have screw caps. Those allergens using petrolatum as the vehicle should have the screw caps replaced with the appropriate numbered friction fit caps enclosed with the kit. The two liquid allergens in this system should retain their screw caps to minimize evaporation.

Polyethylene squeeze bottles allow dispensing of rather standard quantities of the allergen mixtures. The ointment bottles have a 2.0-mm orifice. There are additional unlabeled polyethylene bottles enclosed with the kit. There are extra ointment and liquid plugs for these extra bottles.

The allergens are applied to the paper disk (Al-test patch), either as one full drop of a liquid vehicle-allergen mixture, or as a 2.0-mm diameter, 1.0-cm long cylinder of petrolatum-allergen mixture dispensed from the polyethylene squeeze bottle.

Strips of six or less Al-test units are attached to 2-inch wide Dermicel Hypo-allergenic Cloth Tape (Johnson & Johnson, New Brunswick, NJ) or Scanpor® (Hollister-Stier) (Figs. A19.1 and A 19.2). Long strips of tape do not always adhere well to the backs of children, presumably because of the great mobility and activity of their backs and scapulae. Numerous short strips containing two to four patch test units per strip may be preferable in this age group. Four rows of six patch tests are usually applied to adults. In hot weather, extra adhesion can be obtained by spraying a pressure sensitive silicone adhesive (Hollister Incorporated, 211 East Chicago Avenue, Chicago, IL 60611) to the upper and lower exposed adhesive edges of the tape. This is done after the Al-test has been positioned on the tape. Patch tests should not be applied to the area directly over the vertebrae since false-positive tests from mechanical trauma can result. If one allergen is specifically suspect, it should be applied as a separate test strip so that the patient can remove the patch test if marked itching occurs. The upper arm can be used in this instance to facilitate removal but this site should probably not be used for routine patch tests since false-negative tests are more common in this area.

[a] Patch Test Kit Instructions are reproduced with permission from the American Academy of Dermatology.

During application of patch tests to the upper back, the patient should stand erect with shoulders dorsiflexed in a military "attention" posture. This will allow the tape to fit tightly against the back when the patient assumes normal standing, sitting, and reclining postures. The upper portion of the test strip is adhered first, then very gentle traction is applied to the lower portion of the tape with the fingers of one hand while the tape is smoothed down on the back with the other hand from top to bottom. After the tests

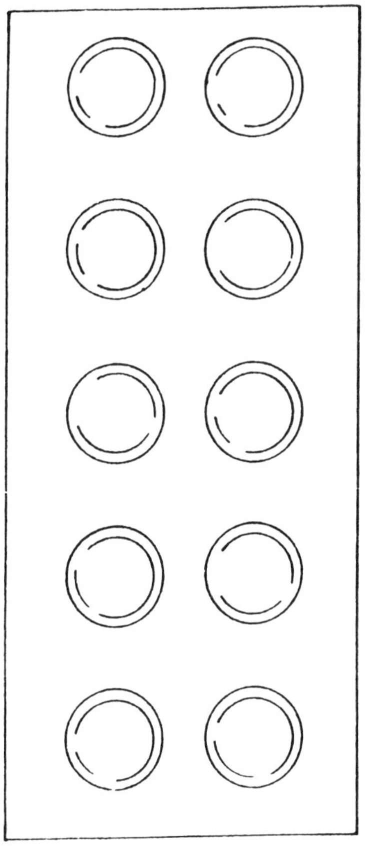

Figure A19.1. Finn Chambers come to you already mounted on Scanpor tape. Simply remove the protective paper backing and they're ready to use. Finn Chambers on Scanpor are available from Hermal Pharmaceutical Laboratories, Inc., Oak Hill, NY 12460.

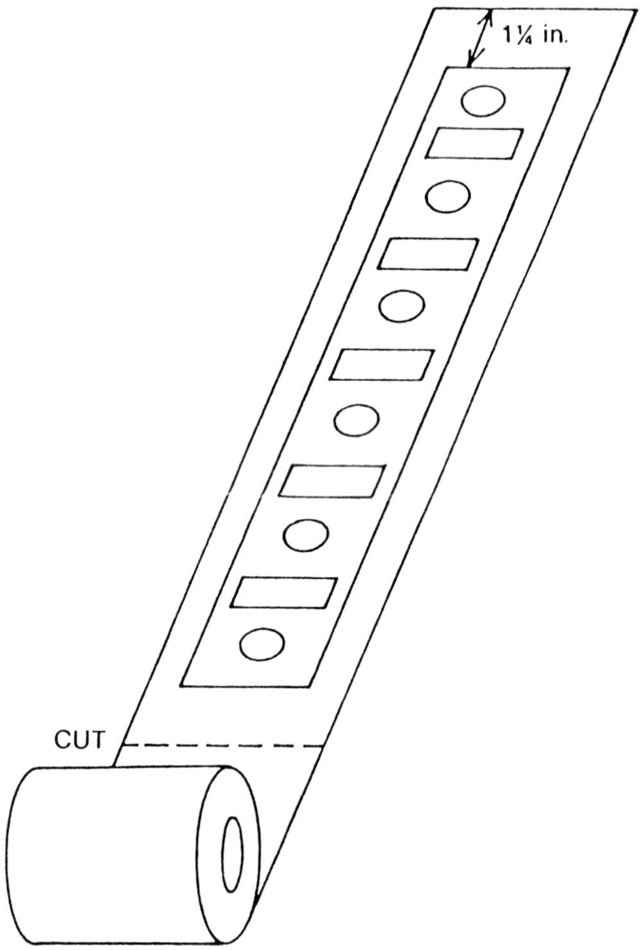

Figure A19.2. Pull tape out about 10 inches leaving the roll attached for stabilization. Place a strip of Al-test (5 to 6 units) on adhesive side of tape so there is approximately 1¼ inches of free tape at either end. Cut tape and prepare other rows as needed. Demicel Hypoallergenic Cloth Tape is available from Johnson & Johnson, New Brunswick, NJ. Order Al-test Patches from Hollister-Stier Laboratories, P. O. Box 19957, Atlanta, GA. 30325.

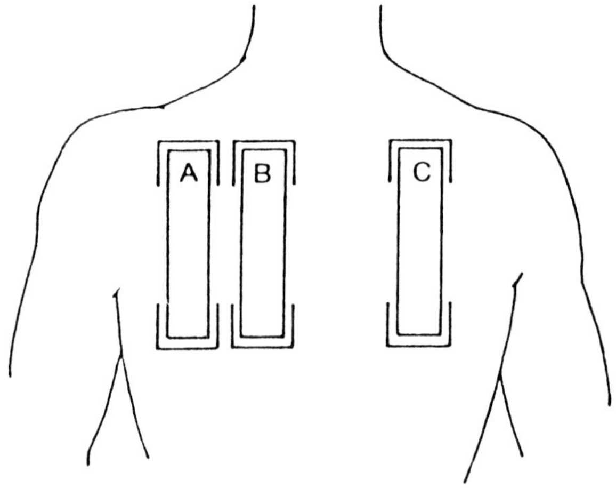

Figure A19.3. 1. With a UV ink saturated cotton swab, paint the skin in staple-like frames as shown. 2. Letter the back of each tape at the top with ordinary pen.

are affixed to the patient's back, the skin around the top and the bottom of each strip is painted with skin ink (Ultraviolet Products Incorporated, 5114 Walnut Grove Avenue, San Gabriel, CA 91778). The best results are obtained by applying the ink with a thoroughly saturated cotton swab as shown in Fig. A19.3. This ink fluoresces a bluish-white under a Wood's light. The back of each tape strip should be marked A, B, C, etc., so that it can be realigned in the proper frame during evaluation (Fig. A19.2). The patient can remove all patch test rows at home after 48 hours. When a single 72-hour reading is performed, the patient should be instructed to bring the patch test rows with him when he returns for his evaluation. The strips may be conveniently wrapped in waxed paper or aluminum foil. During evaluation, each strip will be returned to its original testing site using the upper and lower fluorescent ink outlines for each row. The exact test causing the positive reaction can be ascertained.

CHAPTER 20

Lipid Storage Diseases of the Eyelid

STEPHEN WINFIELD, M.D.
ALAN H. FRIEDMAN, M.D.

HYPERLIPOPROTEINEMIA

The lipoproteins can be separated by electrophoresis into four main groups: chylomicrons, β-lipoproteins, pre-β-lipoproteins, and α-lipoproteins. Five basic phenotypes of hyperlipoproteinemia have been defined (1, 2).

Ocular manifestations of the hyperlipoproteinemias include xanthelasma of the lids, eruptive xanthomas of the lids or mucous membranes (less commonly on the iris and retina), and tuberous xanthomas of the lids (3). Corneal manifestations such as arcus lipoides (4), arcus senilis (5, 6), arcus juvenilis (7, 8), and lipid keratopathy may occur. Lipemia retinalis, the turgidity of plasma associated with hypertriglyceridemia, may be noted (4). The ocular findings are summarized in Table 20.1.

Eruptive xanthomas are yellow papular lesions on an erythematous base, usually indicating a serum triglyceride level over 1,500 mg/100 ml.

Xanthelasma (xanthomas palperbrarum) occurs most commonly in the middle-aged or elderly person with normal serum cholesterol. It can occur in association with primary hypercholesterolemia or in individuals who have nonfamilial serum cholesterol elevation. Xanthelasma is associated with other xanthomas and with hyperlipidemia syndromes in about 5% of patients. They are reported to occur more frequently in individuals with diabetes. One third of patients with xanthelasma have an elevated serum cholesterol level. In children this association is more apparent (9). The lesions are multiple soft, yellowish plaques most commonly found on the inner aspect of the upper and lower lid (Fig. 20.1). Histopathological studies reveal collections of foamy macrophages in the superficial dermis in relation to blood vessels (Fig. 20.2). Esterified cholesterol is the predominant lipid found in the lesion. Surgical excision is usually corrective although less than one half recur (10). Cauterization is sometimes effective for smaller lesions. Recurrence is more likely in patients with systemic disease.

JUVENILE XANTHOGRANULOMA

Juvenile xanthogranuloma (nevoxanthoendothelioma) is a benign histiocytic inflammatory condition of infants and small children. The disease affects both sexes equally. The skin and the eye are most commonly involved (11, 12); visceral involvement is rare (12, 13). The skin lesions are usually round and elevated with a yellowish-orange, tan, or reddish-blue hue. They measure 4–20 mm in diameter and appear on the face, scalp, trunk, or extensor surfaces of the limbs.

Ocular involvement often occurs in the absence of skin lesions and is usually unilateral, most commonly involving the iris and ciliary body. Eighty-five percent of patients with iris involvement are under 1 year of age. This may present as a solitary nodule or the iris may be diffusely thickened and heterochromic. Those lesions may be highly vascular, with thin-walled vessels in the stroma, and may lead to recurrent spontaneous hyphema and glaucoma (14). The iris lesions of juvenile xanthogranuloma may respond to topical treatment with steroids and mydriatics (15). Unlike the cutaneous lesions, spontaneous regression

Table 20.1.
Ocular Manifestations of the Hyperlipoproteinemias

Primary Type	Lipoprotein Abnormality	Raised Lipid Fraction	Eyelids	Cornea	Fundus
I	chylomicrons	triglycerides	eruptive xanthomas	lipid keratopathy	lipemia retinalis
II	β-lipoprotein	cholesterol	xanthelasmata	corneal arcus	
III	broad β-band	cholesterol triglycerides	eruptive xanthomasmata	corneal arcus	lipemia retinalis
IV	pre-β lipoprotein	triglycerides	eruptive xanthomas		lipemia retinalis
V	α-lipoprotein	triglycerides	eruptive xanthomas		lipemia retinalis

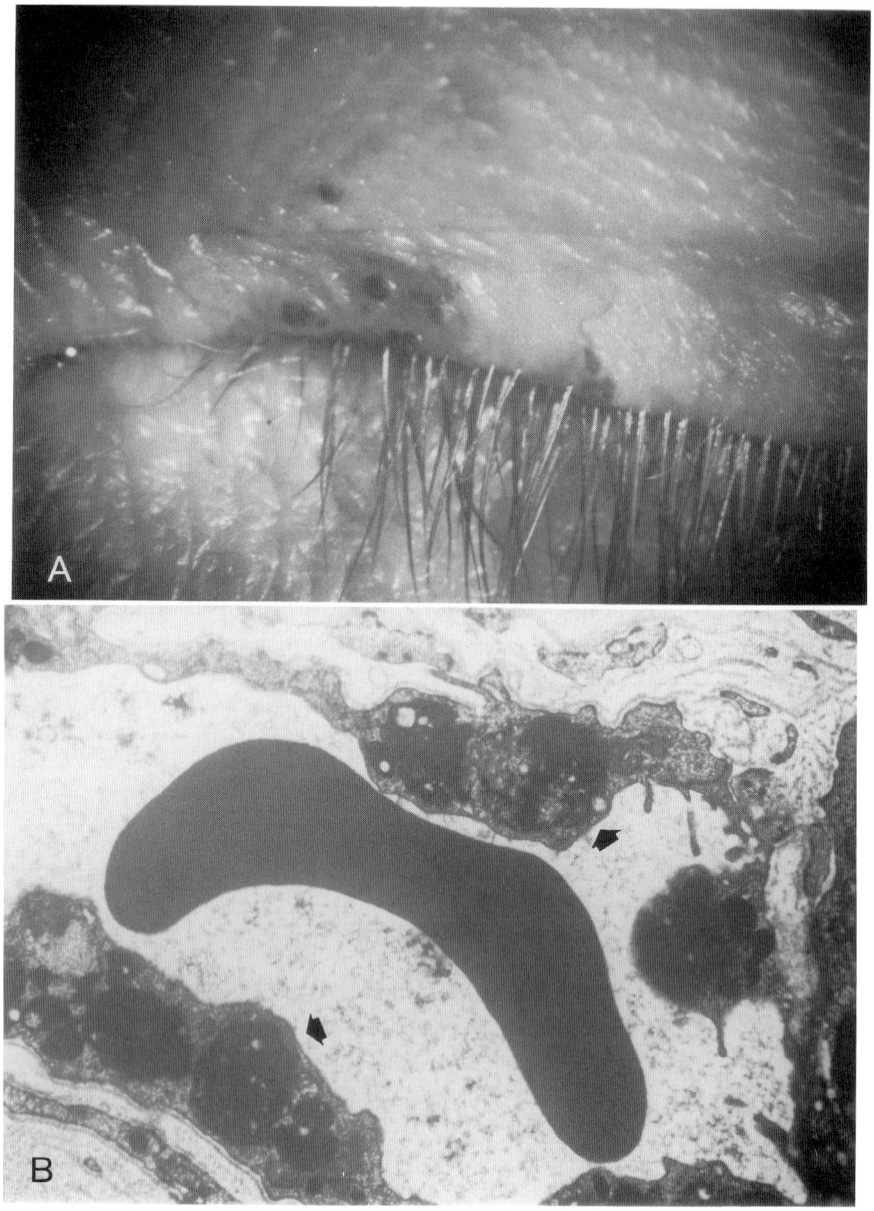

Figure 20.1. *A,* Clinical photograph of male with Fabry's disease. Note angiokeratomas on upper lid. *B,* Electron micrograph of congenital biopsy. Note presence of deposits in endothelial cells (*arrows*). Original magnification, × 18,000.

of iris lesions have not been reported and may require surgical removal or radiation therapy (16, 17).

The eyelids are a common site of cutaneous involvement. Patients with eyelid lesions do not seem to have intraocular involvement (14). Similar to cutaneous lesions at other sites, the eyelid lesions resolve without sequelae in 1 to 2 years (25). Epibulbar lesions involving the sclera, conjunctiva, and cornea are rare. The posterior uveal tract and the retina are rarely involved. Orbital involvement is the rarest form of ophthalmic juvenile xanthogranuloma (14, 18–20). A relationship between juvenile xanthogranuloma and neurofibromatosis has been described (21–23). A rare coexistence of juvenile xanthogranuloma and Niemann-Pick disease has also been reported (24).

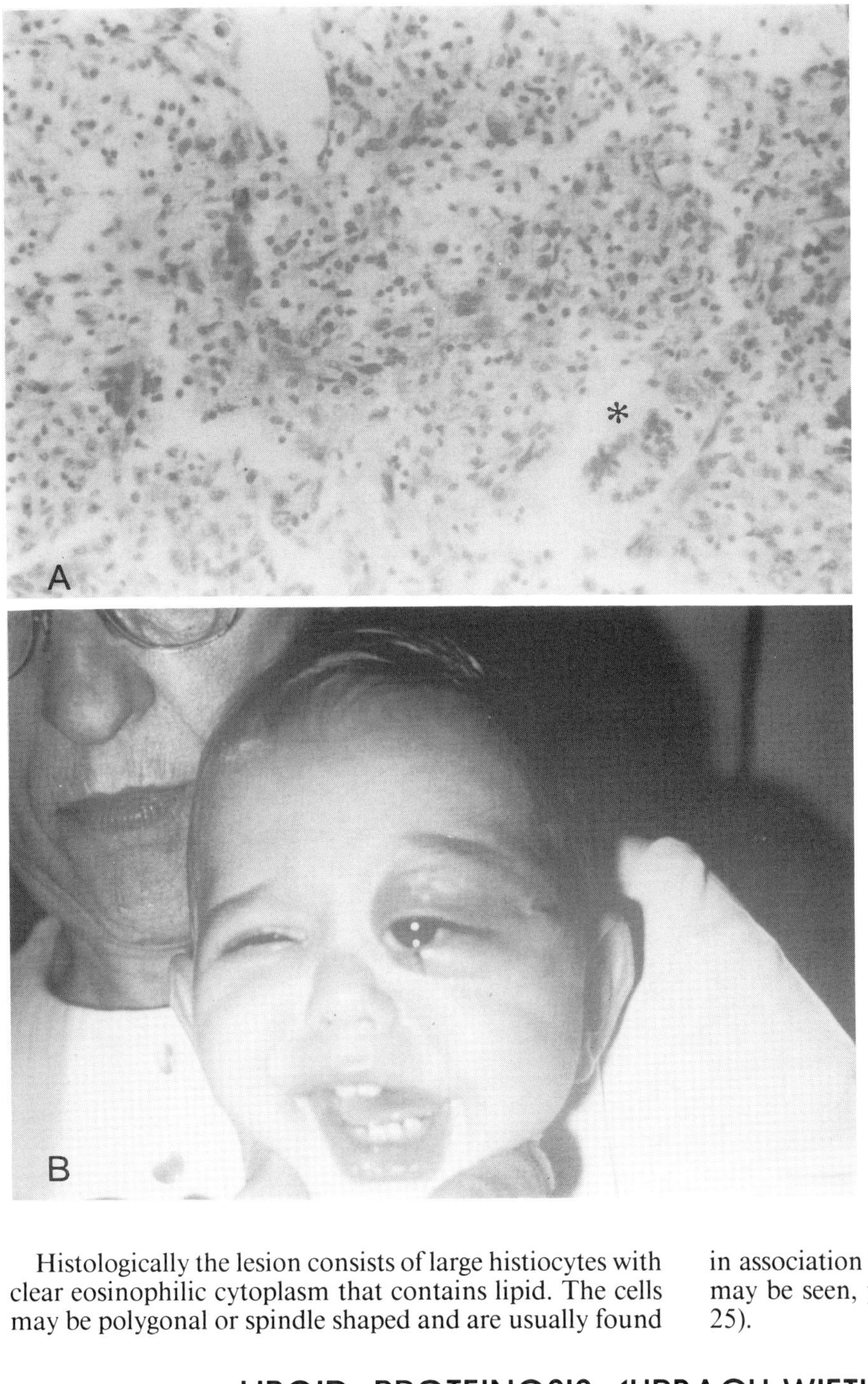

Figure 20.2 *A,* Photomicrograph of JXG lesion showing a diffuse granulomatous inflammation containing histiocytes and Touton giant cells (*asterisk*). Hematoxylin and eosin stain; original magnification × 500. *B,* Clinical photograph of a 1-year-old boy with a xanthogranuloma on the upper lid.

Histologically the lesion consists of large histiocytes with clear eosinophilic cytoplasm that contains lipid. The cells may be polygonal or spindle shaped and are usually found in association with inflammatory cells. Touton giant cells may be seen, particularly with cutaneous lesions (12, 14, 25).

LIPOID PROTEINOSIS (URBACH-WIETHE SYNDROME)

Lipoid proteinosis is a rare condition of the lids and mucous membranes that is characterized by hyaline infiltration of tissues and an autosomal recessive pattern of inheritance (26). Multiple yellow-white pearly nodules about 2–3 mm in diameter occur in linear fashion in the eyelid margins along the roots of the cilia. This lid involvement is highly diagnostic and may lead to chronic blepharitis and madarosis. These lesions can be removed by simple excision (27, 28). Whitish plaque-like lesions are found on mucous membranes and vocal cords. Lesions may also be found on the extensile skin surfaces of the elbows and axillae. The skin papules may become atrophic, hyperkeratotic, or may ulcerate and leave a pitted scar (27, 29).

Histopathological studies reveal papillomatosis of the epidermis with large dermal collections of amorphous eosinophilic PAS positive material. Skin biopsy shows decreased lipid content without an inflammatory response. Electron microscopy reveals large masses of extracellular, finely granular, amorphous material with no fibrillar structure. The enzyme defect is unknown.

FABRY'S DISEASE

Fabry's disease (glycosphingolipid lipidosis, angiokeratoma corporis diffusum) is a systemic disorder of glycosphingolipid metabolism transmitted by an X-linked gene. There is accumulation of the glycosphingolipid galactosylgalactosylglucosyl ceramide secondary to absence of an α-galactosyl hydrolase. Renal and vascular involvement usually leads to death by age 50 (31, 32). Ocular findings include a whorl-like corneal epithelial dystrophy, dilated and tortuous conjunctival and retinal vessels, and feathery opacities of the lens. Papilledema and optic atrophy may be seen (33, 34). Angiokeratoma is an intradermal cavernous hemangioma, over which there is a wart-like thickening of the horny layer of the epidermis. Angiokeratoma of the lids and lid edema have been noted as a relatively common finding in Fabry's disease (35).

WEBER-CHRISTIAN DISEASE

Weber-Christian disease (relapsing febrile nonsuppurative panniculitis) is a condition of unknown etiology affecting predominantly middle-aged or elderly women (36). Symptoms include malaise fever and the appearance of crops of tender nodules and papules in the subcutaneous strap, the trunk, and in the extremities. Inflammation of the mesenteric fat and viscera may lead to abdominal pain and diarrhea (33).

Ocular findings include necrotic eyelid lesions, subconjunctival nodules, and corneal ulcers. Exophthalmos may result from involvement of the orbital fat. There may be recurrent episcleral inflammation and iridocyclitis during the attacks. Macular hemorrhage has been reported. Heparin has been used to treat the ocular symptoms (36, 37).

Histologically three stages of lesions can be seen:

1. Early phase with fat necrosis consisting of an acute inflammatory reaction containing polymorphonuclear leucocytes, lymphocytes, and histiocytes.
2. Granulomatous inflammation with macrophages engulfing the released triglycerides and epitheloid cells.
3. Fibrosis and scarification with clinical depression of overlying skin.

REFERENCES

1. Fredericks DS, Levy RI, Lees RS: Fat transport in lipoproteins: An integrated approach to mechanisms and disorders. *N Engl J Med* 276: 34, 1967.
2. Spaeth GL: Ocular manifestations of lipoprotein disease. *J Contin Ed Ophthalmol* 41: 11, 1979.
3. Vinger PF, Sachs BA: Ocular manifestations of hyperlipoproteinemia. *Am J Ophthalmol* 70: 563, 1970.
4. Bron AJ: Dyslipoproteinemia and their ocular manifestations. *Birth Defects* 12 (3): 257, 1976.
5. Cogan DG, Kuwabara T: Arcus senilis: Its pathology and histochemistry. *Arch Ophthalmol* 61: 553, 1959.
6. Andrews JS: The lipids of arcus senilis. *Arch Ophthalmol* 68: 264, 1963.
7. Forsius H: Arcus Senilis corneae: Its clinical development and relationship to serum, proteins, and lipoproteins. *Acta Ophthalmol* (Suppl 42): 1–78, 1954.
8. Macarneg PVJ Jr, Lasagna L, Snyder B: Arcus not so senilis. *Am Intern Med* 68: 345, 1968.
9. Spaeth GL: Ocular manifestations of the lipidoses. In Tasman W (ed): *Retinal Disease in Children.* New York, Harper & Row, 1971, p 127.
10. Mendelson BC, Masson JK: Xanthelasma: Follow up results after surgical excision. *Plast Reconstr Surg* 58: 535, 1976.
11. Crocker A: The histiocytosis Syndromes. In Fritzpatrick T, Arndt K, Clark, et al (eds): *Dermatology in General Medicine.* New York, McGraw-Hill, 1971, p 1328–1338.
12. Helwig EB: Histiocytic and fibrocytic disorders. In Graham JH, Johnson W, Helwig E (eds): *Dermal Pathology.* New York, Harper & Row, 1972, p 715.
13. Lottsfeldt FI, Good RA: Juvenile xanthogranuloma with pulmonary lesions. *Pediatrics* 33: 233, 1964.
14. Zimmerman L: Ocular lesions of juvenile xanthogranuloma. *Trans Am Acad Ophthalmol Otolargyngol* 69: 412, 1965.
15. Clements D: Juvenile xanthogranuloma treated with local steroids. *Br J Ophthalmol* 50: 663, 1966.
16. Gass JDM: Management of juvenile xanthogranuloma of the iris. *Arch Ophthalmol* 71: 344, 1964.
17. Maumenee A, Longfellow D: Treatment of intraocular nevoxanthoendothelioma. *Am J Ophthalmol* 49: 1, 1960.
18. Gaynes PM, Colon GS: Juvenile xanthogranuloma of the orbit. *Am J Ophthalmol* 63: 755, 1967.
19. Sanders TE: Infantile xanthogranuloma of the orbit: A report of three cases. *Am J Ophthalmol* 61: 1299, 1966.
20. Staple TW, McAlister WH, Sandors TE, Miller JE: Juvenile xanthogranuloma of the orbit: Report of a case with bone destruction. *Am J Roentgenol Rad Nucl Med* 91: 629, 1964.
21. Okisaka S, Ono H, Isamu A: A case of neurofibromatosis with juvenile xanthogranuloma and congenital glaucoma. *Folia Ophthalmol Jpn* 21: 273, 1970.
22. Newell GB, Stone OJ, Mullins JF: Juvenile xanthogranuloma and neurofibromatosis. *Arch Dermatol* 107: 262, 1973.
23. Jensen NE, Sabharwal S, Walher AE: Naevo-xanthoendothelioma and neurofibromatosis. *Br J Dermatol* 85: 326, 1971.
24. Sibulkin D, Olichnoy J: Juvenile xanthogranuloma in a patient with Nieman-Pich disease. *Arch Dermatol* 108: 829, 1973.
25. Sanders T: Intraocular juvenile xanthogranuloma. *Am J Ophthal* 53: 445, 1962.
26. Murphree AL, Mavmanee IH: *The Eye in Genetic Disease: An Atlas.* St. Louis. Mosby.
27. Warburg M: *Diagnosis of Metabolic Eye Disease.* Copenhagen, Manksgaard, 1972, p 16.
28. Blodi FC, Whinory RD, Henricks CA: Lipid proteinosis (Urbach-Wierthe) involving the lids. *Trans Am Ophthalmol Soc* 58: 155, 1960.
29. McKusick VA: *Mendelian Inheritance in Man: Catalogs of Autosomal Dominant, Autosomal Recessive, and X-linked Phenotypes.* Baltimore. Johns Hopkins University Press, 1978, p 570.
30. Newton FH, Rosenberg RN, Lampert PW, et al: Neurologic involvement in Urbach-Wiethe's disease (lipoid proteinosis): A clinical ultrastructural, and chemical study. *Neurology* 21: 1205, 1971.
31. Desnick RH, Kilonsky B, Sweeley CC: Fabry's disease. In Stanbury JB, Wyngaardon JB, Fredrickson DS (eds): *The Metabolic Basis of Inherited Disease*, ed 4. New York, McGraw-Hill, 1978, p 810.
32. Johnson DL, Desnick RJ: Molecular Pathology of Fabry's disease: Physical and Kinetic properties of alpha-galactosidase A in cultured human endothelial cells. *Biochem Biophys Acta* 538: 195, 1978.
33. Sher NA, Letson RD, Desnick RJ: The ocular manifestations in Fabry's disease. *Arch Ophthalmol* 97: 671, 1979.
34. Franceschetti AT: Fabry's disease: ocular manifestations. *Birth Defects* 12: 195, 1976.
35. Spaeth GL, Frost P: Fabry's disease: its ocular manifestations. *Arch Ophthalmol* 74: 760, 1965.
36. Frayer W, Wise R, Tsaltus T: Ocular and adnexal changes associated with relapsing febrile nonsuppurative panniculitis. *Trans Am Ophthalmol Soc* 66: 233, 1968.
37. Milner R, Mitchinson M: Systemic Weber-Christian disease. *J Clin Pathol* 18: 150, 1965.

CHAPTER 21

Eyelid Manifestations of Connective Tissue Disorders

GEORGE B. BARTLEY, M.D.
JOHN D. BULLOCK, M.D., M.S., F.A.C.S.
ROBERT R. WALLER, M.D.

Abnormalities of the eyelids may be found with most of the connective tissue diseases. Although the signs, such as lid edema or erythema, are often nonspecific, several of the disorders affect the eyelids in characteristic patterns. The classic malar and lower eyelid rash of lupus erythematosus, the heliotrope eyelids of dermatomyositis, or the asymptomatic papular eruptions of Degos' disease are almost pathognomonic for these conditions. The eyelid signs of connective tissue disorders often improve with treatment of the systemic disease. Surgery may be necessary in cases in which lid malpositions compromise adequate protection of the globe.

LUPUS ERYTHEMATOSUS

Lupus erythematosus (LE) is a chronic inflammatory disorder that may involve various organs, including the skin and mucous membranes, kidneys, nervous system, joints, heart, lungs, gastrointestinal tract, and retina. No specific cause has been determined; genetic, hormonal, metabolic, and environmental factors all may cause faulty regulation of B-cell function, possibly by defective suppressor T-cell activity. Autoantibodies are produced, particularly to nuclear antigens such as deoxyribonucleic acid, ribonucleic acid, and histones. Antigen-antibody complexes localize in vascular basement membranes, leading to inflammation and tissue damage. The clinical course is usually chronic and marked by exacerbations and remissions.

Lupus erythematosus is more common among women than men; blacks are affected more frequently than whites. The onset of the disease may occur at any age, although presenting signs and symptoms usually first arise during the third or fourth decade of life. The clinical manifestations of LE vary from purely cutaneous involvement (discoid LE) to a potentially life-threatening multisystem disorder (systemic lupus erythematosus, SLE). An overlap syndrome with other connective tissue disorders may occur.

Although discoid LE may appear to involve only the skin, it may be associated with an elevated erythrocyte sedimentation rate or the presence of circulating antinuclear antibodies and may progress to the disseminated form of lupus in a minority of patients (1). Signs and symptoms of SLE range from nonspecific fatigue, malaise, anorexia, photosensitivity, arthralgias, and skin rashes to fatal renal failure, cerebritis, and cardiopulmonary collapse. Systemic lupus erythematosus may develop in response to certain medications, including hydralazine, phenytoin, procainamide, penicillin, the sulfonamides, isoniazid, and methyldopa.

The most common eye findings associated with LE occur in the retina, as either primary effects of the disease and its vascular abnormalities or secondary to the antimalarials often used to treat the condition. Cotton-wool spots, retinal hemorrhages, hard exudates, arteriolar attenuation, retinal edema, and swelling of the optic nerve head may be noted (2, 3). The characteristic retinal pigment epithelial disturbances of hydroxychloroquine toxicity are well-known.

Conjunctivitis, episcleritis, uveitus, and keratopathy have been described in association with LE. Proptosis has been reported in association with SLE (4), and lupus cerebritis may cause a host of neuroophthalmic signs, including nystagmus, visual field defects, internuclear ophthalmoplegia, cranial nerve palsies, ptosis, and blindness.

Cutaneous involvement (5) may be localized solely to the skin (discoid LE) or may be a part of disseminated LE. Discoid LE is primarily an affliction of women in the third to fifth decades of life. The classic discoid lesions are erythematous, well-defined, indurated, elevated plaques (Figs. 21.1 and 21.2). Hyperpigmentation and hypopigmentation, atrophy, telangiectases, scaling, and pruritus are common. The lesions may occur anywhere on the body but are especially frequent in areas exposed to the

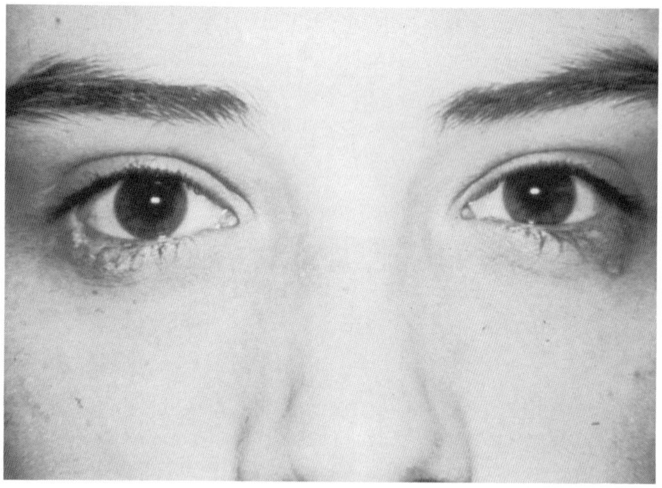

Figure 21.1. Discoid lupus erythematosus. Eyelid lesion is indurated, elevated, and erythematous. (Courtesy of Dr. Thomas J. Liesegang.)

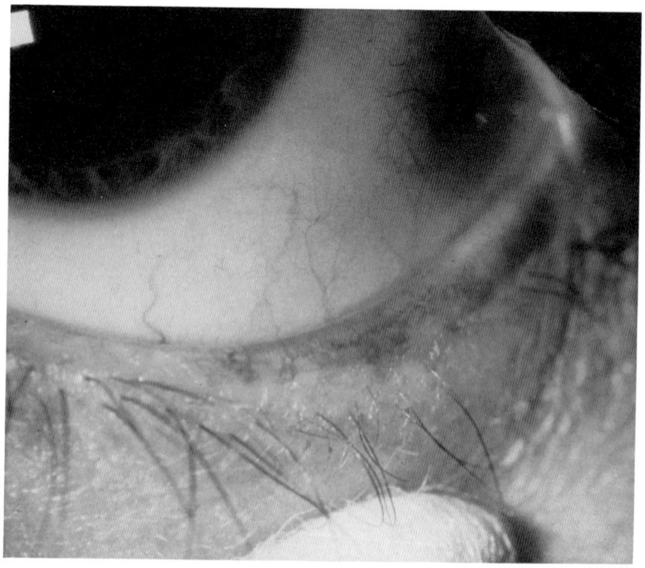

Figure 21.2. Discoid lupus erythematosus. Telangiectases and pigmentary changes are common in discoid lesions. (Courtesy of Dr. Thomas J. Liesegang.)

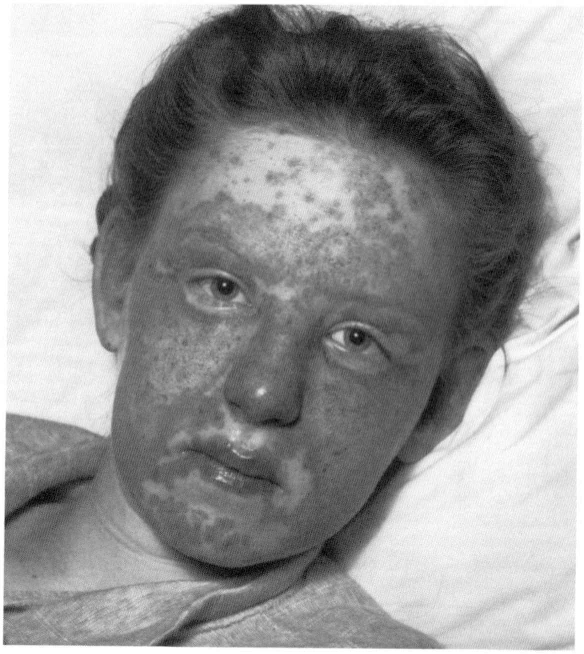

Figure 21.3. Disseminated lupus erythematosus. Eyelids are involved as part of a generalized facial rash. This patient died 2 months later from systemic lupus erythematosus.

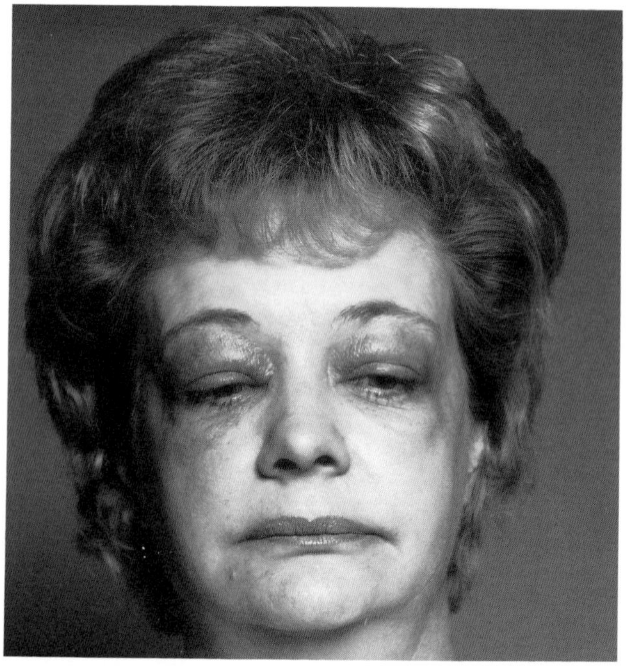

Figure 21.4. Disseminated lupus erythematosus. Eyelids are edematous and erythematous, resembling heliotrope rash often considered "pathognomonic" for dermatomyositis.

sun. In addition to the well-known malar erythematous maculopapular butterfly rash, discoid lesions often occur in the scalp and cause alopecia, on the nasal and oral mucosa, or along the vermillion border of the lip. Nonspecific bullae, verrucae, purpura, urticaria, or angioedema also may be manifestations of cutaneous lupus.

The eyelids may be the only skin areas affected in some cases of discoid LE, although serologic abnormalities may coexist and indicate systemic involvement (1). The clinical presentation may resemble that of chronic blepharitis, with thickening and erythema of the eyelid skin, madarosis, and scaling (6–10). The differential diagnosis of discoid LE involving the eyelids also includes eczema, rosacea, allergic dermatitis, granuloma fasciale, tinea fasciale, polymorphic light eruption, lymphocytic infiltrates, vitiligo, seborrhea, sarcoidosis, and lymphogranuloma venereum (1, 6). Histopathologic evaluation can confirm the diagnosis of discoid LE by immunofluorescent identification of immunoglobulin deposition at the dermoepidermal junction (1). Early diagnosis and treatment are important to prevent cicatricial trichiasis, entropion, and ectropion (11) with secondary corneal abnormalities (1). Discoid eyelid lesions may respond to hydroxychloroquine (1) or corticosteroids (6, 10). Relapses are common and may be precipitated by sunlight, exposure to cold, trauma, or stress (10).

Facial and eyelid involvement may occur in cases of disseminated LE (10, 12) (Fig. 21.3). Blepharitis has been found (13, 14), as has eyelid erythema (15, 16). The appearance of reddish, horizontal lines just above the lashes of the upper lid is due to telangiectases and has been termed "Boston lids" (17). The lines are most prominent when the systemic disease is active. Edema of the lids is common, particularly when a nephrotic syndrome results from lupus renal disease (18).

Although "heliotrope eyelids" have often been considered pathognomonic for dermatomyositis, violaceous, tender, and swollen lids without a malar rash may occur in association with disseminated LE (19) (Fig. 21.4).

Another unusual variant of LE, the profundus form, should be considered in the differential diagnosis of eyelid edema. Panniculitis resulting in lid swelling as the presenting manifestation of LE profundus in the report by Nowinski and associates (20). Antimalarials may be used for treatment, and it is important to recognize that both discoid and systemic LE may coexist with the profundus variant.

SCLERODERMA

Like SLE, scleroderma may be confined to the skin (morphea and variants) or may involve multiple organ systems (progressive systemic sclerosis). Duke-Elder (10) considered these different manifestations to be separate diseases. A specific cause for scleroderma has not been determined, but connective tissue fibrosis results from inflammation, microvascular abnormalities, and an increased rate of collagen synthesis. Females are affected three to four times more frequently than males, and the disease usually first becomes apparent after age 20 years. Clinical manifestations include Raynaud's phenomenon, joint pain, xerostomia, esophageal and intestinal dysfunction, and generalized muscle weakness. Necrotizing arteritis in the kidneys may lead to accelerated hypertension and renal shutdown, whereas cardiac fibrosis may precipitate heart failure.

Symmetric induration of the skin may involve the distal extremities alone (acrosclerosis), or it may be widespread and progressive. Involvement of the facial connective tissue leads to the characteristic appearance of an expressionless mask as the skin becomes tight, shiny, hyperpigmented, and atrophic. Calcification may occur in the subcutaneous tissues.

Ophthalmic abnormalities related to scleroderma predominantly occur in the eyelids, although retinal vascular changes have been reported (21–23). Scleroderma localized to the skin may be classified as morphea (single lesions), generalized morphea (multiple cutaneous lesions with or without muscle atrophy), and linear scleroderma (a unilateral paramedian line of sclerosis) (24). Initially, morphea lesions appear as red or purple plaques; later, the centers become cream-colored but the border appears violaceous ("lilac ring") (24) because of telangiectatic vessels. The lesions usually are asymmetrically distributed on the face, chest and back, extremities, and genitalia. A report of symmetric eyelid morphea emphasized the dif-

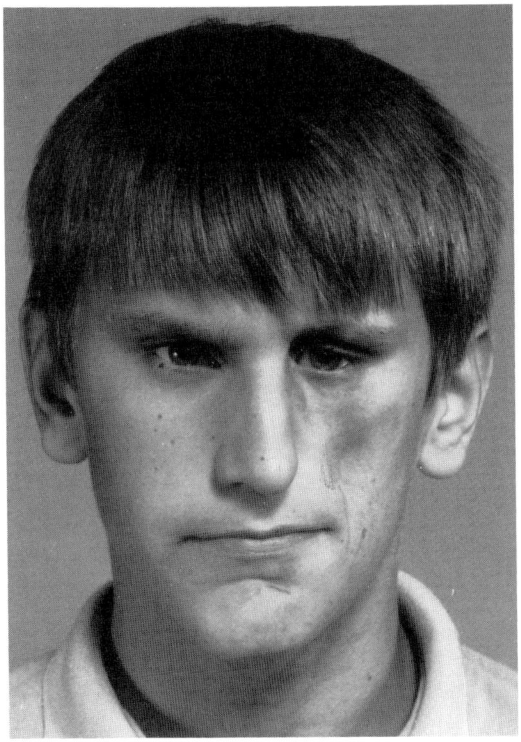

Figure 21.5. Linear scleroderma. Skin of face and eyelids is indurated along "sabre-cut"; mild hemifacial atrophy is also present.

ferential clinical and pathologic features between morphea and lichen sclerosus et atrophicus (24).

The linear (*sclérodermie en coup de sabre*) form of localized scleroderma, in contrast, has been reported in association with various ocular and eyelid abnormalities. In cases of sabre-cut scleroderma, the skin becomes indurated and atrophic and may show areas of hyperpigmentation or hypopigmentation (Fig. 21.5). The tarsal plates may atrophy, as may the orbicularis and levator muscles, resulting in ptosis (25, 26). Heterochromia and pigmentary glaucoma (26) may be associated with linear scleroderma, as may segmental iris atrophy (27). One case of linear scleroderma was heralded only by 8 months of nonspecific, unilateral eyelid swelling (28). Duke-Elder and MacFaul (10) noted iritis, retinal hemorrhages, phthisis bulbi, optic nerve neurocytoma, and extraocular muscle paresis in association with this form of localized scleroderma.

Progressive systemic sclerosis often involves the skin of the eyelids (10, 16–18, 21, 22, 29–36). The connective tissue of the lids initially hypertrophies and becomes edematous, but later scarring and atrophy result in extreme tightness and shortening of the lids with a "woody" texture to palpation. Blepharophimosis results, with reduction in the size of the palpebral aperture and loss of the upper lid folds. Eversion of the lids may be impossible. Tiny telangiectases and areas of pigmentation may be noted on the eyelids. Lagophthalmos is not uncommon, and severe four-lid ectropion may result in corneal infections (36). Treatment is usually symptomatic, but ectropion may require surgical correction.

POLYMYOSITIS/DERMATOMYOSITIS

Polymyositis and dermatomyositis are variants of an inflammatory disease that affects the connective tissue, skin, and skeletal muscle. Familial occurrence is unusual, and both sexes are affected with approximately equal frequency. The age at onset is bimodal—the peak occurrence is at around age 50 years and a smaller peak is in the early teenage years. Approximately 10–20% of the patients have an occult malignancy, most commonly of the breast, and the inflammatory myopathy and dermopathy may improve dramatically with excision of the primary tumor. Although a definitive cause is unknown, a disturbance of cell-mediated immunity is a possible cause for polymyositis/dermatomyositis. Lymphocytes that produce muscle-damaging lymphotoxin have been identified in biopsy specimens. The evidence for a humoral cause is controversial (37).

Symmetric weakness, often without pain, of the hip girdle and proximal leg muscles is the most common presenting symptom. Often an event such as an upper respiratory tract infection, drug reaction, or prolonged exposure to sunlight precedes the onset of the disease (37). Muscles of the shoulder, arm, and pharynx and the neck flexors are involved next, and the characteristic facial rash is a common dermatologic feature. Other systemic manifestations include weight loss, arthritis, myocarditis, Raynaud's phenomenon, interstitial pulmonary fibrosis, and subcutaneous calcification. The prognosis is good, especially for children, and many patients recover complete muscle strength.

As in scleroderma, the eyelids are the most common site of ocular involvement in polymyositis/dermatomyositis. Retinal abnormalities have been found, including hemorrhages, edema, exudate, and optic atrophy (38, 39). Today, the most common ocular manifestations of dermatomyositis are periorbital and facial erythema and edema (40); in the past, "toxic retinopathy" was perhaps the most frequent eye finding (16, 35, 41). Although not pathognomonic (19), the heliotrope rash of dermatomyositis should "immediately suggest the diagnosis" (42). Keil (43) described the characteristic dermatomyositic facies: swollen lids, narrowed eyelid fissures, contiguous edema of the cheek and nose, and background skin that appears faintly rosy, pale blue, or wine-colored because of many closely set telangiectases (Fig. 21.6). The net effect is a "heliotropic bloating of the face, resembling the early stages of cadaveric decomposition" (43). In black patients, the rash appears as a deep purple shadow (37). Eyelid edema may either pit with pressure (38, 43) or be firm (18, 44). Later, the skin of the eyelids may show either dense pigmentation or a reticular pattern with the areas of depigmentation (43). Although relatively rare, ocular muscle weakness (40), ptosis (41), and extraocular and orbicularis tenderness (10, 44) may occur in association with polymyositis/dermatomyositis.

Several features help to differentiate the rash of dermatomyositis from that found in SLE. The dermatomyositic skin discoloration tends to be more violaceous than erythematous, is more likely to involve the eyelids than the face, and is usually more indurated and less discrete than the classic malar butterfly rash of SLE (45). The treatment

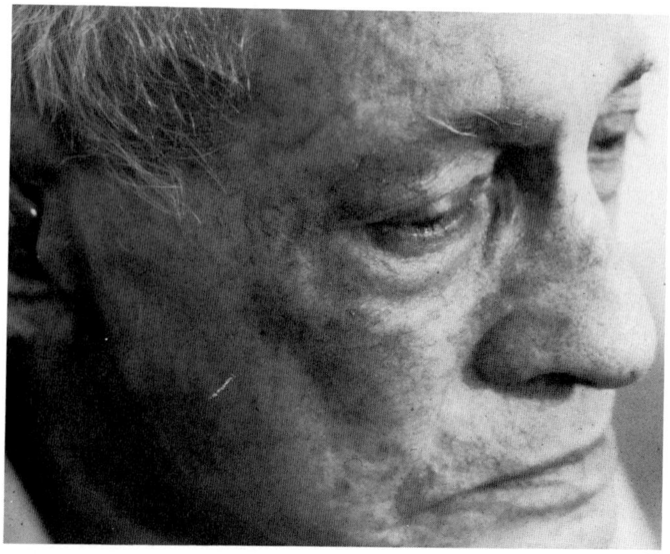

Figure 21.6. Dermatomyositis. The violaceous hue of the eyelids (heliotrope rash) is due to numerous closely set telangiectases. (Courtesy of Dr. W. P. Daniel Su.)

of this disorder is usually systemic corticosteroids or immunosuppressives such as methotrexate and azathioprine. An evaluation for hidden malignant disease should be considered in every adult patient with dermatomyositis.

RHEUMATOID ARTHRITIS

Rheumatoid arthritis (RA) is a chronic inflammatory process that results in a nonsuppurative synovitis and a variety of extraarticular signs and symptoms. Females are more commonly affected than males, and the disease usually first becomes manifest between the ages of 35 and 45 years. The usual clinical course is one of exacerbations and remissions. Although the cause is unknown, an autoimmune disturbance is likely for both the polyarthritis and extraarticular abnormalities. The subcutaneous rheumatoid nodule is the characteristic pathologic lesion and consists of a core of fibrinoid necrosis with peripheral palisading of mononuclear cells. The nodules are firm and nontender, are most commonly found on body surfaces subject to friction or pressure, and are thought to be precipitated by inflammation of small vessels. In addition to rheumatoid nodules, some of the more common extraarticular manifestations include pleuropericarditis, pulmonary nodules, lymphadenopathy, splenomegaly, peripheral neuropathy from both vasculitis and nerve entrapment, dermal infarcts and hemorrhages, and ulcers of the distal extremities. The most common ocular manifestations of RA are inflammation of the sclera and episclera and keratoconjunctivitis sicca.

The presence and severity of episcleritis and scleritis generally parallel other extraarticular manifestations of RA. The onset of ocular inflammation in an otherwise "quiet" patient may indicate increased systemic involvement in general (46). Patients who have RA with scleritis or episcleritis have a significantly higher mortality rate than patients without ocular inflammation (47, 48). Either simple or nodular episcleritis may be found in association with RA. Inflammation of the sclera may localize either anteriorly or posteriorly and may or may not be accompanied by necrosis. The nodules of rheumatoid episcleritis or scleritis are histopathologically similar to subcutaneous rheumatoid nodules (49).

The cornea may be involved in RA in several ways. Limbal furrowing or guttering is not uncommon and may result in corneal perforation (3, 50). A sclerosing peripheral keratitis may be found adjacent to areas of episcleritis or scleritis, but the most common corneal manifestations of RA result from the lacrimal dysfunction of Sjögren's syndrome. Retinal manifestations of RA are rare but may include nerve fiber infarcts (51).

Specific eyelid involvement in RA is also unusual. Carter and associates (52) reported the first example of subcutaneous rheumatoid nodules involving the eyelids. Although the lesions initially resembled chalazia, they eventually broke down and resulted in a full-thickness lid defect. Treatment consisted of surgical debridement and closure. Pathologic examination confirmed the rheumatoid nature of the lid lesions.

Rheumatoid nodules have been reported on the bridge of the nose (53). These lesions simulated basal cell carcinoma and were thought to be secondary to localized pressure from eyeglasses. Conversely, clinically typical subcutaneous nodules may be found in the absence of rheumatic disease. Rao and Font (54) reported a series of eyelid and periorbital subcutaneous nodules that histopathologically resembled those found in association with RA. None of the patients had been affected by or had the subsequent development of RA or rheumatic fever. Simple excision was the only treatment necessary. Similarly, a case was reported in which a mass involving the right orbit and right lower lid resulted in proptosis in a young boy (55). Although histopathologically similar to a subcutaneous rheumatoid nodule, no association with RA or rheumatic fever was found.

WEGENER'S GRANULOMATOSIS

The classic triad of Wegener's granulomatosis (WG) has been considered to be focal necrotizing glomerulonephritis, disseminated vasculitis affecting small and medium-sized vessels, and necrotizing respiratory tract granulomas. Limited forms of the disease without renal involvement have been described (56–58). Males and females are affected with approximately equal frequency. Although the disease may occur at any age, young and middle-aged adults are most commonly affected. A specific cause is unknown, although circulating autoantibodies, immune complex deposition, deficient cell-mediated immunity, and hypersensitivity phenomena have all been implicated at one time or another.

Systemic symptoms include malaise, weight loss, arthralgias, diffuse muscle pain, and depression. Fever, night sweats, otitis, hearing loss, rhinitis, sinusitis, saddle-nose deformity, tracheal stenosis, pneumonitis, myocardial necrosis, pericarditis, proteinuria, chronic renal failure, hemorrhagic skin lesions, focal skin ulcers, subcutaneous nodules, and cranial nerve palsies may all be found (59–61). Untreated WG follows a rapidly fatal course. Cyclophosphamide has emerged as the drug of choice, and improvement or cure can sometimes be accomplished.

Ocular involvement, which may be the initial clinical manifestation of WG, occurs in 30–40% of cases and is often secondary to contiguous nasal or paranasal sinus disease (61–63). Orbital involvement may cause proptosis, chemosis, ophthalmoplegia, dilated retinal veins, and optic nerve compression with visual loss (57, 61, 62). Nasolacrimal duct obstruction, scleritis, episcleritis, keratitis, conjunctivitis, uveitis, and signs of retinal ischemia are not uncommon. Wegener's granulomatosis that manifests as a necrotizing chalazion has also been reported (64).

Eyelid manifestations are nonspecific in WG. Of the 40 patients with ocular and adnexal involvement in the Mayo Clinic study by Bullen and associates (61), eight (20%)

were affected by abnormalities of the eyelids. Four patients had periorbital edema associated with orbital disease; two of these patients had bilateral eyelid swelling even though the orbital involvement was unilateral. Three patients had ptosis, and one patient had lower eyelid retraction.

Lethal midline granuloma is a rare destructive inflammatory process that has been described as a variant of WG (65, 66). Although necrotizing granulomas of the upper respiratory tract may simulate WG, the term "idiopathic midline destructive disease" has been introduced to emphasize that it is a distinct entity (67). Subcutaneous nodules in the eyelids and brow were recently reported in a patient with this disorder (68).

DEGOS' DISEASE

Degos' disease (DD) (malignant atrophic papulosis) is a rare disorder with skin, intestinal, and central nervous system manifestations (69). A necrotizing arteriolitis or endovasculitis with subsequent thrombosis causes characteristic skin changes that may be confused with those found in SLE. Multiple asymptomatic, discrete papules, 2 to 3 mm in diameter, are distributed over the trunk, but they rarely involve the head and extremities. The lesions have a depressed white center surrounded by an erythematous border, and they are the first noticeable sign of the disease in most cases (Fig. 21.7). The lesions have been found on the eyelids and should suggest the diagnosis (70–72).

Ocular manifestations secondary to central nervous system involvement include diplopia, visual field defects, ophthalmoplegia, ptosis, papilledema, and optic atrophy, and tortuous collateral cilioretinal arteries may develop in response to progressive retinal ischemia (69). Intestinal perforation secondary to multiple infarcts is the usual cause of death in patients with Degos' disease (10).

POLYARTERITIS NODOSA

Polyarteritis nodosa (periarteritis nodosa) is a rare multisystem disease characterized by a necrotizing inflammation of small and medium-sized vessels. A hypersensitivity reaction may be the initiating event. Men are affected more commonly than women, and the onset of the disease is usually in young adulthood or middle age. Mild constitutional complaints may be the presenting symptoms, but multisystem failure may rapidly ensue as widespread vascular occlusion develops. Eyelid edema may occur as a result of involvement of the orbital arteries, as a consequence of renal failure, or as a result of exudates within the eyelids themselves (12, 16, 18, 29, 73) (Fig. 21.8).

NODULAR FASCIITIS

Although nodular fasciitis has also been referred to as "subcutaneous pseudosarcomatous fasciitis" or "fibromatosis" because of the often rapid growth and microscopic appearance that mimic a spindle-cell sarcoma, nodular fasciitis is a benign proliferation of the connective tissue of the superficial fascia in response to an unknown stimulus. The lesions are found most commonly on the trunk and arms. Font and Zimmerman (74) described 10 patients with involvement of the eye and adnexa; five of the patients had eyelid lesions. Simple excision of the nodular proliferations gave excellent results.

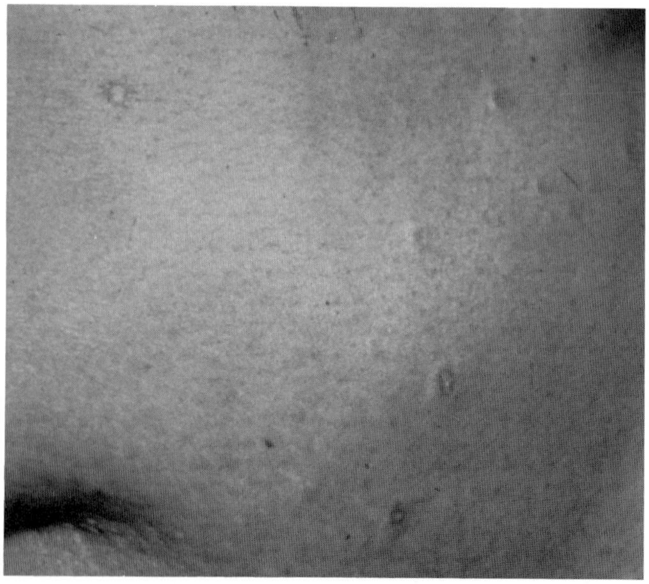

Figure 21.7. Degos' disease. The characteristic lesion has a depressed white center surrounded by an erythematous border and usually measures 2 to 3 mm in size. (Courtesy of Dr. W. P. Daniel Su.)

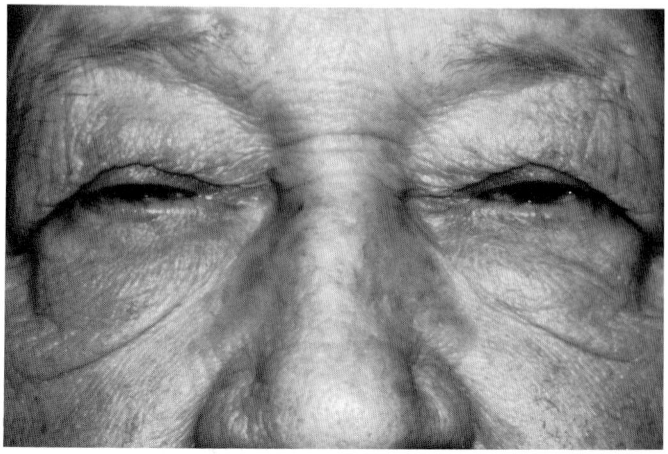

Figure 21.8. Polyarteritis nodosa. Dermatochalasis, blepharochalasis, and bilateral ptosis from levator aponeurosis disinsertion after several episodes of eyelid edema.

CUTIS LAXA

Cutis laxa is an extremely rare condition in which the skin becomes inelastic and hangs in redundant folds. The disease may be congenital or acquired and may result from decreased levels of elastase inhibitor. The eyelids may droop markedly, an effect that results in ectropion. Death often results from pulmonary complications (75, 76).

EHLERS-DANLOS SYNDROME

Ehlers-Danlos syndrome (cutis hyperelastica or fibrodysplasia hyperelastica) is a connective tissue disorder of unknown cause in which the skin is hyperextensible, fragile, and easily scarred. Angioma-like pseudotumors may be found around the knees and elbows, and fatty subcutaneous cysts are found on the legs and buttocks. Hyperextensibility of the joints is a well-known feature. The most common ophthalmic manifestations are epicanthal folds and Méténier's sign (easy eversion of the upper eyelid). Surgery for patients with this condition is frustrating because sutures often pull through the skin and retraction of the wound edge results in gaping incisions (77, 78).

PSEUDOXANTHOMA ELASTICUM

Pseudoxanthoma elasticum (PXE) is an autosomal recessive disorder characterized by loose, yellowish, and inelastic skin over the neck, axillae, inguinal regions, and umbilicus. Arterial degenerative disease may result in claudication, angina, hypertension, and gastrointestinal hemorrhage. The association of PXE and angioid streaks is well-known and is referred to as the "Grönblad-Strandberg syndrome." Eyelid changes are nonspecific, although Duke-Elder and MacFaul (10) cited a report of yellow flecks composed of degenerated elastic tissue at both canthi of each eye.

MUCOPOLYSACCHARIDOSES

The ocular features of this group of hereditary metabolic disorders consist of various combinations of corneal clouding, retinal pigmentary degeneration, and optic atrophy (79). Eyelid manifestations are unusual and nonspecific; mild ptosis and thick lids may be found in Hurler's syndrome (mucopolysaccharidosis I) and ptosis associated with Horner's syndrome can accompany Morquio's disease (mucopolysaccharidosis IV) (80).

SCLEROMYXEDEMA

First described by Dubreuilh (81) in 1906, scleromyxedema (lichen myxedematosus) is a rare disorder of connective tissue acid mucopolysaccharides in which confluent lichenoid papules are found in association with diffuse skin thickening. The characteristic infiltrative skin lesions are caused by the proliferation of fibroblasts and deposition of mucinous material in the upper dermis. Diagnostic criteria also include exclusion of the clinical and laboratory findings of thyroid dermopathy and the demonstration of a monoclonal serum paraprotein (82, 83). This disorder may be found in association with diabetes mellitus (84). Successful treatment has been reported with melphalan (85), radiation therapy (82), and 8-methoxypsoralen and ultraviolet-A radiation (86).

Infiltration of the eyelids with mucinous material results in a clinical picture similar to that found in scleroderma (Fig. 21.9). The lids are indurated, tight, and shortened. Conjunctivitis from exposure may result.

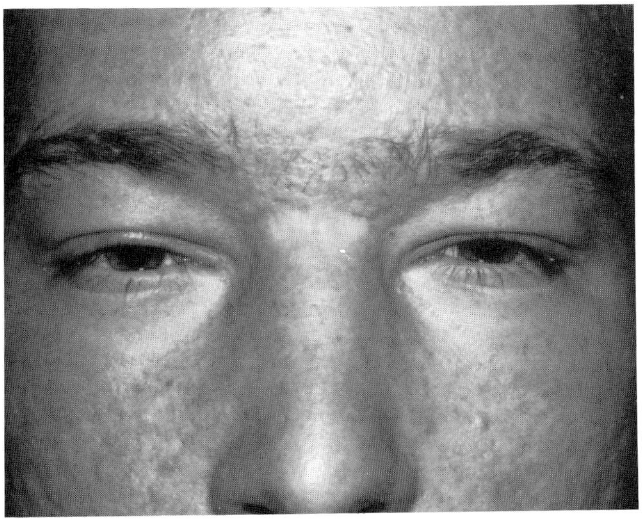

Figure 21.9. Scleromyxedema. Dermal deposition of mucinous material results in tight, indurated skin similar in appearance to scleroderma.

OTHER DISORDERS

Giant-cell arteritis (polymyalgia rheumatica), Marfan's syndrome, ankylosing spondylitis, Reiter's syndrome, and relapsing polychondritis are included in many reviews of connective tissue or rheumatic disorders. No characteristic eyelid findings have been described in association with these diseases.

REFERENCES

1. Donzis PB, Insler MS, Buntin DM, Gately LE: Discoid lupus erythematosus involving the eyelids. *Am J Ophthalmol* 98: 32–36, 1984.
2. Aiello JS: Ocular findings in lupus erythematosus. *Am J Ophthalmol* 35: 837–843, 1952.
3. Henkind P, Gold DH: Ocular manifestations of rheumatic disorders. *Rheumatology* 4: 13–59, 1973.
4. Brenner EH, Shock JP: Proptosis secondary to systemic lupus erythematosus. *Arch Ophthalmol* 91: 81–82, 1974.
5. Tuffanelli DL, Dubois EL: Cutaneous manifestations of systemic lupus erythematosus. *Arch Derm* 90: 377–386, 1964.
6. Huey C, Jakobiec FA, Iwamoto T, Kennedy R, Farmer ER, Green WR: Discoid lupus erythematosus of the eyelids. *Ophthalmology* 90: 1389–1398, 1983.
7. Feiler-Ofry V, Isler Z, Hanau D, Godel V: Eyelid involvement as the presenting manifestation of discoid lupus erythematosus. *J Pediatr Ophthalmol Strab* 16: 395–397, 1979.
8. Klauder JV, DeLong P: Lupus erythematosus of the conjunctiva, eyelids and lid margins. *Arch Ophthalmol* 7: 856–867, 1932.
9. DeLong P, Klauder JV: Lupus erythematosus of the eyelids and conjunctiva. *Arch Ophthalmol* 16: 321–322, 1936.
10. Duke-Elder S, MacFaul PA: The ocular adnexa. In Duke-Elder S (ed): *System of Ophthalmology.* St. Louis, CV Mosby, 1974, vol 13, p 321–338.
11. Kearns W, Wood W, Marchese A: Chronic cutaneous lupus involving the eye lid. *Ann Ophthalmol* 14: 1009–1010, 1982.
12. Maumenee AE: Ocular manifestations of collagen diseases. *Arch Ophthalmol* 56: 557–562, 1956.
13. Spaeth GL: Corneal staining in systemic lupus erythematosus. *N Engl J Med* 276: 1168–1171, 1967.
14. Gold DH, Morris DA, Henkind P: Ocular findings in systemic lupus erythematosus. *Br J Ophthalmol* 56: 800–804, 1972.
15. Cordes FC, Aiken SD: Ocular changes in acute disseminated lupus erythematosus. *Am J Ophthalmol* 30: 1541–1555, 1947.
16. Hollenhorst RW, Henderson JW: The ocular manifestations of the diffuse collagen diseases. *Am J Med Sci* 221: 211–222, 1951.
17. Michels RG: Ocular manifestations in connective tissue disorders (CTD). In Ryan SJ, Smith RE (eds): *Selected Topics on the Eye in Systemic Disease.* New York, Grune & Stratton, 1974, p 301–313.
18. Tassman WS: The eyelid manifestations of internal disease. *Int Ophthalmol Clin* 4: 35–43, 1964.
19. Carr RW, Goldman AS, Travis LB: Heliotropic discoloration of the eyelids. Occurrence in a probable case of disseminated lupus erythematosus. *Am J Dis Child* 112: 585–586, 1966.
20. Nowinski T, Bernadino V, Naidoff M, Parrish R: Ocular involvement in lupus erythematosus profundus (panniculitis). *Ophthalmology* 89: 1149–1154, 1982.
21. Pollack IP, Becker B: Cytoid bodies of the retina. In a patient with scleroderma. *Am J Ophthalmol* 54: 655–660, 1962.
22. Manschot WA: Generalised scleroderma with ocular symptoms. *Ophthalmologica* 149: 131–137, 1965.
23. Maclean H, Guthrie W: Retinopathy in scleroderma. *Trans Ophthalmol Soc UK* 89: 209–220, 1969.
24. El Baba F, Frangieh GT, Iliff WJ, Hood AB, Green WR: Morphea of the eyelids. *Ophthalmology* 89: 1285–1288, 1982.
25. Segal P, Jablonska S, Mrzyglod S: Ocular changes in linear scleroderma. *Am J Ophthalmol* 51: 807–813, 1961.
26. Stone RA, Scheie HG: Periorbital scleroderma associated with heterochromia iridis. *Am J Ophthalmol* 90: 858–861, 1980.
27. Serup J, Alsbirk PH: Localized scleroderma 'en coup de sabre' and iridopalpebral atrophy at the same time. *Acta Derm Venereol (Stockh)* 63: 75–77, 1983.
28. Long PR, Miller OF, III: Linear scleroderma. Report of a case presenting as persistent unilateral eyelid edema. *J Am Acad Dermatol* 7: 541–544, 1982.
29. Vail D: Diffuse collagen diseases with ocular complications. *Trans Ophthalmol Soc UK* 72: 155–169, 1952.
30. Agatston HJ: Scleroderma with retinopathy. *Am J Ophthalmol* 36: 120–121, 1953.
31. Horan EC: Ophthalmic manifestations of progressive systemic sclerosis. *Br J Ophthalmol* 53: 388–392, 1969.
32. Kirkham TH: Scleroderma and Sjögren's syndrome. *Br J Ophthalmol* 53: 131–133, 1969.
33. Velayos EE, Cohen BS: Progressive systemic sclerosis. Diagnosis at the age of 4 years. *Am J Dis Child* 123: 57–60, 1972.
34. West RH, Barnett AJ: Ocular involvement in scleroderma. *Br J Ophthalmol* 63: 845–847, 1979.
35. Kearns T: Collagen and rheumatic diseases: ophthalmic aspects. In Mausolf FA (ed): *The Eye and Systemic Diseases*, ed 2. St. Louis, CV Mosby, 1980, p 123–136.
36. Nancarrow JD, Jawad SM: A rare case of severe bilateral ectropion from scleroderma. *Plast Reconstr Surg* 67: 352–354, 1981.
37. Brooke MH: *A Clinician's View of Neuromuscular Diseases.* Baltimore, William & Wilkins Co, 1977, p 138–147.
38. Munro S: Fundus appearances in a case of dermatomyositis. *Br J Ophthalmol* 43: 548–558, 1959.
39. Tuovinen E, Raudasoja R: Poikilodermatomyositis with retinal haemorrhages and secondary glaucoma. *Arch Ophthalmol* 43: 669–672, 1965.
40. O'Leary PA, Waisman M: Dermatomyositis. A study of 40 cases. *Arch Derm Syph* 41: 1001–1019, 1940.
41. Bruce GM: Retinitis in dermatomyositis. *Trans Am Ophthalmol Soc* 36: 282–297, 1938.
42. Walsh FB, Hoyt WF: *Clinical Neuro-Ophthalmology*, ed 3. Baltimore, William & Wilkins, 1969, vol 2, p 1183.
43. Keil H: The manifestations in the skin and mucous membranes in dermatomyositis, with special reference to the differential diagnosis from systemic lupus erythematosus. *Ann Intern Med* 16: 828–871, 1942.
44. Lisman JV: Dermatomyositis with retinopathy. *Arch Ophthalmol* 37: 155–159, 1947.
45. Wedgwood RJP, Cook CD, Cohen J: Dermatomyositis. *Pediatrics* 12: 447–466, 1953.
46. Lachmann SM, Hazleman BL, Watson PG: Scleritis and associated disease. *Br Med J* 1: 88–90, 1978.
47. Jones P, Jayson MIV: Rheumatoid arthritis: a long-term follow-up. *Proc Roy Soc Med* 66: 1161–1163, 1973.
48. McGavin DDM, Williamson J, Forrester JV, Foulds WS, Buchanan WW, Dick WC, Lee P, MacSween RNM, Whaley K: Episcleritis and scleritis: a study of their clinical manifestations and association with rheumatoid arthritis. *Br J Ophthalmol* 60: 192–226, 1976.
49. Ferry AP: The histopathology of rheumatoid episcleral nodules. An extra-articular manifestation of rheumatoid arthritis. *Arch Ophthalmol* 82: 77–78, 1969.
50. Brown SI, Grayson M: Marginal furrows. A characteristic corneal lesion of rheumatoid arthritis. *Arch Ophthalmol* 79: 563–567, 1968.
51. Meyer E, Scharf J, Miller B, Zonis S, Nahir M: Fundus lesions in rheumatoid arthritis. *Ann Ophthalmol* 10: 1583–1584, 1978.
52. Carter BT, Sanborn GE, Humphries MK, Jr: Rheumatoid nodules of the upper lid. Report of a case. *Arch Ophthalmol* 94: 2127–2128, 1976.
53. Healey LA, Wilske KR, Sagebiel RW: Rheumatoid nodules simulating basal-cell carcinoma. *N Engl J Med* 277: 7–9, 1967.
54. Rao NA, Font RL: Pseudo-rheumatoid nodules of the ocular adnexa. *Am J Ophthalmol* 79: 471–478, 1975.
55. Floyd BB, Brown B, Isaacs H, Minckler DS: Pseudorheumatoid nodule involving the orbit. *Arch Ophthalmol* 100: 1478–1480, 1982.
56. Carrington CB, Liebow AA: Limited forms of angiitis and granulomatosis of Wegener's type. *Am J Med* 41: 497–527, 1966.
57. Cassan SM, Divertie MG, Hollenhorst RW, Harrison EG: Pseudotumor of the orbit and limited Wegener's granulomatosis. *Ann Intern Med* 72: 687–693, 1970.
58. Cassan SM, Coles DT, Harrison EG, Jr: The concept of limited forms of Wegener's granulomatosis. *Am J Med* 49: 366–379, 1970.

59. Wolff SM, Fauci AS, Horn RG, Dale DC: Wegener's granulomatosis. *Ann Intern Med* 81: 513–525, 1974.
60. Hu CH, O'Loughlin S, Winklemann RK: Cutaneous manifestations of Wegener granulomatosis. *Arch Dermatol* 113: 175–182, 1977.
61. Bullen CL, Liesegang TJ, McDonald TJ, DeRemme RA: Ocular complications of Wegener's granulomatosis. *Ophthalmology* 90: 279–290, 1983.
62. Straatsma BR: Ocular manifestations of Wegener's granulomatosis. *Am J Ophthalmol* 44: 789–799, 1957.
63. Haynes BF, Fishman ML, Fauci AS, Wolff SM: The ocular manifestations of Wegener's granulomatosis. Fifteen years experience and review of the literature. *Am J Med* 63: 131–141, 1977.
64. Verrey VF, Landolt E: Augensymptome der Wegenerschen Granulomatose. Bericht über einen Fall. *Ophthalmologica* 153: 309–320, 1967.
65. Cutler WM, Blatt IM: The ocular manifestations of lethal midline granuloma (Wegener's granulomatosis). *Am J Ophthalmol* 42: 21–35, 1956.
66. Byrd LJ, Shearn MA, Tu W: Relationship of lethal midline granuloma to Wegener's granulomatosis. *Arthr Rheum* 12: 247–253, 1969.
67. Tsokos M, Fauci AS, Costa J: Idiopathic midline destructive disease (IMDD): a subgroup of patients with the "midline granuloma" syndrome. *Am J Clin Pathol* 77: 162–168, 1982.
68. Chu FC, Rodrigues MM, Cogan DG, Fauci AS: The pathology of idiopathic midline destructive disease (IMDD) In the eyelid. *Ophthalmology* 90: 1385–1388, 1983.
69. Lee DA, Su WPD, Liesegang TJ: Ophthalmic changes of Degos' disease (malignant atrophic papulosis). *Ophthalmology* 91: 295–299, 1984.
70. Feuerman EJ: Papulosis atrophicans maligna Degos. *Arch Dermatol* 94: 440–445, 1966.
71. Howard RO, Klaus SN, Savin RC, Fenton R: Malignant atrophic papulosis (Degos' syndrome): *Arch Ophthalmol* 79: 262–271, 1968.
72. Howard RO, Nishida S: A case of Degos' disease with electron microscopic findings. *Trans Am Acad Ophthalmol Otolaryn* 73: 1097–1112, 1969.
73. Comberg U: Über Periarteriitis nodosa. *Klin Mbl Augenheilk* 130: 850–854, 1957.
74. Font RL, Zimmerman LE: Nodular fasciitis of the eye and adnexa. *Arch Ophthalmol* 75: 475–481, 1966.
75. Schreiber MM, Tilley JC: Cutis laxa. *Arch Dermatol* 84: 226–272, 1961.
76. Goltz RW, Hult AM, Godfard M, Gorlin RJ: Cutis laxa: manifestation of generalized elastolysis. *Arch Dermatol* 92: 373–387, 1965.
77. Duke-Elder S: Normal and abnormal development. Congenital deformities. In Duke-Elder S (ed): *System of Ophthalmology*. St. Louis, CV Mosby, 1963, vol 3, pt 2, p 1112.
78. Lorincz AL: Ehlers-Danlos syndrome (cutis hyperelastica). In Demis DJ, McGuire J (eds): *Clinical Dermatology*. Philadelphia, Harper & Row, 1984, vol 1, p 1–7.
79. Kenyon KR, Quigley HA, Hussels IE, Wyllie RG, Goldberg MF: The systemic mucopolysaccharidoses. Ultrastructural and histochemical studies of conjunctiva and skin. *Am J Ophthalmol* 73: 811–833, 1972.
80. Geeraets WJ: *Ocular Syndromes*, ed 3. Philadelphia, Lea & Febiger, 1976, p 227–303.
81. Dubreuilh W: Fibromes miliaries follicularies: sclerodermis consecutive. *Arch Dermatol Syph* 7: 569–570, 1906.
82. Hill TG, Crawford JN, Rogers CC: Successful management of lichen myxedematosus. *Arch Dermatol* 112: 67–69, 1976.
83. Lai A, Fat RFM, Suurmond D, Rádl J, Van Furth R: Scleromyxedema (lichen myxoedematosus) associated with a paraprotein, IgG_1 of type Kappa. *Br J Dermatol* 88: 107–116, 1973.
84. Abd EL, Aal H, Salem SZ, Salem A: Lichen myxedematosus: histochemical study. *Dermatologica* 162: 273–276, 1981.
85. Feldman P, Shapiro L, Pick AI, Slatkin MH: Scleromyxedema: a dramatic response to melphalan. *Arch Dermatol* 99: 51–56, 1969.
86. Farr PM, Ive FA: PUVA treatment of scleromyxedema. *Br J Dermatol* 110: 347–350, 1984.

SECTION IV

NEOPLASTIC DISEASES OF THE EYELID

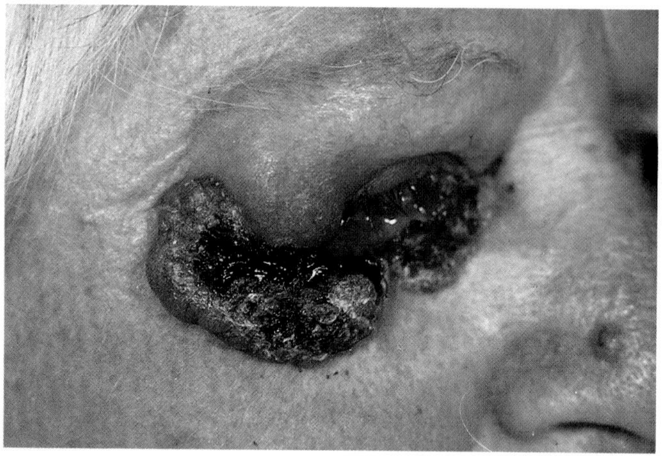

Figure 22.16

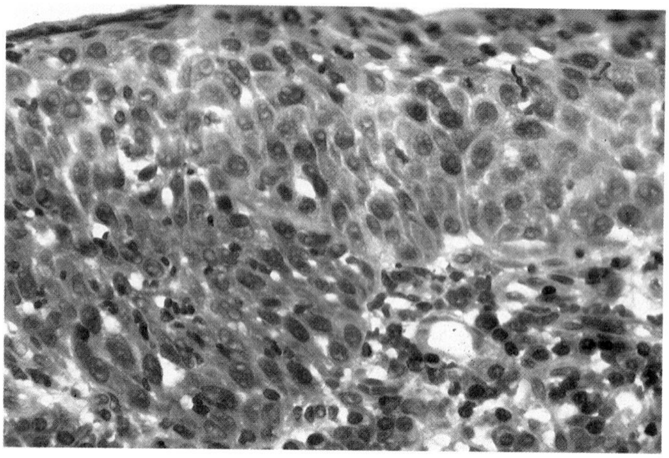

Figure 22.26

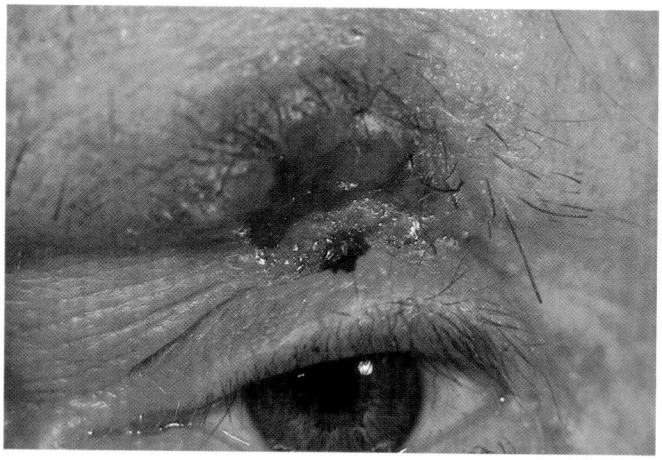

Figure 22.27

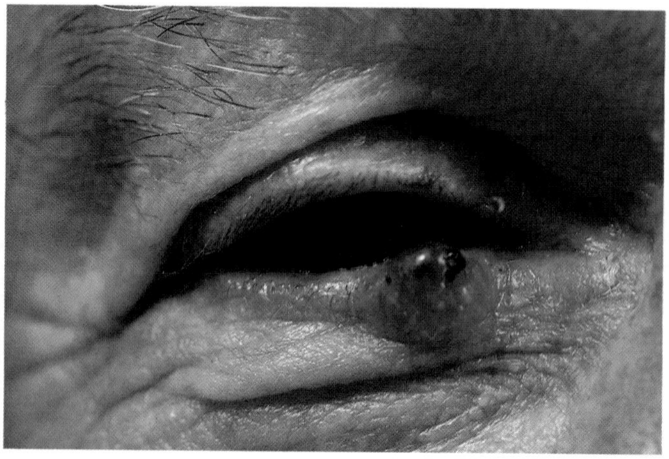

Figure 22.32

CHAPTER 22

Clinical Evaluation of Tumors of the Eyelid and Ocular Adnexa

ALBERT HORNBLASS, M.D., F.A.C.S.

Tumors of the eyelid and ocular adnexa constitute a serious problem because of their proximity to the eye, brain, and paranasal sinuses.

INCIDENCE

The incidence of tumors varies with the investigators, geographic area, and socioeconomic patient population. Henkind and Friedman (1) report that, out of 557 lid lesions studied from 1966 through 1970, 26% were benign tumors, 19.2% malignant tumors, 8.9% melanotic neoplasms, 1.3% adnexal tumors, 3.6% vascular tumors, 1.3% mesodermal tumors, 19.7% cystic lesions, 4.3% metabolic, and 14.6% inflammatory. Basal cell epithelioma is far more common than squamous cell carcinoma, with the ratio on the order of 10:1 (2). Kwitko, Boniuk, and Zimmerman (3) state that the ratio of basal cell to squamous cell carcinoma is closer to 39:1. Basal cell carcinoma constitutes about 90% of malignant tumors in the orbital region (4). According to Martin (5), it is approximately 85%; according to Kwitko and associates (3), it is 91%. A Japanese study of 52 malignant tumors of the eyelid revealed a peak incidence of 70–79 years of age (6). Squamous cell carcinoma was the lesion most frequently seen in 48% of cases. This was followed by basal cell carcinoma, sebaceous adenocarcinoma, malignant melanoma and lymphoma. Skin cancer in general, specifically, basal cell carcinoma, is the most common cancer in the U. S (5).

CLASSIFICATION

Duke-Elder (7) has classified tumors of the eyelids into eight categories:

1. Epithelial Tumors
   - Cutaneous
     - Benign
       - Papilloma (Fig. 22.1)
       - Senile keratosis (Fig. 22.2)
       - Seborrheic keratosis
       - Keratoacanthoma
       - Inverted follicular keratosis (Fig. 22.3)
       - Trichoepithelioma
       - Benign calcifying epithelioma of Malherbe
       - Cornu cutaneum
     - Malignant
       - Carcinoma
         - Squamous cell epithelioma
         - Basal cell epithelioma (rodent ulcer)
         - Intraepithelial carcinoma
       - Xeroderma pigmentosum
   - Tumors of the sebaceous glands
     - Adenoma
       - Sebaceous adenoma of the skin
       - Adenoma of the meibomian glands
       - Adenoma of Zeis' glands
     - Adenocarcinoma
       - Adenocarcinoma of the skin

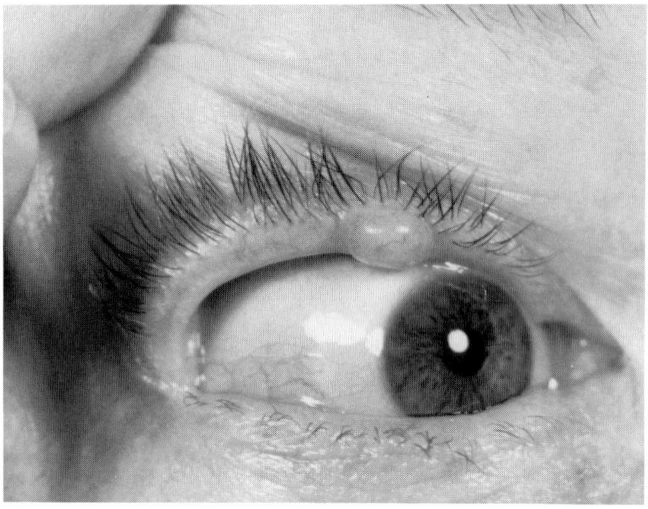

Figure 22.1. Elevated marginal papilloma, right upper eyelid.

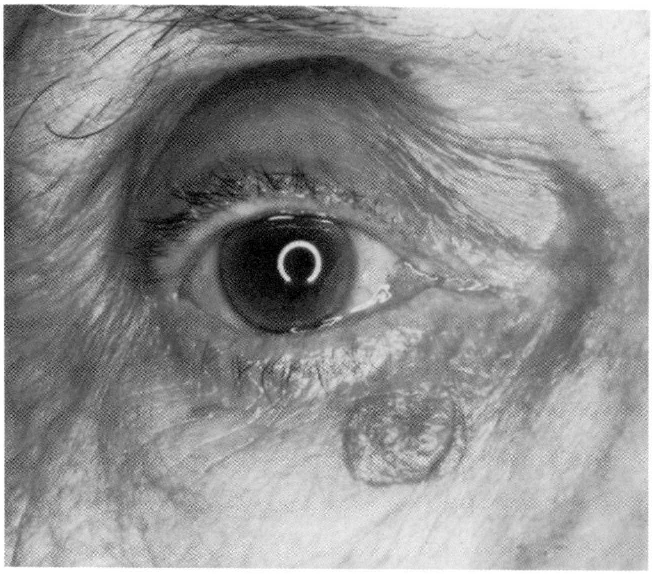

Figure 22.2. Seborrheic keratosis of the right lower eyelid.

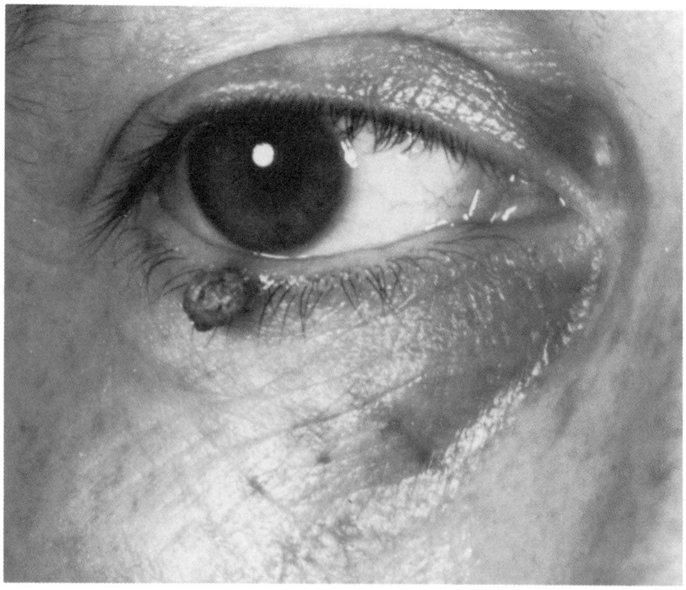

Figure 22.3. Keratotic papilloma on the right lower eyelid.

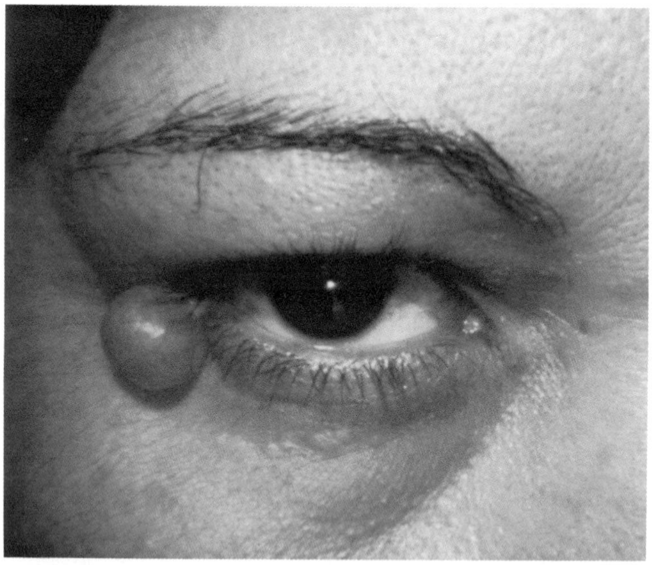

Figure 22.4. Large sudoriferous cyst on margin of right lower eyelid.

Adenocarcinoma of the meibomian glands
Adenocarcinoma of Zeis' glands
Tumors of the sweat glands (Fig. 22.4)
Hidradenoma
Hidradenoma of the skin
Syringoma
Pleomorphic adenoma
Adenoma of Moll's glands
Hidradenocarcinoma
Hidroadenocarcinoma of the skin
Hidroadenocarcinoma of Moll's glands
Papillary cystadenoma lymphomatosum
Oncocytoma

2. Mesenchymal tumors
   Benign fibroma, tuberous sclerosis (78), lipoma, rhabdomyoma, leiomyoma, myxoma, chondroma
   Malignant sarcoma
3. Tumors of the lymphoreticular tissue
   Benign lymphoma
   Lymphosarcoma
   Reticulum cell sarcoma
   Giant follicular lymphoma
   Burkitt lymphoma
   Hodgkin disease
   Mycosis fungoides
   Plasmocytoma
4. Vascular tumors
   Hemangioma (Fig. 22.5)
   Capillary
   Cavernous
   Plexiform

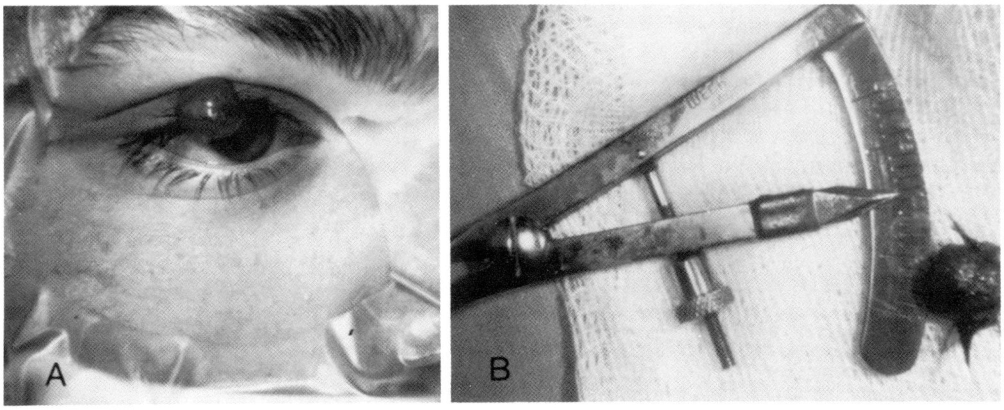

Figure 22.5. *A*, Hemangioma of right upper eyelid in 18-year-old boy. *B*, Specimen of hemangioma excised from patient shown in *A*.

Hemangioendothelioma
Hemangiopericytoma
Spider angioma
Senile angioma
Angioma serpiginosum
Telangiectatic granuloma
Angiokeratoma of Mibelli
Multiple hemorrhagic sarcoma of Kaposi
Glomus tumor
Lymphangioma, lymphangioendothelioma
5. Nervous tissue tumors
Neurofibromatosis (Fig. 22.6)
Plexiform neuroma
Diffuse neurofibromatosis
Molluscum fibrosum
Multiple mucosal neuroma syndrome
Neurilemmoma
Granular cell Schwannoma of Abrikossoff
Ganglioneuroma
Amputation neuroma
6. Pigmented tumors
Nevus
Malignant melanoma
7. Metastatic tumors
8. Developmental tumors
Dermoids
Teratoma
Phakomatos choristoma

According to Font (8), epithelial tumors of the eyelid, lid margins, and lacrimal caruncle are of the following two types:

1. Basal cell type
   Adnexal tumors of hair follicles, sweat glands and sebaceous (meibomian) glands
   Basal cell carcinoma
2. Squamous cell type
   Intraepithelial tumors (Bowen disease)
   Squamous cell (epidermoid) carcinoma

Most malignant tumors are entirely basal cell or squamous cell in type, but, since gradations do occur, the term "basosquamous" sometimes applies.

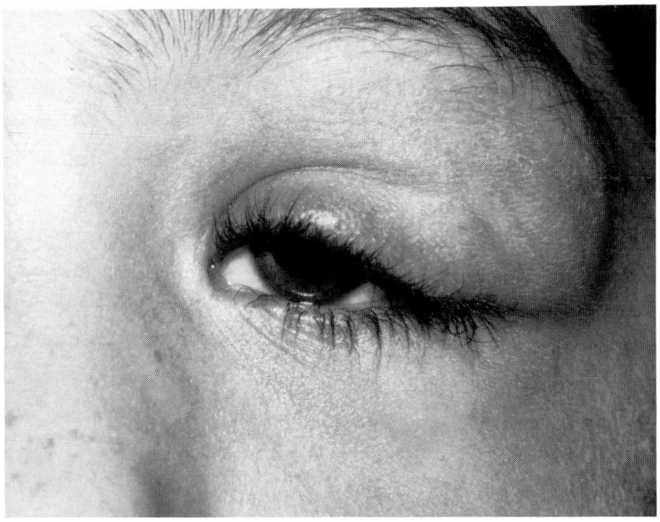

Figure 22.6. Neurofibromatosis of upper eyelid.

RACE

In the Perlman and Hornblass study (9, 10), basal cell carcinoma had a predilection for whites (99%). This was in agreement with Payne and associates (11), who found that, of 270 patients for which race was specified, 100% were white.

AGE

The average age (63 years) of the patients in the Perlman and Hornblass study (9, 10) was consistent with the findings of Hollander and Krugh (11), although Reese (4) and Payne and associates (12) found the highest incidence to be in the fifth decade of life. It should be stressed that malignant tumors of the ocular adnexa can occur at any age. Biggs (13) studied 18 cases of oncocytic lesions of the ocular adnexa and found a predilection for elderly patients (median age, 73), which supports the view that transformation to oncocytes may be related to aging. Diagnoses range from oncocytoma to oncocytic hyperplasia and oncocytic carcinoma.

Sebaceous carcinomas occur predominantly in men 60-

64 years of age. The tumors have a high degree of malignancy; thus, the prognosis is poor.

In a study of 104 cases of sebaceous carcinoma that arose from ocular adnexa, 12 patients died from metastatic disease (13). A bad prognosis was associated with vascular, lymphatic and orbital invasion, multicentric origin, tumor diameter greater than 10 mm, and pagetoid invasion.

SEX

Aurora and Blodi (15) obtained a male-to-female ratio in basal cell carcinoma of 16:1; Hollander and Krugh (11) 17:1; and Cobb, Thompson, and Allt (16) 19:1. Perlman and Hornblass (9, 10) found no sex predilection in their study, and the ratio of males to females was 1.04:1. Aurora and Blodi (15) found that women below the age of 50 years develop the tumor at an earlier age than men. Basal cell carcinoma of the eyelids seemed to be distributed evenly between men and women. Thereafter, many more men were affected than women. In women, the condition is apt to have its onset 6 to 10 years earlier than in men, although there is apparently no notable difference in duration of symptoms in the two sexes.

Aurora and Blodi (15), in their survey of 172 cases of basal cell carcinoma of the eyelids, discovered that the "solid" morphologic type of carcinoma made up 68% of the cases. Its incidence in men was twice as high as its incidence in women, whereas the adenoid variety of tumors occurred more often in women than in men.

ETIOLOGY

Carcinomas arising in the skin of the eyelids and surrounding structures tend to be more prevalent in light-skinned people who are much more exposed to sunlight and perhaps even to wind and rain (17). In the United Kingdom, it is rare to find a squamous epithelioma arising in the lower eyelid; this is not the case in different parts of the world, which leads to the speculation that climatic conditions play a major role in producing the clinical picture found in different countries. In addition to exposure to sunlight (18), exposure to x-rays or chemical carcinogens promotes eyelid cancer. Squamous cell carcinoma is frequently related to some chronic injury or irritation.

Graham and Helwig (19) discuss the incidence and clinical development of precancerous dermatoses, and particularly their relationship to cutaneous and internal cancer. White men with a combination of light complexion, hair, and eyes who had spent most of their lives in the southeastern United States predominated. Among the 144 patients with senile keratosis, 18 showed 26 lesions with histologic evidence of invasion of the corium; none were metastatic. Above-normal levels of arsenic were seen in 10 of 17 lesions.

SYMPTOMS

The presenting symptom reported by patients in the Perlman and Hornblass (9, 10) study was a mass or a growth in 87% of cases. Aurora and Blodi (15) and Payne and associates (12) state that 38% presented with masses. Following are other presenting symptoms:

- Mass or growth
- Irritation
- Ulceration
- Bleeding
- Tearing
- Cosmesis
- Trichiasis
- Blinking
- Asymptomatic condition

Of interest in the review of Perlman and Hornblass (9, 10) was a 61-year-old white man who exhibited tearing as his only symptom. Present for 2 years, with a palpable but not externally visible mass at the medial canthus and with extensive orbital involvement requiring exenteration.

DURATION

Aurora and Blodi (15) obtained a mean duration of symptoms of more than 5 years in their series, whereas Payne and associates (12) found that 10% of their subjects had their lesions for at least 10 years. Perlman and Hornblass (9, 10) found an average duration of 20 months prior to treatment.

LOCATION

Martin (5), Hollander and Krugh (11), Payne and associates (12), Reese (4), and Henkind and Friedman (1) all found the location of the eyelid basal cell carcinoma to be similar in distribution, most commonly affecting the lower eyelid. There is some disagreement as to the second most common location of eyelid tumors. Most authors state that the inner canthus is the second most commonly affected area, but the studies of Henkind and Friedman (1) and Perlman and Hornblass (9, 10) showed the upper lid to be the next most common site for tumors. The outer canthus is affected the least.

SIZE

Cobb, Thompson, and Allt (16) demonstrated that large and small lesions do not favor any particular region of the eyelids, whereas Aurora and Blodi (15) found that extensive lesions involved the medial canthus 1½ times more often than the lower eyelid.

DIFFERENTIAL DIAGNOSIS

The differential diagnosis from benign to malignant conditions can be difficult. Charles (20) has outlined some of the pitfalls in diagnosis and therapy in basal cell carcinoma.

Font (8) suggests that the electron microscope is helpful in establishing the histologic diagnosis, which may be misdiagnosed with light microscopy. In one case, a large cell with acidophilic cytoplasm, previously diagnosed as a ganglion cell by light microscopy, was correctly diagnosed as a rhabdomyoblast after the detection of actin and myosin in bundles under electron microscopy. Weigent and Staley (21) reported a case of a 70-year-old man with a carcinoma of the meibomian glands who had a painless nodule that had been incised and drained on three separate occasions but continued to enlarge. Electron microscopic studies suggested that the tumor arose from sebaceous duct cells rather than from cells composing the sebaceous gland.

Since clinical diagnosis is impossible, sebaceous cell carcinoma must be identified histologically (22). The tumor spreads into the tissues of the eyelid. Pagetoid sliding toward the surface of the skin or conjunctiva from the primary site and lymphatic dissemination commonly occur. The tumor may have a multicentric origin in a single eyelid. This condition is best managed by a team approach involving an oncologist, a radiotherapist, and an ophthalmic plastic surgeon. Many surgeons still recommend exenteration. My own preference is wide excision, followed by either cryosurgery or immunotherapy and possibly radiation therapy. If, however, the tumor is deep or is invading ocular tissues, an exenteration is indicated.

Basal cell carcinoma generally spreads by direct extension to surrounding tissues. However, several cases of metastasis have been reported. Hall, Tappan, and Decker (23) report a man with lung metastasis from basal cell carcinoma of the eyelid that failed to respond to 5-fluorouracil and later to actinomycin D. He died within a year after the first chemotherapy. Aldred and associates (24) described a patient with a basal cell carcinoma arising in the lid of a 53-year-old man with lepromatous leprosy extended through the cornea into the anterior chamber. Hornblass and Stefano (25), in a retrospective study of 100 cases of basal cell carcinoma treated by surgical excision, found nine pigmented lesions. The lesion was clinically misdiagnosed as melanoma.

The differential diagnosis should include nonpigmented (Fig. 22.7) or pigmented nevi (Fig. 22.8), papilloma and keratoacanthomas.

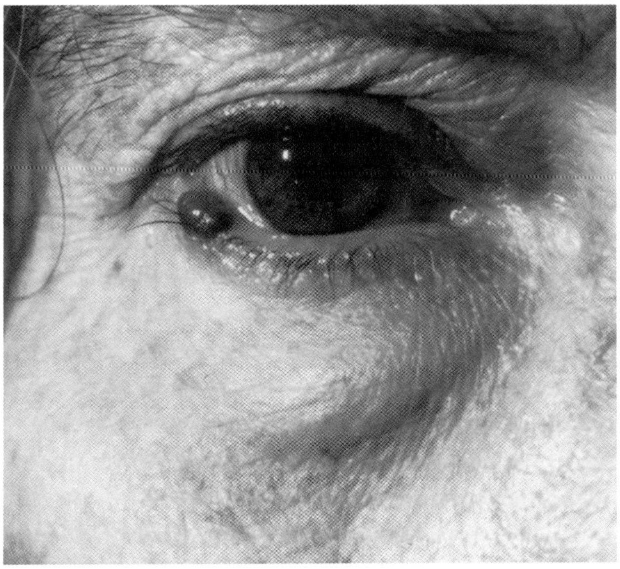

Figure 22.8. Raised pigmented nevus on right lower eyelid.

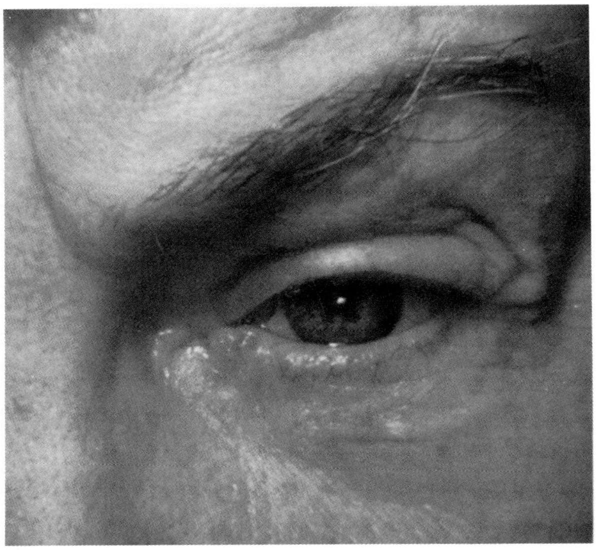

Figure 22.7. Nonpigmented nevus on inferior punctum of left lower eyelid.

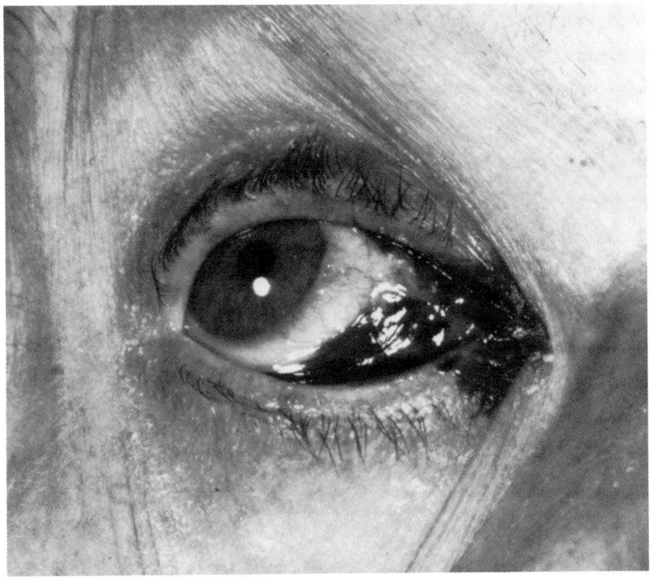

Figure 22.9. A 72-year-old woman with progressive ocular melanosis that progressed to malignant melanoma.

The clinical course of keratoacanthoma is that of a small papillary lesion that enlarges rapidly from 4 to 8 weeks to its maximal size of 1–2 cm and involutes spontaneously, leaving only a faint scar. A characteristic feature of keratoacanthoma (26, 27) is an umbilicated surface with a central keratin core. Trelfall (28) reported a case of a 45-year-old man with squamous cell carcinoma of the eyelid that simulated keratoacanthoma. The treatment was excision with radical unilateral neck dissection. The tumor recurred continuously and was treated with excision and radiotherapy.

Seborrheic keratosis, benign calcifying epithelioma, and inverted follicular keratosis are part of differential diagnosis. Chalazions frequently masquerade as meibomian gland carcinoma and basal cell carcinoma. Leone (27) reviewed five such misdiagnosed cases.

Portney (29) reported an 84-year-old man who underwent surgical excision for meibomian cell adenocarcinoma that started out as a chalzion-like mass. Metastases to the right preauricular area and right parotid gland were evident 6 months later.

Other lesions simulating a malignant tumor can be a trichoepithelioma, melanosis (Fig. 22.9), sudoriferous cysts, molluscum contagiosum, ectopic lymph nodes (30), neurofibroma and other lacrimal gland tumors (31, 32), embryonal sarcoma (33), embryonal adenoides cysticum (34), palpebral myxoma (35), benign lymphocytic lymphoma (36), and lymphangioma (37). Riley and Henderson (38) reported a case of a malignant transformation in an originally benign mixed tumor of the lacrimal gland. Mucoepidermoid carcinoma of the lid can appear like a chronic blepharitis or chalazion. These are potentially lethal lesions. (39).

MANAGEMENT

Dizon and associates (40) stress early diagnosis and aggressive treatment. They studied 20 recurrences of basal cell carcinoma of the lids in 12 patients. Doxanas and associates (41) studied 165 basal cell carcinomas of the eyelids and classified tumors into nodular, ulcerative, morphea, and multicentric. There were no recurrences with frozen sections. In 126 cases treated with frozen section monitoring, 27% were incompletely excised and 5.5% recurred. Surgical margins should always be monitored, particularly in patients with morphea and multicentric types. In view of the unpredictable behavior and difficulty in treatment, the following management was suggested:

1. Perform biopsy of suspicious lesions before treatment to establish early diagnosis and prevent unnecessary radical operations (Fig. 22.10).
2. Perform aggressive surgical excision for aggressive recurrent lesions.
3. Use frozen sections.
4. Provide close, regular follow-up at 6-month intervals, especially for lesions in the medial canthal region and for tumors at the margins of resection.

EXCISIONAL VERSUS INCISIONAL BIOPSIES

All suspicious lesions should be biopsied. If the entire lesion can be removed without any major reconstruction, an excisional biopsy should be performed (Fig. 22.11); otherwise, an incisional biopsy should be performed (Fig. 22.12). Frozen sections are not nearly as accurate as permanent histologic sections; however, I believe they are helpful in surgery.

IMPORTANCE OF CLEAR MARGINS

The difficulty of eradicating the carcinoma while leaving the patient with eyelids that will function normally produces special problems in the management of eyelid tumors (42). The general principle involved in surgical treatment of carcinoma arising in the periphery of the orbit

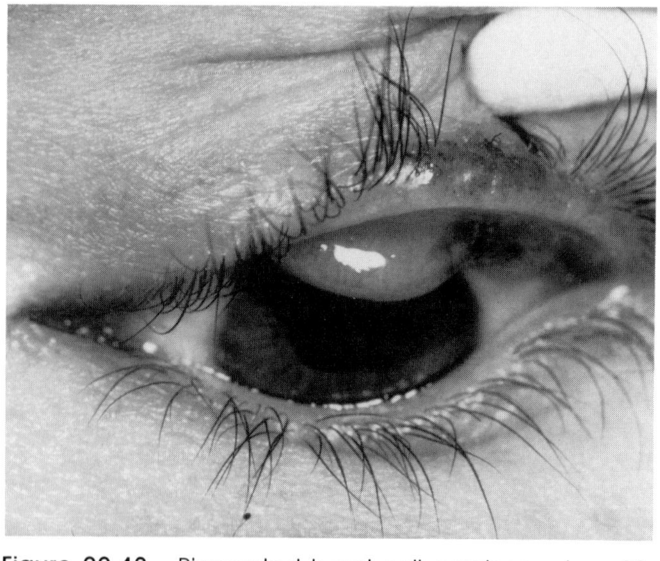

Figure 22.10. Pigmented basal cell carcinoma in a 30-year-old woman. Note invasion on margin and on tarsal conjunctival surface.

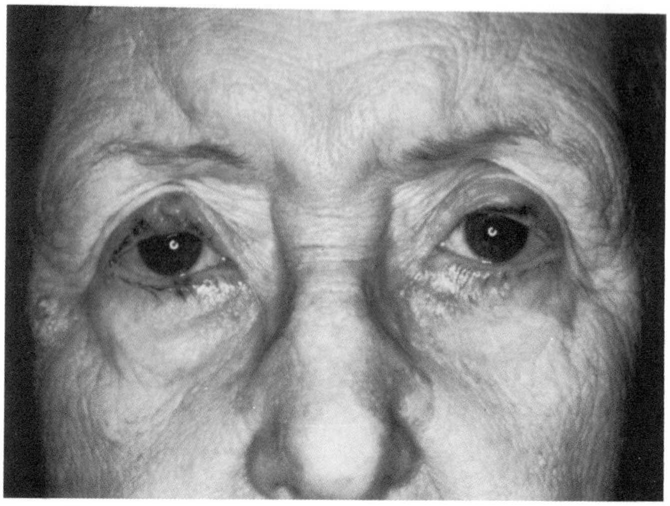

Figure 22.11. Woman, age 66, with 3-month history of squamous cell carcinoma of right upper lid.

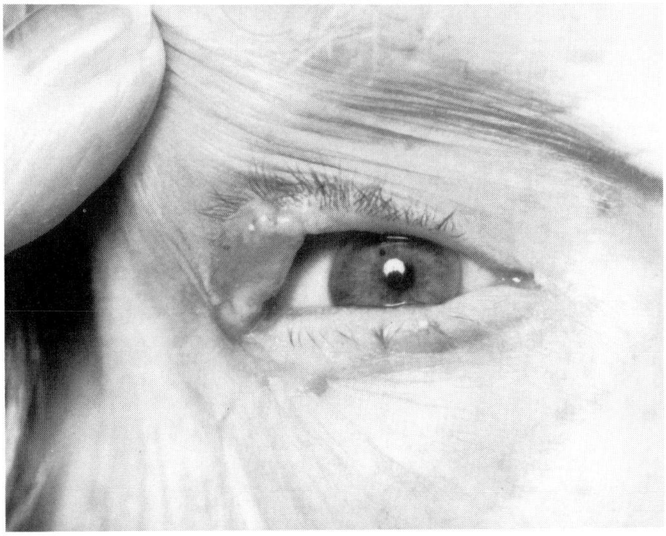

Figure 22.12. Sebaceous adenocarcinoma of upper eyelid.

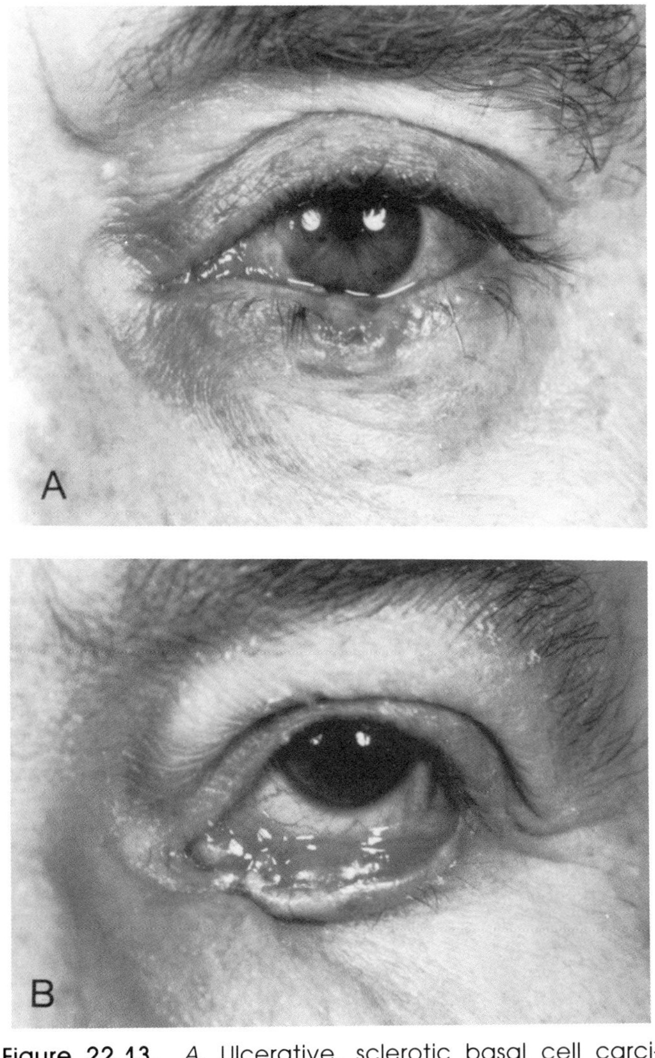

Figure 22.13. *A*, Ulcerative, sclerotic basal cell carcinoma on left lower lid. *B*, 58-year-old man with infiltrative basal cell carcinoma of left lower lid.

and immediately beyond this is to resect the tumor with an adequate margin of normal tissue around it and beneath it and to fill the defect with a skin flap. In some sites around the eyelids, the depth of tissue involved by carcinoma is limited to 2–3 mm. After resection of tumors in these areas, a comparatively shallow defect can be covered with a full-thickness skin graft. The reconstruction problem is much more complicated when the full thickness of the eyelid has been resected and is more difficult in cases involving the upper than the lower eyelid.

Collin (43) studied 226 patients with histologically proven basal cell carcinoma of the eyelids (Fig. 22.13). All lesions were excised with a 3–5 mm macroscopic clearance, and the defect was closed by direct closure (29.8%), skin graft (9.8%), or flap (60.4%) technique. If histologic examination showed incomplete excision, the operation was repeated. Three deaths occurred during the study. The overall recurrence rate for the average follow-up period of 3–6 years was 2.3% for basal cell carcinomas treated with primary surgery and 30% for secondary surgery on lesions that had recurred (Figs. 22.14 and 22.15).

Mustarde (17) states that a free skin margin of at least 5 mm should be carried out in basal cell carcinoma. If the tumor is a squamous epithelioma, the margin of normal skin between the tumor and the edge of the lid should be about 1 cm. Holmstrom, Bartholdson, and Johanson (44) studied 203 eyelid cancers in 193 patients. A 3-year follow-up showed 18 recurrences; no metastases were found.

Older, Quickert, and Beard (45) studied 157 white patients with basal cell carcinoma involving the eyelids. Seventy-two percent had frozen section evaluation at surgery. The tumors ranged from 2 to 30 mm. There were no recurrences. It is suggested that the good results obtained in this study are attributable to the fact that 97.5% of the lesions were free of tumor cells at the surgical margins as determined by histologic examination. Similarly, Perlman and Hornblass (9) showed that, if basal cell carcinomas of the eyelids are fully excised at the first procedure with clear histologic margins, the cure rate is

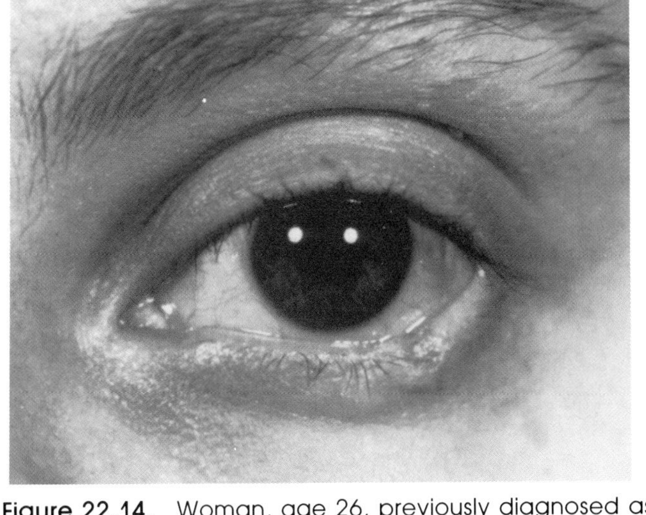

Figure 22.14. Woman, age 26, previously diagnosed as having recurrent chalazion of left lower lid. Note loss of lashes.

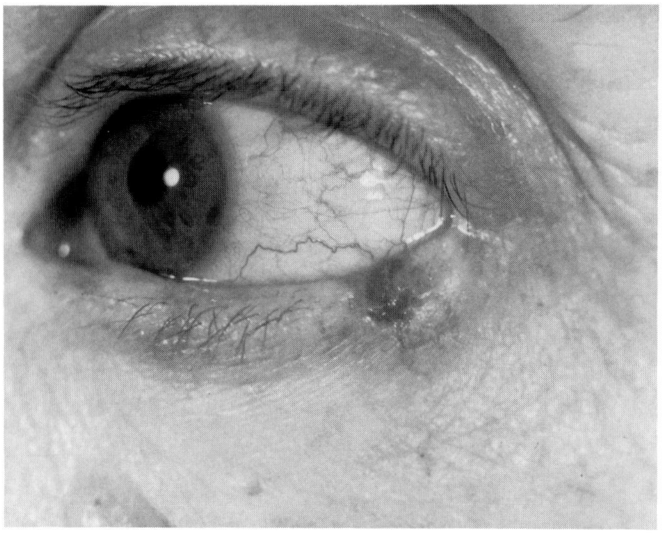

Figure 22.15. Basal cell carcinoma of left lower lid.

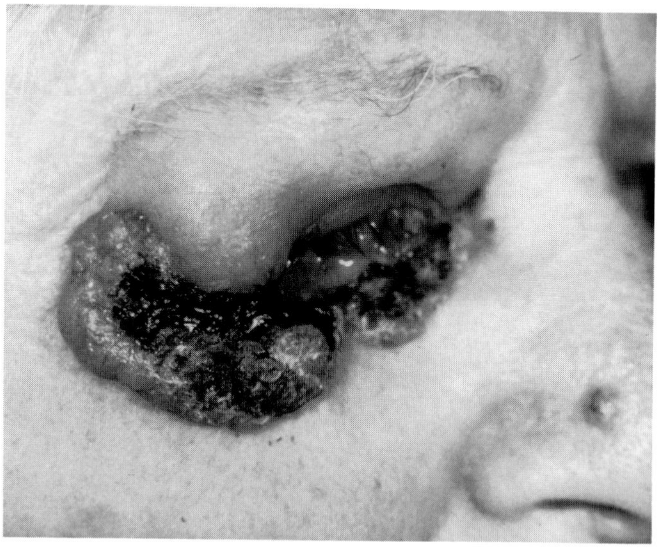

Figure 22.16. Infiltrating periocular basal cell carcinoma.

about 99%. Bedford and Migdal (46) in England reported on the results of 377 patients treated for eyelid neoplasms; they limited their treatment with surgery for simple excision and Wolfe graft or radiotherapy, which appears to offer an excellent treatment. Vickers (47) who studied 272 cases, recommended consideration of tumor type, site, age, and general patient condition before treatment. The decision should be made by a team of radiotherapists, plastic surgeons, and dermatologists consulting together.

ORBITAL EXENTERATION

The necessity for orbital exenteration in basal cell carcinoma is, fortunately, rare. Of 273 cases analyzed by Payne and associates (12) only eight (3%) required such radical treatment; in the Perlman-Hornblass series of patients (9), five of 107 (5%) came to exenteration (Figs. 22.16 and 22.17).

RADIATION

In an Australian study (48), there was a 90% or better recurrence-free rate after irradiation of 896 patients with squamous cell carcinoma and basal cell carcinoma. Complications were lid necrosis, keratinization, corneal ulceration or opacity, corneal abrasion or keratitis, cataract, loss of the eye, telangiectasia, lid deformity, and epiphora. Szabo (49) treated 94 patients with radiation; relapse occurred in four. He states that there was no radiation damage. Lederman (50) studied 689 patients. Basal cell carcinoma was observed in 348 men and 282 women. Squamous cell carcinoma occurred in 44 men and 50 women. The recurrence-free rate for basal cell carcinoma of the lower lid and inner canthus after 4 years was 95% and 90.8%, respectively. There were no recurrences of the upper lid. The recurrence-free rate of squamous cell carcinoma was 87.5%. The overall complication rate was 13.3% for basal cell carcinoma and 10% for squamous cell carcinoma. The use of a therapeutic contact lens as a means of protecting the cornea against damage from secondary changes in the eyelid is also of great value.

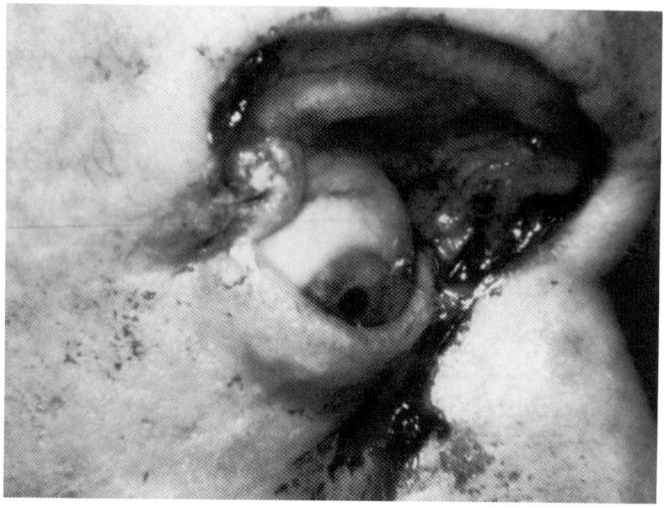

Figure 22.17. Man, age 65, with history of a mental disorder, who had an extensive basal cell carcinoma of the right upper lid.

Tapley (51) states that radiation therapy should be given after excision of any skin carcinoma when the surgical margins are inadequate. Radiation therapy should also be given after excision of a recurrent lesion, especially if there has been more than one recurrence in the same area. Goldschmidt (52) states that sun-exposed areas of patients younger than 40 years should not be treated with irradiation when other methods are available, and that previous radiation treatments to the same skin generally contraindicate radiotherapy. Savar (53) reported on two patients with orbital exenteration for recurrent basal cell carcinoma after multiple courses of radiation to the orbit; postoperatively, there may be sloughing of skin grafts from the bony surface that receives the highest exposure to the radiation, presumably secondary to death of soft tissue elements within the bone.

CRYOSURGERY

Bullock, Beard, and Sullivan (35) state that cryotherapy is an effective modality in the treatment of basal cell carcinoma in the eyelids and periorbital area, which cured 93% of the 29 lesions in 25 patients in their study. This method is especially advantageous in patients with blood clotting disorders, those with medical contraindications, those who refuse classical surgery, those who have had prior radiation or surgery, those with basal cell nevus syndrome or xeroderma pigmentosum, and those with medial canthal tumors. Torre (54) had a 10% recurrence rate around the eyelid with cryotherapy, which he advocates in lesions with multiple multicentric foci, superficial basal cell, sclerosing epithelioma, and epithelioma in scar tissue or near invading bone and cartilage. Fontana and Muti (55) report excellent results in Italy with cryotherapy in skin tumors. Biro and associates (56) reported on 87 basal cell carcinomas of the eyelids, and 155 of the nose treated by cryosurgery; three recurrences were noted on the eyelid and four on the nose. Cosmetic results were excellent (Fig. 22.18).

CHEMOSURGERY

Mohs (57) employs chemosurgery for cancer of the eyelid and suggests that treatment of cancer of the skin consist of chemosurgery, topical chemotherapy, immunotherapy, or systemic chemotherapy. The original chemosurgical technique consisted of application of zinc chloride to produce fixation of the lesion, excision of this tissue with microscopic scanning of underlayers, and repeated excision to remove all of the cancer. He now advocates the use of fresh-tissue techniques (58, 59). Szujewski (60) reports that chemosurgery caused complete tumor regression for 10 years in 65 of 71 patients with basal cell carcinoma and in 6 of 71 with squamous cell carcinoma of the nasolabial or nasolacrimal grooves. Resnick and associates (61) reported on a 59-year-old white man who presented with a darkly pigmented inner canthal tumor. It was a pigmented basal cell epithelioma.

RADIATION VERSUS SURGERY

The controversy of radiation versus surgery persists. In an excellent review, Anderson (62) gives the pros and cons of each modality.

The management of several types of tumors of the orbit in children is discussed by Wybar and Dalley (63). External irradiation, exenteration, chemotherapy, radical radiotherapy, and systemic steroids are modalities to be used. Radical cranioorbital (64) resection is advocated in recurrent orbital rhabdomyosarcoma along with radiation and chemotherapy. It has been useful in treatment of lacrimal gland tumors, squamous cell carcinoma (Fig. 22.15) and invasive hemangiopericytomas.

RECURRENCES

Incomplete excision and recurrence rate are obviously the most important aspects in the treatment of basal cell carcinoma. Einaugler and Henkind (65) found 50% of the tumors to be incompletely excised, whereas Aurora and Blodi's study (15) showed 23% of primary cases to be incompletely excised. Gooding, White, and Yatsuhashi (2) found that 35% of lesions which show marginal extension will recur; Aurora and Blodi (15) had 80% with incomplete excision go on to have one or more recurrences. Rakofsky (66), reporting on 95 basal cell carcinomas, states that of the almost 50% of the specimens showing inadequate excision 23.4% recurred. Most other investigators (10, 15, 16) had significantly less involved margins (Figs. 22.19 and 22.20).

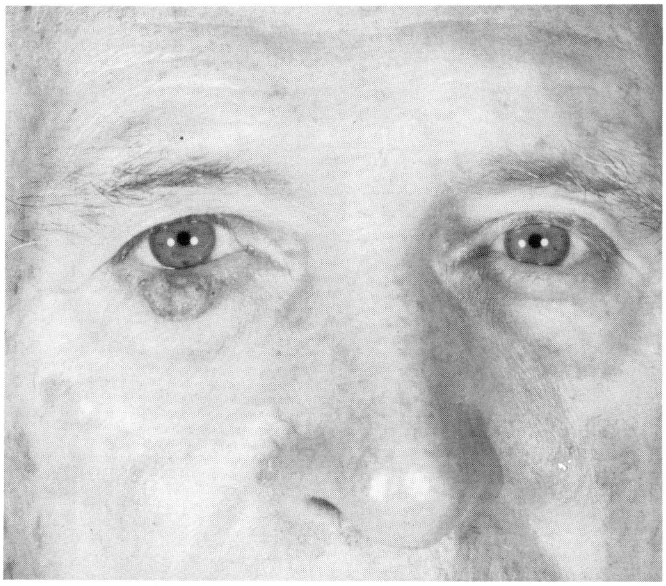

Figure 22.18. Irritative seborrheic keratosis of the right lower lid.

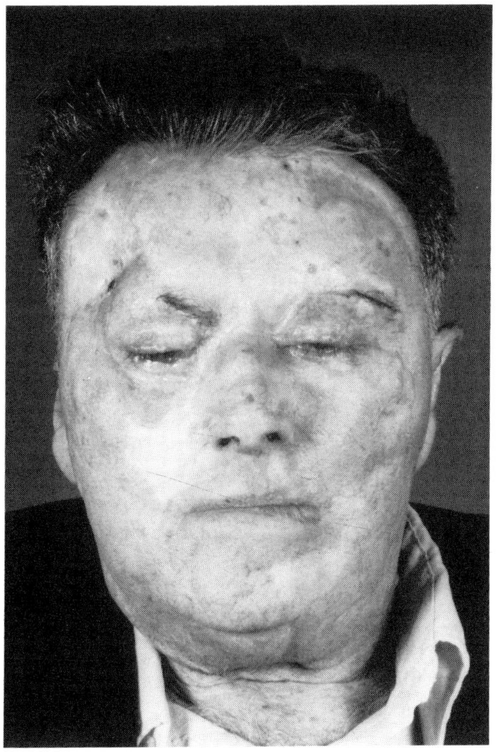

Figure 22.19. Man, age 65, with basal cell nevus syndrome. He had 65 operations on his face and neck.

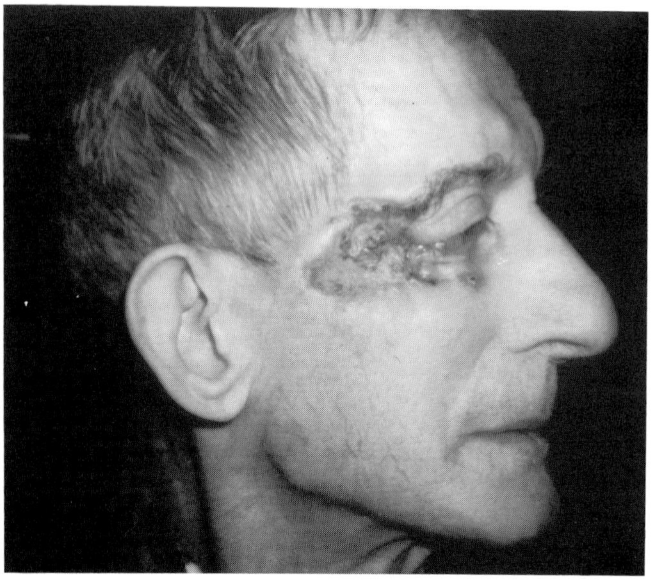

Figure 22.20. Extensive invasive basal cell carcinoma of right periorbital area.

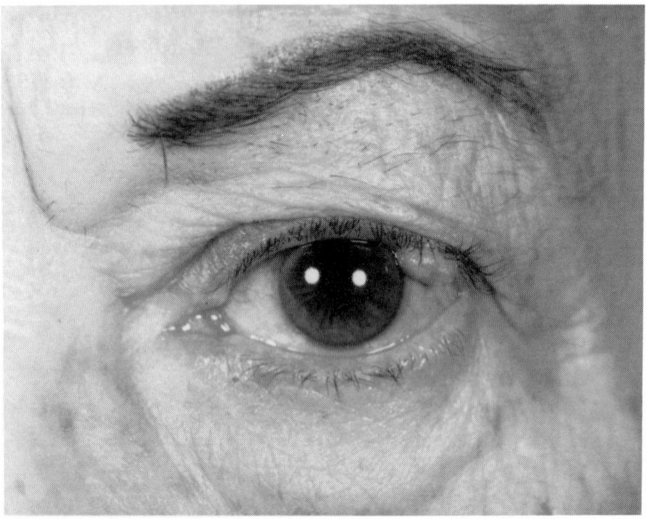

Figure 22.21. Intradermal nevus, left upper lid.

Beard (67), in a review of basal cell carcinoma of the eyelid, states that inadequate excision rates of 5.5–50% have been reported, with a recurrence rate of 12–34%. He advocates a multitreatment approach. Azelaic acid has been used with some success in the treatment of ocular and adnexal malignant melanoma (68), as has extensive cryotherapy.

In an Australian study (48), there was a 90% or better recurrence-free rate after the irradiation of 896 patients. The same article reviewed 261 patients treated by surgical excision, for which the recurrence rate was 23%. This study stressed, as I believe, that the primary treatment should be meticulously performed because the first treatment obviously gives the best chance of success. Radiation therapy is quite successful for conjunctival and orbital lymphoid tumors. In a study by Jereb and associates (69), 24 patients were reported. Between 2400 to 2750 rads in 2 to 3 weeks for eyelid and conjunctiva and about 3500 rads for retrobulbar lesions were given. The eye was shielded by a lead block. Twenty patients who were alive have been free of tumor.

METASTASES TO THE ORBIT

Font and Ferry (70) reviewed 227 cases of carcinoma metastatic to the eye and orbit. The most common signs and symptoms produced by orbital metastasis included exophthalmos in 75% of the cases, pain in 29% of the cases, decreased vision in 29%, periorbital swelling in 25%,

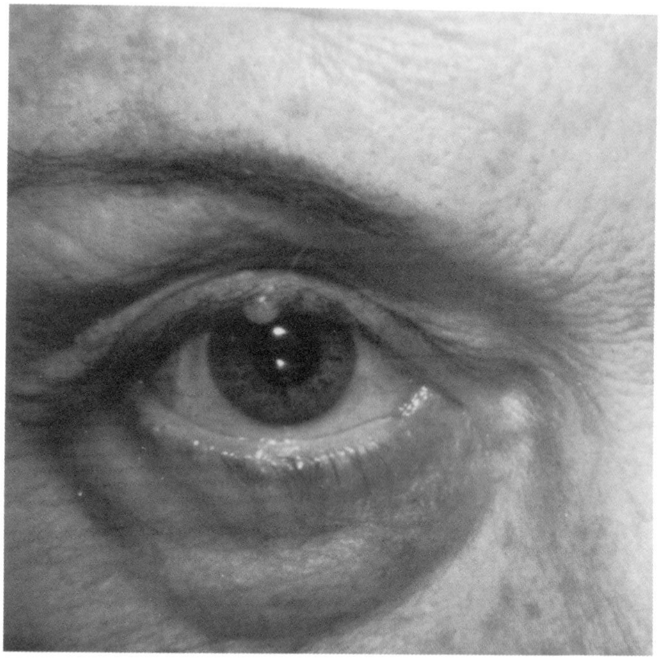

Figure 22.22. Papilloma of right upper eyelid.

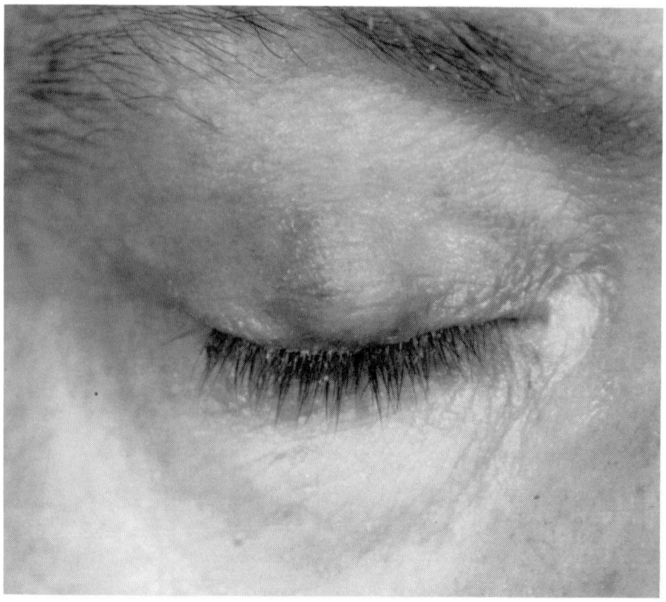

Figure 22.23. Chalazion of right upper lid.

a visible mass in 21%, and ophthalmoplegia and diplopia in 18%. In order of frequency, the sites of the primary tumors were breast, lung, genitourinary tract, pancreas, and ileum. Moltow-Lippa and associates (71) have described the pitfalls of misdiagnosis of metastatic breast carcinoma and inflammatory lesions. Computed tomograph scan and biopsy are critical for diagnosis.

AREAS OF RESEARCH

Hematoporphyrin

Hematoporphyrin (72, 73) derivative has been found to accumulate in tumor cells and can be used to differentiate neoplastic from normal tissue by its ability to fluoresce under violet light. This may help to make frozen-section control of tumor edges outmoded [(79); Fig. 22.21 and 22.22].

Donor Material

Preserved collagen (74) sclera and fascia lata (75) have been used in reconstruction of the orbit. Cadaver eyelids under proper conditions may be practical.

Microsurgical Techniques

Although ophthalmologists were pioneers in the microscope and microinstruments, oculoplastic surgeons have not been in the vanguard of microsurgery of the vascular system. However, a new field of microplastic surgical technique is developing (Figs. 22.23–22.26).

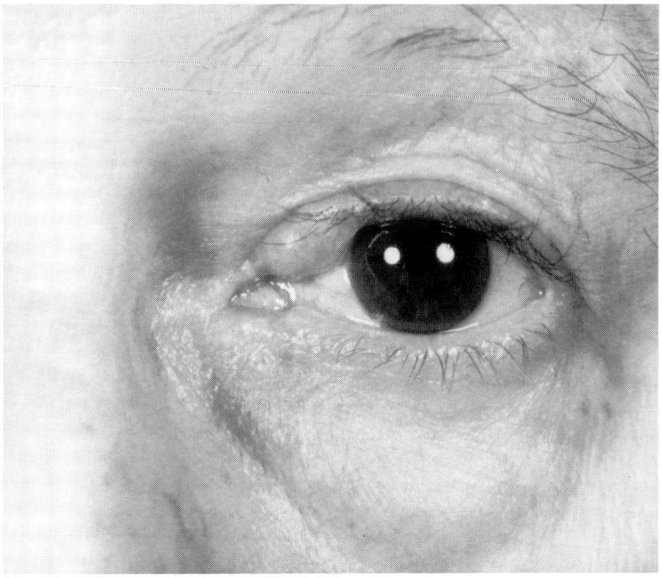

Figure 22.24. Marginal cyst of left upper lid.

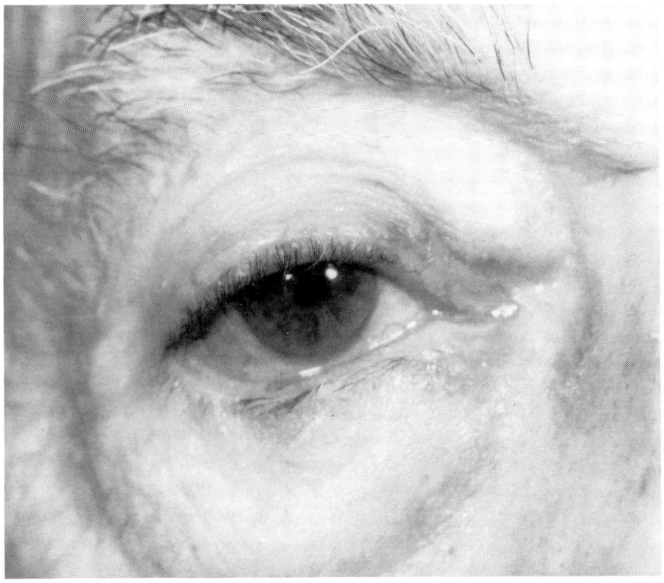

Figure 22.25. Mucoid epidermoid carcinoma of the right lower lid.

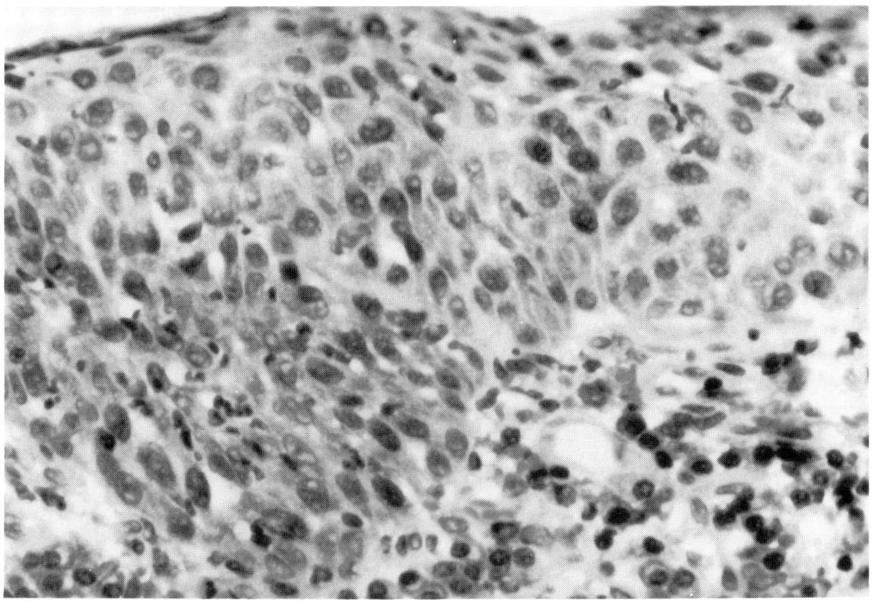

Figure 22.26 Pathology of patient, age 25, who demonstrated mucoid epidermoid carcinoma.

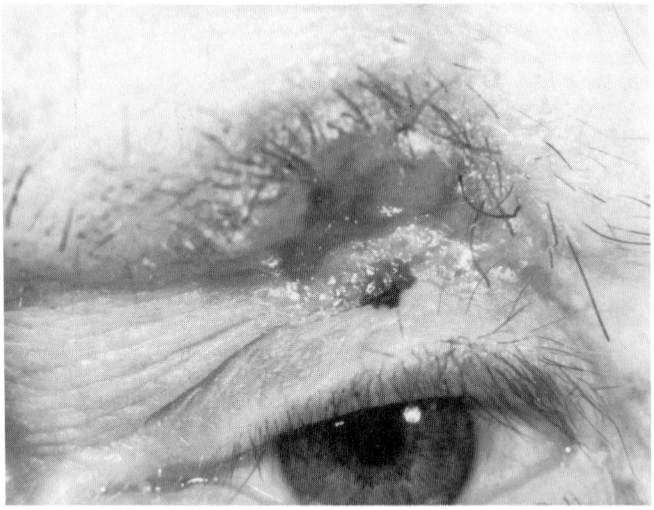

Figure 22.27. Infiltrating basal cell carcinoma of right upper lid.

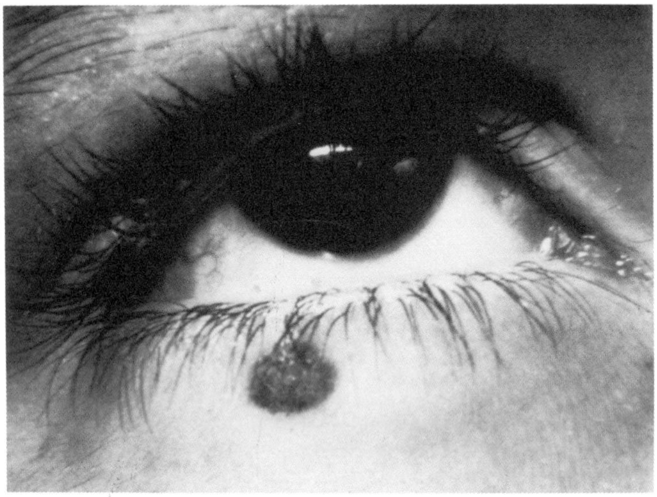

Figure 22.28. Nevus of right lower eyelid, which was removed by excisional biopsy.

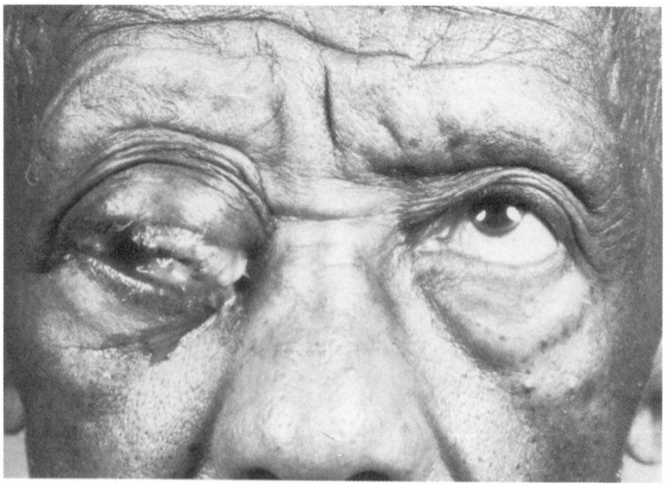

Figure 22.29. Squamous cell carcinoma of conjunctiva and lid. An incisional biopsy was first performed to ascertain the diagnosis, and this was followed by exenteration.

Immunotherapy

This complete wide-open field offers interesting and hopeful modalities in extensive tumors. Dulton and associates (76) reported on three patients with epithelial malignancies of the ocular adnexa that had invasive tumors with scleral involvement. In an attempt to preserve the globe, treatment consisted of local surgical excision without lamellar or full-thickness sclerectomy, followed by cryotherapy utilizing a double-cycle freeze-thaw-refreeze technique to the underlying scleral bed and area of suspected residual tumor. This technique may offer a useful alternative to exenteration or enucleation in selected patients with ocular invasion of tumor in whom more radical

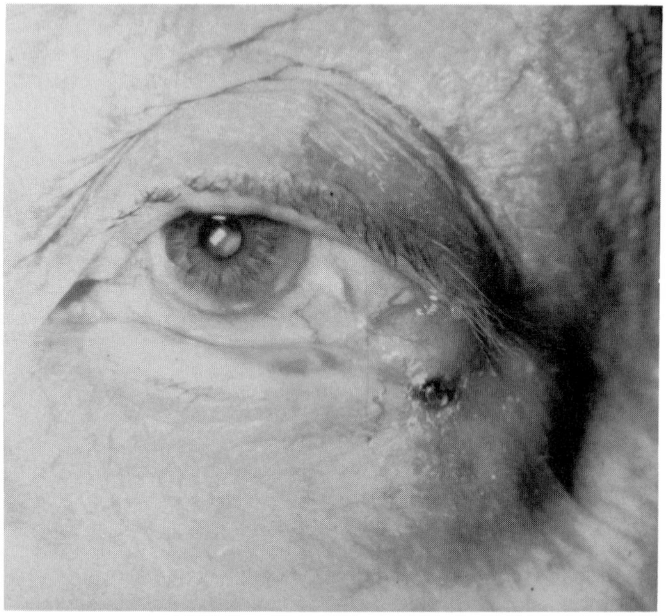

Figure 22.30. Basal cell carcinoma of the left lower lid and left lateral canthus.

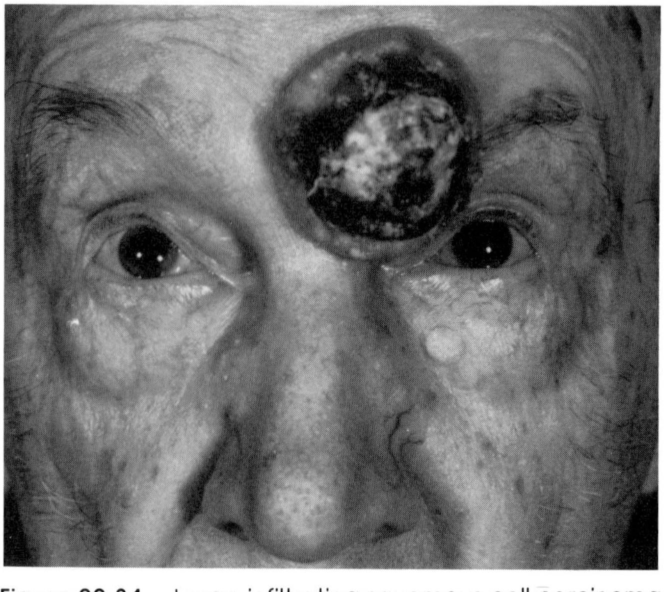

Figure 22.31. Large infiltrating squamous cell carcinoma of left medial canthus and forehead.

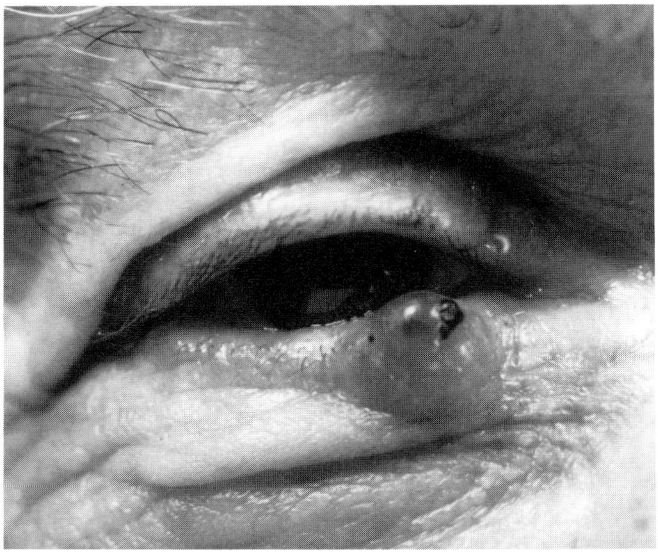

Figure 22.32. Mucinous adenocarcinoma in the right lower lid in a 57-year-old white man.

surgery may be visually incapacitating or not otherwise feasible. A review article by Knowles and Jakobiec (77) analyzed 400 ocular adnexal lymphoid neoplasms. The study focuses on the use of hybridoma-derived monoclonal antibodies, which are capable of detecting maturational stages of B- and T-cell differentiation and functionally distinct T-cell subsets, in order to investigate the interactional and immunoregulatory defects that participate in the generation of the ocular adnexal lymphoid proliferations (Figs. 22.29 and 22.32).

REFERENCES

1. Henkind P, Friedman A: Cancer of the lids and ocular adnexa. In Andrade R, Gumport SL, Popkin GL, Rees TD (eds): *Cancer of the Skin: Biology-Diagnosis-Management*. Philadelphia, WB Saunders, 1976.
2. Gooding CA, White G, Yatsuhashi M: Significance of marginal extension in excised basal cell carcinoma. *N Eng J Med* 272: 923, 1965.
3. Kwitko ML, Boniuk M, Zimmerman LE: Eyelid tumors with recurrence to lesions confused with squamous cell carcinoma. I. Incidence and errors in diagnosis. *Arch Ophthalmol* 69: 693–697, 1963.
4. Reese AB: *Tumors of the Eye*, (ed) 3. New York, Harper & Row, 1976.
5. Martin HE: Cancer of the eyelids. *Arch Ophthalmol* 22: 1–20, 1939.
6. Abe M, Ohnishi Y, Hara Y, Shinoda Y, Jingu K: Malignant tumor of the eyelid. *Jpn J Ophthal* 27: 175–84, 1983.
7. Duke-Elder S (ed): *System of Ophthalmology*. London, Henry Kimpton Ltd, 1974, vol 8, pt 1.
8. Font RL: Electron microscopy of tumors of the eye and ocular adnexa. In Reese AB (ed): *Tumors of the Eye*, ed 3. New York, Harper & Row, 1976.
9. Perlman GS, Hornblass A: Basal cell carcinoma of the eyelids. *Surg Forum* 26: 540–542, 1975.
10. Perlman GS, Hornblass A: Basal cell carcinoma of the eyelids: A review of patients treated by surgical excision. *Ophthalmol Surg* 7(4): 23–27, 1976.
11. Hollander L, Krugh FJ: Cancer of the eyelid. *Am J Ophthalmol* 29: 244–253, 1944.
12. Payne JW, Duke JR, Butner R, et al.: Basal cell carcinoma of the eyelids: A long-term follow-up study. *Arch Ophthalmol* 81: 553–558, 1969.
13. Biggs SL: Oncolytic lesions of the caruncle and other ocular adnexa. *Arch Ophthalmol* 95: 474–478, 1977.
14. Rao MA, Hidayat A, McLean IW, Zimmerman LE: Sebaceous carcinoma of the ocular adnexa: A clinicopathologic study of 104 cases. *Hum Pathol* 13: 113–122, 1982.
15. Aurora AL, Blodi FC: Reappraisal of basal cell carcinoma of the eyelids. *Am J Ophthalmol* 70: 329–336, 1970.
16. Cobb GM, Thompson GA, Allt WEC: Treatment of basal cell carcinoma of the eyelids by radiotherapy. *Can Med Assoc J* 91: 743–748, 1964.
17. Mustarde JC: Basal cell and squamous cell carcinomas in the orbital region. Switzerland, 1975, *Excerpta Med*
18. Siddiqui S: Skin cancer. *Med Trial Tech* 21(2): 163–169, 1974.
19. Graham JH, Helwig EB: Cutaneous precancerous conditions in man. *Ntl Cancer Inst Monogr* 10: 323–333, 1963.
20. Charles NC: Basal cell carcinomas of the eyelids: Pitfalls in diagnosis and therapy. *J Dermatol Surg* 1: 28–32, 1975.
21. Weigent CC, Staley NA: Meibomian gland carcinoma: Report of a case with electron microscopic finding. *Hum Pathol* 7: 231–234, 1976.
22. Wolfe JT, Yeatts RP, Wick MR, Camphale RJ, Waller RR: Sebaceous carcinoma of the eyelid. Errors in clinical and pathologic diagnosis. *Am J Surg Pathol* 8: 597–606, 1984.
23. Hall TE, Tappan WM, Decker JW: Basal cell carcinoma with metastases: Report of two cases. *Rocky Mt Med J* 67: 39–40, 1970.
24. Aldred NVV, Ramirez VA, Nicholson DH: Intraocular invasion by basal cell carcinoma of the lid. *Arch Ophthalmol* 98: 1821–1822, 1986.
25. Hornblass A, Stefano JA: Pigmented basal cell carcinoma of the eyelids. *Am J Ophthalmol* 92: 193–197, 1981.
26. Christensen L, Fitzpatrick TB: Keratocanthoma of the ocular adnexa. *Arch Ophthalmol* 53: 857–859, 1955.
27. Leone CR: Meibomian gland carcinoma. *Ear Eyes Nose Throat Mon* 53: 406–411, 1974.
28. Trelfall GN: Squamous carcinoma of the eyelids simulating keratocanthoma: Report of a case. *Aust NZJ Surg* 44: 357–359, 1974.
29. Portney GL: Meibomian gland adenocarcinoma. *Ann Ophthalmol* 5: 193–196, 1973.
30. Cykiert RC, Albert DM, Cornog JL, Bellows AR: Suspected multiple primary tumors of the lacrimal and parotid glands. *Arch Ophthalmol* 94: 1530–1533, 1976.
31. Faraci RP, Chretien PB: Adenocarcinoma of the lacrimal gland with simultaneous pulmonary metastases. *Arch Surg* 109: 107–110, 1974.
32. Henderson JW, Neault RW: En bloc removal of intrinsic neoplasms of the lacrimal gland. *Am J Ophthalmol* 82: 905–909, 1976.
33. Lederman M, Wybar K: ocular malignant diseases, embryonal sarcoma. *Proc R Soc Med* 69: 895–903, 1976.
34. Howell JB, Anderson EE: Transformation of epithelioma adenoides cysticum into multiple rodent ulcers: fact or fallacy. A historical vignette. *Br J Dermatol* 95: 233–242, 1976.
35. Bullock JD, Beard C, Sullivan JH: Cryotherapy of basal cell carcinoma in oculoplastic surgery. *Am J Ophthalmol* 82: 841–847, 1976.
36. Tabor GL: Benign lymphocytic lymphoma of the right upper eyelid and left plica semilunaris. *Ann Ophthalmol* 5: 694–965, 1973.
37. Pang P, Jakobiec FA, Iwamoto T, Hornblass A: Small lymphangioma of the eyelids. *Ophthalmology* 91: 1278–1284, 1984.
38. Riley, FC, Henderson JW: Report of a case of malignant transformation in benign mixed tumor of the lacrimal gland. *Am J Ophthalmol* 70: 767–770, 1970.
39. Herschorn BJ, Jakobiec FA, Hornblass A, Iwamoto T, Harrison WA: Mucoepidermoid carcinoma of the palpebral mucocutaneous junction. A clinical light microscopic and electron microscopic study of an unusual tubular variant. *Ophthalmology* 90: 1437–1446, 1983.
40. Dizon RV, Shannon GM, Sliguini, JJ: Basal cell carcinoma recurrence: early diagnosis and surgical treatment. *Ophthalmol Surg* 8: 31–39, 1977.
41. Doxanas MT, Green WR, Ilf CE: Factors in the successful surgical management of basal cell carcinoma of the eyelids. *Am J Opthalmol* 91: 726–736, 1981.
42. Char DH: The management of lid and conjunctival malignancies. *Surv Ophthalmol* 24: 679–689, 1980.
43. Collin JR: Basal cell carcinoma in the eyelid region. *Br J Ophthalmol* 60: 806–809, 1976.
44. Holmstrom H, Bartholdson L, Johanson B: Surgical treatment of eyelid cancer with special reference to tarsoconjunctival flaps: A follow-up of 193 patients. *Scand J Plast Reconstr Surg* 9: 107–115, 1975.

45. Older JJ, Quickert MH, Beard C: Surgical removal of basal cell carcinoma of the eyelids utilizing frozen section control. *Trans Am Acad Ophthal Otolaryngol* 79: 658–663, 1975.
46. Bedford MA, Migdal CS: The management of eyelid neoplasms. *Trans Ophthal Soc UK* 102: 116–118, 1982.
47. Vickers HR: Treatment of malignant disease of the orbital region. *Proc R Soc Med* 66: 689–690, 1973.
48. Cancer of the eyelids: Radiation or surgery (editorial)? *Med J Aust* 1: 391, 1977.
49. Szabo P: Clinical characteristics and radiotherapy of eyelid and canthal carcinomas. *Dermatol Monatsschr* 163: 41–47, 1977.
50. Lederman M: Radiation treatment of cancer of the eyelids. *Br J Ophthalmol* 60: 694–805, 1976.
51. Tapley NV: Radiotherapy for basal and squamous cell carcinoma of the skin. *Neoplasms of the Skin and Malignant Melanoma.* Chicago, 1976.
52. Goldschmidt H: Radiotherapy of skin cancer: modern indications and techniques. *Cutis* 171: 253–261, 1976.
53. Savar DE: High-dose radiation to the orbit. A cause of skin graft failure after exenteration. *Arch Ophthalmol* 100: 1755–1757, 1982.
54. Torre D: Cryosurgery. In Andrade R, Gumport SL, Popkin GL, Rees TD (eds): *Cancer of the Skin. Biology-Diagnosis-Management* Philadelphia, WB Saunders, 1976, Vol 2.
55. Fontana AM, Muti E: Results with cryotherapy in skin tumors. *Panminerva Med* 17: 384–389, 1975.
56. Biro K, Price E, Brand A: Cryosurgery for basal cell carcinoma of the eyelids and nose. *Am Acad Dermatol* 6: 1042–1047, 1982.
57. Mohs FE: Prevention and treatment of skin cancer. *Wis Med J* 73: 85–92, 1974.
58. Callahan MA, Monhet GD, Callahan A: Cancer excision from eyelids and ocular adnexa. The Moh's fresh technique and reconstruction. *Cancer* 6: 322–329, 1982.
59. Callahan MA, Monhet GD, Callahan A: Cancer excision from eyelids and ocular adnexa. The Mohs' fresh tissue technique and reconstruction. A five-year study of 109 patients. *Ala J Med Soc* 20: 289–294, 1983.
60. Szujewski HA: Chemosurgical treatments. *Oncology* 23: 265–269, 1969.
61. Resnick KI, Sadun A, and Albert DM: Basal cell epithelioma: an unusual case. *Ophthalmology* 88(12): 1182–5, 1981.
62. Anderson SR: Tumors of the eye and its adnexa. *Acta Ophthal* 54: 1–16, 1976.
63. Wybar K, Dalley V: Other tumors of the eye and orbit in cancer of the children: *Clin Manag (Berlin)* 1975.
64. Murray JE, Matson DD, Habal MB, Geelhoed GW: Regional cranio-orbital resection for recurrent tumors with delayed reconstruction. *Surg Gyn Obstet* 134: 437–447, 1972.
65. Einaugler RB, Henkind P: Basal cell epithelioma of the eyelids: Apparent imcomplete removal. *Am J Ophthalmol* 67: 413, 1959.
66. Rakofsky SI: The adequacy of the surgical excision of basal cell carcinoma. *Ann Ophthalmol* 5: 596–600, 1973.
67. Beard C: Observations on the treatment of basal cell carcinoma of the eyelids. *Trans Am Acad Ophthal Otolaryngol* 79: 664–670, 1975.
68. Willshaw HE, Rubinstein K: Azelaic acid in the treatment of ocular and adnexal malignant melanoma. *Br J Ophthalmol* 67; 54–57, 1983.
69. Jereb B, Lee H, Jakobiec FA, Kutcher J: Radiation therapy of conjunctival and orbital lymphoid tumors. *Int J Radiat Oncol Bio Phys* 10: 1013, 1019, 1984.
70. Font RC, Ferry AP: Carcinoma metastatic to the eye and orbit. A clinicopathologic study of 28 cases metastatic to the orbit. *Cancer* 38: 1326–1335, 1976.
71. Mottow-Lippa L, Jakobiec FA, Iwamoto T: Pseudoinflammatory metastatic breast carcinoma of the orbit and lids. *Ophthalmology* 88: 575–580, 1981.
72. Carpenter RJ, Neel HB, Ryan RJ, Sanderson DR: Tumor fluorescence with hematoporphyrin derivation. *Trans Am Bronch Esoph Assoc*
73. Sanderson DR, Fontana RS, Lipson RL, et al: Hematoporphyrin as a diagnostic tool: A preliminary report of new techniques. *Cancer* 30: 1368–1372, 1972.
74. Soll DB: *Management of Complications in Oculoplastic Surgery.* Birmingham, AL, Aesculapius, 1976.
75. Crawford JS: Nature of fascia lata and its fate after implantation. *Am J Ophthalmol* 67: 900–907, 1969.
76. Dulton JJ, Anderson RL, Tse DT: Combined surgery and cryotherapy for scleral invasion of epithelial malignancies. *Ophthalmol Surg* 15: 289–294, 1984.
77. Knowles DM, Jakobiec FA: Ocular adnexal lymphoid neoplasms: Clinical histopathologic electron microscopic and immunologic characteristics. *Hum Pathol* 13; 148–162, 1982.
78. Boles S, Juhos DA: A case of palpebral myxoma. *Ophthalmologica* 171: 488–492, 1975.
79. Hornblass A: Incidence of tumor. In Hornblass, A (ed): *Tumors of the Ocular Adnexa and Orbit.* St. Louis, Mosby CV, 1979.

CHAPTER 23

Biopsy Techniques in Oculoplastic Surgery

ALBERT HORNBLASS, M.D.
NEIL D. GROSS, M.D.

The biopsy provides the clinician with a powerful method for the diagnosis of "suspicious" lesions. A biopsy should be performed on all growths that bleed easily, spontaneously ulcerate, increase in size, or are otherwise suspected as malignant. All tumors, except those that are easily diagnosed by inspection (e.g., a wart or skin tag), should be removed for histologic examination. Additionally, any inflammatory condition, especially those for which the diagnosis is uncertain, should be biopsied (1).

Physicians are frequently confronted with lesions of the lids, the conjunctiva, and occasionally, the orbit. The individual biopsy technique chosen must be based upon the location of the lesion and its suspected histologic diagnosis. It should minimize the cosmetic defect and interfere the least with subsequent surgery.

This chapter describes both routine and special biopsy techniques. A summary of these methods is compiled in Table 23.1. A listing of the necessary materials for routine biopsy is included in Table 23.2. Selected aspects of tissue preservation are also covered.

GENERAL CONSIDERATIONS

The goal of every biopsy is to remove tissue that is representative of the lesion. The specimen should be of adequate size for histological examination; it must not be crushed and should include some normal tissue, so the pathologist can compare affected and nonaffected areas.

Mature, well-developed lesions are the best type of growth on which to perform a biopsy. Tumors that are complicated by infection or scratching are not likely to be helpful. Secondary changes such as crusting, lichenification, or hyperpigmentation may also complicate histological identification (1).

The clinician should be encouraged to perform a biopsy, without hesitancy, if indicated. Single or multiple biopsies may be done; when in doubt, several areas may be selected for a biopsy.

ROUTINE BIOPSY TECHNIQUES

PUNCH BIOPSY

The punch biopsy is a simple procedure used most frequently by dermatologists. It provides a cylinder of tissue for histopathologic diagnosis. This method was first described by Keyes in 1887 (2).

The punch is the primary instrument utilized in this technique. It has a circular, sharp cutting edge and can be obtained in different sizes varying from 2 to 8 mm in diameter. Typically, a 3- or 4-mm punch is employed. After tissue preparation and injection of local anesthesia, the punch is placed over the lesion. It is then forced through the skin by pushing and twisting its handle. The

Table 23.1
Biopsy Techniques

Routine Methods
Punch biopsy
Shave biopsy
Excisional biopsy
Incisional biopsy
Special Methods
Superficial temporal artery biopsy
Fine-needle aspiration biopsy of the orbit

Table 23.2
Materials for biopsy

Skin Punches:
sizes 3 or 4 mm
Local Anesthetic:
Lidocaine 1% or 2% with or without epinephrine 1:100,000; injectable benadryl may be substituted in patients allergic to lidocaine
Scalpel with No. 15 blade
Forceps with fine teeth
Scissors:
Westcott, Iris, or other sharp scissors.
Syringe and Needle:
1–3 ml syringe with a 27- or 30-gauge needle is preferred for subcutaneous injection[a]
Sutures and needle holders
Properly labeled specimen bottles

[a] For small incisional biopsies, local anesthetic can be omitted at the discretion of the doctor and patient. The injection is often more irritating than the biopsy.

depth of tissue penetration depends upon the amount of force exerted. Epidermis and sections of dermis can be obtained (1).

The punch technique is simple and requires few instruments. However, since the punch is round, orientation of the excised specimen is difficult. In addition, the fine skin of the eyelid and close approximation of the globe and adnexal structures to a lid margin lesion make this technique frequently unsuitable.

SHAVE BIOPSY

The shave, or parallel incision, technique provides a disk of tissue for analysis. This method is primarily used for a lesion whose major component protrudes above the skin (e.g., seborrheic keratosis or a skin tag).

Initially, the scalpel is held parallel to the skin surface. The lesion is then incised flush with the skin, and the elevated portion of the tumor is removed. Deeper tissue can be included by "tenting up" the surrounding area with local anesthetic or by pinching the skin prior to the initiation of the incision.

This method is also simple and minimizes the cosmetic defect after a biopsy. It is recommended for *superficial* lesions that will be subsequently treated by curettage or electrodessication. It is never to be employed if a melanoma is suspected. In this instance, the specimen obtained will be too superficial to allow for definitive histologic grading (1); (Fig. 23.1).

INCISIONAL BIOPSY

The incisional biopsy technique is frequently employed by the surgeon. It is geared to obtain a small but sufficient amount of tissue for a diagnosis (e.g., basal cell carcinoma or keratoacanthoma). This method is relatively simple and frequently does not even require local anesthesia.

After local skin preparation with 10% alcohol, the lesion may or may not be injected with local anesthetic, depending on patient or surgeon preference. Then, a scalpel or Westcott scissors (authors' preference) is directed perpendicularly to the skin surface, and the incision is made across the lesion. An area of clinically appearing normal and affected skin is included. A small triangle is then fashioned with two additional "bites," and the base of the lesion is amputated. Direct digital pressure for 5 minutes with a sterile dressing usually provides adequate hemostasis. Local handheld cautery can be used to treat local bleeding points. A fine-toothed forceps is used to manipulate the specimen. The defect can be left open or sutured.

This method provides fine tissue control and ensures that an adequate sample will be harvested as direct visualization is easily obtained. When correctly performed, this method leaves no significant cosmetic defect.

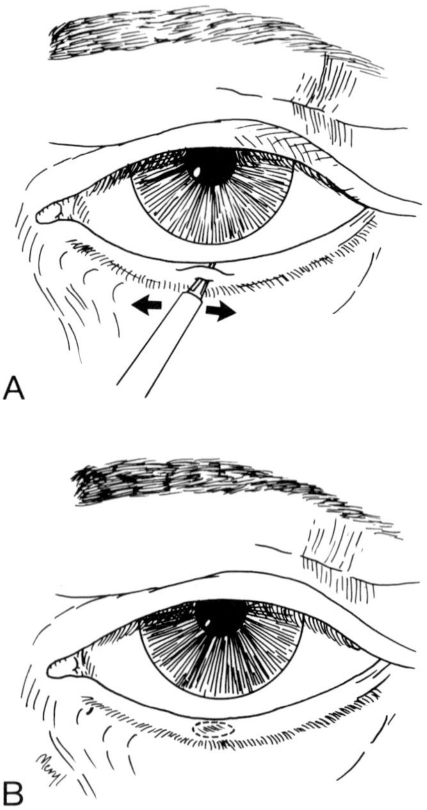

Figure 23.1. An eyelid margin lesion whose major portion lies above the skin. The Shave biopsy: A razor blade knife is inserted in the center of the lid margin lesion at skin level. It is moved from side to side, smoothly "shaving" the suspicious growth off the lid margin. *B*, Resulting epithelial defect on margin of lid. Will granulate in 3 weeks.

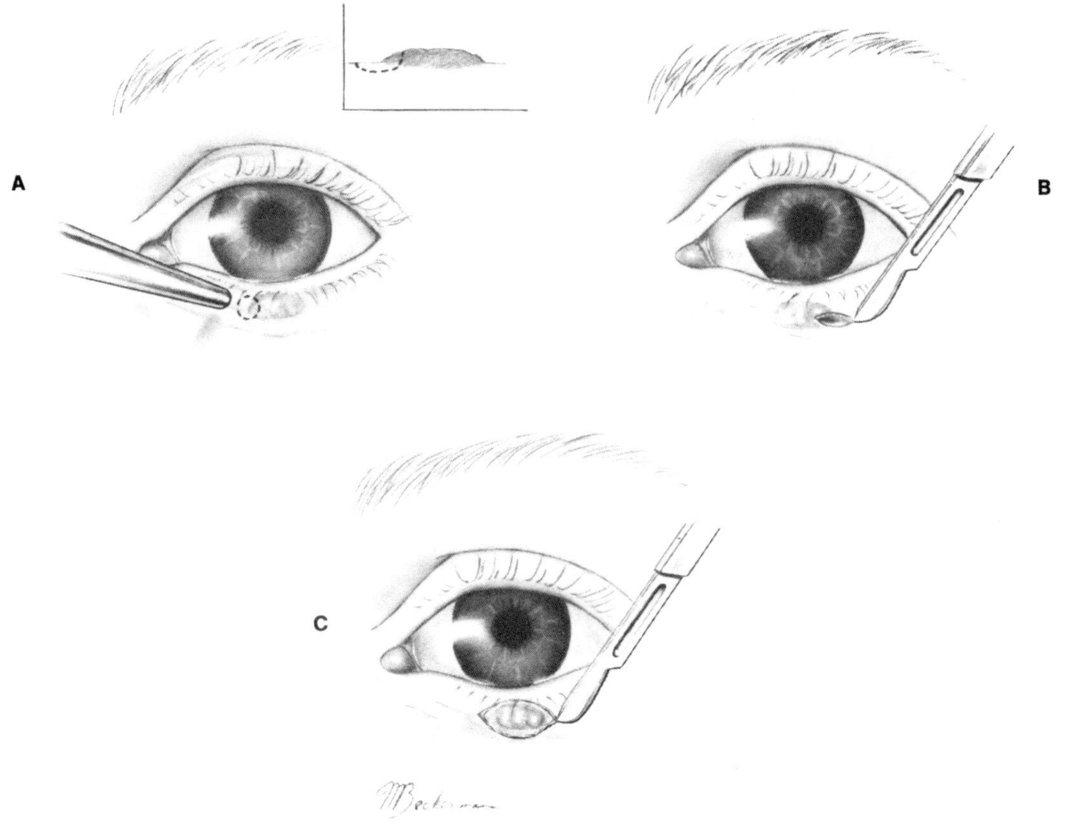

Figure 23.2. *A*, Trephine straddling the nasal portion of tumor on left lower lid incorporating normal skin. *Inset, upper right*, shows depth of trephine incorporating both lesion and normal skin. *B*, No. 15 Bard-Parker blade (or Westcott scissors can be substituted) is used to make elliptical incision through lesion, included in specimen is normal tissue. *C*, Excisional biopsy. No. 15 Bard-Parker blade is used to remove tumor in elliptical incision going approximately 1 mm wide of lesion.

EXCISIONAL BIOPSY

The excisional biopsy technique is the procedure of choice for the surgeon who intends simultaneously to perform a biopsy on a tumor and to completely excise it. It also affords the surgeon the advantages of direct visualization and excellent tissue control, thereby facilitating the preservation of nearby delicate adnexal structures.

To ensure the best cosmetic result, the surgeon utilizes an ellipse that incorporates the lesion and 1 to 2 mm of normal tissue. The area is demarcated initially with a surgical marking pencil after the area has been cleaned and injected with a local anesthetic, as needed. A No. 15 scalpel is used to incise the skin ellipse. A suture may be placed at one end of the specimen to mark a temporal or nasal margin. The base of the ellipse is amputated with a Westcott scissors. A handheld microcautery unit is usually adequate for hemostasis. One or two 6-0 silk sutures may be required to close the defect.

It should be remembered that a closed space is created when the wound is sutured. Drainage is thereby inhibited. Consequently, the surgeon must pay stricter attention to aseptic techniques. This method must also be employed, with caution, when resection of lesions near or at the lid margin are contemplated. Injudicious use of this method can lead to lid notching or ectropion (Fig. 23.2).

SPECIAL BIOPSY TECHNIQUES

SUPERFICIAL TEMPORAL ARTERY BIOPSY

A superficial temporal artery biopsy is performed to confirm suspected cases of giant cell arteritis. The portion of the artery to be removed should be harvested from the same side as the involved eye, if possible. A biopsy is positive up to 2 weeks after the institution of steroid therapy. Therefore, steroids should never be withheld pending biopsy.

The technique for doing a biopsy on the superficial temporal artery is relatively simple. Anatomically, the vessel lies on the superficial aspect of the temporalis fascia (3). It is surrounded by fibrofatty tissue, which is easily dissected. Initially, the temporal artery is palpated within the hairline or above the ear. Its course is delineated with a marking pen. Lidocaine 2% without epinephrine is sparingly used to infiltrate the skin locally. Small volumes of local anesthetic without epinephrine must be used, since the pulsations used to identify the artery are dampened by the injection.

The skin is incised with a No. 15 scalpel blade. The underlying subcutaneous tissue can be separated with a sharp scissors or bluntly divided with skin rakes. A curved hemostat is used for deeper blunt dissection down to the temporalis fascia. The artery is then identified by its visible and, occasionally, palpable pulsations. Blunt dissection must be used in this area while isolating the artery, as the temporalis muscle is in close proximity and will bleed briskly if violated. The artery is then identified; its proximal and distal ends are then ligated with 4-0 chromic or silk suture. Next, a 2- to 3-cm segment of artery is excised. One should avoid crushing the edges that are to be examined. Subcutaneous absorbable sutures can be placed to minimize dead space. No drain needs to be placed. The skin is closed in running fashion, and a dressing is placed over the wound. The skin sutures can be safely removed in 4–5 days (Fig. 23.3).

FINE-NEEDLE ASPIRATION BIOPSY OF THE ORBIT

Orbital lesions that are poorly imaged by computed tomographic (CT) scan, considered to be inoperable, or only incompletely removable may be amenable to fine-needle aspiration biopsy (FNAB). This technique was first described by Martin and Ellis (4) in 1930. Recently, it has been modified for use in the orbit by Kennerdell and associates (5). It has been most helpful in identifying suspected malignant epithelial tumors.

In essence, this technique involves the placement of a needle, under either ultrasound (6) or CT control (7), directly into an orbital lesion; the aspiration of some of its contents are for cytological examination. A syringe pistol with a 20 ml plastic disposable syringe and a 22-gauge, 3.8-cm disposable needle are used. Cells are aspirated via suction created by the surgeon. Aspirated material is immediately stained with the Papanicolaou preparation and evaluated by a cytopathologist familiar with the technique.

Successful use of this method enables the patient to avoid open orbital exploration. Unfortunately, FNAB can provide no information regarding the spread of a tumor. It is also less helpful for diagnosing pseudotumor or other forms of lymphoid dysplasia, since the cellular architecture of the lesion cannot be ascertained from an aspirate. It must be noted that placing a needle in a closed space, such as the orbit, can lead to hemorrhage, which then leads to secondary damage of delicate orbital structures, including the optic nerve. This technique is not to be used in cases of suspected benign mixed tumors of the lacrimal gland, as the protective capsule will be damaged and potentially malignant cells will spill into the orbit. For obvious reasons, one must also avoid placing a needle in a potentially vascular lesion.

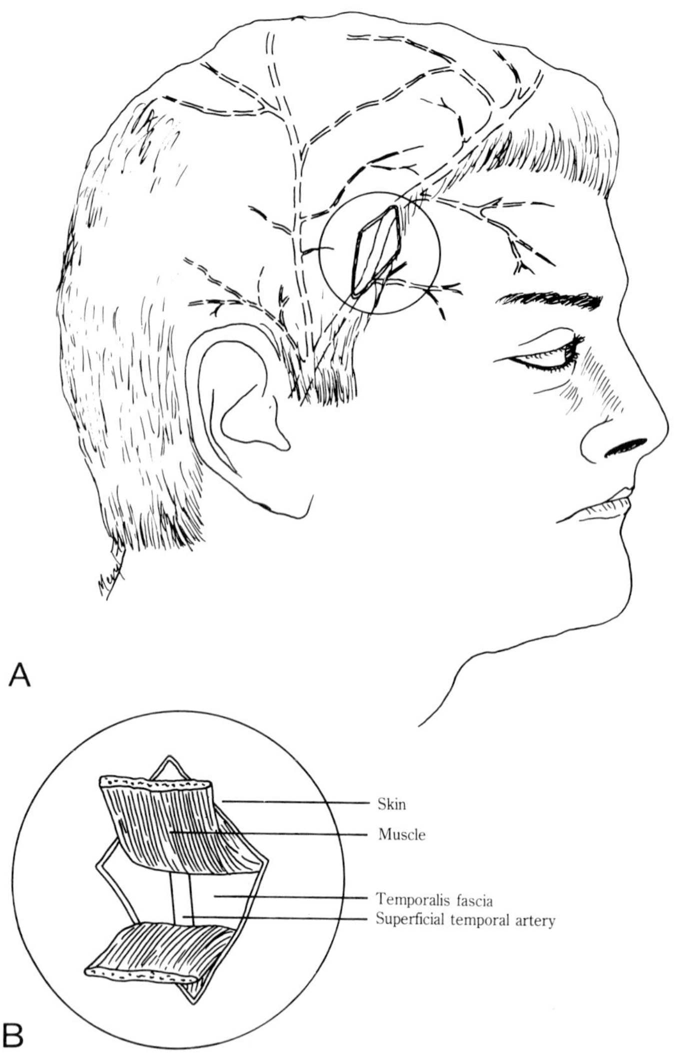

Figure 23.3. *A*, Course of the branches of the superficial temporal artery. The encircled portion, at the hairline, is the most accessible and inconspicuous tributary for biopsy. *B*, Regional anatomy of the superficial temporal artery. Skin and subcutaneous tissue overlying the temporalis fascia. The superficial temporal artery lies on top of this fascia.

TISSUE PROCESSING

To ensure accurate histologic analysis, the surgeon must place the tissue specimens immediately in the appropriate medium to avoid degradation artifact. Specimens for light microscopy studies should be placed in a 10% formalin solution. Examination of tissue by electron microscopy requires tissue preservation in glutaraldehyde. Immunologic marker study specimens should be placed in a solution of RMP 1640 culture media (1).

REFERENCES

1. Pariser DM, Caserio RJ, Eagleston WH: *Techniques for Diagnosis of Skin and Hair Disease*. New York, Thieme, 1986, vol 2, ch 7.
2. Keyes EL: The cutaneous punch. *J Cutan Genitourin Dis* 5: 98–101, 1887.
3. Cullen JF, Coleiro JA: Review: Ophthalmic complications of giant cell arteritis. *Surv Ophthalmol* 20: 251, 1976.
4. Martin HE, Ellis EB: Biopsy by needle puncture and aspiration. *Ann Surg* 92: 169–181, 1930.

5. Kennerdell JE, Dekker A, Johnson B, Dubois PJ: Fine-needle aspiration biopsy: A report of its use in orbital tumors. *Arch Ophthalmol* 97: 1315, 1979.
6. Spoor TC, Kennerdell JS, Dekker A, Johnson BL, Rehkopf P: Orbital fine-needle biopsy with B-scan guidance. *Am J Ophthalmol* 89: 274–277, 1980.
7. Dubois PJ, Kennerdell JS, Rosenbaum AE, Dekker A, Johnson BL, Swink CA: Computerized tomographic localization for fine-needle aspiration biopsy of orbital tumors. *Radiology* 131: 149–152, 1979.
8. Hornblass A: Evaluation and diagnosis of tumors, In Hornblass A (ed): *Tumors of the Ocular Adnexa and Orbit*. St. Louis, CV Mosby 1979.

CHAPTER 24

Benign Lesions of the Eyelid

LASZLO BIRO, M.D.
ELY PRICE, M.D.

The eyelid and periorbital area, although part of the integument, differ in many respects from the rest of the skin. Some benign lesions, such as syringomas and xanthelasma are found primarily on the lid while others, such as warts and seborrheic keratoses are detected elsewhere; management on the lid is somewhat different because of the anatomic location. Dermatologists diagnose and manage lesions of the eyelid as an office procedure. These lesions offer a challenge to dermatologists because of the delicate location, difficulty of diagnosis, and great variety one may encounter (Table 24.1).

DIAGNOSIS

It is often quoted in the ophthalmologic literature that malignant lid lesions are misdiagnosed approximately 50% of the time (1). A relatively common example of such an error is confusion of sebaceous carcinoma with chalazion, and melanoma with deeply pigmented nevus cell nevus. In an attempt to cover our ignorance of distinguishing various benign lesions from one another, the catch-all term "papilloma" has been introduced; this term was originally used to define a virus-induced tumor. Later on histologists defined as an entity a number of clinically different lesions based on histologic appearance of papillomatous changes. As a result, clinicians (2) now apply the term "papilloma" to lesions as varied as warts, skin tags, seborrheic keratoses, actinic keratoses, and nevus cell nevi. However, the term should not be used as a clinical diagnosis but should be reserved for pathologic description. It has been our experience that many of the simple benign lesions that we easily diagnose elsewhere on the face, we often misdiagnose on the eyelid. A few key rules therefore must be strictly observed so that proper diagnosis can be attempted on clinical grounds:

1. It is essential that lid lesions be examined in good light. If at all possible, sunlight serves best in detecting fine details.
2. The surface of lesions must be closely observed and, if it is covered by a crust or scale, it should be properly cleansed either with saline or alcoholic swab. Once this is done, the clean surface must be closely scrutinized. What do we look for? Is it smooth or perhaps studded by indentations like the surface of a berry? If the scale is adherent to the underlying lesion, it should be closely examined and determined whether it is a dry or greasy type of scale. What is the color of the surface? Is it uniform or perhaps variegated? Is there a capillary running through the surface? Is there a fine vellus hair in the lesion? It is often helpful to use a small magnifying glass or loupe to detect some of these fine surface changes. Once the surface has been observed, palpate the lesion to determine whether it is soft, hard, or cystic.
3. History: The onset and duration of the lesion can be extremely important. (Nevus versus seborrheic keratosis.) When taking history, one must pay attention to symptoms such as tenderness, previous treatment, recurrence, and presence of similar lesions elsewhere.
4. Often it is difficult to tell a solid lesion from a cystic one or to detect a central dell in a small lesion on the lid. Freezing with a cryogen while protecting the globe with a shield will reveal a dell quickly (diagnostic of molluscum contagiosum). One may use the same freezing technique in an attempt to differentiate inclusion cysts and hydro-

Table 24.1.
Benign Lesions of the Eyelid

Tumors of the Epidermis	Vascular
Benign	Hemangioma
Epidermal nevus (verrucous)	Lymphangioma
Seborrheic keratosis	Spider nevus
Dermatosis papulosa nigra	Lymphomas
Dermoid cyst	Lymphocytoma cutis
Inclusion cyst—milium	Lymphoma
Inverted follicular keratosis	Mycosis fungoides
Fibroepithelial papilloma (skin tag)	Lymphocsarcoma
Precancerous	Metabolic
Actinic keratosis	Xanthelasma
Cutaneous horn	Amyloidosis
Bowen's disease	Xanthoma
Melanocytic Nevi	Inflammatory
Nevus cell nevus	Viral
Melanotic freckle	Verruca vulgaris
Tumors of the Epidermal Appendages	Molluscum contagiosum
Hyperplasias	Granulomas
Nevus sebaceous	Chalazion
Sebaceous hyperplasia	Foreign body reaction
Adenomas	Sarcoid
Sebaceous adenoma	Granuloma annulare
Hydrocystoma (eccrine)	Granuloma pyogenicum
Syringoma	Miscellaneous
Adenoma of the Meibomian gland	Neurofibroma
Benign Epitheliomas	Traumatic inclusion cyst
Trichoepithelioma	Junvenile xanthogranuloma
Pilomatrixoma	Comedone
Trichofolliculoma	

cystoma from a cystic basal cell carcinoma, however, one may have to use a fine incision.

5. Appearance of dark pigment in a lesion often leads the examiner to consider malignant melanoma. Occasionally the pigment may not be anything more than oxidized keratin such as in the case of an open comedone, or more often, dried crust resulting from earlier bleeding. A comedone can be easily expressed, and crust can be removed as discussed earlier.

In most instances we should not rely solely on clinical impression alone, but we should perform a biopsy. Definitive treatment should be planned only after pathology report has been obtained.

TECHNIQUE OF BIOPSY

Biopsy is performed under local anesthesia using a 30-gauge needle, or, if for some reason one cannot use anesthesia by injection, one may resort to cryoanesthesia with nitrous oxide or liquid nitrogen spray. Short freeze time of 5–6 seconds allows rapid removal of a small portion of the lesion by an Iris scissor. Hemostasis is achieved either by aluminum chloride or Monsel's solution. Cryoanesthesia is used mostly in children and occasionally on some adults who are extremely afraid of injections near the eyelid.

ALTERNATIVE DERMATOLOGIC MANAGEMENT TECHNIQUES TO EXCISION SURGERY

CURETTAGE AND ELECTRODESICCATION

Curettage and electrodesiccation are useful for seborrheic keratoses, actinic keratoses, mollusca and warts. The difficulty with curettage on the eyelids, is that they overlie the ocular globe, and one should not press the curette firmly against this structure.

Technique

The lesion is anesthetized with 2% Xylocaine injected directly beneath it. This also serves to lift it from the tarsus. Larger tumors can be held by thumb and index finger of the left hand while the right hand holds the 2–4 mm curette. If the lesion is located on the lower lid, it may be pulled down over the orbital ridge, which serves as a firm base for curetting (3). The same effect can be achieved with the upper lid, but the upper lid is less mobile. When the benign tumor is close to the palpebral margin, the conjunctiva may also be anesthetized and a Jaeger retractor inserted, which serves as a firm base. The curettage removes the tumor and leaves a base that bleeds

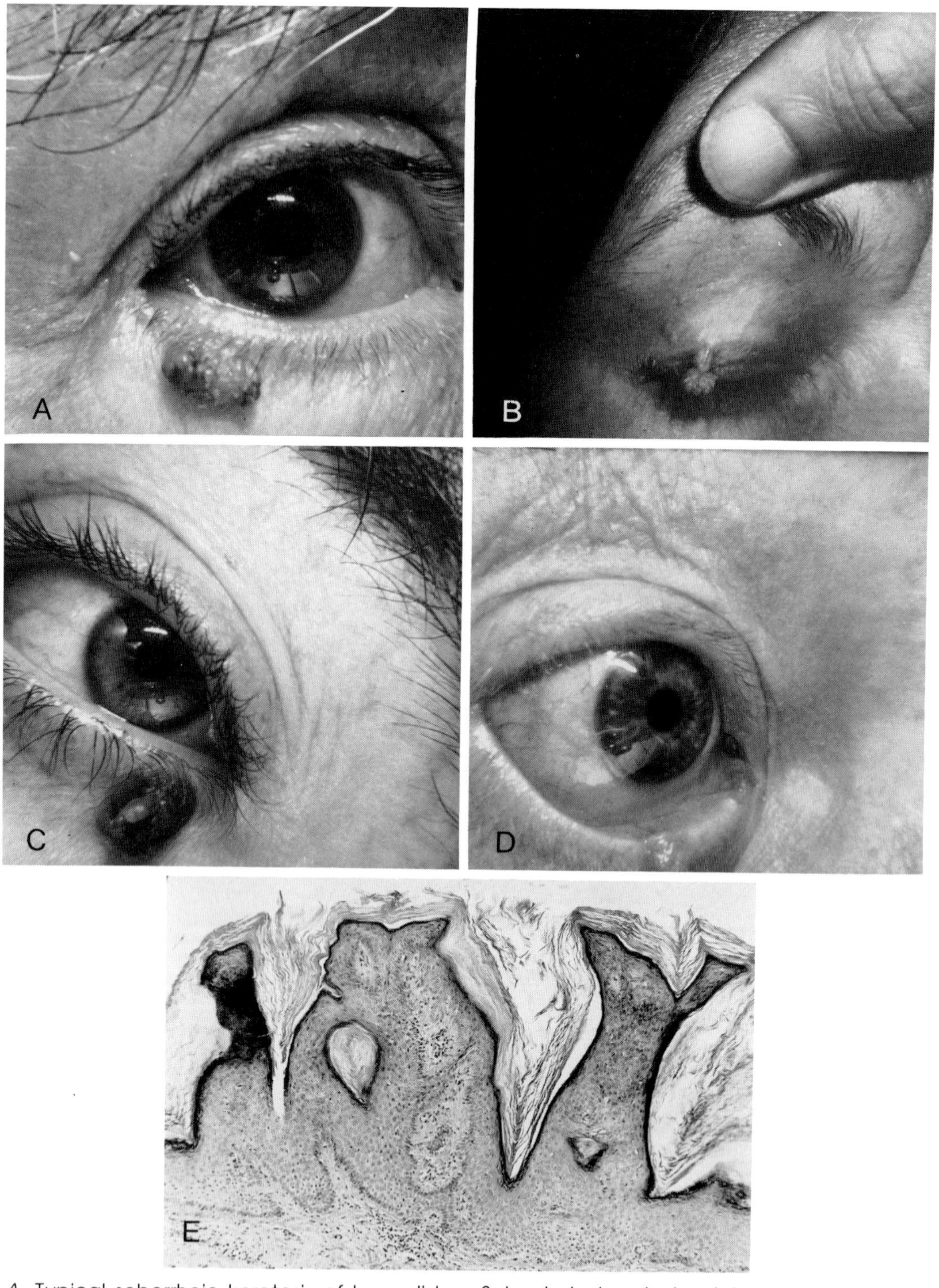

Figure 24.1. *A*, Typical seborrheic keratosis of lower lid near free margin. Observe surface with dotted appearance and spotty pigmentation. *B*, Atypical seborrheic keratosis pedunculated resembling fibroepithelial papilloma. *C*, Seborrheic keratosis of lower lid with deep pigmentation at base. Small skin colored papilloma rising from center. *D*, Seborrheic keratosis of free lid margin. Smooth surface resembling intradermal nevus. *E*, Seborrheic keratosis: There is hyperkeratosis and papillated epidermal hyperplasia with acanthosis. Horn pseudocysts are present. (Courtesy of E. Heilman, M.D. and R. Friedman, M.D.)

slightly. The bleeding may be stopped by electrodesiccation.

Electrodesiccation employs a spark-gap machine that delivers high-frequency, highly damped, high-voltage, low-amperage, unipolar current (4). With a low current setting it may be safely used without causing scarring and its consequences. An alternative technique utilizes light electrodesiccation first to soften the tissue so that it may be curetted easily. Smaller lesions may be treated this way employing a 1-mm cup curette, which is less traumatic for this delicate area. Twenty percent aluminum chloride in alcohol is applied to the base of the lesion to stop the bleeding, which avoids the overuse of electrodesiccation.

CYROSURGERY

Advanced technology in cryosurgery has been developed in the past 10 years. It is especially useful for treating lesions of the eyelid, ranging from malignant tumors such as basal cell carcinomas (5) to benign lesions, e.g., warts, keratoses (6). Depending on the type of lesion, we may use either spray or probe technique. When using spray technique, we generally use a very fine tip such as the D tip with the CryAc machine or 24 gauge tip with CS-76. Occasionally in an attempt to protect the surrounding skin, we use either a truncated or otoscopic cone to confine the spray. Lesions, especially molluscum contagiosum or wart, situated near the free margin of the eyelid respond well to the probe technique. Jaeger retractor serves as a firm base. The probe is lubricated with KY jelly, then placed on the lesion at room temperature. Once freezing begins and the probe is in perfect contact, it can be lightly pulled away from the globe. The size of the probe must correspond to the size of the lesion or could even be a bit smaller. As a rule we use 1–2 mm probe. Occasionally we may not rely on the destructive effect of cryosurgery alone; therefore we use either a fine scissor or curette after a benign lesion has been frozen for 6–10 seconds to remove the raised portion of the growth. The removed tissue serves also for biopsy.

The major advantage of using cryosurgery for benign lesions of the lid is the fact that it does not require anesthesia prior to the procedure. The disadvantage is an instant edema that may last for 24–48 hours. Healing generally takes place in 7–10 days.

TEN BENIGN LID LESIONS

SEBORRHEIC KERATOSIS

The eyelids as well as other areas of the face are common sites for these brownish lesions, which appear as if stuck on to the surface of the lid. They are sharply demarcated and slightly raised and appear in two varieties. Most have a verrucous or waxy surface, but some have a smooth

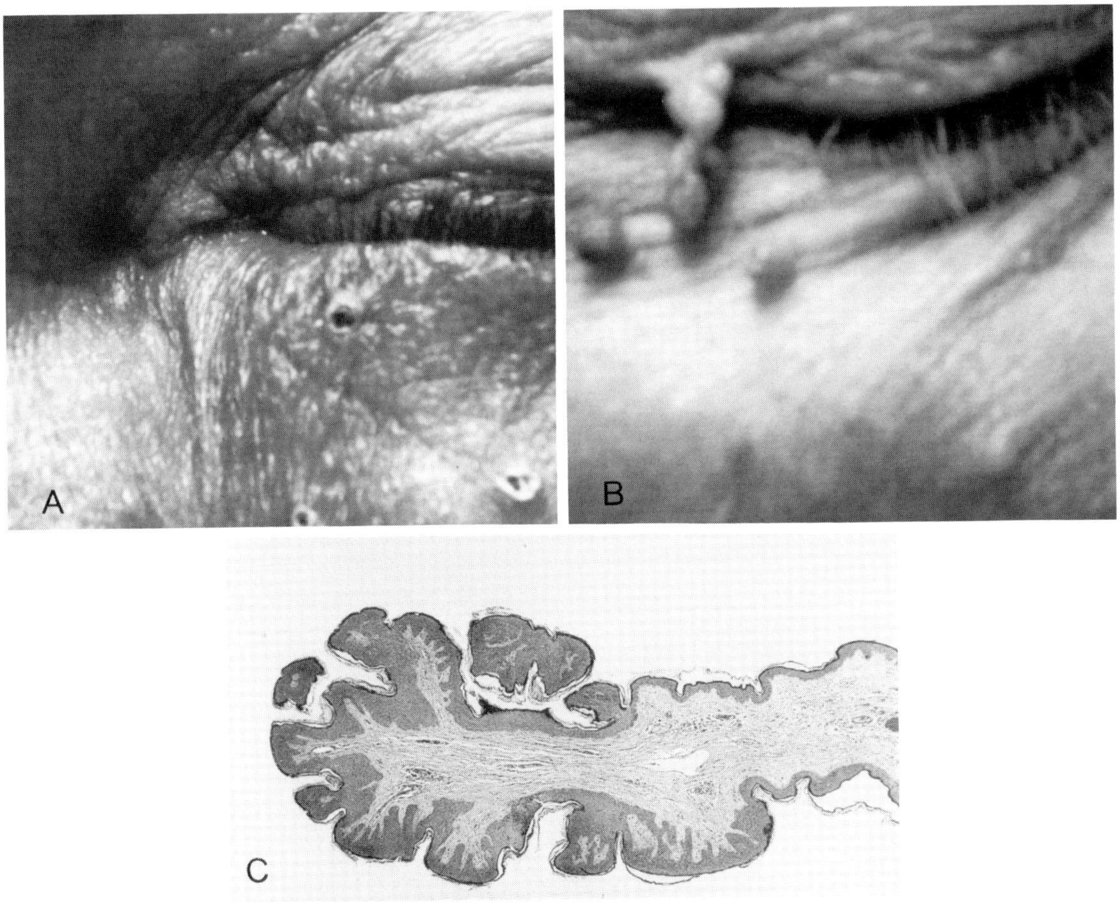

Figure 24.2. *A*, Multiple fibroepithelial papillomas of the upper eyelid. *B*, Fibroepithelial papillomas after treatment by light desiccation. *C*, Fibroepithelial papilloma: The cornified layer shows slight hyperkeratosis and there is gently papillated epidermal hyperplasia. The stroma is made up of interweaving collagen bundles. No skin appendages such as hair follicles or sweat glands are seen. (Courtesy of E. Heilman, M.D. and R. Friedman, M.D.)

surface. The presence of keratotic plugs distinguish the latter from nevi, which they can resemble. They vary in size from a few millimeters to large enough to encompass the entire lid. If the lids are subject to rubbing, the base of these keratoses may be erythematous. A variety of seborrheic keratosis seen in the adult black population is termed dermatosis papulosa nigra. These are often found on the upper cheeks but extend onto the lower and upper lid. They are small pigmented papules a few millimeters in diameter (Fig. 24.1).

Differential Diagnosis. These lesions must be differentiated from nevus cell nevi, fibroepithelial papillomas and actinic keratoses.

Management. Preferred technique is light desiccation with curettage performed under local anesthesia. Cryosurgery is reserved only for flat lesions under 3 mm in size.

FIBROEPITHELIAL PAPILLOMA

Commonly known as "skin tags," these lesions are also called "acrochordon" or "soft fibromas." They may be found on the upper and lower eyelid. They appear as skin-colored, smooth filiform papules often found in multiples in this location. If they are found on the upper lid, they may protrude enough to interfere with vision (Fig. 24.2).

Differential Diagnosis. These lesions must be differentiated from filiform warts, seborrheic keratoses, actinic keratoses, and occasionally intradermal nevi.

Management. Lesions with thin 1–2 mm stalk are easily removed by an iris scissor under local anesthesia. Lesions with a larger stalk must first be anesthetized, then lightly desiccated to avoid bleeding during their removal by iris scissor.

WARTS

There are two types of verrucae found on the eyelid and periorbital area: verruca vulgaris and verruca planus. Verruca vulgaris is generally a firm elevated growth with papillomatous hyperkeratotic surface. Verruca planus, on the other hand, is a slightly elevated smooth papule 1–2 mm in diameter with a brownish tinge; it is often hard to detect this lesion on the eyelid. Both of these are caused

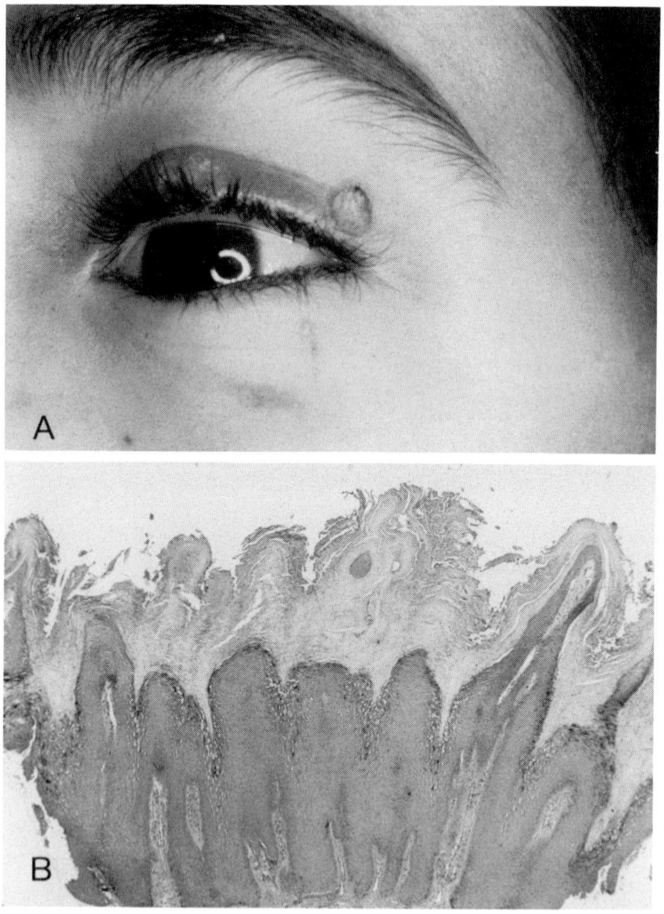

Figure 24.3. *A*, Multiple warts on the upper lid in a 4-year-old child. *B*, Verruca vulgaris: There is compact hyperkeratosis with parakeratosis, papillated epidermal hyperplasia, acanthosis and a prominent granulare layer in the epidermis. The underlying stroma contains an increased number of dilated and tortuous blood vessels. (Courtesy of E. Heilman, M.D. and R. Friedman, M.D.)

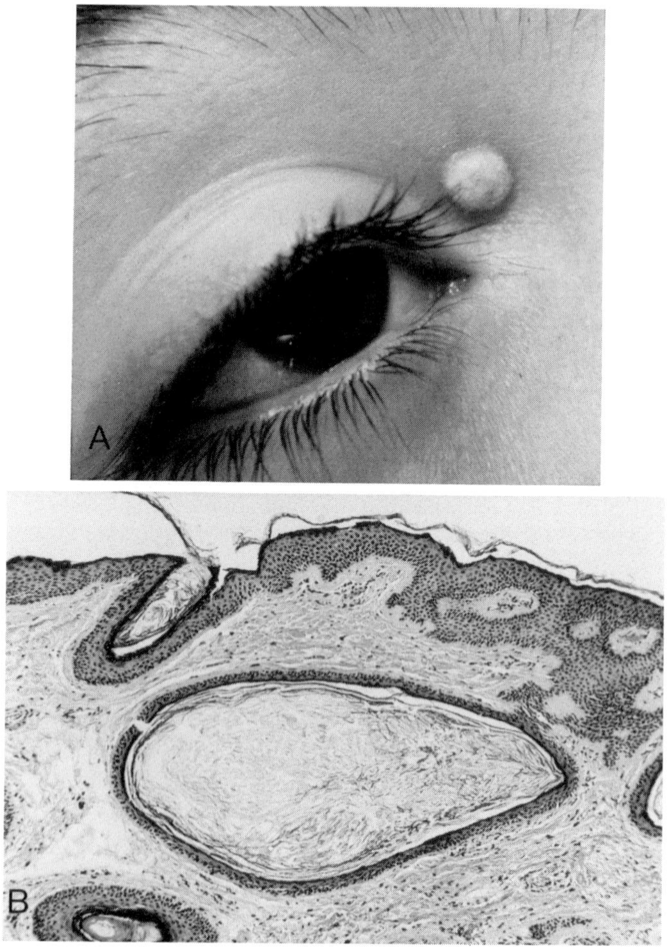

Figure 24.4. *A*, Inclusion cyst of upper lid near medial canthus. *B*, Milium: This is a small epidermal cyst filled with concentric layers of cornified cells lined by a squamous epithelium. (Courtesy of E. Heilman, M.D. and R. Friedman, M.D.)

by human papilloma virus. Recent classification based on antiserum and electromicroscopy indicate that verruca plana (flat wart) are HPV-3 type while the vulgaris type are HPV-2 or HPV-4 with a more aggressive HPV-1 (7) (Fig. 24.3).

Differential Diagnosis. Common warts must be differentiated from fibroepithelial papillomas, seborrheic keratoses; flat warts, on the other hand, from syringomas. It is wise to examine other areas of the body, especially the hands, since their presence will generally weigh in favor of the diagnosis of verruca.

Management. Preferred treatment is cryosurgery, especially for lesions under 3 mm in size. As mentioned earlier, when using cryosurgery no anesthesia is required. Light desiccation under local anesthesia can also be utilized.

INCLUSION CYST AND MILIA

Inclusion cyst generally is a single whitish nodule filled with desquamated keratin. Milia, on the other hand, may be present either as a single lesion or multiple. Milia are 1–2 mm in diameter with a smooth white surface (Fig. 24.4).

Management. Inclusion cyst over 5 mm in diameter is best removed by excision. Small milia (1–2 mm in size) can be easily incised by Hagedorn's needle; dermatologists often use a special comedone extractor (Shalita's comedone extractor).

XANTHELASMA

These yellowish slightly raised plaques may be found on the upper and lower lid. They are traditionally regarded as cutaneous signs of lipid abnormalities, but in only one third of individuals are such findings verified. In the Fredrickson and Lee classifications, they are found in type 2 and type 3 lipoproteinemia, both of which are associated with elevated cholesterol (Fig. 24.5).

Differential Diagnosis. Multiple small papules of xanthelasma at times must be differentiated from syringomas.

Management. While ophthalmologists usually excise these lesions, treatment is often unsatisfactory since they tend to recur in a short period of time. Dermatologists favor careful light application of 100% trichloroacetic acid for a few seconds with prompt neutralization with alcohol swab. These lesions, which initially turn white, become inflamed, erythematous, and form a crust in a few days. After the crust dries and falls off there is a satisfactory flattening of the lesion with loss of the yellowish color. Lesions tend to recur with this method also, but may be retreated.

MOLLUSCUM CONTAGIOSUM

These are small skin-colored dome-shaped papules (2–4 mm) with a umbilicated center. Clinically the umbilication may be seen by light spraying with a cryogen such as Frigiderm. Of course, the eye must be carefully protected. These lesions are discrete and appear waxy and present a particular problem when near the border of palpebral fissure. They are of viral etiology and belong to the pox virus group (Fig. 24.6).

Differential Diagnosis. They are a single giant mollusca and must be differentiated from keratoacanthoma.

Management. We prefer cryosurgery using the probe technique. Alternative technique is light desiccation under local anesthesia.

SYRINGOMA

These small (1–2 mm) skin-colored papules are often limited to the lower lid; however, they may be found in other locations. They often start at puberty and progressively increase in number and size. They represent an adenoma of the intraepidermal eccrine duct (Fig. 24.7).

Differential Diagnosis. These lesions must be distinguished from xanthelasma and flat warts.

Management. Removal especially for multiple lesions is best performed by conservative excision. Occasionally single lesions can be treated by desiccation and curettage, however, they may recur.

MELANOCYTIC NEVI

There are three types of nevus cell nevi on the lid as well as anywhere else on the body. They are *intradermal,*

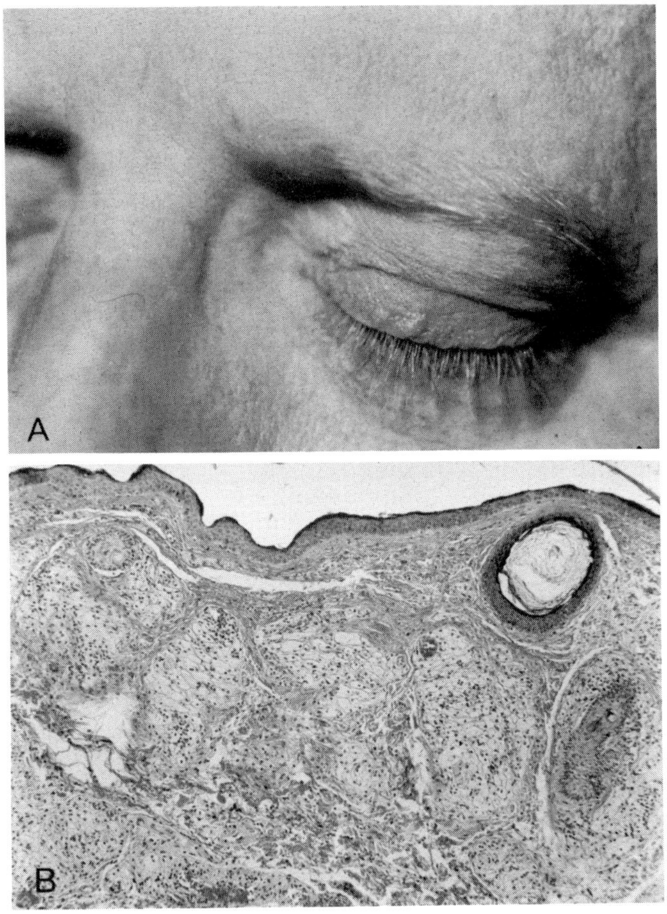

Figure 24.5. *A*, Xanthelasma of medial aspect of upper lid. Notice yellowish discoloration and new lesion developing near free margin. *B*, Xanthalasma: There are numerous foamy histiocytes throughout the dermis and particularly around the blood vessels of the middermis. (Courtesy of E. Heilman, M.D. and R. Friedman, M.D.)

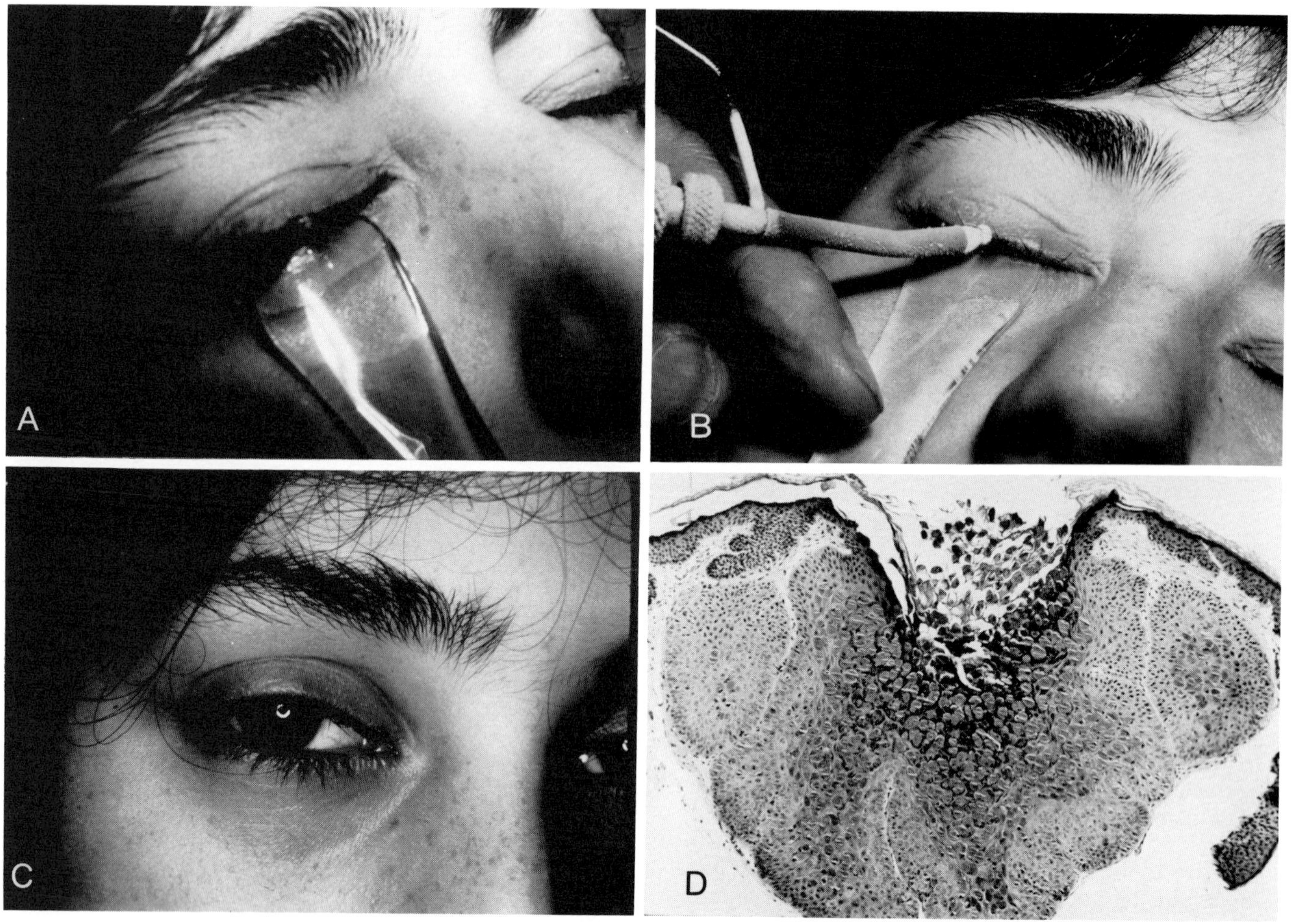

Figure 24.6. *A*, Single molluscum contagiosum on free margin of upper lid. *B*, Same lesion treated with Cry-Ac machine using 2 mm cryoprobe for 12 seconds. *C*, Three weeks after cryosurgery. *D*, Molloscum contagiosum: This shows a small crater-like lesion lined by a thickened squamous epithelium. It is filled with degenerating squamous cells containing characteristic hyalinized intracellular viral inclusions (molluscum bodies). (Courtesy of E. Heilman, M.D. and R. Friedman, M.D.)

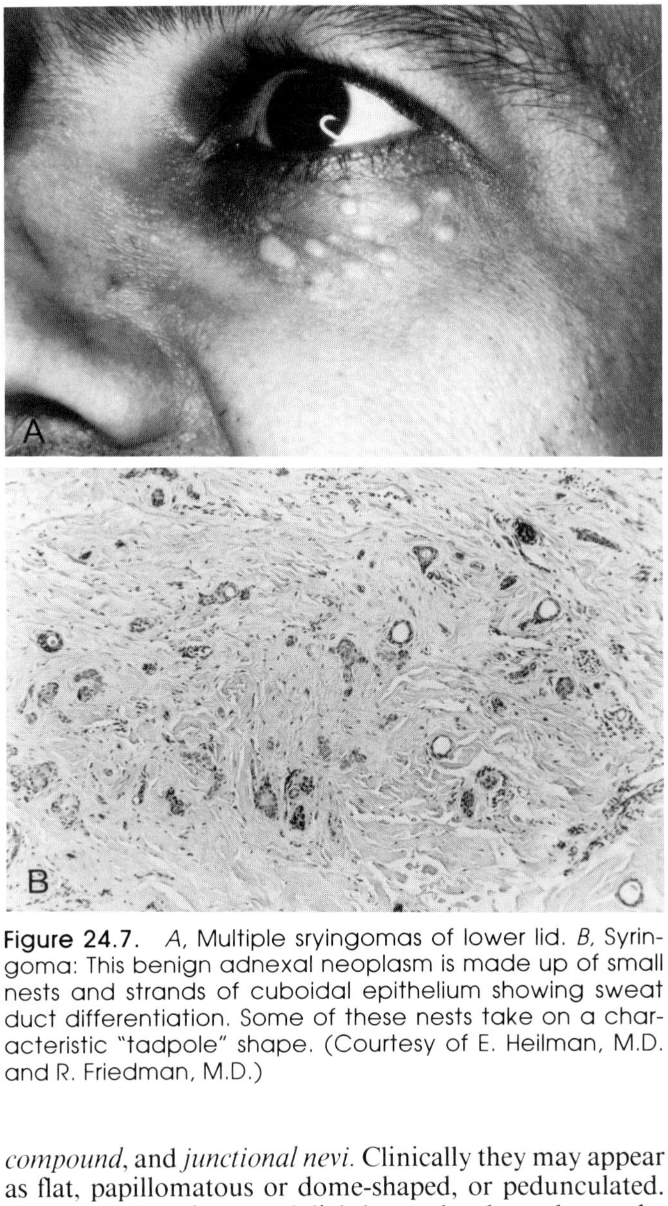

Figure 24.7. *A*, Multiple sryingomas of lower lid. *B*, Syringoma: This benign adnexal neoplasm is made up of small nests and strands of cuboidal epithelium showing sweat duct differentiation. Some of these nests take on a characteristic "tadpole" shape. (Courtesy of E. Heilman, M.D. and R. Friedman, M.D.)

compound, and *junctional nevi*. Clinically they may appear as flat, papillomatous or dome-shaped, or pedunculated. They may be pigmented lightly or deeply and may be occasionally skin colored. Flat-shaped lesions are usually junctional nevi. The elevated and papillomatous types are compound while the pedunculated and dome shaped are intradermal nevi. These are not hard fast rules, however, and combinations of types exist (Fig. 24.8).

Differential Diagnosis. These lesions must be differentiated from seborrheic keratosis, pigmented basal cell carcinoma, and, occasionally, from early melanoma.

Management. Excision is recommended.

HEMANGIOMAS

In childhood, capillary hemangiomas may involve the eyelid and may become large enough to warrant intervention. Capillary hemangioma, or strawberry hemangioma, may consist of bright-red, singular or multiple tumors. It appears in the first months of life. It will grow in early infancy and usually starts to regress and involute spontaneously by age 7 (Fig. 24.9).

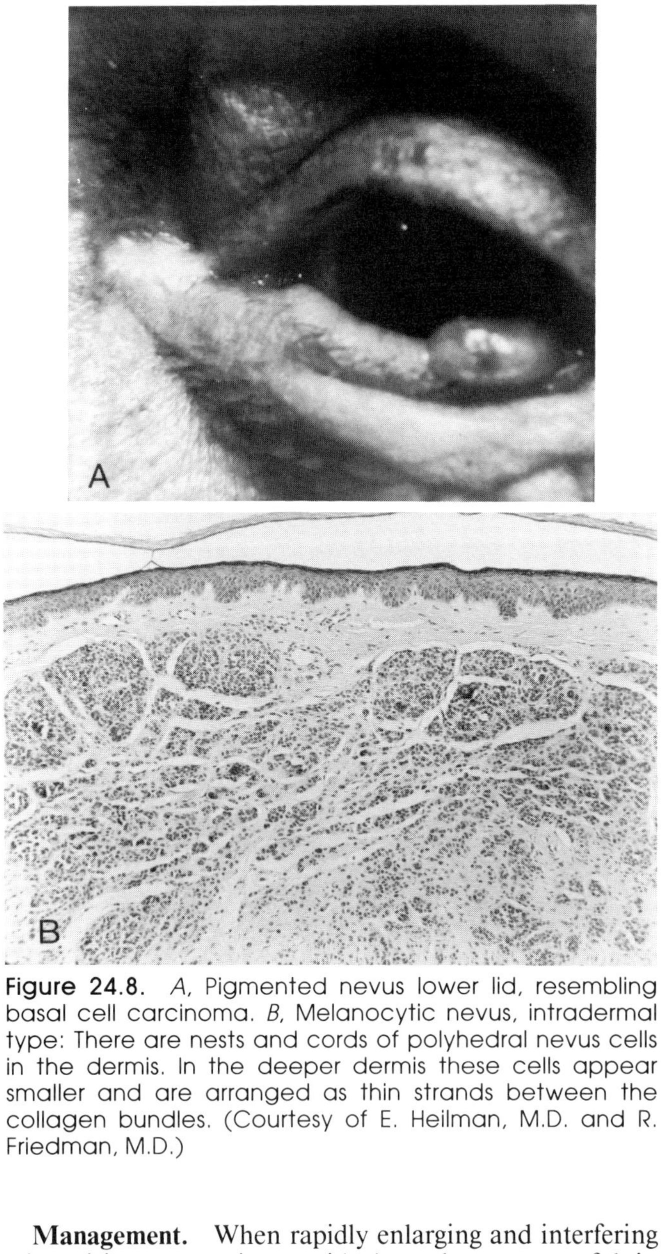

Figure 24.8. *A*, Pigmented nevus lower lid, resembling basal cell carcinoma. *B*, Melanocytic nevus, intradermal type: There are nests and cords of polyhedral nevus cells in the dermis. In the deeper dermis these cells appear smaller and are arranged as thin strands between the collagen bundles. (Courtesy of E. Heilman, M.D. and R. Friedman, M.D.)

Management. When rapidly enlarging and interfering with vision, systemic steroids have been successful in repressing these lesions. Also cryosurgery by the probe technique has been used; results have been satisfactory.

ACTINIC KERATOSIS

Rarely actinic keratoses are seen on the eyelid in persons who are exposed to sunlight for long periods. They are small lesions measuring from a few millimeters to a centimeter. The lesions are erythematous with adherent scales and show little infiltration. When they show pronounced hyperkeratosis they may take on the appearance of cutaneous horn. These are usually limited to the upper lid. They are considered premalignant and contain anaplastic cells but are biologically benign (Fig. 24.10).

Differential Diagnosis. These lesions must be differentiated from seborrheic keratoses, early basal cell, and prickle cell carcinomas. A clinical variant of actinic kera-

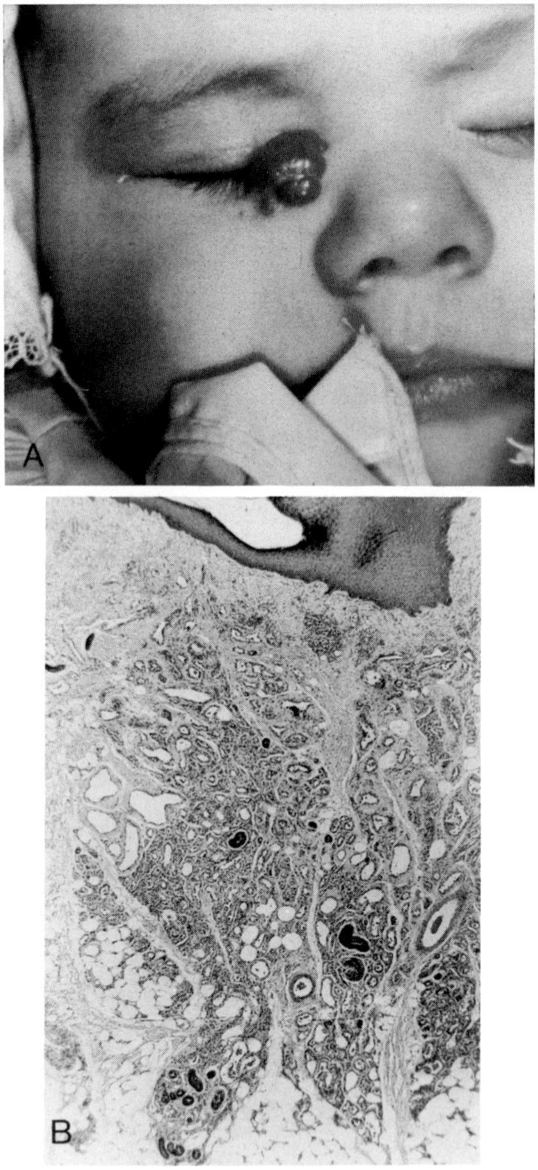

Figure 24.9. *A*, Strawberry hemangioma rapidly enlarging of inner canthus extending to upper and lower lid. *B*, Congenital hemangioma: There is a marked increase in thin walled blood vessels that extend throughout the dermis. These vessels can extend into the deeper subcutaneous fibroadipose tissue. (Courtesy of E. Heilman, M.D. and R. Friedman, M.D.)

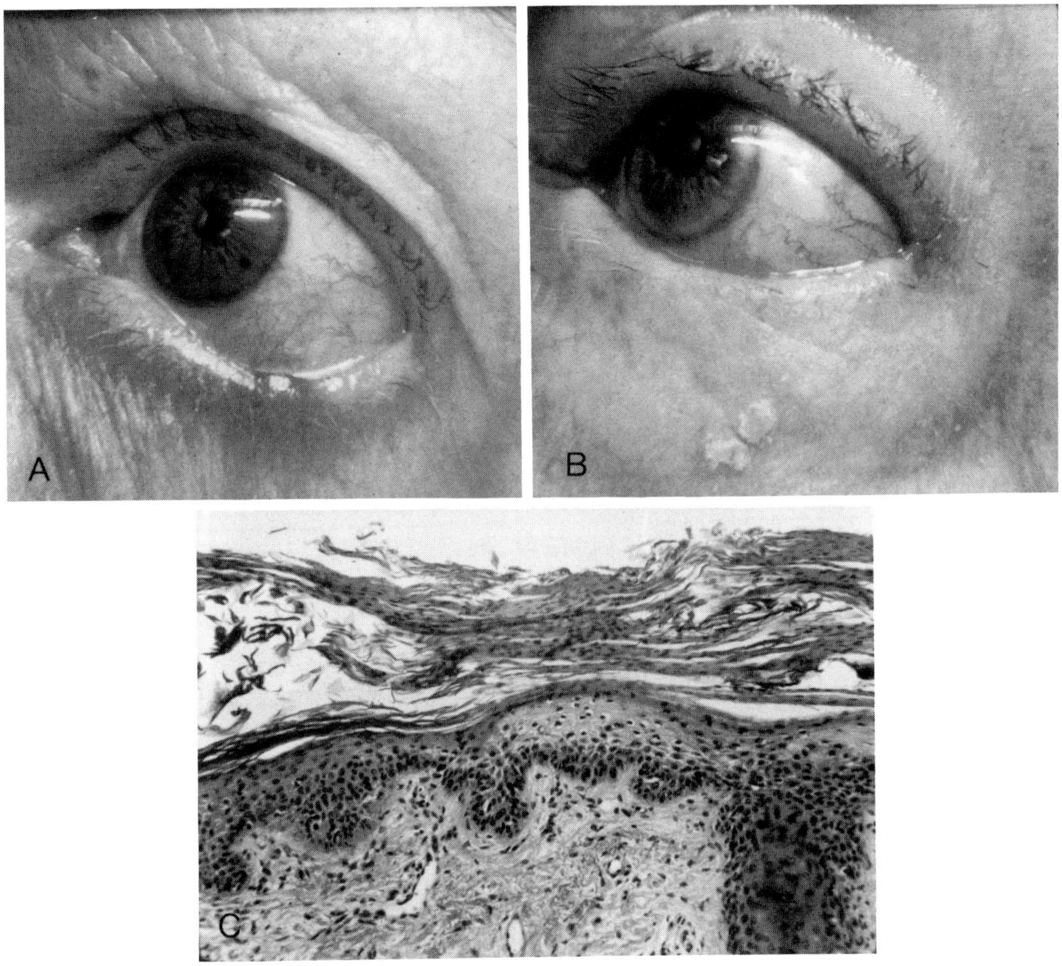

Figure 24.10. *A*, Actinic keratosis of free margin of lid. *B*, Crusted lesion of lower lid resembling actinic keratosis. Under crust, however, typical basal cell carcinoma. *C*, Actinic keratosis: There is hyperkeratosis of the epidermis and an increased number of cytologically atypical keratinocytes arranged mostly along the basal layer. The dermis is altered by an increased amount of abnormal elastic fibers due to chronic ultraviolet exposure (solar elastosis). (Courtesy of E. Heilman, M.D. and R. Friedman, M.D.)

tosis is the cutaneous horn, which should always be submitted to pathology because of the early changes of squamous cell carcinoma often seen at the base of these lesions.

Management. Cryosurgery or desiccation and curettage is equally satisfactory. Of course, when early changes of squamous cell carcinoma are detected, excision or superficial radiation is recommended.

REFERENCES

1. Henkind P: Thoughts on eyelid tumors. In Hornblass A (ed): *Tumors of the Ocular Adenexa and Orbit*. St. Louis, CV Mosby, 1979, p 51.
2. Rodriguez-Sains, RS: Ophthalmologic oncology, common eyelid tumors. *J Dermatol Surg Oncol* 8:247–253, 1982.
3. Biro L, Price E: Dermatologic management of eyelid tumors. In Hornblass A (ed): *Tumors of the Ocular Adenexa and Orbit*. St. Louis, CV Mosby , 1979, p 69.
4. Jackson R: Basic principles of electrosurgery: a review. *Can J Surg* 13:354–361, 1970.
5. Biro L, Price E, Brand A: Cryosurgery for basal cell carcinoma of the eyelid and nose: five year experience. *J Amer Acad Dermatol* 6:1042–1047, 1982.
6. Biro L, Price E, Brand A: Cryosurgery, a complementary modality. *Cutis* 28:520–525, 1981.
7. Jansen AB, et al: *Lab Invest* 47:491–497, 1982.

CHAPTER 25

Squamous Cell Carcinoma of the Eyelid[a]

DAVID M. REIFLER, M.D.
ALBERT HORNBLASS, M.D.

Squamous cell carcinoma [squamous cell epithelioma, epidermoid carcinoma, epithelioma spinocellulare, prickle cell epithelioma, spinalioma (1)] is relatively rare in the eyelids and accounts for 2.4–30.2% of all eyelid malignancies (2–32). Similar to its occurrence elsewhere in the skin, this potentially lethal neoplasm is capable of metastasis to regional lymph nodes (1, 20, 26, 33–36). In this respect, squamous cell carcinoma behaves quite differently than basal cell carcinoma (37, 38). Yet clinically, squamous cell carcinoma may resemble basal cell carcinoma, as well as a variety of other benign and malignant tumors (22, 38–40). In the past, this lesion may have been frequently overdiagnosed by pathologists and confused histologically with other benign entities (22).

Sun exposure (33, 36) and the presence of predisposing factors such as genetic effects (41, 42) and chronic skin damage (33) have been shown to play important roles in the development of squamous cell carcinoma. The lesion is thought to arise with an initial phase of intraepidermal carcinoma in situ (45). Certain clinically diagnosed premalignant dermatoses may also give rise to squamous cell carcinoma in the lid (46). A pathologic study of squamous epithelial skin lesions reveals a broad, continuous spectrum of conditions ranging from mild dysplasia to poorly differentiated, invasive carcinoma (9, 44).

Proper management of squamous cell carcinoma is dependent upon early diagnosis and definitive treatment. Complete surgical extirpation of the tumor has been advocated by many authors (20, 23, 24, 47), including histologic confirmation of the adequacy of the resection by standard frozen sections (45) or Mohs' technique (13, 32, 48–51). Other methods of treatment have been advocated, such as radiation therapy (15, 17, 21, 52, 53) and cryotherapy (28, 54–57).

The treatment advocated by these authors consists of complete excision with frozen-section control (47). The techniques are similar to those used in the management of basal cell carcinoma and other eyelid neoplasms (58–60). The various methods of reconstruction are well outlined elsewhere in this volume. However, because of the potential for metastasis and lethality, wider excision is recommended with close postoperative follow-up.

HISTORY

In 1775, Percivall Pott (61) first recognized soot as a carcinogen in chimney sweeps with cancer of the scrotum. Squamous cell carcinoma was therefore the first malignancy recognized as being caused by external irritation and associated with occupational hazards. Other causes of skin cancers have since been noted, including hydrocarbon (62) and actinic exposure (63).

In 1902, Krompecher distinguished between basal cell carcinoma and epithelioma spinocellulare (squamous cell

[a] This chapter was based upon a thesis prepared for the American Society of Ophthalmic Plastic and Reconstructive Surgery, Inc, and published, in part, under the same title in *Survey of Ophthalmology* 30:349–365, 1986.

carcinoma) (1). In that same year, roentgen radiation–induced squamous cell carcinoma was first reported by Frieben (64), soon after the discovery of x-rays. Within a short time, cutaneous carcinoma appeared in some patients who had been exposed to x-rays (65, 66). In 1961, Forrest (67) reported a case of squamous cell carcinoma of the eyelids following radiation therapy for retinoblastoma. An interval of 20 years between the radiation therapy and the eyelid tumor occurred in this case. The longest reported interval between ocular radiation therapy and the development of squamous cell carcinoma of the lid is 62 years (68).

In 1922, Darier and Ferrand (69) distinguished between squamous cell and basal cell carcinoma as *epithelioma pavimenteux typique* and *epithelioma pavimenteux atypique*, respectively. They also classified "metatypical" forms; i.e., mixed (basosquamous) and intermediate forms referred to as *epithelioma pavimenteaux mixte et intermediary.* The term "basosquamous carcinoma" (basal squamous or basalosquamous cell carcinoma) is still used by some pathologists and refers to basal cell carcinomas that show area of squamous differentiation (27). Because these lesions, even if quite large, behave clinically as basal cell carcinomas, the use of this term has been discouraged by ocular and dermatologic pathologists (36). In fact, squamous differentiation in a basal cell carcinoma may actually be associated with a lower mortality than when this feature is absent (70).

INCIDENCE

Squamous cell carcinoma constitutes 2.4–30.2% of malignant lid lesions, and less than 1 to 2% of all lid lesions (2–32). About 5–9.2% of all skin cancers arise in the eyelid, and cancers in this location account for at least 11% of all mortalities from skin malignancies (11, 71). In one series of 660 cases of squamous cell carcinoma of the skin there were 8 cases of squamous cell carcinomas of the lid, which constituted 1.2% of the total (46). In a large series of squamous cell carcinomas of the skin arising in the head and neck, lesions of the lids and canthi accounted for 2.8% of the total (71).

Because of the tendency in the past, for overdiagnosis of the eyelid squamous cell carcinoma, some authors believe that the incidence of this lesion cannot be accurately judged from the older literature. This view was first set forth in 1963 by Kwitko and associates (22) at the Armed Forces Institute of Pathology. Their series of patients with eyelid malignancies had a lower incidence of squamous cell carcinoma (2.4%) than any series that had previously been reported. In their series, the ratio of basal cell carcinoma to squamous cell carcinoma was 38.6 to 1. In more recent studies reported since 1963, the proportion of squamous cell carcinomas among all eyelid cancers has been higher than that found by Kwitko and associates (22); the proportion ranges widely, from 2.9% to as high as 32.3% (23–32). The data regarding the incidence of squamous cell carcinoma, as reported in the older literature prior to 1963, therefore should not be entirely discounted, and the calculation that squamous cell carcinoma "is seen about 40 times less frequently than basal cell carcinoma of the lid," (36) may be underestimated.

Shulman (20) found that of 195 malignant eyelid tumors, 178 (91.3%) were basal cell carcinomas and 14 (7.2%) were squamous cell carcinomas, a ratio of 12.7 to 1, respectively. Similarly, Aurora and Blodi (26) found 80.3% basal cell carcinomas and 7.0% squamous cell carcinoma, a ratio of 11.4 to 1.

The relative frequency of various eyelid malignancies shows striking differences in different parts of the world. In one Chinese series (31), the relative incidence of squamous cell carcinoma was about 10%, and about 47% were basal cell carcinomas. In Sweden, the incidence of squamous cell carcinoma of the eyelid has been reported to be 2.2 per 1,000,000 population (72). In that country 49.9% of the population are men and 50.1% are women. The relative incidences of squamous cell carcinoma of the lid in men and women in this study was given at 1.3 and 0.93 per 1,000,000 total population, respectively.

ETIOLOGY

In general, squamous cell carcinomas of the skin are most frequent in parts of the world where light-skinned people are exposed to large amounts of total sunlight. Thus, the amount of ultraviolet exposure and the skin type and color are the most important factors (33, 36, 44). Similar skin-damaging factors appear to be operative in so-called precancerous or premalignant keratoses. Those conditions that may spawn a squamous cell carcinoma include Bowen's dermatosis, senile (solar) keratosis, and keratoses resulting from arsenic, tar, or irradiation (33, 36, 43, 73).

Although virtually all types of precancerous dermatoses can occur on the lid, they are observed much less often than other keratotic lesions (34). In addition, squamous cell carcinoma infrequently arises from solar keratosis and in only 3% of Bowen's dermatoses (73). Squamous cell carcinomas originating from actinic keratoses probably have a more benign course than those that arise from other forms of carcinoma in situ (44).

Occupations that entail considerable handling of oils or tar may be associated with an increased incidence of precancerous and cancerous lesions of the skin, including the eyelids (46, 74). Sunlight exposure, however, correlates with occupational hazards in the development of eyelid skin cancers. In one study (75), occupational groups exposed to sunlight and the elements had an incidence of cancer of the eye and eyelids that was about three times that found in all other groups. It is probably for this reason that eyelid squamous cell carcinoma occurs more commonly in males than females (47).

Because total sun exposure in a predisposed individual is of prime importance in the production of squamous cell carcinoma of the lid, this neoplasm is much less common in younger adults and exceedingly rare in children (25, 76). In children, the occurrence of eyelid squamous cell carcinoma is usually associated with a specific premalignant dermatosis such as irradiation or xeroderma pigmentosum (77), or radiation dermatitis (67).

The prototypal disease that is associated with a genetic predisposition to squamous cell carcinoma is xeroderma pigmentosum (41, 42). This rare, premalignant dermatosis is usually inherited in an autosomal recessive manner. Basal cell and squamous cell carcinomas are most frequently encountered lesions (41, 42). In the most acute form of the disease, malignant transformation occurs early and leads to death as early as 3 years of age (42) Similar to the abnormal fibroblasts discovered in patients with retinoblastoma, DNA repair is defective in xeroderma pigmentosum (78).

A genetic predisposition to cancer has been suggested in patients with Bowen's disease, a premalignant dermatosis that may give rise to squamous cell carcinoma. Bowen's disease is associated with other skin tumors, both malignant and premalignant, in up to 50% of cases and with an internal cancer in up to 80% of cases (79, 80). Malignant transformation occurs more frequently in Bowen's disease of mucous membrane (40%) than in Bowen's disease of the skin (73).

CLINICAL PRESENTATION

TOPOGRAPHIC DISTRIBUTION

There have been conflicting reports as to whether squamous cell carcinoma is found more frequently in the upper or the lower lids. Geographic or racial factors may in part be responsible for differences in reported statistics. In the United Kingdom, Mustarde (81) and Shulman (20) found the upper lid to be more commonly affected than the lower lid, while Lederman (30) and McCallum (46) found a lower lid predominance.

In reviewing different series of squamous cell carcinoma of the lid, one finds that its occurrence in the lower lid is actually more common than the upper lid, with a ratio of about 1.1 to 1, respectively. It should be emphasized that any preponderance of lower lid involvement in squamous cell carcinoma is not as pronounced as that seen in basal cell carcinoma, where the ratio of lower lid involvement to upper lid involvement is probably somewhere between 3:1 and 5:1.

Some authors have noted that squamous cell carcinoma of the lids arises at the lid margin (30, 44, 45). Intraepithelial carcinoma also has a predilection for arising at a marginal as opposed to an extramarginal location (46).

There is also a relatively high incidence of squamous cell carcinoma in the canthal areas, particularly the medial canthus. In some series, squamous cell carcinomas of the canthi have outnumbered those confined to the lid (71). These are also frequently situated in an infraorbital location. It is therefore apparent that a significant number of skin cancers, including squamous cell carcinoma, may be found in areas usually scruitinized in a careful ophthalmologic examination.

CLINICAL APPEARANCE AND DIFFERENTIAL DIAGNOSIS

Squamous cell carcinoma of the lid may arise from a precancerous dermatosis or de novo (82, 83). The earliest lesion is most commonly in the form of a roughened scaly patch that tends to develop crusting erosions and fissures over a period of some months (Fig. 25.1) (1, 35, 37, 84). Ulcers that are typically shallow, with a red base and sharply defined, indurated, elevated borders eventually develop beneath the crusting debris (Fig. 25.2). The ulceration tends to occur more rapidly than in basal cell carcinoma and may become extensive if ignored.

Following local extension into dermis, deeper invasion of connective tissue and periosteum are the typical routes of spread into the orbit and lacrimal passages (Fig. 25.3). According to Duke-Elder (1), if left unattended, the entire orbital region and major portion of the face are "destroyed in a fetid-smelling, ulcerating, fungating crater which may eventually reach the cranial cavity." In general, lymphatic spread is to the parotid (preauricular) nodes if the tumor is in the upper lids or lateral canthus, and to the submaxillary nodes if the tumor is in the lower lid or medial canthus (35, 85). Death may occur after a prolonged and painful debilitating illness.

The clinical diagnosis of squamous cell carcinoma of the lid is made difficult by several complicating factors. First, the clinical appearance of this lesion may take several protean forms (1, 84). In addition to the common ulcerative type, squamous cell carcinoma, particularly at the lid margin, may manifest itself as a papillomatous growth, a rounded nodular or cyst-like lesion, or a cutaneous horn

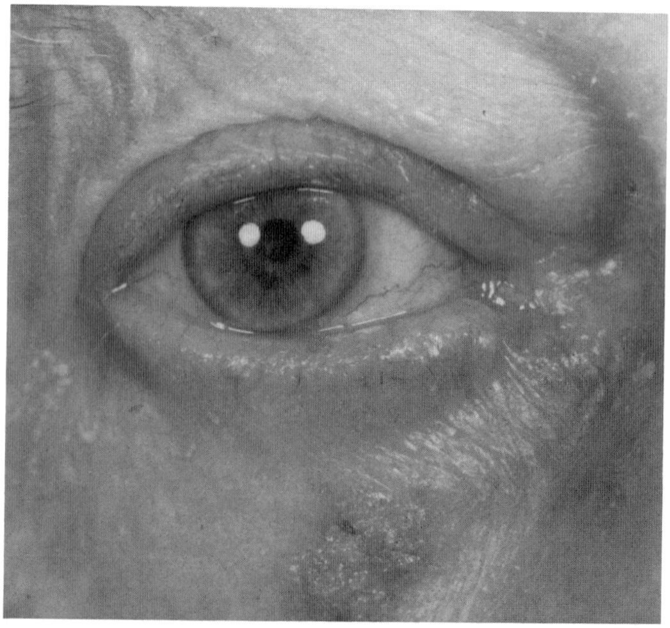

Figure 25.1. Squamous cell carcinoma of the infraorbital region showing scaling and fissuring of the epidermis.

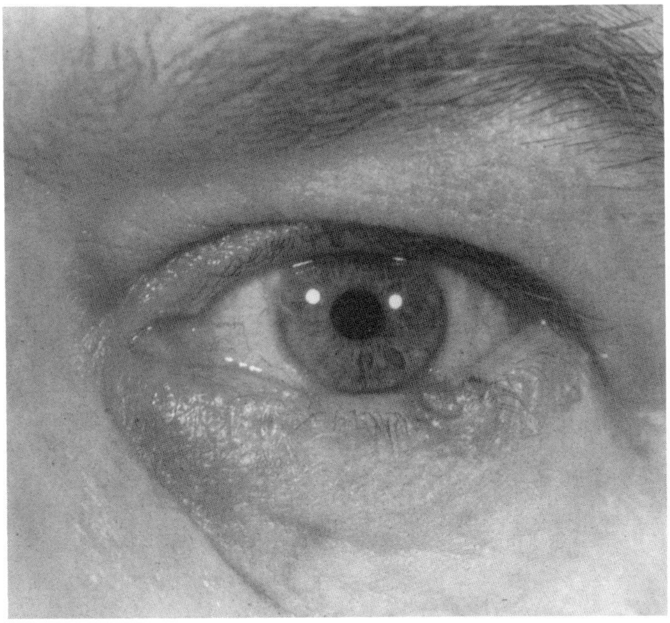

Figure 25.2. Squamous cell carcinoma of the left lower lid margin showing ulceration with heaped up margins.

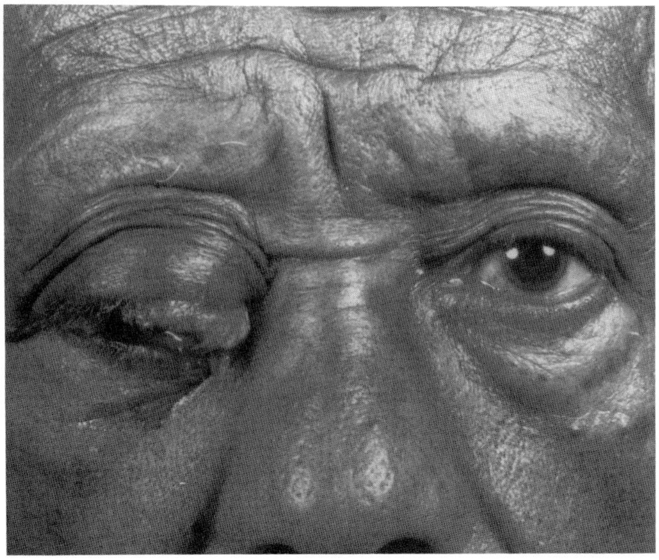

Figure 25.3. Extensive squamous cell carcinoma of the right upper lid that presented with orbital invasion. The patient underwent exenteration of the right orbit and has survived 9 years without metastasis or recurrence.

(39). Benign-appearing lesions, characteristic of verrucae or keratoacanthoma, may actually reveal histologic evidence of invasive squamous cell carcinoma at deeper levels of sectioning (86). Undertreatment of squamous cell carcinoma based on the mistaken diagnosis of keratoacanthoma may result in recurrence and metastasis (87).

Second, other malignant, precancerous, and even benign tumors may mimic squamous cell carcinoma; this phenomenon has resulted in the overdiagnosis of this latter condition (22). According to Reese (37), basal cell and squamous cell carcinomas may present with virtually an identical clinical appearance. However, keratin production may be more evident in squamous cell carcinoma, yielding a translucent pearly-white shagreen (35, 37). Precancerous dermatoses, such as actinic keratosis and Bowen's disease, can be distinguished from squamous cell carcinoma only by careful histologic examination. Benign conditions that may have been both clinically and histologically confused with squamous cell carcinoma include inverted follicular keratosis, keratoacanthoma, and pseudoepitheliomatous hyperplasia (22, 82). Variants of squamous cell carcinoma, such as the less aggressive adenoid type ("adenoacanthoma"), generally show no clinically distinctive features and may likewise resemble other benign or malignant tumors (88).

Finally, patients with squamous cell carcinoma tend to have other tumors of the skin, including Bowen's disease, senile keratosis, and basal cell carcinoma (82). These patients frequently have chronic skin changes from actinic or chemical exposure, with areas of telangiectasias and chronic dermatitis. It is evident that neither the appearance nor the clinical setting of a suspected epidermal malignancy will yield an unequivocal diagnosis of squamous cell carcinoma in any given case. Yet the need for an accurate differentiation between the aforementioned conditions is very important. Because of the dramatic differences in prognosis between a potentially metastasizing and lethal squamous cell carcinoma and other less dangerous tumors, the recommended modes of therapy will vary accordingly (89). An accurate diagnosis of squamous cell carcinoma is dependent upon histopathologic examination that demonstrates consistent cytologic features and evidence of invasion of the dermis (82, 83). Only an adequate biopsy or representative portions of an epidermal tumor will provide the information necessary to make a diagnosis.

PATHOPHYSIOLOGY

While this chapter emphasizes the clinical features and management of eyelid squamous cell carcinoma, a discussion of the pathophysiology is also important. The development of squamous cell carcinoma is thought to progress through different phases as enumerated below. For further details regarding illustrative histopathology, the reader is referred to a review recently published by the authors (89a).

Squamous cell carcinoma of the lid begins with an early epithelial phase referred to as *actinic keratosis* (senile keratosis, solar keratosis) (45). In actinic keratosis, there is subtotal replacement of the epidermis by atypical cells (intraepithelial squamous dysplasia), which are sharply demarcated from hyperplastic but otherwise normal adnexal keratinocytes and from the surrounding epidermis. In this stage of intraepithelial dysplasia, the general scheme of stratified maturation from the basal to the superficial epidermal layers is still preserved.

The process of differentiation may become disorganized with total replacement of the epidermis in a stage referred to as "intraepidermal squamous cell carcinoma" or "squamous cell carcinoma in situ" (35, 36, 83, 90). Clinically, this lesion may arise in a precancerous dermatosis such as actinic keratosis or it may arise de novo (82). Histologically, the epithelium shows complete disorganization, with numerous atypical cells having large hyperchromatic nuclei. Individual cells appear that are large and round and have a homogeneous, eosinophilic cytoplasm. Even though the marked atypicality of the epidermal cells includes cells of the basal layer, the basement membrane remains intact. The dermis is involved only insofar as a chronic inflammatory infiltration is frequently found.

Bowen's disease is a special clinicopathologic example of intraepidermal squamous cell carcinoma. It is histologically indistinguishable from other types of squamous cell carcinoma in situ (36, 83). Clinically, Bowen's disease manifests itself as a slowly enlarging erythematous patch of sharp but irregular outline that shows little or no filtration. Areas of scaling and crusting within the patch, generally are found.

At the lid margin, a relatively frequent site of occurrence, intraepidermal squamous cell carcinoma may behave more aggressively than lesions located away from the lid margin. In one series (46), intraepidermal squamous cell carcinoma located at the lid margin progressed to invasive squamous cell carcinoma in three of 22 cases, resulting in fatality in one case. In the other three cases, there was inadequate excision, which led to recurrence.

Invasion of the dermis is the hallmark for the diagnosis of invasive squamous cell carcinoma (33, 83, 90). The invading cells are not uniform in appearance; they show different degrees of differentiation, hyperchromatic nuclei, and abnormal keratinization (Fig. 25.4). Keratinizing nests of squamous cells may be interspersed within the tumor (Fig. 25.5). Broders (91) developed a system of grading squamous cell carcinoma according to the proportion of maturing (differentiating) cells present (Table 25.1). The degree of keratinization (differentiation) is the essential feature of Broder's system of grading. However, it is now generally recognized that in addition to the number of differentiating cells, the degree of atypicality of the tumor cells, the depth of invasion, and other factors also are important in grading the malignancy (92). Extensive acantholysis, which tends to produce tubular and pseudoglandular patterns that are characteristic of adenoid squamous cell carcinoma ("adenoacanthoma"), is probably associated with a better prognosis (88).

Some pathologists report the degree of malignancy in a semiquantitative way, such as "well," "moderately," or "poorly differentiated" tumor (33). The function of keratin formation is retained in malignant epidermal cells of low grades of malignancy. Individual tumor cells often show dyskeratosis and keratinization as a prominent feature. Most squamous cell carcinomas of the lids are well differentiated, contrasting with those of the nasopharynx or sinuses (44). The more poorly differentiated squamous cell carcinomas of the maxillary antrum are far more likely to cause a secondary invasion of the orbit than tumors arising in the lid (93).

In tumors of higher grades of malignancy, evidence of increasing degrees of cellular anaplasia are manifested by irregularly shaped and sized cells, enlarged nuclei, abnormal mitoses, and loss of intercellular bridges (33, 44, 90). Keratin pearls are less frequent, and keratinization occurs only in small cell groups or in single cells. In the adenoid squamous cell carcinoma variant, extensive acantholysis is observed, but the tendency for keratinization persists (88).

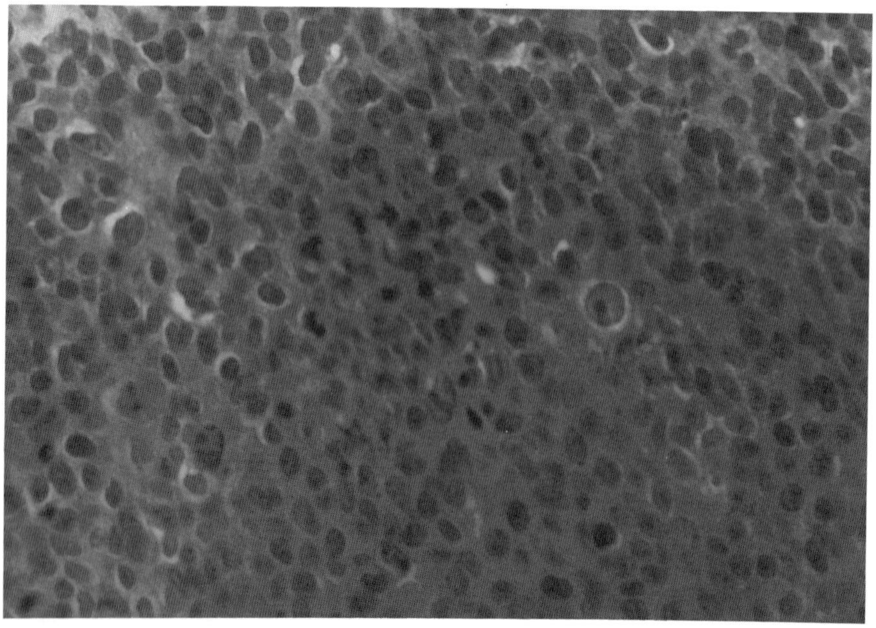

Figure 25.4. Moderately well differentiated invasive squamous cell carcinoma showing cellular pleomorphism and variable degrees abnormal keratinization. Hematoxylin and eosin; original magnification × 40.

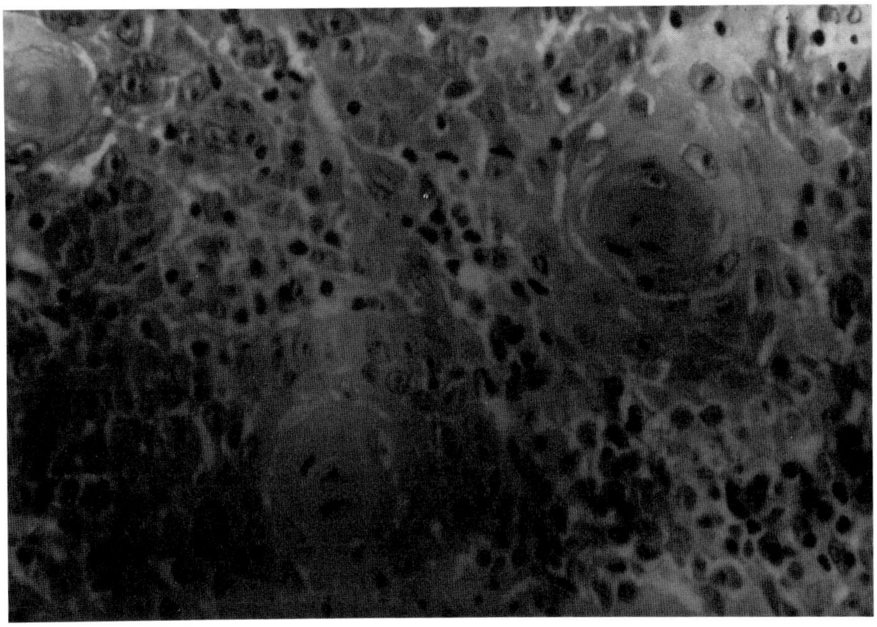

Figure 25.5. Well-differentiated squamous cell carcinoma of the lid with keratin pearls. Hematoxylin and eosin; original magnification × 40.

Table 25.1
Broders' Grading System for Squamous Cell Carcinoma[a]

Grade	Percentage of Cells that are Differentiated
1	> 75
2	$> 50; < 75$
3	$> 25; < 50$
4	< 25

[a] Broders AC: Practical points on the microscopic grading of carcinoma. *NY J Med* 32: 667–671, 1932.

Squamous cell carcinoma may invade the dermis at various levels. Deeper penetration may have some correlation with dissemination through the lymphatic system in a particular area, although it is not nearly as significant as in other lesions, such as malignant melanoma (92). Although the most common specific tissue affinity for invasive squamous cell carcinoma is for the dermis, many different routes of spread exist; squamous cell carcinoma may spread along fascial planes, periosteum, embryologic fusion planes, nerve sheaths, lymphatic vessels, and blood vessels (94).

Early invasion of the orbicularis muscle by a squamous cell carcinoma may occur and is probably related to the unique anatomy of the eyelid. The dermis of the eyelid is very thin, and the underlying orbicularis muscle here is very superficially located (44). Deep penetration of the lash follicles at the lid margin further places the epidermis in an intimate relationship with the tarsus and orbicularis muscle (46).

Squamous cell carcinoma of the lid has the potential for regional lymph node metastasis (1, 20, 22, 26, 31, 33–38, 41, 44). In this respect, squamous cell carcinoma behaves quite differently than basal cell carcinoma. In general, the distribution of lymph node metastasis follows the known lymphatic drainage pathways: (*a*) to the parotid nodes from the lateral canthus and most of the upper lid, and (*b*) to the submaxillary nodes from the medial canthus and most of the lower lid (33, 85). However, parotid node metastasis can also arise from primary tumors in the lower lid.

The reported incidence of regional lymph node metastasis in squamous cell carcinoma has varied widely, from as low as 1.3% (71) to as high as 21.4% (20). In a series of 12 patients who underwent surgical excision with frozen section control, we did not encounter any case of lymph node or distant metastasis (47). This variability is undoubtedly affected by many factors, including histologic characteristics, patient selection, location of the tumor, and etiology (33). In a series of 16 adenoid squamous cell carcinomas of the lid with adequate follow-up, there was not one case of regional lymph node or distant metastasis (88). Considering all sites, the incidence of metastasis has been reported to be as low as 0.1% in squamous cell carcinoma arising from actinic keratoses (34), but as high as 18% in de novo cases, and 26% in roentgen-associated cases (76). Usually metastasis from squamous cell carcinoma of the lid is a late occurrence, and even in neglected tumors, lymph node involvement is more likely to result from secondary infection rather than actual metastasis (1). Since the majority of squamous cell carcinomas of the lid are associated with sun exposure and perhaps less prone to be neglected than lesions arising elsewhere, the incidence of metastasis is probably very low.

In one series of 79 squamous cell carcinomas of the lids and canthi (71), there was only one case of metastasis to parotid nodes, although 26 of these lesions arose in the upper lid and outer canthus. In fact, the one case of parotid node metastasis was associated with a primary lesion in the lower lid. This same series of patients included a total of 2802 cutaneous squamous cell carcinomas of the face, and there was a much higher overall incidence of 19% metastasis to parotid nodes. On the other hand, in another series of 14 cases of squamous cell carcinoma of the lids (20), three patients (21.4%) developed lymph node metastasis that were uniformly fatal within 2 years.

Squamous cell carcinoma is by far the most frequent of the secondary epithelial neoplasms in the orbit (93). However, orbital squamous cell is much more likely to arise in the paranasal sinuses rather than the periorbital skin. Although squamous cell carcinomas occur in the eyelids much less frequently than do basal cell carcinomas, a much greater proportion of the former may reach the orbit. In either case, orbital invasion may take years to occur and is often preceded by several previous operations, irradiations, and recurrences of the tumor.

Orbital invasion of a squamous cell carcinoma of the lid may be associated with an early and severe involvement of the orbital nerves (95). This may cause a complete ptosis and ophthalmoplegia prior to the development of proptosis. Eventually, involvement of the orbital nerves and bony orbit causes severe and constant pain that may hasten the patient's cachexia, debilitation, and ultimate demise (1). Involvement of the orbital nerves may also provide a route for intracranial extension of the neoplasm.

The prognosis of squamous cell carcinoma of the lid may be correlated with several factors including (*a*) the presence of predisposing conditions, such as radiation therapy or xeroderma pigmentosum; (*b*) the histologic grade of malignancy; and (*c*) the site of the lesion. However, neglect of these tumors or lack of available medical care in certain parts of the world, probably has a much greater impact on human suffering caused by this disease.

The reported mortality rates for squamous cell carcinoma of the lid (Table 25.2) have ranged from 0 (23, 47) to 30% (22). Series of cases using nonsurgical methods of therapy, such as radiation therapy and cryotherapy, may have reported lower mortality rates due to patient selection. Duke-Elder (1) estimated the mortality rate of squamous cell carcinoma of the lid to be about 12% after surgical excision.

Table 25.2
Mortality Rates in Various Series of Squamous Cell Carcinoma of the Eyelid

Authors	No. of Squamous Cell Carcinomas of the Lid	No. of Tumor Deaths	Mortality Rate, %
Birge (8)[a]	39	8	28.2
Mohs (13)	19	1	5.3
Shulman (20)	14	3	21.4
Kwitko et al. (22)	13	4	30.7
Aurora and Blodi (26)	10	4	26.6
Lederman (30)	59	3	5.1
Anderson (32)	8	1	12.5
Caya (88)	16	0	0.0
Reifler and Hornblass (47)	12	0	0.0
TOTAL	174	24	13.7

[a] Reference numbers are in parentheses.

Birge (8) collected the rates of mortality, blindness, and exenteration with various grades of squamous cell carcinoma found about the eye. Although the majority of these lesions (39 of 59) arose in the lids and canthi, the rest occurred on the conjunctiva, limbus, or cornea. In spite of this mix of cases, it is clear that higher grades of malignancy were associated with increased rates of mortality and morbidity. Restricting the analysis to squamous cell carcinoma of the lids and canthi, Birge (8) also found an increased rate of mortality and blindness for lesions situated in the upper lid and medial canthus.

TREATMENT AND COMPLICATIONS

A review of the treatment of squamous cell carcinoma of the lids might best begin with a word about prevention. The use of protection clothing and pharmacologic sunblocking agents should be recommended for any patient with a history of precancerous or cancerous skin lesions.

In dealing with eyelid malignancies, the treating physician may not be objective about the various options, but rather prejudiced by his or her training and limited experience (96, 97). However, in the case of squamous cell carcinoma, due respect must be given to the potential for metastasis and lethality (1, 20, 22, 26, 31, 33–38, 41, 44). The methods of microscopically controlled eradication of squamous cell carcinoma should be at least as meticulously applied to this condition as they are in cases of other eyelid neoplasms (13, 32, 48–51, 58–60, 98–100).

EXCISION WITH FROZEN-SECTION CONTROL

The adequacy of excision can be monitored with frozen-section control (47). Using this method, surgeons can perform immediate ophthalmic plastic reconstruction most conveniently. Others have successfully used Mohs' chemosurgical fresh-tissue techniques in the treatment of eyelid squamous cell carcinoma (32). In the presence of some medical contraindication to surgery, consideration may be given to some uncontrolled field-type of therapy, particularly radiation therapy (15, 17, 21, 30, 52, 53, 101), cryotherapy (28, 54, 55, 101–103), or chemotherapy (104–107).

Frozen-section control, either by standard methods or Mohs' technique, is not without its limitations. These methods are probably less precise when the tumor extends into the orbital fat and are virtually impossible in the examination of bone (32). In cases of deep orbital extensions of squamous cell carcinoma, absolute reliance upon the examination of frozen sections is therefore unwarranted. As with more superficial lesions, relatively generous tumor-free margins probably should be excised in cases of squamous cell carcinoma as compared with basal cell carcinoma.

RADIATION THERAPY

Radiation has been used in the treatment of eyelid malignancies for over 70 years. However, early in this century, it was noted that squamous cell carcinoma did not respond to radium therapy as well as basal cell carcinoma (10, 108).

Squamous cell carcinoma is relatively radioresistant. Therefore, in radiotherapy of squamous cell carcinoma of the lid, a great amount of radiation may be administered, and proper shielding of the eye is thus crucial. In one protocol (53), a total dose of 5440 rads is given for squamous cell carcinoma of the lid, as opposed to 3400 rads in cases of basal cell carcinoma. With this higher dose, the total amount of radiation reaching the lens, about 57 rads, is still below the theoretical minimum cataractogenic dose.

Treatment of eyelid cancer with radiation can be administered with contact apparatus (17, 53). Postradiation reactions such as erythema, oozing, and swelling invariably occur, although the complications of late radiation necrosis and ectropion may be reduced with careful selection of patients (17).

CRYOTHERAPY

Most series reporting the cryosurgical treatment of squamous cell carcinoma of the lids have been small (28, 54, 55). Initially, recurrences were common and failures occurred when there was involvement of the conjunctival fornix (54). More recently, a series of 21 patients with squamous cell carcinoma of the lid, in which the therapy consisted of liquid nitrogen spray, was reported (57). In this series of patients, there was reportedly no recurrences, with an average follow-up of 21.6 months. Complications included lacrimal obstruction (16%), permanent loss of eyelashes, and localized skin depigmentation that lasted from 6 months to over 6 years. Another potential complication is the development of eyelid defects that may require plastic reconstruction. The authors noted numerous contraindications to this mode of therapy, including involvement of the fornix, fixation to periosteum, cold intolerance, indistinct tumor margins, and a tumor size greater than 10 mm.

Bowen's disease of the lid has also been treated with liquid nitrogen (55). In a series of patients, recurrences after one treatment were common. In five patients with recurrences, two or three additional treatments were required to effect a cure.

MISCELLANEOUS "FIELD THERAPIES"

In addition to radiation therapy and cryotherapy, other methods of treatment of squamous cell carcinoma that lack histologic control include curettage and electrodessication (10, 24, 27), topical chemotherapy and immunotherapy (108), and photoradiation therapy (110). As a group, all of these methods represent so-called field therapies, and all combinations of these methods within this group have been advocated as adjuncts to surgical excision.

Topical chemotherapy, using 5-fluorouracil cream, has been reported to eliminate squamous cell carcinoma in situ in solar keratoses, arsenical keratoses, and late radiation dermatitis (104). Bowen's type of carcinoma has also been successfully treated with local chemotherapy (105). Although topical chemotherapy has eradicated invasive squamous cell carcinomas in controlled investigational instances, local chemotherapy is believed to be an ineffective method in the routine treatment of invasive squamous cell carcinoma (106). The use of 5-fluorouracil in malignant eyelid tumors is further limited by the side effects of ocular irritation. Even proponents of this therapy have cautioned against getting 5-fluorouracil too close to the eyes (107). Topical chemotherapy may rarely be indicated in unusual cases, such as xeroderma pigmentosum, for the management of large areas of multiple, superficial skin cancers in the periorbital region away from the eyes.

ORBITAL EXENTERATION

In cases of squamous cell carcinoma with secondary orbital invasion, the treatment of choice is orbital exenteration. The incidences of recurrences and tumor deaths have been variously reported. In a series of 48 cases of orbital exenteration reported by Rathbun and associates (111), there were six cases of squamous cell carcinoma, including the sites of origin on conjunctiva (three cases), skin (two cases), and lacrimal sac (one case). In these cases of squamous cell carcinoma, there were no tumor recurrences 5 months to 13 years following exenteration. The cases of basal cell carcinoma also had relatively good results following exenteration. Of 14 patients with basal cell carcinoma, 12 patients had no recurrence and two patients had recurrences but were still alive 7–10 years later. Simons and associates (112) also reported good results in cases of exenteration for basal cell carcinoma. However, in three cases of squamous cell carcinoma, there were two tumor deaths.

REFERENCES

1. Duke-Elder S, MacFaul PA: The ocular adnexa. In Duke-Elder S (ed): *System of Ophthalmology*. St. Louis, CV Mosby, 1974, vol 8, p 423.
2. Regaud C, Coutard H, Monod O, Richard G: Radiotherapie des cancers de la region orbito-palpebrale. Resultat et techniques de l'Institute du Radium de 1919–1923. *Ann Oculist (Paris)* 163: 1–30, 1926.
3. Lavorde S: Les epitheliomas de paupieres et leur traitement par le radium. *Presse Med* 41: 1548–1550, 1933. (abstracted in *Arch Ophthalmol* 12: 451–452, 1934)
4. Geschickler CF, Koehler HP: Ectodermal tumors of the skin. *Am J Cancer* 23: 804–836, 1935.
5. O'Brien CS, Bradly AE: Tumors of the eyelids. *JAMA* 107: 933–938, 1936.
6. Reese AB: In discussion on O'Brien. *JAMA* 107: 937, 1936.
7. Sharp GS: Treatment of cancer of the eyelids. *JAMA* 111: 1617–1622, 1938.
8. Birge HL: Cancer of the eyelids, conjunctiva, and cornea. II. Squamous cell epithelioma. *Arch Ophthalmol* 20: 254–270, 1938.
9. Martin HE: Cancer of the eyelids. *Arch Ophthalmol* 41: 616–624, 1939.
10. Driver JR, Cole HN: Epithelioma of the eyelids and canthi. Report series of 324 cases. *Am J Roentgenol* 41: 616–624, 1939.
11. Hollander L, Krugh JF: Cancer of the eyelid. *Am J Ophthalmol* 27: 244–253, 1944.
12. Hunt HB: Cancer of the eyelid treated with radiation, with consideration of irradiation cataract. *Am J Roentgenol* 57: 160–180, 1947.
13. Mohs FE: Chemosurgical treatment of cancer of the eyelid. A microscopically controlled method of excision. *Arch Ophthalmol* 39: 43–59, 1948.
14. del Regato JA: Roentgen therapy of carcinoma of the skin of the eyelid. *Radiology* 52: 564–573, 1949.

15. Stetson CG, Schulz MD: Carcinoma of the eyelid. Analysis of 301 cases and review of the literature. *N Engl J Med* 241: 725–732, 1949.
16. Roseberg B: Carcinoma of the eyelids. *Am J Roentgenol* 69: 196–207, 1953.
17. Wildermuth O, Evans JC: The special problem of cancer of the eyelid. *Cancer* 9: 837–841, 1956.
18. Welch RB, Duke JR: Lesions of the lids. A statistical note. *Am J Ophthalmol* 45: 415–416, 1958.
19. Fayos JV, Wildermuth O: Carcinoma of the skin of the eyelids. *Arch Ophthalmol* 67: 289–302, 1962.
20. Shulman J: Treatment of malignant tumors of the eyelids by plastic surgery. *Br J Plast Surg* 15: 37–47, 1962.
21. McKenna RJ, Macdonald I: Carcinoma of the eyelid treated by irradiation. *Calif Med* 96: 184–189, 1962.
22. Kwitko ML, Boniuk M, Zimmerman LE: Eyelid tumors with reference to lesions confused with squamous cell carcinoma. I. Incidence and errors in diagnosis. *Arch Ophthalmol* 69: 693–697, 1963.
23. Maumenee AE, Stallard HB, Lederman M, Smith B, Boniuk M: Discussion of carcinomas of the conjuctiva and eyelid. In Boniuk M (ed): *Ocular and Adnexal Tumors. New and Controversial Aspects.* St. Louis, CV Mosby, 1964, p 101.
24. Domonkos AN: Treatment of eyelid carcinoma. *Arch Dermatol* 91: 364–371, 1965.
25. Mortada A: Incidence of lid carcinomata and their stages in U.A.R. *Bull Ophthalmol Soc Egypt* 60: 331–348, 1967.
26. Aurora A, Blodi F: Lesions of the eyelids. A clinicopathologic study. *Surv Ophthalmol* 15: 37–47, 1970.
27. Leventhal HH, Messer RJ: Malignant tumors of the eyelid. *Am J Surg* 124: 522–526, 1972.
28. Zacarian SA: Cancer of the eyelid. A cryosurgical approach. *Ann Ophthalmol* 4: 473–480, 1972.
29. Zacarian SA: Cryosurgery of malignant tumors of the skin. In Zacarian SA (ed): *Cryosurgery of Tumors of the Skin and Oral Cavity.* Springfield, IL, CC Thomas, 1973.
30. Lederman M: Radiation treatment of cancer of the eyelids. *Br J Ophthalmol* 60: 794–805, 1976.
31. Ni C, Searl SS, Kuo PK, Chu FR, Chong CS, Albert DM: Sebaceous cell carcinoma of the ocular adnexa. *Int Ophthalmol Clin* 22: 23–61, 1982.
32. Anderson RL: Results in eyelid malignancies treated with Mohs' fresh-tissue techniques. In: *Symposium on Diseases and Surgery of the Lids, Lacrimal Apparatus, and Orbit.* St. Louis, CV Mosby, 1982, p 380.
33. Stoll HL: Squamous cell carcinoma. In Fitzpatrick TB (ed): *Dermatology in General Medicine*, ed 2. New York, McGraw-Hill, 1979, p 362.
34. Lund HZ: How often does squamous cell carcinoma of the skin metastasize? *Arch Dermatol* 92: 635–637, 1965.
35. Hogan MJ, Zimmerman LE (eds): *Ophthalmic Pathology*, ed 2. Philadelphia, WB Saunders, 1962, p 214.
36. Yanoff M, Fine BS: *Ocular Pathology. A Text and Atlas*, ed 2. Hagerstown, MD, Harper & Row, 1982.
37. Reese AB: *Tumors of the Eye*, ed 3. Hagerstown, MD, Harper & Row, 1976, p 38.
38. Henkind P: Thoughts on eyelid tumors. In Hornblass A (ed): *Tumors of the Ocular Adnexa and Orbit.* St. Louis, CV Mosby, 1974, p 51.
39. Boniuk M, Zimmerman LE: Eyelid tumors with reference to lesions confused with squamous cell carcinoma. II. Inverted follicular keratosis. *Arch Ophthalmol* 69: 698–707, 1963.
40. Boniuk M, Zimmerman LE: Eyelid tumors with reference to lesions confused with squamous cell carcinoma. III Keratoacanthoma. *Arch Ophthalmol* 77: 29–33, 1967.
41. Mortada A: Incidence of lid, conjunctival and orbital malignant tumors in xeroderma pigmentosa in Egypt. *Bull Ophthalmol Soc Egypt* 61: 231–236, 1968.
42. Whitmore PV: Skin and mucous membrane disorders. In Duane TD (ed): *Clinical Ophthalmology.* Hagerstown, MD Harper & Row, 1980, vol 5, ch 27, p 8.
43. Montgomery H: Precancerous dermatosis and epithelioma in situ. *Arch Dermatol Syphilol* 39: 387–408, 1939.
44. Jakobiec FA, Rootman J, Jones IS: Secondary and metastatic tumors of the orbit. In Duane TD (ed): *Clinical Ophthalmology.* Hagerstown, MD, Harper & Row, 1976, vol 2, ch 46, p 30.
45. Jakobiec FA: Tumors of the lids. In *Symposium on Diseases and Surgery of the Lids, Lacrimal Apparatus and Orbit.* St. Louis, CV Mosby, 1982, ch 20, p 264.
46. McCallum DI, Kinmont PDC, Williams DW, Cotton RE, Wroughton MA: Intraepidermal carcinoma of the eyelid margin. *Br J Dermatol* 93: 239–252, 1975.
47. Reifler DM, Hornblass A: Squamous cell carcinoma of the lid. Presented at the 16th Annual Scientific Symposium, American Society of Ophthalmic Plastic and Reconstructive Surgery, San Francisco, October, 1985.
48. Mohs FE: The chemosurgical method for microscopically controlled excision of external cancer with reference to cancer of the eyelid. *Trans Am Acad Ophthalmol Otolaryngol* 62: 335–336, 1958.
49. Robins P: Mohs chemosurgery for tumors in the periorbital area. In Jakobiec FA (ed): *Ocular and Adnexal Tumors.* Birmingham, AL, Aesculapius, 1975, ch 34, p 484.
50. Anderson RL, Ceilley RI: A multispeciality approach to the excision and reconstruction of eyelid tumors. *Ophthalmology* 85: 1150–1163, 1978.
51. Callahan A, Monheit GD, Callahan MA: The Mohs' technique in ophthalmic plastic surgery. In *Symposium on Diseases and Surgery of the Lids, Lacrimal Apparatus, and Orbit.* St. Louis, CV Mosby, 1982, p 364.
52. Halnan KE, Britten MJA: Late functional and cosmetic results of treatment of eyelid tumors. *Br J Ophthalmol* 52: 43–53, 1968.
53. Gladstein AH: Radiotherapy of eyelid tumors. In Jakobiec FA (ed): *Ocular and Adnexal Tumors.* Birmingham, AL, Aesculapius 1978, p 484.
54. Zacarian SA: The cryogenic approach to the treatment of lid tumors. *Ann Ophthalmology* 2: 706–713, 1970.
55. Fraunfelder FT, Wallace RT, Farris HE, Wingfield DL: Cryosurgery for malignancy of the eyelid. *Ophthalmology* 87: 461–465, 1980.
56. Torre D: Cryosurgical treatment of eyelid tumors. In Jakobiec FA (ed): *Ocular and Adnexal Tumors.* Birmingham, AL, Aesculapius, 1978, ch 36, p 517.
57. Fraunfelder FT, Zacarian SA, Wingfield DL, Limmer BL: Results of cryotherapy for eyelid malignancies. *Am J Ophthalmol* 97: 184–188, 1984.
58. Chaflin J, Putterman AM: Frozen section control in the surgery of basal cell carcinoma of the eyelid. *Ophthalmic Surg* 14: 935–940, 1983.
59. Older JJ, Quickert MH, Beard C: Surgical removal of basal cell carcinoma of the eyelids utilizing frozen-section control. *Trans Am Acad Ophthalmol Otolaryngol* 79: 240–244, 1970.
60. Epstein GA, Putterman AM: Sebaceous adenocarcinoma of the eyelid. *Ophthalmic Surg* 14: 935–940, 1983.
61. Potter M: Percivall Potts' contribution to cancer research. *Natl Cancer Inst Monogr* 10: 1–5, 1963.
62. Hueper WC: Chemically induced skin cancer in man. *Natl Cancer Inst Monogr* 10: 377–391, 1963.
63. Elliot JA, Welton DG: Epithelioma, report on 1,742 treated patients. *Arch Dermatol* 53: 307–332, 1946.
64. Frieben A, cited by Stroll HL: Cancroid des rechten Handruckens nach langdauernder Einwirkung von Rontgenstrahlen. *Fortsch Roentgenstr* 6: 106, 1902.
65. Porter CA, White CJ: Multiple carcinomata following chronic x-ray dermatitis. *Ann Surg* 46: 649–671, 1947.
66. Rowntree CW: Contribution to the study of x-ray carcinoma and the conditions which precede its onset. *Arch Middlesex Hosp (London)* 13: 182–205, 1908.
67. Forrest AW: Tumors following radiation about the eye. *Trans Am Acad Ophthalmol Otolaryngol* 65: 649–771, 1961.
68. Albert DM, McGhee CNJ, Seddon JM, Weichselbaum RR: Development of additional primary tumors after 62 years in the first patient with retinoblastoma cured by radiation therapy. *Am J Ophthalmol* 97: 189–196, 1984.
69. Darier J, Ferrand M: L'Epitheliome pavimenteaux mixte et intermediare. *Ann Dermatol Syphiligr* 3: 385, 1922.
70. Birge HL: Cancer of the eyelids. I. Basal cell and mixed basal cell and squamous cell epithelioma. *Arch Ophthalmol* 19: 700–708, 1938.

71. Ridenhour CE, Spratt JS: Epidermoid carcinoma of the skin involving the parotid gland. *Am J Surg* 112: 504–507, 1966.
72. Swanbeck G, Hillstrom L: Analysis of etiological factors of squamous cell skin cancer of different locations. 4. Concluding remarks. *Acta Dermatol Venereol* (*Stockh*) 51: 151–156, 1971.
73. Stout AP: Malignant manifestations of Bowen's disease. *NY J Med* 39: 801–809, 1939.
74. Kennaway EL: The anatomical distribution of the occupational cancers. *J Indust Hygiene* 7: 69–93, 1925.
75. Lane LA: An occupational study of cancer of the eye and adnexa. *Surg Gynecol Obstet* 64: 458–464, 1937.
76. Doxanas MT, Green WR, Arentsen JJ, Elsas F: Lid lesions of childhood. A histopathologic survey at the Wilmer Institute (1923–1974). *J Pediatr Ophthalmol* 13: 7–39, 1976.
77. Gaasterland DE, Rodrigues MM, Moshell AN: Ocular involvement in xeroderma pigmentosum. *Ophthalmology* 89: 980–986, 1982.
78. Cleaver JE: Defective repair replication of DNA in xeroderma pigmentosum. *Nature* 218: 652–656, 1968.
79. Graham JH, Helwig EB: Bowen's disease and its relationship to systemic cancer. *Arch Dermatol Syphilol* 80: 133–159, 1959.
80. Graham JH, Helwig EB: Bowen's disease and its relationship to systemic cancer. *Arch Dermatol Syphilol* 83: 738–758, 1962.
81. Mustarde JC: Basal cell and squamous cell carcinomas of the orbital region. In Chambers RG, et al (eds): *Cancer of the Head and Neck*. Amsterdam, Excerpta Medica, 1975, p 75.
82. Boniuk M: Differentiation of squamous cell carcinoma from other epithelial tumors of the eyelid. In Boniuk M (ed): *Ocular and Adnexal Tumors. New and Controversial Aspects*. St. Louis, CV Mosby, 1964, ch 3, p 75.
83. Pinkus H, Mehregan AH: *A Guide to Dermatohistopathology*, ed 3. New York, Appleton-Century-Crofts, 1981, p 339.
84. Henkind P, Friedman A: Cancer of the lids and ocular adnexa. In Andrade R. Gumport SL, Popkin GL, Rees TD (eds): *Cancer of the Skin. Biology-Diagnosis-Management*. Philadelphia, WB Saunders, 1976, vol 2, p 1345.
85. Jones LT, Wobig JL: *Surgery of the Eyelids and Lacrimal System*. Birmingham, Alabama, Aesculapius, 1976, p 56.
86. Newman Z, Giladi A: Plea for a radical approach in so-called keratoacanthoma of the eyelid. *Plast Reconstr Surg* 47: 231–233, 1971.
87. Sage HH, Casson PR: Squamous cell carcinoma of the scalp, face and neck. In Andrade R, Gumport SL, Popkin GL, Rees TD (eds): *Cancer of the Skin. Biology-Diagnosis-Management*. Philadelphia, WB Saunders, 1976, vol 2, p 899.
88. Caya JG, Hidayat AA, Weiner JM: A clinicopathologic study of 21 cases of adenoid squamous cell carcinoma of the eyelid and periorbital region. *Am J Ophthalmol* 99: 291–297, 1985.
89. Char DH: The management of lid and conjunctival malignancies. *Surv Ophthalmol* 24: 679–689, 1980.
89a. Reifler DM, Hornblass A: Squamous cell carcinoma of the eyelid. *Surv Ophthalmol* 30: 349–365, 1986.
90. Lever WF, Schaumberg-Lever G: *Histopathology of the Skin*, ed 5. Philadelphia, JB Lippincott, 1975, p 537.
91. Borders AC: Practical points on the microscopic grading of carcinoma. *NY J Med* 32: 667–671, 1932.
92. McCord CD, Cavanagh HD: Microscopic features and biologic behavior of eyelid tumors. *Ophthal Surg* 11: 671–681, 1980.
93. Henderson JW: *Orbital Tumors*, ed 2. New York, Thieme-Stratton, 1980, ch 16, p 425.
94. Mohs FE, Lathrop TG: Modes of spread of cancer of the skin. *Arch Dermatol Syphilol* 66: 427–439, 1952.
95. Trobe JD, Hood CI, Parsons JT, Quisling RG: Intracranial spread of squamous cell carcinoma along the trigeminal nerve. *Arch Ophthalmol* 100: 608–611, 1982.
96. Beard C: Observations on the treatment of basal cell carcinoma of the eyelid. *Trans Am Acad Ophthalmol Otolaryngol* 79: 664–670, 1975.
97. Beard C: Management of malignancy of eyelids. *Am J Ophthalmol* 92: 1–6, 1981.
98. Callahan A: Letter. *Surv Ophthalmol* 25: 409, 1981.
99. Dixon RS, Mikhail GR, Slater HC: Sebaceous carcinoma of the eyelid. *J Am Acad Dermatol* 3: 241–243, 1980.
100. Harvey JT, Anderson RL: Management of meibomian gland carcinoma. *Ophthal Surg* 13: 56–61, 1982.
101. Hornblass A (ed): *Tumors of the Ocular Adnexa and Orbit*. St. Louis, CV Mosby, 1979.
102. Fraunfelder FT, Zacarian SA, Limmer BL, Wingfield DL: Cryosurgery for malignancy of the eyelid. *Ophthalmology* 87: 461–465, 1980.
103. Fraunfelder FT: The indications and contraindications of cryosurgery. *Arch Opthalmol* 96: 729, 1978.
104. Klein E: Tumors of the skin. IX. Local cystostatic therapy of cutaneous and mucosal premalignant and malignant lesions. *NY J Med* 65: 888–889, 1968.
105. Fulton JE et al: Treatment of Bowen's disease with topical 5-fluorouracil under occlusion. *Arch Dermatol* 97: 170, 1968.
106. Stoll HL: Squamous cell carcinoma. In Halm F (ed): *Cancer Dermatology*. Philadelphia, Lea & Febiger 1979, p 113.
107. Belisario JC: 5-Fluorouracil (5-FU) and other cytotoxic agents. Topical use. In Maddin S (ed): *Current Dermatologic Management*, ed 2. St. Louis, CV Mosby, 1975.
108. New GB, Benedict WL: Radium in the treatment of diseases of the eye and adnexa. *Am J Ophthalmol* 3: 244–250, 1920.
109. Williams AC, Klein E: Experience with local chemotherapy and immunotherapy in premalignant skin lesions. *Cancer* 25: 450–462, 1970.
110. Dougherty TJ: Photoradiation therapy for cutaneous and subcutaneous malignancies. *J Invest Dermatol* 77: 122–124, 1981.
111. Rathbun JE, Beard C, Quickert MH: Evaluation of 48 cases of orbital exerteration. *Am J Ophthalmol* 72: 191–199, 1971.
112. Simons JN, Robinson DW, Masters FW: Malignant tumors of the orbit and periorbital structures treated by exenteration. *Plast Reconstr Surg* 37: 100–104, 1966.

CHAPTER 26

Sebaceous Gland Tumors of the Eyelid

DAVID M. REIFLER, M.D.
ALBERT HORNBLASS, M.D.

True neoplasms of sebaceous gland origin rarely occur in the eyelid (1–10). This is in direct contrast to inflammatory conditions, such as chalazion (11), that are commonly seen in daily clinical ophthalmologic practice. The different types of sebaceous gland lesions therefore range from the most common to the most rare. The clinical and pathologic features of the entities, eyelid sebaceous carcinoma (1–10, 12–28) and sebaceous adenoma (3, 29), have been well described. Sebaceous carcinoma of the lid is an aggressive, malignant neoplasm with metastatic and lethal potential that accounts for approximately 1–2% of all eyelid malignancies (4, 30, 31). Although sebaceous adenoma has received relatively less attention, the presence of such a lesion may be of significant prognostic importance, particularly when associated with visceral malignancy (Muir-Torre syndrome) (29, 32). The sebaceous glands of the ocular adnexa that may give rise to neoplasms include meibomian glands, the glands of Zeis, and those glands associated with fine hairs of the eyelid surface (5). The meibomian gland is the most common primary site for the occurrence of sebaceous carcinoma among these different locations (9), but the origin may be multicentric (15, 18) or obscured by diffuse growth (6). In most cases, sebaceous carcinoma of the lid is initially misdiagnosed as it may simulate recurrent chalazia (1, 2, 5, 13, 19) or chronic blepharoconjunctivitis (15, 25), basal cell or squamous cell carcinoma (31), or orbital tumor (5, 19).

HISTORY

According to Ginsberg (4), the earliest report of sebaceous carcinoma was given by Thiersch in 1865, although others (1, 3) have generally credited Allaire, whose case report was not published until 1891. Ginsberg noted that "early reports were marked by confusion of terminology, uncertainty of interpretation, and an apparent reluctance to consider the lesion malignant." The first report of a sebaceous carcinoma of the lid in the American literature was probably given by Knapp (33) in 1901. Despite diffuse infiltration that required removal of the patient's entire upper lid, Knapp referred to this lesion as an "adenoma." The view that all meibomian gland tumors should be classified as "adenomas" rather than "carcinomas" was also quite widespread in Europe until the earlier part of this century (4). This is exemplified in von Michel's contribution to the Graefe-Saemisch handbook (1908) in which he expressed his doubts about the existence of eyelid sebaceous carcinoma (34); this opinion was carried over by other authors in subsequent revisions of this text (1). However, the malignant nature of these tumors was soon recognized by others such as Van Duyse (35) and Scheerer (36) in 1914, and later by Morax (37) in 1926. The separation of eyelid sebaceous carcinomas from benign sebaceous adenomas was subsequently emphasized by Lebensohn (38), Hagedoorn (1, 39), and others (4).

The various clinical appearances of sebaceous carcinoma such as chalazion and blepharoconjunctivitis were first emphasized in the 1930s by Hagedoorn (1, 39) and others (2, 4). Recognition of the various clinicopathologic features of sebaceous carcinoma has substantially reduced tumor morbidity and mortality.

The contributions of authors that have stressed the occasional association of sebaceous gland neoplasms with multiple visceral carcinomas should also be noted. This interesting finding was first reported independently by Muir and associates (40) and Torre (41) in 1968. Since these original descriptions, at least 25 more cases of the Muir-Torre syndrome have been reported (32). A predisposition to malignancy in family members of patients with the Muir-Torre syndrome has also been noted (42), and the occurrence of this syndrome with sebaceous gland tumors of the lid was first reported by Jakobiec (29) in 1974 (a case of sebaceous adenoma originating in a meibomian gland). A case of sebaceous carcinoma of the lid that was associated with the Muir-Torre syndrome was recently reported by Finan and Connolly (32). Other investigators, although aware of the Muir-Torre syndrome, have not found an association between sebaceous carcinoma of the lid and multiple visceral carcinoma (7).

INCIDENCE

In series of true sebaceous tumors of the eyelids, sebaceous adenoma comprises a much smaller percentage of cases than sebaceous carcinoma. Rao and associates (6) found 154 sebaceous carcinomas compared with 26 cases of adenomas and hyperplasias of eyelid sebaceous glands. Obviously the incidence of true benign sebaceous eyelid tumors may be higher than reported because of a selection bias for aggressively malignant tumors among the reporting referral institutions.

The relative incidence of sebaceous carcinoma among all eyelid malignancies has been variously reported, although most series in Europe and North America place this figure between 1 and 5.5% (4, 7, 10, 30, 31, 37). The rarity of this lesion may account for its absence even in large series of eyelid carcinomas, either because of statistical chance or a lack of recognition. For example, in a report of 149 eyelid carcinomas reported by Martin (43) in 1939, there was not one case of sebaceous carcinoma.

Sebaceous carcinoma of the lid is worldwide in distribution (3), but there appears to be a significant difference in the reported incidence between the Eastern and Western hemispheres (4, 10). In a collaborative study of eyelid malignancies from Boston, Massachusetts and Shanghai, China (10), the relatively increased incidence of sebaceous carcinoma in Orientals was strikingly emphasized. In the Boston population, sebaceous carcinoma accounted for 1.5% of all eyelid malignancies, while in the Shanghai population, the incidence of eyelid sebaceous carcinoma was 32.7%. The relative incidence of basal cell carcinoma in the Boston group was 92.5%, but in Shanghai the incidence was found to be only 42%.

Sebaceous carcinoma of the lid predominantly occurs in adults between the 4th and 10th decades, with the average age being about 65 years (9). Exceptionally rare cases have been reported in children (1, 3, 44) and adolescents (5, 10, 45). In larger series the lesion has been found to be about 1½ to 2 times more common in women that in men (9, 10), and this appears to be true in both Caucasian and Oriental populations.

PATHOPHYSIOLOGY

ETIOLOGY

The etiology of sebaceous gland tumors is unknown, but the relatively increased incidence of eyelid sebaceous carcinoma in the elderly is a characteristic that is seen in other cutaneous and visceral carcinomas. Genetic factors also appear to be important in view of the increased incidence of sebaceous carcinoma in Orientals (4, 8, 10). A prior history of radiation therapy has been present in some cases (5, 21, 45–47). This may reflect the interaction of both environmental and genetic factors, since these cases have been noted in retinoblastoma survivors (see below). However, in some instances of eyelid sebaceous neoplasms the history of radiation therapy may be remote or vague. In a series of 12 cases of sebaceous carcinoma of the lid that were recently reviewed at the Manhattan Eye, Ear, and Throat Hospital, we found two elderly patients (one male and one female) who had radiation treatments for benign skin conditions many years previously (unpublished data). Schlernitzaur and Font (21) also described a case of eyelid sebaceous carcinoma many years following radiation therapy for a benign condition.

Other cases of sebaceous carcinoma of the lid following prior regional radiation therapy have been reported to occur in younger individuals. Three of these cases were putatively induced by radiation therapy for bilateral retinoblastoma (5, 45, 46). At the time of presentation of the eyelid malignancies, the ages of these retinoblastoma survivors were 12, 13, and 30 years, with a latent period from the initial treatment that ranged from 10 to 19 years. The first of these cases, reported by Boniuk and Zimmerman (5), developed in a 13-year-old girl who previously had local x-ray treatments on the same side for bilateral retinoblastoma at the age of 1 year. These authors also reviewed a similar case of a 30-year-old woman that had been reported previously by Forrest (46). In the latter case, radiation for retinoblastoma had been given at 4 years of age, and the authors were able to reinterpret this "unclassified malignant tumor of the orbit and eyelid" as sebaceous carcinoma. Lemos and associates (45) reported a third case of eyelid sebaceous carcinoma in a 12-year-old boy that followed radiation therapy for retinoblastoma given early in childhood. More recently, Wolfe and associates (47) found a 12% prevalence of a previous exposure to irradiation in patients with sebaceous carcinoma of the eyelid.

As previously mentioned, sebaceous carcinoma of the lid may also be seen many years following radiation therapy for benign conditions. The first such case, reported by Schlernitzaur and Font (21), was that of a 35-year-old woman who received multiple radiation treatments between the ages of 6 months and 15 years for an extensive cavernous hemangioma of the left side of the face. Multiple lesions later developed within areas of radiodermatitis, including squamous cell carcinoma of the labial commissure of the left upper and lower eyelids which required orbital exenteration at the age of 36 years.

CLINICAL PRESENTATION

Sebaceous adenoma of the lid most commonly arises in the meibomian gland (3, 29). Because there are more meibomian glands in the upper than in the lower eyelid, it is not surprising that this lesion more frequently affects the upper lid. Sebaceous adenomas of the lid begin insidiously as a painless nontender lump arising within the tarsus. The gradual enlargement may produce thickening and distortion of the lid that may be misdiagnosed and treated as a chalazion, and incomplete excision may lead to local recurrence (3, 29). Multiple cutaneous lesions or visceral malignancy may also be associated (Muir-Torre syndrome) (29).

The clinical presentation of sebaceous carcinoma of the lid shows great variability and frequently results in misdiagnosis (1, 2, 5, 17, 19, 25, 28). The most common presentation is that of an enlarging mass. In most cases, especially those of meibomian origin, the tarsus and deeper structures of the eyelid are involved and there is little evidence of erosion or ulceration of the skin (Fig. 26.1) (5). Meibomian carcinoma invariably causes a loss of definition of the meibomian gland orifices (Fig. 26.2) (48). When tumors arise entirely or in part from the glands of Zeis, a loss of lashes invariably occurs (Fig. 26.1), sometimes with an ulceration of the lid margin (Fig. 26.3) (5), a papillomatous outgrowth, (10) or, rarely, a cutaneous horn (5, 17). Many sebaceous carcinomas arise simultaneously from both the glands of Zeis and the meibomian glands, and there may even be concurrent involvement of the upper and lower lids (5, 15, 18). On the other hand, involvement of the lid margin may be a sign of an advanced meibomian carcinoma that eventually results in a gross distortion of the lid (3). In the early stages, the pretarsal skin can be freely moved over the lesion.

When viewed through the conjunctiva, the yellow-white color of a sebaceous carcinoma in the meibomian gland may become apparent and a lobular architecture of the tumor may be discerned. Follicular changes are frequently seen adjacent to the mass (23). Ulcerative changes in the conjunctival sac that may occur may also lead to a proliferating mass on the inner surface of the lid (3).

METASTASIS AND EXTENSION

The most frequent evidence of metastasis is enlargement of the preauricular lymph nodes, parotid gland, or cervical lymph nodes (26). The incidence of lymph node metastasis is about 17% (4) to 23% (9) in larger series. Metastasis to preauricular lymph nodes usually occurs 3 months to 6 years after excision of the tumor (6), often associated with recurrence of the primary tumor (4). Even though the primary lid tumor may be small, a huge preauricular mass may develop. Occasionally, parotid lymph nodes with metastasis may present clinically as parotid tumors. Other sites of distant metastases include lung, liver, and brain (9, 12, 50).

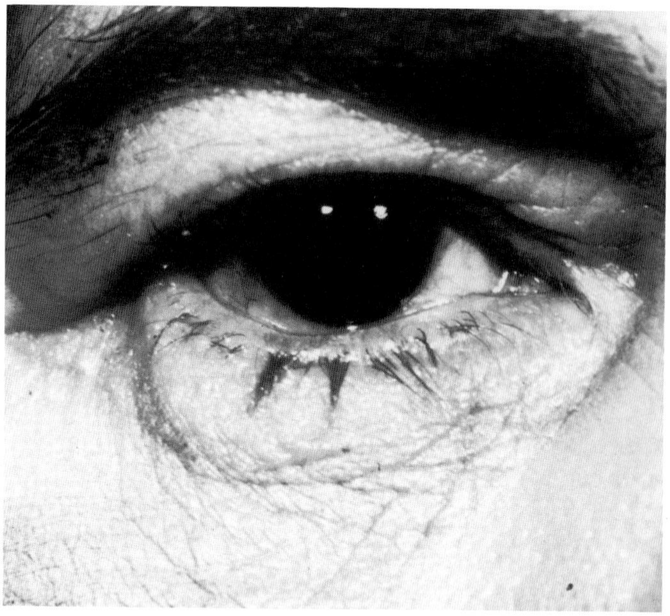

Figure 26.1. A 55-year-old woman with sebaceous carcinoma of the right lower lid. The patient was treated six times for "recurrent chalazion" until a biopsy was taken. The thickened and nontender tissue showed no gross involvement of the overlying epidermis although the lash line showed focal areas of alopecia. (Courtesy of Murray Meltzer, M.D.)

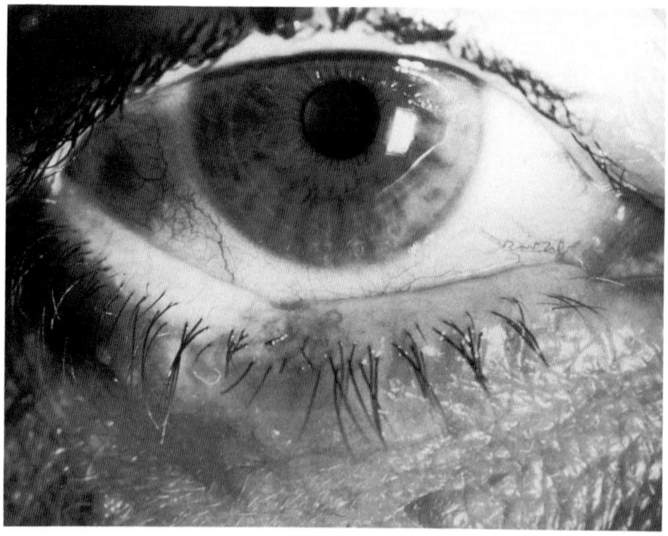

Figure 26.2. A 65-year-old man with sebaceous carcinoma of the right lower lid. Involvement of the lid margin was present with notching and destruction of the meibomian gland orifices.

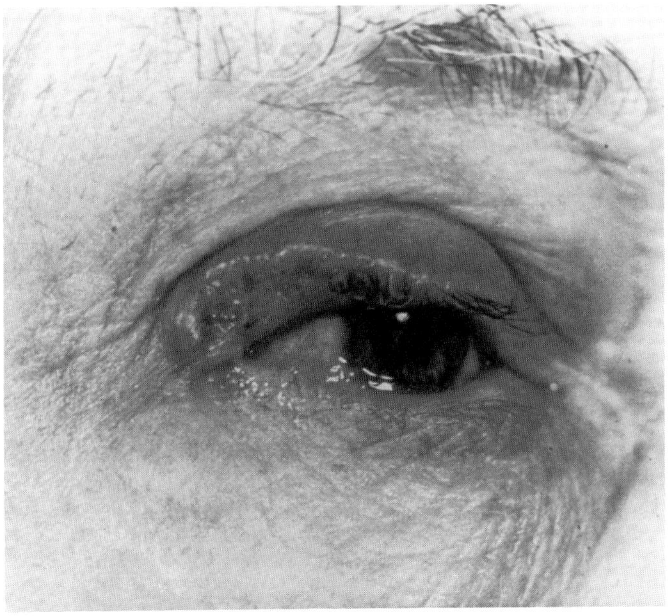

Figure 26.3. A 78-year-old man had had two chalazion excisions of the right upper lid prior to a biopsy which revealed sebaceous carcinoma. There was extensive involvement of the lid margin with ulceration that correlated microscopically with extensive pagetoid spread. (Courtesy of Murray Meltzer, M.D.)

Orbital extension of eyelid sebaceous carcinoma occurs in about 6–16% of cases (4, 9) and may even be the main presenting feature (10, 19). Orbital extension is seen in a high percentage of cases with recurrence and is associated with increased mortality rate of up to 76% (9). Orbital invasion is particularly seen in advanced cases. However, a small primary tumor may be overlooked until it spreads into the orbit or lacrimal gland (19). Intracranial extension may also occur with erosion of the orbit (24).

MORTALITY

Sebaceous carcinoma is perhaps the most lethal of all eyelid neoplasms. Overall mortality rates ranging between 23% (9) and 41% (8) have been reported. The rather high mortality rate of 41% reported by Ni and Kuo (8) probably reflects a higher incidence of advanced cases in their series, or perhaps a more aggressive course in Orientals. Recognition of the various histopathologic features of sebaceous carcinoma and the institution of prompt, definitive therapy have substantially reduced tumor morbidity and mortality. In a series of sebaceous carcinoma from the Wilmer Institute covering a 58-year period, there was a 24% mortality prior to 1970 but no tumor-related deaths in patients seen after 1970 (51).

At the Armed Forces Institute of Pathology (AFIP), Rao and associates (9) identified various clinicopathologic features of sebaceous carcinoma that were associated with a bad prognosis. These included vascular, lymphatic, and orbital invasion; involvement of both upper and lower eyelids; poor differentiation; multicentric origin; duration of symptoms greater than 6 months; tumor diameter exceeding 10 mm; a highly infiltrative pattern; and pagetoid invasion of the overlying epithelia of the eyelids.

In the AFIP series (9), sebaceous carcinoma of the upper lid had a 28% mortality, but none of the patients with lower lid tumors died. In cases with involvement of both the upper and lower lids, the mortality rate rose to 83%, primarily because of the extensive and perhaps multicentric involvement. Although multicentric origin of carcinoma in both the meibomian glands and the glands of Zeis had an extremely high mortality rate, sebaceous carcinomas arising from only the glands of Zeis had an excellent prognosis, with no fatalities among seven cases (9).

The need for prompt recognition of sebaceous carcinoma cannot be overly emphasized, since the prognosis is dramatically affected by the duration of symptoms prior to excision (7, 9). In those patients who had symptoms longer than 6 months, the mortality almost tripled (9). Features that are interrelated to the duration of symptoms include tumor size, extension, and metastasis, and each of these have been correlated with prognosis. Clinical series that have enjoyed the advantages of prompt referral have yielded low incidences of mortality (51, 52).

HISTOPATHOLOGY

While this chapter emphasizes the clinical features of eyelid sebaceous gland tumors, certain histopathologic features are well worth mentioning. The reader is referred to the various standard textbooks on ophthalmic pathology for a more detailed presentation of illustrative photomicrographs. Distinguishing between sebaceous hyperplasia and sebaceous adenoma may be extremely difficult, but in the former case, the architecture of the sebaceous glands remains normal except for increased cellularity in both the ducts and acini with a greatly increased number of acini surrounding each duct (Fig. 26.4) (3). However, the absence of ducts does not necessarily exclude the diagnosis of adenoma (1). The main feature that charac-

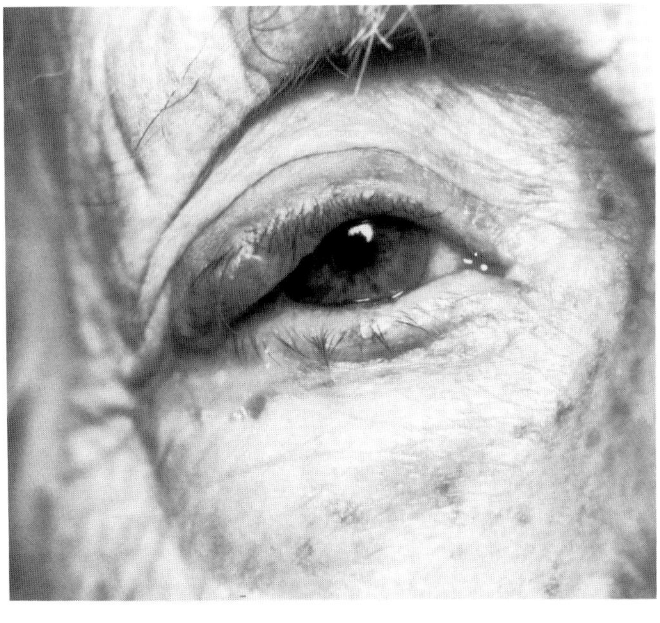

Figure 26.4. A 72-year-old with recurrent chalazion with biopsy proven sebaceous gland carcinoma.

terizes a sebaceous lesion as neoplastic is the loss of central ductules and the loss of the parallel linear organization of the acini. The presence of islands of keratin-producing cells is seen in different types of carcinomas, including squamous cell, basal cell, and sebaceous types (10), but is probably inconsistent with a diagnosis of adenoma (1).

Histologically, sebaceous carcinoma displays a loss of orderly differentiation with excessive mitotic activity and tendency for invasiveness. The constituent neoplastic cells exhibit all degrees of differentiation. In the more differentiated areas, cells continue to be arranged in sheets or acinar formation. Straatsma (3) noted morphologic variations of sebaceous carcinoma including those with (*a*) giant lobules, (*b*) extensive sheets, (*c*) thick cords, or (*d*) diffusely scattered cells. Rao and associates (6) classified histologic patterns as (*a*) lobular, (*b*) comedocarcinoma, (*c*) papillary, and (*d*) combined forms. However, both of these studies found a lack of correlation between these histologic patterns and the prognosis.

In contrast to the relative unimportance of the above morphologic variations, other features of cellular differentiation in sebaceous carcinoma appears to affect the prognosis. Rao and associates (9) classified sebaceous carcinoma as "well differentiated," "moderately differentiated," and "poorly differentiated," and in these three groups of patients, the mortality rates were 9%, 30%, and 60% respectively. These authors did not find a significantly higher mortality among patients with tumors showing squamous or basal cell differentiation. Ni and Kuo (8) also found that better-differentiated tumors were the least malignant, but they also noted that tumors with significant squamous cell or basal cell differentiation were more aggressive. The criteria for grading the degree of differentiation of sebaceous carcinoma as described by Wolfe and associates (47) are listed in Table 26.1.

Table 26.1
Criteria for Grading Degree of Differentiation of Sebaceous Carcinomas[a]

Grade	Criteria
1	Well differentiated; foamy cytoplasm in all cells
2	Large vacuolated nuclei and foamy cytoplasm in most cells
3	Small hyperchromatic nuclei and little cytoplasm in most cells
4	Undifferentiated; small hyperchromatic nuclei and little cytoplasm; diagnosis requires positive fat stain, ultrastructural study, or areas of better differentiation

[a] From Wolfe JT, Yeatts RP, Wick MR, Campbell RJ, Waller RR: Sebaceous carcinoma of the eyelid. Errors in clinical diagnosis. *Am J Surg Pathol* 8: 579–606, 1984.

The tendency for sebaceous carcinoma to invade the overlying epidermis produces a change resembling Paget's disease (5). The pagetoid change of the epidermis resembles intraepidermal squamous cell carcinoma. However, in contrast to squamous cell carcinoma, pagetoid change will show intervening epidermal cells that are benign (11). The pagetoid spread of malignant cells has been reviewed by many authors (5, 15, 19, 24, 31) and is associated with a very poor prognosis (9, 27). Clinically, pagetoid spread may produce a generalized thickening and inflammation of the lids (15), or may even extend onto the corneal epithelium (49). Because of the potential for a multicentric origin and/or pagetoid spread, multiple biopsy sites are recommended in cases where the clinical suspicion is high (48). Even so, the diagnosis may be missed (25, 47, 48) and full-thickness eyelid biopsies may be necessary to make the correct diagnosis (5).

TREATMENT, RESULTS, AND COMPLICATIONS

In most cases of sebaceous carcinoma of the lid (Fig. 26.5), histologically controlled surgical extirpation of the tumor is recommended (7, 23, 48, 52, 53). Wide local excision with standard frozen section control can give excellent results (23, 52), particularly when the tumor is small and the symptoms have been present for less than 6 months. Even with frozen section control, wide local excision should include at least 5–6 mm of normal tissue at the resection margin and may entail the removal of the entire tarsal plate. Using these methods combined with immediate oculoplastic reconstruction in 11 consecutive patients, Epstein and Putterman (52) found no regional or distant metastases and only one instance of local recurrence with an average follow-up of 68 months. The sole patient with local recurrence was one of three in that series who had pagetoid spread identified histologically. Other series, such as those from the AFIP, undoubtedly had a higher incidence of pagetoid change and advanced cases.

Some authors advocate a Mohs' fresh-tissue excision technique in the treatment of eyelid sebaceous carcinoma (7, 48, 53), since a physician experienced with this technique can "examine all tissue planes to determine whether or not a tumor has extended beyond the excision plane" (48). To date, there are no controlled studies comparing the relative effectiveness of wide excision with frozen-section control versus Mohs' fresh-tissue excision technique. With either method, histologic studies of the surgical margins may not be reliable because of the possibility of noncontiguous spread, multicentric origin or subclinical metastasis at the time of excision. In this light, Callahan and Callahan (7) stated that "when sebaceous carcinoma of the upper lid has been present for more than six months and certainly as long as several years, marginal studies are valueless and exenteration is the only safe treatment." Other authors (54) reserve exenteration for tumors not limited to the eyelid. Other methods of treatment including primary radiation therapy (49) and cryotherapy (55) are more controversial and probably should be reserved for those patients who cannot tolerate or who refuse surgery.

According to Doxanas and Green (51), lymph node biopsy should be performed in cases of suspected regional metastasis. This will differentiate instances of inflammatory enlargement from true lymph node metastasis. A radical neck dissection is indicated in the presence of enlarged preauricular or cervical lymph nodes with biopsy-proven metastasis.

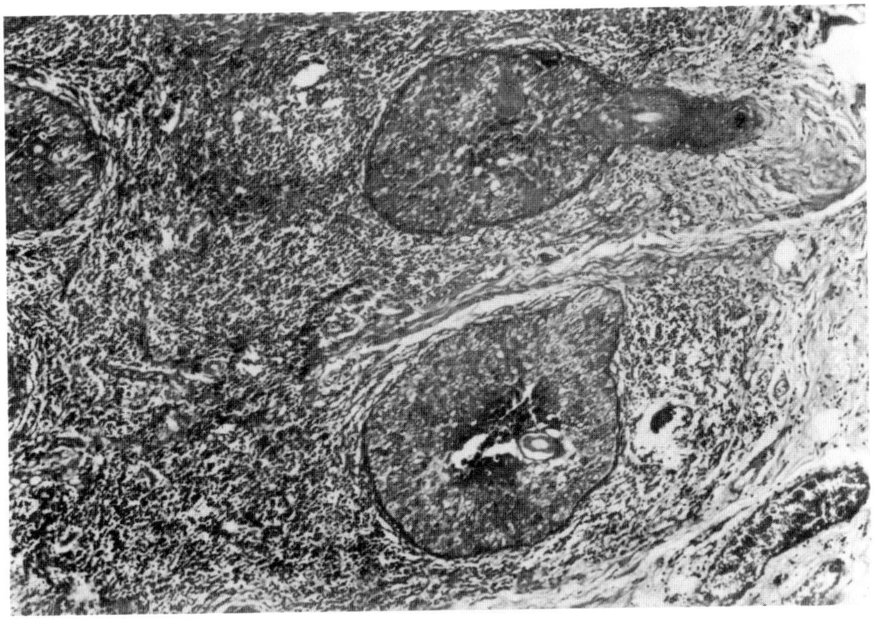

Figure 26.5. Sebaceous carcinoma displays a loss of orderly differentiation with excessive mitotic activity.

Those authors who have advocated radiation therapy in the treatment of sebaceous carcinoma of the eyelid have reserved this mode of therapy for recurrences or metastases following initial surgical excision (26). Other authors have recommended consideration of radiation therapy as a primary treatment (49, 56). Recurrences following radiation therapy are commonly seen and the prognosis following radiation therapy is probably worse than that following surgical excision (6). Nunery and associates (54) reported six cases of meibomian gland carcinoma that had recurrences 2 months to 2 years following primary radiation therapy at a relatively early stage, with dosages ranging from 3300 to 11,400 rads. Radiation therapy for sebaceous carcinoma of the lid should therefore be reserved for patients who refuse surgery and those who cannot withstand anesthesia (48, 54).

Cryotherapy has been mentioned in the treatment of sebaceous carcinoma, with treatment consisting of liquid nitrogen application (55). Apparently, only a few cases of sebaceous carcinoma have been treated in this manner, and none of the cases have been described in detail. Because of the potential for metastasis and lethality, this form of therapy is not recommended.

CONCLUSION

Sebaceous neoplasms of the eyelid may arise in the meibomian glands, the glands of Zeis and those glands associated with fine hairs of the eyelid surface. Sebaceous adenoma is a rare benign neoplasm that typically presents in the lid as a solitary, yellowish nodule and histologically displays increased numbers of sebaceous cells in irregularly shaped lobules.

Sebaceous carcinoma is a rare but aggressive malignant neoplasm with metastatic and lethal potential that accounts for approximately 1–2% of all eyelid malignancies. This tumor may be found with greater frequency in Orientals. Sebaceous carcinoma may masquerade as a blepharoconjunctivitis, blepharitis, chalazion or lacrimal gland tumor, which results in misdiagnosis and delay in definitive treatment. A multicentric origin and pagetoid spread are among the factors that adversely affect the prognosis. Various factors improve the prognosis greatly, including an early diagnosis and excision when the lesion is small and well differentiated. Ophthalmologists must therefore be constantly vigilant and prepared to perform adequate biopsies for all suspected lesions. Stains for fat in fresh-frozen tissue may reveal intracytoplasmic lipid droplets and help to confirm the diagnosis. The treatment of choice is complete surgical extirpation of the tumor with histologically controlled methods.

ACKNOWLEDGMENTS

Dr. Murray Meltzer provided photographs and clinical summaries for Figures 26.1 and 26.3. Cathy H. Reifler reviewed and proofread the manuscript, and Rebecca McCrumb typed the manuscript.

REFERENCES

1. Hagedoorn A: Adenocarcinoma of meibomian glands. *Arch Ophthalmol* 12: 850–866, 1934.
2. Knapp, A: In discussion of O'Brien CS, Braley, AE: Common tumors of the eyelids. *JAMA* 107: 937, 1936.
3. Straatsma BR: Meibomian gland tumors. *Arch Ophthalmol* 56: 71–93, 1956.
4. Ginsberg J: Present status of Meibomian gland carcinoma. *Arch Ophthalmol* 73: 271–277, 1965.
5. Boniuk M, Zimmerman L: Sebaceous carcinoma of the eyelid, eye, caruncle and orbit. *Trans Am Acad Ophthalmol* 72: 619–642, 1968.
6. Rao NA, McLean IW, Zimmerman LE: Sebaceous carcinoma of the eyelid and caruncle: Correlation of clinicopathologic features with prognosis. In Jakobiec FA (ed): *Ocular and Adnexal Tumors*. Birmingham, AL, Aesculapius, 1978, p 461.
7. Callahan M, Callahan A: Sebaceous gland carcinoma. In Jakobiec, FA (ed): *Ocular and Adnexal Tumors*. Birmingham, AL, Aesculapius, 1978, p 477.
8. Ni C, Kuo P: Meibomian gland carcinoma: a clinical pathological study of 156 cases with long-term follow-up of 100 cases. *Jpn J Ophthalmol* 23: 388–401, 1979.
9. Rao NA, Hidayat AA, McLean IW, Zimmerman LE: Sebaceous

carcinoma of the ocular adnexa a clinicopathologic study of 104 cases with a five-year follow-up. *Hum Pathol* 13: 113–122, 1982.
10. Ni C, Searl SS, Kuo PK, Chu FR, Chong CS, Albert DM: Sebaceous carcinomas of the ocular adnexa. *Int Ophthalmol Clin* 23: 23–61, 1982.
11. Yanoff M, Fine BS: *Ocular Pathology: A Text and Atlas.* Hagerstown, MD, Harper & Row, 1975, p 217.
12. Magnus JA: Adenocarcinoma of meibomian gland with secondaries in the liver. *Trans Ophthalmol Soc UK* 67: 432–435, 1947.
13. Rice ML, Lindeke HT: Adenocarcinoma of the meibomian gland. *Am J Ophthalmol* 33: 1434–1437, 1950.
14. Sweebe EC, Cogan DG: Adenocarcinoma of the meibomian gland. A pseudochalazion entity. *Arch Ophthalmol* 61: 282–290, 1959.
15. Scheie HG, Yanoff M, Frayer WC: Carcinoma of sebaceous glands of the eyelid. *Arch Ophthalmol* 61: 282–290, 1959.
16. Taylor RP, Lehman JA: Sebaceous adenocarcinoma of Meibomian gland. Presentation of a case and review of the literature. *Arch Ophthalmol* 82: 66–68, 1969.
17. Brauninger GE, Hood CI, Worthen DM: Sebaceous carcinoma of the lid margin masquerading as a cutaneous horn. *Arch Ophthalmol* 90: 380–381, 1973.
18. Cavanagh HD, Green WR, Goldberg HK: Multicentric sebaceous adenocarcinoma of the meibomian gland. *Am J Ophthalmol* 77: 326–337, 1974.
19. Shields JA, Font RL: Meibomian gland carcinoma presenting as a lacrimal gland tumor. *Arch Ophthalmol* 92: 304–306, 1974.
20. Weigent CE, Staley NA: Meibomian gland carcinoma report of a case with electron microscope findings. *Hum Pathol* 7: 231–234, 1976.
21. Schlernitzauer DA, Font RL: Sebaceous gland carcinoma of the eyelid following radiation therapy for cavernous hemangioma of the face. *Arch Ophthalmol* 95: 2203–2204, 1977.
22. Reese AB: *Tumors of the Eye,* ed 3. Hagerstown, MD, Harper & Row, 1976, p 41.
23. Tenzel RR, Stewart WB, Boynton JR, Zbar M: Sebaceous carcinoma of the eyelid. Definition of surgical margins. *Arch Ophthalmol* 95: 2203–2204, 1977.
24. Bryant J: Meibomian gland carcinoma seeding intracranial soft tissues. *Hum Pathol* 8: 455–457, 1977.
25. Foster CS, Allansmith MR: Chronic unilateral blepharoconjunctivitis caused by sebaceous carcinoma. *Am J Ophthalmol* 86: 218–220, 1978.
26. Maniglia AJ: Meibomian gland adenocarcinoma of the eyelid with neck metastases. *Laryngoscope* 88: 1421–1426, 1978.
27. Russell WG, Page DL, Hough AJ, Rogers LW: Sebaceous carcinoma of meibomian gland origin. The diagnostic importance of pagetoid spread of neoplastic cells. *Am J Clin Pathol* 73: 504–511, 1980.
28. Wagoner MD, Beyer CK, Gonder JR, Albert DM: Common presentation of sebaceous gland carcinoma of the eyelid. *Ann Ophthalmol* 14: 159–163, 1982.
29. Jakobiec FA: Sebaceous adenoma of the eyelid and visceral malignancy. *Am J Ophthalmol* 78: 952–960, 1974.
30. Welch RB, Duke JR: Lesions of the lids: A statistical note. *Am J Ophthalmol* 45: 415–416, 1964.
31. Kwitko ML, Boniuk M, Zimmerman LE: Eyelid tumors with reference to lesions confused with squamous cell carcinoma. I. Incidence and errors in diagnosis. *Arch Ophthalmol* 69: 693–697, 1963.
32. Finan MC, Connolly, SM: Sebaceous gland tumors and systemic disease: A clinicopathologic analysis. *Medicine* 63: 232–242, 1984.
33. Knapp H: A case of adenoma of the meibomian glands with a synopsis of what is known of that kind of tumor. *Trans Am Ophthalmol Soc* 9: 328–331, 1901.
34. Von Michel J: In Saemisch T (ed): *Handbuch der gesamten Augenheilkunde,* ed 2. Leipzig, W. Engelmann, 1908, vol 5, p 321.
35. Van Duyse GM: Carcinome pavimenteux non keratinisant adenomatode de la glande de Meibomius. *Arch Ophthal (Paris)* 39: 355–372, 1914.
36. Scheerer, R: Ein Beitrag zur Kenntnis der Geschwulste der Meibomschen Drusen. *Klin Mbl Augenheilk* 52: 86–99, 1914.
37. Morax V: *Cancer de l'Appareil Visuel.* Paris, Gaston Doin & Cie, 1926, p 101.
38. Lebensohn JE: Primary carcinoma of meibomian gland. *Am J Ophthalmol* 18: 552–554, 1935.
39. Hagedoorn A: Adenocarcinoma of meibomian gland: Report of additional cases. *Arch Ophthalmol* 18: 50–56, 1937.
40. Muir EG, Bell AJY, Barlow KA: Multiple primary carcinomata of the colon, duodenum, and larynx associated with kerato-acanthoma of the face. *Br J Surg* 54: 191–197, 1967.
41. Torre D: Multiple sebaceous tumors. *Arch Dermatol* 98: 549, 1968.
42. Bakker PM, Tjon A Joe SS: Multiple sebaceous gland tumors of internal organs. A new syndrome? *Dermatologica* 142: 50–57, 1971.
43. Martin HE: Cancer of the eyelids. *Arch Ophthalmol* 41: 616–624, 1939.
44. Knapp H: On hypertrophy and degeneration of Meibomian glands. *Trans Am Ophthalmol Soc* 10: 57–63, 1903.
45. Lemos LB, Santa Cruz DJ, Baba N: Sebaceous carcinoma of the eyelid following radiation therapy. *Am J Surg Pathol* 2: 305–311, 1978.
46. Forrest AW: Tumors following radiation about the eye. *Trans Am Acad Ophthalmol Otolaryngol* 65: 694–717, 1961.
47. Wolfe JT, Yeatts RP, Wick MR, Campbell RJ, Waller RR: Sebaceous carcinoma of the eyelid. Errors in clinical diagnosis. *Am J Surg Pathol* 8: 597–606, 1984.
48. Harvey JT, Anderson RL: The management of meibomian gland carcinoma. *Ophthal Surg* 13: 56–61, 1982.
49. Hendley RL, Rieser JC, Cavanagh HD, Bodner BI, Waring GO: Primary radiation therapy for Meibomian gland carcinoma. *Am J Ophthalmol* 87: 206–209, 1979.
50. Gowey RJ, Kern WH: Metastasizing adenocarcinomas of the tarsal glands. *Calif Med* 103: 126–130, 1965.
51. Doxanas MT, Green WR: Sebaceous gland carcinoma. Review of 40 cases. *Arch Ophthalmol* 102: 245–249, 1984.
52. Epstein GA, Putterman AM: Sebaceous adenocarcinoma of the eyelid. *Ophthalmic Surg* 14: 935–940, 1983.
53. Dixon RS, Mikhail GR, Slater HC: Sebaceous carcinoma of the eyelid. *J Am Acad Dermatol* 3: 241–243, 1980.
54. Nunery WR, Welsh MG, McCord CD: Recurrence of sebaceous carcinoma of the eyelid after radiation therapy. *Am J Ophthalmol* 96: 10–15, 1983.
55. Fraunfelder FT, Zacarian SA, Wingfield DL, Limmer BL: Results of cryotherapy for eyelid malignancies. *Am J Ophthalmol* 97: 184–188, 1984.
56. Ide CH, Ridings GR, Yamashita T, Buesseler JA: Radiotherapy of a recurrent adenocarcinoma of the meibomian gland. *Arch Ophthalmol* 79: 540–544, 1968.

CHAPTER 27

Sweat Gland and Skin Appendage Tumors of the Eyelid

JACK CHALFIN, M.D.

Sweat gland tumors are classified according to their origin from either apocrine or eccrine glands. Benign and malignant varieties of each type of sweat gland tumor are found on the eyelids. Neoplasms of the apocrine glands are very rare. Tumors of the eccrine sweat glands and ducts are more common. Most of these tumors are benign.

ECCRINE TUMORS

SYRINGOMA

Description

Syringomas are the most common eyelid eccrine sweat gland tumor (1) (Fig. 27.1).

Syringomas appear as skin-colored or slightly yellow, firm papules 1 to 3 mm in size and are usually multiple. They appear most commonly after puberty and in women.

Syringomas occur more often on the lower eyelids than on the upper eyelids. Only three cases of the malignant variant have been reported (2), and none of these have been on the eyelids.

Differential Diagnosis

Milia and the individual lesions of multiple trichoepitheliomas can be confused, on external appearance, with syringomas. They can easily be differentiated by histological differences. Trichoepitheliomas do have a malignant potential, although this is rare.

Histology

Syringomas occur in the upper and mid dermis. They contain numerous small cystic ducts and solid epithelial strands embedded in a fibrous stroma.

The lesions are definitely of eccrine origin. Electron

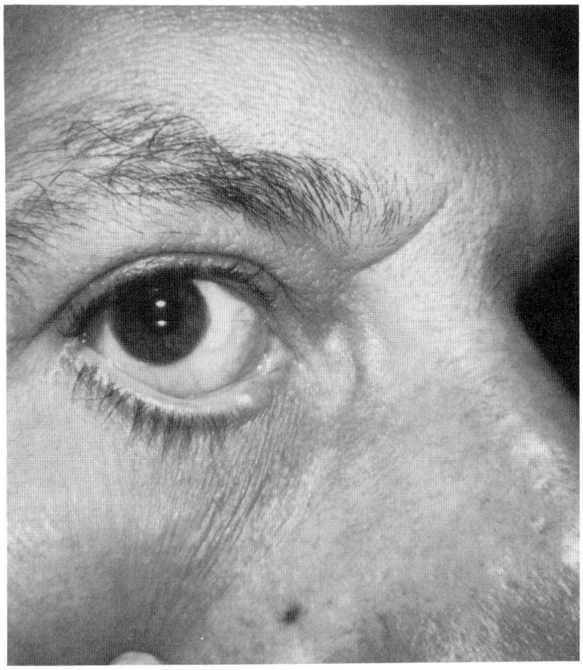

Figure 27.1. Syringoma.

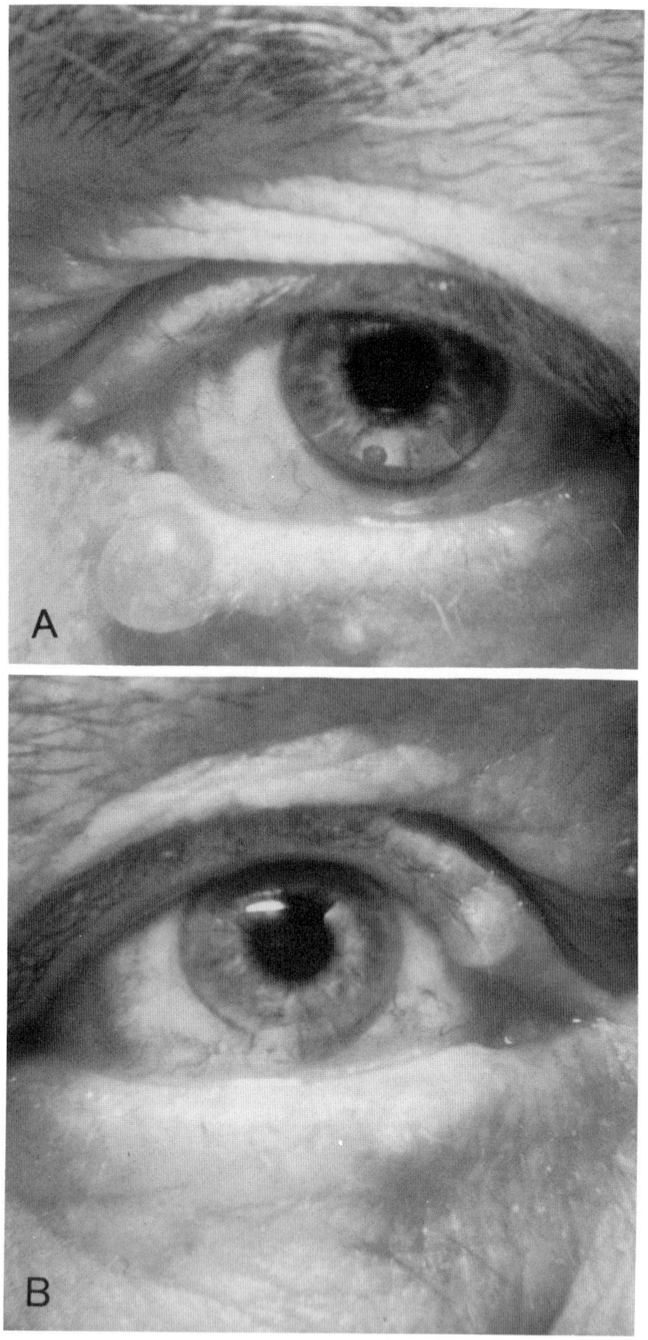

Figure 27.2. *A* and *B*, Apocrine hidrocystoma.

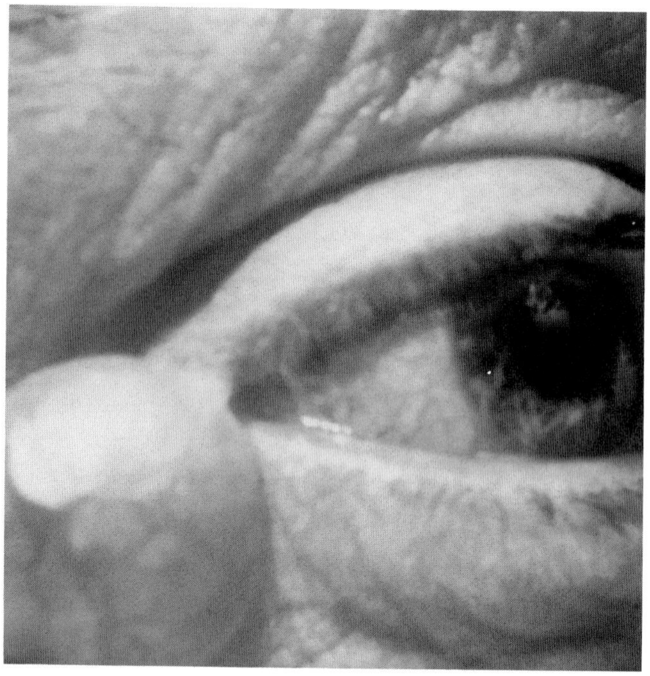

Figure 27.3. Epidermal cysts. *A*, Small, marginal epidermal cyst. *B*, Large, lateral canthal epidermal cyst.

microscopy shows that the cells of the solid strands and of the outer wall of the ducts are identical to the outer cells of the walls of embryonic eccrine sweat glands. The luminal cells are ductal and secretory. Glycogen as well as all of the eccrine types of enzymes are present.

Treatment

These tumors should be excised for tissue diagnosis. Malignant variants that are well differentiated are treated with local excision. More anaplastic tumors and tumor recurrences are treated with radical excision with or without regional lymph node dissection (3).

ECCRINE HIDROCYSTOMA

This is a rare tumor that occurs on the face of older women who have chronic exposure to heat. The tumors appear as translucent vesicles or cysts that are yellow or slightly blue in color. They are benign and can be treated by local excision.

APOCRINE TUMORS

The glands of Moll are modified apocrine glands. Stout and Cooley (4) reviewed 43 sweat gland tumors from all over the body. They reported that only 11 of 43 sweat gland tumors that they examined were of apocrine origin.

APOCRINE HIDROCYSTOMA

These tumors are solid, dome-shaped translucent nodules that appear on the face, ears, and scalp. They range in size from 1 to 10 mm and may have a bluish color. They can be confused, grossly, with blue nevi, hemangiomas, and syringocystadenoma papilliferum (Fig. 27.2).

CYLINDROMA

Description

Clyindromas occur as single or multiple lesions and occur usually on the scalp. Associated lesions can appear on the face and eyelids in the multiple form. The multiple form is dominantly inherited and is frequently associated with trichoepitheliomas, which are also dominantly inherited.

The individual lesion is a small, flesh-colored papule or larger dome-shaped lesion that is usually located on the scalp. There are three reported cases of malignant changes in cylindromas (5).

Differential Diagnosis

The multiple form can be confused with trichoepitheliomas and the lesions of neurofibromatosis. The solitary lesions may resemble a nodular basal cell carcinoma or sebaceous hyperplasia.

TUMORS WITH HAIR DIFFERENTIATION

MULTIPLE TRICHOEPITHELIOMA

Description

These dominantly inherited tumors appear at puberty on the face. They are also seen on the scalp, neck, and upper trunk. The lesions are skin colored or slightly pink and may have telangiectatic vessels running over the surface of the larger ones. Rarely, they can undergo malignant changes.

Differential Diagnosis and Histology

Multiple trichoepitheliomas may be confused with the angiofibromas of tuberous sclerosis.

The characteristic histologic feature of trichoepitheliomas is the "horn cyst." These cysts consist of an outer shell of flattened basophillic cells covering a fully keratinized inner core. A primitive hair papilla is sometimes present. Parts of the lesion often contain islands of basophillic cells (similar to the cells of a basal cell carcinoma) in either lacy or more solid groups.

SEBACEOUS TUMORS

NEVUS SEBACEOUS

These tumors appear at birth on the scalp or face and may involve the brow and eyelids. They begin as hairless plaques that develop verrucous or nodular lesions after puberty.

SEBACOUS EPITHELIOMA

These lesions usually occur as solitary cystic nodules on the faces and upper eyelids of older people. The multiple form can resemble a spreading nodular basal cell carcinoma.

TUMORS WITH EPIDERMAL DIFFERENTIATION

EPIDERMAL CYST

Epidermal cysts are slow-growing, elevated, round, firm lesions that are either intracutaneous or subcutaneous and measure from 2 to 5 mm. They can occur anywhere on the face, neck, and back. The content is semisolid (Fig. 27.3).

MILIUM

Milia are white, globoid, small, firm lesions usually measuring 1 or 2 mm in size (Fig. 27.4). They arise either spontaneously, after mild dermabrasion, or in bullous diseases of the skin.

These lesions are always benign and are removed by simple surgical excision or cauterization for cosmetic purposes.

MALIGNANT TUMORS OF SWEAT GLAND ORIGIN

CARCINOMA OF THE ECCRINE GLANDS

Description

These are rare tumors with no characteristic appearance or location (6). Although they are radiosensitive, metastases are frequent. Once the metastases extend beyond the regional lymph nodes, the disease is usually fatal. Surprisingly, malignant eccrine gland tumors are found least on the palms of the hands and the soles of the feet where eccrine glands abound.

Differential Diagnosis and Histology

These tumors are histologically similar to adenoid basal cell carcinomas, malignant clear-cell hidradenoma, and metastatic adenocarcinomas.

The tumors vary from fairly well-organized glandular structures to diffuse anaplastic aggregates of vacuolated cells. These differences in differentiation can occur even in the same tumor. Glycogen and eccrine enzymes are present proportional to the amount of differentiation.

CARCINOMA OF THE APROCRINE GLANDS

Description

These tumors are mainly found in the axillae but also on the nipples, vulva, and glands of Moll of the eyelids.

These tumors are extremely rare (7, 8). Apocrine tumors are thought to be slow growing and can be treated with block excision, in which case careful attention should be given to obtaining tumor-free margins. Cases have been reported of metastases, death, and recurrence (7) but these have all had unclear or unavailable histology.

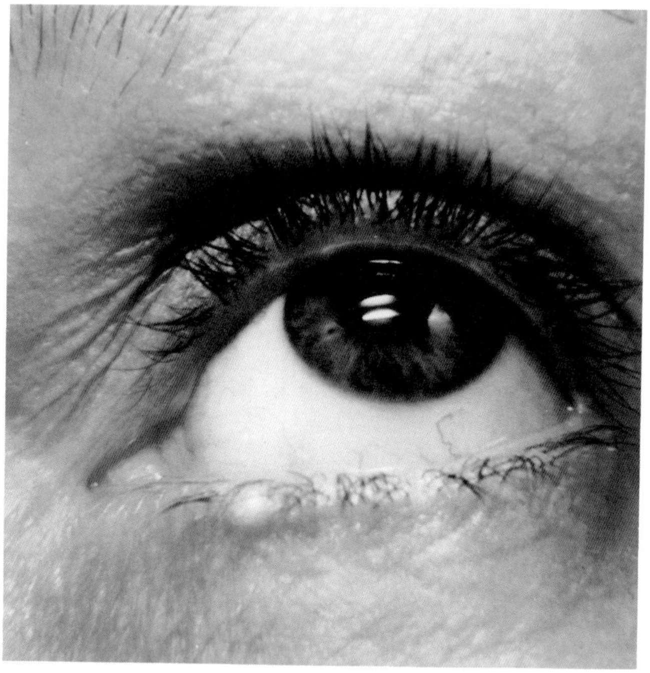

Figure 27.4. Milium.

CARCINOMA OF THE MEIBOMIAN GLANDS

Aurora and Blodi (8) reviewed all of the eyelid tumors at their institution over a 37-year period. There were 892 eyelid tumors in this group of which 214 were carcinomas (23.99%). Seven patients (3.27%) had sebaceous gland carcinomas, but only two could be shown to have definitely arisen from meibomian glands.

REFERENCES

1. Boniuk M: Tumors of sweat gland origin. *Int Ophth Clin* 2: 239, 1962
2. Lipper S, Peiper SC: Sweat gland carcinoma with syringomatous features. A light microscopic and ultrastructural study. *Cancer* 44: 157–163, 1979.
3. Fakhery B, Fishman LN: Sweat gland carcinoma: Report of a case in an unusual location and a review of the literature. *J Maine Med Assoc* 65: 80–81, 1974.
4. Stout AP, Cooley SGE: Carcinoma of sweat glands. *Cancer* 4: 521, 1951.
5. *Dermatology In General Medicine*. New York, McGraw Hill, 1971, p 452.
6. Rodriguez MM, Lubowitz RM, Shannon GM: Mucinous (adenocystic) carcinoma of the eyelid. *Arch Ophthamol* 89: 493–494, 1973.
7. Aurora AL, Luxenberg MN: Case report of adenocarcinoma of glands of Moll. *Am J Ophthalmol* 70: 984–990, 1970.
8. Aurora AL, Blodi FC: Lesions of the eyelids: a clinicopathological study. *Surv Ophthalmol* 15: 94–104, 1970.

CHAPTER 28

Capillary Hemangiomas of the Adnexa in Infants

BURTON J. KUSHNER, M.D.

NATURAL COURSE

Capillary hemangiomas in infants are occasionally present at birth, however, more frequently appear within the first several weeks of life. There is a subsequent rapid phase of growth lasting about 6 months and then a relative quiescent period (11, 12). Subsequently, they tend to undergo involution, with approximately 30% having completed the involution by 3 years of age, 60% by 4 years of age, and 70% by 7 years of age (3). They are a relatively common tumor in infants with an estimated incidence of 1–2% (4).

DIAGNOSIS

The diagnosis of an infantile capillary hemangioma can usually be made by clinical observation. The presence of a bluish or a strawberry-colored mass that is soft and spongy to the touch and tends to increase when the child is crying or in a dependent position is usually diagnostic. Frequently there may be multiple hemangiomas present on the child's body, and there is often a positive family history for infantile hemangiomas. Congenital hydrops of the nasolacrimal sac can be confused easily with an infantile hemangioma because of the frequent bluish discoloration of that lesion. Congenital hydrops of the nasolacrimal sac should be suspected if the mass is located in the region of the nasolacrimal sac. It can be differentiated from a hemangioma by its presence at birth, a concomitant obstruction of the nasolacrimal drainage system, and its firmess when palpated. The port-wine stain (nevus flammeus) that is associated with the Sturge-Weber syndrome is histopathologically different from an infantile hemangioma. Jakobiec and Jones (4) feel it is more appropriately referred to as a "telangiectasia." It differs from a capillary hemangioma in that it is a flat and a noncompressible lesion.

Ultrasonography is usually not necessary to diagnose an infantile capillary hemangioma; however, it may be helpful in determining the extent of the tumor, as well as its cell type (Fig 28.1) Similarly, computerized axial tomography may be helpful in determining the extent of orbital or retrobulbar involvement (Fig. 28.2).

Walsh (5) has observed a peculiar tendency for orbital hemangiomas to be fed by anomalous branches of the internal or external carotid artery and found them to involute after ligation of the feeder vessel. In his 16 cases he found that arteriography was usually necessary to document this anomaly.

Usually there are no systemic manifestations of hemangiomatosis in infants. Very large or multiple tumors can cause thrombocytopenia due to the tendency for platelets to get trapped in the tumor. Also cardiac failure can result from the high-velocity shunting (4, 6, 7). Hemangiomas of the orbit also have an unusual predilection for being associated with hemangiomas in the subglottic region, which can cause respiratory obstruction (8, 9).

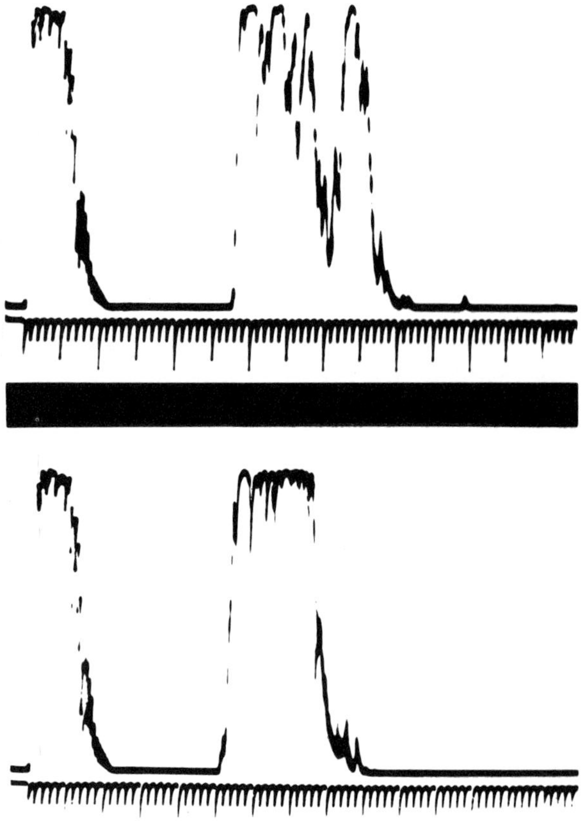

Figure 28.1. Scan echogram of an infantile-type hemangioma (cavernous/capillary). Typical echogram showing high and low spikes. *Top,* before pressure with probe. *Bottom,* during pressure. Note the marked decrease in the width of the tumor during pressure due to its soft consistency. The low reflective area in the *top* echogram indicates a large cavernous space. If it was predominantly capillary, it could not be as easily compressed. (Courtesy of Dr. Karl Ossoinig).

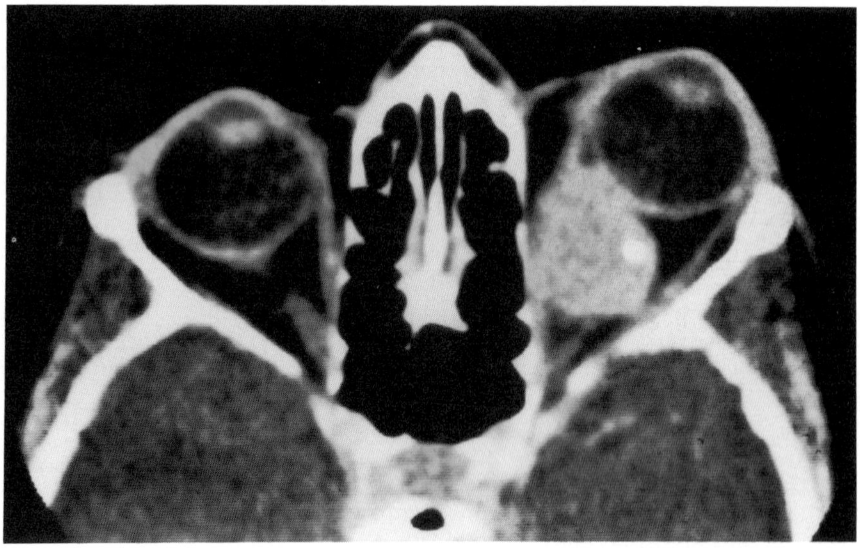

Figure 28.2. Computerized axial tomogram of infant with hemangioma of right orbit. Proptosis secondary to retrobulbar hemangioma is present.

PATHOLOGY

Infantile capillary hemangiomas consist mainly of a proliferation of endothelial cells supported by a fibrous tissue stroma. The amount of encapsulation is variable. Vascular channels of varying sizes and amount may be present (Fig. 28.3). Some authorities use the term "capillary" to refer to infantile hemangiomas with few vascular spaces, and "mixed capillary-cavernous" to refer to those lesions with larger vascular channels. Jakobiec and Jones (4) prefer to use the term "cavernous" for those tumors occurring in older individuals. They feel that infantile capillary hemangiomas are more approximately described as "hamartomas" rather than "neoplasms."

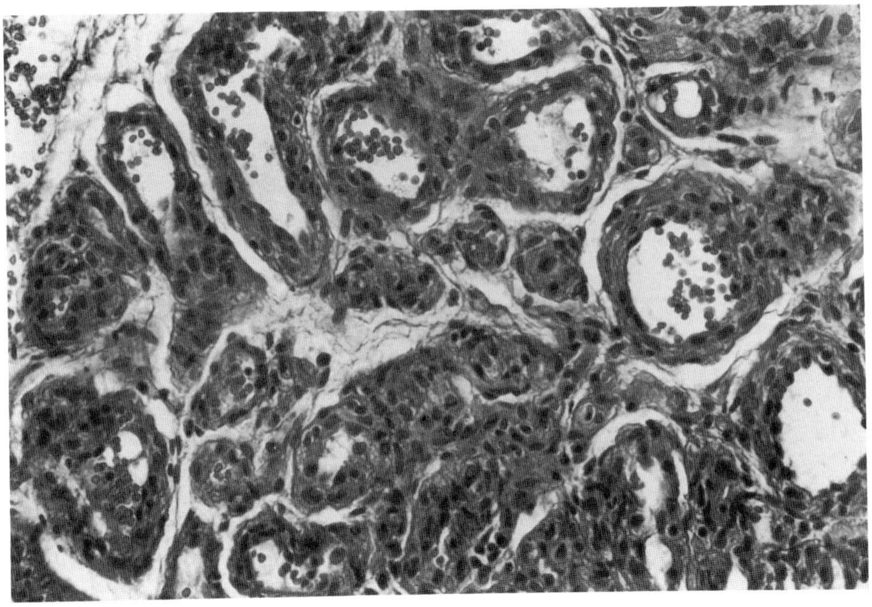

Figure 28.3. Infantile hemangioma. Note proliferation of endothelial cells with a rich fibrous stroma. Numerous vascular channels are present. Original magnification, × 25.

INDICATIONS FOR TREATMENT

Infantile capillary hemangiomas have a high spontaneous involution rate and therefore some authorities have recommended treating them with "intelligent neglect" (3). Hemangiomas that occur around the eye, however, pose very special problems. Complication rates of between 41–80% in the form of amblyopia or strabismus have been reported in several large series of infantile adnexal hemangiomas (10–12). Therefore an active approach to treatment of infantile capillary hemangiomas has been recommended when they involve the adnexa (13). Indications for active treatment include occlusion of the visual axis, the inducement of strabismus, or the presence of anisometropia sufficient to cause amblyopia. In addition, a rapidly growing tumor that may be threatening to cause any of these three events should be taken as an indication for treatment.

In addition to causing amblyopia by occlusion of the visual axis or inducing strabismus, soft tissue masses around the eye, such as hemangiomas, can cause marked refractive errors. Robb (12) found that 46% of 37 patients with adnexal hemangiomas had asymmetric refractive errors, with the involved eye tending to be the more myopic and astigmatic eye. He found that the axis of the cylinder typically tended to point toward the mass of the tumor if one used plus cylinder convention. Hoyt and coworkers (14) found that neonatal eyelid closure in human infants tended to cause an axial myopia. It is therefore critical that a child being followed with an adnexal hemangioma undergo frequent retinoscopy with the use of cycloplegia if the decision is made to defer active treatment. The fact that the visual axis is not occluded or that strabismus is not developing is not a guarantee that amblyopia due to anisometropia is not present (Fig. 28.4). I have found that early treatment of adnexal hemangiomas in the presence of high astigmatic refractive errors can result in a reversal of the induced astigmatism if the hemangioma is successfully eliminated (15).

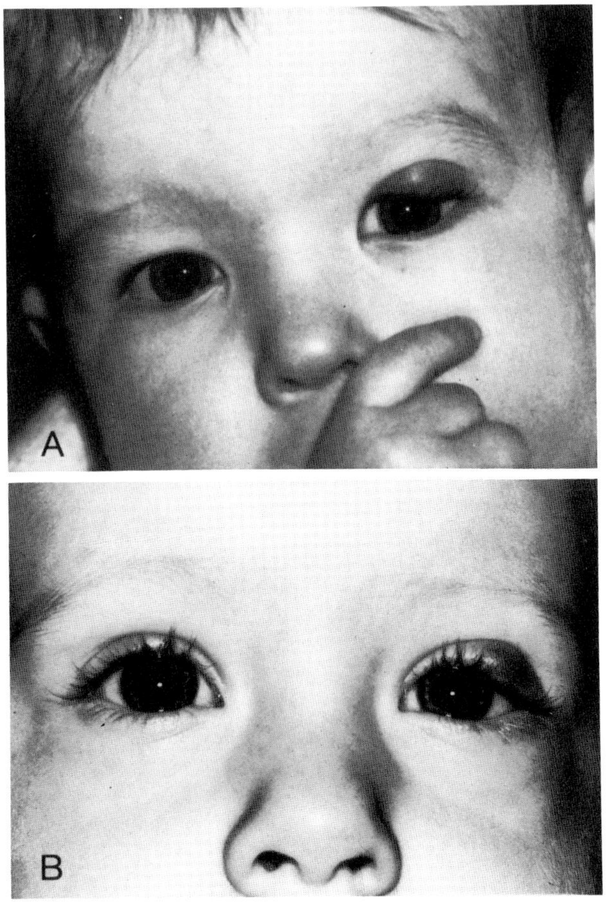

Figure 28.4. Two children with almost identical hemangiomas of the left upper lid. *A*, Refraction is OD, +.50 sphere; OS, +100+2.50 × 80°; and the anisometropia is sufficient to cause amblyopia. *B*, Refraction is OD, +.75+.25 × 180° and OS, +1.00 sphere. Without cycloplegic retinoscopy the potential threat to vision of the hemangioma in panel *A* is not evident.

Figure 28.5. Injection is carried out directly into the substance of the tumor using a tuberculin syringe.

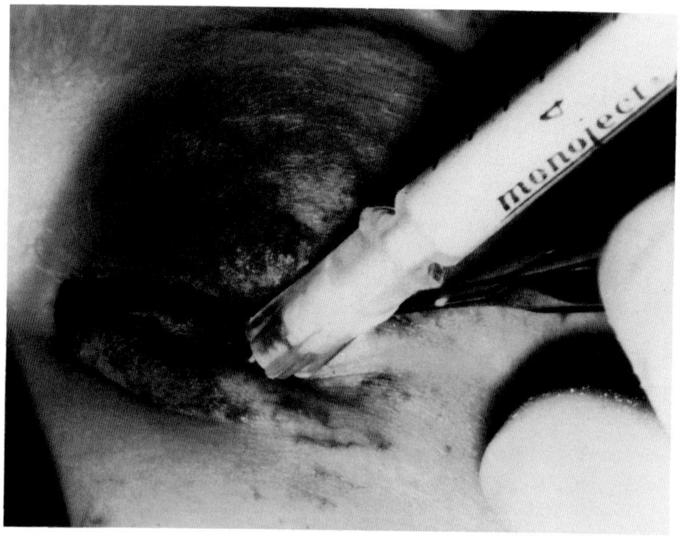

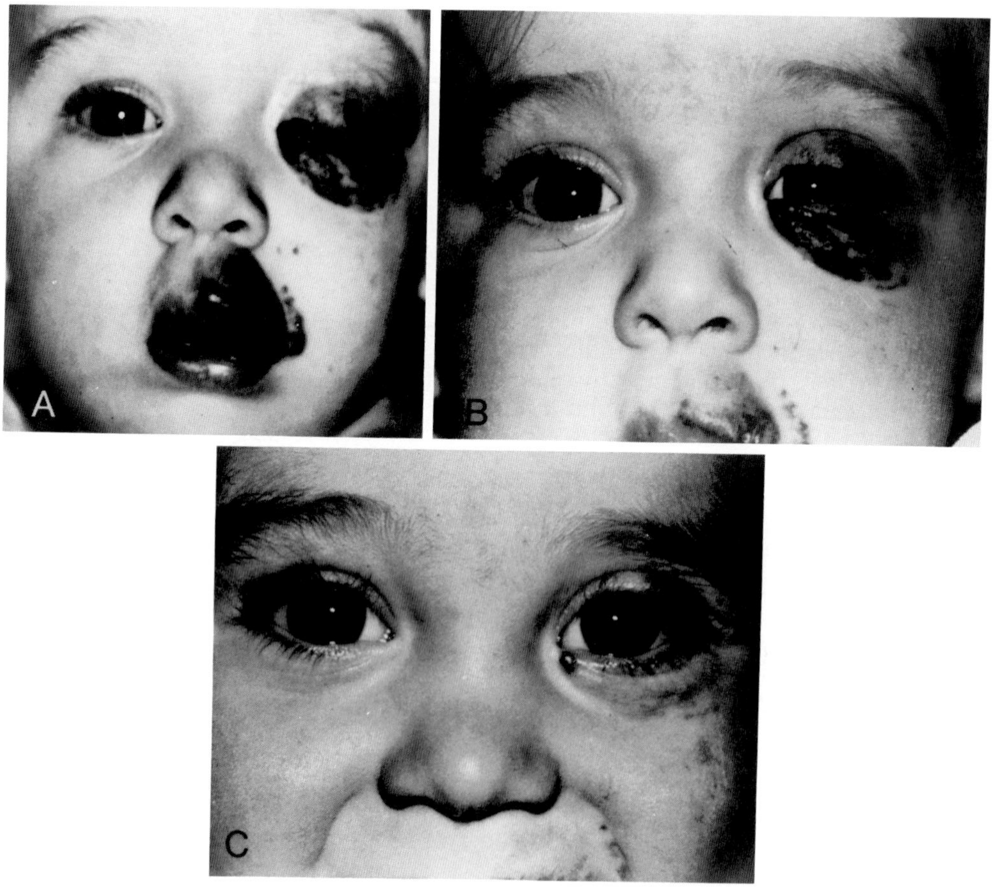

Figure 28.6. *A*, Four-month-old child just prior to corticosteroid injection. *B*, Same child in panel *A* 9 days after corticosteroid injection. *C*, Same child at 10 months of age, 3 months after second injection; neither amblyopia nor strabismus is present. (From Kushner BF: Intralesional corticosteroid injection for infantile adnexal hemangioma. *Am J Ophthalmol* 93: 496–506, 1982. Published with permission from the American Journal of Ophthalmology. Copyright by the Ophthalmic Publishing Co.)

TREATMENT MODALITIES

Reviews of different methods of treating infantile adnexal capillary hemangiomas indicate numerous problems (15). Surgery can result in extensive scarring, as well as cause a tendency for rebound growth. Jakobiec (4) feels that rebound is particularly likely to occur if surgery is undertaken during the active phase of growth and feels it is more appropriately performed between 3 to 5 years of age. If amblyopia is developing, however, this delay could result in irreversible deprivation amblyopia. Cryotherapy has been associated with cutaneous atrophy. Schlerosing injections can cause severe scarring and are unpredictable. Henderson (13) advocates the use of radon seeds for treating infantile hemangiomas. Jakobiec (4) feels that radon seeds are hard to retrieve and can impair orbital bone growth. He recommends superficial radiotherapy, 80–120 kV given as 100–200 rads monthly for 4–6 months up to 500–600 rads. For deeper tumors he advocates orthoradiation.

In 1967, Zarem and Edgèrton (16) reported the successful treatment of a series of infants with hemangiomas using prednisone. Subsequently, others found this treatment method successful (17–20). The use of systemic corticosteroids in infants requires careful monitoring of their metabolic status as there is a tendency to induce growth delay and cushingoid characteristics.

INTRALESIONAL CORTICOSTEROID INJECTION

In their original classic report, Zarem and Edgerton (16) briefly mentioned as an addendum that two patients were treated with intralesional corticosteroid injection. It was unclear whether this was in addition to, or instead of, systemic corticosteroids. Subsequently, Mazzola (21) reported a large series of infantile hemangiomas treated with intralesional corticosteroids with good results. I have found that the use of intralesional corticosteroids in infantile adnexal capillary hemangiomas substantially decreases my complication rate with respect to amblyopia and strabismus (15, 22). Subsequently, others have reported its use with similar good results (23, 24).

My preferred technique consists of injecting 40 mg of

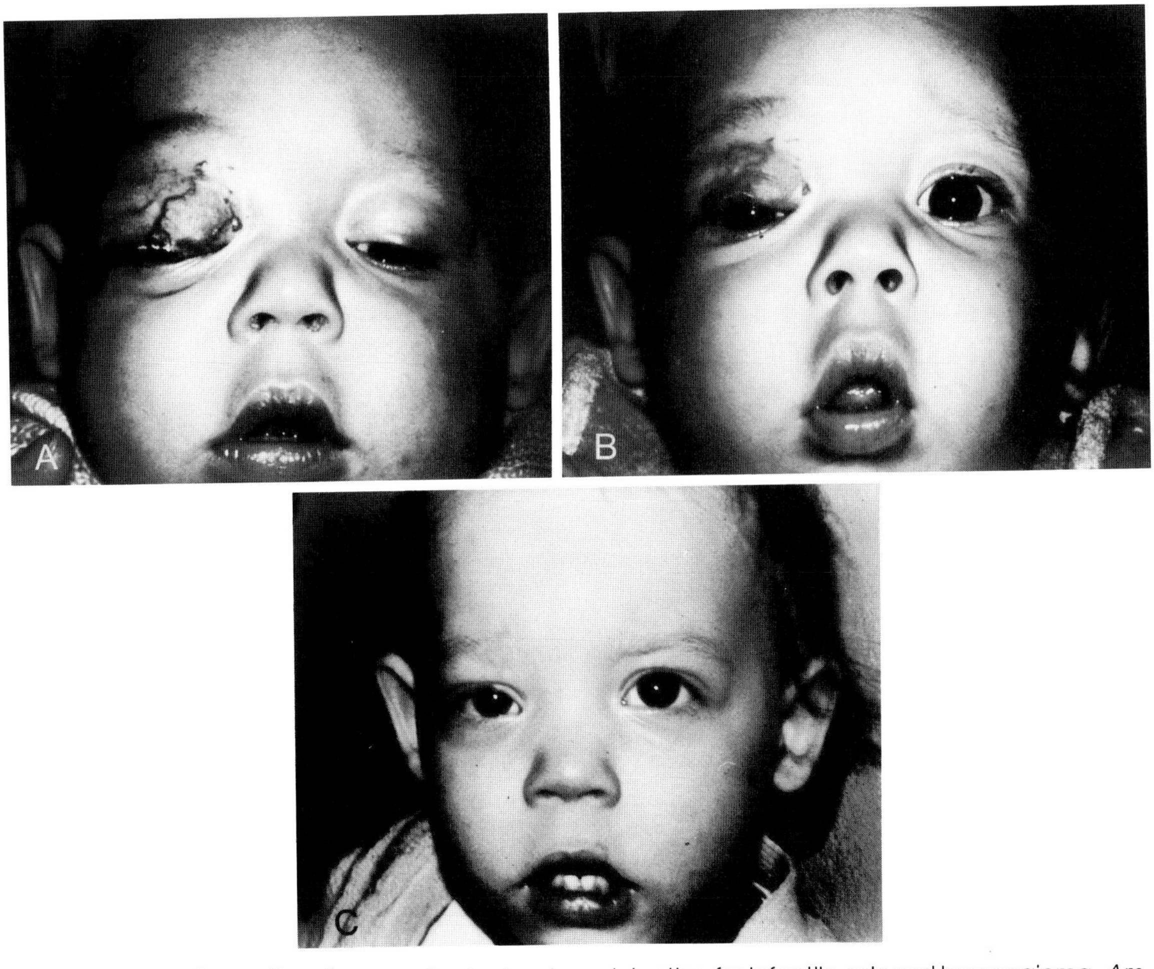

Figure 28.7. *A,* Child, 4½ months of age, prior to treatment. *B,* Ten days after initial injection, marked resolution of the lesion is evident. *C,* By 7 months of age, resolution is complete. (From Kushner BF: Intralesional corticosteroid injection for infantile adnexal hemangioma. *Am J Ophthalmol* 93: 496–506, 1982. Published with permission of the American Journal of Ophthalmology. Copyright by the Ophthalmic Publishing Co.)

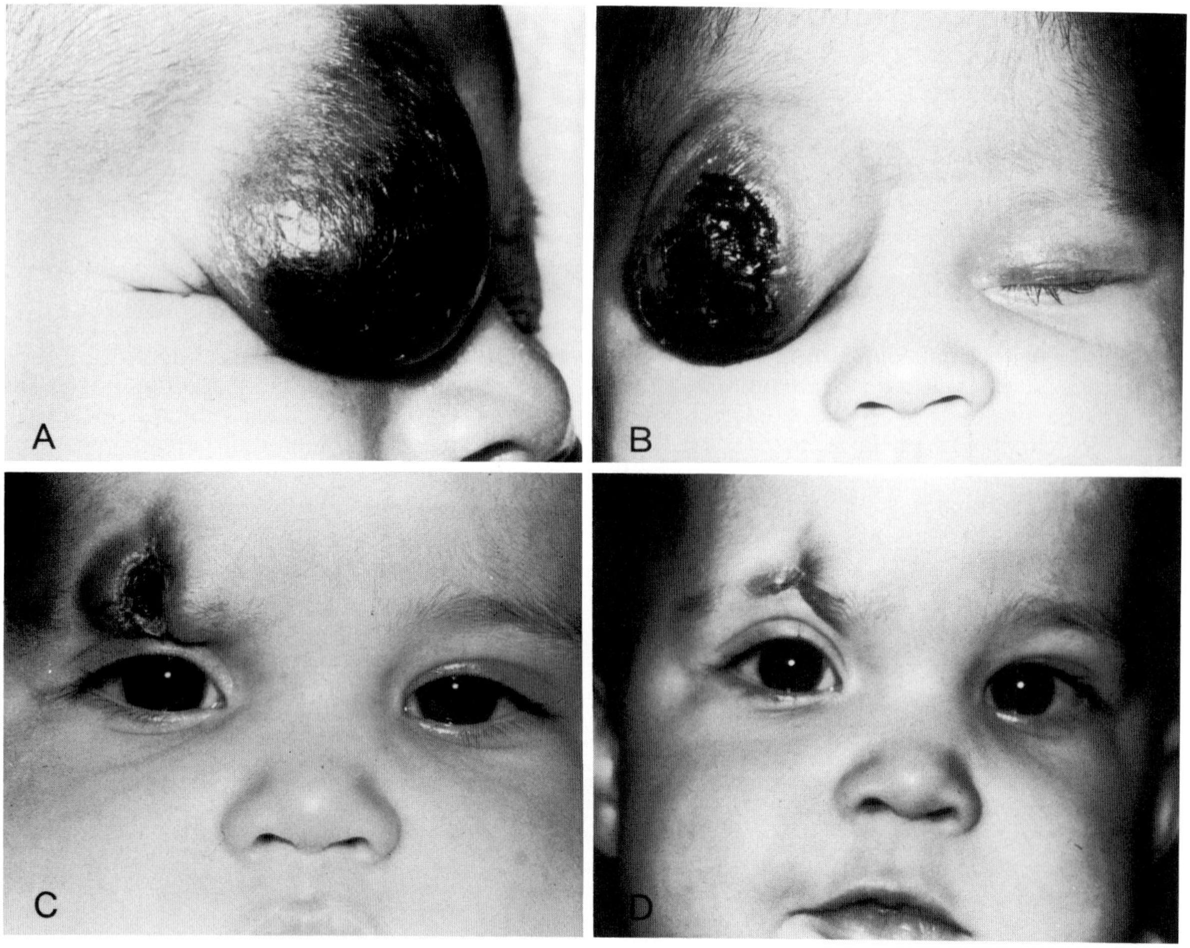

Figure 28.8. Child with large orbital hemangioma at 8 days of age. *C,* At 4 months of age, 1 week after second injection, there is marked resolution of the tumor. *D,* At 8 months of age, the resolution is complete. Neither amblyopia nor strabismus is present. (From Kushner BF: Intralesional corticosteroid injection for infantile adnexal hemangioma. *Am J Ophthalmol* 93: 496–506, 1982. Published with permission of the American Journal of Ophthalmology. Copyright by the Ophthalmic Publishing Co.)

triamcinolone and 6 mg of a preparation consisting of equal parts of betamethasone sodium phosphate and betamethasone acetate directly into the lesion. It is done under a light general anesthetic to avoid the complication of a large hematoma or inadvertent damage to the globe. I attempt to distribute the medications evenly throughout the tumor either in one or multiple percutaneous punctures using two separate tuberculin syringes (Fig. 28.5). Usually the volume of liquid injected into the tumor results in a marked swelling of the lesion that lasts for about 8 hours. A light patch is used to cover the eye until the swelling goes down. Parents are advised to avoid having the child immunized with any vaccine containing live virus for 1 week prior to or after injection. For large tumors, I have given up to twice the usual dose safely. Typically a response is noted within several days of injection. Initially, a blanching of the vessels can be noted, which is followed by a rapid decrease in tumor size. The most rapid involution occurs within the first 1–2 weeks. Further regression can occur up to 4–5 weeks. If regression is incomplete, a second injection is given 6–8 weeks after the first (Figs. 28.6 and 28.7). My series is now up to 24 patients (25). I have found total, or near total, involution of the tumor in 16 cases after one or two injections. Only one child required a third injection for a rebound 6 months after the second injection. In seven cases, the tumor remained but was less than 50% of the original size and involution was sufficient to prevent amblyopia, anisometropia, or strabismus. In three patients there was minimal or no response. Early treatment even resulted in the preservation of vision in several patients who had total occlusion of the visual axis prior to treatment (Fig. 28.8). In many patients there was reversal of the pretreatment anisometropia if involution was obtained (Fig. 28.9).

Apt advocates the use of intralesional corticosteroids for infantile adnexal capillary hemangiomas but uses a different injection protocol (L. Apt, personal communication). He uses weekly injections for 4 weeks and a lower dosage of corticosteroid. He recommends using 0.4–0.5 mg/kg of body weight of a medication consisting of equal parts of betamethasone sodium phosphate and betamethasone acetate. If for some reason injection cannot be given weekly, he recommends the use of 2.5 mg/kg of triamcinolone in addition to the previously mentioned medication,

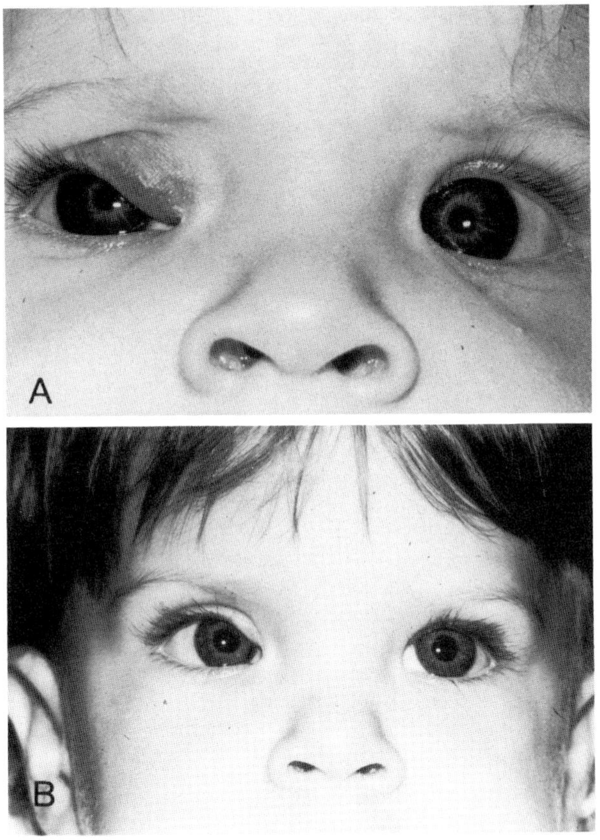

Figure 28.9. *A,* This medial hemangioma is associated with a +3.00 cylinder × 10 as seen at 6 weeks of age. *B,* After intralesional corticosteroid injection, and resolution of the lesion, the cylinder has reduced to + .50 × 35. Neither amblyopia nor strabismus is present. (From Kushner BF: Intralesional corticosteroid injection for infantile adnexal hemangioma. *Am J Ophthalmol* 93: 496–506, 1982. Published with permission of the American Journal of Ophthalmology. Copyright by the Ophthalmic Publishing Co.)

with the two being given every 2 weeks for two injections. If incomplete involution occurs, the course may be repeated in 1–3 months.

I have not observed any complication in my 25 patients (unpublished data). Care should be taken to draw back on the syringe before injecting the medication to prevent it from going into the vascular compartment. Occasionally whitish deposits of the solid steroid material can be seen subcutaneously; these usually absorb in several months. Mazzola (21) indicated that several of his patients developed transient cushingoid characteristics. This may be more likely to occur when the treatment is carried out weekly as he recommends as opposed to intervals of approximately 2 months as I have utilized.

Injecting retrobulbar hemangiomas with corticosteroids carries the possible risk of a severe retrobulbar hemorrhage. In addition, there have been reports of occlusion of the central retinal artery after retrobulbar corticosteroid injection without hemorrhage occurring (25, 26). Also, intranasal injection of corticosteroid has resulted in optic nerve neuropathy and retinal and choroidal microvascular embolism due to what has been postulated as retrograde

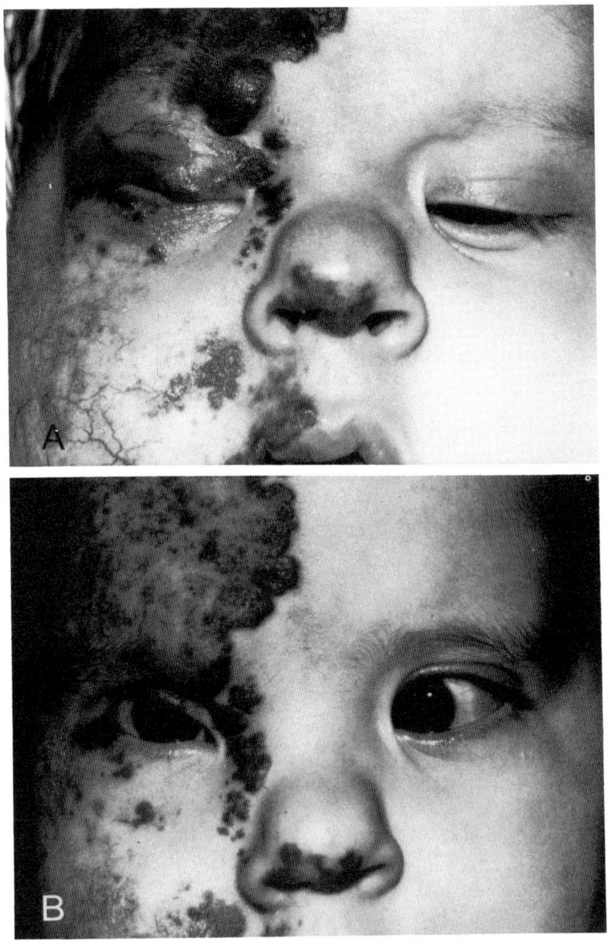

Figure 28.10. *A,* Child with extensive hemangiomas involving the face and lids. *B,* After intralesional injection of the right lids, the visual axis was opened sufficiently to prevent amblyopia, as evidenced by child fixating with the involved eye while on a program of occlusion therapy. Subsequent manifestation of the subglottic hemangioma resulting in respiratory distress necessitated the institution of systemic corticosteroid.

flow through the vascular tissue or anomalous collateral circulation (27, 28). For this reason, if a tumor extends at all into the orbit, injection should be carried out slowly with simultaneous indirect ophthalmoscopic monitoring of the optic nerve during injection. If the tumor is retrobulbar, or far posterior in the orbit, other treatment modalities should be considered.

Systemic corticosteroid therapy should be considered if systemic factors such as subglottic hemangioma with airway obstruction, or cardiac failure are present (Fig. 28.10).

Not all infantile adnexal capillary hemangiomas are sensitive to corticosteroids. It has been suggested that responsiveness to corticosteroids appears inversely related to the encapsulation of the tumor and the cavernous component [B. J. Kushner, unpublished data; R. L. Anderson, personal communication; (29)].

The mechanism of action of corticosteroids on hemangiomas is thought to be due to a vasoconstricting property rather than an antiinflammatory effect. Frequently, a blanching of the lesion is seen shortly after injection, which suggests vasoconstriction. Zarem and Edgerton (16) found only minimal inflammatory activity in hemangioma biopsy specimens that they studied. It has been shown that corticosteroids increase vascular sensitivity to circulating vasoconstricting agents (30). Studies in humans and animals have shown that cortisone produces arteriolar constriction and narrowing of precapillary sphincters (31, 32).

REFERENCES

1. Walsh T, Tompkins V: Some observations on the strawberry nevus of infancy. *Cancer* 9: 869–904, 1956.
2. Bowers RE, Graham EA, Tomlinson KM: The natural history of the strawberry nevus. *Arch Dermatol* 82: 667–680, 1960.
3. Margileth A, Museles M: Cutaneous hemangiomas in children: Diagnosis and conservative management. *JAMA* 194: 523–526, 1965.
4. Jakobiec FA, Jones IS: Vascular tumors, malformations and degenerations. In Duane TD (ed): *Clinical Ophthalmology.* Philadelphia, Harper & Row, 1981, vol 2, p 1–40.
5. Walsh TS Jr: Giant strawberry nevi of the orbital arteries: Treatment by ligation. *Surgery* 65: 659–667, 1969.
6. Goldberg SJ, Fonkalsrud E: Successful treatment of hepatic hemangioma with corticosteroids. *JAMA* 208: 2473–2474, 1969.
7. Jackson C, Greene HL, O'Neill J, Kirchner S: Hepatic hemangioendothelioma. *Am J Dis Child* 131: 74–77, 1977.
8. Yee RD, Hepler RS: Congenital hemangiomas of the skin with orbital and sublottic hemangiomas. *Am J Ophthalmol* 75: 876–879, 1973.
9. Lee MH, Ramanathan S, Chalon J, Turndorf H: Subglottic hemangioma. *Anesthesiology* 45: 459–462, 1976.
10. Haik GR, Jakobiec FA, Ellsworth RM, Jones IS: Capillary hemangioma of the lids and orbit. An analysis of the clinical features and therapeutic results in 101 cases. *Ophthalmology* 86: 760–789, 1979.
11. Stigmar G, Crawford JS, Ward CM, Thomson HG: Ophthalmic sequelae of infantile hemangiomas of the eyelids and orbit. *Am J Ophthalmol* 85: 806–813, 1978.
12. Robb RM: Refractive errors associated with hemangiomas of the eyelids and orbit in infancy. *Am J Ophthalmol* 83: 52–58, 1977.
13. Henderson JW: *Orbital tumors*, ed 2. New York, Decker, 1980, p 117.
14. Hoyt CS, Stone RD, Fromer C, Billson FA: Monocular axial myopia associated with neonatal eyelid closure in human infants. *Am J Ophthalmol* 91: 197–200, 1981.
15. Kushner BJ: Intralesional corticosteroid injection for infantile adnexal hemangioma. *Am J Ophthalmol* 93: 496–506, 1982.
16. Zarem HA, Edgerton MT: Induced resolution of cavernous hemangiomas following prednisolone therapy. *Plast Reconstr Surg* 39: 76–83, 1967.
17. Fost ND, Esterly NB: Successful treatment of juvenile hemangiomas with prednisolone. *J Pediatr* 72: 351–357, 1968.
18. Hiles DA, Pilchard WA: Corticosteroid control of neonatal hemangiomas of the orbit and ocular adnexa. *Am J Ophthalmol* 71: 1003–1008, 1971.
19. Katz HP, Askin J: Multiple hemangiomata with thrombopenia. *Am J Dis Child* 115: 351–357, 1968.
20. de Venecia G, Lobeck CC: Successful treatment of eyelid hemangiomas with prednisolone. *Arch Ophthalmol* 84: 98–102, 1970.
21. Mazzola RF: Treatment of hemangiomas in children by intralesional injection of steroids. *Chir Plastica (Berlin)* 4: 161–171, 1978.
22. Kushner BJ: Local steroid therapy in adnexal hemangioma. *Ann Ophthalmol* 11: 1005–1009, 1979.
23. Zak TA, Morin DJ: Early local steroid therapy of infantile eyelid hemangiomas. *J Pediatr Ophthalmol Strab* 18: 15–27, 1981.
24. Brown BZ, Huffaker G: Local injection of steroids for juvenile hemangiomas which disturb the visual axis. *Ophthal Surg* 13: 630–633, 1982.
25. Kraushar MF, Seelenfreund MH, Freilich DB: Central retinal artery closure during orbital hemorrhage from retrobulbar injection. *Trans Am Acad Ophthalmol Otolaryngol* 78: 65–70, 1974.
26. Ellis PP: Occlusion of the central retinal artery after retrobulbar corticosteroid injection. *Am J Ophthalmol* 85: 352–356, 1978.
27. Evans DE, Zahorchak JA, Kennerdell JS: Visual loss as a result of primary optic nerve neuropathy after intranasal corticosteroid injection. *Am J Ophthalmol* 90: 641–644, 1980.
28. Whiteman DW, Rosen DA, Pinkerton RMH: Retinal and choroidal microvascular embolism after intranasal corticosteroid injection. *Am J Ophthalmol* 89: 851–853, 1980.
29. Sasaki GH, Pang CY, Wittliff JL: Pathogenesis and treatment of infant skin strawberry hemangiomas: Clinical and in vitro studies of hormonal effects. *Plast Reconstr Surg* 74: 359–368, 1984.
30. Zweifach BW, Shore E, Black MM: The influence of the adrenal cortex on behavior of the terminal vascular bed. *Ann NY Acad Sci* 56: 626–633, 1953.
31. Wyman LC, Fulton GP, Shulman MH: Direct observations on the circulation in the hamster cheek pouch in adrenal insufficiency and experimental hypercorticalism. *Ann NY Acad Sci* 56: 643–656, 1953.
32. Stuttgen G: Vasoconstriction in response to corticosteroids observed in human lips. *Dermatologica* 152 (Suppl 1): 91–100, 1976.

CHAPTER 29

Benign Eyelid Tumors of Neurogenic Origin

JANET M. NEIGEL, M.D.

Most neurogenic tumors occurring in the eyelids are derived from Schwann cells, which are the supporting structure of axons, the peripheral nervous system counterpart of the central nervous system oligodendrocyte. These cells, which migrate from the neural crest, may give rise to the schwannoma (neurilemoma), neurofibroma (Table 29.1), and probably the granular cell tumor. The neural crest not only can differentiate into the Schwann cell but also into the sympathicoblast, which can subsequently differentiate into paraganglionic and ganglionic tumors. The neural crest also gives rise to the melanocyte.

Neurogenic tumors of the eyelids produce varied signs and symptoms depending on the involved site. They may be asymptomatic, or they may cause occasional pain, blepharoptosis, and/or paresthesias.

TRAUMATIC NEUROMA

Synonyms for traumatic neuroma include amputation neuroma, pseudoneuroma, neuroma, neurinoma, hyperplastic scar of nerve, and hypertrophic neuroma.

Occasionally, traumatic neuroma is a late complication of both eyelid surgery and traumatic wounds (1). It has been reported to have occurred in the orbit following enucleation (2, 3) and also in the conjunctiva following pterygium excision; the latter most likely occurs from a severed intrascleral nerve loop of Axenfeld (4).

The traumatic neuroma is not a true neoplasm but rather a regenerative proliferation of a peripheral nerve at the site of a laceration, amputation, or compression injury of a nerve. It represents a reactive hyperplasia caused by an abortive attempt at regeneration. The Schwann cell and its axon of the proximal stump grow toward the distal stump. If they fail to fuse, the axon becomes entangled in soft tissue, forming spirals and producing a collection of axons, fibroblasts, and Schwann cells in a dense collagenous matrix. According to Reese (5), the time interval between severance of a nerve and the appearance of a traumatic neuroma can range from several months to more than 50 years.

Grossly traumatic neuromas are oval, fusiform, or oblong; semimobile; gray-white; and firm or rubbery, circumscribed masses without a capsule. Histologically, they consist of a combination of tangled proliferations of endoneural and perineural connective tissue, neurilemmal cells, and regenerating axons (Fig. 29.1). They are surrounded by dense fibrous tissue. The cut surface appears as a dense fibrous structure with no vascularity. Clinically, a neuroma is tender and sensitive to pressure. Pain may be present at the site of the neuroma, or it may be referred to the area originally innervated by the nerve. Since these lesions can occur in previous surgical sites of tumor excision, recurrent tumor must be ruled out. Once the traumatic neuroma is identified, it does not require any formal method of treatment. These lesions bear a superficial resemblance to the lesions in the multiple mucosal neuromas syndrome, which are characterized by a loosely fibrous matrix.

Table 29.1
Comparison of Schwannoma and Neurofibroma

Feature	Schwannoma	Neurofibroma
Classification	tumor	hamartoma
Proliferation	solitary	multiple
Capsule	encapsulated	nonencapsulated
Color	pleomorphic gray	homogeneous gray
Associated with von Recklinghausen's	almost never	usually
Degenerative changes	usually present	less common
Neurites	do not traverse tumor	pass through tumor
Axons	push axons aside	incorporate axons
Arrangement of cells	compact	loose, myxomatous
Distribution	centrifugally	centripetally
Symptomatology	painful and tender	asymptomatic
Mast cells	rare	frequent
Alcian blue stain for mucopolysaccharide	negative	positive
Tumor mass	Schwann cell	Schwann cell, endoneural cell and axons
Malignant change	almost never	8–15%

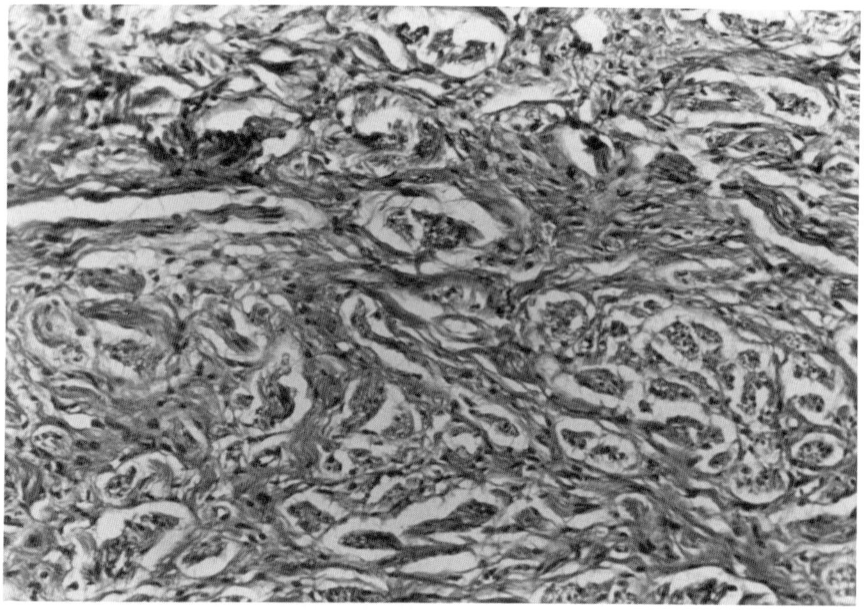

Figure 29.1. Traumatic neuroma. Photomicrograph shows a tangle of nerve fibers in a dense fibrous matrix. (Courtesy of Leroy R. Sharer, M.D.)

SCHWANNOMA (NEURILEMOMA)

Schwannoma, which is a benign tumor of the peripheral nervous system, is derived from neuroectoderm and was first described in 1908 by Verocay (6). Schwann cells derived from the neural crest have been determined to be the cells of origin of the schwannoma (7). This tumor, which is usually solitary, is found in all age groups but occurs predominantly in the 3rd and 4th decade (Fig. 29.2). Schwannomas have been reported to occur in association with von Recklinghausen's disease in approximately 10% of patients, in which case they may be multifocal (5).

A schwannoma is an encapsulated tumor usually attached to, or surrounded by, a nerve. The capsule consists of fibroblasts and collagen and is associated with Schwann cells, which make up the bulk of the tumor. Axons are found only at the periphery and do not traverse the tumor. The tumor is usually round, oval, or sometimes fusiform and milky-white, tan, or gray with irregular yellow areas. On gross cut section, one may see whorling with cystic spaces and areas of mucinous material. Histologically, this tumor tends to have two types of presentation (Fig. 29.3). In the Antoni A, or "solid type", tumor cells are elongated and spindle-shaped and are arranged in parallel sheets with palisading nuclei. The cytoplasm is pale and eosinophilic. There are delicate connective tissue fibers with a high reticulum content. These cells may also be grouped into nodules to produce an organoid unit of cells and fibers known as Verocay bodies, which show some resemblance to tactile corpuscles. The texture is compact. The Antoni B, or "soft type," shows cell pleomorphism with irregular cell types scattered in loose connective tissue with microcysts that may coalesce to form cystic spaces. Here the texture is loose. Degenerative changes may occur secondary to vascular thrombosis. Blood vessels show hyaline thickening of their walls, which results in areas of necrosis and hemorrhage. Lymphocytes, mast cells, lipid-filled foam cells, and hemosiderin-laden macrophages may also be present, usually around blood vessels. The Antoni A pattern is commonly intermixed with the Antoni B pattern.

Clinically, schwannomas may cause pain due to compression of the nerve of origin. Schwannomas may also masquerade as a recurrent chalazion (8). Schwannomas are usually slow growing and almost never undergo sarcomatous transformation, although it has been reported

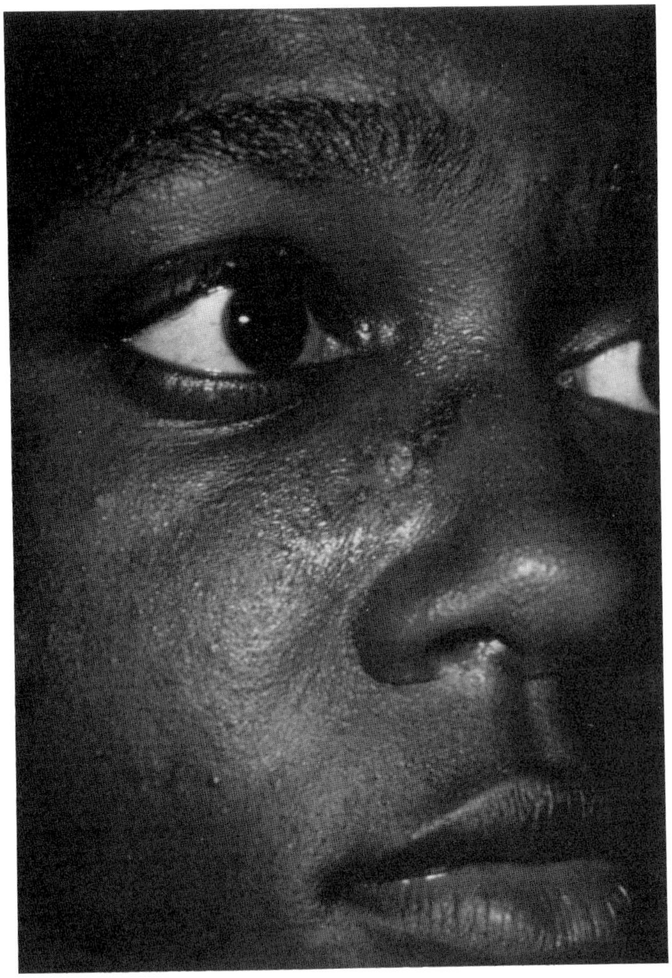

Figure 29.2. Schwannoma of right lower lid in a 19-year-old black female.

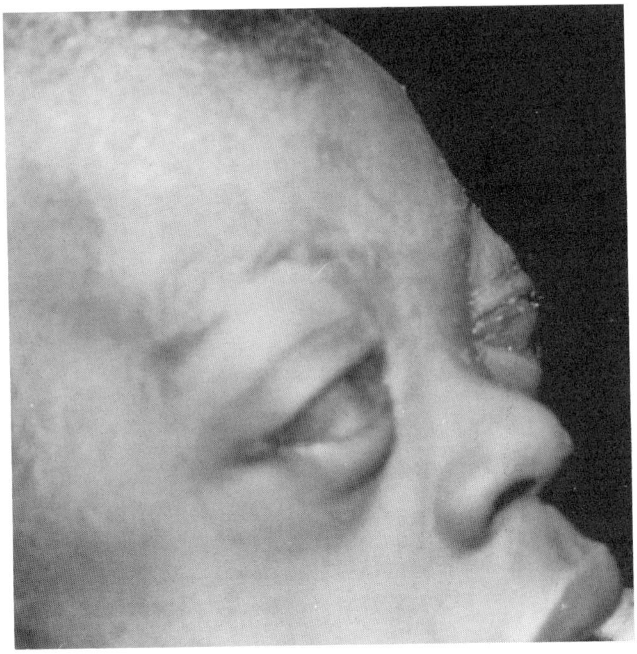

Figure 29.4. Neurofibromas of the eyelids. (Courtesy of Anthony R. Caputo, M.D.)

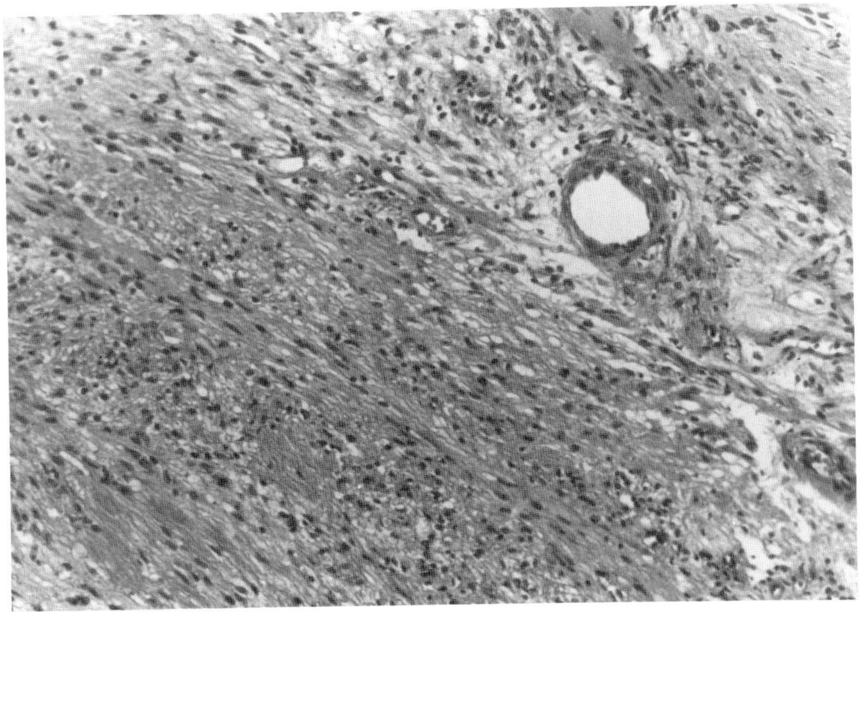

Figure 29.3. Schwannoma. Photomicrograph shows an admixture of Antoni A and Antoni B tissue. (Courtesy of Leroy R. Sharer, M.D.)

in a case of a documented benign schwannoma in a patient with von Recklinghausen's disease (9). There has been a report of an increased frequency of unrelated malignant tumors in patients with solitary schwannomas (10).

Treatment of this tumor consists of surgical excision, which is easily accomplished due to its encapsulation. The tumors rarely recur after excision, and the prognosis is excellent. These tumors are insensitive to radiation or chemotherapy.

SOLITARY NEUROFIBROMA

An isolated or solitary neurofibroma is not a true neoplasm but a hamartoma that may occur in the eyelids and is unassociated with von Recklinghausen's disease (Fig. 29.4). It is a diffuse tumor arising from both the nerve trunk and sensory terminals and may be associated with pigment production (5). The tumor is gray and movable, firm, and rubbery in consistency. It is slow growing and well circumscribed. Clinically, it has been reported to have presented as solid lid edema unassociated with neurofibromatosis (11). A neurofibroma is caused by diffuse proliferation of the Schwann cell, neurites, and endoneural fibroblasts that distorts the nerve's internal architecture. Neurites pass through the tumor and retrogressive changes are uncommon. Well-formed tactile corpuscles may be present. Histologically, (Fig. 29.5) it is characterized by elongated and spindled Schwann cells in a hypertrophied matrix with serpentine nuclei. The cells are fusiform and arranged in thin cords. There are numerous collagen fibrils oriented in a loose pattern that is often referred to as "wire-like." Mast cells are often present along with lymphocytes, fibrocytes, and histiocytes. The cut surface is pale gray, homogeneous, and translucent.

The solitary neurofibromas that are unassociated with neurofibromatosis tend to be more compact and tend to develop in both young and middle-aged adults. Treatment is by excision; even if the tumor is not completely excised it does not tend to recur. This is in contrast to the neurofibromas found in von Recklinghausen's disease, in which the tumor tends to be larger and more likely to recur. When associated with von Recklinghausen's disease, they are the prototype tumor, and in approximately 8–10% one of these tumors undergoes malignant change (12).

PLEXIFORM NEUROMA (NEUROFIBROMA)

A plexiform neuroma may occur alone or in association with other manifestations of von Recklinghausen's disease. According to Harkin and Reed (13), a patient presenting with a plexiform neuroma, even when it is a solitary lesion, is considered to have neurofibromatosis even though it may be the sole clinical manifestation. It is caused by a proliferation of Schwann cells and nerve fibers inside the nerve sheath, which results in fusiform swelling and marked thickening and tortuosity of the nerves. It is usually unilateral and first seen between the ages of 2 and 5. It most commonly involves the supraorbital branch of the trigeminal nerve (14). In the lids it is sometimes associated with thickening and pigmentation of the skin which produces folds (elephantiasis neuromatosis) and is movable over the mass.

The typical plexiform pattern is the result of the bizarre arrangement of the Schwann cells, endoneurium, and axons in a mucinous matrix surrounded by a perineural sheath (Fig. 29.6). Palisading and whorls are not found. Neurofibrils can be seen passing through the tumor; many

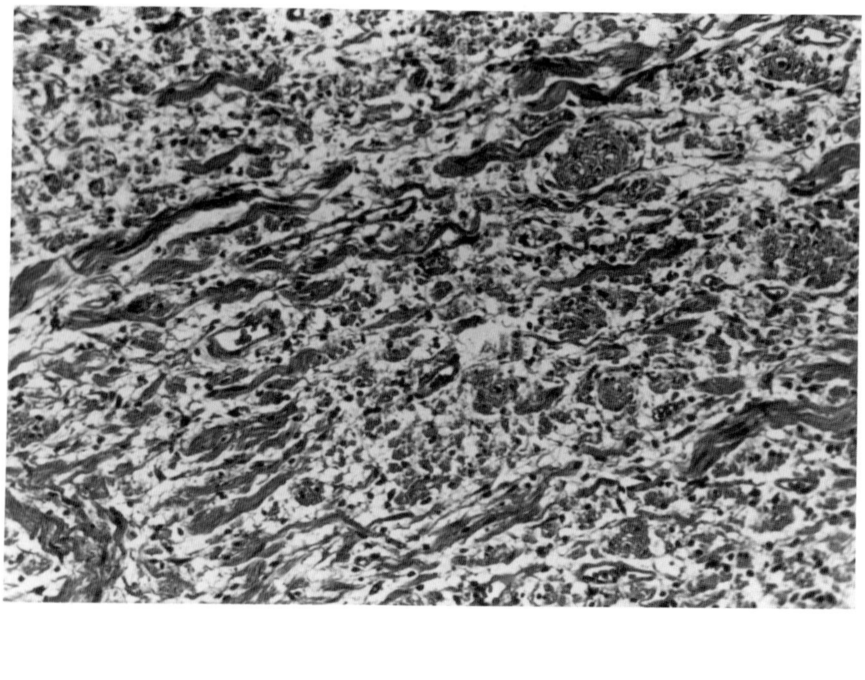

Figure 29.5. Solitary neurofibroma. Photomicrograph shows Schwann cells in a myxomatous matrix. (Courtesy of Leroy R. Sharer, M.D.)

are irregularly swollen. On cut section, these neurofibrils have scattered, pale, translucent, gray cords or nodules. The texture of this tumor has been compared to a "bag of worms" and is the most striking lid manifestation of neurofibromatosis (Fig. 29.7). It is soft, occasionally tender, and has a predilection for the upper lid, thereby causing ptosis. The lid margin often assumes a characteristic S-shaped configuration (15). A plexiform neuroma does not metastasize but may be locally aggressive. There is no known treatment, but surgery can be employed for cosmesis.

GRANULAR CELL TUMOR (SCHWANNOMA OR MYOBLASTOMA)

The granular cell tumor was originally described by Abrikossoff (16) in 1926, who believed it to have originated from immature striated muscle cells. Although controversial, this concept has been replaced by the neurogenic theory which states that the cell of origin is the Schwann cell (17). This cannot be regarded as conclusive since other studies (18, 19) have suggested the cell of origin may be an undifferentiated mesenchymal (fibroblast-like) cell. Rarely, it has been reported to have occurred in the eyelid (20–23). The tumor is usually benign, well circumscribed, and easily removed; although some tumors reported were poorly demarcated and infiltrated adjacent stroma (21). It is found in intimate relationship with striated muscle and peripheral nerves.

Granular cell tumor is twice as common in females and can occur at any age but usually occurs in the fourth to sixth decade. It is usually solitary, although it can be multifocal; in either case it is usually slow growing, firm, and asymptomatic. This nodular lesion is composed of sheets of plump polygonal cells arranged in clusters or cords with small, round vesicular and hyperchromatic nuclei with little supportive stroma. The granular cells contain no glycogen. These cells have abundant cytoplasm that contain eosinophilic granules which are periodic acid-Schiff positive and Sudan black B positive. Myelin stains are equivocal, and phosphatase activity is negative. A slender reticulin and fibrous framework within the tumor can be seen. The cut surface is firm and homogeneous and often has a yellowish tint.

The overlying epidermis is nonulcerated but may show pseudoepitheliomatous hyperplasia, which has been mistaken for squamous cell carcinoma. This has never been reported to have occurred in the eyelid, but there has been one case reported of pseudoepitheliomatous hyperplasia of the conjunctiva (24). Treatment of this slow-growing tumor is wide surgical excision as this tumor is insensitive to radiation or chemotherapy.

GANGLIONEUROMA

The ganglioneuroma is an extremely rare benign tumor that is most often found in the brain of children and young adults between the ages of 6 and 20. It also has been reported as a solitary lesion of the face and in the upper eyelid (14). It presents as a smooth, firm, slow-growing encapsulated mass. Twenty-five percent of the incompletely differentiated cases undergo malignant transformation with local spread and metastases. Most arise from immature ganglion cells that differentiate into mature ganglion cells. Histologically, one finds well-formed, large ganglion cells with abundant cytoplasm and glial tissue surrounded by Schwann cells. On section the tissue is pale yellow-white. This tumor is insensitive to radiation and should be surgically excised since there is a tendency to develop malignant change.

MULTIPLE MUCOSAL NEUROMAS SYNDROME

The multiple mucosal neuromas syndrome is similar to neurofibromatosis (13) in that both are genetically determined disorders of neural crest derivatives. The lesions in this syndrome, however, are true neuromas and resemble traumatic neuromas rather than neurofibromas. The syndrome is autosomal dominant and is frequently associated with carcinoma of the thyroid and pheochromocytoma, also known as the "multiple endocrine neoplasia type 2b." Numerous small nodules likened to "grains of rice" occur on the eyelids, lips, and tongue (Figs. 29.8–29.10). Histologically, the myelinated nerves are hypertrophied and tortuous with a thickened perineurium. Ganglion are sometimes present within the enlarged nerves.

The multiple system involvement of this syndrome consists of thickened eyelids and tarsal plates. The cilia may be displaced cutaneously secondary to neuromas in the grayline. Mucosal neuromas may also occur in the bulbar and palpebral conjunctiva as well as at the limbus. Heavy eyebrows and prominent orbital ridges are also common.

Highly visible corneal nerves, ectopic lacrimal punctum, lacrimal hyposecretion, bilateral pheochromocytomas, medullary carcinoma of the thyroid, intestinal ganglioneuroma, a marfanoid habitus, and characteristic facies are also associated with this syndrome. An absent flare response to intradermal histamine also occurs (25, 26). Riley and Robertson (27) found no involvement of the lacrimal gland on an autopsy specimen and postulated that the keratoconjunctivitis sicca often found probably represents autonomic dysfunction secondary to the neuromas. Since the ophthalmologist may be the first one to see these patients, it is important that this syndrome be recognized to facilitate early diagnosis and treatment of the potentially fatal associated carcinomas.

MELANOCYTIC LESIONS

There are some primary melanocytic lesions that arise from descendants of the neural crest. They give rise to melanocytic hamartomas and tumors of the eyelids. It is generally agreed that these cells arise from the Schwannian sheaths of dermal nerves and are neuroectodermal in origin (14). These benign lesions range from ephelis and lentigo to the five types of nevi. Rare pigmented tumors (e.g., storiform neurofibroma and melanotic schwannomas) may represent mixtures of Schwann cells and melanocytes, Schwann cell tumors producing melanin, or variant melanomas (28). These tumors are sometimes indistinguishable from blue nevi (29).

An *ephelis* (freckle) is found normally on areas of sun-exposed skin. It is a well-circumscribed macular area that is yellow, brown, or black due to increased melanin in the basal cell layer of the epidermis. Similar to this but larger in size is lentigo, which may be found on nonexposed skin. Here there are increased numbers of melanocytes present in the basal layer of the rete ridges.

Lentigo maligna (melanotic freckle of Hutchinson or precancerous melanosis of Dubreuilh) is an acquired premalignant lesion. It is a slow-growing pigmented macule on sun-exposed skin found in adults older than age 50. These lesions may wax and wane over many years. Histologically, there are hyperpigmented and pleomorphic melanocytes in the basal layer of the epidermis with some melanophages present. It is often indistinguishable from a junctional nevus. An underlying chronic nongranulomatous inflammatory infiltrate is common. Approximately one-third will become invasive lesions (30).

The *nevus* is a hamartomatous tumor consisting of atypical dermal melanocytes. It is a flat or elevated and usually well-circumscribed lesion. Histologically, the nevus cell is a small cell with scanty cytoplasm and a deeply staining nucleus. The nevus cells may occasionally resemble epitheloid cells, fibroblasts, or Schwann cells. Depending on the location of the nevus cells within the dermis, the pigmented nevus may be subclassified into the junctional nevus, the compound nevus, or the intradermal nevus.

The *junctional nevus* is common in the prepubertal age group. The nevus cells are located at the dermal-epidermal junction. This nevus has a low potential for malignancy. The compound nevus has both junctional and intradermal components. It is usually elevated and may be papillomatous. It has a low malignant potential. The common mole is the intradermal nevus. The nevus cells are entirely within the dermis. In some pigmented nevi there are spindled cells mixed with melanocytes which are considered to be Schwann cells, in addition to the usual nevus cells. When the neurogenous components predominate,

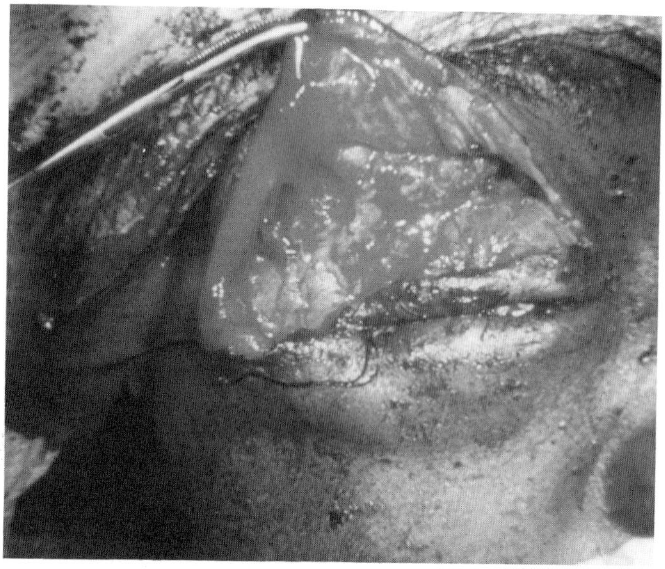

Figure 29.6. Plexiform neuroma of right upper lid. (Courtesy of Christine Zolli, M.D.)

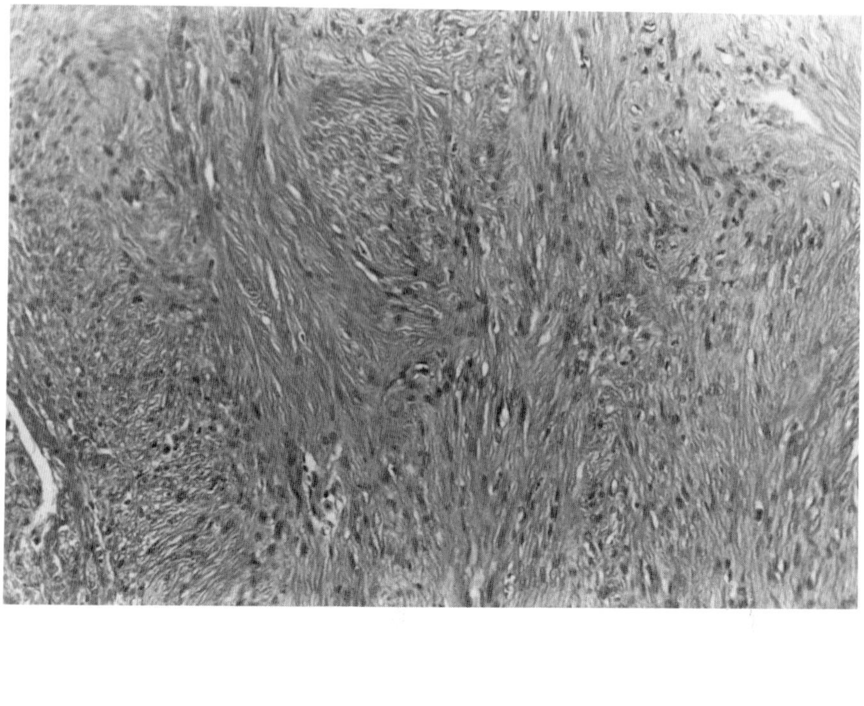

Figure 29.7. Plexiform neuroma. (Courtesy of Leroy R. Sharer, M.D.

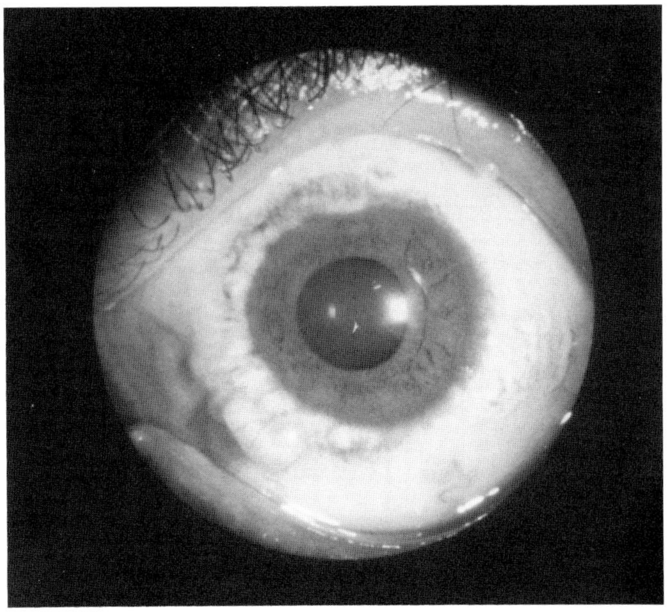

Figure 29.8. Multiple mucosal neuromas at limbus and on grayline of upper eyelid in a patient with multiple mucosal neuromas syndrome. (Courtesy of Rudolph S. Wagner, M.D.)

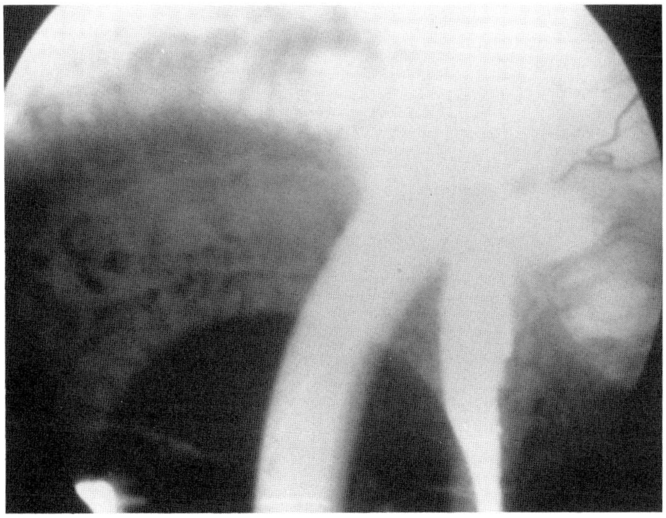

Figure 29.9. Slitlamp photomicrograph demonstrates thickened corneal nerves in multiple mucosal neuromas syndrome. (Courtesy of Rudolph S. Wagner, M.D.)

the lesions are termed "neurofibromatoid nevi" and may be part of the rare neurocutaneous melanosis syndrome.

The *blue nevus* is usually a flat and well-circumscribed nodule present early in life. The nevus cells are in the deep dermis and are spindle shaped and elongated. There may be melanophages present. This lesion becomes malignant only rarely.

Oculodermal melanocytosis (nevus of Ota) is a blue-gray pigmentation of the eyelid and conjunctiva following the distribution of the ophthalmic, maxillary, and sometimes the mandibular branches of the trigeminal nerve. It is usually present at birth, although it may appear later. It

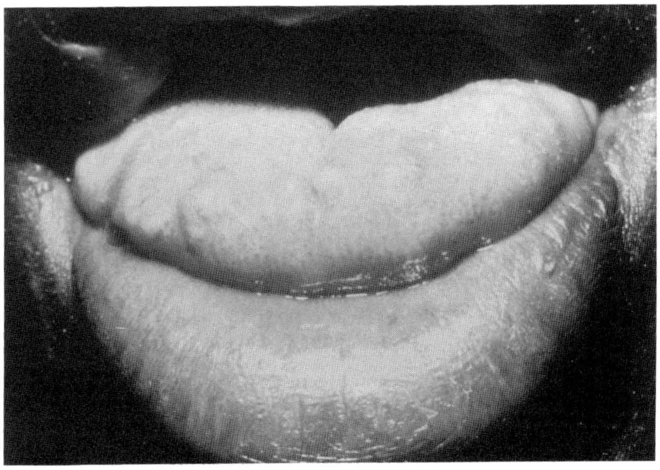

Figure 29.10. Neuromas on tongue and thickened lips. (Courtesy of Rudolph S. Wagner, M.D.)

is more common in females and is more commonly found in blacks and Orientals (31). Approximately 5% are bilateral (32). Histologically, there are groups of dendritic or fusiform-shaped cells containing large granules of melanin scattered deep within the dermis. Malignant change has only been reported in white patients.

REFERENCES

1. Boniuk M: Tumors of the eyelids. *Int Ophthalmol Clin* 2: 239–317, 1962.
2. Blodi FC: Amputation neuroma in the orbit. *Am J Ophthalmol* 32: 929–932, 1949.
3. Messmer EP, Camara J, Boniuk M, Font RL: Amputation neuroma of the orbit: report of two cases and review of the literature. *Ophthalmology* 91: 1420–1423, 1984.
4. Johnson R, Preston R, Newton JC: Amputation neuroma following pterygium excision. *Am J Ophthalmol* 62: 569–572, 1966.
5. Reese AB: *Tumors of the Eye*, ed 3. Hagerstown, MD, Harper & Row, 1976, pp 156–172.
6. Verocay J: Multiple Geschwulste als Systemerkrankung am Nervosen Apparate Festschrift Hans Chiari. *W Braumuller Wien und Leipzig*, 378–415, 1908.
7. Stout AP: Peripheral manifestations of the specific nerve sheath tumor (neurilemmoma). *Am J Cancer* 24: 751–796, 1935.
8. Shields JA, Guibor P: Neurilemoma of the eyelid resembling a recurrent chalazion. *Arch Ophthalmol* 102: 1650, 1984.
9. Schatz H: Benign orbital neurilemmoma: sarcomatous transformation in von Recklinghausen's disease. *Arch Ophthalmol* 86: 268–273, 1971.
10. DasGupta TK, Brasfield RD, Strong EW, Hajdu SI: Benign solitary schwannomas (neurilemmomas). *Cancer* 24: 355–366, 1969.
11. Mortada A: Benign tumors of lid dermis presenting as solid edema. *Arch Ophthalmol* 70: 369–371, 1963.
12. Saxen E: Tumors of sheaths of peripheral nerves- studies on their structure, histiogenesis and symptomatology. *Acta Pathol Microbiol Scand* 26 (Suppl. 79): 1–135, 1948.
13. Harkin JC, Reed RJ: Tumors of the peripheral nervous system. In *Atlas of Tumor Pathology*. Washington, D.C., Armed Forces Institute of Pathology, 1969, 2nd series, Fascicle 3.
14. Duke-Elder S, McFaul PA: The ocular adnexae. In Duke-Elder S (ed): *System of Ophthalmology*. St. Louis, CV Mosby, 1974, vol 13.
15. Smith B, English FP: Classical eyelid border sign of neurofibromatosis. *Br J Ophthalmol* 54: 134–135, 1970.
16. Abrikossoff A: Uber Myome, ausgehend von der quergestreiften willkurlichen Muskulatur. *Virchows Arch (Pathol Anat)* 260: 215–233, 1926.
17. Sobel HJ, Marquet E: Granular cells and granular cell lesions. *Pathol Annu* 9: 43, 1974.
18. Sobel HJ, Marquet E, Schwarz R: Is schwannoma related to granular

cell myoblastoma? *Arch Pathol* 95: 396–401, 1973.

19. Pour P, Althoff J, Cardesa A: Granular cells in tumors and in nontumorous tissue. *Arch Pathol* 95: 135–138, 1973.
20. Dunnington JH: Granular cell myoblastoma of the orbit. *Arch Ophthalmol* 40: 14–22, 1948.
21. Strong EW, McDivitt RW, Brasfield RD: Granular cell myoblastoma. *Cancer* 25: 415–422, 1970.
22. Friedman Z, Eden E, Neumann E: Granular cell myoblastoma of the eyelid margin. *Br J Ophthalmol* 57: 757–760, 1973.
23. Rubenzik R, Tenzel RR: Granular cell myoblastoma of the lid: a case report. *Ann Ophthalmol* 8: 421–422, 1976.
24. Ferry AP: Granular cell tumor (myoblastoma) of the palpebral conjunctive causing pseudoepitheliomatous hyperplasia of the conjunctival epithelium. *Am J Ophthalmol* 91: 234–238, 1981.
25. Baum JL, Adler ME: Pheochromocytoma, medullary thyroid carcinoma, multiple mucosal neuroma; a variant of the syndrome. *Arch Ophthalmol* 87: 574–584, 1972.
26. Robertson, DM, Sizemore GW, Gordon H: Thickened corneal nerves as a manifestation of multiple endocrine neoplasia. *Trans Am Acad Ophthalmol Otolaryngol* 79: 772–787, 1975.
27. Riley FC, Robertson DM: Ocular histopathology in multiple endocrine neoplasia type 2b. *Am J Ophthalmol* 91: 57–64, 1981.
28. Jakobiec FA, Jones IS: Neurogenic tumors. In Duane TD, Jaeger EA (eds): *Clinical Ophthalmology*. Philadelphia, Harper & Row, 1984, vol 2, pp 1–19.
29. Russell DS, Rubinstein, LJ: *Pathology of Tumors of the Nervous System*, ed 4. Baltimore, Williams & Wilkins, 1977.
30. Naidoff MA, Bernardino, VB, Clark WH: Melanocytic lesions of the eyelid skin. *Am J Ophthalmol* 82: 371–382, 1976.
31. Gonder JR, Ezell PC, Shields JA, Augsburger JJ: Ocular melanocytosis: a study to determine the prevalence rate of ocular melanocytosis. *Ophthalmology* 89: 950–952, 1982.
32. Skalka HW: Bilateral oculodermal melanocytosis. *Ann Ophthalmol* 8: 565–567, 1976.

CHAPTER 30

Pigmented Eyelid Lesions

ROBERT FOLBERG, M.D.
VITALIANO B. BERNARDINO, JR., M.D.
EVALINA A. BERNARDINO, M.D

A patient with a pigmented eyelid lesion presents a particular problem to the ophthalmologist. The differential diagnosis of a pigmented eyelid lesion is lengthy and ranges from innocent nevi and seborrheic keratosis to pigmented basal cell carcinoma, squamous cell carcinoma, and malignant melanoma. Of this list, malignant melanoma is the chief concern: some pigmented lesions are purely cosmetic problems (such as seborrheic keratosis); some may cause extensive tissue destruction and, if advanced, may be life threatening (such as basal cell carcinoma); some have the potential for regional node metastasis but are only rarely the cause of a patient's demise (such as cutaneous squamous cell carcinoma). However, RF malignant melanoma has the potential for widespread dissemination.

From the perspective of histogenesis, it is important for the reader to understand that most nevi and melanomas are derived from epidermal melanocytes. By contrast, lesions such as pigmented seborrheic keratosis, pigmented basal cell carcinoma, pigmented actinic keratosis, and pigmented squamous cell carcinoma are all derived from the nonmelanocytic epidermal cells: the pigmentation is a secondary phenomenon. Cutaneous lesions that are secondarily pigmented tend to behave like their nonpigmented counterparts.

Even if it is clear that a pigmented eyelid lesion is not currently a melanoma—as in the case of a giant hairy nevus of the eyelid—the ophthalmologist must consider the likelihood of a melanoma developing at some future date in that lesion. Also, the ophthalmologist must consider the ophthalmic morbidity (possible amblyopia) associated with such a lesion.

It is curious that the death rate from malignant melanoma is declining even as the incidence is increasing (1). Clearly, this paradox must be attributed to early diagnosis and management of melanomas and melanoma precursors. Many ophthalmologists are aware of the need for early diagnosis of melanoma, so that there is a tendency to divide all pigmented eyelid lesions into two groups: (*a*) melanomas and melanoma precursors (lesions of great concern) and (*b*) other pigmented eyelid lesions (lesions of lesser concern). This bipartite classification is admirable for its emphasis on the early detection of melanoma and melanoma precursors, but it overlooks other important lesions (pigmented squamous cell carcinoma and pigmented basal cell carcinoma) that, although not directly derived from melanocytes, are nevertheless secondarily pigmented and can cause significant morbidity.

The emphasis on early diagnosis and management of cutaneous melanoma may lead to another type of error: overdiagnosis of melanoma with overtreatment of totally innocuous lesions such as pigmented seborrheic keratosis. Each of the authors has seen examples of eyelid resections performed for pigmented eyelid lesions with no potential for evolution into melanoma.

The reader will note that many fine points in the differential diagnosis of pigmented eyelid lesions require careful attention to the surface topography, lesion edges, and color. For this purpose, most dermatologists carry a pocket magnifying lens and examine pigmented lesions under excellent illumination. Ophthalmologists may use their indirect ophthalmoscopy lenses for magnification and should examine cutaneous lesions in well-lighted examining rooms. Jakobiec (2) has recommended studying cutaneous eyelid lesions at the slitlamp, an instrument that provides both excellent magnification and illumination, and we heartily endorse his suggestion.

The reader will note that the clinical setting will help to narrow the differential diagnosis. For example, the patient's age may limit certain diagnostic considerations. Additionally, while melanomas (generally of the acral lentiginous type) do occur in black patients, they are exceedingly rare in sun-exposed areas such as the eyelid.

In the discussion that follows, references to differential diagnosis refer to the clinical differential diagnosis, not the differential diagnosis considered by the pathologist. Pathologists may refer to texts devoted to the pathology of melanomas and other pigmented lesions (3, 4) for a more complete discussion of the pathology differential diagnosis.

As a final note of introduction, this chapter deals only with pigmented cutaneous eyelid lesions. Conjunctival melanoma and its precursors have been the subject of recent reviews (5–7). In order to aid in the early detection of eyelid melanomas and also to provide a reference for other pigmented eyelid lesions, the topic of melanoma and melanoma precursors is presented first.

EYELID MELANOMAS

It is somewhat comforting to realize that malignant melanoma of the eyelid skin is extremely rare. In fact, the largest clinicopathologic series of eyelid melanomas described only five cases (8). Since eyelid melanoma is rare, it is necessary to borrow information gleaned from the study of melanomas in other body sites and apply these concepts to the eyelid.

There are four commonly accepted clinicopathologic forms of cutaneous melanoma: *lentigo maligna* melanoma, *superficial spreading* melanoma, *acral lentiginous* melanoma, and *nodular* melanoma (9). Despite the recent suggestion that this subclassification may be artificial (10), there is ample evidence to suggest that the varieties of melanoma are distinctive clinically as well as histologically (9, 10). Additionally, the differential diagnosis of each type of melanoma is somewhat different.

LENTIGO MALIGNA MELANOMA

Lentigo maligna melanoma is perhaps the most common form of eyelid melanoma. It accounts for 91% of head and neck melanomas (11) and tends to develop in older patients (beyond middle age) on sun-damaged skin. Most reported cases have involved either the lower eyelid or the canthi (8, 12, 13) and occur in the same distribution as basal cell carcinomas, which is also attributed to the ultraviolet light carcinogen.

Clinical Features

Lentigo maligna melanoma begins as a flat, freckle-like tan spot that enlarges progressively over many (5–10 or more) years. This spot tends to have irregular edges (indented or notched) and tends to acquire flecks of dark-brown and black pigmentation as it enlarges (Fig. 30.1). If a skin biopsy is obtained at this stage of development, cytologically atypical melanocytes are seen within the basal-most layer of the epidermis. These atypical melanocytes tend not to resemble one another and may be separated from each other by normal epidermal keratocytes (Fig. 30.2). The atypical melanocytes also have the tendency to be dispersed along adnexal structures. Since lentigo maligna develops on sun-damaged skin, solar elastosis and epidermal atrophy may be prominent features.

Since the lesion described in the preceding paragraph is confined to the epidermis, most authors do not designate it as a melanoma. Instead, it is called a "lentigo maligna" (14). The term *lentigo maligna* may be used interchangeably with the term *Hutchinson's* (melanotic) *freckle.* Since lentigo maligna does not involve the dermis histologically, clinically observed normal skin markings are visible (see Figure 30.1 and compare with superficial spreading melanoma discussed below).

Within the lentigo maligna lesion, portions of the tan pigmentation may appear to "break up" or disappear, only to be replaced by a slightly gray or blue discoloration (15). The focal loss of pigmentation within the lesion may reflect focal immunologically mediated regression. It is important to remember that the arrangement of color in lentigo maligna is disorderly or haphazard.

The lentigo maligna lesion may persist with gradual centrifugal (or radial) growth for many years. It has been estimated that in 30% of untreated lesions, a focal nodule may appear (16). This nodule corresponds histologically to the downward (vertical) growth into the dermis of malignant melanoma.

When malignant melanoma occurs in the context of the

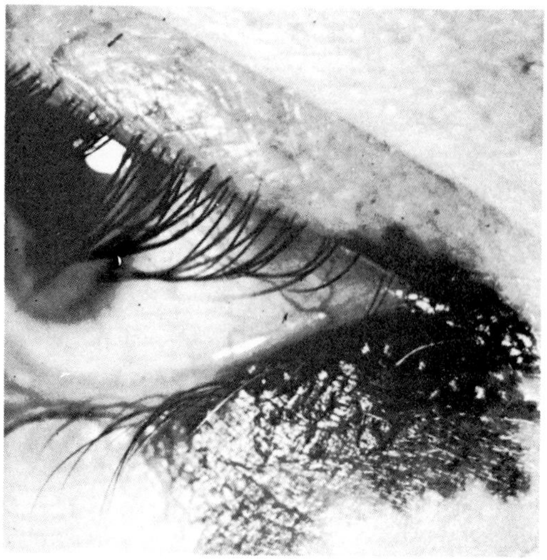

Figure 30.1. Clinical appearance of lentigo maligna. Note that the borders show irregular notching. The lesion is flat and skin markings are retained. (From Naidoff MA, Bernardino VB Jr, Clark WH Jr: Melanocytic lesions of the eyelid skin. *Am J Ophthalmol* 82: 371–382, 1976. Published with permission from the American Journal of Ophthalmology. Copyright by the Ophthalmic Publishing Co.)

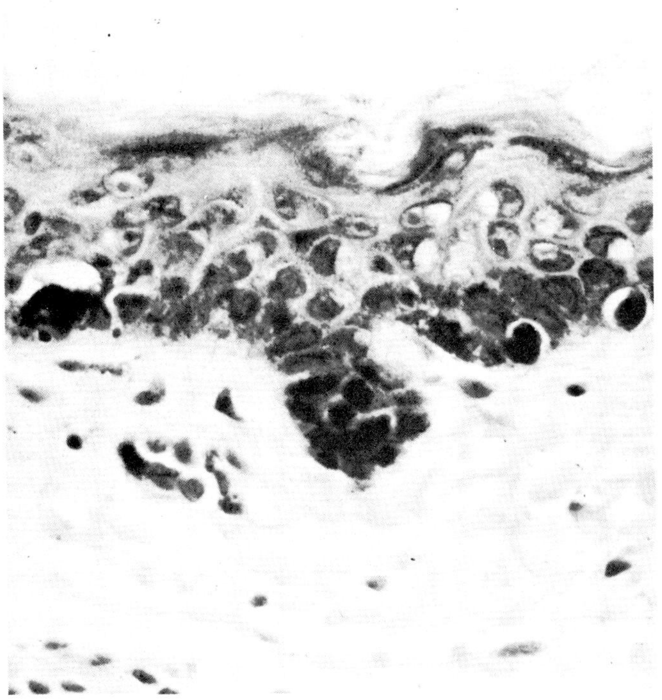

Figure 30.2. Histopathology of lentigo maligna illustrated in Figure 30.1. Atypical melanocytes are present along the basilar layers of the epidermis. (From Naidoff MA, Bernardino VB, Jr, Clark WB Jr: Melanocytic lesions of the eyelid skin. *Am J Ophthalmol* 82: 371–382, 1976. Published with permission from the American Journal of Ophthalmology. Copyright by the Ophthalmic Publishing Co.).

radial growth of lentigo maligna, the entire lesion is known as *lentigo maligna melanoma* (17). Lentigo maligna, therefore, is the early stage of lentigo maligna melanoma, however, it is not inevitable that lentigo maligna will evolve into lentigo maligna melanoma (13).

The key to the management of lentigo maligna melanoma is the recognition of its earliest stage, lentigo maligna. Lentigo maligna should be distinguished from other pigmented eyelid lesions occurring in older patients: common lentigo (sometimes known as "senile lentigo"), pigmented actinic keratosis (13, 14), pigmented squamous cell carcinoma in situ (14), and seborrheic keratosis (14).

Differential Diagnosis

Common ("senile") lentigo tends to be smaller than lentigo maligna. Unlike lentigo maligna, common lentigo is uniformly tan and has smooth borders. Common lentigo may enlarge slightly, but a history of progressive enlargement should raise suspicions of lentigo maligna.

Actinic keratosis, a possible precursor of squamous cell carcinoma, may present rarely as a spreading pigmented lesion that simulates lentigo maligna (13). The pigmented actinic keratosis, like lentigo maligna, tends to involve sun-exposed skin. While pigmented actinic keratosis has not been reported as a distinct entity on the eyelid skin, it does tend to involve the face. Pigmented actinic keratosis appears to be a relatively flat tan or brown lesion but, unlike lentigo maligna, the edges of pigmented actinic keratosis may be slightly palpable. Also unlike lentigo maligna, pigmented actinic keratosis tends to have a uniform distribution of pigment. The pathology of pigmented actinic keratosis is identical to the nonpigmented variety except that there is an excessive accumulation of melanin within cytologically normal melanocytes. This accumulation suggests a block in the normal transfer of melanin to squamous epithelial cells (17). Pigmented actinic keratosis should be treated to prevent the appearance of squamous cell carcinoma. It is not known if pigmented actinic keratosis evolves into pigmented squamous cell carcinoma.

For the same reasons as mentioned above, squamous cell carcinoma in situ may be pigmented (18). Squamous cell carcinoma in situ tends to be associated with excess keratin production (hyperkeratosis), which appears clinically as a gray-white scale atop the lesion. Hyperkeratosis usually is not a feature of lentigo maligna. Squamous cell carcinoma in situ may be found on sun-exposed skin and on nonexposed skin. In nonexposed skin, the differential diagnosis is with superficial spreading melanoma (see next section) rather than with lentigo maligna.

Seborrheic keratosis may be confused very infrequently with lentigo maligna and lentigo maligna melanoma. By histopathology, seborrheic keratosis involves a focal thickening of the epidermis (acanthosis), thus elevating the lesion above the plane of unaffected epidermis (the seborrheic keratosis appears to be stuck onto the skin). Occasionally, the same block in transfer of melanin to the squamous cells of the epidermis may occur in seborrheic keratosis imparting pigment to this "stuck on" lesion. Normally, the elevated pigmented seborrheic keratosis would not be confused with the flat lesion of lentigo maligna, but on rare occasion, epidermal thickening may be seen in lentigo maligna, making clinical differentiation between pigmented seborrheic keratosis and lentigo maligna very difficult (18). On the other hand, seborrheic keratosis may itself be rather flat and if pigmented, may resemble lentigo maligna. The frequently greasy texture of seborrheic keratosis may be removed by gentle scraping with the edge of a scalpel blade or a fingernail. The reader should note that nevus is not in the differential diagnosis of lentigo maligna. As is discussed in detail later in this chapter, nevi are either congenital or acquired, and if acquired, they tend to make their appearance from childhood and adolescence through the 3rd decade of life. Toward the seventh decade of life, at about the time that lentigo maligna becomes a clinical concern, many pigmented cutaneous nevi begin to "disappear" clinically (9). Therefore, a pigmented lesion that first appears after middle age and continues to enlarge should not be considered clinically to be a nevus.

Treatment

The management of lentigo maligna and lentigo maligna melanoma is discussed at the conclusion of the section on eyelid melanomas. It is important to emphasize that while the differential diagnosis presented above appears to be easy, there may be times when the only way to distinguish among the possibilities is a skin biopsy. There should be no difficulty in separating lentigo maligna from its "look alikes" by histology.

SUPERFICIAL SPREADING MELANOMA

Unlike lentigo maligna and lentigo maligna melanoma, which appear only on sun-exposed skin and therefore have a tendency to affect the face, superficial spreading melanoma appears also on skin that is not exposed. This distinction is somewhat important since it is said that superficial spreading melanoma is the most common variant of melanoma, whereas lentigo maligna–lentigo maligna melanoma is an uncommon variant. Statements assigning the frequency of melanoma subtypes are generally based on *all* anatomic sites. Since lentigo maligna and lentigo maligna melanoma have a distinct predilection for the face (11), they are probably found on the eyelid in higher proportions relative to other variants of melanoma.

Clinical Features

Superficial spreading melanoma tends to affect a somewhat younger population than lentigo maligna and lentigo maligna melanoma (11). We hesitate to be dogmatic about the median ages of onset for the various types of melanoma because of a great deal of overlap; however, certain generalizations may be helpful. A patient in the fourth decade of life is unlikely to have lentigo-maligna or lentigo maligna melanoma, but a patient in the seventh decade of life may have either superficial spreading melanoma or lentigo maligna–lentigo maligna melanoma.

Recall that lentigo maligna melanoma begins as a centrifugally (radially) enlarging spot that is flat, and that the appearance of a nodule (invasive disease) qualified the lesion as a melanoma (lentigo maligna melanoma). Superficial spreading melanoma also begins as an enlarging pigmented spot, also with haphazard arrangement of colors and irregular, notched borders, but the neoplastic melanocytes tend to invade the superficial dermis (papillary dermis) rather early in the course (Fig. 30.3). This superficial dermal invasion correlates with the observation that the centrifugally (radially) enlarging spot of superficial spreading melanoma is frequently palpable, whereas the enlarging spot of lentigo maligna, in which the atypical melanocytes are confined to the epidermis, is totally flat (18, 19). In addition, the early invasion of the papillary dermis in the radial growth phase of superficial spreading melanoma may lead to obliteration of the normal, clinically observed skin markings. Recall that skin markings are usually preserved in lentigo maligna, the intraepidermal precursor of lentigo maligna melanoma (Fig. 30.4).

There is no special name, equivalent to lentigo maligna, applied to the early lesion of superficial spreading melanoma, but the early lesion of superficial spreading melanoma may be distinguished histologically from lentigo maligna. Unlike lentigo maligna and lentigo maligna melanoma, the atypical melanocytes in superficial spreading melanoma are not confined to the most basal layer of the epidermis but instead have the distinct predilection for invasion upward into the epidermis, either as individual cells (mimicking Paget's disease of the breast) or in nests. Also, the atypical intraepidermal melanocytes of superficial spreading melanoma do not have any particular tendency to spread along adnexal structures.

The progressively enlarging spot of superficial spreading melanoma may reach a size exceeding 10 mm, at which time areas of pigmentation may disappear, and be replaced by pink or blue-gray zones. These zones of pigment breakup correspond to zones of immunologically mediated lesion regression (14). The phenomenon of focal lesion regression frequently precedes the *focal* appearance of a nodule within the enlarging spot. By the time that a nodule appears, the lesion may have reached the size of 3 to 5 cm. The nodule corresponds to a collection of tumor cells that have invaded more deeply than the superficial (papillary) dermis into the deeper (reticular) dermis or into the subcutaneous fat.

The development of a nodule in either lentigo maligna or in the early phase of superficial spreading melanoma constitutes a radical change in the appearance and behavior of the lesion. The prenodule radial growth phase of

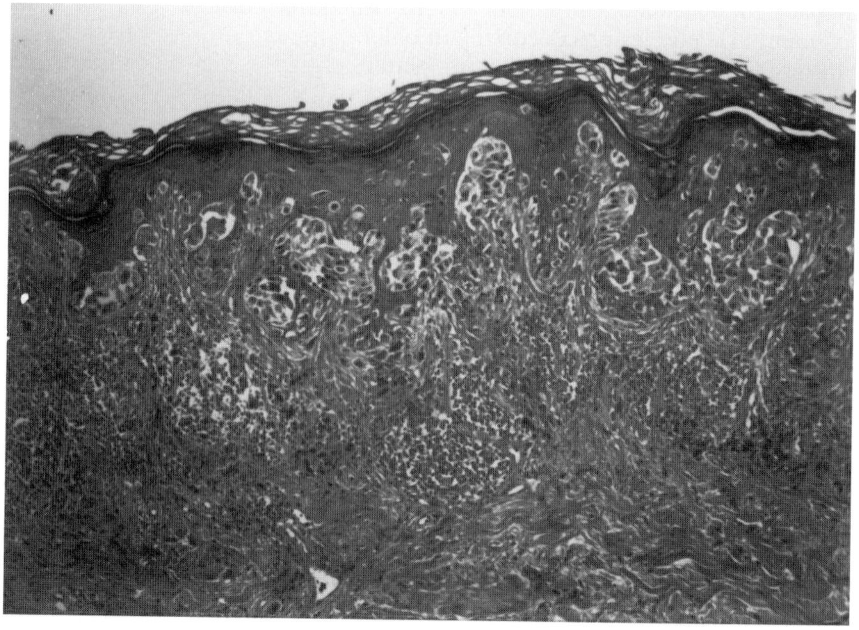

Figure 30.3. Histology of malignant melanoma of the superficial spreading type, invasing to level II (see text). Atypical epithelioid melanocytes invade into the epidermis singly and in nests, resembling Paget's disease (Pagetoid spread). The same cells invade into the papillary dermis. Even though the tumor is superficially invasive, the lesion is in the radial growth phase, a stage of "indolent growth." Tumors excised at this stage do not metastasize. Hematoxylin-eosin stain; original magnification × 25.

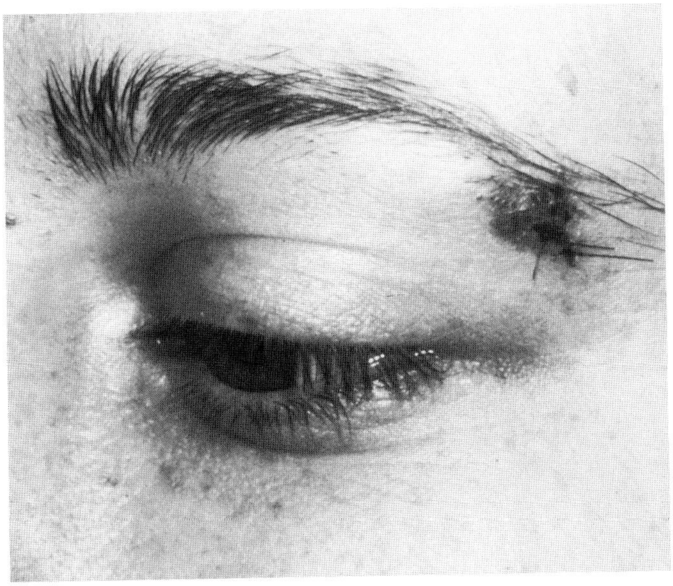

Figure 30.4. Clinical appearance of a small superficial spreading melanoma of the eyebrow. The sutures within the lesion indicate a recent incisional biopsy. The lesion is elevated (clinically palpable) and skin markings are obliterated. Note the haphazard arrangement of pigment.

both lentigo maligna and early superficial spreading melanoma, if totally treated, should result in total cure for the patient: tumors in the radial growth phase (even thin, superficially invasive superficial spreading melanomas) are incapable of spawning metastases. It is only when the vertical growth phase supervenes—a nodule develops, which reflects tumor invasion into deeper cutaneous layers—that the tumor is capable of spawning metastases (11). There are definite histologic criteria for designating a lesion as in a "biologically indolent phase" (radial growth phase) or "biologically virulent phase" (vertical growth phase) for lentigo maligna melanoma and superficial spreading melanoma; these criteria are discussed below. It is important, however, that the clinical radial growth phase (prenodule) be recognized early and treated definitively so that tumor death can be prevented. It is the early recognition of the radial growth phase that has permitted a decline in the mortality from melanoma despite its increasing incidence (1).

Differential Diagnosis

The clinical differential diagnosis of a suspected superficial spreading melanoma includes pigmented squamous cell carcinoma, pigmented seborrheic keratosis, pigmented basal cell carcinoma, cutaneous hemorrhage and cutaneous hemangioma. An innocent pigmented nevus that has been subjected to shave biopsy may recur as a nevus but may simulate superficial spreading melanoma clinically as well as histologically (20).

The key to distinguishing between pigmented squamous cell carcinoma and superficial spreading melanoma is color and contour: the pigment in a pigmented squamous cell carcinoma is not nearly as haphazard as is seen in superficial spreading melanoma; the presence of excessive keratin (hyperkeratosis) overlying the pigmented squamous cell carcinoma lends a thin gray covering to this lesion, which is not seen in superficial spreading melanoma; and the edges of pigmented squamous cell carcinoma are not nearly as irregular as those seen in superficial spreading melanoma (18) (Fig. 30.5).

While it is true that even early superficial spreading melanoma may have palpable edges, superficial spreading melanoma usually is not nearly as elevated above the plane of the adjacent epidermis as is pigmented or nonpigmented seborrheic keratosis, (Fig. 30.6). The haphazard distribution of color in superficial spreading melanoma is another important distinguishing point.

Clark and co-workers (18) cite two forms of pigmented basal cell carcinoma that may be mistaken for cutaneous melanoma. Pigmented nodular basal cell carcinoma may be mistaken for nodular melanoma (see "Differential Diagnosis"), while the flatter type of pigmented basal cell carcinoma may be mistaken for superficial spreading melanoma (Fig. 30.7). The flatter type of pigmented basal cell carcinoma tends to contain dots of pigmentation in contrast to superficial spreading melanoma, which is pigmented (although chaotically) throughout. The irregular edges of pigmented basal cell carcinoma may resemble superficial spreading melanoma.

Although resolving hemorrhage theoretically may resemble a primary pigmented cutaneous lesion, the history should serve to separate these entities. Cutaneous hemangiomas are often present since birth or young childhood, so an adequate history should serve to distinguish these from superficial spreading melanoma. In addition, mild pressure on the surface of a capillary hemangioma (as with a glass microscopy slide), a procedure known as "diascopy", may blanch the color but will not significantly change the color of a melanoma. The nevus flammeus of

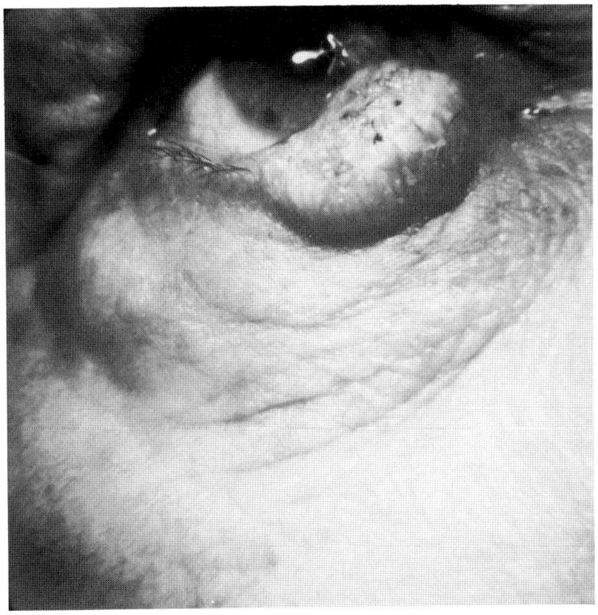

Figure 30.5. Squamous cell carcinoma of the eyelid. Note the flecks of pigmentation over the surface. Note also the gray-white scales, reflecting hyperkeratosis. Hyperkeratosis is not expected in melanomas.

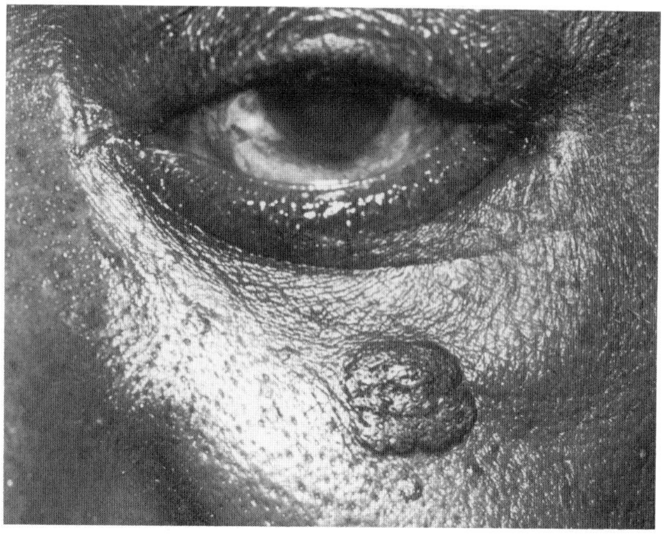

Figure 30.6. Pigmented seborrheic keratosis. The lesion appears "stuck onto" the eyelid skin. The surface is deeply grooved, typical for seborrheic keratosis but not for melanoma. The pigmentation is evenly distributed in contrast to melanoma (see Figure 30.4). Although the patient is black, melanomas are uncommon in blacks.

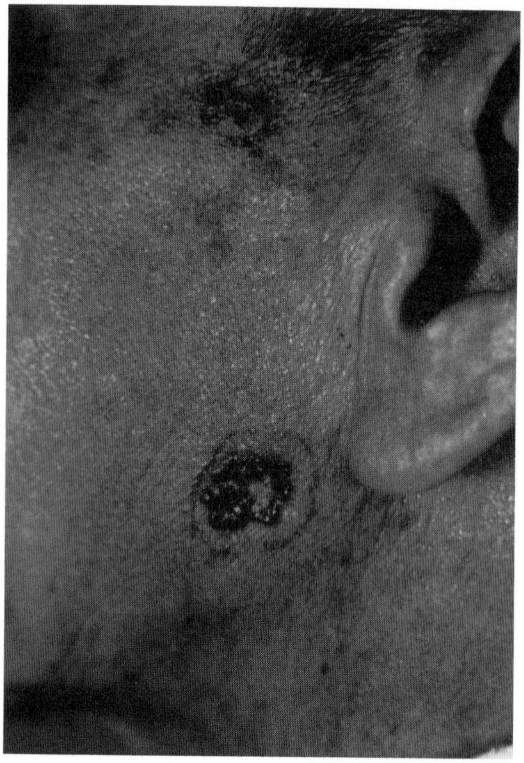

Figure 30.7. Pigmented basal cell carcinoma. Note the raised pearly edges, which is characteristic of basal cell carcinoma.

the Sturge-Weber syndrome, however, does not blanch on pressure.

The entity of recurrent nevus following shave biopsy (20) is discussed in "Eyelid Nevi."

ACRAL LENTIGINOUS MELANOMA

Like lentigo maligna melanoma and superficial spreading melanoma, acral lentiginous melanoma begins as a spot and if untreated in its radial growth phase, a focal nodule may appear. This type of melanoma has a distinctive histology for its radial growth phase (21) and tends to occur in the volar, subungual regions, and commonly in mucosal sites (11). It is seen infrequently in the conjunctiva (7). It is not known if melanomas with the histologic features of acral lentiginous melanoma may be found on the cutaneous portion of the eyelid.

NODULAR MELANOMA

Lentigo maligna melanoma, superficial spreading melanoma, and acral lentiginous melanoma each have a radial growth phase: a phase of a centrifugally enlarging zone of pigmentation within which a focal nodule may develop (the vertical growth phase). In effect, each of the three previously discussed forms of melanoma progresses indirectly toward a virulent form of the disease, through the pathway of a radial growth phase. In nodular melanoma, there is direct progression toward virulent disease: there is no radial growth phase. As the name implies, in nodular melanoma, a nodule simply appears. The vertical growth phase is the initial and only growth phase of nodular melanoma (14).

Clinical Features

The nodule appears typically over a course of 1 year. The edges of the nodule are discreet. The nodule tends to be uniformly pigmented and is commonly brown or black. Nodular melanoma is very uncommon on the eyelid (2). Amelanotic nodular melanomas may be seen, but careful inspection with good magnification (hand magnifying lens or slitlamp) usually reveals flecks of pigmentation (Fig. 30.8).

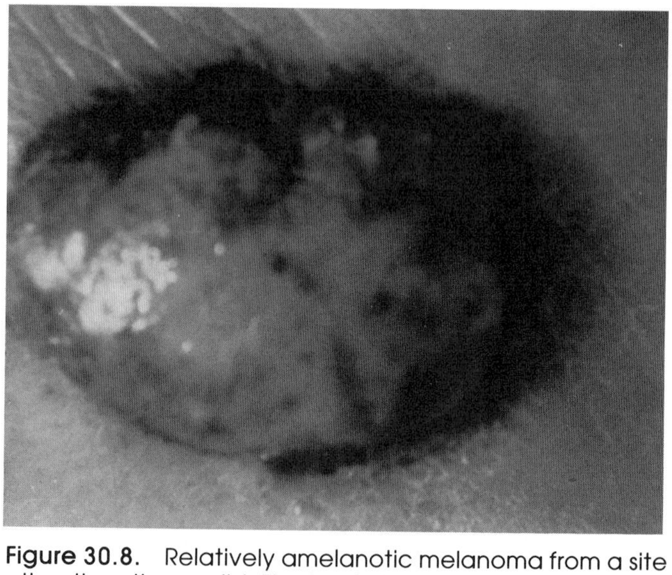

Figure 30.8. Relatively amelanotic melanoma from a site other than the eyelid. Flecks of pigmentation are present. Note the obliteration of skin markings over the surface of the tumor.

Differential Diagnosis

The differential diagnosis of nodular melanoma includes Spitz tumor, blue nevus and cellular blue nevus, pigmented nodular basal cell carcinoma, pigmented seborrheic keratosis, pigmented inverted follicular keratosis, and pyogenic granuloma.

The *Spitz tumor* (also known as a spindle-epithelioid nevus and by the confusing and inaccurate term "benign juvenile melanoma") occurs commonly on the face. While it is seen most frequently in children and adolescents, it may appear in adults. It presents as a globoid pink (infrequently tan) nodule that shows rapid growth over a period of 9 to 12 months, achieving a size of 6 to 10 mm. After a spurt of rapid growth, the lesion stabilizes in size and no further growth is seen. This is in contrast with nodular melanoma, which does not stabilize in size and continues to grow. It must be emphasized that the Spitz tumor is benign. Histologically, the Spitz tumor has a distinctive appearance that in many cases permits separation from nodular melanoma (22, 23).

Blue nevus and *cellular blue nevus* may present as nodular lesions. Histologically, the melanocytes that comprise these lesions are located within the dermis. The blue appearance of a nodular blue or cellular blue nevus is the clue to the distinction between these entities and nodular melanoma: nodular melanomas are most commonly brown or black, rarely pink, and do not show evidence of blue coloration. Patches of blue may be seen in the radial growth phase of lentigo maligna melanoma (lentigo maligna) and superficial spreading melanoma; these patches represent focal regression of the lesion. The blue appearance of partially regressed melanoma results from the presence of melanin in macrophages (melanophages) in the dermis. The blue color seen in blue and cellular blue nevi results from the presence of heavily pigmented spindled melanocytes within the dermis. In the case of partial regression of melanoma or blue nevus, the Tyndall effect explains the blue appearance of melanin viewed through layers of epidermis and dermis.

Pigmented nodular basal cell carcinoma may be confused clinically with nodular melanoma (18) although differences in the quality of pigmentation may permit separation of these entities. The pigmentation of nodular melanoma is usually uniformly brown or black—unless one is dealing with an amelanotic nodular melanoma, which, of course, is not likely to be confused with pigmented nodular basal cell carcinoma (see the discussion of pyogenic granuloma below)—while the small flecks of dark pigmentation may be seen in pigmented basal cell carcinoma.

Pigmented seborrheic keratosis (24) and *pigmented inverted follicular keratosis* (25) have each been confused clinically with nodular melanoma of the eyelid. The surface topography of the lesions should permit clinical separation of these entities. The histopathologic basis for the irregular surface contour of both seborrheic keratosis and inverted follicular keratosis is undulating epidermal hyperplasia, frequently accompanied by increased production of keratin (hyperkeratosis, represented clinically as a scale). By contrast, the surface of a nodular melanoma is smooth as the overlying epidermis is stretched over the nodule of melanoma cells in the dermis. In fact, loss of skin markings is seen commonly in nodular melanoma; ulceration, also seen in advanced nodular melanoma, is unexpected in either pigmented seborrheic keratosis or inverted follicular keratosis unless the lesion has been traumatized.

Rarely, *pyogenic granuloma* may be confused with amelanotic nodular melanoma. Fortunately, most amelanotic nodular melanomas show evidence of small flecks of pigment upon careful examination with magnification; such pigmentation is unexpected in pyogenic granuloma (18).

CUTANEOUS MELANOMA

Of the many factors that have been shown to be associated with prognosis in cutaneous melanoma, the depth of invasion is the most important. The depth of invasion is measured by two different but complementary techniques: levels of invasion (26, 27) and tumor thickness (28, 29). Levels of invasion describe the path that a melanoma takes through zones of the skin:

Level I. Lesion is confined to the epidermis (Fig. 30.2).

Level II. Lesion extends into the papillary (superficial) dermis (Fig. 30.3).

Level III. Tumor fills and expands the papillary dermis to the margin of the reticular dermis.

Level IV. Is the same as level 3 but the tumor cells permeate into the reticular dermis.

Level V. Tumor extends into the subcutaneous fat.

Melanoma limited to no deeper than level II is designated histologically as "radial growth phase disease;" this is a stage of melanoma in which the tumor has no capacity for metastasis. With level III (expansile growth within the papillary dermis down to the margin of the reticular dermis), the tumor is in "the vertical growth phase;" this is a stage in which the melanoma has the capacity to spawn metastases (11).

Since a large series of cutaneous eyelid melanomas, described by tumor leveling, has not been reported, it is difficult to comment critically on the applicability of this system to this anatomic region. The skin of the eyelid is exquisitely thin and a sharp demarcation between papillary dermis (level II) and reticular dermis (level III) is ill defined.

Tumor thickness is measured directly from the glass microslide. With the aid of an ocular micrometer that is installed in the pathologist's microscope, the distance between the top of the epidermis and the most deeply situated melanoma cell is measured. The commonly accepted guidelines regard melanomas measuring less than 0.76 mm in thickness to have an excellent prognosis, tumors measuring greater than 1.50 mm to have a poor prognosis, and tumors measuring between 0.76 and 1.50 mm to have an indeterminate prognosis (28, 29).

There are other features that add prognostically important information to the study of a cutaneous melanoma. Among these secondary factors is the location of the lesion. It is claimed that melanomas of the face seldom metastasize (30), but it is not certain if this claim considers the fact that most facial melanomas are of the lentigo maligna melanoma type and therefore carry a better prognosis. Additional clinical and histologic features related to prognosis are the presence and extent of ulceration of the tumor, the number of mitotic figures within the tumor, and the presence and nature of an inflammatory response at the base of the tumor (11).

CLINICAL APPROACH TO A PATIENT WITH SUSPECTED PIGMENTED EYELID LESION

The clinical differential diagnosis of pigmented eyelid lesions presented above may assist with the preoperative evaluation of a patient. If there is any doubt, and total removal of the lesion (excisional biopsy) would require extensive surgery, removal of a portion of the lesion to its complete depth (incisional biopsy) should be performed (31). Under no circumstances should a pigmented cutaneous lesion be treated by a destructive technique (electrodessication, cautery, or cryosurgery) without first obtaining a tissue diagnosis. Furthermore, if a lesion is excised, it must be sent to the pathology laboratory for study.

If the lesion is in fact a melanoma, a preoperative incisional biopsy not only confirms the clinical impression but also aids in determining the extent of surgery to be performed (i.e., the extent of the surgical margins and the need to perform lymph node dissection). While there is considerable controversy concerning the role of manipulation of an eye harboring *uveal* melanoma (32), dermatologists consider incisional biopsy into a suspicious pigmented cutaneous lesion to be a standard patient evaluation technique (Fig. 30.4). Finally, the initial diagnosis of a pigmented cutaneous lesion should not be rendered from a frozen section since the fine cytologic details that permit separation of lesion which histologically simulate melanoma from melanomas and melanoma precursors cannot be appreciated properly on frozen section. Many experienced pathologists simply refuse to interpret frozen section material on a primary (never-before biopsied) pigmented cutaneous lesion.

A patient with a suspected eyelid melanoma of the lentigo maligna or superficial spreading type should have a careful slitlamp examination with eversion of the eyelids to exclude simultaneous cutaneous and conjunctival involvement. Likewise, because so many melanomas are related to excessive exposure to ultraviolet light, a patient with a suspected eyelid melanoma should have a careful total body skin examination to exclude the presence of other actinic-induced lesions.

Cutaneous melanoma tends to spread first to regional lymph nodes, unlike uveal melanoma, which has a predilection for initial metastasis to the liver. With an eyelid melanoma, the nodal groups deserving attention are the parotid nodes (preauricular nodes) and the submandibular nodes. The indications for performing prophylactic lymph node dissections for eyelid melanomas are not well established since this tumor appears so rarely in this location. Prophylactic lymph node dissection has been recommended for eyelid melanomas that are greater than 1.5 mm thick or that have achieved level 4 or 5 invasion (13).

TREATMENT OF EYELID MELANOMAS

If a pigmented eyelid lesion should prove histologically to be one of the lesions that mimics melanoma (e.g., pigmented squamous cell or basal cell carcinoma or pigmented seborrheic keratosis), treatment of the lesion should consist of whatever modality is best used to treat the more common nonpigmented variety. There is no evidence that secondary pigmentation of a nonmelanoma eyelid lesion changes its biological course.

If a pigmented eyelid lesion should prove histologically to be lentigo maligna or one of the varieties of melanoma, treatment should be directed first toward total extirpation of the lesion. After the lesion has been removed totally, one should worry about reconstruction of the area. All too often, ophthalmologists tend to render less radical treatment to the eye or adnexae because the treatment may compromise vision. There are, however, a number of techniques available for reconstruction of the lids (which may need to be performed in stages), and the possibility of lid tissue loss should not weaken the resolve of the surgeon to totally remove the malignancy.

With regard to surgical excision of cutaneous melanoma, it had been taught that a 5 cm margin of normal tissue be removed around the tumor (33). In the area of the face, this has devastating consequences. Recently, it has been suggested that tumors less than 0.85 mm thick may be completely resected with margins of 1 to 1.5 cm of normal skin; thicker lesions may be treated with margins of 2 to 3 cm of normal skin (30). Mohs' chemosurgery offers no advantage to traditional surgical excision because the same amount of normal tissue must be sacrificed as an adequate margin (30).

The treatment of lentigo maligna is also problematic. The lentigo maligna lesion is by definition confined to the epidermis and is therefore not malignant melanoma. Nevertheless, since malignant melanoma develops in nearly 30% of untreated lentigo maligna lesions (16), it is appropriate to completely extirpate these lesions. In order to conserve eyelid tissue, cryotherapy (34) and low-dose radiation (35, 36) may be used, however, experience with a large number of lentigo maligna and lentigo maligna melanoma lesions suggests that surgical excision is the best modality to prevent recurrence and subsequent metastasis (37).

If the melanoma is advanced to the point that total excision precludes reconstruction to permit useful vision or a comfortable eye, a more radical procedure such as orbital exenteration may be considered. For advanced melanomas that have invaded into the orbit, orbital exenteration may be considered as a palliative procedure. Orbital exenteration for conjunctival melanomas that have invaded or recurred within the orbit has yielded disappointing results (5).

EYELID NEVI

Concepts concerning the nature of nevi and the relationship of these lesions to malignant melanoma are changing rapidly (11). For example, ophthalmologists have been taught that all nevi are congenital (38). According to this view, the major difference between nevi that are present at birth and those that appear in later life is the time at which pigment appears in the lesion. However, there is now substantial evidence that nevi present at birth (congenital) have a different clinical and histologic appearance from nevi that appear (are acquired) later in life (39). Additionally, congenital nevi may be more prone to the subsequent development of melanoma than the "common" acquired nevus (40, 41). Finally, certain types of nevi (dysplastic nevi) have been identified in patients with a familial tendency to develop malignant melanoma (42).

The question of whether or not nevi are precursors of melanoma cannot be avoided. If, for example, it is important to recognize early the radial growth phase of superficial spreading melanoma and lentigo maligna melanoma (i.e., lentigo maligna), is it not also important to recognize the precursors of the melanoma? Since most patients have multiple nevi scattered over the body, it is not feasible to excise all of these to "prevent" the later development of melanoma. Which nevi, then, are worrisome?

The incidence of a precursor lesion of melanoma varies with the biologic subtype of melanoma. Precursor lesions (such as nevi) are rarely seen in association with lentigo maligna melanoma—unless one considers the radial growth phase, lentigo maligna, to be a precursor lesion. Likewise, precursor lesions are rarely seen in acral lentiginous melanoma. By contrast, 55% of a series of 150 cases of superficial spreading melanoma and 35% of a series of 31 nodular melanomas have been seen in association with a precursor lesion (11).

The precursor lesions seen in association with superficial spreading and nodular melanoma may be identifiable histologically and clinically, although information continues to accumulate regarding the nature of these precursors. The reader should pay careful attention to the clinical description of the natural history "common" acquired nevus, because a deviation from the anticipated history of this lesion may trigger the recognition of a precursor of melanoma. In addition, the true congenital nevus, both the small type, less than 10 cm, (40) and large type (41) may be prone to the subsequent development of melanoma. Finally, the clinical and histologic characteristics of dysplastic nevi have been described. Dysplastic nevi may be seen commonly in patients with the predisposition to multiple melanomas and with a heritable form of melanoma (42). The nevus of Ota, while not predisposing to cutaneous melanoma, may predispose to uveal melanoma in white patients (43).

The discussion that follows describes the clinical features of a variety of nevi commonly found on the eyelid skin. The Spitz tumor (nevus), blue nevus, and cellular blue nevus have been described briefly under the differential diagnosis of nodular melanoma. The reader is referred to specialized texts (e.g., 3, 4) for a detailed description of the histologic features of these types of nevi.

COMMON ACQUIRED NEVI

By traditional description, nevi are described as *junctional* (histologically involving the interface of the epidermis and dermis), *compound* (involving both the epidermis and dermis), or *dermal* (involving the dermis alone). According to this traditional classification, nevi are derived from epidermal melanocytes and progressively drop off into the dermis as the lesion ages. Therefore, according to this view, "common" acquired nevi begin as flat lesions that may enlarge to a slight degree in a centrifugal direction but that acquire a component of elevation that reflects the appearance of a dermal component to the lesion. This traditional view of the development of nevi may be oversimplified, as the clinical and histologic appearance of nevi may be different for different body sites (11). For the purposes of this discussion the concepts of junctional, compound, and dermal nevi will be retained.

Common acquired nevi begin to appear between the ages of 6 months and 1 year and may continue to appear through the third decade of life. They are first noticed as flat, regularly pigmented spots measuring between 1 and 2 mm in diameter. Over the course of months to years, they may enlarge to a diameter of 4–6 mm. Note that the maximum diameter of the common acquired nevus is much less than the average diameter of lentigo maligna or the radial growth phase of superficial spreading melanoma. Also, nevi lack the notched borders and the haphazard arrangement of color seen in melanomas.

While in the clinically flat stage, most common acquired nevi are histologically junctional or compound nevi. Nevi may persist in this state for an indefinite period of time (11). In many nevi, a slight elevation in the lesion may appear over a course of 5–10 years as the nevus undergoes transition from the junctional and compound state to an intradermal state. Eventually, such nevi may lose color and become globoid nodules. Note that the appearance of elevation in a nevus is much slower than the dramatic development of a nodule within a progressively enlarging pigmented lesion of superficial spreading or lentigo maligna melanoma. Also, the evolution of a dermal nevus as a small nodule gradually evolving from a flat, uniformly bordered, and colored spot is different from the rapid and progressive evolution of the lesion of nodular melanoma.

Intradermal nevi are found commonly on the margin of eyelids (Fig. 30.9). Some patients will recall the presence of a lesion at that site for many years and may even be able to relate its development from a flat spot. Other patients may not be so observant or historically accurate and may suddenly discover the lesion. Even for the patient who is historically inaccurate, the lack of progressive growth of this small (generally less than 6 mm) nodule on the eyelid serves to distinguish the lesion from nodular basal cell carcinoma and nodular melanoma. Jakobiec (2) has noted that the posterior surface of an intradermal nevus of the lid margin molds to the contour of the underlying globe. In the authors' experience, intradermal nevi of the lid margin are misdiagnosed either as nodular basal cell carcinomas or papillomas. It is a bit difficult to

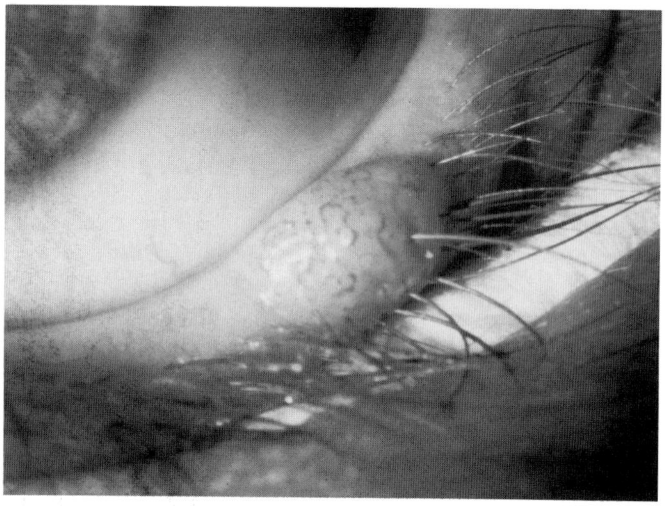

Figure 30.9. Nevus of the eyelid margin. Note the hair protruding from the lesion, a not uncommon feature of eyelid nevi.

understand why a papilloma, with its characteristic undulating surface, would be mistaken for the smooth surface of a nevus.

In summary, there are two main pathways for the development of common acquired nevi: (*a*) the lesion may persist indefinitely as a small flat spot or (*b*) the lesion may evolve gradually into a small, elevated nodule (11). Deviations from these patterns should raise the suspicion that the nevus is atypical and should prompt an excisional biopsy for histologic examination. Examples of deviation from the two accepted evolutionary pathways include the spreading of pigment centrifugally in a flat lesion that has remained quiescent over a period of time or adjacent to the intradermal nevus. As stated simply and elegantly in the American Cancer Society advertisement, "a change in a mole (that has been stable) should prompt concern."

Common acquired nevi of the eyelid margin may be removed by a shave technique without destroying lashes or creating a lid notch. Nevi of the eyelid skin not associated with the lid margin may be excised by a small ellipse (44). As stated before, all lesions removed should be sent to the pathology laboratory for histologic confirmation.

Since many nevi are removed by a shave biopsy technique, it is possible that the lesion may be incompletely excised either at the lateral margins or at the base. Such an incomplete excision does not require further treatment to the area, but surgeons should be aware of the possibility of recurrence of a pigmented lesion at the site of excision of a nevus. The recurrence of pigmentation after incomplete excision of a benign nevus may be alarming to both the patient and surgeon, who may question the pathologist's original diagnosis. Under these circumstances, the recurrent zone of pigmentation may be subjected to repeat excision. Unfortunately, the histologic appearance of benign, recurrent nevi following incomplete primary excision may mimic the early radial growth phase of superficial spreading melanoma, without implying actual evolution into melanoma (20). Both surgeon and pathologist must be aware of the pitfalls in the diagnosis of "pseudomelanoma." It is very helpful to the pathologist if the surgeon relates a history of excision of a benign nevus in the zone of recurrent pigmentation as a means of alerting the pathologist to this potential histologic trap.

DYSPLASTIC NEVI

Dysplastic nevi are also a form of acquired nevi, but they differ from "common" acquired nevi in clinical and histologic appearance as well as in biologic behavior (11, 42). Dysplastic nevi are somewhat larger than common acquired nevi (larger than 5–6 mm). Unlike the common acquired nevus, the outline of the dysplastic nevus is irregular. Dysplastic nevi begin to appear to adolescence on the scalp and on covered body sites. There has been no reported predilection for the eyelids, although the authors have seen two cases of dysplastic nevi of the conjunctiva.

Dysplastic nevi were identified originally in patients with multiple primary melanomas and in patients with a history of familial melanoma. Dysplastic nevi may occur sporadically in patients with no familial history of melanoma.

Dysplastic nevi may be recognized histologically (42) and may be considered to be a formal histogenetic precursor of malignant melanoma, usually of the superficial spreading type (11).

CONGENITAL NEVI

Nevi that are truly visible at birth, congenital nevi, are divided somewhat arbitrarily into small (less than 10 cm) and large or garment types (greater than 10 cm) (39). It should be emphasized that even "small" congenital nevi are larger than the common acquired nevus discussed previously. An "average" small congenital nevus may measure 3–5 cm in diameter whereas a common acquired nevus generally measures less than 6 mm in diameter.

Congenital nevi have a variable appearance. Most lesions are tan with flecks of darker pigmentation within. Long, coarse hairs may protrude from the lesion. Most lesions are palpable and have a velvety texture. Marked thickening of the eyelid skin may result in ptosis, which may, in turn, be a cause of amblyopia (45). Over a period of time, focal nodules may appear within the lesion, which may cause concern. Biopsy of these nodule, however, may reveal all types of benign melanocytic proliferations, so that change in a congenital nevus does not necessarily indicate melanoma.

The histologic appearance of congenital nevi biopsied in childhood may distinguish these lesions from common acquired nevi. In congenital nevi, there is a tendency for nevus cells to permeate throughout the deeper layers of the dermis (reticular dermis) (37). In congenital nevus of the eyelid, nevus cells may be found within the tarsus. It is important for surgeons as well as pathologists to remember that the histologic appearance of congenital nevi biopsied in early infancy may be quite worrisome and may be indistinguishable from melanoma. Congenital melanoma, however, is exceedingly rare. With time, it is likely that the immature histologic appearance of many congenital nevi resolves into the more typical histologic pattern of congenital nevus described above (46).

There is some increased risk for the development of melanoma in both large and small congenital nevi (41, 42) although the exact risk factor is difficult to estimate. It should also be mentioned that large congenital nevi that involve the scalp may be associated with leptomeningeal pigmentation and intracranial melanoma (47).

Congenital nevi of the eyelids present the difficult problem of cosmesis, possible amblyopia and the possible risk of subsequent melanoma. If the eyelid skin is not excessively thickened, cosmetics may be used to mask the blemish. Since the nevus cells permeate into the deeper layers of the dermis, superficial dermabrasion may not produce satisfactory results. Surgical excision of congenital eyelid nevi is difficult and may require split-thickness skin grafting (48) or reconstruction in several stages by means of Z-plasties and flaps (49).

A congenital nevus may span both the upper and lower eyelids (Fig. 30.10) to form a so-called split or kissing nevus (50). The "split" nature of the lesion results from the population of eyelid skin by melanocyte precursors in utero while the lids are still fused; subsequent separation of the lids results in splitting of the nevus. While the split nevus is considered to be a congenital nevus, too few cases have been followed to permit a discussion of the tendency for melanoma to develop in these split congenital nevi. The same management considerations that apply to other types of congenital nevi that affect the eyelid apply to the split nevus.

NEVUS OF OTA

The combination of slate-gray periocular skin pigmentation with a slate-gray scleral pigmentation (Fig. 30.11) and corresponding uveal hyperpigmentation is well known to ophthalmologists. Patients with the nevus of Ota are not at a particular risk for the development of cutaneous melanoma, but white patients with nevus of Ota may be at risk for the development of uveal melanoma (43).

Nevus of Ota, together with blue nevus and cellular blue nevus, are considered to be lesions of deep melanocytes, whereas other forms of nevi and most forms of malignant melanoma are considered to be derived from superficial melanocytes. When neural crest cells, destined to become melanocytes, migrate to the skin, they usually find a final resting place in the epidermis. Most nevi (common acquired, dysplastic, congenital, or Spitz) are derived from epidermal (superficial) melanocytes. Likewise, malignant melanoma of the four major varieties discussed previously are derived from epidermal melanocytes. In the case of lesions of deeper melanocytes, the neural crest cells are thought to have been "hung up" in their path to the epidermis and were therefore trapped within the dermis. The presence of melanin deep in the dermis is responsible for the slate-gray or bluish color of these lesions of deep melanocytes.

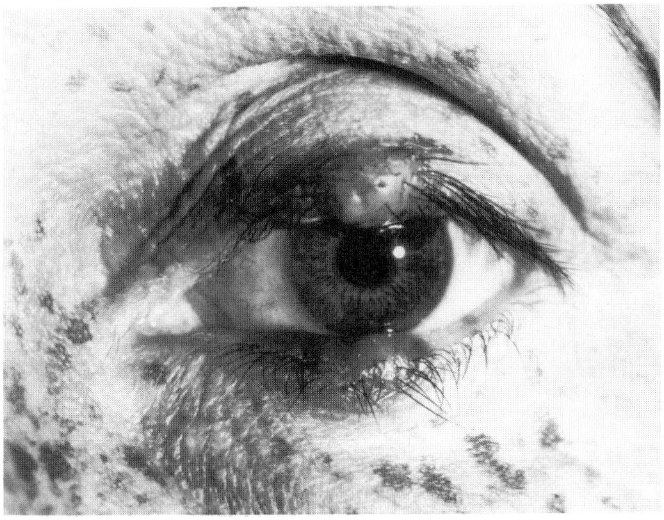

Figure 30.10. Congenital split nevus of the eyelid.

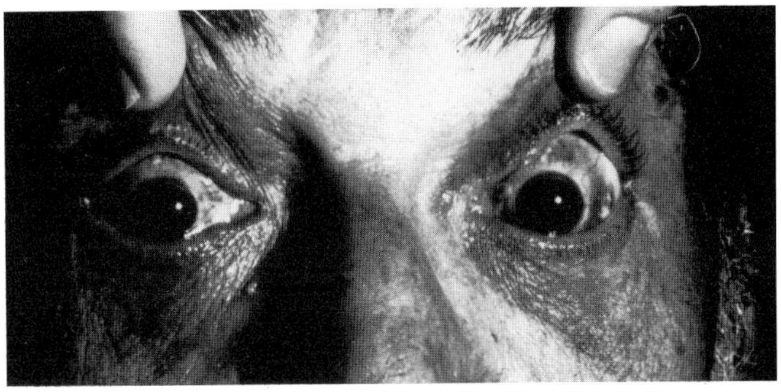

Figure 30.11. Nevus of Ota affecting the left eye.

SUMMARY

While this chapter is concerned with all pigmented eyelid lesions, its main focus is malignant melanoma. Melanoma is the prime concern in the differential diagnosis of eyelid lesions, and the eventual development of melanoma is a concern in many other pigmented lesions. Careful attention to the clinicopathologic features may permit accurate diagnosis of these lesions. Histopathologic confirmation of clinical diagnoses is an essential part of management.

Fortunately, pigmented cutaneous lesions are the focus of much research and investigation. Many long-term prospective studies are now in progress to determine the best methods of classifying, rendering prognoses, and treating these lesions.

REFERENCES

1. Shafir R, Hiss J, Tsur H, Bubis J: The thin malignant melanoma: changing patterns of epidemiology and treatment. *Cancer* 50: 817–819, 1982.
2. Jakobiec FA: Tumors of the lids. In Transactions of the New Orleans Academy of Ophthalmology: *Symposium on Diseases of the Lids, Lacrimal Apparatus and Orbit* St. Louis, Mosby, 1982, pp 264–307.
3. Clark WH Jr, Goldman LI, Mastrangelo MJ (eds): *Human Malig-*

nant Melanoma. Grune & Stratton, 1978.
4. Ackerman AB (ed): *Pathology of Malignant Melanoma.* New York, Masson, 1981.
5. Folberg R, McLean IW, Zimmerman LE: Conjunctival acquired melanosis and malignant melanoma. *Ophthalmology* 91: 673–678, 1984.
6. Folberg R, McLean IW, Zimmerman LE: Primary acquired melanosis of the conjunctiva. *Hum Pathol* 16: 129–135, 1985.
7. Folberg R, McLean IW, Zimmerman LE: Conjunctival malignant melanoma. *Hum Pathol* 16: 136–143, 1985.
8. Naidoff MA, Bernardino VB Jr, Clark WH Jr: Melanocytic lesions of the eyelid skin. *Am J Ophthalmol* 82: 371–382, 1976.
9. Elder DE, Jucovy PM, Tuthill RJ, Clark WH Jr: The classification of malignant melanoma. *Am J Dermatopathol* 2: 315–320, 1980.
10. Ackerman AB: Malignant melanoma: a unifying concept. *Hum Pathol* 11: 591–595, 1980.
11. Clark WH Jr, Elder DE, Guerry D, Epstein MN, Greene MH, Van Horn M: The development and subsequent cellular evolution of the primary human cutaneous melanomas. *Hum Pathol* 15: 1147–1165, 1984.
12. Blodi RC, Widner RR: The melanotic freckle (Hutchinson) of the lids. *Surv Ophthalmol* 13: 23–38, 1969.
13. Rodriguez-Sains RS, Jakobiec FA, Iwamoto T: Lentigo maligna of the lateral canthal skin. *Ophthalmology* 88: 1186–1192, 1981.
14. Clark WH Jr, Mihm MC: Lentigo maligna and lentigo maligna melanoma. *Am J Pathol* 113: 457–463, 1967.
15. Clark WH Jr, Folberg R, Ainsworth AM: Tumor progression in primary human cutaneous malignant melanomas. In Clark WH Jr, Goldman LI, Mastrangelo MJ (eds): *Human Malignant Melanoma.* New York, Grune & Stratton, 1978, pp 15–31.
16. Davis J, Pack GT, Higgins GK: Melanotic freckle of Hutchinson. *Am J Surg* 113: 457–463, 1967.
17. Subrt P, Jorizzo JL, Apisarnthanarax P, Head ES, Smith EB: Spreading pigmented actinic keratosis. *J Am Acad Dermatol* 8: 396–404, 1983.
18. Clark WH Jr, Ainsworth AM, Mihm MC: The clinical manifestations of primary cutaneous malignant melanomas. In Clark WH Jr, Goldman LI, Mastrangelo MJ (eds): *Human Malignant Melanoma.* New York, Grune & Stratton, 1978, pp 33–53.
19. Mihm MC Jr, Fitzpatrick TB, Brown MML, Ruker JW, Malt RA, Kaiser JS: Early detection of primary cutaneous malignant melanoma: a color atlas. *N Engl J Med* 289: 989–995, 1973.
20. Kornberg R, Ackerman AB: Pseudomelanoma: recurrent melanocytic nevus following partial surgical removal. *Arch Dermatol* 111: 1588–1590.
21. Arrington Jr, Reed RJ, Ichinose H, Krementz ET: Plantar-lentiginous melanoma: a distinctive variant of human cutaneous malignant melanoma. *Am J Surg Pathol* 1: 131–143.
22. Kernen JA, Ackerman LV: Spindle cell nevi and epithelioid cell nevi (so-called juvenile melanoma) in children and adults: a clinicopathologic report of 26 cases. *Cancer* 13: 612–625, 1960.
23. Ecchevarria R, Ackerman LV: Spindle and epithelioid nevi in the adult: clinicopathologic report of 26 cases. *Cancer* 20: 175–189, 1967.
24. Mather S, Narang JB, Gupta AK: Seborrheic keratosis. *Ind J Ophthalmol* 31: 37–38, 1983.
25. Scheie HG, Yanoff M, Sassani JW: Inverted follicular keratosis clinically mimicking malignant melanoma. *Ann Ophthalmol* 9: 949–952, 1977.
26. Clark WH Jr: A classification of malignant melanoma in man correlated with histogenesis and biologic behavior. In Montagna W, Hu F (eds): *Advances in Biology of Skin. VIII The Pigmentary System.* Oxford, UK, Pergamon Press, 1967, pp 621–647.
27. Clark WH Jr, From L, Bernardino EA, Mihm MC: The histogenesis and biologic behavior of primary human malignant melanomas of the skin. *Cancer Res* 29: 705–727, 1969.
28. Breslow A: Thickness, cross-sectional area and depth of invasion in the prognosis of cutaneous melanoma. *Ann Surg* 172: 902–908, 1970.
29. Breslow A: Tumor thickness, level of invasion and lymph node dissection in stage I cutaneous melanoma. *Ann Surg* 182: 572–575, 1975.
30. Day CL, Lew RA: Malignant melanoma prognostic factors 3: surgical margins. *J Dermatol Surg Oncol* 9: 787–801, 1983.
31. Goldman LI: The surgical treatment of malignant melanoma. In Clark WH Jr, Goldman LI, Mastrangelo MJ (eds): *Human Malignant Melanoma.* New York, Grune & Stratton, 1978, pp 285–293.
32. Zimmerman LE, McLean IW, Foster WF: Does enucleation of an eye containing a malignant melanoma prevent or accelerate the dissemination of tumor cells? *Br J Ophthalmol* 62: 420–425, 1978.
33. Handley WS: The pathology of melanotic growths in relation to their operative treatment. *Lancet* 1: 927–933, 996–1003, 1907.
34. Graham GR, Steward R: Cryosurgery for unusual cutaneous neoplasms. *J Dermatol Surg Oncol* 3: 437–422, 1977.
35. Kopf AW, Bart RS, Gladstein AH: Treatment of melanotic freckle with x-rays. *Arch Dermatol* 112: 801–807, 1976.
36. Storck H: Treatment of melanotic freckles by radiotherapy. *J Dermatol Surg Oncol* 3: 292–294, 1977.
37. Pitman GH, Kopf AW, Bart RS, Casson PR: Treatment of lentigo maligna and lentigo maligna melanoma. *J Dermatol Surg Oncol* 5: 727–737, 1979.
38. Yanoff M, Fine BS: *Ocular Pathology: A Text and Atlas,* ed 2. Philadelphia, Harper & Row, 1982, p 787.
39. Mark GJ, Mihm MC, Liteplo MG, Reed RJ, Clark WH: Congenital melanocytic nevi of the small and garment type. *Hum Pathol* 4: 395–418, 1973.
40. Rhodes AR, Melski JW: Small congenital nevocellular nevi and the risk of cutaneous melanoma. *J Pediatr* 100: 219–224, 1982.
41. Kopf AW, Bart RS, Hennessy P: Congenital nevocytic nevi and malignant melanoma. *J Am Acad Dermatol* 1: 123–130, 1979.
42. Elder DE, Greene MH, Bondi EE, Clark WH Jr: Acquired melanocytic nevi and melanoma: the dysplastic nevus syndrome. In Ackerman AB (ed): *Pathology of Malignant Melanoma.* New York, Masson, 1981, pp 185–215.
43. Gonder JR, Shields JA, Albert DM, Augsberger JJ, Lavin PT: Uveal malignant melanoma associated with ocular and oculodermal melanocytosis. *Ophthalmology* 89: 953–960, 1982.
44. Putterman AM: Intradermal nevi of the eyelid. *Ophthal Surg* 11: 584–587, 1980.
45. Antinone RL, Helveston EM, Bennett JE, Keener P: Giant hairy nevus: preventable cause of amblyopia. *J Pediatr Ophthalmol* 13: 192–195, 1976.
46. Ainsworth AM, Folberg R, Reed RJ, Clark WH Jr: Melanocytic nevi, melanocytomas, melanocytic dysplasias and uncommon forms of melanoma. In Clark WH Jr, Goldman LI, Mastrangelo MJ (eds): *Human Malignant Melanoma.* New York, Grune & Stratton, 1978, pp 167–208.
47. Reed WB, Becker SW Sr, Becker SW Jr: Giant pigmented nevi, melanoma and leptomeningeal melanocytosis. *Arch Dermatol* 91: 100–119, 1965.
48. Hirshovitz B, Mahler D: Plastic surgery for pigmented hairy naevus of the eyelids: by excision and masquerade graft. *Br J Ophthalmol* 53: 343–345, 1969.
49. de Dulanto R, Camacho-Martinez F, Sanchez-Muros J, de Cosme L: A giant hairy pigmented nevus on the face: excision and reconstruction in stages. *J Dermatol Surg Oncol* 5: 215–218, 1979.
50. Ehlers N: Divided nevus. *Acta Ophthalmologica* 47: 1009–1011, 1969.

CHAPTER 31

Basal Cell Nevus Syndrome

ANDREW S. MARKOVITS, M.D.

The basal cell nevus syndrome is a rare, genetically transmitted disease. The ophthalmologist should be aware of this entity, even though he or she may pass through an entire career without seeing a case. The incidence is less than 0.4% of all basal cell carcinomata (1), but since the first tumors often appear on the eyelids, the ophthalmologist can be instrumental in making the initial diagnosis and instituting therapy (2).

The triad of multiple basal cell carcinomata, mandibular bone cysts, and skeletal anomalies was first integrated into a distinct syndrome in 1960 by Gorlin (whose name has been linked eponymically with the syndrome) and Goltz (3). The association of basal cell nevi and jaw cysts was described as early as 1939 (4), but case reports prior to those of Gorlin grouped these findings with those of epithelioma adenoides cysticum, rather than as a discrete entity.

Basal cell nevus syndrome is transmitted by autosomal dominant inheritance with variable penetrance (5–8). Linkage studies have not identified specific chromosomal loci (8). The sexes are equally affected, and incidence is relatively unpredictable. Gorlin considered the syndrome to be an inborn error of metabolism, while others classify it as a phakomatosis (9, 10). Categorizing the lesion as a "nevus" is actually a misnomer; we associated the word *nevus* with a "circumscribed, stable malformation of the skin," although the original Latin word means a mole or "shapeless mass" (11). Efforts at more correctly titling the disease seem to have failed (3, 8, 12–15).

The syndrome's chief threat is multiple basal cell carcinomata, which are histologically indistinguishable from sporadic basal cell carcinoma. The tumors are characteristically smooth-surfaced, elevated, round papules, which may be flesh-colored or pigmented. They may appear quite benign prior to microscopic examination, sometimes resembling melanocytic nevi, von Recklinghausen's neurofibromatosis, or skin tags (Figs. 31.1–31.3). For this reason, one should be alerted to the associated abnormalities and family history.

The lesions are most frequently on the eyelids, nose, cheek, and trunk, and less frequently on other parts of the face, scalp, and neck. Unlike ordinary basal cell carcinomata, they are independent of actinic exposure (5, 6, 8, 12). The distribution is typically bilateral and roughly symmetrical, and the size is variable. The tumors usually become noticeable in adolescence but may be present at birth or during infancy. Patients diagnosed in the fourth decade are likely to have been missed previously (7, 13, 16–20). Thus, early diagnosis and treatment are of particular importance to these patients, who are typically much younger than the usual patient with isolated basal cell carcinoma (age 50 to 80) (28).

Histologic studies indicate small multifocal centers in the basal cells of the rete ridges. As they enlarge, they produce either a filigreed or a reticular pattern, or sometimes larger solid islands of cells. In the early phases, there is little invasion of the reticular part of the dermis. The tumor cells induce a fibrous stroma (desmoplastic reaction), and the lesion may become papular or pendunculated (7). There may be pigment in and around the tumor masses. The behavior of basal cell nevus syndrome carcinomata is peculiar in that they may be less invasive, and remain confined to the epidermis for unusually long periods of time (21). They later demonstrate invasion and ulceration and may exhibit all categories of basal cell differentiation; they may rarely metastasize to the cerebrum, cerebellum and lung (13). For this reason, basal cell nevus syndrome is a clinical, rather than a pathologic, diagnosis (1, 3, 12, 16).

The chief differential diagnoses are also autosomal dominant, genetically transmitted diseases: von Recklinghausen's neurofibromatosis and adenoid cystic epithelioma

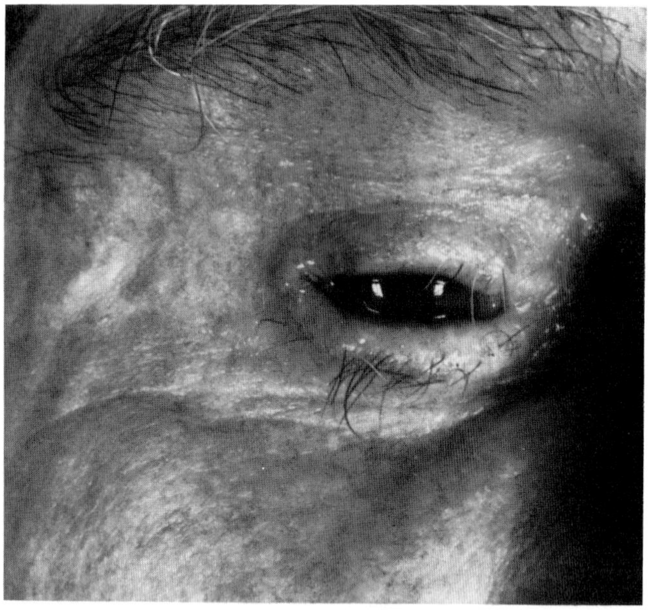

Figure 31.1. *A, B,* Father of patient in Figures 31.5–31.7 showing apparent tumor-free lids after multiple local excisions and plastic repairs.

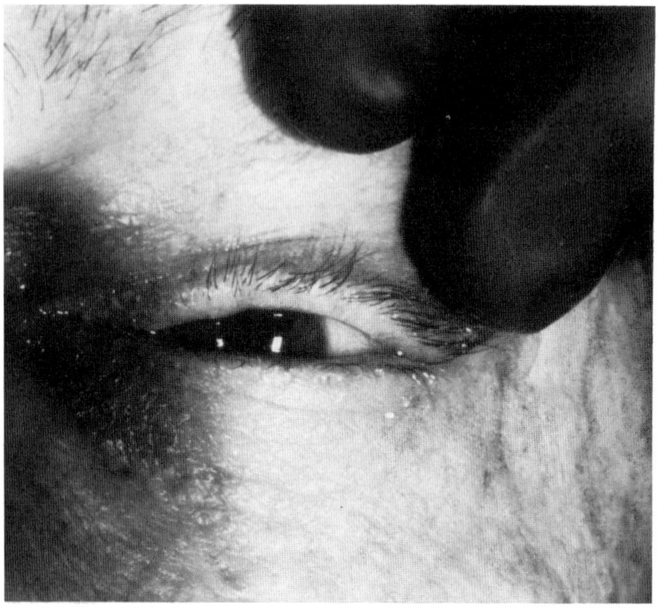

Figure 31.1. *B*

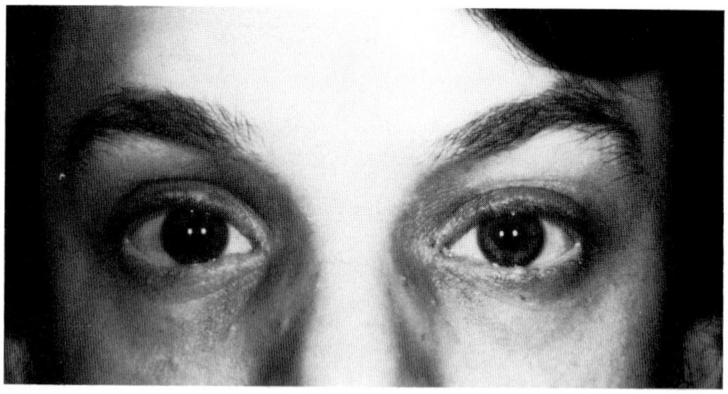

Figure 31.2. Youthful patient with basal cell nevus syndrome, demonstrating sublety of lesions to cursory inspection.

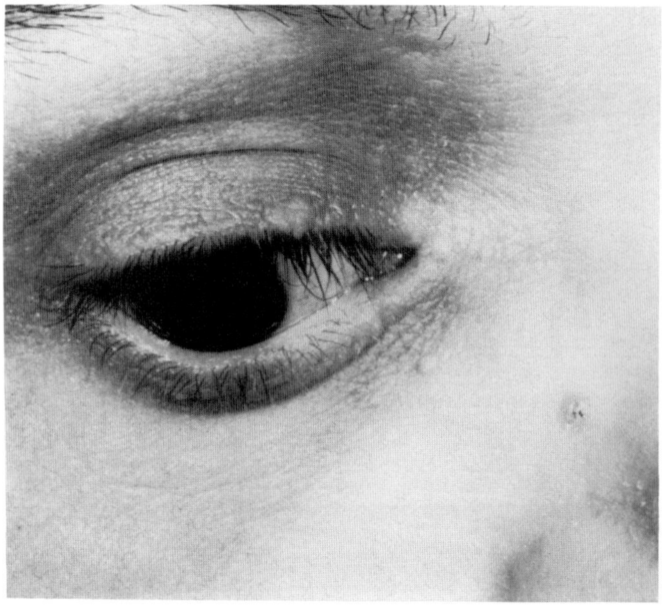

Figure 31.3. Close-up right eye of patient in Figure 31.2 showing basal cell carcinomata medial portion upper lid, medial canthus lower lid inferior to punctal area, another below this at orbital rim, and one in nasojugal crease area.

(Brooke's tumor). The former may be excluded clinically by the presence of cafe au lait spots, as well as different histology. Brooke's tumor is more difficult to differentiate clinically, but occurs chiefly in the nasolabial folds, whereas it occurs mainly in the lids in basal cell nevus syndrome. Histologic differentiation may be difficult, with as high as 30% of Brooke's lesions being misdiagnosed as basal cell carcinomata in one series (10).

At least one-third of patients afflicted with basal cell nevus syndrome manifest ophthalmic abnormalities, chiefly tumors of the eyelids, which may invade the orbit (5, 12, 13, 18, 19) and strabismus (5–7, 14). Less frequent ophthalmic abnormalities include congenital cataract, congenital glaucoma (3), retinal and optic nerve head colobomata (3), iris malignant melanoma (20), retinitis pigmentosa (22), orbital rhabdomyosarcoma (15), and epicanthal folds, hypertelorism, and retinal atrophy (6, 23). Additional skin findings include dyskeratosis of the palm and sole and epithelial cysts. Fine telangiectasia and milia may be found just beneath the skin surface.

The other common components of basal cell nevus syndrome are jaw cysts (3, 5–7) and skeletal abnormalities. The cysts may be multiple and recurrent, presenting in the first decade and causing jaw swelling and pain. They may generate fibrosarcoma (18, 23). Skeletal anomalies occur in 75% of these patients (3) and most frequently include bifid ribs and other costal malformations (3, 5–7, 12 16–18). Other less frequent skeletal anomalies include kyphoscoliosis, shortened metacarpals, and spina bifida. A characteristic facies may be present, including frontal and temporoparietal bossing, mandibular prognathism, and lower facial hypoplasia and hypertelorism (Figs. 31.5–31.7) (5–7). These findings, combined with the presence of ectopic calcification (Figs. 31.4–31.6) of the ovary, uterus, and dura (5–7, 14) suggest an abnormal calcium metabolism in these patients and an impaired renal response to parathyroid hormone with resulting deficit in tubular resorption of phosphate has been demonstrated (5).

Central nervous system abnormalities include partial agenesis of the corpus callosum (23); medulloblastoma, which may be transmitted to the descendents (12, 13, 14); hydrocephalus (6, 14, 18); mental retardation with characteristic lamellar calcification of the falx cerebri and tentorium (24); electroencephalographic abnormalities (7); and schizophrenia (7). Genital anomalies include hypogonadism in males and ovarian fibromata (6).

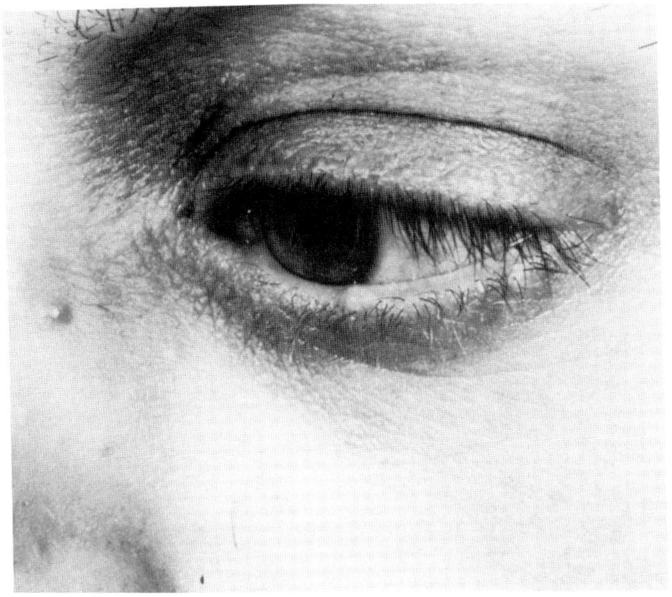

Figure 31.4. Close-up left eye of patient in Figure 31.2 showing lesions medial and above upper lid crease, three on lower lid margin, and one pigmented lesion at area of nasojugal crease.

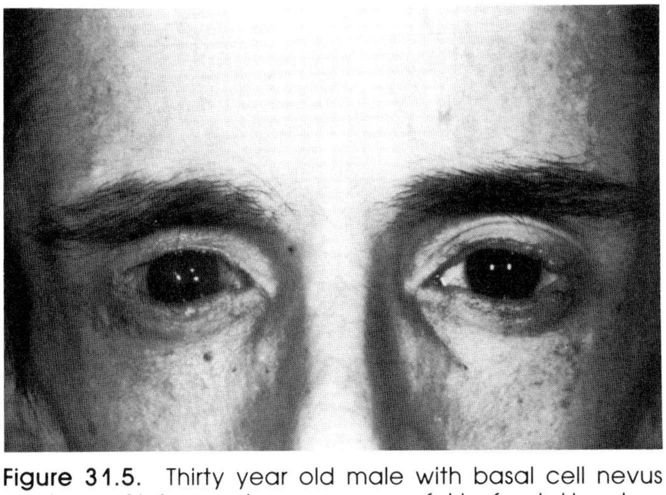

Figure 31.5. Thirty year old male with basal cell nevus syndrome. Note aged appearance of skin, frontal bossing.

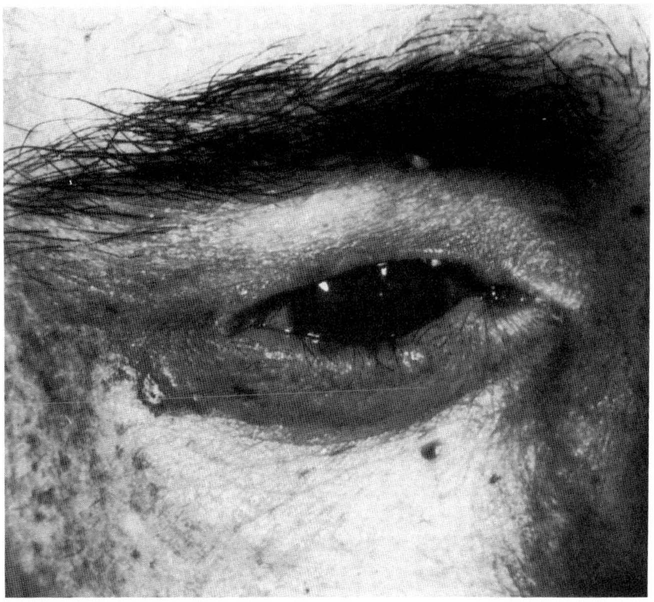

Figure 31.6. Close-up right eye of patient in Figure 31.5 showing multiple lesions of both lids, brow, and nose, almost all of which were biopsy-positive for basal cell carcinoma.

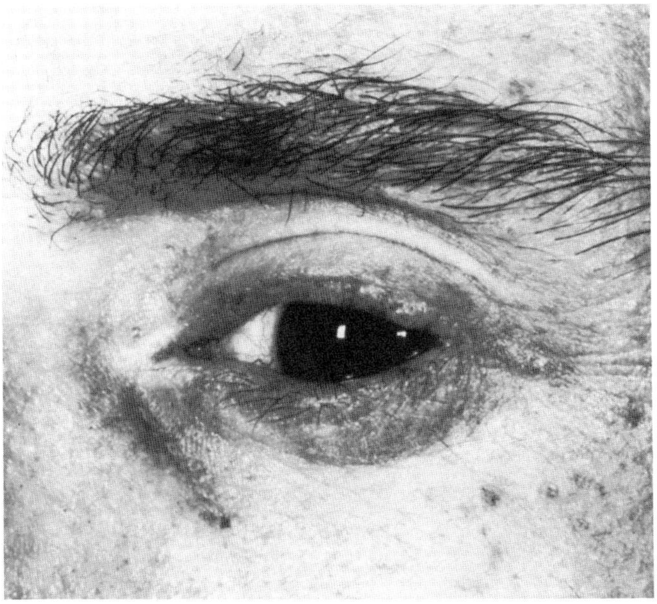

Figure 31.7. Close-up of left eye of patient in Figure 31.5 showing multiple lesions both lids, lateral and medial canthi, and above medial brow: biopsy-positive for basal cell carcinoma.

The management of these patients is difficult, especially when lesions are very numerous. One should biopsy any lesion of any patient suspected of having this syndrome. Once the diagnosis of basal cell nevus syndrome has been made, one must decide which lesions to watch and which to treat (Figs. 31.7 and 31.8). Clinically, elevation, pedunculation, and ulceration are indicative of lesion activity and therefore are indications for treatment (2).

As with conventional basal cell carcinomata, surgical excision with frozen section monitoring of the borders remains the treatment of choice. The place of cryotherapy in this disease has not been clearly defined, but it may be an appropriate alternative for patients with hundreds of lesions or who lack prospective skin graft donor sites due to disease involvement or previous surgical intervention (25). In view of the apparent success of freezing in squamous cell carcinoma, malignant melanoma, and basal cell carcinoma even incompletely excised lesions might benefit from this admittedly new and uncontrolled modality (26). Finally, orthovoltage radiation would be the last choice, but one that could possibly be lifesaving in an advanced case (27).

The astute clinician is in a unique position vis-a-vis this disease, in that early diagnosis can vastly improve the quality of life for victims, increase their longevity, and provide the opportunity for realistic genetic counseling to prevent further tragedy in these unfortunate patients' lives.

REFERENCES

1. Maddox WD, Winkelmann RK, Harrison EG, Devine KD, Gibilisco JA: Multiple nevoid basal cell epitheliomas, jaw cysts, and skeletal defects. *JAMA* 188: 106, 1964.
2. Markovits AS, Quickert MH: Basal cell nevus. *Arch Ophthalmol* 88: 397, 1972.
3. Gorlin RJ, Goltz RW: Multiple nevoid basal cell epitheliomas, jaw cysts, and bifid ribs. *N Engl J Med* 262: 908, 1960.
4. Straith FE: Hereditary epidermoid cysts of the jaw. *Am J Ortho Oral Surg* 25: 673, 1939.
5. Berlin NJ, Van Scott EJ, Clendenning WE, Archard HO, Block JB, Witkop CJ, Haynes HA: Basal cell nevus syndrome. Combined conference at the National Institutes of Health. *Ann Intern Med* 64: 403, 1966.
6. Gorlin RJ, Vickers RA, Kelln E, Williamson JJ: The multiple basal cell nevi syndrome. *Cancer* 18: 89, 1965.
7. Clendenning WE, Block JB, Radde IC: Basal cell nevus syndrome. *Arch Dermatol* 90: 38, 1964.
8. Anderson DE: Linkage analysis of the nevoid basal cell carcinoma syndrome. Ann Hum Genet, 32: 113, 1968.
9. Nover AV, Korting GW: Zur Kenntnis des Familiarsen Basalzell-naevus. *Klin Mbl Augenheilk* 156: 621, 1970.
10. Gray HR, Helwig EB: Epithelioma adenoides cysticum and solitary trichoepithelioma. *Arch Dermatol* 87: 102, 1963.
11. Dorland's Illustrated Medical Dictionary, ed 25. Philadelphia, W B Saunders, 1974, 975, 1046.
12. Mason JK, Helwig EB, Graham JH: Pathology of the nevoid basal cell carcinoma syndrome. *Arch Pathol* 79: 401, 1965.
13. Taylor WB, Anderson DE, Howell JB, Thurston CS: The nevoid basal cell carcinoma syndrome. *Arch Dermatol* 98: 612, 1968.
14. Neblett CR, Waltz TA, Anderson DE: Neurological involvement in the nevoid basal cell carcinoma syndrome. *J Neurosurg* 35: 577, 1971.
15. Schweisguth O, Gerard-Merchant R, Lemerle J: Naevomatose base-cellulare association a un rhabdomyosarcome congenital. *Arch Fr Pediatr* 25: 1083, 1968.
16. Howell JB, Caro MR: The basal cell nevus. *Arch Dermatol* 79: 67, 1959.
17. Davidson F: Multiple naevoid basal cell carcinomata and associated congenital abnormalities. *Br J Dermatol* 75: 439, 1962.
18. Tamoney HJ: Basal cell nevus syndrome. *Am Surg* 35: 279, 1969.
19. Shelley WB, Rawnsley HM, Berrman H: Quadrant distribution of basal cell nevi. *Arch Dermatol* 100: 741, 1969.
20. Kedem A, Even-Paz Z, Freund M: Basal cell nevus syndrome associated with malignant melanoma of the iris. *Dermatologica* 140: 91, 1970.
21. Zion VM, Duane T: *Clinical Ophthalmology*. New York, Harper & Row, 1981, vol 5, chap 13, p 10.
22. Happle R, Mehrle G, Sander LZ, Hohn H: Basalzellnevus-Syndrom. *Arch Dermatol Forsch* 241: 96, 1971.
23. Binkley GW, Johnson HH: Epithelioma adenoides cysticum basal cell nevi, agenesis of the corpus callosum and dental cysts. *Arch Dermatol Syph* 63: 73, 1951.
24. Pollard J, New P: Hereditary Cutaneomandibular Polyoncosis: A syndrome of myriad basal cell nevi of the skin, mandibular cysts, and inconstant skeletal anomalies. *Radiology* 82: 840, 1964.
25. Bullock JD, Beard C, Sullivan JH: Cryotherapy of basal cell carcinoma in oculoplastic surgery. *Am J Ophthalmol* 82: 841, 1976.
26. Sutton JJ, Anderson RJ, Tse DT: Combined surgery and cryotherapy for scleral invasions of epithelial malignancies. *Ophthal Surg* 15: 4, 1984.
27. Feman SS, Apt T, Roth AM: The basal cell nevus syndrome. *Am J Ophthalmol* 78: 222, 1974.
28. Henderson JW: *Orbital Tumors*. Philadelphia, W B Saunders, 1973, pp 444–494.

SECTION V

DISORDERS OF EYEBROWS AND EYELASHES

CHAPTER 32

Eyebrow and Eyelash Manifestations of Dermatologic and Systemic Disorders

DAVID S. ORENTREICH, M.D.
NORMAN ORENTREICH, M.D.

The hair of the eyebrows and eyelashes may be affected by dermatologic and systemic disorders. Since many structures of the eye share with the skin a common ectodermal origin, there are hereditary, infectious, and systemic conditions that exhibit both dermatologic and ophthalmologic pathology. Recognition of characteristic symptoms and signs can provide early clues to the presence of systemic disease.

The eyelash or ciliary follicles are the only hair follicles free of arrectores pilorum muscles and grow in five or six imperfect rows in the upper eyelid and three or four in the lower (1). This arrangement allows for the simultaneous shedding of any random number without leaving gaps in the eye's protection. Sebaceous glands of Zeis and apocrine glands of Moll open into the pilary canal infundibula. These pilosebaceous units are richly invested with capillaries and nerves. The eyelashes exit the skin at right angles, unlike all the rest of the hairs of the body, which exit at varying slanting angles. The cilia of the upper eyelid are curved upwards and are longer than those of the lower eyelid where they curve downwards. Curiously, the eyelashes rarely become gray until late in life.

About 30 large meibomian (or tarsal) glands nearly fill the tarsal plate of the upper lid and are oriented perpendicular to the lid margin. The lower lid, which has a more rudimentary tarsus, has about half as many meibomian glands. They are histologically similar to sebaceous glands. With aging, the proximal portion of the meibomian gland often degenerates. In distichiasis there is an additional inner row of eyelashes derived from the meibomian glands, which normally contain no piliary apparatus.

The eyebrows ordinarily grow to a length of approximately 1 cm. They lie just above the orbits, and their outline depends on the shape of the orbital arch of the frontal bone. In youth and middle age the eyebrow hairs are thick, stiff, and short. With advancing age the eyebrows become longer, curly, and assume a bushy appearance. Other hair follicles that increase, rather than decrease, in length with age are situated in the internal nares and on the helix of the ear.

COMMON DERMATOSES AFFECTING THE EYEBROWS AND EYELASHES

SEBORRHEIC DERMATITIS

Seborrheic dermatitis is a chronic, sometimes pruritic, inflammatory disease of the skin with a predilection for the scalp, forehead, eyebrows (Fig. 32.1), eyelids, nasolabial folds, lips, and postauricular, presternal, and intertriginous areas. The clinical picture is characterized by dry, moist, or greasy scales and by erythematous or yellowish-pink patches, usually with indistinct borders.

Patients with seborrheic blepharitis complain of irrita-

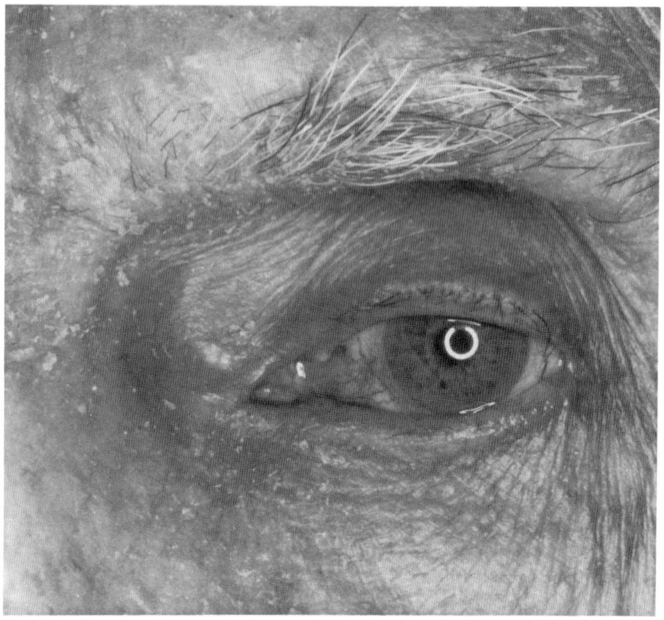

Figure 32.1. Seborrheic dermatitis of eyebrow and periorbital area.

tion, burning, and itching of the lid margins. The margins of the lids may be erythematous and granular (marginal blepharitis) with fine adherent scales between the eyelashes and a tendency to painful fissuring. In severe cases there may be destruction and replacement of cilia by scar tissue. The conjunctivae are at times injected.

Seborrheic dermatitis occurs from birth to old age. In the adult, stressful events such as myocardial infarction may be associated with the precipitation or exacerbation of seborrheic dermatitis. Seborrheic dermatitis is also associated with Parkinson's disease. Although the specific etiology is unknown, hypersecretion of sebum and the presence of the lipophilic fungus *Pityrosporum ovale* are thought to play a role in pathogenesis.

The clinical presentation may at times blend with that of psoriasis. Lupus erythematosus may also involve the eyelids and should be considered in the differential diagnosis. Seborrheic dermatitis can usually be differentiated from lupus erythematosus by clinical criteria: the latter is characterized by margination, atrophy, follicular dilation and plugging, a greater degree of alopecia, and the absence of yellowish scales in the seborrheic areas. Seborrheic dermatitis-like lesions may be seen in Leiner's disease (infants with diarrhea and dysfunctional fifth component of complement), Letterer-Siwe disease (a form of histiocytosis X in children), pemphigus erythematosus, and in reaction to the administration of arsenic, gold, or methyldopa.

Seborrheic dermatitis usually responds rapidly to topical corticosteroid creams; nonfluorinated steroids, such as hydrocortisone and hydrocortisone acetate, are preferable for chronic use. Blepharitis may be managed by warm compresses of normal saline. The scalp, eyebrows, and lip margins should be kept clean by cleansing with a nonirritating baby shampoo. Careful application of 0.5% selenium sulfide cream to the eyelid margins is also helpful in the control of seborrheic blepharitis (2). Scales should be removed from the lid margins daily with a damp cotton applicator.

Therapy should include attempts to control seborrhea elsewhere as well. The scalp should be treated daily for seborrheic dermatitis with antidandruff shampoos [containing either selenium sulfide (3); zinc pyrithione (3, 4), sulfur, and salicylic acid (4); or tar] and, if necessary, topical antiinflammatory steroid preparations. While shampooing the scalp, the patient can also carefully wash the face including the eyebrows and eyelashes. Adequate control of scalp involvement frequently facilitates a remission of seborrheic blepharitis. Intralesional triamcinolone acetonide, 2.5 mg/ml, administered in 0.05 ml aliquots at 0.5 to 1 cm intervals, is helpful in resistant cases. Seborrheic blepharitis may coexist with staphylococcal blepharitis and can be managed by the application of sodium sulfacetamide ophthalmic ointment at bedtime.

Potential sequelae of prolonged (improper) use of high-potency (especially fluorinated and conjugated), topical cutaneous corticosteroids in the periorbital area are cutaneous atrophy, hypopigmentation, telangiectasia, and facial hypertrichosis; glaucoma and cataract are potential sequelae from prolonged leakage of these steroids into the conjunctival sac. The characteristic steroid cataract is posterior subcapsular in location; there is no evidence that the development of nuclear or cortical cataract is influenced by clinical use of corticosteroids (V. L. Lubkin, personal communication). Chronic use *in* the eye may predispose to candidal overgrowth, herpes simplex infection, and severe corneal complications when used in the treatment of herpes simplex keratitis.

It is unlikely that absorption of topical cutaneous hydrocortisone medications applied chronically and carefully to the eyelid and periorbital skin can induce glaucoma, cataracts, or ocular herpes simplex infection (V. L. Lubkin, personal communication); steroid applied to the external eyelid skin is absorbed in the dermis and subcutaneous tissues of the lid before it can diffuse through to the internal conjunctival lid surface. However, either injudicious application or a wicking effect may allow medication to reach the conjunctival and corneal surfaces by seeping through the palpebral fissures (5). Although it is estimated that only 1% or less of epicutaneously applied hydrocortisone will be absorbed into the epidermis (6), more potent corticosteroids and penetration-enhancing vehicles increase the percent dose absorbed by eyelid skin. Absorption of corticosteroid through inadvertent conjunctival contact poses a greater danger when the more potent corticosteroids and penetration-enhancing vehicles are used to treat dermatoses of the eyelids and periorbital area.

It is well established that glaucoma, cataract (7), and herpes simplex keratitis may be seen following topical ocular and systemic treatment with corticosteroids. Corticosteroids applied to skin can cause disturbances in the hypothalamic-pituitary-adrenal axis (8), particularly if large doses are applied to large areas or if occlusion is employed. It is therefore theoretically possible—but to the best of our knowledge undocumented—that glaucoma and cataracts could result from chronic systemic absorption of pharmacologic quantities of high-potency corticosteroids applied to large areas of dermatitic integument. However, the chronic application of low-potency topical steroids, e.g., hydrocortisone, to a small area of skin, such as the periorbital region, would be unlikely to induce glaucoma or cataracts; the same may also hold true of high-potency corticosteroids, provided they do not reach the conjunctival surface. Since several cases of glaucoma following the prolonged use of high-potency topical cutaneous corticosteroids [e.g., dexamethasone (9), flurandrenolone (10), fluocinolone acetonide 0.1% (11), triamcinolone acetonide 0.1% (9, 12, 13), prednisolone (13), fluocortolone 0.5% (14), and betamethasone 0.1% (15)] to treat eyelid dermatoses have been reported, it would seem prudent to admonish against careless use and to suggest periodic measurements of intraocular pressures in patients treated over a long period of time, especially if there is a family history of glaucoma (16).

It is relevant to analyze whether intralesional corticosteroid therapy possibly relates to the development of glaucoma or steroid cataract. In general, the oral use of prednisone in a dose above 10 mg/day for 1 year (3650 mg/yr) is, in susceptible individuals, a legitimate related possible cause of steroid cataract (7). The equivalent dose of triamcinolone acetonide is 2 mg/day for 1 year (730 mg/yr) because it is five times more potent than predisone. In our practice, the therapeutic dose of intralesional triamcinolone acetonide is limited to a *total* of 50 mg/month (equivalent to 3000 mg of prednisone per year), even when multiple distant sites are injected. To the best of our knowledge there are no reported cases of glaucoma or steroid cataract associated with the intralesional *cutaneous* (in contradistinction to subconjunctival) administration of corticosteroids. The monthly treatment of chronic severe atopic, seborrheic, or contact dermatitis in the periorbital area with triamcinolone acetonide 1 mg/ml (our preference), would not require more than a total volume of 0.5 ml for each side, or 12 mg/yr. The above regimen is equivalent to administering 60 mg/yr of systemic prednisone, which is far below the threshold dose for steroid cataract development. Additionally, intralesional therapy obviates the misuse of topical preparations and their leakage through the palpebral tissues into the conjunctival sac. The therapeutic use of intralesional triamcinolone acetonide is discussed further under "Alopecia Areata."

PSORIASIS

Psoriasis is a chronic recurrent disease of exaggerated epidermal proliferation that exhibits dry, erythematous scaling and slightly raised papules that enlarge and coalesce to form plaques. The characteristic individual lesions may be localized or widespread. Involvement is frequently symmetrical with a predilection for knees, elbows, intergluteal and sacral areas, nails, trunk, and scalp. Psoriasis occurs in all races, affects both sexes with equal frequency, and may appear at any age. Psoriasis may appear at sites of injury (isomorphic or Koebner phenomenon) and has no known etiology; there is a strong familial predisposition. In some patients (6%) there is an associated inflammatory arthritis (41% have HLA-B27) that usually involves the distal joints; it is in these patients that anterior uveitis and keratoconjunctivitis sicca may occur (17).

The face is usually spared; however, about 10% develop ocular symptoms and signs (18, 19). The clinical features of ocular psoriasis include pruritus, epiphora, and photophobia. On examination there may be fine, scaly, erythematous patches affecting the eyelids and eyebrows. The lids may be swollen, edematous, and thickened. If such changes are located in the vicinity of the eyelashes, there is a marginal blepharitis, often with partial alopecia. Uncommonly, after a particularly severe marginal blepharitis, inflammatory ectropion, madarosis, or trichiasis may develop. Psoriasis may extend to the conjunctiva and appear as demarcated yellowish-red plaques that cause irritation, mattering of the lids on awakening, foreign-body sensation, tearing, and conjunctivitis. Rarely, a severe conjunctivitis may lead to scarring and symblepharon. Keratitis is uncommon (18, 20), and lenticular opacities have been described (21). The severity of ocular lesions seems to coincide with cutaneous activity.

Psoriasiform lesions may be seen in seborrheic dermatitis, drug eruptions (especially with beta-blockers, gold, and methyldopa), pityriasis rosea, secondary syphilis, subacute lupus erythematosus, glucagonoma syndrome (necrolytic migratory erythema), and the rare acrodermatitis paraneoplastica (Bazex's syndrome).

Therapy for psoriasis of the lids includes topical 1% hydrocortisone and intralesional triamcinolone acetonide, 2.5 mg/ml, administered in 0.05 ml aliquots at 0.5 to 1 cm intervals. Phototherapy is not efficacious in the periorbital area since the eyes are typically shielded with photoprotective goggles during this form of treatment.

FUNGAL INFECTIONS

The dermatophytoses are ringworm infections by fungi of the genera *Microsporum*, *Trichophyton*, and *Epidermophyton*. Ringworm often occurs in epidemics and may be carried by pets. Dermatophytes occasionally infect the skin of the eyelids (22), eyelashes (23–25), eyebrows (22), and face adjacent to the lids (26, 27), especially in children who frequently have an associated tinea capitis (23, 25, 28). The eyelashes are rarely involved (24, 25, 28, 29), but when they are, there is usually a nearby ringworm of the face (27, 29) or scalp (25, 28). Dermatophytes rarely produce systemic disease unless there are extenuating circumstances, e.g., inherited or acquired immunodeficiency.

Ringworm on the face or scalp is typically a pruritic, erythematous, scaling, circular or irregular, well-demarcated patch with a microvesicular border and a variable tendency toward central clearing. Alopecia may be present. Commonly implicated organisms include *M. audouini* (23–25, 27), *T. mentagrophytes* (22, 26), *M. lanosum* (29), and *M. canis*. A dermatophytosis may be responsible for a chronic blepharitis with thickening of the lids, erythematous lid margins, loss of cilia, and an injected conjunctiva covered with follicles. Culturing a plucked cilium is a good means of identifying the infecting organism (24).

T. mentagrophytes ringworm affecting the brow and eyelids can resemble the clinical picture of pyoderma (22). Human infection by the zoophilic fungi *T. mentagrophytes* and *T. verrucosum* is distinguished clinically by a more marked inflammatory reaction than that produced by anthropophilic fungi. Zoophilic fungi often produce suppurative folliculitis with kerion formation in the scalp. In contiguous areas, such as the face and eyelids, a suppurative folliculitis may occur with indolent cutaneous and subcutaneous infiltration or kerion celsi (30). These infections are rare, are seen mostly in rural areas, and are usually acquired from animals; cattle are the most common source.

Eyebrow infection without involvement elsewhere has been noted particularly in children, and *M. canis* is frequently the etiologic agent (30). Fluorescence of involved hairs under a Wood's light can usually be demonstrated if the causative agent is *M. canis*.

A diagnosis of dermatophyte infection is most easily confirmed by direct microscopic examination of skin scrapings in a 10% potassium hydroxide slide mount. Also, specimens should be cultured on appropriate media (e.g., Sabouraud's cycloheximide-chloramphenicol agar) since the culture may be positive when the potassium hydroxide mount is not, and valuable epidemiologic information is obtained by identifying the etiologic agent. For example, if the zoophilic dermatophyte *M. canis* is isolated, a search should be made for an infected cat or dog (28, 29). Treatment modalities include oral griseofulvin or ketoconazole. Therapy should be continued for 2–3 weeks following resolution. Topical antifungal creams containing either clotrimazole, miconazole nitrate, or haloprogin may also be effective.

PEDICULOSIS

Pediculosis palpebrarum, usually caused by *Phthirus pubis*, the pubic or crab louse, may be seen in conjunction with pediculosis pubis, usually transmitted during sexual intercourse. In addition to its infestation of eyelash, eyebrow, and pubic hair, *Phthirus pubis* may also inhibit the beard, moustache, and axillary hair. Because of its width, *Phthirus pubis* requires widely spaced hairs to hold on to, thus accounting for its infestation of these areas. Infestation of the eyelashes occurs more often in children, probably conveyed through the intimate contact between an infested mother and her child; the child's absence of pubic, axillary, and secondary sexual facial hair may explain the louse's preference for the eyelashes (31).

An intensely pruritic blepharoconjunctivitis usually accompanies eyelid involvement. It is due to mechanical puncture of the skin and irritation from the insect's salivary secretions and fecal excrement. Occasionally, pediculosis palpebrarum may be caused by the lice responsible for pediculosis capitis or pediculosis corporis, i.e., *Pediculus humanus capitis* or *Pediculus humanus corporis*, respectively. This occurs particularly in children who have had contact with an infected adult.

Finding an adult louse or the oval grayish nits containing ova securely attached to the cilia is diagnostic. Nits are elliptical and fixed to the hair shaft. The ova of live nits fluoresce under Wood's light. The nits must be differentiated from the scaling seen in seborrheic blepharitis. Occasionally, an extruded intact keratin hair sheath of the internal and external root layers will mimic a nit on the hair shaft. However, hair sheaths are cylindrical and can be manually slid distally but not proximally on the hair shaft.

Pediculosis of the eyebrows and eyelashes may be treated solely by thorough removal of nits and lice with a fine forceps; this is more commonly performed in conjunction with medical therapy. Pediculosis palpebrarum may be treated by a thick application of any of the following two times a day for 8 days: petrolatum ophthalmic ointment, 0.025% physostigmine ophthalmic ointment, 5% sulfur ointment, or yellow oxide of mercury (32). Undesirable effects of physostigmine on vision, pupillary size, and accommodation have limited its usefulness (33). Isoflurophate drops or ointment (Floropryl) or 3% ammoniated mercury ointment applied to the eyelid margins have been reported to be effective (2). However, isoflurophate, a potent long-acting cholinesterase inactivator and miotic used occasionally to treat primary open-angle glaucoma, probably should not be used for infestations of eyelashes by lice. The patient should bathe and shampoo with lindane, also known as gamma benzene hexachloride (Kwell or Scabene), to remove body lice; however, its use is contraindicated during pregnancy and for infestation of the periocular area since it is irritating to the eyes and mucous membranes. Other pediculicides to be avoided in the ocular region are chlorophenothane (DDT), pyrethrins, and malathion (33).

HYPERTROPHIES

Familial hypertrichosis may be generalized or only localized to the eyebrows (hyperplasia superciliorum). Generalized hypertrichosis, or *congenital hypertrichosis lanuginosa*, is a rare condition characterized by persistence and excessive growth of lanugo hair. Sometimes double eyebrows (duplicata superciliorum) have been noted (34). The eyebrows, or eyebrows and eyelashes, may be extraordinarily long and thick in the localized forms of hypertrichosis.

Synophrys is a condition in which the medial portion of the eyebrows grow together over the glabella making the eyebrows confluent. This may occur idiopathically or in kwashiorkor, congenital hypothyroidism (metabolic cretinism) (34), Waardenburg's syndrome, Touraine's centrofacial lentiginosis, Down's syndrome, and the Brachmann-de Lange (Cornelia de Lange) syndrome. Children born to mothers using trimethadione or paramethadione during pregnancy express a constellation of defects including mental deficiency, brachycephaly, tetralogy of Fallot, and mild synophrys with an unusual upslant to the eyebrows (35).

Trichomegaly, or excessively long and thick eyelashes, may occur in the Brachmann-de Lange syndrome, in kwashiorkor, and as a familial trait. Two patients, in whom B-cell lymphoma was treated with recombinant leukocyte A interferon, noted increased growth of eyelashes after approximately 4 months of therapy (36). Over the next few months thick curly eyelashes grew to lengths of 2–6.5 cm. This abnormality persisted well into the second year of therapy. Other documented causes of drug-induced generalized hypertrichosis include minoxidil, dilantin, diazoxide, and androgenic agents.

Hypertrichosis of the temple and lateral zygomatic arch areas is characteristic of *porphyria cutanea tarda* and may extend to the lateral eyebrows. Facial hirsutism of the newborn is a characteristic feature of the fetal alcohol syndrome which occurs in the offspring of chronically alcoholic women (35). In the periorbital area, the excess hair may extend to and merge with the eyebrows. Additional ophthalmologic findings in the fetal alcohol syndrome include short palpebral fissures, strabismus, and ptosis of the eyelid (35).

Distichiasis, *tristichiasis*, and *tetrastichiasis* describe the presence of double, triple, and quadruple eyelashes respectively. These are extremely rare hereditary defects. In the autosomal dominant distichiasis-lymphedema syndrome an extra row of eyelashes replacing the meibomian glands is associated with lymphedema, predominantly from the knees downward (35). Like trichiasis, distichiasis may cause considerable irritation to the conjunctiva and cornea with similar consequences (see "Trichiasis").

MALPOSITION

CONGENITAL

In 1984, one of us (DSO) observed a peculiar, congenital malposition of the eyebrows in a 39-year-old black man who presented to the dermatology clinic at the Mount Sinai Medical Center (New York City) for an unrelated condition. The abnormality consisted of a bilateral, symmetric, abrupt discontinuity of the eyebrow arch at a point approximately two-thirds lateral to the medial border of the eyebrow (Fig. 32.2). He reported that this malposition had been present since birth and that his father, sister, and daughter were similarly affected.

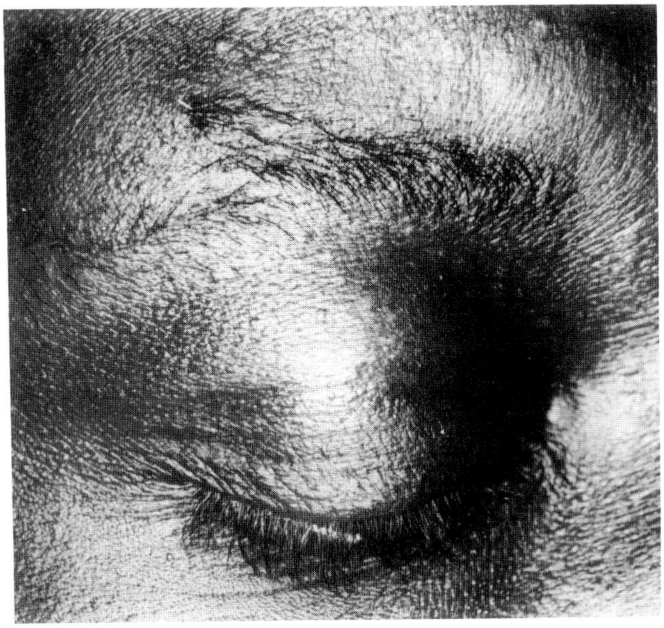

Figure 32.2. Congenital malposition of the eyebrow.

TRICHIASIS

Trichiasis is a condition in which the eyelashes are misdirected toward the globe either as a sequela of senile entropion, degeneration of fascial attachments to the lower lid, or diseases that cause scarring of the eyelid margin or conjunctiva. As a consequence, the lashes rub against and irritate the cornea and conjunctiva, sometimes inducing conjunctivitis, secondary infection, corneal ulceration, and even perforation. Some cases of trichiasis are pemphigus vulgaris, cicatricial pemphigoid, toxic epidermal necrolysis, psoriasis, lepromatous leprosy, and trachoma. Treatment entails surgical reconstruction or permanent destruction of the aberrant ciliary follicles, and is discussed elsewhere in this volume.

ALOPECIA

ALOPECIA AREATA

Alopecia areata is ususally a patchy, circumscribed, nonscarring alopecia that features pathognomonic exclamation-point hairs and typically involves the scalp but can involve the eyebrows or eyelashes alone (Fig. 32.3). Involvement of eyebrows, especially before puberty, usually portends a worse prognosis. There is also a variety of alopecia areata in which the shedding is diffuse rather than localized. The eyebrows and eyelashes are frequently lost in cases of alopecia totalis and alopecia universalis. Other ocular abnormalities that may be associated with alopecia areata include lens opacities, Horner's syndrome, ectopias of the pupil, iris atrophy, and tortuosity of fundus vessels (37).

Pathophysiologically, the anagen growth phase is interrupted because of perifollicular lymphocytic inflammation. Immunologic abnormalities in patients with alopecia areata indicate that an immunopathologic mechanism is involved (38).

Characteristic grid-like pitting of the fingernails, fingerprint arches (39), and premature graying may be associated with alopecia areata. Sometimes epilating a small stub hair from an affected site may show the characteristic atrophic hair root. Eyebrow and eyelash loss does not occur in common male-pattern or androgenetic alopecia. Trichotillomania, atopic dermatitis, seborrheic dermatitis, secondary syphilis, and, rarely, fungal infections (favus) should be considered in the differential diagnosis of alopecia areata.

Collecting hairs and examining the roots can be very helpful in differentiating alopecia areata from trichotillo-

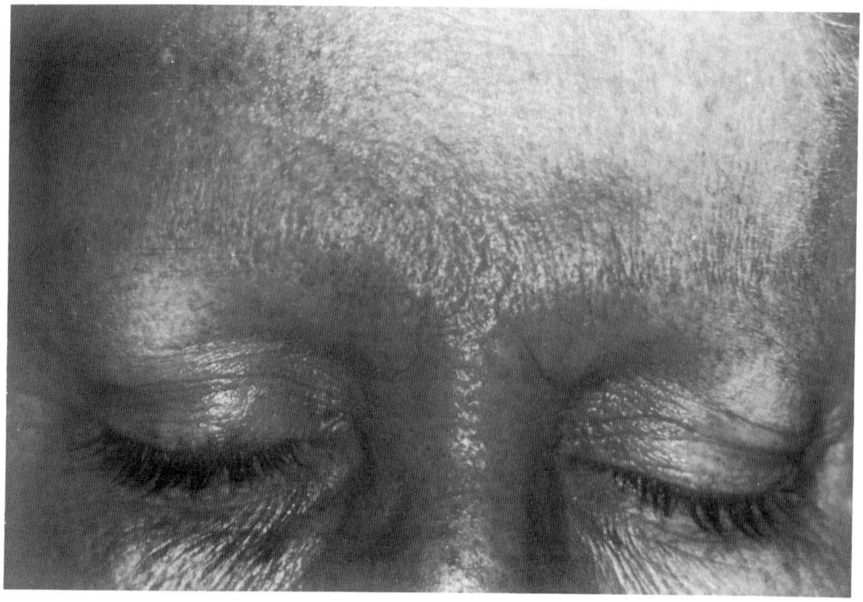

Figure 32.3. Alopecia areata of the eyebrows.

mania. The anagen (growing) hair root neurotically extirpated in trichotillomania is readily distinguished from the naturally shed normal telogen (resting) hair root and from the abnormal hair root seen in alopecia areata. In alopecia areata, examination of shed hairs will show bayonet hairs in large numbers. Bayonet hairs have no visible hair root but show a tapered proximal end produced by the interruption of the anagen phase of the hair cycle (40).

Association of hair loss (especially patchy) with atopy, vitiligo, diabetes mellitus, pernicious anemia, Hashimoto's thyroiditis, Addison's disease, or ocular and testicular abnormalities (41) favors alopecia areata rather than trichotillomania. In addition, loss of eyebrows or lashes associated with hair loss of the scalp, beard, axillae, arms, legs, and pubic area also supports the diagnosis of alopecia areata.

Hair regrowth in response to the injection of antiinflammatory corticosteroids into an alopecic site is both diagnostic and therapeutic in alopecia areata (42). Failure to respond to this treatment occurs only in the most severe active phases of this disorder or where there has been inflammatory destruction of the hair papillae. When hair regrowth fails to occur after treatment with intralesional corticosteroids, an underdosage or overdosage may be causative (42).

For the treatment of alopecia areata, the antiinflammatory corticosteroid of choice is triamcinolone acetonide. Triamcinolone acetonide, 2.5 to 5 mg/ml, is the usual concentration for treating alopecic eyebrows or eyelashes. Our therapeutic schedule is to inject no more frequently than monthly intervals. The total volume is usually 0.5 ml for each side. The higher concentration of 5 mg/ml for 1 month would be equivalent to 300 mg of prednisone administered per year, which is quite below the threshold dose for developing steroid cataract.

Lidocaine is not an optimal diluent; it creates a more painful injection and may produce vasospasm. A steroid suspension should be diluted with isotonic (0.9%) sodium chloride containing 0.9% benzyl alcohol as a preservative. Diluents containing phenol or one of the parabens may cause flocculation of the steroid suspension. Flocculation interferes with the injectability and biological action of the suspension and has been associated with embolism and amaurosis (43). Dilutions should be used before crystal growth occurs. Particle size can be checked under a microscope. Steroid suspensions containing crystals 50 μm or larger should be discarded unless the crystals can be sonicated to less than 10 μm in size.

The prompt use of a prediluted suspension avoids growth of large crystals that, if accidentally injected into a vessel, can cause amaurosis, which is the most serious immediate adverse side effect when injecting the eyebrows, face, or scalp (43). This potential embolic complication can be minimized by using a 30-gauge needle, injecting not more than 0.05 to 0.1 ml aliquots of steroid suspension with each puncture, using a 1.0 ml tuberculin-type syringe, and injecting at 0.5 to 1.0 cm intervals using a multiple discrete puncture technique. The single-injection fanning technique, not recommended by the authors, increases the risk of amaurosis, especially if one does not draw back the plunger of the syringe to determine whether the needle has entered a blood vessel.

To administer reproducible doses of the suspension, uniform distribution of the steroid particles is required. To ensure an even suspension in the syringe, the bottle of steroid suspension should be thoroughly agitated before the suspension is withdrawn through a large bore needle. It should be injected before the suspension settles in the syringe. If immediate injection is not possible, the settled particles may be resuspended by drawing an air bubble into the syringe and inverting the syringe several times. The air bubble is then expelled prior to injection.

If triamcinolone acetonide 5 mg/ml is used, hair regrowth at the sites of injection will usually be evident within 3 weeks. A total dose of 50 mg is typically the maximum administered per month to adults with extensive alopecia areata of the scalp (44). Previously injected sites that are actively regrowing hair do not require reinjection so long as growth continues, and to do so would incur the risk of steroid-induced atrophy and hair loss.

Alternate modalities for treating alopecia areata include the application of contact allergens, such as diphenylcyprone, dinitrochlorobenzene, or squaric acid dibutylester (45). In addition, the topical application of anthralin as well as photochemotherapy (employing topical or oral 8-methoxypsoralen followed by exposure to ultraviolet-A light) have been tried.

TRICHOTILLOMANIA

Self-inflicted hair loss can be brought about by hair pulling; rubbing; twisting; cutting; shaving; sucking; biting; mutilating with a comb, brush, or other instrument; and by applying noxious substances. Indeed these activities are not always self-inflicted, but may be performed by a "partner in neurosis" (46).

The bizarre configuration of hair loss in trichotillomania will often engender suspicion if not outright diagnosis on the part of the clinician. These bizarre configurations differ from patterned androgenetic or male-pattern alopecia, from the often circular patches of hair loss in alopecia areata, and from diffuse hair loss observed following infection, high fever, and exposure to certain chemicals and drugs (e.g., rodenticides such as thallium, anticoagulants such as warfarin and heparin, and antimetabolites such as methotrexate). Patients will often and persistently deny the artifactual cause of their blemish (46).

Trichotillomania appears clinically as irregularly shaped, partially alopecia areas containing hairs broken off at different lengths (Figs. 32.4 and 32.5). The involved areas may show erythema, edema, and postinflammatory hyperpigmentation. Persistent, localized, usually upper eyelash loss of prolonged duration (approximately 1 year) accompanied by low-grade blepharitis, residual small stubs of hair, and onychophagia in a young female favor a diagnosis of the self-inflicted neurotic manifestation called *trichotillomania* (47). Although impractical in the periorbital area, histopathology can differentiate alopecia areata and trichotillomania (48).

The "trichotillo test" enables confirmation of the clinical diagnosis; it may also stop or decrease the vehemence of the patient's (and/or parents') denials and lead to cessation of the neurotic behavior. This test was devised to differentiate between self-inflicted alopecia and organic causes of hair loss such as alopecia areata. A small bandage is carefully sutured over the alopecic region (e.g., eyebrow or scalp). The patient, who is advised to leave this area alone, usually manages to comply. Removal of the bandage in 1 month will reveal hair regrowth (47).

INFLAMMATORY ALOPECIAS

Cicatricial pemphigoid (benign mucous membrane pemphigoid or essential skrinkage of the conjunctiva) is a chronic progressive subepidermal bullous disease related to bullous pemphigoid. Most patients are 60 years of age or older. Since the blisters on the conjunctiva are evanescent, the initial ophthalmological symptoms are usually burning; excessive tearing; foreign-body sensation; photophobia; and a chronic, recalcitrant, exudative, ulcerative conjunctivitis, which in time progresses to symblepharon, synechiae, cicatricial alopecia, trichiasis, ankyloblepharon, entropion, xerophthalmia, and neovascularization of the cornea with visual loss.

Erythema multiforme is an acute, self-limited, nonspecific, hypersensitivity reaction pattern to a multitude of circumstances. The major or bullous variety, also known as the Stevens-Johnson syndrome, typically involves cutaneous and mucosal surfaces and presents with stomatitis, balanitis, conjunctivitis, keratitis, and iridocyclitis. Subsequent visual impairment may develop. The eyelids may be involved, and as the lesions heal, cicatricial shrinkage of the lids and conjunctivae may cause lid distortion, alopecia, trichiasis, tear deficiency, corneal damage, and symblepharon. Some of the most commonly associated precipitating factors are herpes simplex infection, infectious mononucleosis, mycoplasma pneumonia, and drugs (especially the sulfonamides). Treatment is supportive and usually includes systemic corticosteroids.

Toxic epidermal necrolysis, or Lyell's disease, is widely regarded as a variant of severe erythema multiforme. There is rapid development of a widespread tender erythema that progresses to large flaccid bullae and detachment of the epidermis in large sheets, which leaves the

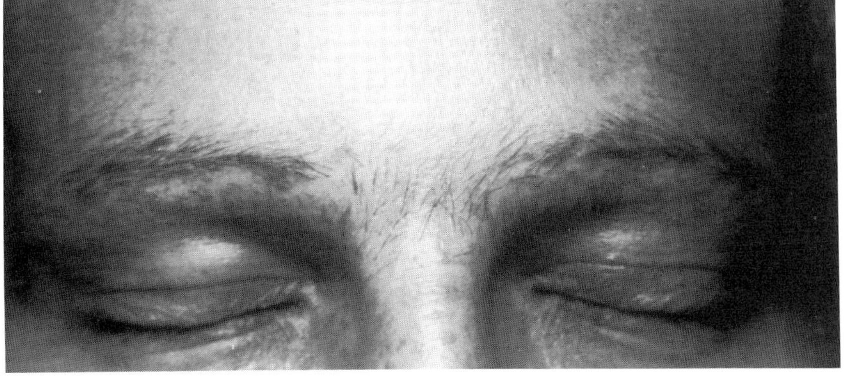

Figure 32.4. Trichotillomania of eyebrows and eyelashes.

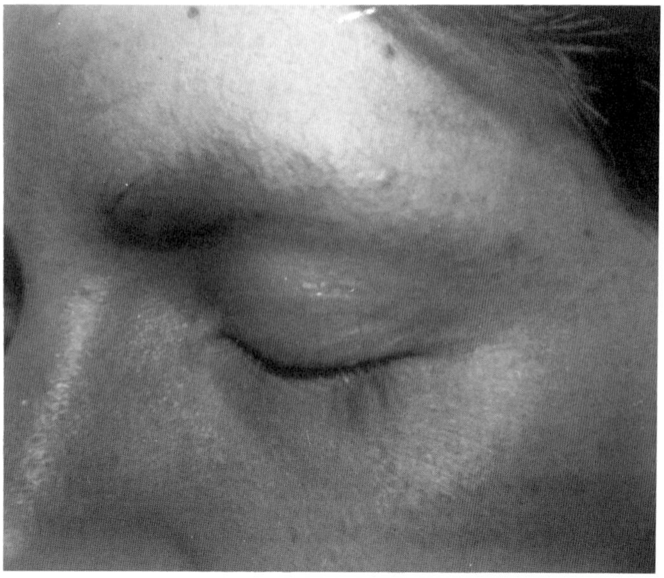

Figure 32.5. Trichotillomania of eyebrow and eyelashes.

dermis exposed. As a rule, mucous membranes are severely involved. There may be a prodromal conjunctival burning sensation and periorbital edema followed by shedding of eyebrows and cilia together with the epidermis of the eyelids and periorbital area. A mucopurulent conjunctivitis may occur in about 50% of cases. Sequelae due to scarring include symblepharon, entropion, trichiasis, ectropion, and cicatricial alopecia.

Cicatricial alopecia of the eyelashes and eyebrows may also occur in the recessive or dominant forms of dystrophic epidermolysis bullosa, bullous impetigo, lamellar ichthyosis, herpes simplex, varicella, and herpes zoster. In herpes zoster, a common pattern of cutaneous involvement is a concomitant eruption along the frontal, lacrimal, and nasociliary branches of the ophthalmic division of the trigeminal nerve. The eyelids may be involved with grouped, frequently umbilicated vesicles on an erythematous base, that undergo crusting and may heal with scarring, alopecia, ectropion, entropion, and trichiasis.

Moderately severe seborrheic or atopic blepharitis with pruritus and chronic rubbing of the eyelids and brows can also cause alopecia of the eyebrows and eyelashes. A permanent, postinflammatory, cicatricial alopecia may be a sequelae of any severe chronic blepharitis, including lupus erythematosus, lupus vulgaris, tertiary syphilis, and folliculitis decalvans. A chronic contact blepharitis as well as a chronic bacterial blepharitis may produce hair loss, but ordinarily this should present no diagnostic difficulty. Permanent alopecia of the eyelashes or eyebrows frequently occurs after radiotherapy of malignant eyelid tumors.

ALOPECIA MUCINOSA

Also referred to as "follicular mucinosis," alopecia mucinosa is characterized clinically by grouped, occasionally pruritic, follicular papules; erythematous, raised, infiltrated plaques; and loss of hair from the involved areas. The lesions are distributed mostly on the face, neck, and scalp but may appear elsewhere as well. Histologically, there are mucinous changes in the outer root sheaths and sebaceous glands. In the primary or idiopathic benign form, the lesions tend to be localized and to resolve spontaneously. When alopecia mucinosa occurs secondary to lymphoma, the individual is usually elderly, the lesions are more widespread, and the histologic appearance is that of mycosis fungoides or lymphoma.

TRAUMATIC OR TRACTION ALOPECIA

Traumatic or traction alopecia can be associated with the misuse of eyelash curlers or the improper removal of artificial eyelashes and their adhesives. Chronic plucking of eyebrows for aesthetic purposes can produce permanent alopecia. It is estimated that for every 100 hairs plucked, one dermal papilla will be epilated, which produces permanent alopecia for that follicle. Because over 60% of the eyebrow hairs are in the telogen (resting) phase and because plucking of a telogen hair induces onset of the anagen (growing) phase will prompt regrowth, it follows that women who regularly pluck their eyebrows complain of the need to repluck on a weekly basis. Microscopic examination of eyelashes lost by trauma usually shows some anagen roots that never are shed spontaneously or with gentle traction.

Shaving the eyebrows, on the other hand, does not induce the onset of anagen, and there ensues a prolonged period of "alopecia." This phenomenon was responsible for the misconception in the early days of head surgery that shaving the eyebrows produced permanent hair loss. The prolonged period before regrowth is explained by the high proportion of eyebrow hairs that are normally in the resting phase; they grow for only 30 to 60 days and rest for about 100 days; in addition, the eyebrows grow more slowly than scalp hair: 0.16 mm/day compared with 0.35 mm/day, respectively (49). Clearly, within the period of most hospitalizations little hair regrowth will occur. The opposite circumstance holds true for hairs with long anagen periods, such as scalp and beard hair, which grow for about 1000 days (3 years) and rest for 100 days. In their case, plucking produces 3 months of alopecia (telogen), and shaving or cutting is followed by immediate regrowth. When reconstructing a traumatic or surgically created wound involving the eyebrow, one can facilitate realignment by not shaving the eyebrow preoperatively.

MADAROSIS

Hair loss of the periorbital area may take the form of madarosis (Hertoghe's sign), or loss of the lateral portions of the eyebrows and eyelashes, which results in the appearance of a greater hair density medially. Some causes of madarosis are hypothyroidism, alopecia areata, trichotillomania, atopic dermatitis, psoriasis, ulerythema ophryogenes, secondary syphilis, measles, small pox, lepromatous leprosy, amyloidosis, mycosis fungoides, follicular mucinosis, and drug reactions. The numerous causes of madarosis make it a nonspecific physical finding.

CUTANEOUS ALBINISM (ALBINOIDISM)

Tietz (50) described a pedigree in which complete deaf-mutism was invariably associated with generalized albinism, which, however, did not involve the eyes. The irides were blue, and there were no associated ocular abnormalities such as nystagmus or photophobia. All the involved individuals had hypoplasia of the eyebrows with only a few sparse albino hairs where the eyebrows normally are. The inheritance was autosomal dominant.

ALOPECIA ASSOCIATED WITH GENODERMATOSES

Alopecia of the eyebrows or eyelids may be a component of other rare genodermatoses. In anhidrotic ectodermal dysplasia there is a thinning of the lateral portions of the eyebrows and a decreased number of eyelashes. Alopecia is also observed in hidrotic ectodermal dysplasia, pachyonychia congenita, dyskeratosis congenita, xeroderma pigmentosum, and progeria. Sparseness of lower eyelashes may occur in mandibulofacial dysostosis. The eyebrows are absent in less than 50% of patients with trisomy 13 syndrome (35).

The Rothmund-Thomson syndrome (poikiloderma congenitale) is an autosomal recessive dermatosis characterized by poikiloderma of the face, ears, and limbs. It is frequently accompanied by juvenile cataracts, congenital bone defects, hypogonadism, and disturbances of hair growth. Absence or sparseness of eyebrows and eyelashes occurs in 50% of cases (34), and trichiasis may be present. Scalp, axillary, and public hair may also be involved.

In the autosomal dominant hereditary hypotrichosis of Marie Unna (51) there is an often patchy, scarring alopecia (more severe in males) in which eyebrows, eyelashes, and body hair are absent or scant from birth. After puberty the axillary, pubic, and beard hair is also sparse. Facial milia may be present; otherwise, affected individuals are normal.

In Tay's syndrome, the hair of the scalp, eyebrows, and eyelashes is short, sparse, and brittle. Examination of the hairs reveals pili torti and trichorrhexis nodosa–like changes. These individuals are affected with diffuse, red, scaling skin; keratoderma of the palms and soles; and a progeria-like appearance with close-set eyes, beaked nose, and sunken cheeks (52).

In monilethrix, the hair shaft can be normal at birth, but by adolescence it develops a characteristic beaded appearance and brittle quality. It is an autosomal dominant developmental defect of hair shaft formation, and the eyebrows and eyelashes may be affected. In some cases present from birth, improvement has occurred with puberty.

Pili torti is a structural defect in which the hair shaft is twisted on its own axis. Eyelashes and eyebrows may be affected alone or in association with the scalp hair. Examination may reveal only stumps of broken hair. Pili torti is found in Bjornstad's syndrome, Menkes's kinky hair syndrome, and in familial hypotrichosis of the Marie Unna type (34).

Ulerythema ophryogenes, or keratosis pilaris rubra atrophicans (keratosis pilaris atrophicans faciei), is a rare autosomal dominant dermatosis occurring mostly in young men. Onset occurs a few months after birth; the lateral one-third of the eyebrow develops small horny follicular red papules (53). It may spread to the neighboring skin of the cheeks and forehead. The lesions heal with pitted scarring, atrophy, and alopecia. The eyelashes may be lost as well. Pathogenically, follicular hyperkeratosis is believed to form a barrier to the outgrowing hair, thereby inducing a chronic inflammatory reaction. Ulerythema ophryogenes is associated with atopy, while some affected patients may have various ectodermal defects (54). It has also been reported in association with Noonan's syndrome (55).

The closely related keratosis follicularis spinulosa decalvans is characterized by similar lesions (follicular red papules) that may affect the face (including the eyebrows and eyelashes), trunk, and extremities (53). Onset is in infancy. Additionally, this entity is associated with widespread keratosis pilaris, scarring alopecia of the scalp, hyperkeratosis of the palms and soles, atopy, photophobia, and corneal abnormalities. Involvement of the eyelashes may lead to blepharitis and punctate corneal defects (53).

SURGICAL CORRECTION OF EYEBROW AND EYELASH ALOPECIA

Hair transplantation to repair hair defects was described by Okuda in 1839 (56, 57) for the treatment of alopecia of the eyebrows and moustache areas as well as the scalp; he used cylindrical metal punches. Fujita reported eyebrow reconstruction in leprosy patients by means of punctiform hair grafting in 1953 (58). In this technique, a free skin graft with hairs is divided into small pieces, each containing from two to 10 hairs. Utilizing a thick injection needle or a slender scalpel, the surgeon inserts these pieces into holes that have been prepared in the recipient site (59). Fujita further reported eyebrow reconstruction in traumatic scarring, in a scar due to x-ray therapy for hemangioma, and in a patient with a pigmented nevus around the eyelids accompanied by defects of eyebrow and eyelashes (59).

Many causes of eyebrow and eyelash alopecia have been covered in the preceding discussion. These causes fall into broad categories: autoimmune (alopecia areata), inflammatory, traumatic, self-inflicted, neoplastic, congenital, and postoperative. Surgical correction is appropriate for definitively permanent alopecias that have not responded to medical therapies or that have not resolved spontaneously. For example, the myriad of medical modalities to treat alopecia areata in addition to its tendency for spontaneous recovery or spontaneous progression obviates surgical correction.

In general, strip grafts (60) are suitable for total alopecia of the eyebrows; punch grafts are probably best for partial alopecia. The donor site is ordinarily chosen from a parietooccipital area of the scalp that contains coarse hair. Since a hair follicle's growth characteristics are genetically determined, the follicle will retain these characteristics wherever it is transplanted, i.e., donor dominance. Therefore, scalp hair transplanted to the eyebrow will, after a several month lag period, grow to the long length it attained when situated on the scalp and thus require trimming. Eyebrow hair follicles are probably the most suitable but not necessarily the most feasible substitute for lost eyelashes.

POLIOSIS (CANITIES)

Premature graying (poliosis) of the eyelashes and eyebrows may develop in sympathetic ophthalmia and iridocyclitis (61). Poliosis may occur when hair regrows in areas previously affected by alopecia areata or following x-irradiation. Poliosis may also involve the eyelashes and eyebrows in vitiligo and in the Vogt-Koyanagi-Harada and Alezzandrini syndromes.

Leukotrichia of the eyebrows and/or eyelashes may also be seen in piebaldism, which is a congenital defect of the pigmentary system that may occur alone or in association with other abnormalities of neural crest derivation, such as in Waardenburg's syndrome.

VITILIGO

Vitiligo is a common, acquired, idiopathic hypomelanosis that is often familial. The typical lesion is a round or oval, amelanotic macule or patch that is several millimeters to several centimeters in diameter and that enlarges with time. The margins may be convex and hyperpigmented. Hair in involved areas may become gray (poliosis). Perifollicular repigmentation within the macule may be observed. The extent of involvement is extremely variable. Commonly involved areas include the eyelids (Fig. 32.6), face, extensor bony surfaces, periorificial areas, anterior tibial areas, flexor wrists, axillae, and lower back. Mucosal involvement is not uncommon. Vitiligo exhibits the Koebner (isomorphic) phenomenon, i.e., lesions develop at sites of injury. This may account for the typical distribution of vitiligo in areas of repeated subliminal local trauma.

No race is spared, and the sexes are equally affected. Onset may occur at any age; however, in 50% of cases, vitiligo appears before the age of 20. Patients often report onset during summer months; this is probably because the previously unnoticed amelanotic patch has been accentuated by tanning of the surrounding normal skin.

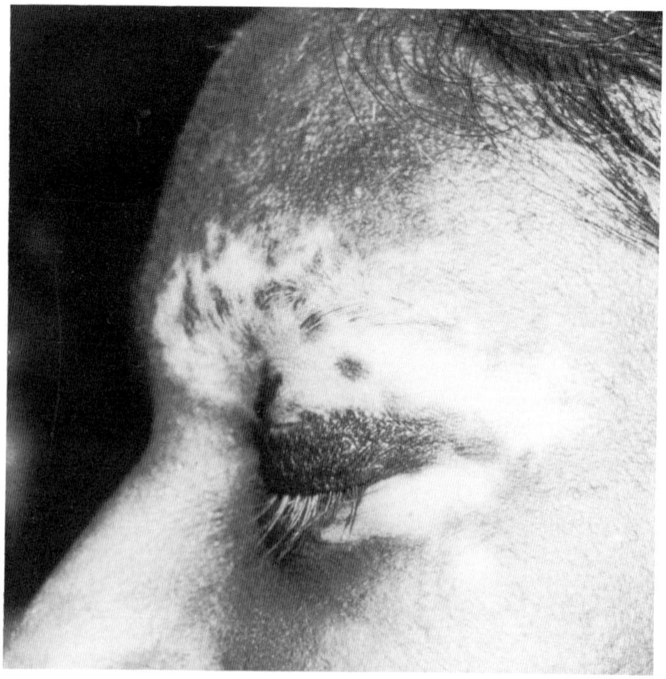

Figure 32.6. Vitiligo of periorbital skin and poliosis of eyebrows and eyelashes.

Although most patients with vitiligo appear to be in good health, the condition has been associated with such autoimmune endocrine disorders as diabetes mellitus, Grave's disease, Hashimoto's thyroiditis, and Addison's disease. In addition, vitiligo is associated with such immunologic illnesses as pernicious anemia (62), thymomas, myasthenia gravis, and autoimmune hemolytic anemia. Vitiligo has also been associated with a variety of dermatoses, e.g., premature graying, alopecia areata, halo nevi, morphea, systemic scleroderma, and advanced malignant melanoma. Sudden onset of vitiligo in the elderly should prompt an examination for the presence of a neoplasm, such as malignant melanoma, or an autoimmune disorder.

Occasionally, there is an increased tortuosity of retinal blood vessels, depigmentation of the iris, and atrophy of retinal pigment epithelium (63). Amelanotic macules frequently involve the lids and periocular skin; additionally, the eyebrows and eyelashes may become depigmented. Vitiligo may occur in patients with uveitis (64) and as part of the Vogt-Koyanagi-Harada and Alezzandrini syndromes.

Routine histopathology shows normal skin except for absence of melanocytes; the dopa reaction for melanocytes is also negative. Routine laboratory investigation is usually unremarkable, but further testing may reveal antithyroid cell, antithyroglobulin, antimicrosomal (smooth muscle), antiparietal cell, and antiadrenal cell antibodies (65).

The course of vitiligo is unpredictable and may be characterized alternatively by slow progression, stabilization, or exacerbation. Complete spontaneous repigmentation is unusual. Vitiligo must be distinguished from piebaldism, Waardenburg's syndrome, albinism, pityriasis alba, tinea versicolor, idiopathic guttate hypomelanosis, postinflammatory hypomelanosis, chemical depigmentation, scleroderma, and nevus depigmentosus.

Treatment modalities include the oral administration or topical application of psoralen followed by exposure to longwave ultraviolet light (PUVA). Topical and intralesional corticosteroids, such as triamcinolone acetonide, 2.5 mg/ml, are sometimes effective. When other modalities fail, cosmetic makeup such as Covermark (Lydia O'Leary), and full- (59, 66, 67) or split-thickness skin grafts are worth trying. Another successful technique is epidermal grafting in which pigment-bearing epidermis is obtained by producing a suction blister; it is then grafted onto a prepared recipient bed within an achromic area (68).

Patients with vitiligo comprise a heterogeneous group, and not all may be responsive to grafting. There are two general types of vitiligo: the localized, segmental, or dermatomal variety, which may have a neurogenic pathogenesis; and the generalized variety, which likely has an autoimmune pathogenesis. In a study of vitiligo, type unspecified, the disorder-manifested recipient dominance, i.e., normal, pigmented skin grafted into an area of vitiligo became vitiliginous, and vitiliginous skin grafted into a normal site became pigmented (69). It remains to be established whether both or only one of these general types show recipient dominance. Autologous minigrafting was successful in three cases of segmental vitiligo, while in one case of generalized vitiligo it was not (66). These findings suggest that segmental vitiligo demonstrates donor dominance and generalized vitiligo is recipient dominant; however, appropriate controls (69) are required before a definite conclusion can be reached.

Complete depigmentation by the administration of monobenzylether of hydroquinone 20% (Benoquin) for patients with extensive vitiligo is rarely recommended. Vitiliginous areas must be protected from sunburn with strong sunscreens since these areas have lost their innate protection. Sunscreen application to the normal skin surrounding vitiligo will prevent accentuation of the color contrast between these two areas.

VOGT-KOYANAGI-HARADA SYNDROME

The Vogt-Koyanagi-Harada syndrome is characterized by chronic bilateral uveitis, meningeal irritation (aseptic meningitis), poliosis (including the eyebrows and eyelashes), vitiligo, alopecia areata–like hair loss (often involving the eyebrows and eyelashes), and dysacousia. Choroiditis, optic neuritis, and retinal detachment are less often associated.

ALEZZANDRINI SYNDROME

The Alezzandrini syndrome is characterized by a unilateral degenerative retinitis that is followed after several months by facial vitiligo and poliosis on the same side. The latter often involves the eyelashes. Perceptual deafness may also be present (70).

PIEBALDISM

Piebaldism designates a cutaneous condition of dual coloration, usually white and black or shades of brown, in the form of spots or patches of one color on a background of the other. In man, piebaldism (partial albinism) is an unusual, autosomal dominant trait that may involve large areas of skin but typically and most commonly manifests itself as a white forelock.

The hypomelanosis of piebaldism is congenital; sometimes, in fair-skinned Caucasians, the anomaly may not be apparent at birth. Consistency in the pattern of hypomelanosis is especially characteristic on the face—a white macule in the center of the chin and hypopigmentation of the supraglabellar region in a wedge-shaped configuration, the base of which follows the frontal hairline (usually including a white forelock) and the apex of which points to the bridge of the nose, where it is associated with poliosis of the medial portions of the eyebrows and eyelashes.

The usual finding in piebaldism is paucity or absence of normal, pigment-forming melanocytes. If melanocytes are present, it may be possible to stimulate them to produce pigment. Perhaps this is why photochemotherapy is sometimes partially successful. Alternatively, one may try to repopulate or "seed" the hypopigmented areas with normal melanocytes. This was the rationale for pigmentary correction of piebaldism by autografts (71). Correction was possible because piebaldism is donor dominant and not recipient dominant.

WAARDENBURG SYNDROME

This dominantly inherited pattern of developmental anomalies features lateral displacement of the inner ocular canthi; high, broad, nasal root; synophrys; heterochromic irides; deafness and mental retardation; white forelock; and congenital graying of the hair, which may include the eyebrows and eyelashes.

COSMETICS

Eyebrows and eyelashes receive a great deal of attention in an attempt to enhance beauty. A spectacular variety of complexly formulated and colored mascaras and eyelid and eyebrow pencils have been developed. Reactions to these eye area cosmetics include contact dermatitis, infection by contamination, conjunctivitis, and conjunctival pigmentation. Probably the most common complaints are stinging and burning of the eyes and lids on application of eye area cosmetics, caused by the evaporation of irritating volatile components in some of these products (72).

Contact dermatitis is of two types: irritant and allergic. An irritant contact dermatitis may occur within hours after the skin comes in contact with sufficient quantities of the inciting substance. Allergic contact dermatitis usually occurs 24 to 48 hours after a sensitized individual, with the appropriate cell-mediated immune response, comes in contact with even minute amounts of allergen. It may be impossible to distinguish irritant from allergic contact dermatitis by morphologic and histologic criteria.

Contact dermatitis of the periorbital area may be caused by cosmetics applied either to the eye area or used on the hair, face, or fingernails, and conveyed by the fingers to the eyelids (72). The upper eyelids are the most commonly affected site. Frequently, the causative agent is nail polish or the phosphoric acid sesquisulfide used in matches and matchboxes. Rubbing the eyes after handling cosmetics, soaps, detergents, hair products, ophthalmic ointments, or chemicals may also provoke a contact dermatitis reaction. In the majority of patients with allergic contact dermatitis to nail cosmetics the dermatitis involves the eyelids, face, and neck, while the paronychial areas are usually spared.

Mascara, eyebrow pencils, eyeliners, and false eyelash adhesive may contain allergens and such potentially sensitizing ingredients as pigments, parabens, antimicrobial preservatives, lanolin, balsam of Peru, synthetic resins, or bleaching materials, i.e., mercury and hydroquinone. Particles of some of these products (mascara flakes, eyeshadow dust, and mascara extenders such as nylon or rayon fibers) may also induce a physical irritant conjunctivitis if they become lodged on the conjunctiva. Conjunctival tattooing may be caused by applying eyeliner to the conjunctival side of the lid margin (73).

Dyeing of eyelashes is performed by some skin care and beauty salons predominantly for blond-haired women who wish to accentuate their eyes. The Federal Drug and Cosmetic Act forbids the use of permanent oxidation–type dyes containing paraphenylenediamine on eyelashes and eyebrows because an allergic reaction could cause corneal damage and blindness (74). However, metallic dyes (rare sensitizers) and semipermanent azo and aniline dyes, not requiring oxidation, are relatively safe. Nevertheless, prudence dictates performing a patch test for sensitivity on the inner forearm days prior to eyelash application. Patients with allergic hypersensitivity to paraphenylenediamine should be warned of the possibility of cross-reaction dermatitis from immunologically related compounds, including azo and aniline dyes (74).

The extremely thin skin of the eyelids is especially susceptible to contact dermatitis. Acute contact dermatitis is characterized by unilateral or bilateral pruritus, erythema, edema, vesiculation, and exudation. The skin around the eyes tends to react with massive edema so that in many cases there is a clinical similarity to erysipelas. Chronic lesions show erythema, scaling, crusting, lichenification, and dyschromia. In addition to blepharitis, contact sensitizers may independently or concomitantly produce a conjunctivitis characterized by a papillary response, hyperemia, chemosis, and a watery mucoid discharge.

Treatment requires identifying and eliminating the responsible agent. The mainstays of therapy are application of soothing cool compresses of either physiologic saline, aluminum acetate 5% (Burow's solution) diluted 1:40, or equal parts whole milk and water, in conjunction with judicious use of topical or systemic intralesional corticosteroid preparations. In addition, antihistamines to control pruritus and antibiotics to treat secondary infection may be indicated. Finally, to prevent recurrence, patch testing after convalescence and avoidance of the established inciting substances are essential.

Eye infections, resulting from the use and misuse of mascara, eyeliner, and their applicators, are uncommon but may be serious. Inadequately preserved cosmetics may become contaminated with *Staphylococcus epidermidis* and *S. aureus*, which may cause conjunctivitis and blepharitis. Keratitis and corneal ulceration has been attributed to mascara and applicators contaminated with *Pseudomonas aeruginosa* (75) and occasionally *Fusarium solanae* (76).

A modern procedure for tattooing the base of the eyelashes has appeared in the plastic surgical literature (77) and has received attention in the lay press. Eyelash tattooing is an ancient technique that is still practiced, usually by women, in many cultures. Today, for example, women in Morocco tattoo their eyelid margins. Women apply eyeliner to emphasize the contour of the eyes and enhance their beauty. The modern method of implanting permanent eyeliner was developed for the handicapped or elderly woman who finds it difficult or impossible to neatly and safely apply eyeliner, and for other women who feel the need to liberate themselves from the daily task of applying eyeliner (77).

After local anesthesia and with a specially designed instrument, the sterile tattoo pigment mixed with equal parts glycerin is implanted at the base of and in between the lashes in a dot-like fashion. Penetration depth is set at 1.2 mm; a penetration of greater than 1.5 mm will enter the tarsus and produce fan-shaped pigment spread. Anticipated potential complications such as loss of eyelashes, pigment spread, infection, hypertrophic scarring, or allergic reaction were not observed in a report of 125 persons (77).

The major disadvantage of this procedure, for women who are not elderly or handicapped, is its permanency. In today's world of rapidly changing styles, women enjoy the freedom to change their appearance depending upon the occasion. Furthermore, what is considered esthetically appealing today may be very different in the future.

There is also a small but very definite incidence of allergy to red (mercury), green (chromium), yellow (cadmium), and blue (cobalt) tattoo pigments (74). However, the predominantly iron-based pigments used for tattooing the base of eyelashes are considered "hypoallergenic." Allergic reaction to simple carbon is exceedingly rare. Glycerin is a very rare sensitizer (74).

Attempts to physically remove the pigment, either to treat an allergic reaction or to accommodate a patient who elects to have it removed for nontherapeutic reasons, could be destructive to the eyelids and eyelashes.

SUMMARY

The eyebrows and eyelashes may exhibit a surprising diversity of abnormalities, many of which offer clues to the presence of illness elsewhere while others provide confirmation of a particular diagnosis. Furthermore, their prominent position and integral role in appearance make eyebrows and eyelashes the object of attention, adornment, admiration, anxiety, and abuse.

ACKNOWLEDGMENT

We thank Dr. Virginia Lubkin for her helpful comments.

REFERENCES

1. Montagna W, Ford DM: Histology and cytochemistry of human skin. XXXIII. The eyelid. *Arch Dermatol* 100: 328–335, 1969.
2. Ellis PP: *Ocular Therapeutics and Pharmacology*, ed 6. St. Louis, C.V. Mosby, 1981.
3. Orentreich N, Taylor EH, Berger RA, Auerbach R: Comparative study of two antidandruff preparations. *J Pharm Sci* 58: 1279–1280, 1969.
4. Orentreich N: A clinical evaluation of two shampoos in the treatment of seborrheic dermatitis. *J Soc Cosmet Chem* 23: 189–194, 1972.
5. Howell JB: Eye diseases induced by topically applied steroids: the

thin edge of the wedge. *Arch Dermatol* 112: 1529–1530, 1976.
6. Malinson FD, Ferguson EH: Percutaneous absorption of hydrocortisone-1-C^{14} in human subjects. *J Invest Dermatol* 25: 281–283, 1955.
7. Lubkin VL: Steroid cataract—A review and a conclusion. *J Asthma Res* 14: 55–59, 1977.
8. Gell KA, Baxter DL: Plasma cortisol suppression by steroid creams. *Arch Dermatol* 89: 734–740, 1964.
9. Hales RH: Glaucoma induced by careless use of steroids. *J Pediatr Ophthalmol* 10: 206–207, 1973.
10. Brubaker R, Halpin J: Open-angle glaucoma associated with topical administration of flurandrenolide to the eye. *Mayo Clin Proc* 50: 322–326, 1975.
11. Cubey RB: Glaucoma following the application of corticosteroid to the skin of the eyelid. *Br J Dermatol* 95: 207–208, 1976.
12. Zugerman C, Saunders D, Levit F: Glaucoma from topically applied steroids. *Arch Dermatol* 112: 1326, 1976.
13. Nielsen NV, Sorensen PN: Glaucoma induced by application of corticosteroids to the periorbital region. *Arch Dermatol* 114: 953–954, 1978.
14. Vie R: Glaucoma and amaurosis associated with long-term application of corticosteroids to the eyelids. *Acta Dermatol Venerol (Stockh)* 60: 541–542, 1980.
15. Eisenlohr JE: Glaucoma following the prolonged use of topical steroid medication to the eyelids. *J Am Acad Dermatol* 8: 878–881, 1983.
16. Larsen WG: Corticosteroids and glaucoma. *Arch Dermatol* 95: 645–646, 1967.
17. Wilson LA: *External Diseases of the Eye*. Hagerstown, MD, Harper & Row, 1979.
18. Kaldeck R: Ocular psoriasis. *Arch Dermatol Syphilol* 68: 44–49, 1953.
19. Vaughan D, Asbury T: *General Ophthalmology*, ed 8. Los Altos, CA, Lange Medical Publications, 1977.
20. Stuart JA: Ocular psoriasis. *Am J Ophthalmol* 55: 615–617, 1953.
21. Korting GW: *The Skin and Eye*. Philadelphia, WB Saunders, 1973.
22. Ostler HB, Okumoto M, Halde C: Dermatophytosis affecting the periorbital region. *Am J Ophthalmol* 72: 934–938, 1971.
23. Franks AG, Mandel EH, Sternberg AS: Endemic infection with *Microsporum audouini* in a family of eight persons. *Arch Dermatol Syphilol* 62: 54–57, 1950.
24. Hopkins WG, Krause AC: Infection of the eyelashes with *Microsporum audouini*. *Am J Ophthalmol* 33: 1793–1794, 1950.
25. Montgomery RM, Walzer EA: Tinea capitis with infection of the eyelashes. *Arch Dermatol Syphilol* 46: 40–43, 1942.
26. Shapiro L: Tinea facialis. *Arch Dermatol* 99: 504–505, 1969.
27. Silvers SH: Microsporon audouini infection of the eyelashes. *Arch Dermatol Syphilol* 49: 436, 1944.
28. Costa OG: Microsporon infection of the palpebral and ciliary regions. *Arch Dermatol Syphilol* 48: 65–69, 1943.
29. Franks AG, Mandel EH: Microsporon lanosum infection of the eyelashes. *Arch Dermatol Syphilol* 62: 708–713, 1950.
30. Rippon JW: *Medical Mycology*, ed 2. Philadelphia, WB Saunders, 1982.
31. Alexander JO: Phthirus pubis infestation of the eyelashes. *JAMA* 250: 32, 1983.
32. Arndt KA: *Manual of Dermatologic Therapeutics*, ed 3. Boston, Little, Brown & Co, 1983.
33. *AMA Drug Evaluations*, ed 5. Chicago, American Medical Association, 1983, p 1855.
34. Butterworth T, Ladda RL: *Clinical Genodermatology*. New York, Praeger, 1981, vol 2.
35. Smith DW: *Recognizable Patterns of Human Malformation*, ed 3. Philadelphia, WB Saunders, 1982.
36. Foon KA, Dougher G: Increased growth of eyelashes in a patient given leukocyte A interferon. *N Engl J Med* 311: 1259–1260, 1984.
37. Rook A, Dawber R: *Diseases of the Hair and Scalp*. Oxford, Blackwell Scientific Publications, 1982.
38. Safai B, Orentreich N, Good RA: Immunological abnormalities in patients with alopecia areata (AA). *Clin Res* 27: 244A, 1979.
39. Selmanowitz VJ, Victor S, Warburton D, Orentreich N: Fingerprint arches in alopecia areata. *Arch Dermatol* 110: 570–571, 1974.
40. Orentreich N: Hair loss in young boy: trichotillomania or alopecia areata? *JAMA* 234: 761, 1975.
41. Brown AC, Pollard ZF, Jarrett WH II: Ocular and testicular abnormalities in alopecia areata. *Arch Dermatol* 118: 546–554, 1982.
42. Orentreich N, Sturm HM, Weidman AI, Pelzig A: Local injection of steroids and hair regrowth in alopecias. *Arch Dermatol* 82: 894–902, 1960.
43. Selmanowitz VJ, Orentreich N: Cutaneous corticosteroid injection and amaurosis: analysis for cause and prevention. *Arch Dermatol* 110: 729–734, 1974.
44. Orentreich N: Treatment of alopecia areata. *JAMA* 238: 347, 1977.
45. Case PC, Mitchell AJ, Swanson NA, Venderveen EE, Ellis CN, Headington JT: Topical therapy of alopecia areata with squaric acid dibutylester. *J Am Acad Dermatol* 10: 447–451, 1984.
46. Selmanowitz VJ, Orentreich N: Cosmetic treatment of factitial defects. *Cutis* 6: 549–552, 1970.
47. Orentreich N: Etiology of loss of eyelashes in a child. *JAMA* 207: 961, 1969.
48. Ackerman AB, Niven J, Grant-Kels JM: Differential diagnosis in dermatopathology. Philadelphia, Lea & Febiger, 1982.
49. Johnson E: Cycles and patterns of hair growth. In Jarrett (ed): *The Physiology and Pathophysiology of the Skin*. London, Academic Press, 1977, vol 4, p 1249.
50. Tietz W: A syndrome of deaf-mutism associated with albinism showing dominant autosomal inheritance. *Am J Hum Genet* 15: 259–264, 1963.
51. Rook A, Wilkson DS, Ebling FJG: *Textbook of Dermatology*, ed 3. Oxford, Blackwell Scientific Publications, 1979, vol 1.
52. Tay CH: Ichthyosiform erythroderma, hair shaft abnormalities, and mental and growth retardation. *Arch Dermatol* 104: 4–13, 1971.
53. Rand R, Baden H: Keratosis follicularis spinulosa decalvans. *Arch Dermatol* 119: 22–26, 1983.
54. Davenport DD, Wash L: Ulerythema ophryogenes. *Arch Dermatol* 89: 74–80, 1964.
55. Pierini DO, Pierini AM: Keratosis pilaris atrophicans faciei (ulerythema ophryogenes): a cutaneous marker in Noonan syndrome. *Br J Dermatol* 100: 409–416, 1979.
56. Okuda S: Clinical and experimental studies of transplantation of living hairs. *Jpn J Dermatol Urol* 46: 135–138, 1939.
57. Okuda S: Klinische und experimentelle Untersuchungen uber die Transplantation von lebenden Haaren. *Jpn J Dermatol* 40: 537, 1939.
58. Fujita K: Reconstruction of eyebrow. *La Lepro* 22: 364, 1953.
59. Fujita K: Hair transplantation in Japan. In Kobori T, Montagna W (eds): *Biology and Diseases of the Hair*. Baltimore, University Park Press, 1976, p 519–527.
60. Lewis LA, Resnik SS: Strip and punch grafting for alopecia of the eyebrow. *J Dermatol Surg Oncol* 5: 557–559, 1979.
61. Bruno MG, McPherson SD Jr: Harada's disease. *Am J Ophthalmol* 32: 513–522, 1949.
62. Bor S, Feiwel M, Chanarin I: Vitiligo and its aetological relationship to organ-specific autoimmune disease. *Br J Dermatol* 81: 83–88, 1969.
63. Albert DM, Nordlund JJ, Lerner AB: Ocular abnormalities occurring with vitiligo. *Ophthamlology* 86: 1145–1158, 1979.
64. Nordlund JJ, Taylor NT, Albert DM, Wagoner MD, Lerner AB: The prevalence of vitiligo and poliosis in patients with uveitis. *J Am Acad Dermatol* 4: 528–536, 1981.
65. Brostoff J, Bor S, Feiwel M: Autoantibodies in patients with vitiligo. *Lancet* July 26, 1969, p 177–178.
66. Falabella R: Repigmentation of segmental vitiligo by autogenous minigrafting. *J Am Acad Dermatol* 9: 514–521, 1983.
67. Orentreich N, Selmanowitz VJ: Autograft repigmentation of leukoderma. *Arch Dermatol* 105: 734–736, 1972.
68. Falabella R: Epidermal grafting: an original technique and its application in achromic and granulating areas. *Arch Dermatol* 104: 592–600, 1971.
69. Orentreich N: Autografts in alopecias and other selected dermatological conditions. *Ann NY Acad Sci* 83: 463–479, 1959.
70. Butterworth T, Ladda RL: *Clinical Genodermatology*. New York, Praeger, 1981, vol 1.
71. Selmanowitz VJ, Rabinowitz AD, Orentreich N, Wenk E: Pigmentary correction of piebaldism by autografts. I. Procedures and clinical findings. *J Dermatol Surg Oncol* 3: 615–622, 1977.
72. Pascher F: Reactions to eye area cosmetics. In Frost P, Horwitz SN (eds): *Principles of Cosmetics for the Dermatologist*. St. Louis, CV

Mosby, 1982.
73. Zuckerman BD: Conjunctival pigmentation due to cosmetics. *Am J Ophthalmol* 62: 672–676, 1966.
74. Fisher AA: *Contact Dermatitis*, ed 2. Philadelphia, Lea & Febiger, 1973.
75. Wilson LA, Ahearn DG: *Pseudomonas*-induced corneal ulcers associated with containated eye mascaras. *Am J Ophthalmol* 84: 112–119, 1977.
76. Kuehne JW, Ahearn DG: Incidence and characterization of fungi in eye cosmetics. *Develop Ind Microbiol* 12: 177, 1971.
77. Angres GG: Eye-liner implants: a new cosmetic procedure. *J Plast Reconstr Surg* 73: 833–836, 1984.

CHAPTER 33

Eyebrow Reconstruction

RUSSELL S. GONNERING, M.D., F.A.C.S.

The eyebrows constitute a major component of the orbital aesthetic unit. Alterations in their form and appearance are readily detectable to even the casual observer. Although cultural differences have dictated varying concepts of their ideal form, their presence is almost universally accepted by all peoples, in all times.

It is therefore rather surprising that, until recently, little attention has been given to them in the disciplines of medicine that deal with the orbital aesthetic unit. The awareness of their importance in preoperative evaluation of blepharoplasty patients has sparked interest in eyebrow anatomy, physiology, and pathology.

ANATOMY

SURFACE TOPOGRAPHY

The visible portion of the eyebrow is made up primarily of the cilia, which are contained in the skin of the eyebrow region. Close observation reveals that these hairs are of three distinct types. More than half of the brow hairs are either of two types: fine, fleece-like vellus hairs, or slightly larger, pigmented small hairs (1). Vellus hairs are fine, nonmedullated hairs that are present over almost the entire body in very large numbers. The presence of these hairs is responsible for the fact that human skin has more hair follicles per unit of area than that of the chimpanzee (2, 3).

The proportion of the third type, large medullated terminal hairs, is what determines whether the brows appear sparse or dense [Fig. 33.1 (4)]. This proportion, hair color density, and growth pattern are determined by polygenetic inheritance patterns (5). Human hair and skin color are probably related to at least four different allelic gene loci (5, 6). The eyebrows are generally more pigmented than the scalp hair and retain this pigmentation longer (6).

In general, the brows take the form of an elongated comma and are separated by a smooth region, the *glabella*. At times, the brows united in the midline, which is a condition known as *synophrys*. The medial head of the brow is usually situated slightly below the orbital margin. The midportion parallels the margin, whereas the tail lies slightly above the margin (7).

"Ideal" aesthetic proportions have been developed, relating the position of the brow to its surrounding structures in both the male and the female (8, 9). The female brow follows a rounded curve, uniting medially with the dorsal radix-dome line of the nose (Fig. 33.2). The medial brow begins at a point directly above the ala of the nose, slightly below the orbital rim. From there, it arcs laterally to end at a point on a line drawn from the ala through the lateral canthus. In this ideal female brow, the highest point is directly above the lateral limbus. The male brow starts and ends at the same spot, but is not as arched; it more closely follows the orbital rim and meets the dorsal radix-dome line closer to a 90° angle.

The follicles of the brow have particular slants in various regions, with individual follicles within those regions lying roughly parallel to each other (10). Medially, the hairs are directed upward or upward and medially. In the body of the brow, they are directed laterally, and in the tail, laterally and slightly downward (4). Incisions made in the brow must recognize this follicle slant, otherwise adjacent follicles will be damaged by the scalpel (11).

The terminal hairs of the brow are crescent shaped, tapered, angular in cross section, and wider than terminal hairs elsewhere on the body (4). They average 1 cm in length (12) but in older males may reach 8–10 cm (4).

The skin of the eyebrow region shows interesting and functionally significant differences from the skin elsewhere

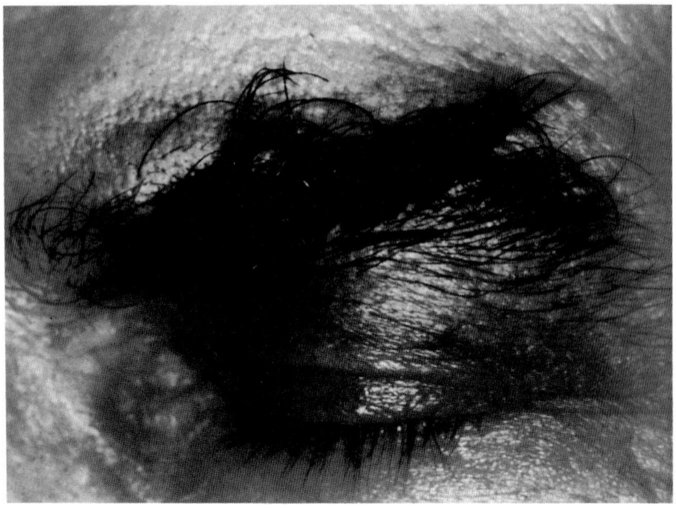

Figure 33.1. Large medullated terminal eyebrow hairs in an elderly male.

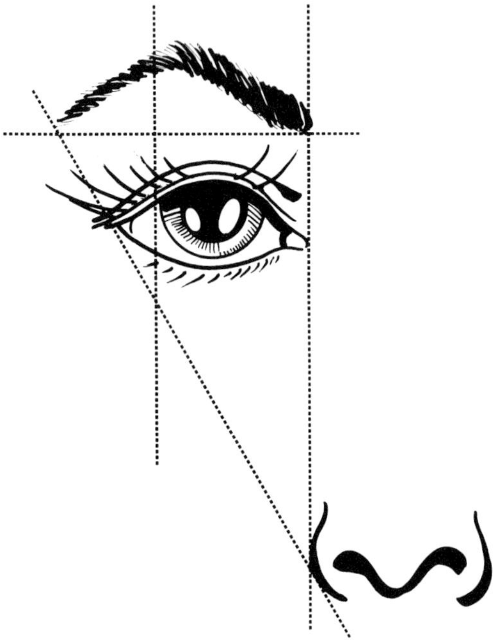

Figure 33.2. "Ideal" aesthetic proportions of female brow. (Adapted from Powell N, Humphreys B: *Proportions of the Aesthetic Face.* New York, Thieme-Stratton, 1984, pp 16–19.)

on the upper face. Numerous large sebaceous glands are present in the glabella and eyebrow region, while eccrine sweat glands are few or absent (4, 10). When injured by trauma or surgery, these sebaceous glands respond with hypertrophy and increased secretion (13, 14). Arrectores pilorum muscles are present surrounding follicles in the glabella, but are absent from follicles in the brow. A particularly rich vascular and nerve supply to the brow follicles is present (10).

The combination of numerous small vellus hairs, heavy sebaceous gland secretion, and minimal sweat production provide an excellent barrier to divert the flow of liquids down the face and away from the eyes (4).

SUBSURFACE TOPOGRAPHY

The skin of the eyebrow region and the accompanying cilia are firmly bound to the underlying muscular layer, making the eyebrow a functional unit of surface and subsurface anatomy (15).

Four muscles operate in this area. They are the frontalis, procerus, orbicularis oculi, and corrugator superciliaris. These are felt to originate from the infraorbital lamina of the premuscle mass of the second branchial arch and reach their definitive locations between weeks 11 and 15 (crown-to-rump length 37–80 mm) of development (16).

The frontalis muscle is the anterior portion of the epicranius, with the occipitalis as the posterior portion. They are connected over the dome of the calverium by the thick galea aponeurotica. The frontalis has no direct bony insertions but rather terminates in an interdigitation with the orbital portion of the orbicularis, which is firmly attached to the skin. The frontalis is supplied by the frontal branch of the facial nerve and functions to raise the brow and produce the horizontal furrows of the forehead.

The procerus is a small muscle that extends from the central portion of the frontalis and inserts on the base of the nasal bones near the lateral cartilages (7). Comparative anatomy studies indicate that this is not part of the frontalis but is derived from muscles that raise the lip (17). Accordingly, this is supplied by the superior buccal branch of the facial nerve (7). Its action draws the medial end of the brow down, creates horizontal creases in the glabella, and has been termed the "muscle of aggression" by Duchenne (18).

The orbital portion of the orbicularis oculi mingles with, but lies mainly superficial to, the frontalis (17). The most peripheral portion has been termed the "musculus superciliaris" by Merkel (19). The orbital portion is composed of fibers that are thicker and more red in color. It circles the orbit in horseshoe fashion, inserting on the bone of the medial orbital margin. It is supplied by the temporal and upper zygomatic branches of the facial nerve in the upper portion and the lower zygomatic branches in the lower portion (7). In forced lid closure, the orbital portion draws the skin of the forehead, cheek, and temple toward the medial canthus.

The corrugator superciliaris lies deep to the orbicularis and frontalis and is varyingly described as a "separate muscle" (7, 15) or a "specialized fasciculus of the orbicularis" (17). It is the last of the facial muscles to develop in the human (16, 20). Its origin is the medial end of the superciliary ridge, and it extends obliquely up and laterally for 2–3 cm to blend with the frontalis-orbicularis-skin complex (15). Its action is to draw the eyebrow toward the nose, thereby producing vertical glabellar furrows. In Wolff (7) this is called the "muscle of trouble," as it is used to express opposition to anything uncomfortable, as well as to shield the eyes from sun. Its nerve supply is the superior zygomatic branch of the facial nerve.

A complicated fascial network is the next element of the functional unit. At the origin of the frontalis, the galea splits to invest the muscle with a thin anterior sheath and a thicker, more defined posterior sheath (15). This deep galea further divides beneath the brow, investing the brow fat pad (11). The denser, posterior portion of the fat-pad capsule attaches tightly to the bone of the supraorbital ridge in the medial one-half to two-thirds of the brow. Laterally, a less tight attachment accounts for the earlier appearance of lateral brow ptosis (11). This posterior sheath of the fat pad is continuous with the orbital septum.

The anterior sheath of the fat pad continues on to become the "postorbicular fascia" (11, 21). The fat pad itself can extend into the lid in this layer as preseptal fat (11).

PHYSIOLOGY

This complex functional unit of skin and cilia, muscle and fat-fascial support provides a mobile brow that is capable of contributing an important component of facial expression and providing protection from sun and perspiration. Failure of the eyebrow to grow after shaving is mentioned anecdotally (22, 23), and discussion of the mechanism of eyebrow growth is in order. Human hairs from all regions have a growth phase (anagen) that is followed by a resting phase (telogen). During the resting phase, the lower portion of the follicle degenerates and the proximal tip of the hair acquires a keratin stump, becoming a "club hair" (24). Reactivation of the follicle by a new hair pushes this club hair out as its replacement reaches the surface. In the brow, two or more of these club hairs are often present and are anchored high in the follicle (1).

In the scalp, the growth phase lasts up to 3 years and is followed by a resting phase of 4 months (25). The brows have a shorter growth phase of 30–60 days, which is followed by a resting phase of 105 days (24, 25). Thus, if shaven, the majority of the hairs in the brow are resting and may take months to begin regeneration. The fact that most of the follicles are in the resting phase also explains why regeneration of hairs in the brow following plucking occurs much more rapidly than in the scalp, as these follicles are more susceptible to the stimulation of new hair formation than those in the active growth phase (26). In either case, the eyebrow hairs are among the slowest growing in the body, growing only 0.16 mm/day as opposed to the 0.35 mm/day seen in the scalp (26).

The abundant sensory innervation surrounding the terminal hairs of the brow may serve a function analogous to the vibrissae of nonhuman primates (1). Unexpected stimulation of the hairs will cause a reflex closing of the eye and turning of the head (4).

Under normal conditions, the frontalis and orbicularis exhibit reciprocal innervation, with the two not contracting at the same time (4). However, in hemifacial spasm, elevation of the brow will cause forced contraction of the orbicularis. This is most likely due to the antidromic passage of the nerve impulses back to the facial nerve trunk and ephaptic transmission to other branches (27). In extreme upgaze, contraction of the frontalis occurs synkinetically with contraction of the levator and superior rectus (4).

The frontalis can act as an accessory muscle of lid elevation by raising the lid 3–5 mm (4). It has been suggested that the headache sometimes present in refractive errors is due to the traction of the frontalis on the galea that occurs during prolonged squinting (4, 15).

RECONSTRUCTION TECHNIQUE

Pathological conditions affecting the eyebrows can be subdivided into disorders affecting texture, density, position, or color. Further subdivision is possible based upon whether the condition is congenital or acquired. Most of these disorders are covered elsewhere in this volume.

The most common malposition affecting the brow is ptosis, which is more pronounced in the lateral portion because of the laxity of the underlying fascial structures (11). Brow ptosis may also be seen following damage to the facial nerve, or more peripherally, its frontal branch. The treatment of brow ptosis is discussed elsewhere in this volume.

More complex or obscure alterations in the fascial system may also alter the position of the brow. Prior neurosurgical procedures may distort the galea to produce either retraction (Fig. 33.3) or ptosis (Fig. 33.4). Correction of such a malposition must take such possible distant causes into consideration. The relief of brow retraction from traction on the galea in the parietal area may involve scalp surgery, just as the relief of brow ptosis may be best handled with a coronal lift.

Distortion of the brows is a common result of lacerations in the area, unless meticulous care is given to the primary repair (Figs. 33.5–33.7). The repair may be complicated by loss of cilia, which are easily shaved from the skin by glass fragments in a windshield injury. Lacerations of the brow are commonly deep, with transection of the skin, orbicularis-frontalis complex, corrugator muscle, and the supraorbital neurovascular bundle. Repair should commence with the careful exploration of the wound to remove foreign material. Possible posterior injury to the globe itself must be ruled out.

First, the wound must be closed in layers, starting with the periosteum. Consideration may be given to a microsurgical perineural repair of the severed supraorbital nerve if one hopes to avoid permanent scalp anesthesia or a painful neuroma. Next, the muscular layer must be repaired; at this point particular attention should be given to the correct alignment of the corrugator to avoid asymmetry of facial expression postoperatively. The use of fine subcuticular absorbable sutures is of utmost importance to avoid skin contour irregularities. Debridement should be kept to a minimum to avoid damage to the surrounding hair follicles. Even grossly devitalized flaps can partially survive as grafts, particularly if intensive postrepair hyperbaric oxygen therapy (100% oxygen at 2 atmospheres twice

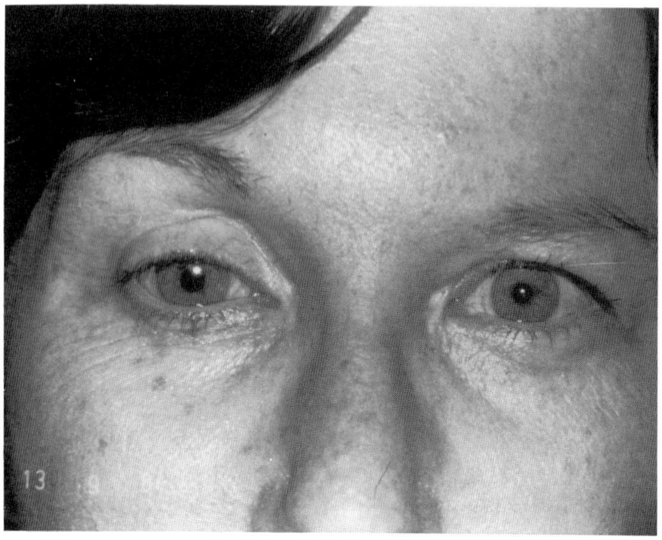

Figure 33.3. Retraction of right brow following craniotomy.

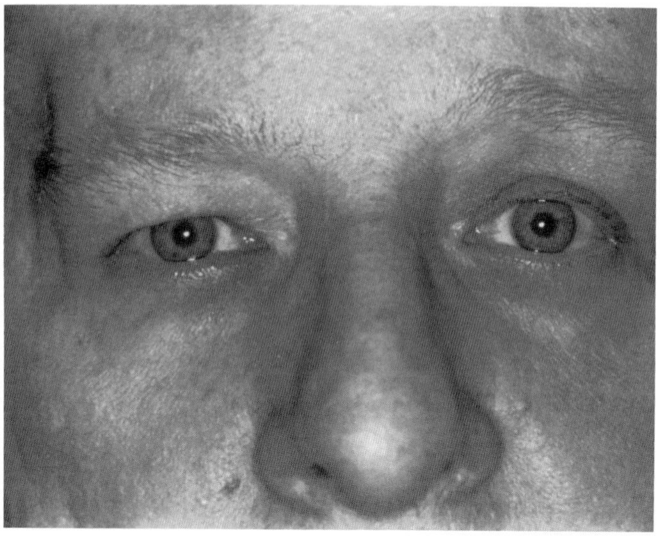

Figure 33.4. Ptosis of right brow following craniotomy.

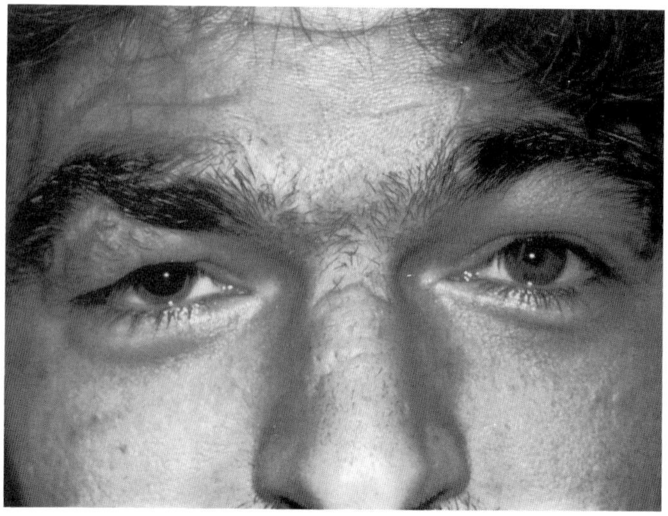

Figure 33.5. Distortion of right brow following repair of laceration.

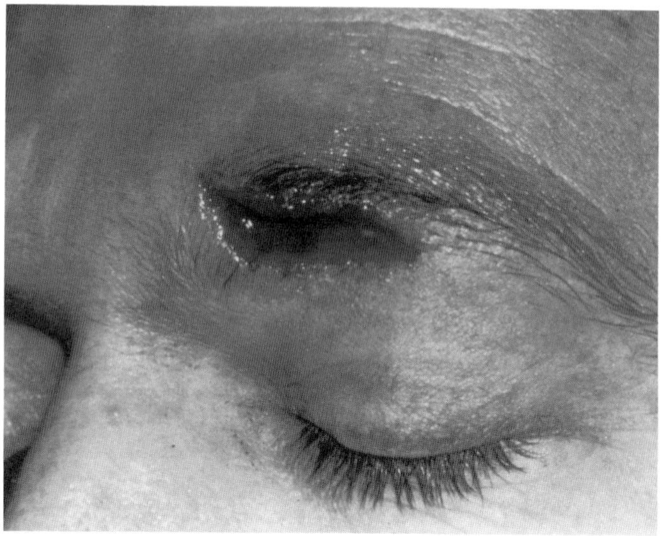

Figure 33.6. Laceration of brow, with transection of neurovascular bundle and corrugator muscle.

a day for 3 days) is available (Figs. 33.8–33.10). Repair of the subcuticular and cutaneous layers should first involve anatomically aligning the borders of the hair-bearing portion of the brow and then proceeding peripherally from there.

Either all or a significant part of the hair-bearing region of the eyebrow may be lost by trauma, surgical removal of neoplasms, thermal or ionizing radiation, or dermatologic disease. Satisfactory reconstruction of this region is limited by alterations in the host bed, such as the poor vascularity seen in burns, and by the lack of suitable physiologic donor material. As outlined under "Anatomy" and "Physiology," the hair of the eyebrow region is unlike the hair of any other region of the body. The only way to duplicate such hair is through the use of the same donor material: either from adjacent normal brow or from the contralateral brow. Both methods have significant limitations and disadvantages, however, and are not suitable in most cases.

Small defects of the brow, especially if they are located centrally and are smaller than 5–7 mm, may be satisfactorily reconstructed by the use of advancement flaps from adjacent normal brow. Judgement must be exercised and care taken not to injure the hair follicles that penetrate the dermis. Such a technique may produce acceptable results in a thick, lush brow but may cause severe foreshortening in a thin brow.

In larger central defects, the use of a free graft from the contralateral brow has been described (28). In defects of the medial third, a small flap based on the head of the opposite brow has also been described (29, 30). The use of both of these techniques carries the risk of damage and

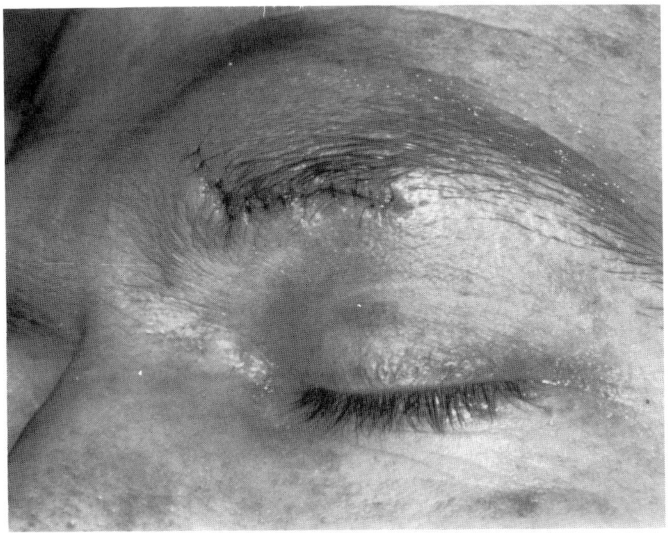

Figure 33.7. Same patient as in Figure 33.6, following meticulous repair.

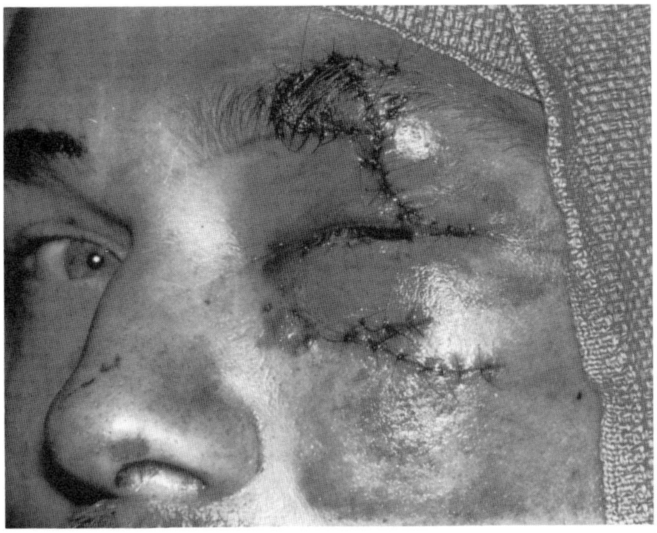

Figure 33.9. Impaired vascularity of brow flap, following repair of patient in Figure 33.8.

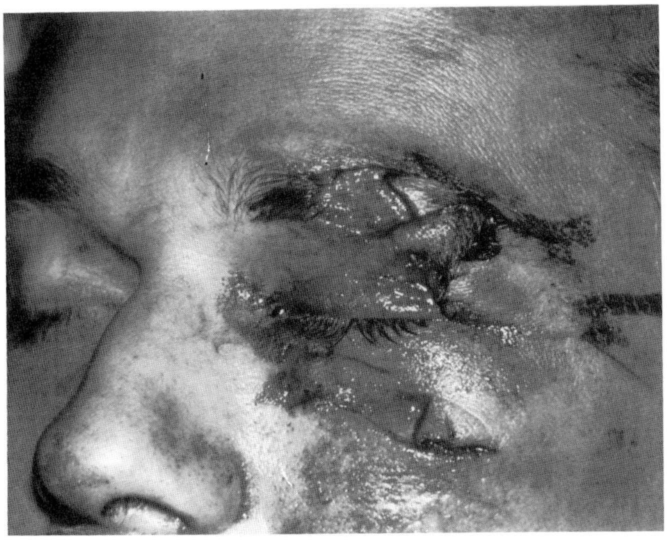

Figure 33.8. Severe laceration of brow following motorcycle accident.

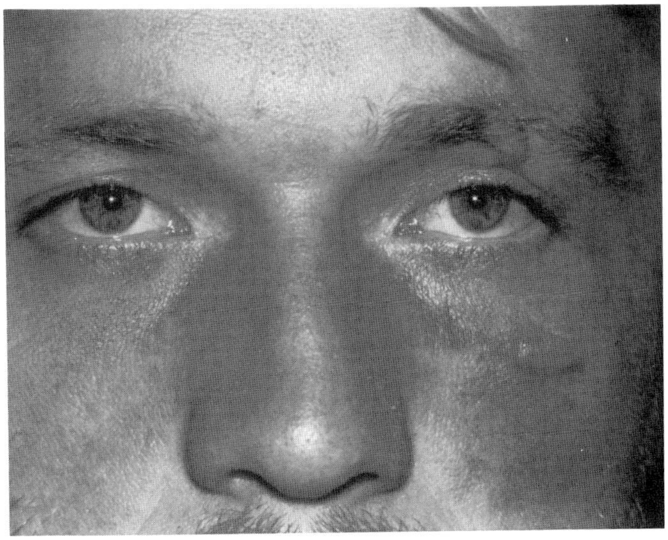

Figure 33.10. Final result of patient in Figure 33.8, following hyperbaric oxygen therapy for ischemic brow flap.

unsightly appearance to the donor brow, which must be considered by both the patient and the surgeon during preoperative planning.

An alternative for reconstruction of partial loss of the brow is the use of multiple, small punch grafts of scalp hair, transplanted in stages (31, 32). Techniques of classic hair transplantation are utilized (33, 34). The donor site is the parietooccipital portion of the scalp. The hair is clipped to about 2 mm to allow for accurate determination of direction of hair growth. Both donor and recipient sites are anesthetized with 2% lidocaine with 1:100,000 dilutions of epinephrine. A hand punch 2–4 mm in size is used to remove plugs from the recipient site. Care is taken to remove the plugs at an angle, so that the grafted hair will lie flat against the skin of the brow. The recipient sites are scattered sufficiently to allow for maximum revascularization. Plugs are then removed from the donor site at corresponding angles and carefully trimmed to prevent damage to the hair follicles. No sutures are used, but the grafts are held in place with a pressure dressing. Donor sites may be closed with sutures. The procedure is repeated after an interval of 2–3 months to allow for adequate revascularization.

Reconstruction of larger areas, or the entire brow, may be attempted with strip grafts taken from behind the ear [Figs. 33.11–33.14 (29, 35, 36)]. A pattern may be made from the contralateral eyebrow and reversed, or a freehand pattern may be constructed. Best results are obtained when the width of the graft is 4–6 mm. The graft is only minimally defatted to avoid damage to the hair follicles, and vascularization most likely occurs from the skin edges.

Brent (41) has described a technique in which medial accentuation of the brow is obtained by transplantation of an additional smaller strip at the medial portion of the

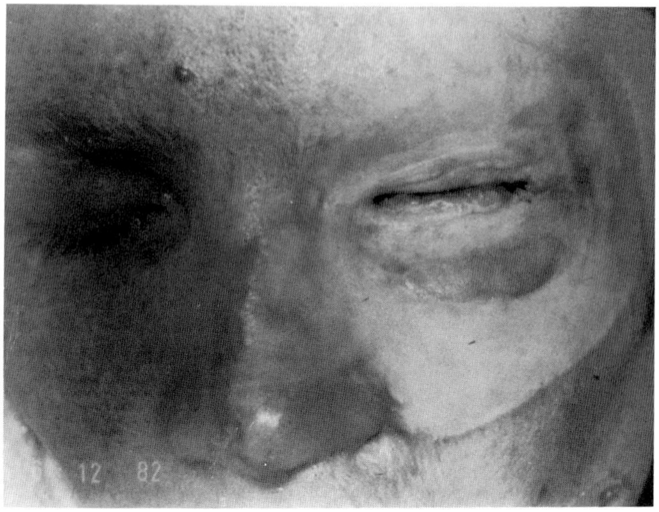

Figure 33.11. Destruction of left brow following third-degree thermal burn.

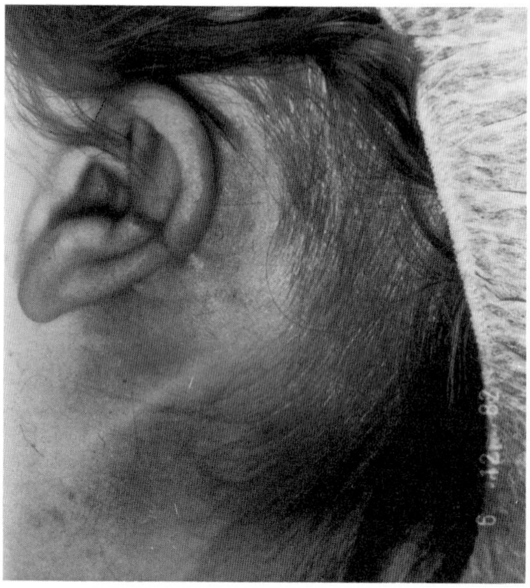

Figure 33.12. Donor site for reconstruction of brow with hair-bearing strip graft.

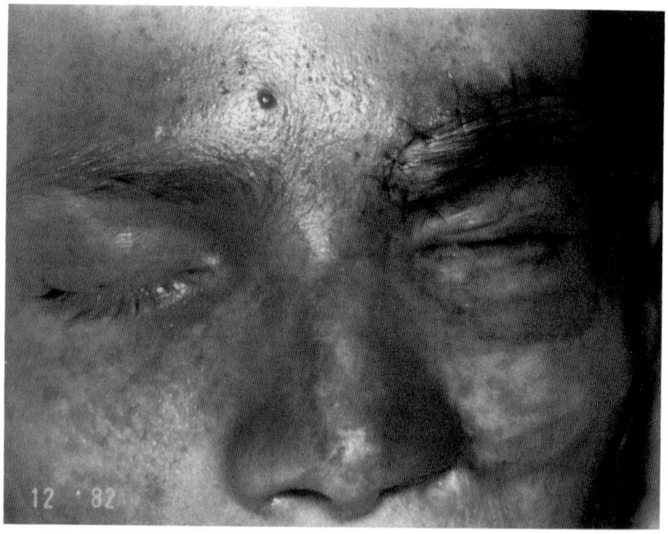

Figure 33.13. Graft sutured into position in patient in Figure 33.11.

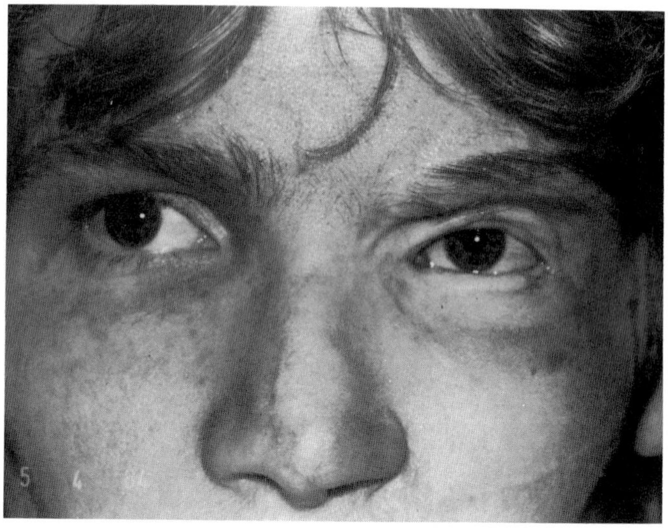

Figure 33.14. Final result of patient in Figure 33.11, following therapy with topical minoxidil.

brow, inferior to the main graft. It is separated from the main graft by an intervening strip of unoperated tissue, which is removed at a later procedure (35).

In instances of loss of the eyebrow secondary to thermal burns or in other situations in which the vascular bed is compromised, the most reliable method of eyebrow reconstruction is the island pedicle flap [Fig.33.15 (29, 37)]. However, such a technique must be used with caution in young males with a positive family history for male-pattern baldness. If the flap is taken from an area that will be involved later in life with such male-pattern baldness, loss of the reconstructed brow will occur.

The hair of the temporal area is trimmed to a length of 1 or 2 mm, and a pattern from the contralateral brow is made. The length of the vascular pedicle must be of sufficient length to allow for rotation and placement in its subcutaneous tunnel without kinking. The course of the artery is palpated and marked on the skin. The artery is then exposed through a preauricular skin incision. The artery is carefully followed distally until the desired length is attained. To avoid vascular embarrassment, the artery is left in a pedicle of soft tissue about 1 cm in width. The hair-bearing portion is then cut, and the flap is introduced through a subcutaneous tunnel into the donor site. This tunnel should be 1–1.5 cm wide to allow for atraumatic passage and to prevent compression. It must be made directly subcutaneous, to avoid injury to the frontal branch of the facial nerve, the path of which the flap will necessarily cross. The flap is sutured into position with multiple, fine skin sutures, and the donor site closed in two layers. The main postoperative problem is lack of venous return. Supportive measures such as elevation of

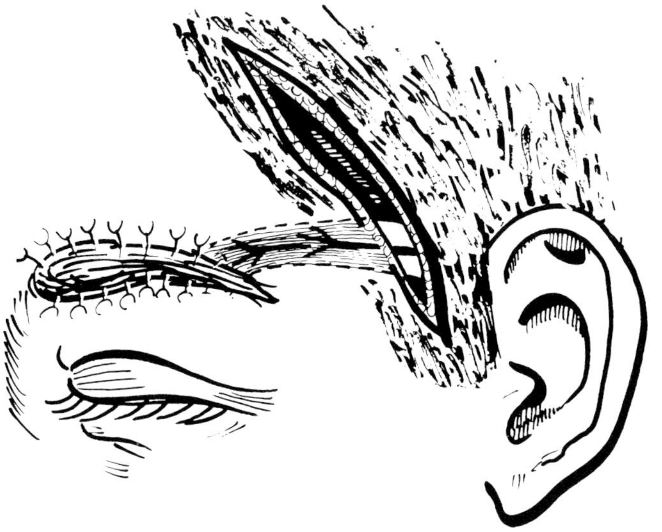

Figure 33.15. Brow reconstruction with island flap based upon the superficial temporal artery.

the head and "milking" of the flap during the first 36 hours should be employed.

The transplanted hair of grafts or flaps may be temporarily lost and will regrow after approximately 3 months (29, 32). Topical minoxidil therapy may be useful in reactivating the follicles (Fig. 33.15). This drug was initially introduced as a systemic antihypertensive but was found to cause hirsutism as a side effect. In topical form, it has been beneficial in treatment of alopecia of the scalp and brow (38) and probably acts either by altering cutaneous blood flow or the immune system (39). Finally, with all procedures that bring scalp hair to the brow, periodic trimming of the hair will be necessary.

REFERENCES

1. Szabo G: The regional frequency and distribution of hair follicles in human skin. In Montagna W, Ellis RA (eds): *The Biology of Hair Growth*. New York, Academic Press, 1958, pp 33–39.
2. Schultz AM: The density of hair in primates. *Hum Biol* 3: 303–321, 1931.
3. Records RE: Eyebrows and eyelids. In Duane TD, Jaeger EA (eds): *Biomedical Foundations of Ophthalmology*. Philadelphia, Harper & Row, 1983, vol 2, ch 1, pp 1–21.
4. Rook A: The skin and the eyes. In Rook A, Wilkinson DS, Ebling FJG (eds): *Textbook of Dermatology*, ed 3. Oxford, Blackwell Scientific Publications, 1979, pp 1923–1924.
5. Livingstone FB: Polygenic models for evolution of human skin color differences. *Hum Biol* 41: 480–493, 1969.
6. Spearman RIC: The genetics of hair growth and coloration. In Jarrett A (ed): *The Physiology and Pathophysiology of the Skin. The Hair Follicle*. New York, Academic Press, 1977, vol 4, pp 1457–1494.
7. Warwick R: *Eugene Wolff's Anatomy of the Eye and Orbit*, ed 7. Philadelphia, WB Saunders, 1976, pp 23, 202–204.
8. Powell N, Humphreys B: *Proportions of the Aesthetic Face*. New York, Thieme-Stratton, 1984, pp 16–19.
9. Ellenbogen R: Transcoronal eyebrow lift and concomitant upper blepharoplasty. *Plast Reconstr Surg* 71: 490–499, 1983.
10. Montagna W: Histology and cytochemistry of human skin. XXXIV: The eyebrows. *Arch Dermatol* 101: 257–263, 1970.
11. Lemke BN, Stasior OG: The anatomy of eyebrow ptosis. *Arch Ophthalmol* 100: 981–986, 1982.
12. Garn SM: Types and distribution of the hair in man. *Ann NY Acad Sci* 53: 498–507, 1951.
13. Hunt TK, Dunphy JE: *Fundamentals of Wound Management*. New York, Appleton-Century-Crofts, 1979, p 44.
14. Ordman LJ, Gilman T: Studies in healing of cutaneous wounds. I. Healing of incisions through the skin of pigs. *Arch Surg* 93: 857–882, 1966.
15. Doxanos MT, Anderson RL: *Clinical Orbital Anatomy*. Baltimore, Williams & Wilkins, 1984, pp 57–62.
16. Gasser RF: The development of the facial muscles in man. *Am J Anat* 120: 357–376, 1967.
17. Whitnall SE: *Anatomy of the Human Orbit and Accessory Organs of Vision*, (facsimile of 1921 ed). Huntington, NY, Krieger, 1979, p 111.
18. Duchenne GBA, cited by Warwick R: *Eugene Wolff's Anatomy of the Eye and Orbit*, ed 7. Philadelphia, WB Saunders, 1976, p 204.
19. Merkel F, cited by Whitnall SE: *Anatomy of the Human Orbit and Accessory Organs of Vision*, (facsimilie of 1921 ed). Huntington, NY, Krieger, 1979, p 132.
20. Futamura R: Ueber die Entwicklung der facialismuskulatur des Menschen. *Anat Hefte* 30: 433–516, 1906.
21. Anderson RL, Dixon RS: Aponeurotic ptosis surgery. *Arch Ophthalmol* 97: 1123–1131, 1979.
22. Krohel GB: Letter to the editor. *JAMA* 241: 2207, 1979.
23. Sebben JE: Letter to the editor. *JAMA* 243: 121, 1980.
24. Butcher ED: Development of the pilary system and the replacement of hair in mammals. *Ann NY Acad Sci* 53: 508–516, 1951.
25. Johnson E: Cycles and patterns of hair growth. In Jarett A (ed): *The Physiology and Pathophysiology of the Skin. The Hair Follicle*. New York, Academic Press, 1977, vol 4, pp 1237–1254.
26. Myers RJ, Hamilton JB: Regeneration and rate of growth of hairs in man. *Ann NY Acad Sci* 53: 562–568, 1951.
27. Nielsen VK: Pathophysiology of hemifacial spasm: I. Ephaptic transmission and ectopic excitation. *Neurology* 34: 418–426, 1984.
28. English FP, Forster TDC: The eyebrow graft. *Ophthal Surg* 10: 39–41, 1979.
29. Wang MKH, Macomber WB, Elliott RA: Deformities of the eyebrow. In Converse JM (ed): *Reconstructive Plastic Surgery*, ed 2. Philadelphia, Saunders, 1977, pp 956–961.
30. Mustarde JC: *Repair and Reconstruction in the Orbital Region*, ed 2. Edinburgh, Churchill Livingston, 1980, pp 204–214.
31. Nordstroem REA: Eyebrow reconstruction by punch hair transplantation. *Plast Reconstr Surg* 60: 74–76, 1977.
32. Lewis LA, Resnik SS: Strip and punch grafting for alopecia of the eyebrow. *J Dermatol Surg Oncol* 5: 557–559, 1979.
33. Nordstroem REA: Hair transplantation. *Scand J Plast Reconstr Surg Suppl* 14: 1–37, 1976.
34. Farber GA: The punch scalp graft. *Clin Plast Surg* 9: 207–220, 1982.
35. Brent B: Reconstruction of ear, eyebrow and sideburns in the burned patient. *Plast Reconstr Surg* 55: 312–317, 1975.
36. Sloan DF: Reconstruction of eyelid and eyebrows in burned patients. *Plast Reconstr Surg* 58: 340–346, 1976.
37. McConnell CM, Neale HW: Eyebrow reconstruction in the burn patient. *J Trauma* 17: 362–366, 1977.
38. Fenton DA, Wilkinson JD: Alopecia areata treated with topical minoxidil. *J Roy Soc Med* 75: 963–965, 1982.
39. Weiss VC, West DP, Fu TS, Robinson LA, Cook B, Cohen RL, Chambers DA: Alopecia areata treated with topical minoxidil. *Arch Dermatol* 120: 457–463, 1984.

CHAPTER 34

Trichiasis, Distichiasis, Madarosis, and Poliosis

JOHN NORRIS HARRINGTON, M.D., F.A.C.S.

TRICHIASIS AND DISTICHIASIS

Trichiasis has been defined as a single row of eyelashes growing in a misdirected fashion, and distichiasis, as a second row that grows along the posterior margin of the lid and replaces the sites of the meibomian glands. More accurately, trichiasis is defined as a misdirection of the eyelashes normally growing from the anterior lamella (Fig. 34.1). Normally, there are three or four rows of eyelashes (Fig. 34.2). Distichiasis is defined more precisely as an accessory row of abnormal lashes in the tarsal portion of the lid that occupies the site of the meibomian glands (1) (Fig. 34.3). Distichiasis is usually congenital and is characterized by abnormal lashes stemming from meibomian gland orifices. It also occurs in Stevens-Johnson Syndrome, ocular pemphigoid, and severe chemical injuries in which metaplasia of the meibomian glands gives rise to the production of aberrant lashes from their orifices.

In trichiasis, the lashes are of normal texture and consequently are irritating to the cornea. In distichiasis, the accessory lashes are often fine and lanuginous in infants and cause little if any irritation; they may become more coarse in older children and produce ocular irritation. In entropion, the lashes rub against the eye, but this is due to an abnormal position of the lid margin and not an abnormality of the lashes themselves, and consequently is dealt with in the chapter on entropion.

TRICHIASIS

Trichiasis may involve only a single eyelash or two, it may segmental, or involve an entire lid or lids. If the eyelashes touch the conjunctiva, the patient experiences a foreign-body sensation, the conjunctiva becomes irritated and inflamed, and epiphora may result. If, however, the lashes are in contact with the cornea, the patient experiences pain and epiphora, the corneal epithelium becomes abraded, and corneal irregularities, ulceration, vascularization, or scarring and opacification may result.

Trichiasis may occur as the result of various etiologies. It can follow any mechanical disruption of the eyelid margin, such as the improper approximation of a lid laceration (Fig. 34.4), an incision with secondary notching or irregularity, or simply from disruption of the hair follicles following injury or surgery of the lid margin, including shave biopsies. Trichiasis may be caused mechanically by a tumor distorting the lid margin. These all generally result in localized trichiasis.

Cicatricial changes as seen in pemphigoid or alkali burns may cause diffuse or localized trichiasis. Trichiasis may also occur in the vertical kinking of the lid, such as a manifestation of ulcerative colitis (2). Although usually acquired, trichiasis may be congenital, as in cases of epiblepharon in which the lashes are mechanically pressed toward the eye by the skin.

Although trichiasis would seem to be relatively simple to treat, this is not always so; satisfactory management requires proper evaluation and the correct approach, depending on the extent of the lid involved. The lashes at fault may, of course, be epilated if patience of the doctor and the patient permit. After epilation, a new lash will usually regrow within 6 weeks. Consequently, successful management by this approach requires countless treatments through the years to keep the patient comfortable.

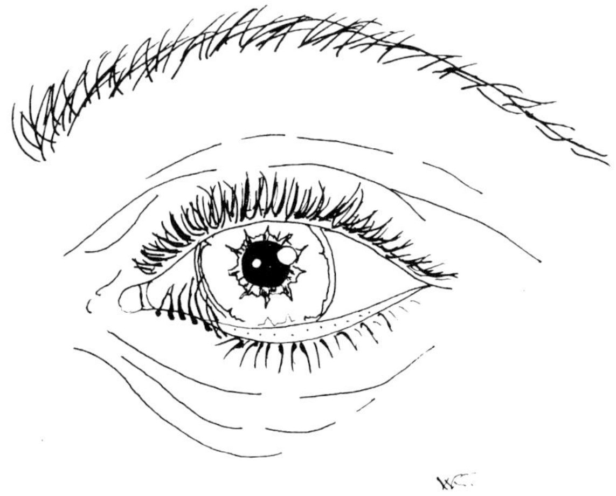

Figure 34.1. Trichiasis. Misdirected lashes growing from the normal lash line.

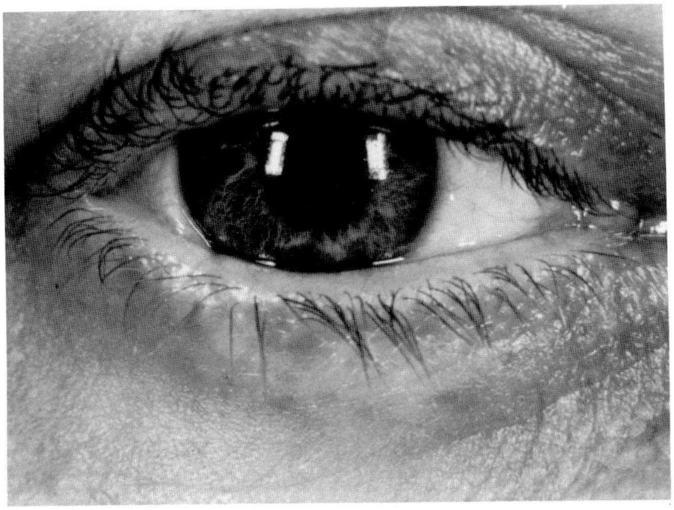

Figure 34.2. Normal lashes growing in rows.

Fluidless, hard scleral contact lenses have been recommended as a means of protecting the cornea from the constant abrasion caused by the inturned eyelashes in trichiasis (3). More commonly, soft contact lenses have been used (4). Others feel that soft contact lenses offer only partial protection because the lens does not cover all of the conjunctiva and as the eye moves, that part left uncovered is inflamed by the inwardly turned lashes. The resulting chemosis can change the fit of the contact lens (5).

Electrolysis may be used to destroy the lash root of an involved lash; however, as only one follicle may be treated at a time, this method is most useful for those cases in which only a few lashes are misaligned. Electrolysis units are available (Fig. 34.5), or a small wire may be attached to hyfrecator set on a very low power setting. As only a

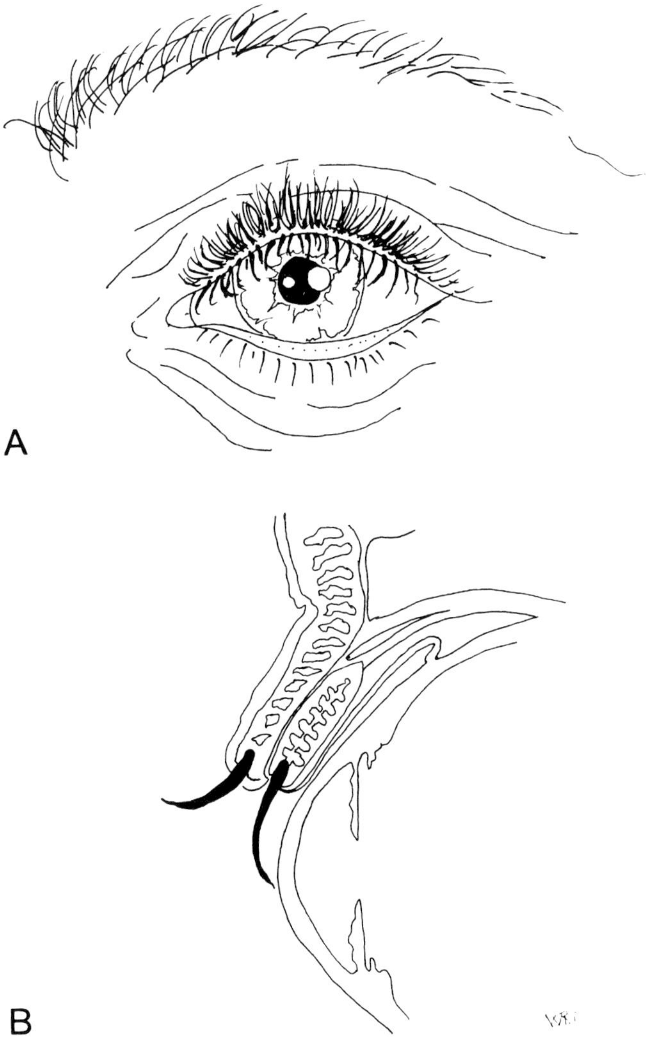

Figure 34.3. Distichiasis. Cilia growing abnormally from the site of the meibomian glands.

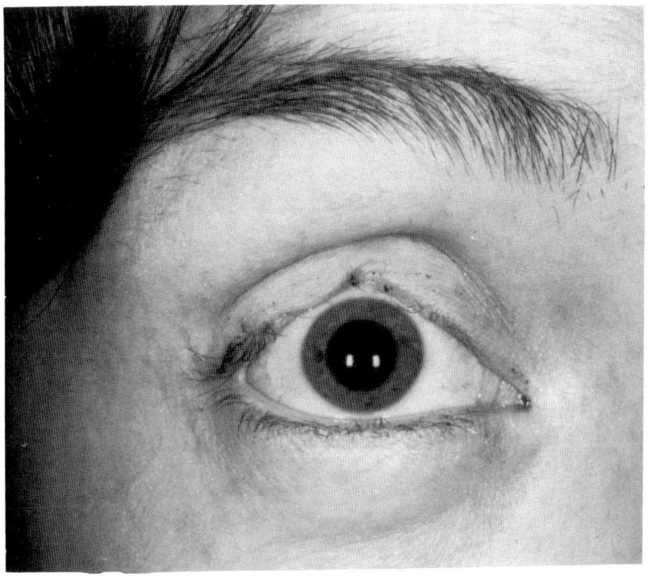

Figure 34.4. Trichiasis occurring on the upper lid due to improper closure of a vertical lid laceration.

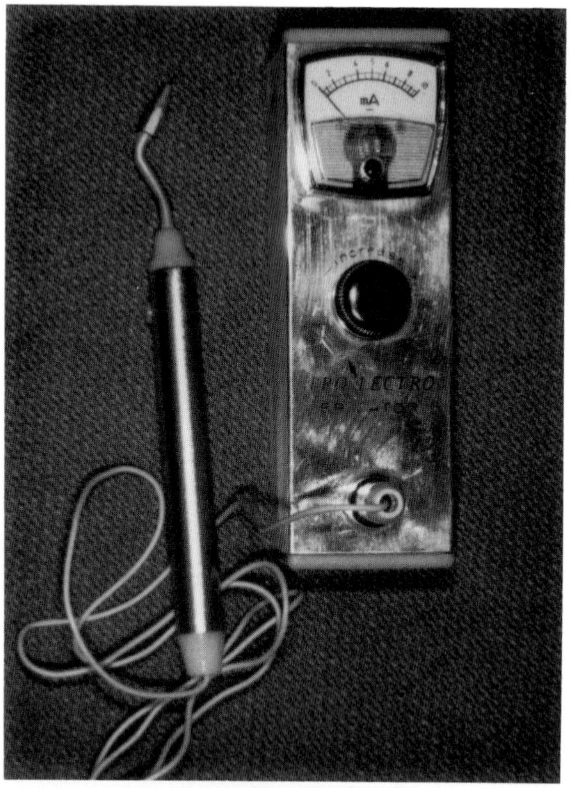

Figure 34.5. Example of a small electrolysis unit. The rectangular portion is held in the hand of the patient as the wire at the tip of the handle is inserted along the shaft of the hair and the current activated.

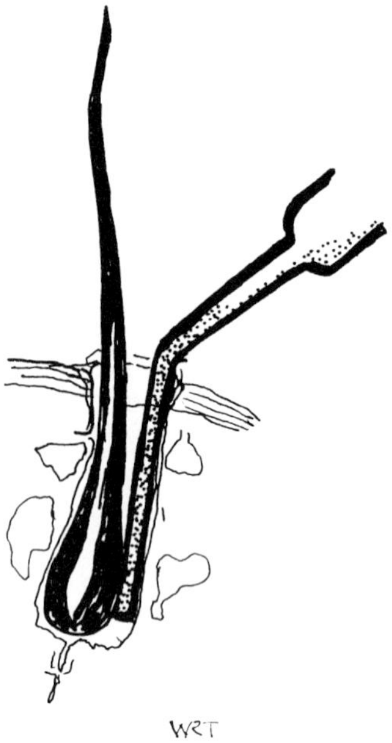

Figure 34.6. It is essential that the electrolysis wire be inserted adjacent to the cilium and to the estimated depth of the lash bulb.

few lashes are generally treated in this manner, it is usually done without anesthesia, although local anesthesia can be used. The current is applied with the wire tip inside the follicle along side the lash root until bubbles appear at the opening of the follicle (Fig. 34.6). The lash can be easily removed with forceps if the root has been killed. This technique has only a 30–50% success rate and may be repeated as needed, although multiple treatments or excess current may lead to scarring and deformity of the lid margin, which worsens the trichiasis.

If more than a few lashes are involved, a surgical approach is more practical and successful. When there is a localized area of inturned lashes, for example with scarring or notching after faulty repair of a lid laceration or incision, a full-thickness wedge resection of the area of the lid involved may be performed. However, when the trichiasis is not localized and involves a more extensive amount of the eyelid, wedge resection is not possible. In such cases, cryotherapy is the best form of treatment.

Cryotherapy is best performed under local anesthesia utilizing an anesthetic agent containing epinephrine, which facilitates the freezing with its vasoconstrictive action. It is essential to use a thermocouple to achieve adequate freezing without overtreating. During treatment, the area immediately adjacent to the application freezes first. From this area, the freeze expands in all directions and forms a hemispherical iceball within the tissue. The temperature within the iceball varies as the freezing progresses (6). Because of this variation in the temperature, the complications that can be encountered with overtreatment, and the inadequate results that can be obtained with undertreatment, it is essential to use a properly placed thermocouple. The thermocouple is placed in the lid at the level of the lash root.

Either a cryoprobe cooled by nitrous oxide gas or liquid nitrogen sprayed through a small nozzle, such as an 18-gauge intracath cut to about 1 inch in length, may be used. If the spray is used, the globe is protected with a bone plate and the surrounding normal skin is walled off with tape. The spray is directed from the tarsal aspect of the lid outward as the lid is held away from the globe. In either case a double freeze-thaw cycle is used by taking the follicle temperature to −20°C rapidly, then allowing a slow thaw, and then repeating the process. This temperature has been found to be the least cold temperature to be consistently effective (7). Cryotherapy has approximately a 90% success rate.

Freezing is not without its side effects. Cryotherapy may cause a complete loss of lashes or a loss of skin pigment, both of which can be cosmetically disfiguring; depigmentation is especially disfiguring in a dark-skinned patient. Cicatricial changes in the eyelids may be made worse, particularly in pemphigoid. Cryotherapy is likely to cause a slough if applied to previously placed grafts of skin or mucous membrane. Moderate to severe edema with bullae may occur following cryotherapy, thus creating a ready site for infection. Consequently, sterile techniques should be used and a broad-spectrum antibiotic ointment should be applied for several days after treatment. In addition, a slough of the lid, particularly the lid margin, may occur with excessive freezing. All these complications are usually prevented by the use of proper technique in application.

There is a great deal of variation in the reaction to cryotherapy by various lid structures. For example, the hair follicle is destroyed at −20°C, whereas −40 to −70°C must be reached to destroy other parts of the lid, such as the punctum, canaliculus, and tarsal plate. At temperatures less cold than −20°C, hair growth may actually be stimulated (8). In cases of pemphigoid or previous graft sites, cryotherapy should be done with caution and the temperature taken to only −10°C and repeated if necessary. Melanocytes in the skin are sensitive to temperatures lower than about −15°C; therefore the possibility of depigmentation must be considered when cryotreatment of a dark-skinned patient is contemplated.

The mechanics by which freezing destroys cells have been well documented (9, 10). Cell necrosis due to cryotherapy is the result of a complex reaction in which there is a change of tissue solute concentration, ice formation, and vascular stasis (11). These effects are enhanced by epinephrine-induced vasoconstriction (12). Survival of the cell is greatly reduced by a slow thaw, as this exposes the cell to the toxic effects of electrolyte imbalance and osmotic pressure changes for a longer period of time. Also, any intracellular ice crystals that may have formed will enlarge as a result of recrystallization during slow thawing, which further damages the cell (13). Therefore, rapid freezing and slow thawing without any effort to speed the thawing process give the best result.

Other techniques for the treatment of trichiasis have been used, for example, laser photocoagulation (14). However this is not in widespread use at this time.

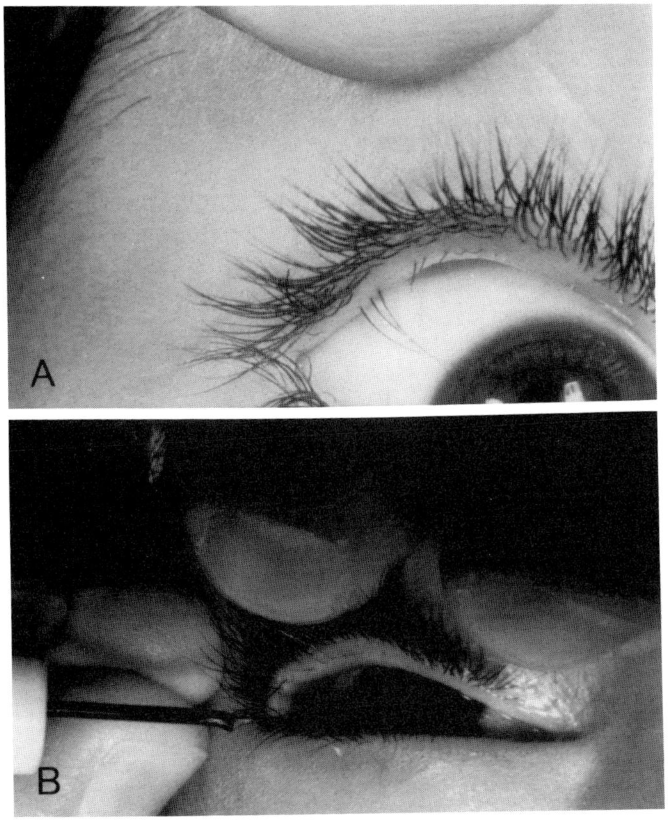

Figure 34.7. *A*, Distichiasis of the upper lid. Note the cilia growing from the meibomian gland orifices. *B*, An electrolysis wire is inserted at the site of the distichiatic lashes.

DISTICHIASIS

Epilation and electrolysis may be used in the treatment of distichiasis (Fig. 34.7), but distichiasis is generally not localized, and these techniques have a high recurrence rate. When distichiasis is localized it may be treated, like localized trichiasis, by full-thickness wedge resection of the lid and primary closure (Fig. 34.8). Distichiasis may also be treated with cryotherapy, particularly if just the lower lids are involved; it is not as satisfactory a method in the upper lids because cryoablation is not selective and will ablate normal lashes as well as the abnormal ones. This causes a problem with cosmesis, as well as with the increased exposure of the eye to dust and debris (15). Hence, when cryotherapy is used in the treatment of distichiasis, it is best combined with surgery. The lid is divided or split along the gray line and the cryoprobe is applied only to the posterior lamella of the lid, which contains the tarsal plate including the meibomian glands from which the lashes grow in distichiasis (16) (Fig. 34.9). This is best accomplished with a nitrous oxide cryoprobe rather than liquid nitrogen spray. Great care must be taken not to damage the normal lash roots in the anterior lamella

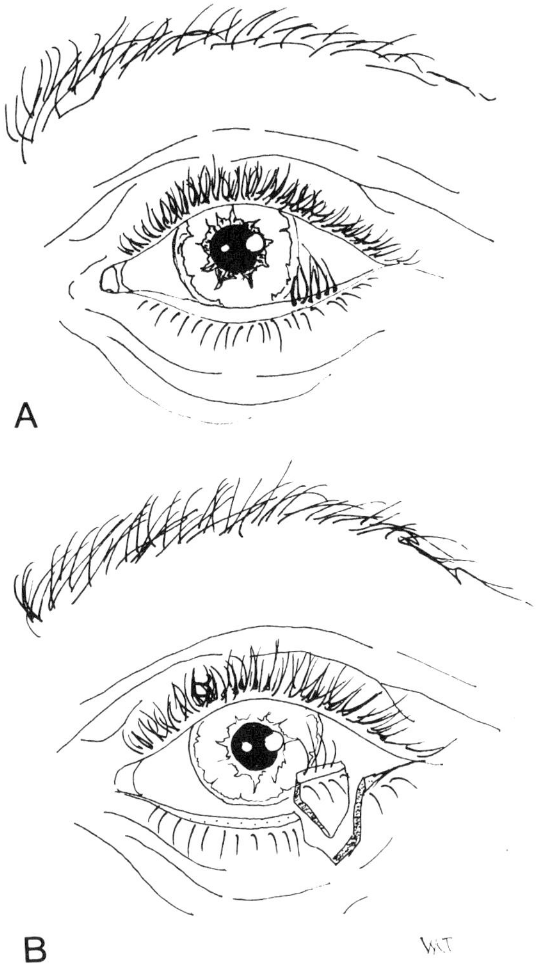

Figure 34.8. *A*, Although distichiasis is usually more generalized, it may occur in a localized manner. *B*, When distichiasis is localized, it can be excised by full-thickness wedge resection and the defect closed primarily.

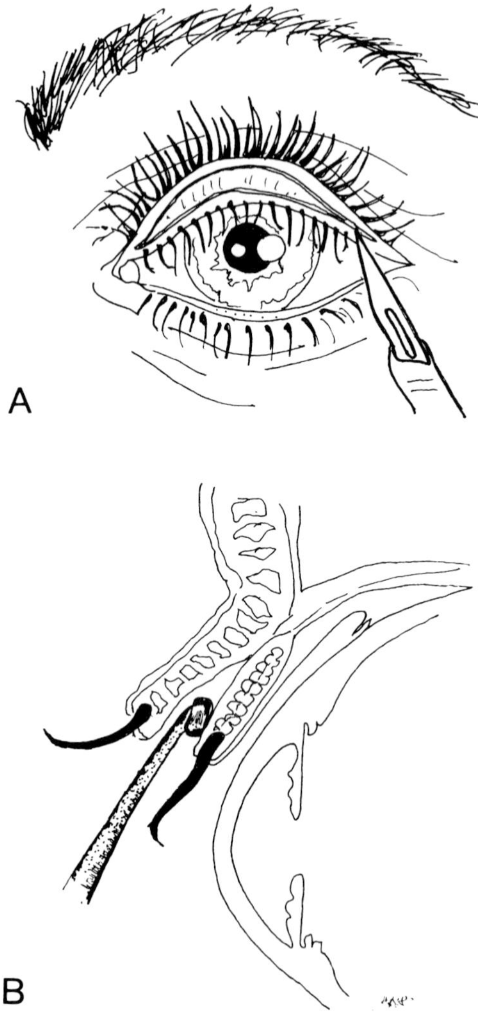

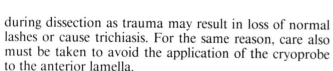

Figure 34.9. *A*, The lid is divided along the gray line. *B*, Cryopexy is applied only to the posterior lamella of the lid to protect and preserve the normal lashes in the anterior lamella.

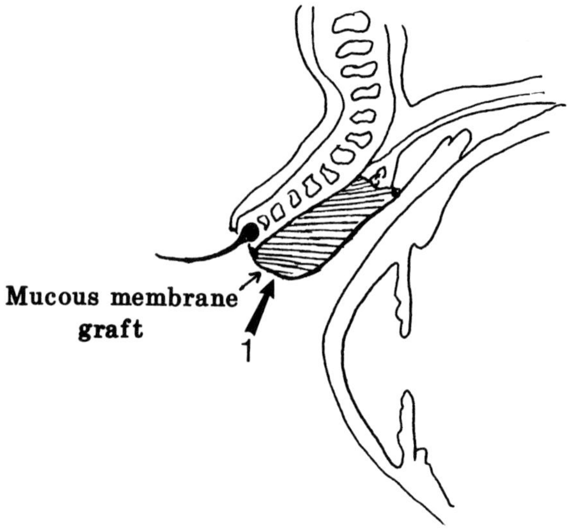

Figure 34.10. The posterior lamella containing the distichiasis metaplastic meibomian glands is excised and replaced with a full-thickness mucous membrane graft (*1*).

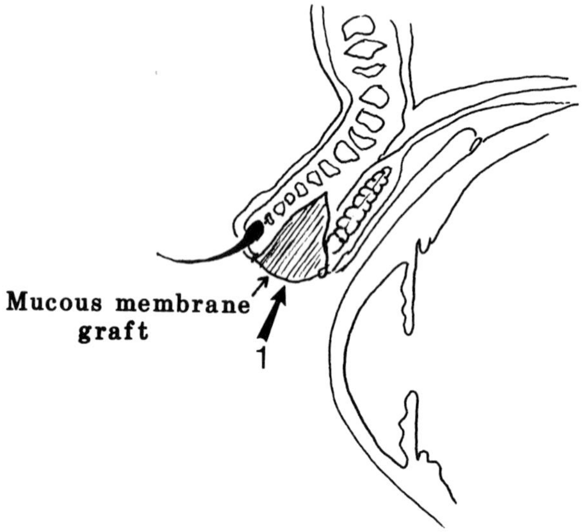

Figure 34.11. A wedge-shaped portion of the lid including the distichiasis is excised from the margin of the lid and replaced with a full-thickness mucous membrane graft (*1*).

during dissection as trauma may result in loss of normal lashes or cause trichiasis. For the same reason, care also must be taken to avoid the application of the cryoprobe to the anterior lamella.

The technique of treatment most often used involves splitting the lid as described above, then excising the posterior lamella, including the abnormal lashes and the metaplastic meibomian glands, and then replacing the excised area with full-thickness mucous membrane grafts (Fig. 34.10). An alternative is to excise a wedge-shaped portion of the lid from along the lid margin, so that the resulting defect is on the lid margin rather than posterior to the margin, and to place a graft of buccal mucosa within the resulting groove (Fig. 34.11). Either technique is a tedious surgery and is best done with the operating microscope, as all offending lashes must be completely excised and the suturing of the graft with a small-caliber suture requires adequate visualization. This technique often leaves the patient with irregular lid margins, trichiasis, and entropion, even though the patient is quite often satisfied with the resulting cosmetic defect in light of the increased comfort that the surgery has provided.

In an effort to prevent the distortion of the lid margin, a technique that avoids an incision or graft at or near the lid margin has been described. An incision is made 2 mm from the lid margin on the tarsoconjunctival aspect of the lid and a partial-thickness flap of tarsus and conjunctiva

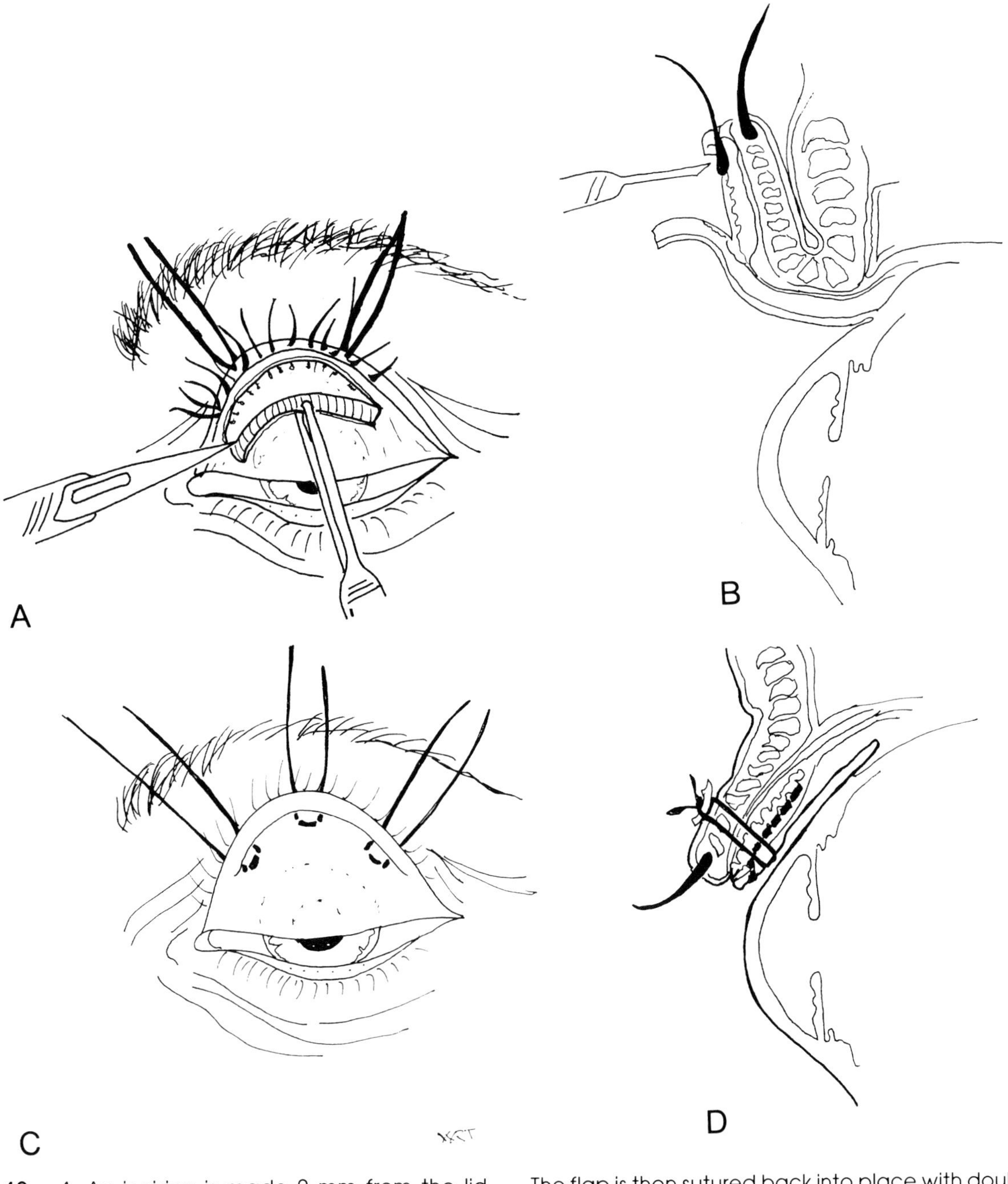

Figure 34.12. *A*, An incision is made 2 mm from the lid margin on the posterior surface of the lid through conjunctiva and partial thickness of the tarsus. *B*, Through the resulting flap that is created, the aberrant lashes and associated metaplastic meibomian gland are excised. *C*, The flap is then sutured back into place with double-armed 6-0 plain gut sutures that are buried on the anterior surface of the flap. *D*, Sutures then are tied over small stents on the anterior aspect of the lid.

is undermined. A flap is thus created, through which the metaplastic meibomian glands, along with the aberrant lashes, can be excised and the flap sutured back into place (17) (Fig. 34.12). As the lid margin is not incised or violated, the chance of lid margin deformity, trichiasis, and entropion are greatly reduced. The flap is sutured back into position with 6-0 or 7-0 nylon sutures, which are passed through the anterior lamella of the lid. The

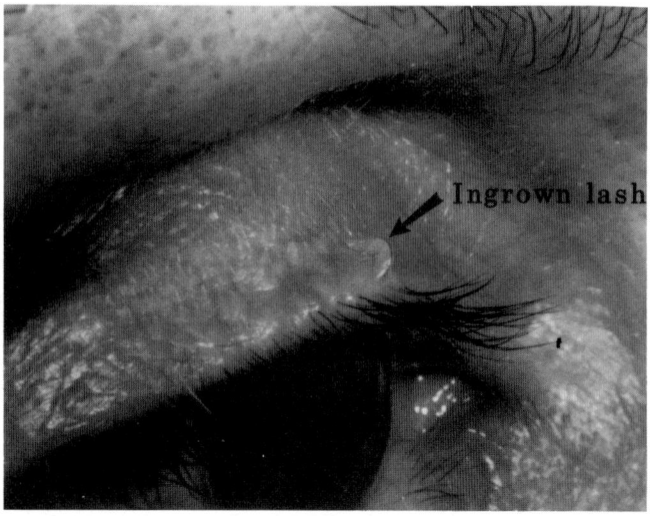

Figure 34.13. An ingrown lash, growing from a normal lash follicle but remaining underneath the skin surface, creating a small cyst-like defect (*arrow*).

suture is then placed through partial thickness of the tarsal flap so that no suture is exposed to the cornea and bulbar conjunctiva, and then the suture is returned through the anterior lamella to exit through the skin, where it is tied and left for about 5 days prior to removal. This also requires the use of an operating microscope.

There are two other types of ciliary malposition that deserve mention here. One is the "ingrown" hair, which is a single cilium that grows from a normal hair follicle generally in a normal direction but whose shank remains under the skin as the hair leaves the follicle. This causes a small cyst-like growth to appear on the lid (Fig. 34.13). It can be relieved by simply uncovering the lash with a needle or knife tip to allow the lash to return to a normal position; this malposition usually does not recur.

The other type of ciliary malposition is one in which fine hairs originating from a skin graft grow in the wrong direction: toward the eye instead of away from it. This can be avoided by keeping in mind the direction of normal hair growth when placing grafts. If it does occur, however, the hairs tend to be so fine that they cause no problems. Should there be a problem, however, careful cryotherapy is the best management. As has been previously stated, in freezing grafts, it is best to undertreat and later re-treat if necessary, rather than to overtreat and cause a slough of the graft.

MADAROSIS

Madarosis is the absence or loss of eyelashes from the lid, which may occur as the result of several etiologies. It may be secondary to inflammation and infection of the lids as seen in seborrheic blepharitis or staphylococcal blepharitis; in such cases, madarosis may often be treated by controlling the inflammation or infection with lid soaks

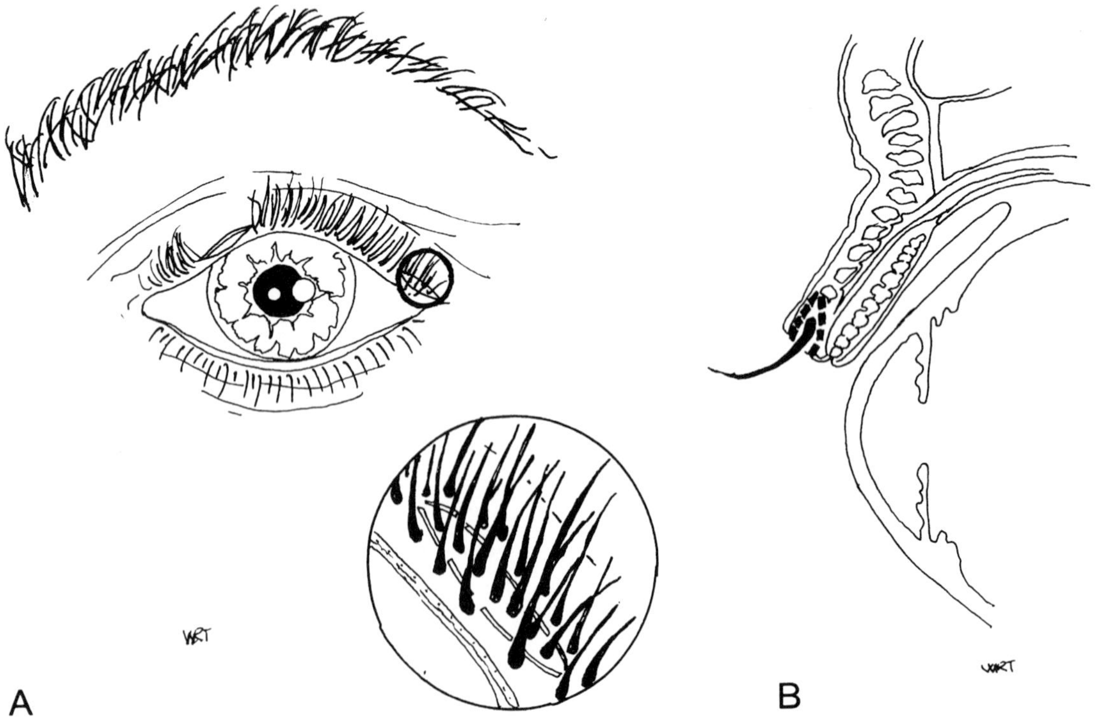

Figure 34.14. *A*, A 4-mm segment of lid containing one row of normal lash follicles is excised from the lateral aspect of the lid where the lashes are the most numerous. The segment of the lid containing the donor lashes is inserted into an incision at the recipient site and sutured in place with 9-0 monofilament nylon. *B*, Individual follicles may be transplanted in a similar manner if desired in a "post hole" area created at the recipient site with an 18- or 19-gauge needle.

and scrubs, along with appropriate topical antibiotic and antiinflammatory medication. It is easiest to give the patient a sheet of instructions detailing how to use compresses of cotton and warm water twice daily, which are followed with scrubs of the lid margin with baby shampoo on applicators and ultimately by the application of a sulfasteroid-combination drop. Other infectious or inflammatory causes of madarosis include herpes zoster, vaccinia, and mycotic infections. Madarosis may be associated with some chronic skin diseases such as psoriasis, acne, neurodermatitis, lichen planus, exfoliative dermatitis, ichthyosis, lupus erythematosus, and alopecia areata.

Madarosis can also result from scarring secondary to trauma or surgery such as tumor excision, although this tends to be more localized. Radiation, prolonged use of topical epinephrine, and intoxication with vitamin A, gold, arsenic, barbiturates, propylthiouracil, and quinine may also cause madarosis. Endocrine disorders such as hypothyroidism and pituitary insufficiency, as well as tuberculosis, syphillis, sickle cell anemia, and other debilitating systemic diseases may cause the loss of lashes. Madarosis may also be seen with uveitis, as in Vogt-Koyanagi-Harada disease.

The loss of lashes is not only a cosmetic defect but also removes one of the mechanisms for keeping dust, debris, and perspiration out of the eye. If only a small localized area of the lid is involved, the area may be excised by a full-thickness pentagonal wedge resection and the remaining lash-bearing portions of the lid anastomosed. Lash grafts may be performed; however, this often results in the transplanted lashes, if the graft takes, growing at bizarre angles and causing trichiasis. Of the techniques for lash grafting, the author's opinion is that the best technique is to transfer a few cilia from areas of dense lashes such as the lateral aspect of the lids (Fig. 34.14) as described by Naugle (18).

Under local anesthesia, an approximately 4-mm segment of lid that includes the lash follicles is excised from the lateral aspect of the lid under the operating microscope with a No. 75 Beaver blade and small scissors. It is essential not to damage the follicle. A similar incision is made at the recipient site, and the donor plug is inserted into the recipient site and sutured with 9-0 monofilament nylon. If desired, individual follicles may be transplanted by "post holing" a small site between the tarsus and skin of the lid at the recipient site with an 18- or 19-gauge needle. The needle is then retracted so the bevel is exposed; the cilium then is inserted with jewelers forceps. The needle is removed, leaving the graft in place. The patient is placed on a broad-spectrum antibiotic drop and seen frequently over the next several weeks to help readjust the direction of growth of the cilia.

Hair grafted from other areas such as the brow or hairline do not do as well as lash grafts because of their difference in length and quality as well as their direction of growth. Many times the use of artificial eyelashes is the best solution, particularly on the upper lid in a female.

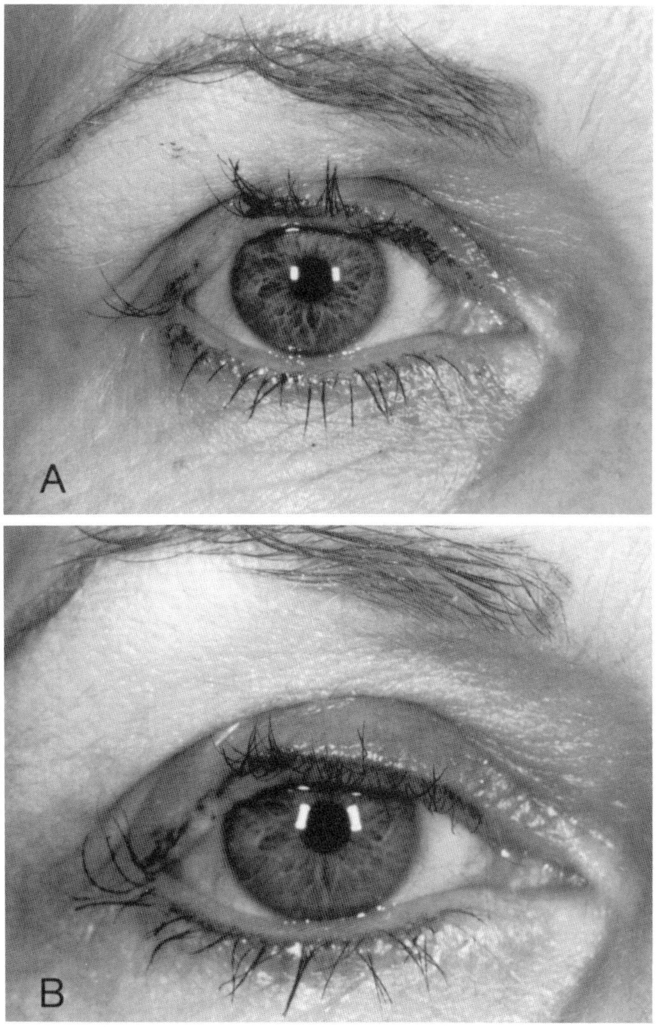

Figure 34.15. *A*, An area of absence of lashes on the upper lid as the result of scarring after excision of a lid lesion. *B*, The same area following the application of subepithelial pigment implantation. In this case the pigment was applied in a series of dots to simulate lashes.

Another cosmetic help may be the application of tattooed pigment along the line of the lashes as is done with the placement of permanent lash enhancer (19) (Fig. 34.15). In this procedure, pigment is placed in the outer dermis with a tattoo needle, and it can be applied as either a solid line of pigment or as linear dots.

POLIOSIS

Eyelashes may lack pigment. This may be congenital, which is termed *leukotrichia*, or acquired. The term *canities* refers to generalized decolorization, whereas the term *poliosis* refers to localized loss or absence of color. Senile canities is the most common form of acquired decoloration of the lashes and brows; it is the manifestation of the normal maturation process in which the hair, typically beginning at the temples, turns gray or white with age. It may progress to involve all the body hair, including the brows and lashes. This decoloration may be masked with dyes and cosmetics, or simply accepted as one of the side effects of birthdays, heredity, worry, or wisdom. In fact, it is due to a progressive deficiency of tyrosinase activity in the melanocytes of the hair bulb.

Poliosis, or localized decoloration of the lashes, is more of a cosmetic defect because of its contrast to the adjacent normal lashes. Poliosis may be seen with vitiligo or with areas of depigmentation of the skin of the lids; Vogt-Koyanagi-Harada syndrome, in which the poliosis is associated with uveitis, vitiligo, retinal detachment and dysacousia; Waardenburg's syndrome, where it is associated with albinism, deafness, hypertelorism, heterochromia iridis, and white forelock; Werner's syndrome (20); lepromatous leprosy; and following the use of certain drugs such as systemic chloroquine or topical thiotepa. Duke-Elder (21) also reports such rare causes as migraine, cataract extraction, hysteria, trachoma, poliosis neurotica, and injury. Albinism, although usually generalized, does affect the eyelids and lashes.

The best treatment of poliosis may be with cosmetics. If only a few lashes are involved, they may be removed by epilation, electrolysis, or wedge resection of the lid as previously discussed under "Trichiasis."

REFERENCES

1. Anderson R: Letter to the editor. *Arch Ophthalmol* 95: 1977.
2. Wright P: Conjunctival changes associated with inflammatory disease of the bowel. *Trans Ophthalmol Soc UK* 100: 96–97, 1980.
3. Cogger T: *Clinical Ophthalmology.* Philadelphia, Harper & Row, 1982, vol 1, Chap 54, p 4.
4. Black C: The Bausch and Lomb soflens. In Gossett A, Kaufman H (eds): *Soft Contact Lens: Proceedings, Symposium, and Workshop of the University of Florida Gainesville.* St. Louis, Mosby, 1972, p 224.
5. Rosen J, Brown S: Other uses of soft contact lenses. In Duane T, Jaeffe E (eds): *Clinical Ophthalmology.* Philadelphia, Harper & Row, 1982, vol 1, Chap 56, p 2.
6. Taylor A: Survival of rat skin and changes in hair pigmentation following freezing. *J Exp Zool* 110: 77, 1949.
7. Sullivan J, Beard C: Cryosurgery for the treatment of trichiasis. *Am J Ophthalmol* 82: 117–121, 1976.
8. Wilkes D, Frawnfelder F: Principles of cryosurgery. *Ophthal Surg* 10: 21–30, 1978.
9. Farrant J: Cryobiology. The basis for cryosurgery. In von Laden H, Cohan W (eds): *Cryogenesis in Surgery.* Flushing, Medical Examination Publishing, 1971, p 15.
10. Karow A, Webb W: Tissue freezing. A theory for injury and survival. *Cryobiology* 2: 99, 1965.
11. Sullivan J, Beard C, Bullock J: Cryosurgery for treatment of trichiasis. *Trans Am Opthalmol Soc* 64: 189–202, 1976.
12. Zacarrion S: *Cryosurgery of Tumors of the Skin and Oral Cavity.* Springfield, IL, Charles C Thomas, 1973, p 16.
13. Collier J, Coster D, Sullivan J: Cryosurgery for trichiasis. *Trans Ophthalmol Soc UK* 98: 81–83, 1978.
14. Berry J: Recurrent trichiasis: Treatment with laser photocoagulation. *Ophthal Surg* 10: 36–38, 1979.
15. Faulk B: Treatment of distichiasis with cryotherapy. *Ophthal Surg* 12: 100–102, 1981.
16. Anderson R, Harvey J: Lid splitting and posterior lamellar cryosurgery for congenital and acquired distichiasis. *Arch Ophthalmol* 99: 631–634, 1981.
17. Dortzbach R, Butera R: Excision of distichiasis eyelashes through a tarsoconjunctival trap door. *Arch Ophthalmol* 96: 111–112, 1978.
18. Naugle T: Eyelash loss corrected by ciliary transplantation. *Ophthalm Times* Feb: 51–53, 1982.
19. Angres G: Angres permalid liner method: a new surgical procedure. *Ann Ophthalmol* 16: 145–148, 1904.
20. Bullock J, Howard R: Werner's syndrome. *Arch Ophthalmol* 90: 53–56, 1973.
21. Duke-Elder S: Diseases of the Eyelids. *System of Ophthalmology.* St. Louis, CV Mosby, 1974, vol 12, Chap 2, p 390.

SECTION VI

ACQUIRED EYELID MALPOSITIONS

CHAPTER 35

Entropion

J. EARL RATHBUN, M.D.

Entropion is the turning in of the eyelid margin against the globe. It may be subclassified as congenital, including epiblepharon, involutional (senile), or cicatricial. The pathophysiology of each is different as is the approach to treatment. The most successful procedures for the correction of each type of entropion are directed at the specific anatomic defects present. A thorough knowledge of eyelid anatomy and the physiologic role of each tissue is essential to the successful correction of entropion.

CONGENITAL ENTROPION (INCLUDING EPIBLEPHARON)

Congenital entropion is an extremely rare condition. It is differentiated from the more commonly occurring epiblepharon by the fact that the entire tarsus and lid margin invert, causing the skin and lashes to abrade the eye; in epiblepharon the tarsus remains in a normal position and the lashes and skin roll over the tarsal edge to come in contact with the eye. Since congenital entropion is so rare, descriptions of the entity are scarce and varied. Fox (1) felt the commonest cause was hypertrophy of the marginal fibers of the orbicularis muscle and advised excision of skin and muscle to evert the lid to normal position. With our current knowledge of the role of the lower eyelid retractors in entropion it appears that disinsertion of the retractors may be an etiological cause, which allows the tarsus to rotate inwards. Thus surgical exploration of the retractors and repair as will be described for involutional entropion would be a logical approach. A more severe form of congenital entropion involving the upper eyelid is characterized by a horizontal tarsal kink in the midportion of the tarsus. This is seen in the newborn and is frequently associated with corneal ulceration. Treatment has included excision of the angulated portion of tarsus and reapposition of the tarsal edges (2), tarsal splitting (3), and lamellar tarsoplasty that involved reversal and replacement of the resected tarsus to equalize vector forces (4).

Epiblepharon is the in-rolling of the eyelid margin and lashes, which involves the nasal one-third or one-half of the lower eyelid (Fig. 35.1). It usually occurs bilaterally. The tarsus remains in a normal position with the pretarsal orbicularis muscle and skin over the superior tarsal edge. The contact of the lashes with the globe may result in tearing, conjunctivitis, or keratitis. The keratitis is usually punctate in nature and is often asymptomatic. Epiblepharon is seen most commonly in Oriental or Indian races during infancy and early childhood. Many cases correct themselves as the full cheeks of childhood decrease and the eyelid skin becomes relatively tighter, which pulls the lashes into a normal position. Asymptomatic cases may be observed without surgical correction if corneal scarring is not developing.

The anatomic defect in epiblepharon is the absence of the adhesion between the lower eyelid retractors and the anterior lamella (orbicularis muscle and skin), which allows the anterior lamella to roll inward. The eyelid crease, which results from this adhesion, particularly in downgaze, is poorly formed or absent. The object of surgical treatment, if it becomes necessary, is to form an adhesion between the anterior lamella of the eyelid and the lower eyelid retractors. This may be accomplished by placing full-thickness eyelid sutures or excising a strip of skin and orbicularis muscle and closing the defect by direct attachment to the tarsus or lower eyelid retractors.

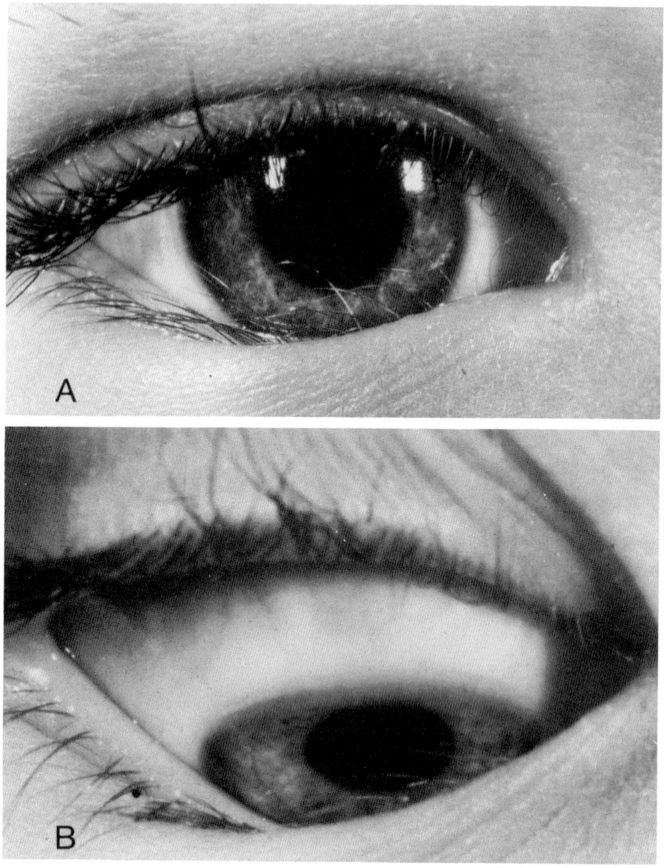

Figure 35.1. *A*, Epiblepharon in primary gaze. *B*, In downgaze.

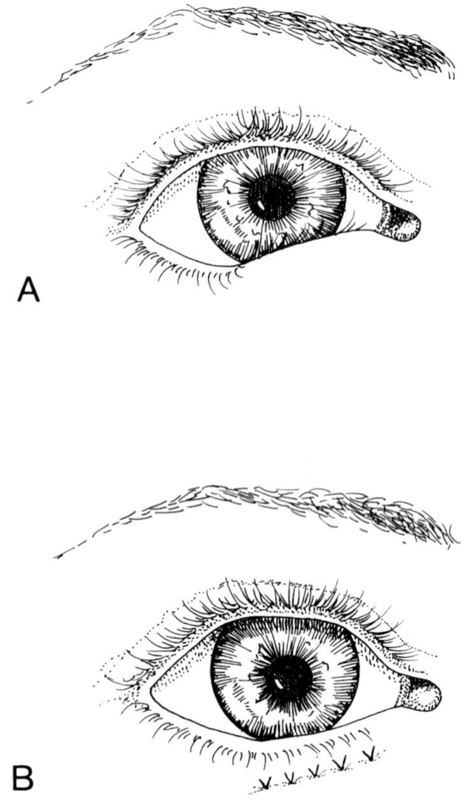

Figure 35.2. *A*, Epiblepharon preoperatively. *B*, Immediately following full-thickness eyelid suture placement.

SUTURE CORRECTION OF EPIBLEPHARON

This procedure (Fig. 35.2) is done under general anesthesia in young children but local anesthesia may be used in older children and adults. After skin preparation the line for suture placement is marked bilaterally with a marking pen. This is to assure symmetry of suture placement, which will result in postoperative symmetry of the newly created lower eyelid creases. This line usually starts 2–3 mm inferior to the punctum and extends slightly inferiorly as it is drawn laterally to the junction of the middle and lateral thirds of the eyelid. If local anesthesia is used, subcutaneous and subconjunctival injections are then made. Three to five sutures are equally spaced along the previously drawn line. One needle of a double-armed 5-0 or 6-0 chromic gut suture is passed just inferior to the inferior tarsal border on the conjunctival side and is brought out through the skin in the previously drawn line. The skin should be pulled inferiorly with light traction as the needle penetrates the orbicularis muscle and skin so that the lashes and eyelid margin are pulled into a normal or slightly overcorrected position. The second needle is similarly placed on the same horizontal plane 3 mm from the first. The suture is tied tightly as tissue necrosis and inflammatory reaction to the suture material aid scar formation and better adhesion between the anterior and posterior lamellae of the eyelid. The sutures are left in position for 3 weeks. Antibiotic ointment is placed on the sutures twice daily to minimize infection.

There are minimal complications with this technique; the most likely problem is the premature loss of the suture and recurrence of the epiblepharon. Reoperation should then be done using the following technique:

EXCISION OF SKIN AND ORBICULARIS MUSCLE TO CORRECT EPIBLEPHARON

Excision of skin and orbicularis muscle is the preferred technique when there is marked epiblepharon, especially with prominence or hypertrophy of the pretarsal orbicularis muscle. This procedure may be done using local anesthesia but requires a general anesthetic in children. After skin preparation and the administration of appropriate anesthesia, the skin of the medial two-thirds of the eyelid is pulled inferiorly and the line of the proposed lower eyelid crease is drawn with a marking pen. This line is the upper incision line. The amount of tissue to be excised is then determined by placing the upper arm of a toothed forceps on this line, grasping sufficient tissue vertically to return the lashes and eyelid margin to a normal position. The inferior incision line is thus determined after repeating this maneuver in several locations across the eyelid (Fig. 35.3*A*). The strip of skin and orbicularis muscle outlined is then excised and hemostasis is obtained. Multiple, interrupted 6-0 catgut sutures are placed to close the skin and orbicularis muscle defect and to establish adherence to the underlying tarsus or lower

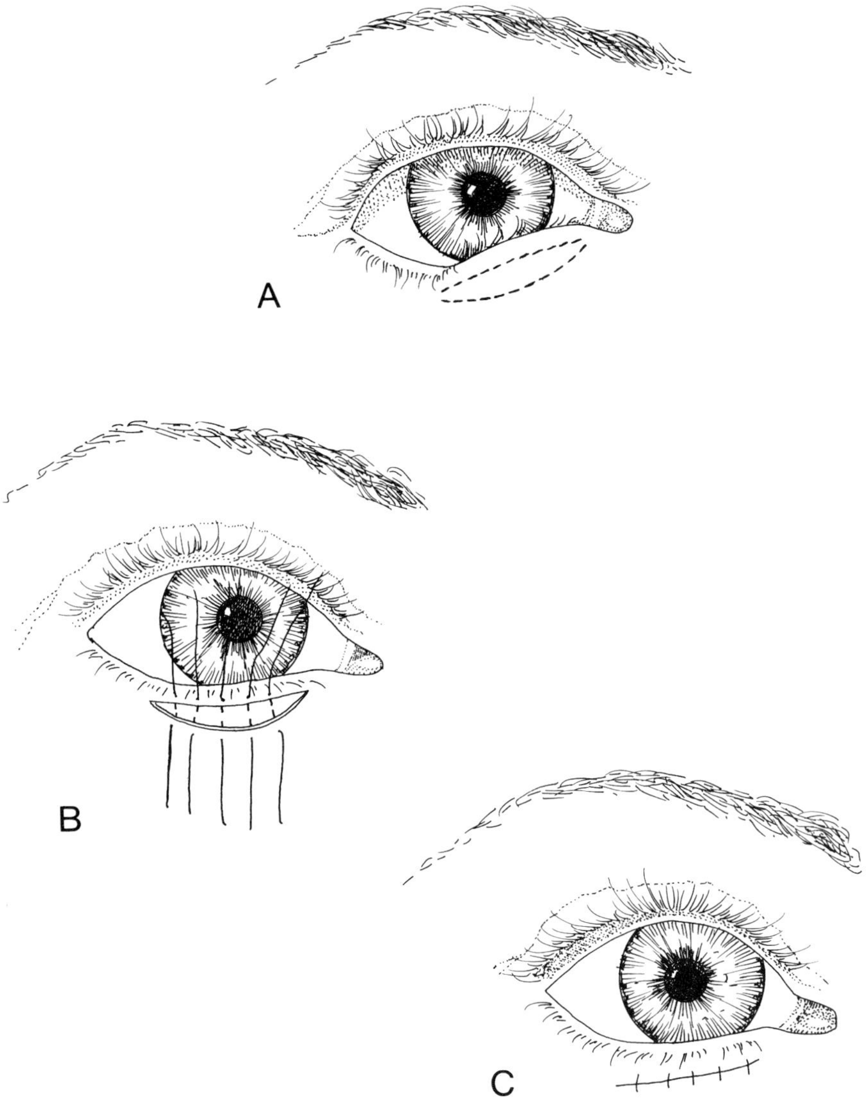

Figure 35.3. Epiblepharon. *A*, After amount of skin and orbicularis muscle excision has been determined by pinching with forceps. *B*, Suture placement. *C*, Immediately postoperative.

eyelid retractors (Fig. 35.3*B*). The suture is passed through the superior edge of the skin and orbicularis muscle, pulled inferiorly enough to bring the lashes and eyelid margin into a normal or slightly everted position, passed through the underlying tarsus or retractors, brought through the inferior orbicularis muscle and skin edges, and tied. Five or six similar sutures are placed along the defect (Fig. 35.3*C*). If a less definite eyelid crease is desired, the deep closure of orbicularis muscle to the lower lid retractors can be closed without including the skin and the skin can be closed in a separate layer by direct approximation. The lower eyelid crease should be discussed with all patients or their families preoperatively as many Orientals prefer to minimize the visibility of a crease (Fig. 35.4).

INVOLUTIONAL ENTROPION

Involutional entropion is caused by aging changes that affect the eyelid tissues and orbital contents. It is characterized by the intermittent or constant turning in of the entire lower eyelid margin, which causes the lashes and eyelid skin to rub against the globe. This is very symptomatic and causes ocular irritation, foreign-body sensation, tearing, recurrent conjunctivitis, and/or keratitis. In cases of intermittent ocular irritation where entropion is suspected, the entropion often may be demonstrated by having the patient look down and squeeze the eyes closed. A number of pathophysiologic aging changes occur that contribute to entropion. The combination of these changes occur in most entropion cases.

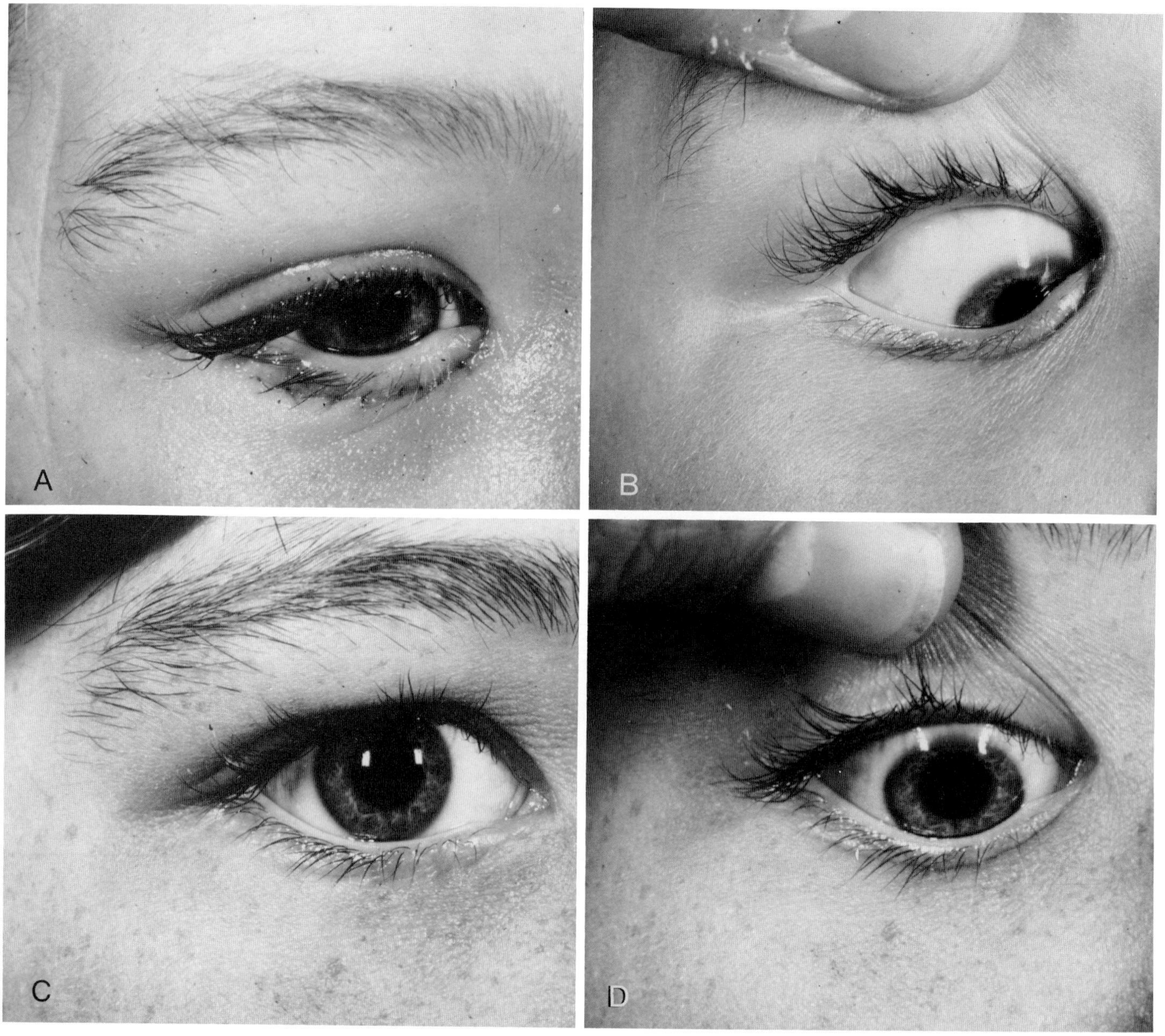

Figure 35.4. Same patient as shown preoperatively in Figure 35.1. *A*, Three weeks postoperative with sutures still in place in primary gaze. *B*, In downgaze. *C*, Eight years postoperative in primary gaze. *D*, In downgaze showing permanency of adhesion.

CONTRIBUTING FACTORS

Enophthalmos

Enophthalmos occurs as part of the aging process due to orbital fat atrophy. This loss of orbital volume results in retrodisplacement of the globe in relation to the eyelid. Fuchs (5) brought attention to the role of enophthalmos in entropion by noting the association of microphthalmos and anophthalmos with entropion. Bick (6) demonstrated that entropion can be temporarily corrected by the injection of 2–4 ml of saline solution into the muscle cone, which causes forward globe displacement. However, enophthalmos by itself will not cause entropion when the eyelid tissues are normal. This was demonstrated by Collin and Rathbun (7), who created enophthalmos in monkeys by different methods without producing entropion. While enophthalmos results in decreased eyelid support, involutional eyelid tissue changes are also necessary for entropion to occur.

Orbicularis Muscle

The role of the orbicularis muscle in involutional entropion has been exaggerated by the previously popular term "senile spastic entropion". The upward and forward movement of the preseptal orbicularis muscle over the lower edge of the tarsus in involutional entropion was demonstrated with radiographic markers by Dalgleish and Smith (8). This movement occurs because of the connective tissue laxity associated with aging. Fox (9) eliminated "reflex spasm" by using topical anesthesia of the cornea and local anesthetic paralysis of the orbicularis muscle. The entropion, however, was not relieved. Radnot (10) showed that entropion can occur in the presence of severe myopathy with histological lesions of the orbicularis muscle. Sisler and associates (11) showed histologically hypertrophy of the orbicularis and Riolan's muscle in entropion. Thus while primary spasm is not a cause of entropion in most cases, the orbicularis muscle is able to contract and will lead to entropion if there is any upward movement over the tarsus due to tissue laxity.

Lower Eyelid Retractors

The role of the lower eyelid retractors as a factor in involutional entropion has received considerable attention in recent years. DeRoetth (12) demonstrated that involutional entropion could be temporarily corrected by an adrenergic drop that stimulated the inferior tarsal smooth muscle. Jones (13) demonstrated that anatomy of the lower eyelid retractors and theorized that laxity of the retractors would allow the lower border of the tarsus to rotate upward and forward, thus resulting in entropion. Laxity or dehiscence of the lower eyelid retractors has been observed by many surgeons and has been demonstrated histologically with repair of the defect, which corrected the entropion. Laxity of the retractors manifests itself clinically by a shallow lower fornix since the retractors insert both into the tarsus and into the conjunctival fornix (Fig. 35.5). A disinsertion of the retractors clinically has a deep lower fornix (Fig. 35.6) with a subconjunctival redness inferior to the tarsal border, which is in contrast with the whitish appearance of a normal eyelid where the retractors are attached. The preseptal muscle is seen subconjunctivally when the retractors are disinserted and a

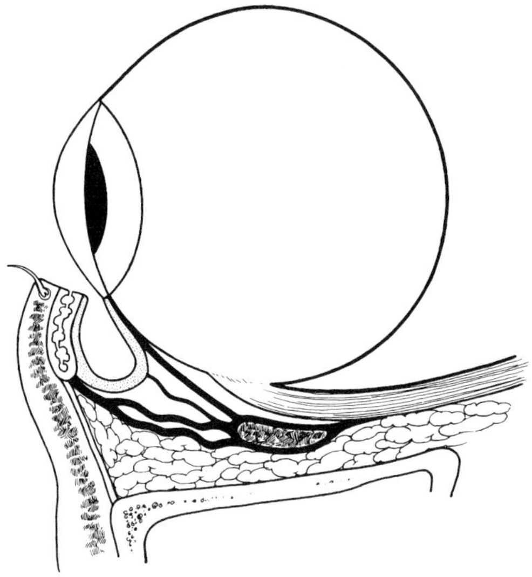

Figure 35.5. Shallow lower fornix that is due to laxity of lower eyelid retractors. (From Collin JRO, Rathbun JE: Involutional entropion. *Arch Ophthalmol* 96: 1058–1064, 1978.)

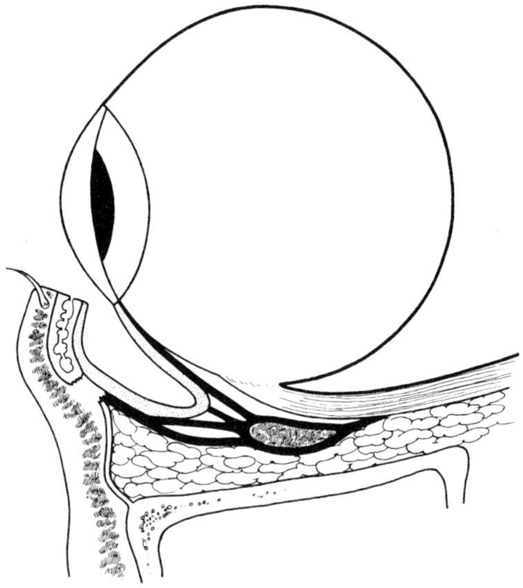

Figure 35.6. Deep lower fornix with disinsertion of lower eyelid retractors. (From Collin JRO, and Rathbun JE: Involutional entropion. *Arch Ophthalmol* 96: 1058–1064, 1978).

white line representing the edge of the retractors may be identified.

Tarsal Plate

The tarsal plate undergoes involutional changes that contribute to the development of eyelid malpositions. Sisler and associates (11) demonstrated tarsal thinning histologically. Dalgleish and Smith (8) demonstrated histologically that the tarsal plate buckles around its horizontal axis and that the upper tarsal border turns inwards four times the upward and outward movement of the lower border. Transfer of the downward traction forces to the upper border of the tarsus or to the anterior lamella of the lid, high on the lid close to the margin, will stabilize this inward rotation of the tarsus. This procedure is utilized in a number of successful entropion procedures.

INVOLUTIONAL ENTROPION PROCEDURES

The history of entropion surgery is of many procedures with treatment of almost all tissues of the lower eyelid. An analysis of the various procedures provides an historical perspective as well as a better understanding of currently highly successful entropion surgery. The procedures can be grouped broadly into procedures that treat the anterior lamella (skin and orbicularis muscle), procedures that treat the posterior lamella (tarsus and conjunctiva with retractors attached inferiorly), and procedures that control tarsal rotation.

Anterior Lamella Procedures

Celsus (14), in the 1st century AD, described the excision of an ellipse of skin and orbicularis muscle, which thus shortened the anterior lamella in relation to the posterior lamella and everted the lid margin. This was modified by Hotz (15), who sutured the upper skin edge directly to the lower border of the tarsus, creating an almost full-thickness scar.

The creation of a full-thickness scar is a characteristic of many successful entropion procedures: Gaillard (16) passed three sutures subcutaneously from the lid margin to the tissues at the inferior orbital rim and then tied them over bolsters and left them in place sufficiently long to create fibrosis in the suture tracts. Quickert and Rathbun (17) placed three sutures through the full eyelid thickness at the lower tarsal border to induce full-thickness fibrosis. Feldstein (18) and Iliff (19) have described more complex methods of suture placement attempting to pass the sutures through the lower lid retractors posteriorly and then passing through the orbicularis muscle and skin close to the eyelid margin. These suture techniques create a scar tissue barrier to upward movement of the preseptal muscle and transfer the pull of the lower lid retractors to the anterior lamella of the lid. Fibrosis has also been produced by Elschnig (20) using the injection of alcohol and by Zeigler (21) using cautery punctures through the skin that are deep enough to create scarring into the tarsus (21). Bodian (22) modified the cautery technique by excising a strip of skin and applying two rows of cautery to the lower pretarsal and upper preseptal orbicularis muscle, thus creating fibrosis as well as shortening the anterior lamella.

Posterior Lamella Procedures

Techniques that mechanically hinge or rotate the superior portion of the tarsus in relation to the inferior portion have been used. In 1857, Streatfield (23) devised an operation to angle the upper portion of the tarsus forward by grooving the anterior tarsus. Wies (24) used a full-thickness horizontal eyelid incision 4 mm inferior to the lid margin that extended across the lid and was repaired to create a mechanical buckling of the tarsus. This procedure angles the upper portion of the lid forward in relation to the lower portion, creates a full thickness scar tissue barrier, and tightens the lower eyelid retractors.

Horizontal eyelid shortening has been utilized in a number of procedures, thereby correcting the relative enophthalmos component and probably creating a scar between the anterior and posterior lamellae in at least one portion of the lid. Butler (25) described the excision of an inverted wedge of tarsus from the lower tarsal border to shorten the lower portion of the tarsus. Fox (26) modified this by also excising a spindle of skin and muscle laterally. Foulds (27) excised a rectangle of tarsus under a skin muscle flap to shorten the eyelid in separate layers. Dalgleish (8) excised a full-thickness pentagonal figure of eyelid in the middle one-third, and Bick (6) advocated full-thickness eyelid resection laterally.

Control of Tarsal Rotation

Rotation of the tarsus can be controlled by preventing the lower border of the tarsus from rotating forward. Jones (13) was the first to demonstrate the detailed anatomy of the lower eyelid retractors by pointing out their analogous counterparts in the upper eyelid. He proposed the concept of retractor dehiscence or laxity in upper eyelid ptosis as well as in lower eyelid entropion. He undertook to devise a procedure to shorten the lower eyelid retractors that would prevent the upward and forward rotation of the inferior tarsal border. In 1963, Jones and associates (28) described tucking of the orbital septum that indirectly shortened the retractors. This was modified to a tucking of the inferior lid retractors, which decreased the recurrence rate and eliminated the restriction of lower lid elevation in upgaze (29). The procedure has been further modified by Dryden and associates (30); they sutured the dehisced retractors directly to the lower border of the tarsus and added eyelid crease sutures. Fibrosis between the anterior lamella and posterior lamella appears to be a necessary part of the lower retractor operations. The only two cases done by Quickert of retractor shortening (personal communication) through a conjunctival incision without a skin incision or full-thickness sutures resulted in rapid recurrence, which encouraged him to abandon this approach.

The orbicularis muscle has been approached and utilized to stabilize the tarsus. Wheeler (31) described the "orbicularis strip advancement" operation in which a 4 mm strip of orbicularis was pulled temporally and sutured to the periosteum of the lateral orbital wall. This creates a fibrotic band as well as a posterior force on the tarsus. Wheeler (31) also described shortening a strip of orbicularis and tightening it below the inferior tarsal border to prevent forward rotation. Hill and Feldman (32) modified this procedure by curretting the anterior surface of the tarsus and the undersurface of the skin overlying the tarsus and then suturing the upper skin edge to the lower border of the tarsus as described by Hotz (15). The shortened orbicularis strip is sutured to the lower border of the tarsus and not below, as was done by Wheeler. Hill and Feldman (32) also advocated the excision of a pentagonal wedge of tarsus to correct horizontal laxity if present. Sisler (33) has advocated a procedure in which strips of preseptal orbicularis muscle are brought superiorly and sutured to the upper portion of the tarsus, thus exerting an anterior pull on the superior tarsus.

Many other procedures to correct entropion have been described. The procedures mentioned here are representative of the approaches used and show how the pathophysiologic defects have been corrected directly or indirectly. One recurring result of almost all the procedures is the formation of a full-thickness eyelid scar, thus reestablishing the pull of the lower eyelid retractors on the anterior lamella of the eyelid and preventing the inward rotation of the eyelid (i.e., entropion).

DESCRIPTION OF FOUR PROCEDURES

While many procedures have been used for entropion, the author prefers to limit his approach to this problem to four procedures with some modification depending on the particular clinical presentation. With these four procedures used in appropriate circumstances, excellent results can be uniformly obtained and recurrences will occur only rarely. In acute entropion temporary relief can be obtained by taping the lower eyelid so that a horizontal pull is exerted (Fig. 35.7). This serves to correct horizontal laxity and stabilize the anterior lamella. Repeated trials may be necessary to determine the configuration needed for each patient.

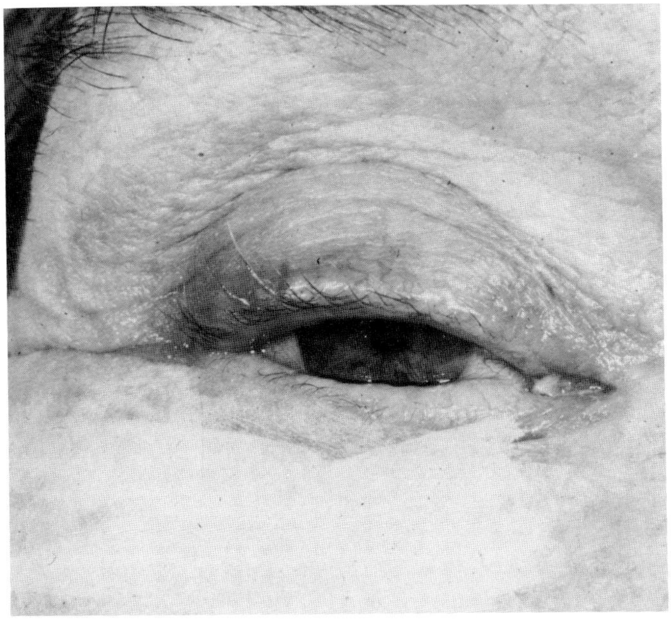

Figure 35.7. Technique of taping lower lid entropion for temporary relief.

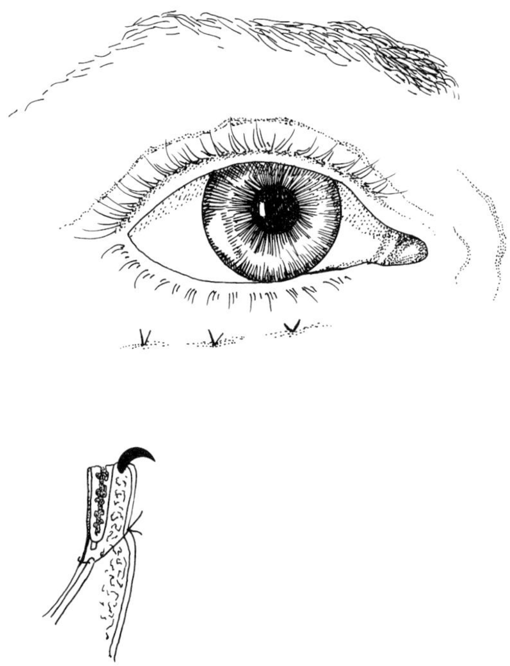

Figure 35.8. Suture repair of entropion showing suture placement.

Suture Technique

This procedure (Fig. 35.8) is effective in cases where there is minimal horizontal eyelid laxity and in cases of intermittent entropion. It is a quick preventative procedure for the patient who must undergo intraocular or retinal detachment surgery and who first manifests entropion when lying supine in the operating room. Since the edema related to the surgery is likely to enhance the entropion problem and have devastating effects on the cornea, the suture technique will allow effective prevention during the postoperative period. This procedure is also useful in providing comfort to a severely ill patient who experiences the irritating effects of entropion while lying supine.

The procedure can be done at the bedside with 4-0 nylon sutures that can usually be left in placc for several weeks or months with a low incidence of infection. This is in contrast to the use of 5-0 chromic gut sutures in the usual technique where significant reaction and scar formation are desired in the early postoperative period.

The suture placement technique is done with local anesthesia with subcutaneous and subconjunctival infiltration. The sutures are evenly spaced in the lateral two-thirds of the eyelid; they are placed so as to exit through the skin in the normal position of the lower eyelid crease (Fig. 35.8). Thus the horizontal plane of the lateral-most suture is approximately 2 mm inferior to that of the medial-most suture. The needle of a double-armed 5-0 chromic gut suture is passed through the conjunctiva below the inferior tarsal border and angled inferiorly to attempt to pick up the lower eyelid retractors. The needle is then redirected anteriorly and superiorly to pass the inferior border of the tarsus. With the skin pulled inferiorly so as to bring the eyelid and margin into a normal position, the needle is then passed anteriorly through the orbicularis muscle and skin. The second needle of the double-armed suture is passed in the same manner 2–3 mm away on the same horizontal plane and the two arms of the suture are tied as tightly as possible to promote necrosis and inflammatory reaction, which will aid scar formation and permanent adhesion between the anterior and posterior lamellae (Fig. 35.8). With the three sutures in place, downgaze should demonstrate prompt inferior movement of the lid and lid margin and should show the definite formation of the lower eyelid crease (Fig. 35.9). The sutures are removed 3 weeks if they have not been extruded before that time. Antibiotic ointment is placed on the sutures twice daily to minimize infection.

Complications are minimal and anatomy is not altered, which makes other procedures less difficult if the entropion recurs. The chief complication is recurrence. This may occur because of inaccurate suture placement, postoperative edema preventing good tissue adhesion, early suture extrusion with inadequate scar formation, or other factors such as horizontal eyelid laxity or enophthalmos, which are not addressed by this procedure.

Wies Procedure

In 1954, Wies (24) reported a procedure that employs a full-thickness horizontal eyelid incision that serves to produce a more definite full-thickness scar than either sutures or cautery. This has been an effective procedure in cases with minimal horizontal lid laxity.

After sterile preparation and the subcutaneous and subconjunctival injection of local anesthetic, a horizontal line 4 mm inferior to the eyelid margin is made with a marking pen. A full-thickness lid incision is made; one must make certain that the conjunctival incision is made equidistant

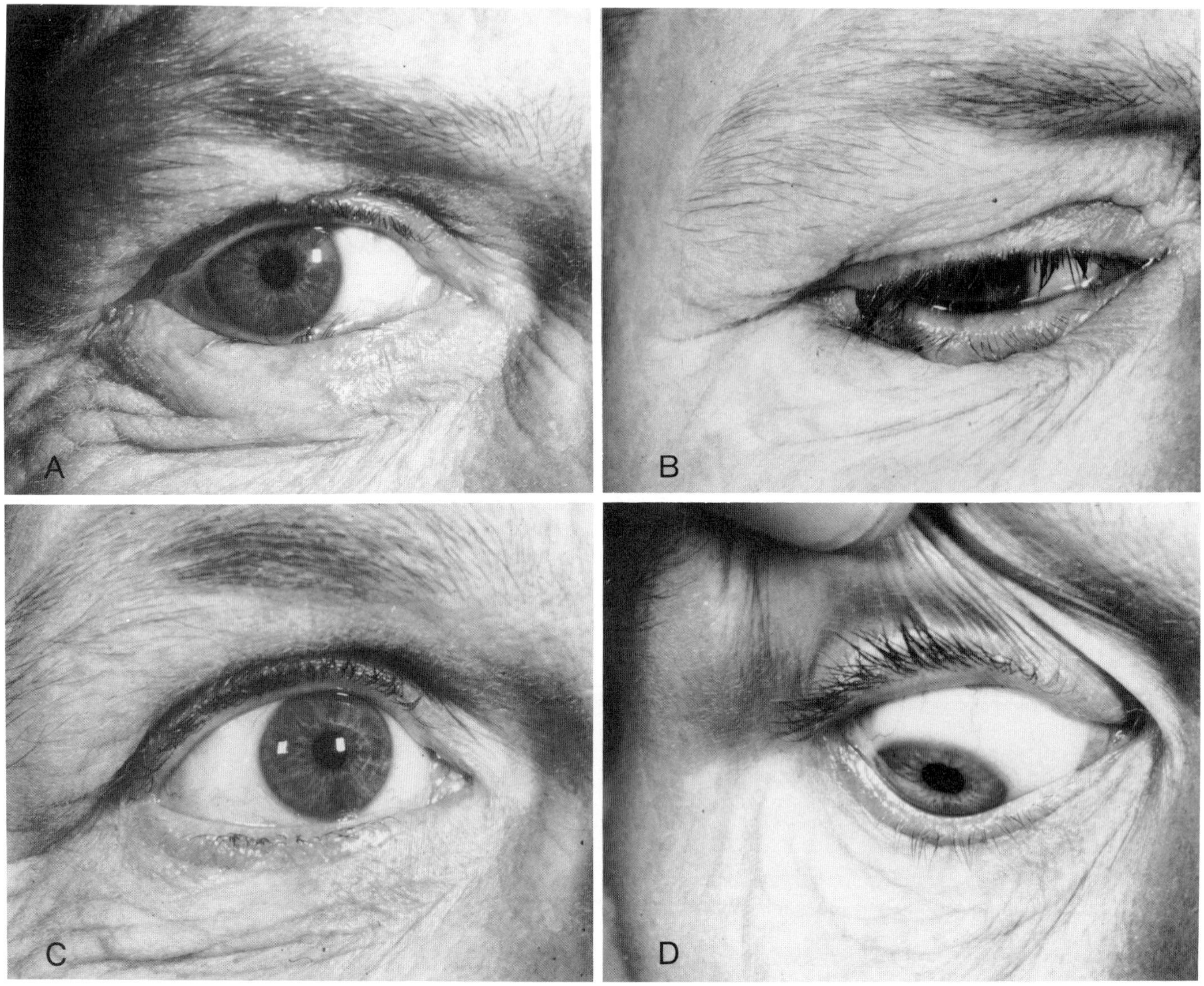

Figure 35.9. Suture repair of entropion. *A*, Preoperative. *B*, Immediately postoperative with lid crease formation on downgaze. *C* and *D*, Four months postoperative.

from the eyelid margin as the skin incision (i.e., 4 mm). This incision is made from inferior to the punctum medially to inferior to the lateral canthus laterally. Several techniques of making this incision have been used. A full-thickness knife incision may be made laterally with the globe being protected with a bone plate and then the remainder of the full thickness incision made with scissors. One must be careful not to allow the lid to buckle or turn inward, which results in a wandering incision. A second method is to make a skin incision across the length of the lid 4 mm below the margin and then to make a separate conjunctival incision 4 mm below the margin. These two incisions are then joined by a knife incision laterally, and scissors are then used to complete the lateral incision using the two incisions as a guide. Note that this horizontal incision is made *through the tarsus* so that tarsus is present superior and inferior to the incision. If the tarsus is narrow, the incision may need to be made closer to the lid margin than 4 mm. A 4-0 doubly armed silk suture is then placed through the inferior conjunctival and tarsal segment and then brought out through the orbicularis muscle and skin superior to the incision, thus not passing through tarsus superiorly (Fig. 35.10). Both arms of the suture are passed in similar fashion 3 mm apart and tied firmly. A small, rolled moistened cotton bolster is placed under each suture knot. Three sutures are spaced across the eyelid and the skin edges are then closed with interrupted or running 7-0 silk suture. The skin sutures are removed in 5-7 days while the mattress sutures are left in place for 14 days. This procedure results in a buckling of the tarsus as well as in the formation of a full-thickness scar. Even with this surgical distortion of tissue, there is very little distortion or scarring, which is clinically apparent after the immediate postoperative period (Fig. 35.11).

When this procedure is done accurately, complications are minimal. Ectropion may occur if significant horizontal

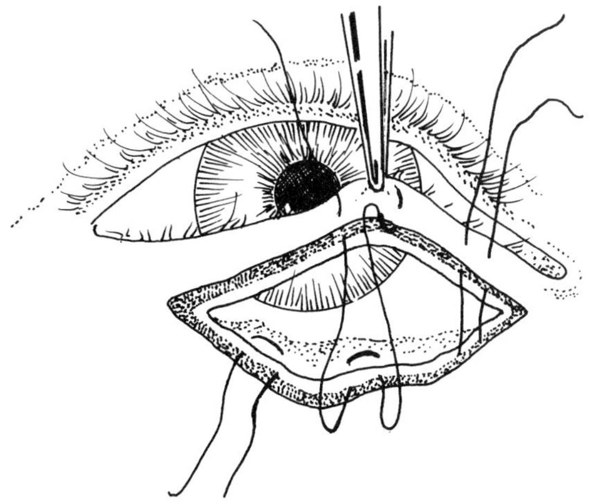

Figure 35.10. Suture placement through conjunctiva and tarsus inferior to the incision and through orbicularis and skin superior to the incision.

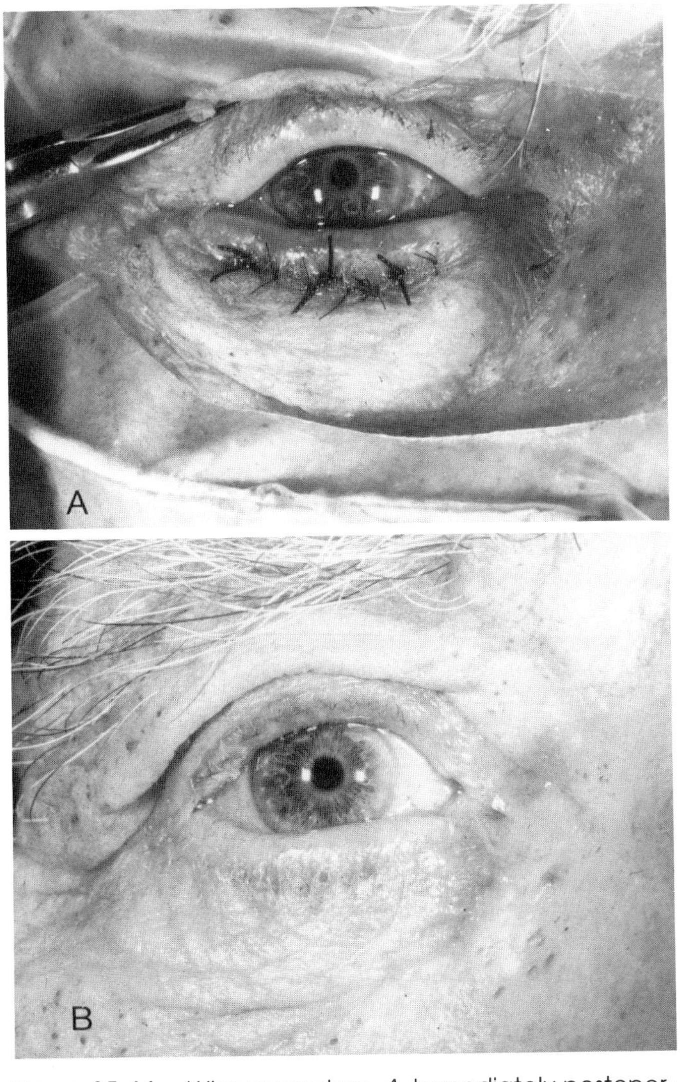

Figure 35.11. Wies procedure. *A*, Immediately postoperative. *B*, Two months postoperative.

eyelid laxity is present or if the eyelid margin is excessively everted with suture placement. In the former the entropion will usually resolve but may require horizontal lid shortening. In the latter the sutures should be removed early and the lid massaged in an attempt to decrease scar formation. Hemorrhage may be a problem if the peripheral arcade is compromised. Irregularity of the eyelid margin may result from uneven cutting of the full-thickness incision. The eyelid margin may slough if it becomes devascularized.

Quickert Entropion Procedure

Quickert's entropion procedure (Figs. 35.12 and 35.13; Ref. 34) combines the effect of the Wies procedure with horizontal eyelid shortening. Also, with our more recent knowledge of the role of lower eyelid retractors, the Quickert procedure has been used to repair the defect in the retractors. The logic behind the procedure is to attempt to correct as many factors that contribute to entropion as possible.

After the subcutaneous and subconjunctival injection of local anesthetic, a full-thickness vertical incision is made perpendicular to the eyelid margin 5 mm medial to the lateral canthus (Fig. 35.12*A,a*). This incision is extended to the inferior border of the tarsus. While the eyelid margin incision may be started with a knife, scissors are preferred for the entire incision. The second full-thickness eyelid incision is made horizontally from the inferior end of the initial incision (Fig. 35.12*A,b*). This incision follows the inferior tarsal border and is carried medially to a point inferior to the punctum. The third incision is made directly lateral, starting at the inferior aspect of the first incision, and is carried to the lateral orbital rim (Fig. 35.12*A,b*). This incision does not follow the inferior tarsal border. The medial flap of eyelid created is then pulled laterally over the lateral flap, which is pulled medially, placing moderate tension on each flap (Fig. 35.12*A,c*). The flaps must be kept in a normal position in relation to the globe and not be allowed to drift inferiorly, which will result in the resection of an excessive amount of lid margin. The point where the lid margin of the medial flap meets the cut lid margin of the lateral flap is marked. The fourth incision is made at this point perpendicular to the eyelid margin and carried to the inferior tarsal border, where it joins the second incision (Fig. 35.12*A* and *B,c*). Thus a rhomboid shape of full-thickness eyelid is excised.

The tarsal borders are approximated and sutured with 5-0 chromic gut (Fig. 35.12*C,1*). The skin and eyelid margin as well as the vertical skin defect are sutured with interrupted 7-0 silk sutures. The horizontal full-thickness incision that now remains is closed with three 5-0 chromic gut, double-armed, mattress sutures. One arm of the suture is placed through the conjunctiva and lower eyelid retractors of the inferior incision line and then brought through the orbicularis muscle and skin superior to the incision line (Fig. 35.12*D,4*). The second arm of the suture is passed in similar fashion 2–3 mm apart on the same horizontal plane. The two arms are tied tightly without bolsters.

If the lid margin is excessively everted, the suture should

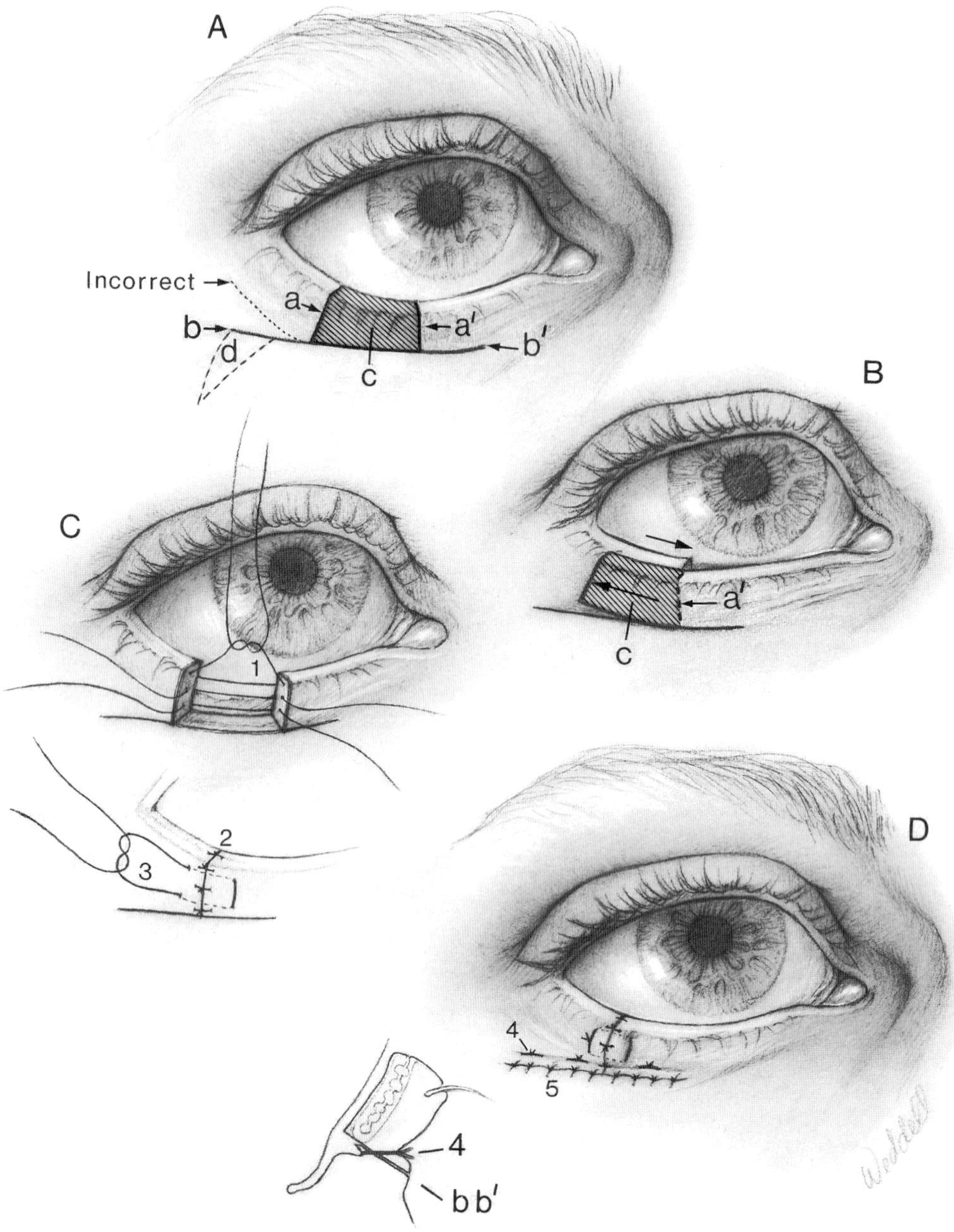

Figure 35.12. Quickert entropion procedure. *A*, *a* to *a*¹, Vertical incision. *b* to *b*¹, Horizontal incision. *c*, Full-thickness excision. *d*, Redundant skin excision. *B*, Lid margin edges overlapped for excision of block *c* at *a*¹. *C*, Tarsoconjunctival closure at *1*. Skin closure at *2*. Horizontal mattress suture at *3*. *D*, Full-thickness sutures similar to Wies operation at *4*. Final skin closure at *5 bb*¹, Plane of horizontal incision. (From Quickert MH, in Sorsby A(ed): *Modern Ophthalmology*, ed 2. London, 1972, vol 4, p 941.)

be replaced with narrower tissue bites both inferiorly and superiorly. If the orbicularis muscle is hypertrophic, a strip may be excised along the inferior skin edge. If an excess amount of skin is present, it can be excised in a blepharoplast fashion by extending the skin incision inferolaterally at a 45° angle, undermining the skin, overlapping the excess skin, and excising a triangle. The skin incision is closed with 7-0 silk sutures (Fig. 35.12*D*,*5*). A moderate-pressure dressing is applied for 24 hours and a metal shield is worn at night for 2 weeks; this is done with all patients who have eyelid margin incisions to prevent inadvertent self-trauma that may lead to wound separation and notch formation. Antibiotic ointment is used twice daily. The skin sutures are removed at 5-7 days and the gut sutures removed at 3 weeks if they have not fallen out before then (Fig. 35.13).

In my experience complications have been rare with this procedure. While wound breakdown has not occurred, the complications that may occur with a full-thickness lid margin incision may occur with this procedure. Recurrence of entropion has only been seen in patients who had had inaccurate placement of incisions and sutures. The determination of the amount of eyelid laxity requires some judgment and may result in entropion if laxity remains.

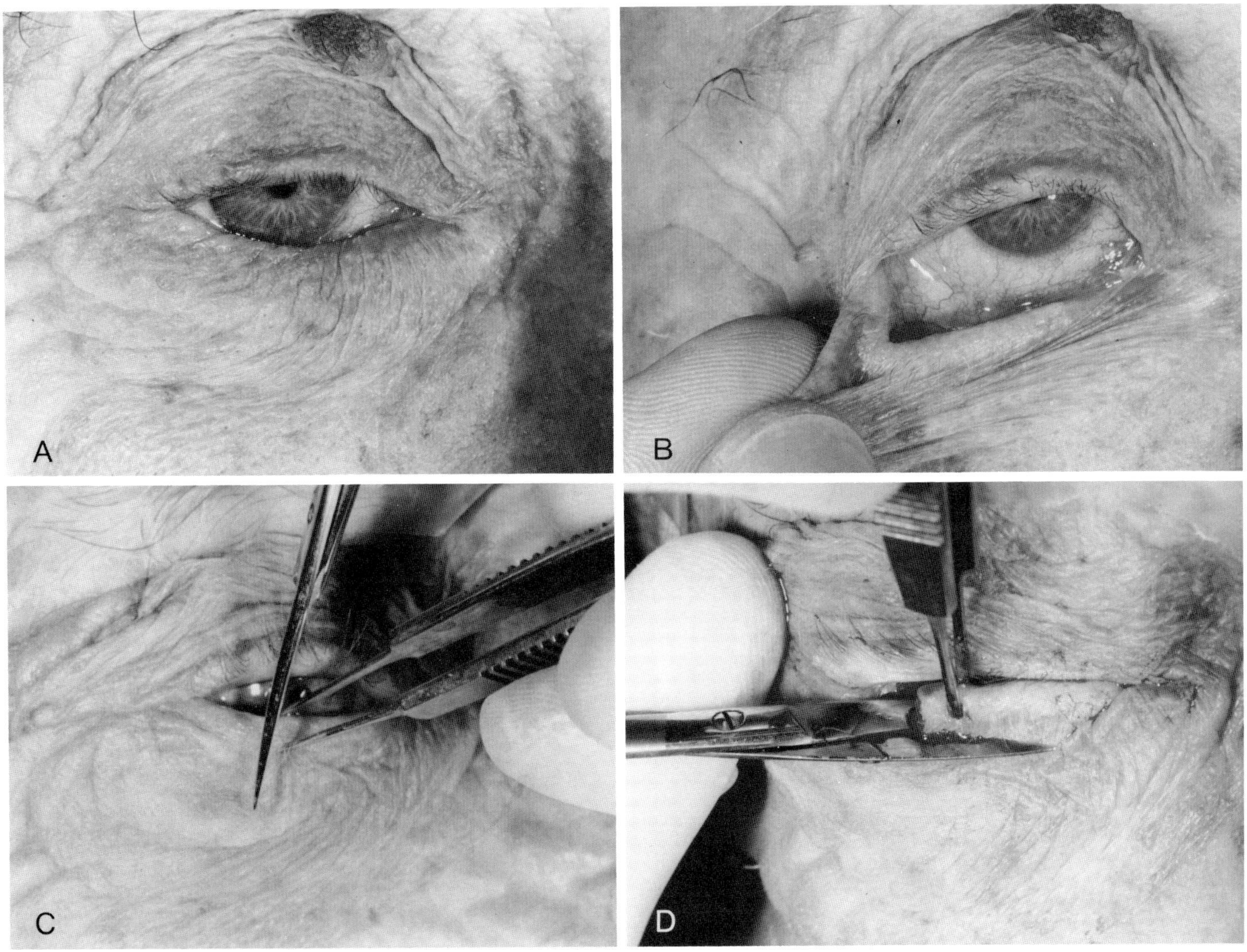

Figure 35.13. Quickert entropion procedure. *A*, Preoperative. *B*, Horizontal eyelid laxity. *C*, Initial vertical full-thickness eyelid incision. *D*, Second incision made medially along lower tarsal border. *E*, Third incision made directly laterally. *F*, Flaps overlapped. *G*, Fourth incision to excise excess eyelid. *H*, After repair of flaps and eyelid margin. *I*, Three Wies-type sutures in position. *J*, Immediately postoperative.

Repair of Lower Eyelid Retractors

This procedure may be used alone or may be combined with a technique of horizontal shortening if horizontal lid laxity is present. I prefer this technique coupled with a lateral canthal tendon tuck or tarsal strip procedure in patients with lateral canthal tendon laxity and entropion. In these cases the Quickert procedure would result in distortion and medial migration of the lateral canthal tendon and an unpleasant shortening of the horizontal fissure length. This procedure is more difficult for the surgeon who performs entropion cases infrequently since it requires a knowledge of lower eyelid anatomy and skill in identifying the variable findings in dehisced lower eyelid retractors.

After subconjunctival and subcutaneous injection of local anesthesia, an incision is made in the lower eyelid crease across the width of the eyelid. This is carried through the orbicularis muscle to the orbital septum. Incision through the orbital septum exposes preaponeurotic fat. The inferior portion of the tarsus is then exposed superior to the orbicularis muscle incision. The dehiscence of the aponeurosis of the lower eyelid retractors is usually seen as inspection is done starting at the inferior tarsal border and moving inferiorly. Confirmation is obtained by feeling a pull when the patient looks inferiorly. The aponeurotic edge is then brought superiorly and sutured to the inferior tarsal border with three 6-0 Prolene mattress sutures (Fig. 35.14*A*). The eyelid margin should now be in a normal or slightly overcorrected position and should move with upgaze and downgaze. The skin and orbicularis muscle are then closed with several interrupted 7-0 silk sutures, which are followed by a running 7-0 silk suture to complete skin closure. A variation in suture closure described by Dryden and associates (30) is to pass the skin closure sutures through the aponeurosis, which increases

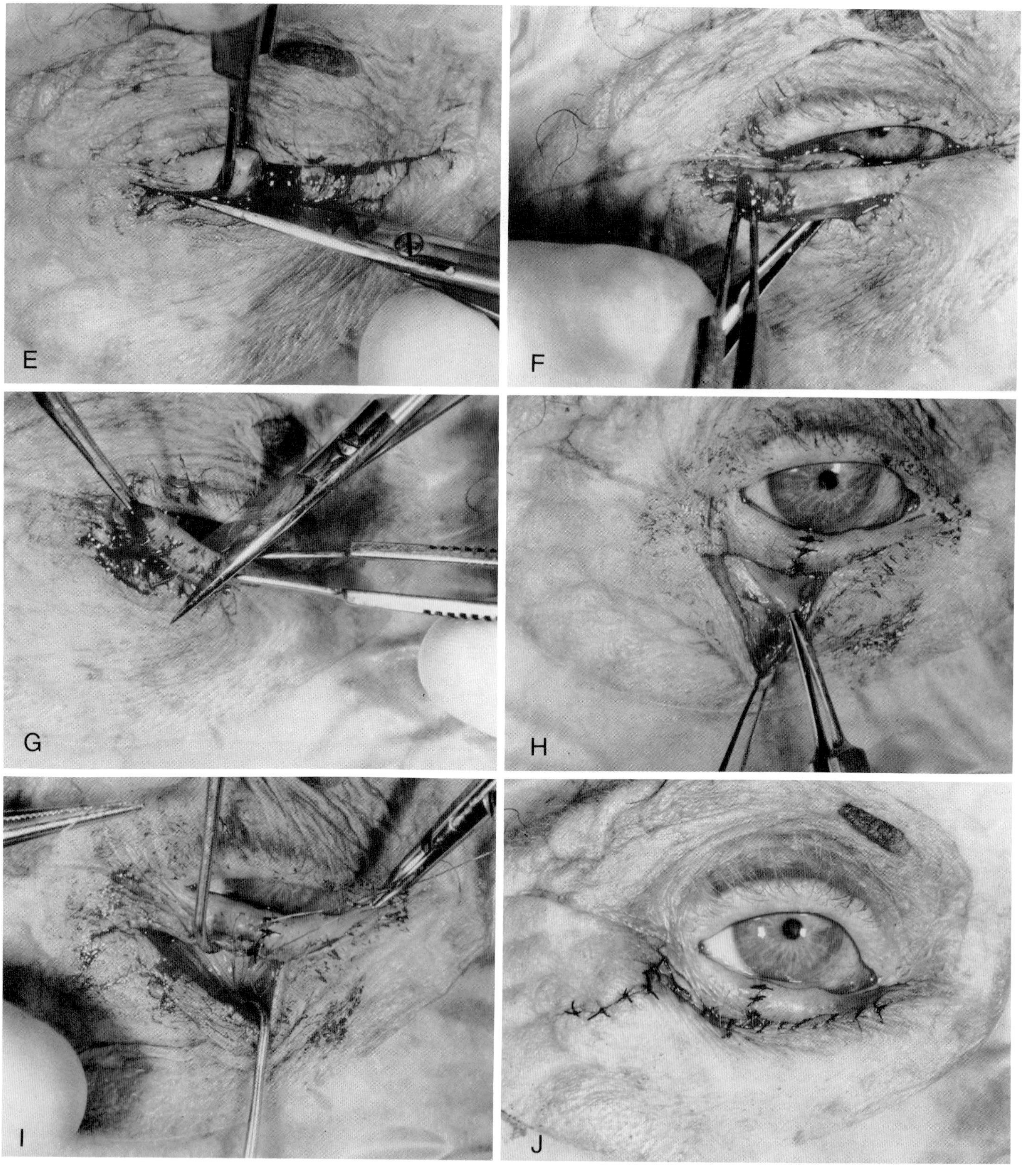

Figure 35.13. *E–J*

the adhesion between the anterior and posterior lamellae and forms a more definite lower eyelid crease Fig. 35.14*B*. An eyepad pressure dressing is used overnight postoperatively. Use of the lateral canthal tendon tucking or tarsal strip procedures in conjunction with lower eyelid retractor repair involves making a separate lateral canthal incision.

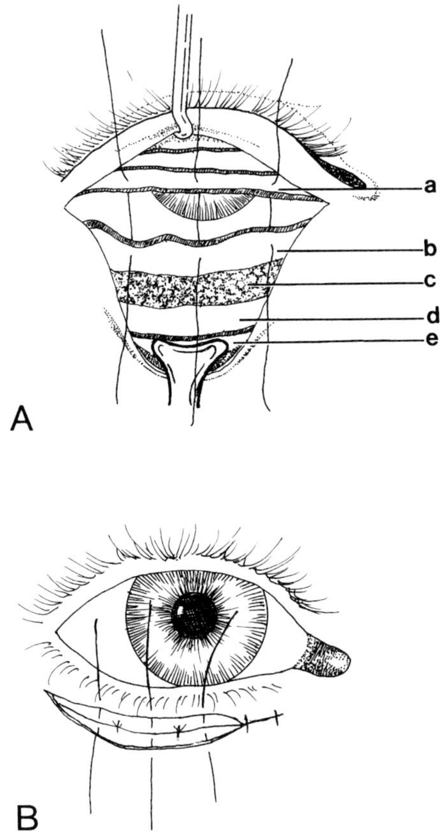

Figure 35.14. Lower eyelid retractor repair: *A,* Suture placement attaching aponeurosis to lower tarsal border: *A,* Tausus. *b,* Intact conjunctiva and inferior tarsal muscle. *c,* Detached retractor aponeurosis. *d,* Orbital fat. *e,* Orbital septum. *f,* Orbicularis muscle. *B,* Skin repair with inclusion of aponeurosis and inferior tarsal border.

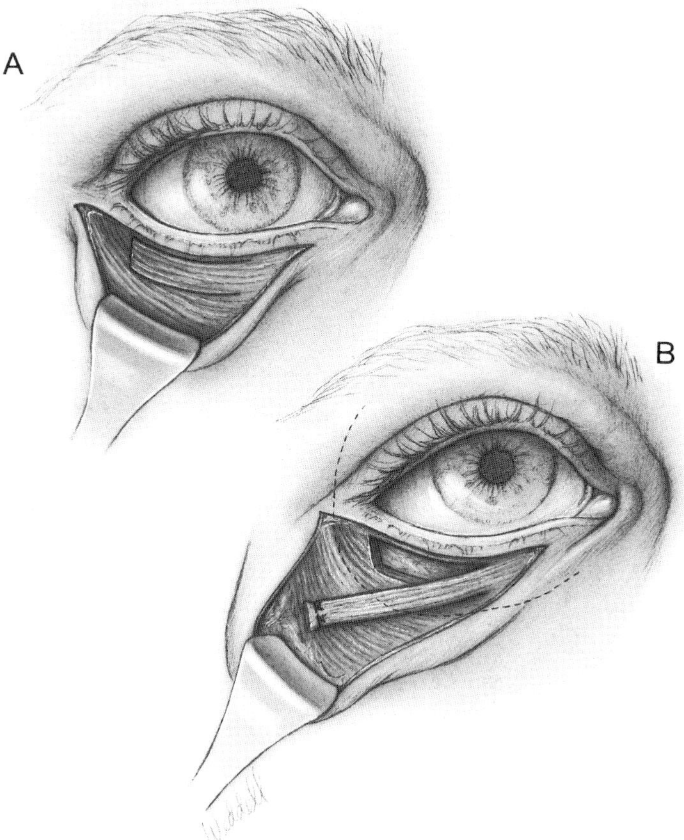

Figure 35.15. Wheeler orbicularis transplant. *A,* Orbicularis strip dissected. *B,* Strip repositioned inferiorly and laterally and sutured to periosteum. *Dotted line* is orbital rim. (From Quickert MH: In Sorsby A (ed): *Modern Ophthalmology,* ed 2. London, Butterworth, 1972, vol 4, p 940.)

The procedure may be combined with blepharoplasty in the form of removal of excess skin by extension of the skin incision.

OTHER PROCEDURES

Two other procedures for the repair of involutional entropion are used by a significant number of opthalmic surgeons; these procedures are discussed here briefly.

Wheeler Orbicularis Transplantation

The Wheeler orbicularis transplantation procedure redirects a dissected strip of orbicularis muscle, which serves as a barrier to prevent the preseptal orbicularis from overriding the pretarsal orbicularis. Subcutaneous local anesthesia is placed on the lateral two-thirds of the eyelid. A skin incision is made inferior to the lash line in the lateral two-thirds of the eyelid and extended several millimeters beyond the lateral canthus. The skin is undermined beyond the inferior tarsal border inferiorly and to the orbital rim laterally. A strip of orbicularis muscle 4–5 mm wide that is centered over the inferior tarsal border and extends over the lateral two-thirds of the eyelid is dissected (Fig. 35.15*A*). The lateral end of this orbicularis strip is cut free; it is dissected free from the underlying tarsus and orbital septum along the length of the strip. The strip is then moved inferiorly and laterally and is sutured at or beyond the orbital rim with sufficient tension to bring the eyelid margin into a slightly overcorrected position (Fig. 35.15*B*). A 4-0 or 5-0 chromic gut suture is used as a mattress suture. If there is excessive muscle beyond the suture, the excess muscle is excised. Skin closure is made with interrupted or running 7-0 silk. A light dressing is used for 24 hours. Variations include the excision of orbital fat through the exposed orbital septum and the extension of the skin incision into a blepharoplasty incision with excision of excess skin.

Base-Down Triangular Tarsal Resection

Base-down triangular tarsal resection results in horizontal tarsal shortening that is maximal inferiorly and minimal superiorly and in a small segment of scar adhesion between the anterior and posterior lamellae. After subconjunctival and subcutaneous injection of local anesthetic, a chalazion clamp is placed for hemostasis. An incision is made at the inferior tarsal border and is centered at the junction of the middle and lateral thirds of the lower eyelid. The length of the incision is 7–10 mm, depending on the degree of tissue laxity. This forms the base of the triangular segment of tarsus that will be excised. Two

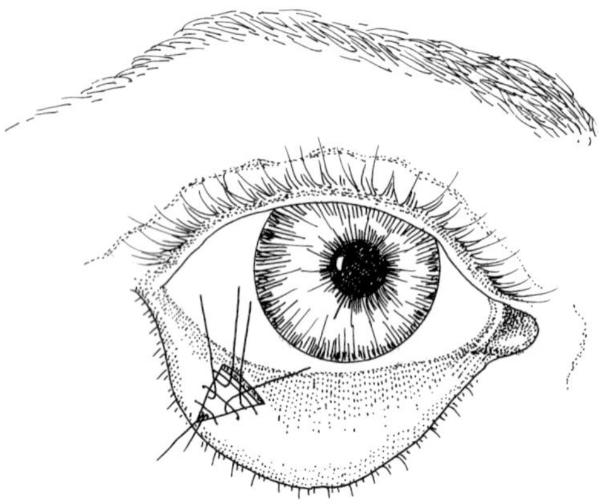

Figure 35.16. Base-down triangular tarsal resection.

incisions extend toward the lid margin; these begin at each end of the horizontal incision and end in an apex just below the superior tarsal border without involving the eyelid margin (Fig. 35.16). This triangular tarsoconjunctival segment is excised, which leaves the pretarsal orbicularis muscle intact. Four interrupted 6-0 chromic gut sutures are preplaced so that the knots will be on the anterior tarsal surface when tied. The chalazion clamp is removed and the sutures tied. The bunched excess of tissue inferior to the tarsal resection is then excised.

CICATRICIAL ENTROPION

Cicatricial entropion presents a more difficult management problem than involutional entropion. By definition, there is a vertical shortening of the posterior lamella (conjunctiva and tarsus) of the eyelid with secondary inward rotation of the eyelid margin and lash line. The constant abrasion of the cornea by the usually stiff eyelid margin and frequently aberrant irregular lashes causes these cases to be more threatening to vision especially if the upper eyelid is involved. Cicatricial entropion, depending upon the disease process, may involve all four eyelids and is particularly devastating if there is generalized conjunctival disease resulting in blockage of the lacrimal secretory ducts and damage to the glands responsible for basic tear secretion. A wide variety of conditions may lead to cicatricial entropion including Stevens-Johnson syndrome, erythema multiforme, ocular pemphigoid, trachoma, essential conjunctival shrinkage, alkali or other chemical burns, chronic allergies, and trauma. Some of these, such as Stevens-Johnson syndrome, present as acute inflammatory conditions that must be controlled by appropriate medical therapy prior to surgical repair. Conditions such as ocular pemphigoid with severe chronic inflammatory problems that will cause progressive scarring require medical control prior to, during, and after surgical repair. Conditions that cause generalized conjunctival damage or disease with compromise of the secretion of tear components will require careful attention to maintenance of moisture during the entire management period.

Treatment varies with the etiology and extent of involvement. Segmental areas of cicatrix may be corrected by segmental excision of full-thickness eyelid. Conjunctival symblepharon may be treated by Z-plasty, conjunctival flap, free conjunctival graft, or buccal mucosal graft. Treatment of generalized cicatricial entropion depends on the severity of the problem. Mild to moderate cicatricial entropion may be treated with procedures that incise the tarsus and rotate the lid margin out. More severe cicatrix may require mucous membrane graft or tarsal lengthening with nasal septum–mucosa, ear cartilage, tarsus, or sclera. Excision of scar tissue may be indicated with severe lid distortion (35).

MARGINAL INCISION WITH RECESSION OR GRAFT

Marginal incision with recession or graft is useful in mild to moderate cicatricial entropion when the mucocutaneous junction of the lid margin is relatively well defined and the tarsal conjunctiva is not keratinized. After the subconjunctival and subcutaneous injections of local anesthesia, an incision is made at the mucocutaneous junction and carried the entire width of the eyelid margin. From this point three different options may be taken. The first option is to extend the incision several millimeters, thus allowing a separation of the anterior lamella (lash line, orbicularis muscle and skin) from the posterior lamella (posterior lid margin, tarsus and conjunctiva). A wedge of buccal mucosa taken from the dentate line of the mouth or a strip of nasal septal mucoperichondrium may be taken and sutured into the defect with running 7-0 chromic gut sutures tied at each end of the graft and knots tied on the skin surface (Fig. 35.17). The second option is to dissect the orbicularis muscle away from the entire anterior surface of the tarsus, thus allowing for a total recession of the anterior lamella in relation to the posterior lamella. This is recessed 3 or 4 mm and anchored to the posterior lamella using full-thickness sutures (6-0 silk) at the superior tarsal border and placing an additional row just above the recessed lash line into the anterior two-thirds of the tarsus (Fig. 35.18*A*,*B*). The strip of tarsus exposed inferiorly may be left uncovered. By 2 to 3 weeks

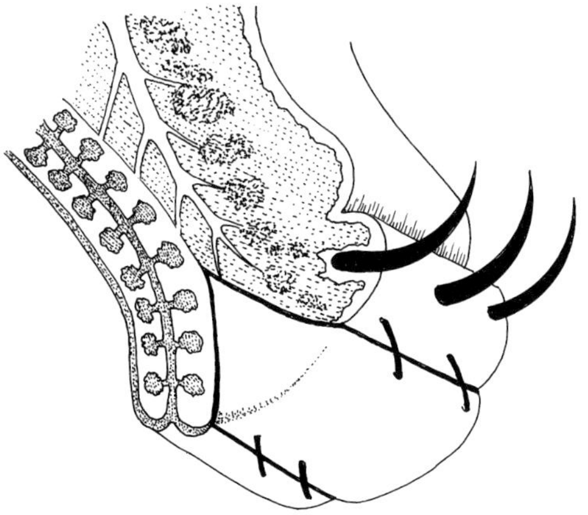

Figure 35.17. Cicatricial entropion with anterior lamella separated from posterior lamella at the lid margin and buccal mucosal graft inserted.

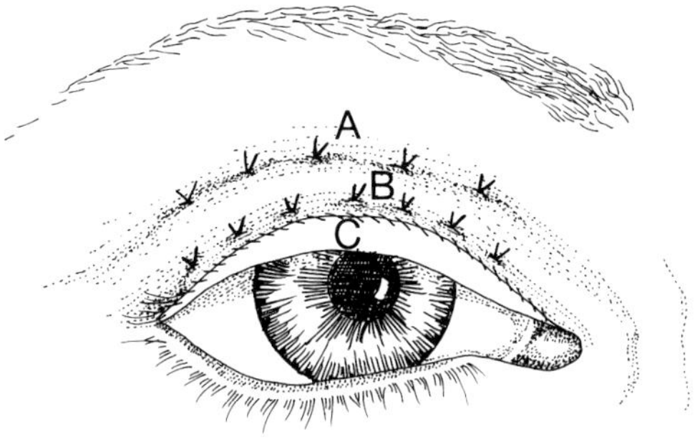

Figure 35.18. Cicatricial entropion with recession of the anterior lamella relative to the posterior lamella. Buccal mucosal graft in place though tarsus may be left exposed. *A*, Full-thickness eyelid suture superior to tarsus. *B*, Suture through anterior two-thirds of tarsus anchoring skin at lid margin. *C*, Buccal mucosal graft.

the skin edge will migrate inferiorly and the conjunctival edge at the tarsal margin will migrate superiorly, thus giving some eversion of the original lid margin. This option is useful when there is generalized mucous membrane disease with no available graft material. A third option is to cover this exposed strip of tarsus with buccal mucosa from the dentate line of the mouth (Fig. 35.18*C*). While there is some graft shrinkage, migration of the wound edges is retarded and the mucosa provides a new lining for the lid margin.

TARSAL FRACTURE PROCEDURES

Rotation of the entire eyelid margin is effective when the disease process causes in-rolling of the margin without severe generalized conjunctival involvement or severe tarsal buckling. In the tarsal fracture procedure, an incision is made through the tarsus 2 mm superior to and parallel to the upper eyelid margin. The entire lid margin can then be rotated outward and kept in position by 6-0 silk mattress sutures; a total of five are usually placed horizontally across the lid. These double-armed sutures are passed through one-half to two-thirds of the thickness of the superior segment of tarsus close to the inferior border; the sutures are then passed through the orbicularis muscle

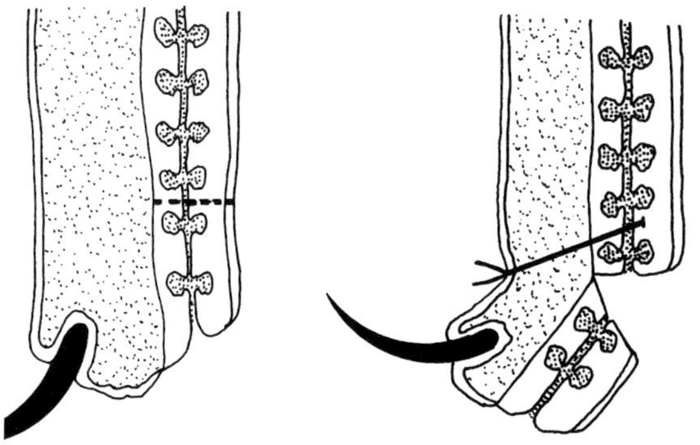

Figure 35.19. Cicatricial entropion: tarsal fracture and lid margin rotation.

and skin being placed near the lash line so as to rotate the margin outward (Fig. 35.19). These sutures are left in place 2–3 weeks to prevent inward rotation of the everted margin. The Wies procedure, as described under "Involutional Entropion," is more effective because it uses a full-thickness eyelid incision. However, there is more probability of damaging the vascular supply to the segment of rotated lid margin in a diseased eyelid with the full-thickness incision of the Wies procedure than with the tarsal fracture incision.

TECHNIQUES FOR TARSAL REPLACEMENT

When there is severe vertical tarsoconjunctival shortening or extensive distortion and scarring of the tarsus that requires excision, a substitute for the diseased tarsus is needed. As the tarsus provides the rigidity of the eyelid, the substitute must provide structure for the support function of the posterior lamella of the lid as well as provide the base for a smooth mucosal lining. If a horizontal strip of tarsus and conjunctiva from another procedure such as a ptosis repair is available or if a flap of tarsus and conjunctiva can be obtained from an opposing, nondiseased eyelid, it can be used and will usually take well. If such tissue is not available, nasal cartilage with its overlying mucosa may be used. While not lined with mucosa, preserved eye-bank sclera may be used to increase vertical lid height being placed as a horizontal strip between tarsal fragments after tarsal incision or excision. The sclera will shrink somewhat but will epithelialize if any viable conjunctiva is available adjacent to the graft. The scleral rigidity will gradually decrease as the graft is replaced by fibrous tissue.

In all cases where either conjunctival grafts or tarsal-conjunctival substitutes are used, sutures must be placed and tied so as to avoid corneal damage, the bed of the graft must be dry after meticulous hemostasis, and the eyelid must be kept on a vertical stretch with sutures taped to the cheek or forehead to keep the graft flat and immobile and avoid buckling or hematoma formation. Procedures to correct cicatricial entropion are used in conjunction with other appropriate oculoplastic surgery procedures, as each case presents a different situation and challenge. In chronic conjunctival diseases with recurrent scarring and shrinkage, multiple procedures will be required over time.

The treatment of entropion requires careful preoperative evaluation to identify and differentiate involutional changes from cicatricial changes. After this the appropriate surgical procedure may be selected. Careful surgical technique with anatomical treatment of the various components present will result in excellent results and minimal recurrences or complications (36).

REFERENCES

1. Fox SA: Primary congenital entropion. *Arch Ophthalmol* 56: 839–842, 1956.
2. Callahan A: *Reconstructive Surgery of the Eyelids and Ocular Adnexa.* Birmingham, AL, Aesculapius, 1966, pp 37–40.
3. Biglan AW, Buerger GF: Congenital horizontal tarsal kink. *Am J Ophthalmol* 1980, 89: 522–524.
4. McCarthy RW: Lamellar tarsoplasty - a new technique for correction of horizontal tarsal kink. *Ophthal Surg* 15: 859–860, 1984.
5. Fuchs E: *Textbook of Ophthalmology*, ed 5. Philadelphia, JB Lippincott, 1917, p 679.
6. Bick MW: Surgical management of orbital tarsal disparity. *Arch Ophthalmol* 75: 386–389, 1966.
7. Collin JRO, Rathbun JE: Involutional entropion. *Arch Ophthalmol* 96: 1058–1064, 1978
8. Dalgleish R, Smith JLS: Mechanics and histology of senile entropion. *Br J Ophthalmol* 50: 79, 1966.
9. Fox SA: The etiology of senile entropion. *Am J Ophthalmol* 48: 607–611, 1959.
10. Radnot M: Mitochondrial crystals in muscles of a patient with spastic entropion. *Am J Ophthalmol* 75: 713–719, 1973.
11. Sisler HA, Labay GR, Finlay JR: Senile ectropion and entropion: A comparative histopathological study. *Am J Ophthalmol* 8: 319–322, 1976.
12. De Roetth A: Mechanism of the senile entropion. *Trans Pac Coast Otoophthal Soc* 44: 173, 1963.
13. Jones LT: The anatomy of the lower eyelid and its relation to the cause and cure of entropion. *Am J Ophthalmol* 49: 29–36, 1960.
14. Celsus, cited by Arruga H: *Ocular Surgery*, ed 3. New York, McGraw-Hill, 1962, p 90.
15. Hotz FC: Eine neue Operation fur entropium und trichiasis. *Arch Augenheil* 9: 1879–1880, pp 68–80.
16. Gaillard, cited by Arruga H: *Ocular Surgery*, ed 3. New York, McGraw-Hill, 1962, p 92.
17. Quickert MH, Rathbun JE: Suture repair of entropion. *Arch Ophthalmol* 85: 304–305, 1971.
18. Feldstein M: Correction of senile entropion. *Ophthalm Surg* 1: 20–23, 1970.
19. Iliff CE, Iliff WJ, Iliff NT: *Oculoplastic Surgery*, Philadelphia, WB Saunders, 1979, pp 135–139.
20. Elschnig HH: Akinesie bei chronischem blepharospasmus. *Med Klin* 18: 1641, 1922.
21. Zeigler SL: Galvanocautery puncture in ectropion and entropion. *JAMA* 53: 183, 1909.
22. Bodian M: A simple operation for senile spastic entropion. *Am J Ophthalmol* 44: 67, 1957.
23. Streatfield JF: On grooving the fibro-cartilage of the lid in cases of entropion and trichiasis. *R London Ophthalmol Hosp Rep* 1: 121, 1857.
24. Wies FA: Surgical treatment of entropion. *J Int Coll Surg* 21: 758–760, 1954.
25. Butler JBV: A simple operation for entropion. *Arch Ophthalmol* 40: 665–667, 1948.
26. Fox SA: Relief of senile entropion. *Arch Ophthalmol* 46: 424–431, 1951.
27. Foulds WS: Surgical cure of senile entropion. *Br J Ophthalmol* 45: 678–682, 1961.
28. Jones LT, Reeh MJ, Tsujimura JK: Senile entropion. *Am J Ophthalmol* 55: 463–469, 1963.
29. Hargiss JL: Inferior aponeurosis versus orbital septum tucking for senile entropion. *Arch Ophthalmol* 89: 210–213, 1973.
30. Dryden RM, Leibsohn J, Wobig JL: Senile entropion: pathogenesis and treatment. *Arch Ophthalmol* 96: 1883–1885, 1978.
31. Wheeler JM: Spastic entropion correction by orbicularis transplantation. *Am J Ophthalmol* 22: 477–483, 1939.
32. Hill JC, Feldman F: Tissue barrier modifications of a Wheeler II operation for entropion. *Arch Ophthalmol* 78: 621–623, 1967.
33. Sisler HA: A biomechanical and physiological approach to corrective surgery for senile entropion. *Am J Ophthalmol* 5: 483–495, 1973.
34. Quickert MH: In Sorsby A (ed): *Modern Ophthalmology*, ed 2. London, Butterworth, 1972, vol 4, p 940.
35. Bercovici E, Hornblass A, Smith B: Cicatricial entropion. *Ophthal Surg* 8: 112, 1977.
36. Hornblass A, Bercovici E, Smith B: Senile entropion. *Ophthal Surg* 8: 47, 1977

CHAPTER 36

Facial Palsy

RALPH E. WESLEY, M.D., F.A.C.S.
C. GARY JACKSON, M.D., F.A.C.S.

Facial nerve palsy can be more devastating than the loss of any other single cranial nerve. The mask-like facial appearance becomes most exaggerated when only half the face laughs or smiles. Any facial expression accentuates the immobile half-face. Drooling or spillage of food from poor apposition of the buccal area to the lower teeth can force the individual to withdraw from social contact.

Brow droop and ectropion are frequently compounded by constant tearing. Or, the patient may have a dry eye so severe that artificial tears must constantly be within reach. The red, painful eye with blurred vision from poor eyelid closure may require that a portion of the eyelids be sewed closed.

Facial palsy constitutes such a severe assault upon that patient's function and appearance that depression, and even suicide, are imminent considerations. Early, accurate diagnosis combined with appropriate multidisciplinary medical and surgical therapy offer the best chance to spare patients the miseries of facial palsy.

This chapter provides information to understand and manage the multitude of ophthalmic derangements from facial palsy. With knowledge of the anatomy and pathophysiology of the facial nerve the ophthalmologist can also assist in reaching primary facial nerve diagnoses that might otherwise be overlooked or delayed.

ANATOMY AND FUNCTION OF THE FACIAL NERVE

Of the twelve cranial nerves, three are purely sensory nerves (I, II, and VIII) and five are purely motor nerves (III, IV, VI, IX, and XII). The four cranial nerves with mixed motor and sensory functions are cranial nerves V, VII, IX, and X. The facial nerve is perhaps the most complex of the cranial nerves. The separate functions of the facial nerve must be appreciated to understand the mechanisms of eye injury from facial nerve palsy.

The facial nerve has four major functions supplied by separate central nuclei: (*a*) *Facial motor nucleus* innervates muscles of facial expression including the orbicularis oculi. (*b*) *Superior salivatory nucleus*, via the pterygopalatine and submandibular ganglia, provides innervation to the lacrimal gland and the palatine glands. (*c*) *The nucleus solitarius* controls taste of the anterior two-thirds of the tongue. (*d*) *Trigeminal sensory nucleus* receives fibers of sensation to a small portion of the external ear. Of the estimated 7000 fibers of the facial nerve, motor fibers are said to comprise 58%, preganglionic fibers for tearing and salivation 24%, and fibers for taste 18% (1, 2).

The major functions of the facial nerve are mediated through four separate branches (Fig. 36.1): (*a*) the greater superficial petrosal nerve from the geniculate ganglion with parasympathetic innervation for tear secretion of the lacrimal gland, (*b*) a branch to the stapedius muscle from the mastoid segment, (*c*) chorda tympani from distal mastoid segment with combined functions of taste of the anterior two-thirds of the tongue and preganglionic parasympathetic fibers to the submandibular ganglion; (*d*) facial nerve at the stylomastoid foramen to innervate the muscles of facial expression, the platysma, stylohyoid, and posterior digastric muscles.

The functions of importance to the eye are the facial motor branch, which affects closure of the eye, and the greater superficial nerve required for lacrimation. After facial nerve injury, regenerating fibers of the chorda tym-

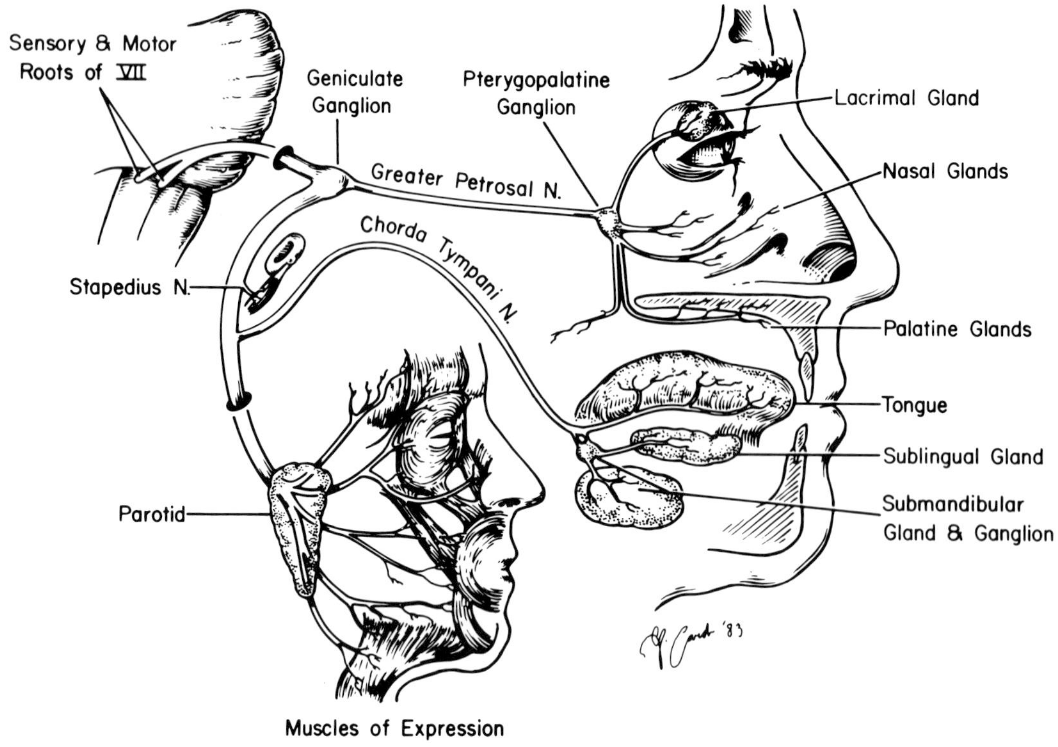

Figure 36.1. Functional anatomy of the facial nerve.

pani for salivation can become misdirected to the lacrimal gland, which causes gustatory tearing, or "crocodile tears", with chewing.

The facial nerve leaves the cerebellopontine angle just caudal to the trigeminal nerve and adjacent to the nervus intermedius to enter the internal auditory canal ensheathed by a finger of meninges for a variable length (3–5). The facial nerve and the nervus intermedius become completely integrated (6) within the internal auditory canal but separated from the vestibular nerve by a ridge of bone, "Bill's bar", an important anatomical landmark for the otoneurosurgeon.

The facial nerve traverses the the longest intraosseous course of any cranial nerve. Within the temporal bone the nerve travels 30 mm, makes two distinct bends, and gives off three branches prior to exiting at the stylomastoid foramen. The *labrinthine segment* runs from the fallopian canal to the geniculate ganglion where a sharp posterior genu occurs. The greater and lesser superficial petrosal nerves arise from this first segment and proceed anteriorly. The *tympanic segment*, beginning at the geniculate ganglion runs posteriorly, remaining in the same horizontal plane and forming the superior landmark of the oval window. Posteriorly the tympanic segment makes a gentle change from horizontal to vertical, forming the final segment called the *mastoid (vertical) segment*, which courses vertically down to exit the temporal bone at the stylomastoid foramen. From the mastoid segment arises the nerve to the stapedius muscle and the chorda tympani to the anterior tongue and the submandibular ganglion.

The stylomastoid foramen lies between the mastoid tip and the styloid process, a site used for injection of local anesthesia to block the facial nerve during intraocular surgery. Outside the temporal bone the facial nerve courses through the parotid gland to innervate temporofacial and cervicofacial musculature with numerous anastomoses and terminal contacts.

Within the brainstem, the facial motor nucleus supplying the upper facial musculature receives innervation from both sides of the brain. The facial motor nucleus controlling the lower face receives innervation only from the contralateral cerebral cortex. Lesions involving upper motor lesions of the cortex classically spare the upper face since that part of the facial motor nucleus has bilateral innervation. Lower motor neuron lesions involving the facial nucleus involve both upper and lower face. Disease within the mastoid segment, however, can cause a facial palsy sparing the upper face that can be misinterpreted as an upper motor neuron lesion (7).

CLINICAL DIAGNOSIS OF FACIAL NERVE PROBLEMS

The evaluation of facial nerve paralysis requires more than a search for the nature and location of the offending lesion. The crucial decision for the neurootologist is the physiologic condition of the facial nerve. The prognosis for return of the facial nerve function has been a major determinant with regards to the controversial subject of surgical facial nerve decompression. Radiologic techniques are particularly useful in defining the location and etiology of neoplastic lesions; electrodiagnostic and topognostic testing best reflect the physiologic condition of the facial nerve.

A battery of tests are required to accomplish all the objectives of facial nerve diagnosis. The evaluation of a patient with Bell's palsy may require an initial radiologic evaluation to rule out tumor, electrophysiologic or topognostic testing to prognosticate return of function, and serial electrophysiologic testing to verify a clinical course expected of Bell's palsy.

RADIOLOGY

Radiologic techniques are most helpful in evaluation for tumor. An experienced radiologist using high-resolution computerized axial tomography (CT) with and without contrast can demonstrate gross anatomy and pathology of the facial nerve from brainstem to the face in exquisite detail. In our center, CT has completely supplanted pleuridirectional polytomography of the temporal bone as the main diagnostic inquisitor of this area. Though plain films (Schuller, Townes, and Stenvers projections) can be used for screening, CT scanning can evaluate areas within the temporal bone such as the geniculate ganglion.

ELECTRODIAGNOSIS

Since first introduced in 1872 (8), electrodiagnostic testing of nerve excitability has become the dominant format in physiologic testing to form a prognosis for return of function versus deterioration of the nerve. Of the many electrophysiologic facial nerve tests, the maximum stimulation test (MST) has been favored based on accuracy in predicting nerve denervation.

With the MST, the maximum stimulation that the patient can tolerate (based on pain) is qualitatively compared with the contralateral side. Even with a completely transsected facial nerve, peripheral nerve excitability characteristics do not begin to deteriorate for some 48–72 hours. The MST can then estimate facial nerve function with serial testing.

Electroneurogonography (ENOG), which has been a major advance, utilizes elaborate computerized analysis of compound action potentials (CAP) generated by suprathreshold stimulation. The comparison of the CAP amplitudes to the healthy side can be used for quantitative analysis of the degree of nerve degeneration. However, the requirement for elaborate test equipment with carefully controlled conditions have caused test-retest variability and controversy regarding the validity of the test.

TOPOGNOSTIC TESTS

The site of a facial nerve lesion can be implied by evaluating the separate facial nerve functions. These tests can be used to assess both the location and the degree of nerve injury. The most commonly employed are the lacrimation test, salivary flow, taste, and audiologic tests.

Lacrimation (Schirmer) Test

Of most importance, the Schirmer test determines the location of the lesion relative to the geniculate ganglion, a site of predilection for tumors. Intact lacrimation indicates a lesion beyond (distal to) the geniculate ganglion where parasympathetic fibers destined for the lacrimal gland leave the facial nerve via the greater superficial petrosal nerve. Reduced or absent tearing suggests a poor prognosis for return of facial nerve function; this prognosis has a reliability of greater than 90% (9, 10).

Salivary Flow

The salivary flow test, which involved cannulating Wharton's ducts to monitor the flow from the submandibular glands stimulated by lemon juice (11), can be used to localize the injury to VII between the geniculate ganglion and the origin of the chorda tympani from the mastoid segment of the facial nerve. The chorda tympani carries parasympathetic fibers to the salivary glands via the submandibular ganglion. The test can be painful, and the results inconsistent. Salivary flow testing remains in use because it senses facial denervation earlier than electrodiagnostic tests (12–16).

Taste

A history of smoking and the gender of the patient affect the test. The topognostic relationship to the facial nerve involves the entrance of taste fibers through the chorda tympani into the mastoid segment of the facial nerve.

Audiologic Tests

The nerve to the stapedial muscle, which dampens the excursions of the stapes in the middle ear, arises from the mastoid segment of the facial nerve. Standard audiologic impedance techniques can easily and objectively measure changes from loss of this nerve. The stapedial reflex test has localizing but not prognostic value (10, 17). Note, however, that dysacousis with facial palsy, formerly thought due to loss of the stapedial reflex, probably occurs as result of cochlear nerve involvement (10, 17, 18).

Auditory brainstem responses (ABR) have been employed in the diagnosis of facial nerve neoplasm (19), facial paralysis in the newborn (20), and in hemifacial spasm (21).

DISORDERS OF THE FACIAL NERVE

Understanding the diagnostic evaluation, natural history, and management of conditions that affect the facial nerve allows the ophthalmologist to tailor eye care to the needs of the individual patient. Clearly a facial palsy of short duration can be managed differently from a prolonged or permanent palsy. Conditions likely to affect lacrimation or interrupt corneal sensation will be more threatening to the eye than facial nerve lesions that cause simple facial motor palsy. This section describes the most important pathologic entitles causing facial palsy.

IDIOPATHIC FACIAL PARALYSIS (BELL'S PALSY)

Bell's palsy, the most frequent category of facial paralysis regardless of age or sex, has an incidence of approximately 20 cases per 100,000 persons per year (22–24). Bell's palsy by definition means an idiopathic facial palsy. When a diagnosis can be made, the condition is no longer considered Bell's palsy.

More females are affected during the second decade of life, and more males over 40 years of age are affected. Overall, both sexes are affected equally (22). The incidence in females increases threefold during pregnancy, with the highest risk occurring during the third trimester (25). No population or ethnic groups appear immune.

Bell's palsy usually occurs as a unilateral facial palsy of sudden onset that slowly improves over the following 6 months. Because Bell's palsy is a clinical diagnosis, variations from the natural history of the disease may suggest another etiology, such as occult neoplasm.

Peiterson (26) has reported experience with over 1000 patients over 15 years. None of his patients remained completely paralyzed though complete remission occurred in only 71% of his patients. Seven percent of patients achieved remission after 1 week, an additional 32% by the 2nd week, and 15% more by the 3rd week. Remission was rare between 3 weeks and 3 months after onset. Absence of remission by 6 months suggests a poor prognosis. Patients under 40 years had better recovery than older patients (33% remission in patients over 60 years of age).

Peculiar clinical features of Bell's palsy should be noted. Idiopathic facial palsy can occur as a polyneuropathy with pain (62%) (27), decreased lacrimation (11%), vestibular involvement (22–43%), and other trigeminal nerve signs (10–48%) (10). Nine nerve palsies can be seen in 19% of Bell's palsies. Sparing of forehead movement does not indicate a supranuclear lesion.

May (10) found an etiology of facial palsy in 20% of patients previously considered idiopathic. Slowly progressive palsy beyond 3 weeks with no return of function beyond 6 months should be considered tumor until proved otherwise. Facial hemispasm, myokymia, blepharospasm and other forms of hyperkinesia suggest neoplasm. A bilateral facial palsy rules out Bell's palsy, though in 6% of May's cases the palsy recurred on the other side. Cranial nerve VIII deficits can occur with Bell's palsy but suggest lesion of the internal auditory canal. Concomitant sixth nerve palsy occurs with lesions of the petrous apex; the jugular foramen syndrome (loss of IX, X, XI with or without XII) implicates a skull base tumor.

Theories regarding the etiology of Bell's palsy have not been accompanied by clinicopathologic corroboration. For many years ischemia was considered (28–32), but many investigators suspect a virus-induced inflammation of the facial nerve to be the etiology of Bell's palsy (9, 10, 33–42). The evidence remains largely circumstantial. Neurologic sequelae arise from viral illnesses such as polio, mumps, and Epstein-Barr viruses. Herpes zoster virus is a known cause of paralysis of the facial nerve (Ramsey-Hunt syndrome).

The higher prevelance of herpes simplex virus antibodies in Bell's palsy patients as measured by complement fixation and radioimmune assay (38) may indicate a reactivation of the simplex virus infection with transient demyelination of the facial nerve. Mulkeus, Bleeker, and Shroder (43) isolated herpes simplex virus from a nerve biopsy of a Bell's palsy patient. On the other hand, Adour (44) found an association of diabetes mellitus in 11% of 6384 patients studied. Other investigators have suggested a hypersensitivity phenomenon as the cause of Bell's palsy (45). Theories combining several etiologies have even been proposed (46). The etiology of Bell's palsy remains controversial and the subject of considerable investigation.

No therapy has been proved efficacious. The dispute rages between surgical decompression and medical corticosteroid treatment. The trend is from surgical decompression in favor of steroid therapy for idiopathic facial paralysis.

NEOPLASM

Between 5 and 15% (47–49) of facial palsy comes from tumors of the facial nerve or from extrinsic neoplasms such as meningiomas. The slow progression of facial palsy, fluctuating palsy, or facial hyperkinesis suggests neoplasm. Sudden onset similar to Bell's palsy has been described (50), however. Early tumor diagnosis depends upon a high index of suspicion; delay in diagnosis occurs frequently.

Facial nerve neoplasms have a predilection for the geniculate ganglion (50–53). Surgical exploration serves to establish a diagnosis as well as to extirpate the lesion. In one study, only 40% of patients (50) had a correct preoperative diagnosis. Benign intratemporal processes include meningioma (50–53), glomus tumors (54, 55), and primary neural tumors (49–53, 56–61). Loss of nerves IX, X, XI, with or without loss of XII (jugular foramen syndrome), suggests meningioma, glomus tumor, or other skull base lesion. Decreased corneal reflex indicates cerebropontine angle involvement of the trigeminal nerve.

The facial nerve impedes access to glomus tumors during skull base surgery. Nerve transposition or selective severance with reanastomosis are common options. Transposing the facial nerve from the fallopian canal disrupts the intrinsic blood supply and causes a brief paralysis that is followed by recovery. With intentional surgical severance and reanastomosis, the palsy is more prolonged. In rare instances, the facial nerve must be sacrificed and reanimation accomplished by direct repair or by interpositional nerve grafting.

Acoustic neuroma rarely causes facial palsy preoperatively. Surgical exposure for complete removal of the acoustic neuroma may require manipulation of the facial nerve, mobilization of the facial nerve out of the bony canal, severance of the facial nerve with direct reanastomosis, partial removal of the facial nerve followed by a segmental nerve graft, or excision of an amount of nerve with the acoustic tumor that precludes any type of facial nerve repair.

With small-to medium-sized (1–2.9 cm) acoustic tumors, facial function can be preserved in over 90% of cases; with tumors larger than 7 cm facial nerve function remains in only 66% (62, 63). The occasional paralysis with smaller tumors tends to be short term and is followed by good recovery. With large tumors, the palsy tends to be prolonged, the recovery of function less satisfactory, and the association with decreased lacrimation and reduced corneal sensation more frequent.

Malignant tumors of the external auditory canal, squamous cell carcinoma, and adenoid cystic carcinoma can extend into the temporal bone and cause facial palsy. Metastic lesions from the orbit, lung, breast, and kidney occur much less commonly (50–53). Facial palsy from malignant gland tumors carries a grave prognosis and requires radical therapy.

Facial paralysis from tumor tends to be long term. Nerve reanastomosis, interposition grafting, or facial reanimation is often necessary.

HERPES ZOSTER OTICUS (RAMSEY-HUNT SYNDROME)

Herpes zoster can cause a painful facial palsy called the *Ramsey-Hunt syndrome.* The palsy usually occurs with greater severity and a more frequent association with generalized central nervous system effects than Bell's palsy. Exposure keratits from ectropion and lagophthalmos are common. Herpetiform vesicles at the external ear canal establish the diagnosis. Due to the severity of the palsy, surgical decompression of the facial palsy has been more popular than treatment with corticosteroids.

MELKERSON-ROSENTHAL SYNDROME

Vasomotor instability from autonomic dysfunction has been postulated (64–67) to cause episodes of facial paralysis with nonpitting facial edema, swelling of the lip, and a fissured tongue known as the *Melkerson-Rosenthal syndrome.* Migraine headaches and other cranial nerve palsies are associated with this syndrome (64–67). The clinical presentation can mimic Bell's palsy, except the facial paralysis may recur on the same or opposite side.

TRAUMA

Injuries to the facial nerve usually arise iatrogenically during surgery or from catastrophic head trauma. Electrodiagnostic testing can suggest the extent of injury with temporal bone fracture. Immediate onset of paralysis after injury indicates a poor prognosis for return of facial nerve function. Exploration of the nerve for primary repair may be necessary.

INFECTION

Facial nerve palsy from acute otitis media has become a rarity with the advent of antibiotic therapy—occurring in less than 1% or less of cases (68–70). Prompt resolution can be expected with antibiotic therapy.

Chronic otitis media causes facial palsy four to five times more commonly than acute otitis media (71–73). Bone destruction from cholesteotoma can affect the facial nerve by infiltration, compression, and infection. Surgical excision is most often required.

A condition known as *malignant external otitis*, with a mortality rate as high as 50% (74, 75), arises in patients compromised by metabolic, hematologic, or immunologic conditions. Medical treatment with antibiotics is the recommended therapy. The facial nerve function can recover in 50% of the survivors.

PEDIATRIC FACIAL PARALYSIS

Bell's palsy is the most common diagnosis when facial palsy occurs in children from newborn to age 18. In one study 42% of cases (76) were idiopathic. Etiologies of pediatric facial palsies include wide-ranging categories, though a diagnosis can be reached more frequently than with adults (77, 78). Hematopoietic derangements, neoplasms, birth trauma, and immune disorders can cause loss of facial function.

Traumatic neonatal facial palsy occurs most often with an uncomplicated forceps delivery. The lateral anatomy of the stylomastoid foramen makes the nerve vulnerable to intrauterine compression injury from the maternal sacrum on the involved face (79, 80) during prolonged, difficult labor. Physical findings may include ecchymosis, tics, synkinesis without other craniofacial abnormalities. Temporal bone x-rays demonstrating a fracture confirm the diagnosis. Neonatal facial palsy from congenital malformation has a poor prognosis since no treatment exists. However, Smith (81) reported 41 of 45 neonates with traumatic facial palsy had complete return of function.

Osseous disorders such as McCune-Albright syndrome, monostotic fibrous dysplasia, and osteopetrosis can cause an acquired, progressive facial palsy in children (82). Congenital cholesteotoma can cause facial palsy. Voorhees and associates (83) have reported the association of pediatric facial palsy and hypertension. The most common congenital facial palsy seen by the ophthalmologist is the *Möbius syndrome* due to a hypoplasia of the facial motor nucleus and the abducens nucleus. These children, who have mask-like faces and esotropia without diplopia from the congenital lateral rectus palsies, may have cardiac defects as well (82).

CEREBROVASCULAR ACCIDENTS

Most nuclear and supranuclear facial paralysis comes from cerebrovascular abnormalities though neoplasms and trauma can produce similar effects. Most strokes are supranuclear, involving the corticobulbar tracts. Since that part of the facial motor nucleus innervating the upper face has innervation from both sides of the brain, facial palsy from cerebrovascular accident usually produces a lower facial weakness and spares the forehead and upper eyelid orbicularis muscle. Consequently, facial palsy from stroke may be much better tolerated by the patient with regard to ocular symptoms than a transient Bell's palsy involving both the upper and lower half of the face.

With an upper motor lesion and intact facial motor nucleus, involuntary contraction of the muscle of facial expression may be accomplished by extrapyramidal tracts. A patient with complete hemifacial palsy may have an intact spontaneous grin through extrapyramidal circuits.

FACIAL NERVE REPAIR AND FACIAL REANIMATION

The size and location of a tumor may prevent even the most skilled surgeon from achieving the goal of complete tumor removal without damage to the facial nerve. Direct microsurgical repair of the cut ends of the nerve should be performed during the initial procedure. If the nerve ends cannot be rejoined, possibly because some of the facial nerve was removed with the tumor, a segment of nerve graft can be interposed microsurgically to reconstitute the facial nerve. In cases in which nerve repair cannot be accomplished, techniques of facial reanimation such as facial-hypoglossal anastomosis can be performed as described below.

NERVE REGENERATION

With injured facial nerves six major factors (84) affect the outcome of regeneration: the cause of the paralysis, the location of the lesion, the cross-sectional area and length of the damaged segment, the duration between injury and treatment (or regeneration), problems with faulty regeneration, and surgical technique. During regeneration, the proximal axons must grow distally within appropriate endoneurial sheaths to function effectively.

If axons originally innervating secretion of the submandibular glands grow down endoneurial sheaths to the lacrimal gland, the patient will have inappropriate tearing during mastication. With nerve repair or nerve grafting, regenerating axons may be misdirected into epineurial or perineurial tissue, which constitutes wasted regeneration and causes neuroma formation. Return of nerve function can easily require 6–12 months even after meticulous nerve repair. With prolonged delay in nerve repair, scarring and shrinkage of the distal neural segment reduces the likelihood of axons growing properly into the distal endoneurial tubes.

When the facial nerve cannot be repaired, dynamic rather than static techniques are recommended. The ideal results of facial reanimation would include facial tone, symmetry both at rest and with voluntary motion, functional control of eye and oral musculature, mimetic function, and minimal fiber misdirection. At 18 months after a facial nerve injury, nerve repair should generally be deferred in favor of facial reanimation techniques (85). Reanimation techniques combined with procedures such as masticatory muscle transfer and reimplantation can give good functional recovery in cases with poor prognosis from excessive delay in nerve repair.

NERVE SUBSTITUTION

With nerve substitution techniques, a normal nerve is completely or partially excised and reanastomosed to the distal facial nerve segment to innervate the facial musculature. In the spinal accessory–facial anastomosis, the posterior half of the eleventh cranial nerve is attached to the distal facial segment. Preserving the anterior portion of the spinal accessory nerve prevents total denervation of the trapezius muscle. Synkinetic movements with shoulder contractions are difficult to attain; lower face recovery is better than upper, and best results are obtained if performed with 2–3 months after injury (86).

The facial-hypoglossal anastomosis can reliably provide reinnervation of the facial nerve (87–90). The nerves match well in size. The nerves can be reapproximated without tension. Tongue atrophy may occur to varying degrees, though effects on chewing, speaking, and swallowing are usually minimal. Facial tone and balance return reliably. Forehead reanimation is least satisfactory.

Patients with the facial-hypoglossal anastomosis may experience a learning or functional adaptation spontaneously. Substitution of XII for VII occurs through some poorly understood brainstem mechanisms linking the facial and hypoglossal nuclei (87). The patients seem to develop spontaneous facial expression not associated with conscious, voluntary tongue movement on the involved side.

Cross facial nerve grafting, neuromuscular island pedicles, muscle transfer, free muscle grafting, and free muscle nerve grafts with neurovascular anastomosis may be used alone or in combination with procedures such as the facial-hypoglossal anastomosis to correct an individual's deficits.

OPERATIVE EXPOSURE OF VII

The definitive management of facial nerve pathology requires surgical exposure from the brainstem to the peripheral musculature. This section describes the techniques of facial nerve exploration and the application of each method.

Transmastoid Exposure

The mastoid approach through a postauricular incision can expose the mastoid (vertical) and/or tympanic (horizontal) facial nerve segments while still preserving hearing. The nerve can frequently be exposed from the geniculate ganglion to the mastoid foramen during a procedure as brief as 45 minutes. Most otolaryngologists perform this procedure.

Middle Fossa Exposure

Exposure proximal to the geniculate ganglion requires the special skills of the neurootologist. The middle cranial fossa approach can be used to expose the meatal (internal auditory canal), labyrinthine, and intracranial segments while preserving hearing. This approach combined with the mastoid exposure can provide access to the whole nerve and still preserve hearing.

With a middle fossa craniotomy through the squamous portion of the temporal bone, the facial nerve is exposed from above rather than from below. The temporal lobe is elevated, and the temporal bone overlying the proximal segments of the proximal facial nerve is drilled away with the use of microsurgical technique. Operating in the middle fossa, one of the most complex areas of human anatomy, is extremely difficult though this procedure in experienced hands is technically elegant. This technique provides limited exposure of the cerebellopontine angle.

Translabyrinthine Surgery

The transmastoid approach with labyrinthinectomy can expose the proximal segments of the facial nerve in cases in which hearing cannot be preserved: acoustic nerve tumor surgery or following trauma. With microsurgical drilling through the vestibular labyrinth, the meatal segment of the facial nerve can be identified and the lateral internal auditory canal used for precise orientation of the facial nerve anatomy. With the posterior fossa dura excised and the cerebellum retracted, this approach provides excellent exposure of the cerebellopontine angle.

Retrolabyrinthine Exposure

Using a postauricular incision and transmastoid approach, the surgeon can expose cranial nerves V–XII. The procedure involves limited risks to the patient and preserves hearing. This approach provides better exposure to the cerebellopontine angle than the middle cranial fossa approach in cases in which hearing can be preserved.

MECHANISMS OF OCULAR SYMPTOMS FROM FACIAL PALSY

Several interrelated mechanisms cause ocular symptoms from facial palsy. Most ocular deterioration after facial palsy comes from drying and exposure. Interruption of the facial motor fibers to the orbicularis oculi muscle causes exposure via ectropion, poor closure with attempted eyelid closure, and a poor blink that inadequately spreads tears across the cornea. Interruption of fibers to the greater superficial petrosal nerve reduces secretion of tears.

With exposure and drying of the eye, the cornea develops painful keratitis with associated conjunctival injection, and decreased vision. The increased mucous production that accompanies a dry eye forms a stagnant culture medium that is undisturbed by the normal cleansing action of flowing tears and blinking eyelids. Patients with dry eyes have decreased resistance to infection due to reduced lysozymes and betazymes (91) found in natural tears. If the cornea dries, breaks in the epithelium leave the cornea vulnerable to bacterial and fungal ulceration.

Epiphora can occur by several mechanisms. A dry eye can cause reflex hypersecretion. Ectropion of the lower eyelid can leave the conjunctiva exposed, which results in a watery eye. Outward rotation of the lacrimal punctum prevents tears from entering the lacrimal system. Failure of the lacrimal system to drain tears frequently comes from weakened orbicularis muscle rather than lacrimal obstruction. A paralyzed or weakened orbicularis muscle fails to provide the dynamic pumping action required for the canaliculus to drain tears.

After proximal injuries to the facial nerve, fibers to submaxillary glands may regenerate in a misdirected fashion to innervate the lacrimal gland. Upon mastication, the patient experiences profuse tearing, sometimes called "crocodile tears."

Eye pain usually comes from drying of the cornea and the conjunctiva. Pain can also come from a secondary iritis. The patient with facial palsy can develop anterior uveitis in which the pain, decreased vision, and photophobia may be misdiagnosed as arising from exposure keratitis. The most dreaded complication is the corneal ulcer. In chronically irritated eyes, a corneal ulcer may not cause sufficient symptoms to alert the patient that a drastic deterioration has occurred.

Acoustic neuromas do not frequently cause facial palsy preoperatively, but patients with facial palsy after removal of acoustic neuroma frequently require ophthalmic care. The cardinal ophthalmic signs of acoustic neuroma, nystagmus, decreased corneal reflex, and papilledema correlate with tumor size (92). Tumors causing nystagmus were at least 2 cm, those causing a diminished corneal reflex were at least 2.5 cm, and neoplasms causing subjective symptoms of papilledema were at least 4.0 cm. The size of the tumor also correlates with the prognosis for return of facial function (61, 62).

Patients with cerebellopontine angle tumors, such as acoustic neuromas, may have corneal anesthesia from loss of trigeminal nerve function. Though this may spare the patient the sensation of the irritated eye, the combination of absent fifth and seventh nerve function eliminates most ocular protective mechanisms. The patient with facial palsy with decreased tearing and absent corneal sensation is the highest-risk patient for corneal ulceration, perforation, and loss of the eye.

The loss of trigeminal nerve function reduces corneal viability as well as corneal sensation much like a muscle loses with motor paralysis. The denervated cornea is more easily damaged. Healing is slower, Defenses to infection are reduced and there is reduced tear production.

Decreased vision from exposure keratitis can severely affect the patient's vocation. Patients who use ointments to prevent ocular drying nearly always have some blurring of vision. Even with ointment applied only at bedtime, the next day vision may fluctuate abruptly as ointment floats across the optical axis.

The patient may be without symptoms for several days or weeks after the onset of facial paralysis. Then irritation and keratitis develop to the full extent. Levine (91) has postulated that with anesthetic cornea some nutritive factor may be present that is eventually exhausted. Regardless of the cause, the full degree of decompensation may take a few weeks to develop. Many months later, the cornea may adjust partially to the exposure and drying much like the cornea adjusts to a contact lens.

OPHTHALMIC EXAMINATION

Certain aspects of the ophthalmic examination deserve particular emphasis to obtain most significant information for the diagnosis and management of facial palsy. The essentials include the patient's complaints, the clinical setting of the facial palsy, and the physical findings of most significance: visual acuity, degree of facial palsy, fullness of closure during sleep and on blinking, presence of corneal sensation, existence of a Bell's phenomenon, ocular motility with emphasis on lateral rectus function, and corneal or conjunctival inflammation.

In the hospital setting, the eye examination must frequently be modified according to the patient's condition and the available equipment. An ophthalmoscope set at +20.00 allows for close corneal examination. A cotton-tipped applicator substitutes for the anesthesiometer. A near card may replace the distant visual-acuity chart.

The clinical history determines management; a patient with Bell's idiopathic facial palsy, a congenital palsy, and facial palsy after tumor removal must have different treatment regimens. With palsy after tumor removal, information from the operating surgeon can be helpful in understanding the prognosis for return of facial function. Was the nerve simply stretched at surgery? Was the facial nerve difficult to separate from the tumor? Was the nerve resutured primarily? Was a nerve graft interposed? Will additional procedures such as facial nerve–hypoglossal reanastomosis be required? Management of eye manifestations will reflect the otologist's appraisal of prognosis.

In consulting on patients with Bell's palsy, an assessment should be made as to whether the facial palsy is consistent with idiopathic facial palsy, or could occult tumor be a reasonable suspicion? Facial palsy progressing beyond 3 weeks, no return of function by 6 months, recurrence of the facial palsy, facial hyperkinesis or dyskinesis, and jugular foramen or apex syndromes suggest tumor.

The patient's complaints help focus the examination into particular problem areas. The most serious pitfall, however, is the patient who has no symptoms due to lack of corneal sensation. Changes in vision usually come from exposure keratitis, but ophthalmic ointment can blur vision to hand motion. A more accurate visual acuity can be obtained after the patient blinks several times to clear ointment from the visual axis.

Evaluation of eyelid closure should include the completeness of the blink. Eyelid closure in postoperative patients can be deceiving. Facial swelling and the pressure of a head dressing on the brow can temporarily increase lid closure. A friend or relative can be asked to observe whether the degree of lagophthalmos during sleep varies from that observed with voluntary closure. The Bell's phenomenon should be determined to assess how well the eye may be protected from lagophthalmos. Corneal sensation should be noted.

Note should be made of brow droop, ectropion, lower punctum position, tearing, lacrimal lake configuration, and fissure size. Motility evaluation should include particular attention to possible nystagmus or sixth nerve weakness after tumor resection.

Corneal drying usually becomes most noticeable along the inferior cornea where the eyelid fails to blink during the day or fails to provide full closure at night. Fluorescein dye can highlight the area when viewed through a slitlamp with a blue light. With keratitis sicca, rose bengal will show severity of the problem much better than fluorescein. Fluorescein stains only break in the epithelium. Rose bengal stains devitalized cells of both the cornea and conjunctiva. The Schirmer test of tear secretion can be used to predict the severity and duration of the keratitis sicca as well as the prognosis for the facial palsy (9, 10).

Redness and discharge can occur with external infection or keratitis sicca. Occasionally, the persistent reddened eye comes from iritis. Anterior uveitis can be difficult to diagnose without a slitlamp. Pupil inequality, photophobia, and decreasing visual acuity may be minimal and go unnoticed in a patient with exposure keratitis. Failure to recognize the patient requiring topical steroid treatment for iritis may allow the painful uveitis to result in anterior synechiae.

The comprehensive evaluation of patients with tearing should include a Schirmer's test to rule out reflex tearing from a dry eye, observation of eyelid and punctual position, and Jones testing to determine lacrimal physiology and patency.

MANAGEMENT OF OPHTHALMIC MANIFESTATIONS OF FACIAL PALSY

Patient education and patient compliance determine the success or failure of treatment in numerous cases. The patient must become a part of the treatment team—titrating the amount of artificial tears or ointment necessary for protection of the eyes, identifying environmental factors that may cause ocular irritation, and recognizing problems that may require immediate attention of the ophthalmologist.

Some patients have an eye that remains red and irritated with blurred vision despite medical and surgical therapy. These patients need compassion and encouragement to face perhaps the most demanding physical and emotional threat of their lives. The Acoustic Neuroma Association[a] can be a valuable source of information and support for patients with facial palsy. The association newsletter provides patients with helpful information and valuable emotional support.

The most frequent pitfall in management of facial palsy is failure to recognize involvement of the lacrimal secretory fibers. The individual develops ocular problems out of proportion to the decreased closure or reduced blink excursion. The greatest frustration comes from the variable results of treatment, similar to the frequent variance between objective ophthalmic findings and subjective patient complaints in facial palsy. The most feared complication is corneal ulceration, which can occur early or late despite reasonable follow-up.

The ophthalmologist managing eye care with facial palsy should be familiar with the numerous medical and surgical options for treatment. Ideally, therapy should be approached with a logical progression, but the problem patient who suddenly responds to punctal occlusion or to the simple addition of a bedside humidifier at night underscores the need to prevail in trying all reasonable alternatives.

NONSURGICAL OPHTHALMIC MANAGEMENT OF FACIAL PALSY

Therapy for facial palsy involves methods to add more moisture to the eyes or techniques to prevent dissipation of existing tear film. The first and most important part of

[a] Acoustic Neuroma Association, Box 398, Carlisle, PA, 17013-0398.

eye care with facial palsy consists of artificial tears and lubricating ointments. Ointments provide longer-lasting effects, but blur the vision. Artificial tears allow for clear vision but may require application as often as every 15 minutes. Frequently the use of ointment at bedtime provides lasting coverage from exposure during sleep, and the use of tears during the day allows the patient to function.

The most common mistake in medical management is failure to educate patients that they can use the artificial tears and ointments as often as necessary rather than follow a schedule of application. A low Schirmer test identifies patients who will likely have prolonged, severe problems from exposure. With increased mucous production in cases of keratitis sicca, infection frequently occurs, which requires topical administration of antibiotics intermittently.

Some patients have such severe irritation with the dry exposed eye that topical steroids must be used for relief. Steroids are used reluctantly, with close supervision due to the risk of bacterial and fungal infections in patients with compromised ocular defenses: decreased blink, decrease tear film, and decreased closure.

Modification of the patient's occupation or living situation may help, i.e., eliminating a dusty, dry, or windy environment. A humidifier may reduce ocular drying. Pateints should avoid ocular irritants such as aerosol sprays, eyelid cosmetics, chlorinated swimming pool water, and air conditioners.

Lacriserts, a wafer inserted into the cul de sac that slowly releases artificial tears, can be used in patients with minimal to moderate dry eye. Lacriserts usually provide improvement for a few months until the patients reject them. Still, the short-term relief can be refreshing to the patient.

Therapeutic soft contact lenses can also provide dramatic short-term relief, though patients eventually find them intolerable. The lenses, easily lost or damanged, are expensive to replace. The therapeutic contact lens can serve as a temporary bandage in patients with neurotropic keratitis (91).

Occlusive bubble shields can be worn at night to reduce evaporation of natural or artificial tears. Bubbles become difficult to replace after adhesive has worn out; patients have difficulty finding a source of supply. Bubbles that attach onto the patient's glasses to prevent drying or reflex tearing during the day are also available. This attachment can allow many individuals to return to occupations they otherwise could not tolerate.

Tinted lenses can reduce the photophobia from keratitis. The tint required for bright light outdoors may require a separate set of lenses from that which will allow the patient relief of photophobia indoors under fluorescent lighting.

Taping the eyelids can correct irritation from ectropion. The tape should be applied across the lower eyelid, which can then be pulled upward and outward in a sweeping motion with the tape (Fig. 36.2).

Applying tape to the upper eyelid will reduce retraction and lagophthalmos. A ½ inch wide piece of steri strip can be applied vertically across the lid crease with the lid closed (Fig. 36.3, *A* and *B*). The tape will prevent the lid from opening fully (Fig. 36.3*C*). The blink will sweep over more of the cornea. At night lagophthalmos will be reduced. Tape procedures work best for short-term improvement, but some conscientious patients can obtain long-term relief.

When all else fails, the patient can usually find relief with a properly applied semipressure eyepad. Patching provides complete coverage of the conjunctiva and cornea, which prevents evaporation of natural tears. To prevent applying the patch directly onto the cornea, one must hold down the paralyzed upper eyelid while taping the patch in place.

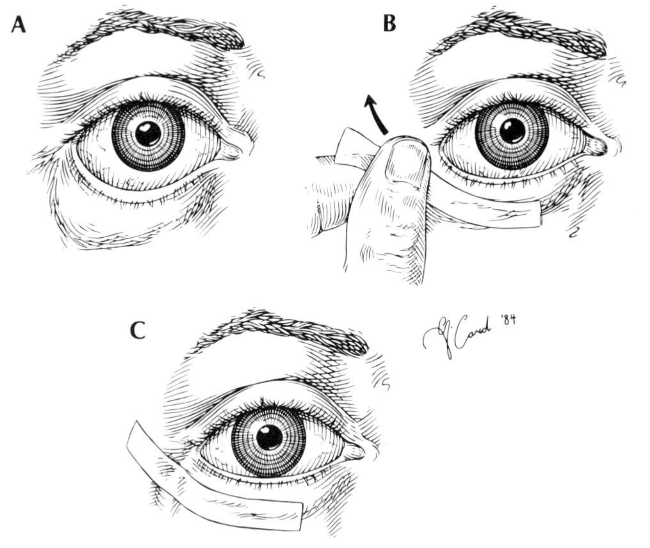

Figure 36.2. *A*, Ectropion and exposure from facial palsy. *B*, Tape applied to lower lid and pulled outward and upward past lateral canthus. *C*, Correction of ectropion with tape (From *Laryngoscope*).

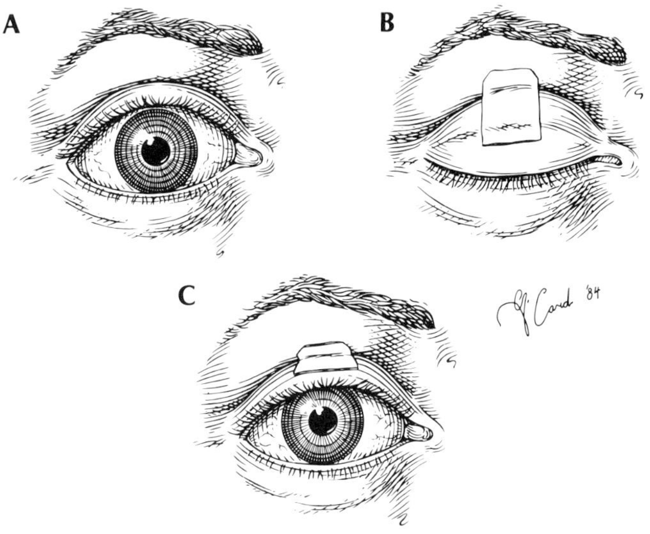

Figure 36.3. *A*, Eye with retraction and exposure from facial palsy. *B*, With eyelid pulled downward, ½ inch piece of Steri strip applied to eyelid. *C*, Reduced exposure and fissure after placement of tape.

SURGICAL MANAGEMENT OF OPHTHALMIC MANIFESTATIONS OF FACIAL PALSY

Tarsørrhaphy

The most conservative management of ophthalmic manifestations of facial palsy may require early surgical intervention. For the patient with facial palsy after acoustic tumor removal who has corneal anesthesia and decreased tearing, performing a lateral tarsorrhaphy provides a considerable margin of safety. The patient with Ramsey-Hunt syndrome (facial palsy from herpes zoster) deserves immediate ectropion repair due to the prognosis for prolonged facial palsy and severe exposure conjunctivitis and keratitis.

For short-term protection of the patient with decreased consciousness after surgery or trauma, nonreactive monofilament suture can be passed through the upper eyelid (Fig. 36.4*A*) and taped down onto the lower eyelid (Fig. 36.4*B*) for complete closure. The tape can be loosened for ocular examination or the administration of medication.

For longer-term closure, a mound of steri strips can be applied to the upper and lower eyelids with enough bulk that sutures can be placed through the steri strips rather than the patient's eyelid. This eliminates inflammation or infection from prolonged closure with sutures. The strips should be applied horizontally to build a mound much like a pyramid (Fig. 36.5*A*). Once several layers are applied, three 4-0 silk sutures can be passed through the tape, but not the patient's skin, for a tarsorrhaphy eyelid closure (Fig. 36.5*B*). The strips can be removed and resutured as needed. Applying benzoin lightly to the eyelid helps the tape to adhere firmly. Gluing the lids together has been reported (93). Cyanoacrylate functions better for total closure of the fissure than for partial closure such as a lateral tarsorrhaphy.

For the patient with lagophthalmos who cannot obtain relief from medical therapy, the lateral tarsorrhaphy can be a simple, effective procedure to reduce ocular discomfort. A 5 mm wide tarsorrhaphy at the lateral canthus generally reduces lagophthalmos by 70–80% and has a minimal cosmetic effect. The lateral tarsorrhaphy can be performed in the office or at the bedside. With return of facial function, the tarsorrhaphy can be separated (94).

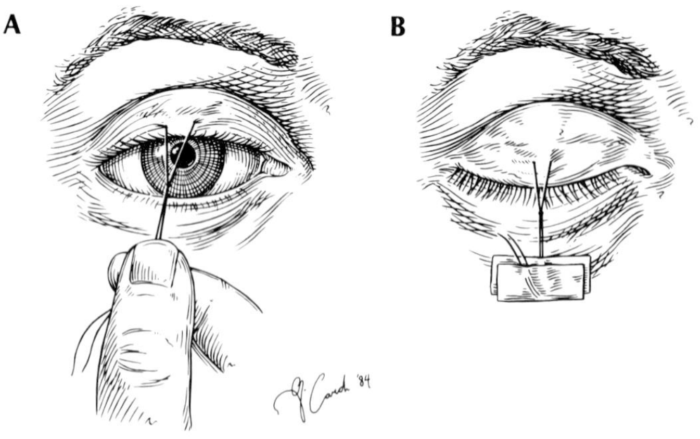

Figure 36.4. *A*, Suture passed through upper eyelid. *B*, Suture taped to lower eyelid accomplishes complete ocular protection; can be released for medication or examination.

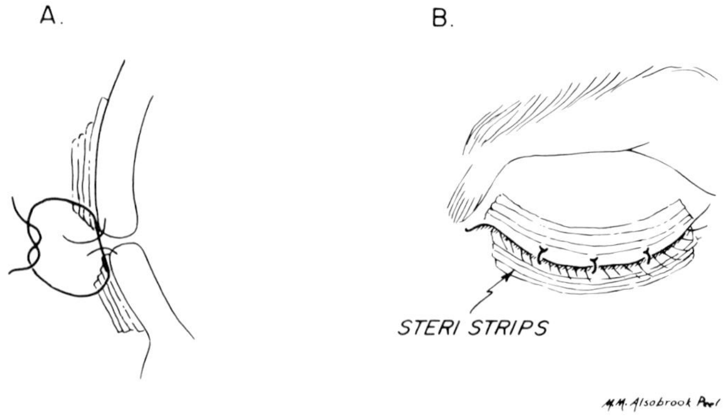

Figure 36.5. *A*, Steri strips applied horizontally to upper and lower eyelids to form mound of tape. *B*, 4-0 silk sutures passed through the tape require no anesthesia in performing temporary tarsorrhaphy.

To perform a lateral tarsorrhaphy, the surgeon applies corneal anesthetic drops and injects lidocaine with epinephrine through a 30 gauge needle into the lateral canthus. Approximately 5 mm from the lateral canthus, a No. 15 blade is used to incise the lid margin to a depth of 1 mm; then all the lid margin lateral to this mark is excised with Wescott scissors (Fig. 36.6*A*). Spatula needles on a doubled-armed 5-0 vicryl suture are then passed into the upper and lower tarsus from medial to lateral (Fig. 36.6*B*) to form a mattress suture to pull the lids together with the knot away from the cornea (Fig. 36.6*C*).

After tying the vicryl suture to bring the cut edges of tarsus together, the surgeon uses 6-0 plain gut running or interrupted sutures (Fig. 36.6*D*) for skin closure. No wound care or suture removal is required. This technique eliminates unsightly, inflammatory rubber bolsters commonly used for this procedure. With more severe keratitis or exposure, a larger tarsorraphy can be performed but results in a less pleasing cosmetic appearance.

If facial function returns, separating the tarsorrhaphy can be considered. The Schirmer test is used before performing this procedure to identify those patients that may be better off not undergoing the tarsorraphy separation in stages and those patients that would benefit from it. With a large lateral tarsorrhaphy, a partial separation can be performed to see how the patient tolerates the severance of the lid adhesions. Usually local infiltration with anesthesia and a generous snip with scissors will separate the previously formed adhesions. If a tarsorrhaphy tends to zipper close, the cut edge of mucous membrane should be sewed to the cut skin edge of the upper and lower lateral lids to prevent the lids from rejoining.

Management of Ectropion

Ectropion can be repaired with a lateral canthoplasty to avoid full-thickness eyelid resections that can cause lid notching and misdirected lashes. The lateral canthal approach provides more tightening of the lid per millimeter of tissue resected (95) and can be combined with a lateral tarsorrhaphy in patients with both ectropion and lagophthalmos.

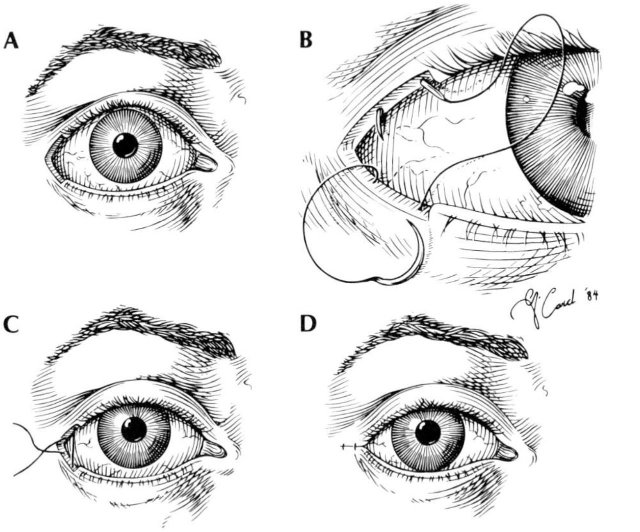

Figure 36.6. *A*, Eyelid with sag of lower lid and retraction of upper eyelid from facial palsy: Lateral lid margin excised. *B*, Double-armed 5-0 vicryl passed through upper and lower tarsal plates. *C*, Knot to be tied laterally. *D*, Final closure and position of eyelids after lateral tarsorrhaphy.

Lidocaine with epinephrine is injected into the lateral canthus, and incisions marked (Fig. 36.7*A*) and performed with a scapel splitting the upper and lower eyelids at the lateral canthus down to the periosteum and out 1 cm onto the skin (Fig. 36.7*B*). Remnants of the lower canthal tendon should be incised to loosen the lower eyelid (Fig. 36.7*C*). The lid should be pulled toward the lateral canthus to determine the necessary tightening. With ectropion from facial palsy at least 5 mm of lower lid should be excised (Fig. 36.7*D*).

The excess lower lid should be excised (Fig. 36.8*A*) and a permanent suture such as 4-0 polydek should be placed through the cut edge of tarsus and the remnants of the lateral canthal tendon-periosteum (Fig. 36.8*B*). The suture should be tied to tighten the lid (Fig. 36.8*C*), and the skin should be closed. The lid should be extremely tight at that conclusion of the procedure as the tissue will relax, giving functional and cosmetic correction of the ectropion (Fig. 36.8*D*).

Management of Lacrimal System

Patients with symptomatic drying sometimes achieve relief if the lacrimal system is occluded to prevent existing tears from draining away. These few patients can be provided dramatic relief by punctal occlusion. A hot spatula or cautery applied to the punctum on the affected side will provide temporary punctal occlusion. During the period of temporary closure, the patient determines whether the keratitis sicca is relieved. If successful, deep cautery can be applied to the punctum to provide permanent occlusion of the lacrimal drainage. An alternate method uses cyanoacrylate glue dropped into the punctum to provide a temporary occlusion of the lacrimal system, thus avoiding the use of cautery or the need for anesthesia (96).

When tearing or conjunctival inflammation arises from

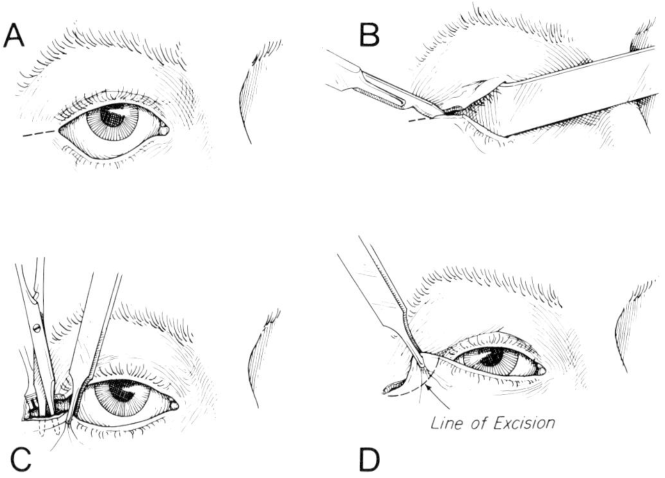

Figure 36.7. *A*, Sagging lower lid from facial palsy. *B*, Canthotomy carried down to periosteum. *C*, All remnants of lower canthal tendon incised. *D*, Lid on stretch to determine amount of resection.

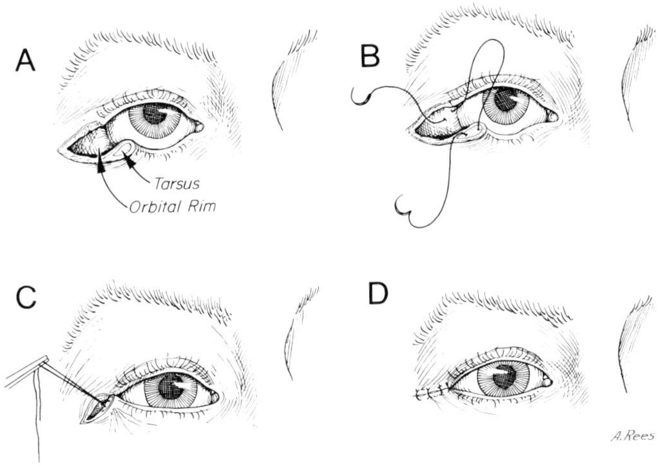

Figure 36.8. *A*, Exposed tarsus after excess lower eyelid excised. *B*, Suture passed through periosteum of lateral orbital rim and tarsal plate of lower eyelid. *C*, Suture tied to tighten eyelid. *D*, Final correction of ectropion.

ectropion in the medial lid segment, special procedures must be used to tighten the lid and rotate the lid inward. The Z-T plasty procedure can be performed with local anesthesia to tighten the lid, relax the skin at the medial canthus, and rotate the punctum inward to permit lacrimal drainage.

A Z-plasty is drawn at the medial canthus (Fig. 36.9*A*). The flaps are incised and undermined. With the posterior lamella of the lid exposed, a vertical full-thickness lid incision and a horizontal spindle of conjunctival lid retractors are marked for excision (Fig. 36.9*B*) similar to the "lazy T" operation (97). The resection is performed with scalpel and scissors, and edges are rejoined with 6-0 vicryl suture to tighten the lid and rotate the punctum inwardly (Fig. 36.9*C*). Finally the flaps of the Z-plasty are transposed, which causes vertical relaxation of the skin at

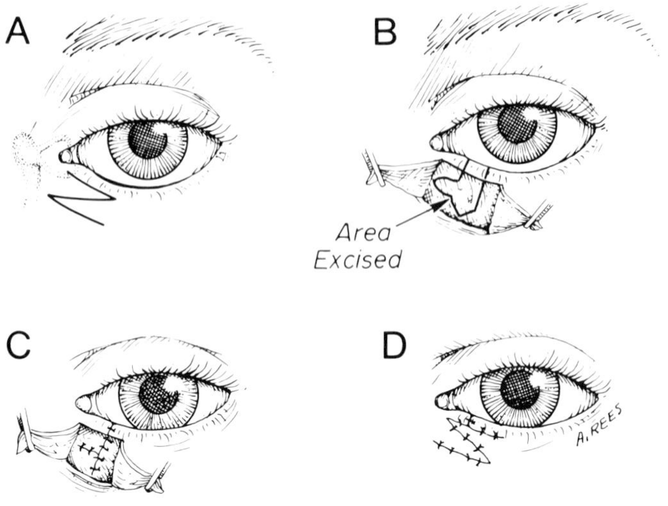

Figure 36.9. *A*, Z-plasty drawn on eyelid with medial ectropion with moderate vertical skin shortage. *B*, With Z-flaps prepared, full-thickness eyelid excision lateral to punctum and spindle of conjunctiva-lid retractors to be excised. *C*, Lid in normal position after horizontal tightening and inward rotation. *D*, Z-plasty flaps transposed for vertical relaxation of skin after correction of medial ectropion.

the medial canthus to facilitate inward rotation of the punetum (Fig. 36.9*D*).

The constant tearing that can occur after facial palsy may be corrected by procedures that eliminate ocular irritation from lagophthalmos or by eliminating lower eyelid malposition from ectropion. In some instances the tearing comes from the weakness or paralysis of the orbicularis muscle failing to provide physiologic suction for the lacrimal drainage system. The upper lacrimal system does not function as a passive drain; active suction induced by eyelid blinking carries tears away. In permanent or prolonged facial palsy with incapacitating epiphora, the lacrimal system must be bypassed with a Jones tube conjunctivodacryocystorhinostomy (CDCR) (98).

The original CDCR described by Jones has stood the test of time as the only effective, predictable lacrimal bypass procedure. The blown-glass drainage tubes may seem archaic, but successful drainage comes from the hydrophilic nature of glass to suck tears into the system. Numerous plastic and silicone tubes have been suggested, but the hydrophobic nature of these materials results in failure.

Prior to CDCR procedure a Schirmer test can identify patients with low tear secretion who have tearing on a reflex, irritant basis. These patients will be worsened with a device that drains existing tears away more quickly. Patients with facial palsy submitting to CDCR have a high rate of success because the medial canthus has a normal configuration that is undisturbed by tumor or trauma.

Two modifications of the original procedure are recommended: First, the tract for the glass tube should be made with a 3 mm dermatology punch. A large tract makes placement easier and reduces the tendency for late migration of the tube. Second, wrapping the tube with an epithelial structure such as a full-thickness buccal mucous membrane graft (99) reduces contraction around the tube. After 6 months the tube can be removed with an intact, epithelialized drainage path to the nose. Removal of the inferior portion of the caruncle, placing the tube at a 45° angle, and opening a large rhinostomy help to make the procedure successful.

Management of Lagophthalmos

The surgical treatment of lagophthalmos can be accomplished with several procedures. These techniques should be considered based upon the length of time the procedure may be required to function, the tightness of closure required for ocular comfort and safety, the action required to activate closure, and the cosmetic effect.

The *lateral tarsorrhaphy* may not provide complete closure but can be used well for short-term palsy as a reversible procedure or left permanently with no cumulative complications. The *palpebral spring procedure* provides a much tighter closure but has an increasing rate of extrusion with passage of time. The *temporalis muscle transposition procedure* uses autogenous material to provide tight closure without problems of late extrusion or infection, but a chewing action must be performed to activate the eyelids.

The *cerclage procedure* provides better closure than the lateral tarsorrhaphy but less effectively than the palpebral spring. The cerclage, though more complicated than a lateral tarsorrhaphy, is much simpler than the palpebral spring. For minimal lagophthalmos gold weights are easily applied to the upper eyelid. Lagophthalmos can be reduced with methods applied to other forms of eyelid retraction such as recessing the retractors of the upper eyelid, Müller's muscle, and the levator aponeurosis. The injection of botulinum toxin near the levator muscle will create a temporary, protective ptosis.

Patients with long-standing facial palsy who fail to obtain adequate closure from a lateral tarsorrhaphy can frequently benefit from a cerclage procedure that uses a 1 mm silicone rod. At surgery the cerclage spring should be tightened so the upper eyelid overrides the lower lid by 1–2 mm; postoperatively, the lid will most likely have 1–2 mm of lagophthalmos. Tighter closure will result in a higher extrusion rate. The technique described below provides medial and lateral fixation, which is important to providing good closure with reduced extrusion of the spring device.

With a protective lens in place, an incision is carried through the medial canthus to the external head of the medial canthal tendon. A lateral incision exposes the lateral orbital rim (Fig. 36.10*A*). First, the silicone rod is sewed into the medial canthal tendon using a small "eye needle" (Fig. 36.10*B*) and fixed with a separate nonabsorbable suture to secure the spring medially. A Wright fasciae needle is used to pass the silicone from the medial canthus to the lateral incision (Fig. 36.10*C*). Passage in the lower lid should be within a millimeter of the lid margin. Incisions in the mid portion of the lid will allow each arm of the silicone to be passed in shorter passes instead of all the way from lateral to medial canthus in one insertion.

After passage of the ends of the silicone rod to the lateral

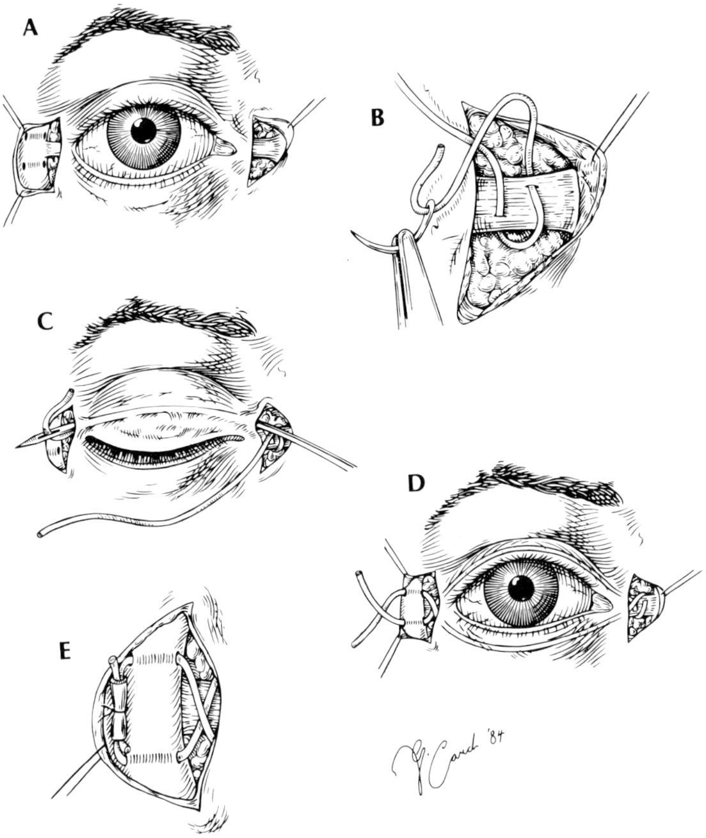

Figure 36.10. *A*, Lateral incision to expose orbit rim. Holes drilled horizontally through orbit rim above and below lateral canthal tendon. Medial incision exposes external head of medial canthal tendon. *B*, Silicone passed through medial canthal tendon. *C*, Fascia needle used to pass silicone to lateral incision. *D*, Silicone crossed at lateral canthus and passed through drill holes. *E*, Watzke sleeve and permanent suture used to fix silicone rod with enough tension that upper eyelid overrides lower eyelid 1–2 mm.

canthus, two holes are drilled through the lateral orbital rim just above and below the lateral canthal tendon. The upper silicone rod should be threaded through the lower hole and the lower rod through the upper hole (Fig. 36.10*D*). This crossing fixation at the lateral canthus establishes an upward and inward pull to the lower eyelid and a downward and inward pull to the upper eyelid.

The ends of the silicone rod are passed through a Watzke sleeve that is tightened so that the upper lid overrides the lower lid by approximately 2 mm. A permanent suture is tied in a clove hitch around the sleeve to prevent loosening (Fig. 36.10*E*).

The cerclage procedure provides immediate improvement in lagophthalmos. The sling can be adjusted under local anesthesia by opening the lateral canthal incision and adjusting the silicone at the Watzke sleeve. Complications include extrusion of the silicone, infection, granuloma formation, loosening, and ectropion. The cerclage can be used in patients who have had previous lateral tarsorrhaphies.

In patients requiring tigher closure than the cerclage a full, tight closure can be accomplished with a palpebral spring. Levine (91) has reported encouraging results; he used 0.011 inch orthodontic wire twisted with round-nosed pliers to form a loop fulcrum 5 mm in diameter. The spring can be implanted through incisions at the lateral orbital rim and the upper tarsus. A 16-gauge needle can be passed from the tarsal incision to the lateral orbital rim to advance the spring into place (Fig. 36.11*A*). The spring is formed to the curvature of the eyelids and fixed superiorly with permanent sutures at the fulcrum and superior end of the spring (Fig. 36.11*B*). A 0.4-mm thick Dacron velour fixed with a Gelform press is placed around the lower end of the spring (Fig. 36.11*C*) and sewed into the eyelid (Fig. 36.11*D*).

The spring can be adjusted under local anesthesia to correct tightness or laxity. Levine (91) has recommended these implants only on patients available for adequate follow-up as the springs have some risk of extrusion and ocular damage (100, 101). The spring can be an extremely effective method of providing relief for a year or so in cases suffering severely from exposure with facial palsy, though McCord (102) observes implanted devices eventually extrude.

To avoid the risk of extrusion of foreign material with long-term facial palsy, surgeons can produce closure of the eyelids using a transposition of temporalis muscle fasciae. In the long term this technique avoids infection, inflammation, or extrusion of the fasciae, but a chewing action is required for eyelid closure, the spring can loosen, and adjustment is more difficult than implanted springs.

A vertical incision at the hairline is carried down to expose the temporalis fascia (Fig. 36.12*A*). The strips of fascia for the sling are marked with methylene blue such

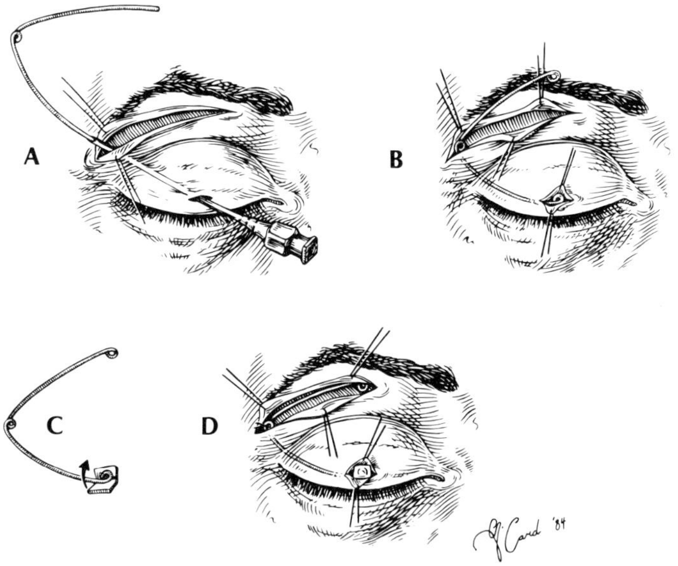

Figure 36.11. Insertion of palpebral spring. *A*, No. 16 gauge needle used to advance palpebral spring from lateral rim incision into central eyelid incision. *B*, Position of spring prior to fixation and adjustment of tension. *C*, Dacron velour placed over eyelid portion of spring to prevent extrusion. *D*, Final fixation of spring with sutures superiorly and velour inferiorly.

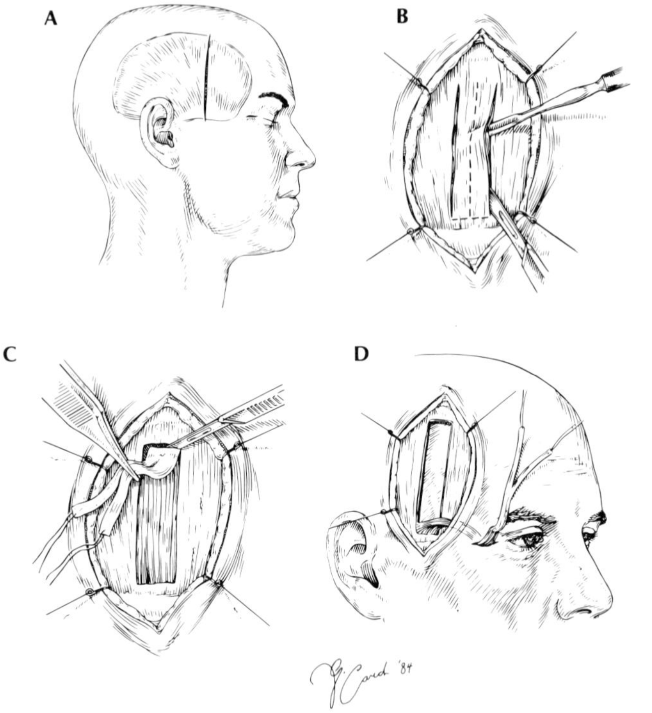

Figure 36.12. *A*, Incision for access to temporal fasciae. *B*, Temporalis fasciae incised to form with base still attached to temporalis muscle superiorly. *C*, Temporalis muscle flap prepared with fasciae still attached. *D*, Muscle and fasciae passed through tunnel to lateral canthal incision.

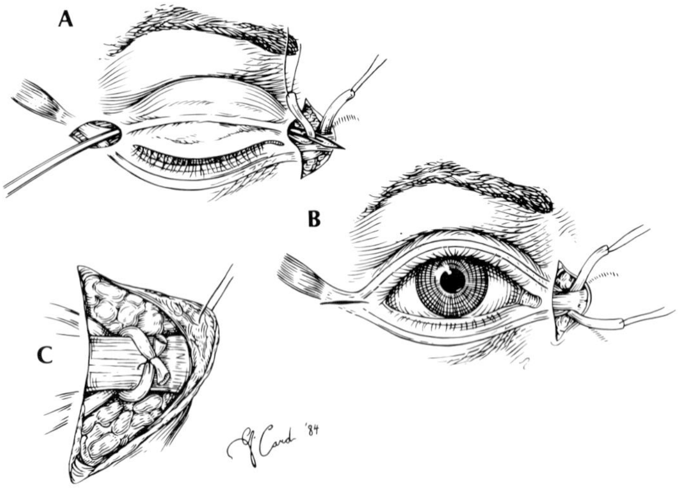

Figure 36.13. *A*, Fasciae should be passed closer to the lid margin in the lower eyelid. *B*, Fasciae passed behind medial canthal tendon. *C*, Final fixation of fasciae to medial canthal tendon after adjusting tautness of the sling.

that the attached base of the fascia will be left superiorly (Fig. 36.12*B*). Once the strips of fascia have been freed inferiorly, the frontalis muscle should be freed from the epicranium (Fig. 36.12*C*). An incision is made at the lateral canthus for passage of the temporalis muscle-fascia complex (Fig. 36.12*D*).

A separate incision should be made at the medial canthus to expose the external head of the medial canthal tendon. A Wright fascia needle is used to pass the separate ends of the fascia from the lateral canthal incision to the medial canthus (Fig. 36.13*A*). The inferior pass should be near the lid margin; the superior pass should be one-third to one-half way up the upper tarsal plate. The fascia should be passed behind the medial canthal tendon (Fig. 36.13*B*) and tightened to produce full closure of the eyelids. The fascia should be fixed to the medial canthal tendon with permanent suture (Fig. 36.13*C*).

Patients learn closure with a chewing motion. This procedure has excellent long-term success except for possible loosening of the fascia. Better long-term stability of the fascia can be accomplished by additional fixation sutures at the lateral canthus and fixation to the tarsal plates made through scalpel stab incisions at the middle and lateral thirds of the eyelid.

Other procedures used in patients with facial palsy include those for both functional and cosmetic improvement: rhytidectomy, brow lift, and blepharoplasty. The rhytidectomy is a true "face-lift" rather than removal of wrinkles since the side with the palsy lacks wrinkles. Brow lift and blepharoplasty can be performed years after onset of facial palsy to provide not only better appearance but also improved peripheral vision. Preoperative photographs and visual field testing help to document the patient's claim to the insurance company that surgery has been undertaken for functional correction.

The blepharoplasty must be performed cautiously in patients with facial palsy because excess removal of skin causes problems of corneal exposure. The safest blepharoplasty technique removes preseptal orbicularis muscle and preaponeurotic fat along with a minimal amount of upper eyelid skin. A high lid fold created with supratarsal fixation stitches plicates excess skin safely up into the orbit rather than plastering the brow down to the eyelids, as can happen with simple, aggressive skin removal.

If brow ptosis accentuates the dermatochalasis, a brow plasty reduces the amount of skin excision required during blepharoplasty. The direct brow incision usually leaves no scar on the side with facial palsy. Excision of an ellipse of skin above the brow will help stabilize the brow. Best long-term results of brow plasty come from fixation to the periosteum with a permanent suture.

SUMMARY

Facial palsy affects the eye primarily by facial motor palsy of the orbicularis muscle. The failure of the eye to close or blink properly may be accompanied by unsuspected keratitis sicca from involvement of parasympathetic fibers to the lacrimal gland that travel through the facial nerve.

Most facial palsy occurs from idiopathic Bell's palsy. Failure of the palsy to improve or resolve after 3–6 months should arouse suspicion of occult neoplasm. A reduced Schirmer test indicates patients likely to have a prolonged palsy with difficult ocular complications from exposure and keratits sicca. Facial palsy after removal of large acoustic neuromas may be accompanied by poor closure, poor tear secretion, and decreased corneal sensation—the triad most likely to result in corneal ulceration.

Facial palsy can affect all age groups and arise from numerous causes. Ophthalmic management tries to provide increased closure and increased moisture through a wide variety of medical and surgical therapies, which must be tailored to the individual patient's facial nerve disorder and personal circumstance.

Depression may come from the patient's severe ocular problems combined with changes in facial appearance and function. The loss of no single cranial nerve can affect patients more than complete seventh nerve palsy. This chapter provides a comprehensive approach to facial nerve mangement from brain to eye, to foster the most effective, multispecialty management.

REFERENCES

1. Esselen E: *The acute Facial Palsies*, Berlin, Springer Verlag, 1977, p 7.
2. Van Buskirk C: The seventh nerve complex. *J Comp Neurol* 82: 303–333, 1945.
3. Guerrier Y: Surgical anatomy, particularly vascular supply of the facial nerve. In Fisch U (ed): *Facial Nerve Surgery*. Birmingham, AL, Aesculapius, 1977, p 13.
4. Esslen E: *The acute facial palsies*. Berlin, Springer Verlag, 1977, p 3.
5. Miehlke A: *Surgery of the Facial Nerve*, ed 2. Philadelphia, WB Saunders, 1973, p 9.
6. Sunderland S, Cesar DF: The structure of the facial nerve. *Anat Rec* 116: 147–165, 1953.
7. May M: Anatomy of cross section of facial nerve in the temporal bone: clinical application. In Fisch U (ed): *Facial Nerve Surgery*. Birmingham, AL, Alesculapius, 1977, p 40.
8. Duchene GB: *De I Electrisation Localisee*, ed 3. Paris, Bailere, 1872, p 864.
9. May M: Facial nerve disorders: update 1982. *Am J Otol* 4: 77–88, 1982.
10. May M, Hardin WB: Facial palsy: interpretation of neurologic findings. *Laryngoscope* 88: 1352–1362, 1978.
11. May M, Blumenthal F, Taylor FH: Bell's palsy: surgery based upon prognostic indicators and results. *Laryngoscope* 91: 2092–2105, 1981.
12. May M, Hawkins CD: Bell's palsy—results of surgery: salivation test versus nerve excitability test as a basis of treatment. *Laryngoscope* 82: 1337–1348, 1973.
13. Diamant H, Ekstrand T, Wiberg A: Prognosis of idiopathic Bell's palsy. *Arch Otolaryngol* 95: 431–433, 1972.
14. May M: Facial paralysis peripheral type. A proposed method of reporting. *Laryngoscope* 80: 331–390, 1970.
15. May M, Harvey JE: Salivary flow, a prognostic test for facial paralysis. *Laryngoscope* 81: 179–192, 1971.
16. Blatt IM: The prognostic reliability of provocative sialometry in Bell's palsy: a 25-year study of 703 patients. In Graham J, House WF (eds): *Disorders of the Facial Nerve: Anatomy, Diagnosis and Management*. New York, Raven Press, 1982, p 85.
17. Citron D, Adour KK: Acoustic reflex and loudness discomfort in acute facial paralysis. *Arch Otolaryngol* 104: 303–306, 1978.
18. Adour KK, Wingard J: Idiopathic facial paralysis (Bell's palsy) factors affecting severity and outcome in 446 patients. *Neurology* 24: 1112–1116, 1974.
19. Brackman DE, House JW, Selters W: Auditory brainstem responses in facial nerve neurinoma diagnosis. In Graham J, House WF (eds): *Disorders of the Facial Nerve: Anatomy, Diagnosis and Management*. New York, Raven Press, 1982, p 87.
20. Harris JP, Davidson TM, May M: Management of a two-and-a half year old with traumatic facial paralysis noted at birth. *Am J Otolaryngol* 4: 183–4, 1982.
21. Moller MB, Moller AR, Janetta PJ: Brainstem auditory evoked potentials in patients with hemifacial spasm. *Laryngscope* 92: 848–852, 1982.
22. Logan WPD, Cushion AA: *Morbidity Statistics from General Practice*. London, Her Majesty's Stationery Office, vol 1, 1858.
23. Mellotte G: Idiopathic paralysis of the facial nerve. *Practioner* 187: 349–353, 1961.
24. Brewis M, Paskenzer DC, Rolland C: Neurologic disease in an english community. *Acta Neural Scand.* (Suppl 42) 24: 89, 1966.
25. Hillsinger RL, Adour KK, Doty HE: Idiopathic facial paralysis, pregnancy, and the menstrual cycle. *Ann Otol Rhinol Laryngol* 84: 433–442, 1975.
26. Peitersen E: The natural history of Bell's palsy. *Am J Otol* 4: 107–111, 1982.
27. Adour KK, Byl FM, Hilsinger RL, Kahn ZM, Sheldon MI: The true nature of Bell's palsy: analysis of 1000 consequentive patients. *Laryngoscope* 88: 787–811, 1978.
28. Worms G, Chams: Angiospasma retiniens au cous de quelques affectiones du sugment ceptalique en particuler dans le paralysis facial "a frigore." *Bull Soc Ophal* 43: 67, 1931.
29. Hilger J: The nature of Bell's palsy. *Laryngoscope* 59: 228–235, 1949.
30. Blunt MJ: The blood supply of the facial nerve. *J Anat* 88: 520, 1954.
31. Kettel K: Pathology and surgery of Bell's palsy. *Laryngoscope* 73: 837, 1963.
32. Esseln E: *The Acute Facial Palsies*. Berlin, Springer Verlag, 1977, p 61.
33. Aminoff MJ: Bell's palsy and its treatment. *Postgrad Med J* 49: 46–51, 1973.
34. Djupesland G, Berdal P, Johannessen TA, Degre M, Stein R, Skrede S: The role of viral infection in acute peripheral facial palsy. *Acta Otolaryngol* 79: 221–227, 1975.
35. Hennebert PE: Traitement precoce de la paralysie faciale site a frigore par des chelateurs. *Acta Otolaryngol (Belg)* 27: 75–78, 1973.
36. Adour KK: Cranial polyneuritis and Bell's palsy. *Arch Otolaryngol* 102: 262–264, 1976.
37. Blatt IM, Freeman JA: Bell's palsy. II. Pathogenetic mechanism of idiopathic peripheral facial paralysis. *Trans Am Acad Ophthal Otolaryngol* 70: 381–397, 1966.
38. Vahlne A, Edstrom S, Arstila P, Beran M, Ejnell H, Nylen O, Lycke E: Bell's palsy and herpes simplex virus. *Arch Otolaryngol* 107: 79–81, 1981.
39. Djupseland G, Berdal P, Johannsen TA, Degre M, Stein R, Skrede S: Virus infection as a cause of acute peripheral facial palsy. *Arch Otolaryngol* 102: 403–406, 1976.
40. Brodie SW: Virology studies and Bell's palsy. *J Laryngol Otol* 93: 563–568, 1979.
41. Yanagihara H, Kisimoto M: Electrodiagnosis in facial palsy. *Arch Otolaryngol* 95: 376–382, 1972.
42. Overend W: Preliminary note on a new cranial reflex. *Lancet* 1: 619, 1896.
43. Bumm P: Registrierung antidromer aktianspotentiale am facialis nerven des manchen. *Arch Otorhinolaryngol* 210: 262–263, 1975.
44. Adour KK, Wingard S, Doty HE: Prevalence of concurrent diabetes mellitus and idiopathic facial paralysis. *Diabetes* 24: 449–451, 1975.
45. McGovern: Panel discussion no. 10. Etiology and pathogenesis of Bell's palsy: Experimental study. *Laryngoscope* 82: 1, 594–601, 1972.
46. Gates G, Mikiten TM: Idiopathic facial paralysis (Bell's palsies). In Graham J, House WF (eds): *Disorders of the Facial Nerve: Anatomy, Diagnosis and Management*. New York, Raven Press, 1982, p 279.
47. Shambaugh GE, Clemis JD: Facial nerve paralysis. In Paparella MM, Shumrick DA (eds): *Otolaryngology*. Philadelphia, WB Saunders, 1973, vol 2, p 263.
48. Devriese PP: Herpes zoster causing facial; paralysis. Panel discussion No. 12. Treatment of facial palsy of infection origin. In Fisch U (ed): *Facial Nerve Surgery*. Birmingham, AL, Aesculapius, 1977, p 419.
49. Saito H, Baxter H: Undiagnosed facial nerve neuroluminenias. *Arch Otolaryngol* 95: 415–419, 1972.
50. Jackson CG, Glasscock ME, Hughes GB, Sismanies A: Facial

paralysis of neoplastic origin: diagnosis and management. *Laryngoscope* 90: 1581–1595, 1980.
51. Neeley GJ, Alford BR: The facial nerve in lesions of the temporal bone: clinical considerations. In Graham J, House WF (eds): *Disorders of the Facial Nerve: Anatomy, Diagnosis and Management.* New York, Raven Press, 1982, 191.
52. Kishimoto S, Saito H: Facial nerve neurolemmoma. A case report and review. *Pract Otolaryngol (Jpn)* 71: 817–824, 1978.
53. Fisch U, Ruttner J: Pathology of intratemporal tumors involving the facial nerve. In Fisch U (ed): *Facial Nerve Surgery.* Birmingham, AL, Aesculapius, 1977, p 448.
54. Alford BR, Gilford FR: A comprehensive study of the tumors of the glomus jugulare. *Laryngoscope* 72: 765–787, 1962.
55. Glasscock ME, Jackson CG, et al: Panel discussion: Glomus jugulare tumors of the temporal bone. The surgical management of glomus tumors. *Laryngoscope* 89: 1640–1651, 1979.
56. Pulec JL: Facial nerve tumors. *Ann Otolaryngol* 78: 962–982, 1969.
57. Janetta PJ, Abbasy M, Maroon JC, Rama FM, Albin MS: Etiology and definitive microsurgical treatment of hemifacial spasm. *J Neurosurg* 47: 321–328, 1977.
58. Conley J, Janecka I: Schwann cell tumors of the facial nerve. *Laryngoscope* 84: 958–962, 1977.
59. Neely JG: Neoplastic involvement of the facial nerve. *Otolaryngol Clin North Am* 7: 385–396, 1974.
60. Pulec JL: Symposium on ear surgery. II. Facial nerve neuroma. *Laryngoscope* 82: 1160–1176, 1972.
61. Avery AP, Sprinkle PM: Benign intraparotid schwanmous. *Laryngoscope* 82: 199–203, 1972.
62. Glasscock ME, Hays JW, Jackson CG, Steenerson RL: A one-stage combined approach for the management of large cerebellopontine angle tumors. *Laryngoscope* 88: 1563–1575, 1978.
63. Glasscock ME, Jackson CG: Surgery of cerebellopontine angle tumors: difficulties, complications and results of translabyrinthine approach. *Rev Laryngol Otol Rhinol* 100: 91–95, 1979.
64. Aderhold K, Kranke E, Pawlik HJ: Melkerson-Rosenthal syndrome mit megacolon Congenitum. *Deut Ges H* 12: 513, 1957.
65. Schroder H, Hartmann G: Melkerson-Rosenthal syndrome und idiopathesches megakolan. *Brun Beitr Klin Chir* 205: 208, 1962.
66. Scott GA, cited by Graff-Radford SB: Melkerson-Rosenthal syndrome: a review of the literature and a case report. *S Med J* 11: 71–74, 1981.
67. Saberman MN, Tenta LT: The Melkerson-Rosenthal syndrome. *Arch Otolaryngol* 84: 292–296, 1966.
68. Pollock Ra, Brown La: Facial paralysis in otitis media. In Graham J, House Wf (eds): *Disorders of the Facial Nerve: Anatomy, Diagnosis, and Management.* New York, Raven Press, 1982, p 221.
69. Persky AH: Facial paralysis of otitic origin. *Arch Otolaryngol* 27: 395–401, 1938.
70. Kettel K: Facial palsy of otitic origin. *Arch Otolaryngol* 27: 395–401, 1938.
71. Cawthorne T, Jongkees LBW: A surgical classification of the paralysis of the facial nerve with guidelines for differential diagnosis and therapy. In Miehlke A (ed): *Surgery of the Facial Nerve*, ed 2. Philadelphia, WB Saunders, 1973, p 52.
72. Shambaugh GE, Glasscock ME: Facial nerve decompression and repair. In Shambaugh GE, Glasscock ME (eds): *Surgery of the Ear.* W.B. Saunders, Philadelphia, 1980, p 530.
73. Sheehy JL, Brackman DE, Graham MD: Complication of cholesteotema: a report of 1024 cases. In McCade BF, Sade J, Abramson M (eds): *Cholesteotema First International Conference.* Birmingham, AL, Aesculapius, 1977, p 429.
74. Meltzer P, Kelemen G: Ryocyaneus osteomyelitis of the temporal bone, mandible, zygoma. *Laryngoscope* 69: 1300–1316, 1959.
75. Chandler JR: Malignant otitis externa. *Laryngoscope* 78: 1257–1294, 1968.
76. May M, Fria TJ, Blumenthal F, Curtain H: Facial paralysis in children: differential diagnosis. *Otolaryngol Head Neck Surg* 89: 841–848, 1981.
77. Alberti MB, Biogioni E: Facial paralysis in children. *J Pediatr* 19: 303, 1957.
78. Shuring AG, Gunter JP: Paralysis of the facial nerve in children. *Clin Pediatr* 9: 105–109, 1970.
79. Linthicum FH: Facial nerve paralysis in children. *Otolaryngol Clin North Am* 7: 433–436, 1974.
80. Kaplan JM, Quintant P, Samson J: Facial nerve palsy with anaphylateral purymia. *Am J Dis Child* 119: 452–453, 1970.
81. Smith JD, Crumley RL, Harker LA: Facial paralysis in the newborn. *Otolaryngol Head Neck Surg* 89: 1021–1024, 1981.
82. Bergstrom L, Baker B: Syndromes associated with congenital facial paralysis. *Otolaryngol Head Neck Surg* 89: 336–342, 1981.
83. Voorhees RL, Zietzer LD, Ross M: Hypertension and associated peripheral facial paralysis. *Laryngoscope* 82: 899–902, 1972.
84. Langly JN, Anderson HK: The union of different kinds of nerve fibers. *J Physiol Lond* 31: 365, 1904.
85. Tucker HM: The management of facial paralysis due to extracranial injuries. *Laryngoscope* 88: 348–354, 1978.
86. Brogdan FH, Gray GH: Differential spinal accessory facial anastomosis with preservation of function of trapezius. *J Neuro Surg* 4: 981–985, 1962.
87. Glasscock ME, Jackson CG, Hays JW: Facial hypoglossal anastomosis for treatment of facial paralysis. In Silverstein H, Norrell H (eds): *Neurologic Surgery of the Ear.* Birmingham, AL, Aesculapius, 1979, vol 88, p 189.
88. Conley J, Baker DB: Hypoglossal-facial anastomosis for reinnervation of the paralyzed face. *Plast Reconstr Surg* 63: 63–72, 1979.
89. Kessler IA, Moldaver J, Pool JL: Hypoglossal facial anastomosis for treatment of facial paralysis. *Neurology* 9: 118–125, 1959.
90. Panel Discussion No. 6: Rehabilitation of the face by VIIth nerve substitution. In Fisch U (ed): *Facial Nerve Surgery.* Birmingham, AL, Aesculapius, 1977, p 234.
91. Levine RE: Management of the eye after acoustic tumor surgery. In House WF, Luetje CM (eds): *Acoustic Tumors. Management.* Baltimore, University Park Press, 1979, vol 2, p 105.
92. Van Meter WS, Younge Br, Harner SG: Ophthalmic manifestations of acoustic neurinoma. *Ophthalmology* 90: 917–922, 1983.
93. Schimek RA, Ballou GS: Eastman 910 monomer for plastic lid procedures. *Am J Ophthalmol* 62: 104, 1966.
94. Mausolf FA: Techniques for repair of orbicularis oculi palsy. *Ophthal Surg* 9: 67, 1978.
95. Wesley RE, Collins JW: McCord procedure for ectropion repair. *Arch Otolaryngol* 109: 319–322, 1983.
96. Hornblass A: Punctal occlusion with cyanoacrylate glue. In Wesley RE (ed): *Techniques in Ophthalmic Plastic Surgery.* New York, Wiley & Sons, 1985.
97. Smith B: The lazy "T" correction of ectropion of the lower punctum. *Arch Ophthalmol* 94: 1149, 1976.
98. Jones LT: Conjunctivodacryocystorhinostomy. *Am J Ophthalmol* 59: 773, 1964.
99. Campbell CB III, Shannon GM, Flanagan JC: Conjunctivodacryocystorhinostomy with mucous membrane graft. *Ophthal Surg* 14: 647–562, 1983.
100. English BS, English KP: The palpebral spring in facial palsy. *Med J Austr* 1: 223, 1972.
101. Moran LR, Rich AM: Four years experience with Morel-Fatio palpebral spring. *Plast Reconstr. Surg.* 33: 446, 1964.
102. McCord CD Jr: Surgery of the eyelids. In Duane TD, Jaeger EA (eds): *Clinical Ophthalmology.* Hagerstown, MD, Harper & Row, 1984, vol 5, p 28.

CHAPTER 37

Acquired Ptosis

J. JUSTIN OLDER, M.D.

Acquired ptosis constitutes a heterogeneous group of conditions. It, essentially, is made up of all types of ptosis that are not present at birth. In the past 20 years, changes in attitude towards acquired ptosis and advancement in the treatment of acquired ptosis have occurred. In the third edition of his excellent text on ptosis, Beard (1) classifies ptosis into "congenital" and "acquired" but uses these terms in quotation marks to "show [his] disapproval" with the classification of ptosis (1). Nevertheless, he breaks down acquired ptosis into *neurogenic, myogenic, traumatic*, and *mechanical*. Dortzbach and Sutula (2) go a step further and add *aponeurogenic* to the other four classifications of acquired blepharoptosis. Frueh (3) challenges the traditional acquired versus congenital classification and feels that all ptosis should be classified into four groups: neurogenic, myogenic, aponeurotic, and mechanical.

One of the advantages of classifying ptosis is to arrive at appropriate treatment for the various conditions. This chapter will present a treatment approach to acquired ptosis. In some cases a particular classification will suggest a specific treatment approach, but in many instances one technique may be used to treat several types of ptosis.

In 1974, Duke-Elder (4) stated, "In contradistinction to congenital ptosis, the acquired condition should not be corrected surgically until all other means have been exhausted." He then proceeds to list two methods of nonsurgical correction: lid crutches and a haptic contact lens fitted with a shelf on which the margin of the upper lid rests.

In the past 15 years, techniques have advanced to such a degree that surgery is usually preferable to the methods discussed in Duke-Elder's test. Even the ptosis of myasthenia gravis, traditionally treated with medication, can respond well to surgical techniques if the medical treatment is not completely satisfactory. This chapter will first present the surgical techniques and then discuss the various types of ptosis and their treatment based on the already understood surgical approaches.

GENERAL SURGICAL CONSIDERATIONS

Only two muscles elevate the upper eyelid: the levator palpebrae superioris, which is innervated by the superior ramus of the third nerve, and Müller's muscle, which is innervated by the sympathetic nervous system. A weakness in either the nervous component or the muscular aponeurotic component of these structures may result in some degree of ptosis. If these neuromuscular systems are intact, ptosis can occur if a tumor or edema overcomes the normal forces keeping the eyelid in its proper position.

The repair of ptosis can be accomplished by eliminating the mechanical force (removing a large tumor), strengthening the neuromuscular force surgically or medically, or bypassing the neuromuscular component by suspending the eyelid to the brow.

If one thinks of the neuromuscular elevating forces of the upper lid as a rubber band and the amount of elevating force as comparable to the amount of tensile strength of the rubber band, then shortening the rubber band by a certain amount should elevate the upper eyelid to some degree. If the rubber band has good elasticity, less shortening should be required than if the rubber band has poor elasticity. If the rubber band has essentially no elasticity, then a brow suspension is probably required. Methods available to tighten the rubber band are shortening the levator muscle aponeurosis complex, shortening Müller's muscle, taking a horizontal section of the tarsus, or a combination of these approaches.

Measuring the amount of eyelid droop and the levator function is the usual way to determine which surgical approach would be most effective in correcting the ptosis. (Refer to the chapter on congenital ptosis for full discussion of measurements of levator function.) Some surgeons instill phenylephrine drops into the eye to see if the ptosis is temporarily corrected by the eye drops. This maneuver helps them determine which surgical procedure to use for ptosis correction (5).

For a small amount of ptosis with good levator function, many surgical procedures will be effective. As the ptosis becomes more severe and the levator function lessens, fewer procedures will be effective.

LEVATOR APONEUROSIS SURGERY

In the author's experience, levator aponeurosis surgery can be effective in all types of acquired ptosis with good to moderate function regardless of the severity of the ptosis. Most cases that will not respond to levator aponeurosis surgery usually require a tarsofrontalis suspension. In aponeurosis surgery, the levator aponeurosis is repaired if a dehiscence is found or the aponeurosis is advanced onto tarsus. Since the aponeurosis and Müller's muscle are adherent to one another, Müller's muscle is also advanced onto the tarsus and thereby shortened to some degree. The surgery is done with the patient awake and alert. Therefore, the amount of levator aponeurosis advancement can be decided upon at the time of surgery. If the aponeurosis is truly intact and Müller's muscle is at fault, as in Horner's syndrome, the aponeurosis and Müller's muscle combination can also be advanced or tucked to the degree that will correct the ptosis at the surgical table (6–9).

TECHNIQUE

The patient is given little or no preoperative sedation in order that he or she may cooperate at surgery by opening the eyes and looking upward and downward. A sedated patient will obviously have droopy eyelids from the sedation, and the accuracy of the surgical procedure will then be limited.

A line is drawn where the lid crease is to be created. This line should match the opposite lid crease for unilateral surgery or should be approximately 10 mm above the lash line in the center of both lids (Fig. 37.1). If the excess skin is to be removed as part of the ptosis procedure, the excess skin should be gathered in a forceps and a second line drawn indicating the amount of excess skin to be removed.

Local anesthetic is then given subcutaneously in the upper lid; 1–2 ml of 2% lidocaine with epinephrine is usually sufficient. Bupivacaine can be added to this mixture, but in most cases the anesthetic without bupivacaine will last for the duration of the procedure. The epinephrine will often stimulate Müller's muscle and partially correct the ptosis. It is, therefore, necessary to evaluate the amount of ptosis correction that the injection may have given. One should assume that some ptosis correction is accomplished by the epinephrine, and the surgical end point is usually a lid height, which is 1 mm above the desired end point. If no epinephrine is used in the anesthetic, then overcorrection is not necessary.

A frontal block can also be used, but care must be taken not to allow infiltration of the anesthetic into the superior orbit. If this occurs and the branch of the third nerve to the superior rectus muscle is anesthetized, the surgical procedure as described must be aborted since the patient can no longer elevate the eyelid.

An incision is then made in the line for the lid crease. If excess skin is to be removed, the excess is removed at this point (Fig. 37.2). If excess skin is not removed, dissection is continued superiorly between the skin and orbicularis muscle for about 8–10 mm (Fig. 37.3). If excess skin has been removed, then dissection continues about 8 mm above the tarsus in a posterior direction (Fig. 37.4). It is necessary to dissect posteriorly about 8 or 10 mm above the tarsus if one is expecting to find a levator disinsertion or dehiscence. If the levator is disinserted and dissection continues posteriorly just above the tarsus, the conjunctiva may be reached without ever seeing the levator aponeurosis. By dissecting 10 mm above the tarsus, the likelihood of reaching the levator aponeurosis prior to reaching the conjunctiva is much greater. Dissection proceeds through the orbicularis muscle until the orbital septum is reached. The septum is teased apart to expose the preaponeurotic

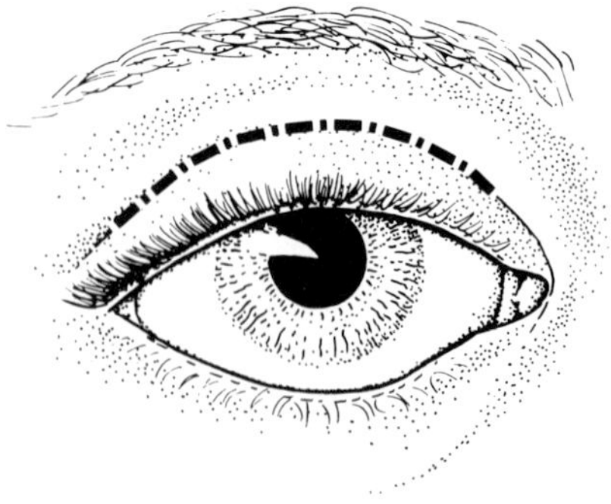

Figure 37.1. Lid crease incision.

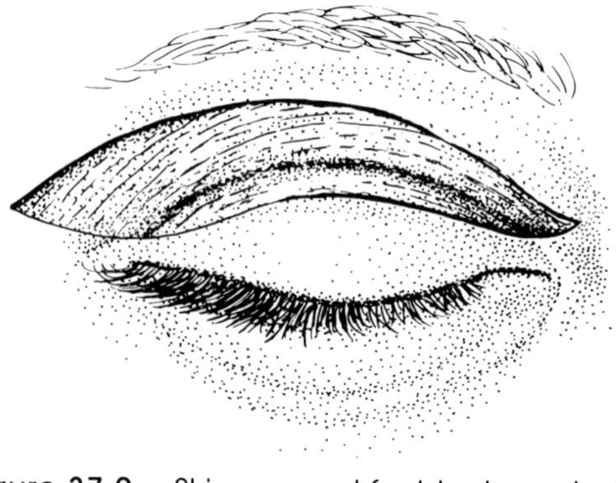

Figure 37.2. Skin removal for blepharoplasty.

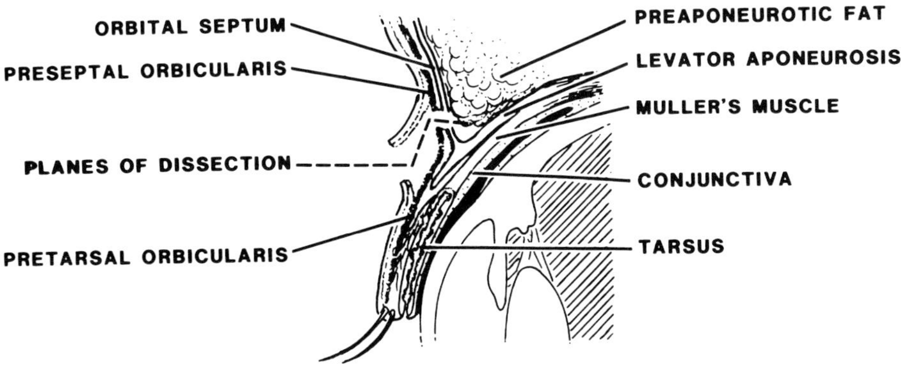

Figure 37.3. Planes of dissection for approach to levator aponeurosis when blepharoplasty is not combined with aponeurosis advancement.

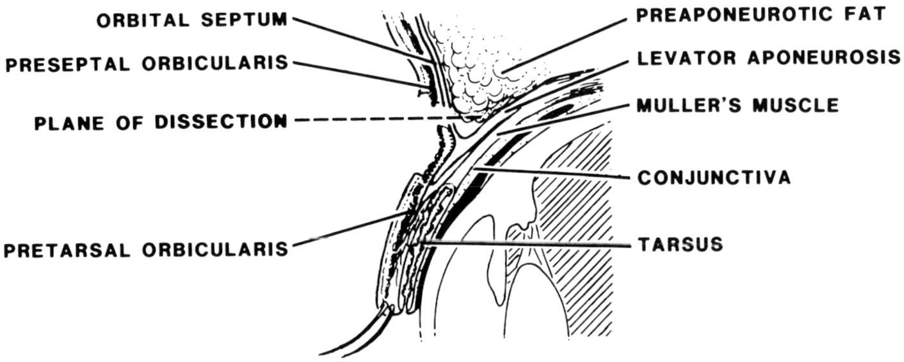

Figure 37.4. Planes of dissection when blepharoplasty is combined with aponeurosis advancement.

fat, which is then reflected away from the underlying aponeurosis. There is a fat capsule that surrounds the fat and separates it from the orbital septum anteriorly and the levator aponeurosis posteriorly. The fat can be reflected within this capsule. If the capsule is broken, the fat will then flow more freely into the surgical field.

As dissection proceeds through the orbicularis muscle and the orbital septum, the patient can be asked to look up and down. This maneuver will assist the surgeon in finding the landmarks. The levator aponeurosis will retract into the orbit as will the attached preaponeurotic fat. The orbicularis and the orbital septum will not move when the patient is asked to look up. This maneuver plus the obvious appearance of preaponeurotic fat will be of significant assistance to the surgeon as he or she looks for the surgical landmarks.

If a blepharoplasty is to be combined with the surgical repair, fat may be removed at this time. In these circumstances, the fat capsule can be incised and the preaponeurotic fat allowed to flow in the field. The fat can then be clamped, cut, and cauterized. The medial fat pad can also be found and surgically excised in the same manner. In some instances, the levator aponeurosis will be infiltrated or replaced by adipose tissue, and care must be taken not to confuse this fatty infiltration with the preaponeurotic fat.

The aponeurosis is then examined, and the inferior border, as well as the superior border, should be found. The patient is asked to look up, and the most superior point of the upper lid curve is identified. The aponeurosis should be advanced into the tarsus at this superior point.

Dissection proceeds to expose the upper one-third to one-half of the tarsus. The pretarsal orbicularis muscle and some of the epitarsal fascia can be reflected away so that there will be a firm attachment between the advanced aponeurosis and the tarsus. A suture is then passed through the levator aponeurosis and, possibly, also Müller's muscle in a vertical direction. The author prefers 5-0 Vicryl, because it has a slow absorption rate. The suture is then passed through tarsus in a horizontal direction and passed back through levator aponeurosis in a mattress fashion. The amount of advancement expected with this first suture is determined arbitrarily. A small amount of ptosis with good levator function would need a small advancement, possibly 8 mm. A large amount of ptosis with poor function might need 12–14 mm. This measurement is taken with the patient keeping the eyes closed and with no tension on the structures. A firm knot is tied in this suture rather than a slipknot since the patient is asked to look up, and the knot might slip during this maneuver. The amount of correction is evaluated, and the curve of the lid is also evaluated as the patient looks up and straight ahead. The patient is then asked to close the eyes. If the ptosis appears to be corrected, the curve of the upper lid appears proper, and the patient has no more than a 2–3 mm palpebral opening upon closure, then the end point is reached.

If the ptosis is undercorrected with this suture, the suture is removed and replaced. Further correction can be obtained by placing the suture higher within the aponeurosis, or by placing it lower onto the tarsus, or by a combination of both of these maneuvers. If the aponeurosis is to be advanced well onto the tarsus, care should be taken that the lash follicles are not injured. If the levator aponeurosis is thin and friable and the sutures need to be placed on the superior border of the aponeurosis or into the levator muscle itself, bleeding might be encountered since this is a very vascular area. A significant hemorrhage at this point can cause swelling of the tissues and difficulty in completing the operation. If a hemorrhage occurs, the suture should be tied immediately in an attempt to stop the bleeding. Bipolar cautery of the bleeding vessels can also be effective.

When the first suture has satisfactorily corrected the ptosis, two additional sutures are placed. Both are similar in configuration to the first one. One suture is placed approximately 5 mm medial to the first. The other is placed 5 mm lateral to the first (Fig. 37.5). If a large aponeurotic advancement has been made, excess levator aponeurosis should be excised.

If a blepharoplasty was not performed in association with the surgery and there appears to be an excess of skin that overlaps the wound, this excess skin can be removed as an elliptical strip. It should be realized that when ptosis surgery is performed, there may be an overlap of skin because the lid has been shortened. Another cause for apparent excess skin is the fact that the patient may no longer need to elevate the brows in order to elevate the eyelids. With relaxation of the brows postoperatively, there may be an excessive amount of skin on the upper lid which was previously stretched because of the brow elevation. This fold of upper lid skin may be unacceptable to the patient postoperatively.

After removal of the appropriate amount of skin, lid crease sutures are placed. Three lid crease sutures of 6-0 mild chromic gut are used. Each suture includes a bite of advanced aponeurosis within the lid closure (Fig. 37.6). After the lid crease sutures are placed, the skin is closed with a running nylon suture. Antibiotic ointment and wet sterile soaks are placed on the eye. These soaks are changed periodically for 12–24 hours. Skin sutures are removed in 6 days.

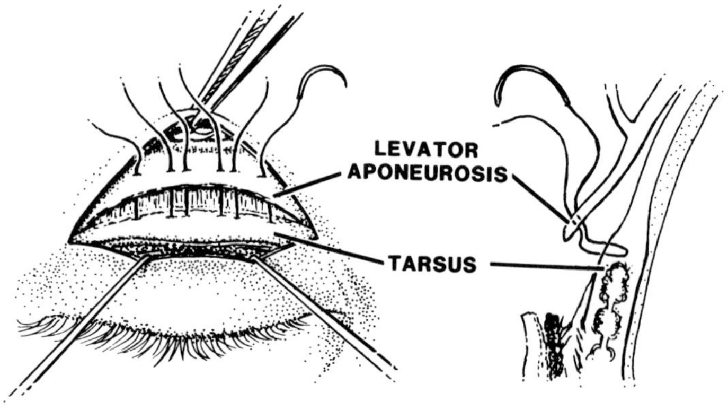

Figure 37.5. Advancement of levator aponeurosis to anterior surface of the tarsus.

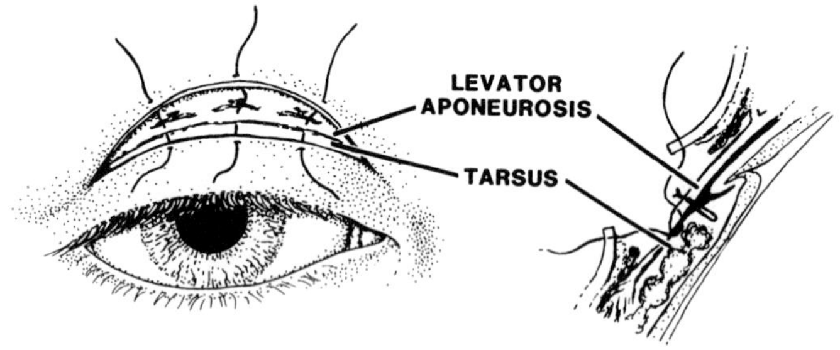

Figure 37.6. Lid crease sutures including a bite of aponeurosis with the skin closure.

COMPLICATIONS

As with any type of ptosis repair, undercorrection, overcorrection, and eyelid notching are possible complications. In the author's experience, 5% of the surgical procedures resulted in undercorrection, and there were no instances of overcorrection (8). The undercorrections occurred when there was a hemorrhage into the muscle at surgery or the aponeurosis appeared too friable or was heavily infiltrated with adipose tissue and could not be sutured properly.

Since the patient is asked to close the eyes after the sutures are placed, the surgeon can determine if there is any degree of overcorrection or inability to close the eyes. Therefore, a significant postoperative overcorrection with poor closure should be a very unlikely complication.

FASANELLA-SERVAT PROCEDURE

In this procedure, the upper 2–3 mm of tarsus along with the lower 2–3 mm of levator aponeurosis, Müller's muscle, and conjunctiva are theoretically resected. However, in practice, if the levator aponeurosis is disinserted to any degree, it will not be included in the resection. Therefore, the resected tissues will include the lower 2–3 mm of Müller's muscle with its associated conjunctiva and the upper 2–3 mm of tarsus. The procedure has been very popular because of its simplicity, lack of significant complications, and need for only a minimal understanding of the upper lid anatomy. The technique herein described is a modification proposed by Crowell Beard (10).

After injection with local anesthetic, the upper lid is everted. The upper part of the tarsus is fixed with two small curved hemostats placed 2–3 mm from the upper border of the tarsus. The bases of the hemostats are forced further than the tips toward the lid margin. This is done to prevent central peaking. The jaws of the hemostat should then contain tarsoconjunctiva, tarsus, Müller's muscle, possibly levator aponeurosis, and palpebral conjunctiva. A 6-0 plain catgut suture is placed in running mattress fashion between the temporal and nasal aspects of the lid proximal to the hemostat. The hemostats are removed and scissors are used to excise the tissue previously included in the hemostats. A scissor cut is made along the crush mark. A running suture of 6-0 plain catgut is then used to sew up the wound made by the scissors. The ends of all of the sutures are brought out through the skin so that the knots are tied above the skin. Antibiotic drops or ointments are used. Dressings may or may not be used.

MÜLLER MUSCLE–CONJUNCTIVA RESECTION

Putterman and Urist (5) described a modification of the Fasanella-Servat operation and called it the "Müller muscle-conjunctiva resection." In this procedure, Müller's muscle and conjunctiva are resected but the tarsus is left intact. The authors tested blepharoptosis patients with 10% phenylephrine hydrochloride eye drops. If the eye drops elevated the eyelid to an acceptable position, it was felt that resection of 8 mm of Müller's muscle and conjunctiva would duplicate the effect on the phenylephrine.

Either local or general anesthesia is acceptable. After the lid is everted on a Desmarres' retractor, the caliper is set at 8 mm. With one arm at the superior tarsal border, a 6-0 black silk suture is then placed through the conjunctiva 8 mm above the superior tarsal border. Placement of this suture may vary from 7 to 9 mm. The 6-0 silk sutures take bites through the center of the conjunctiva and also 7 mm medial and 7 mm lateral to the central bite. This is done at different sites across the eyelid between the superior tarsal border and the marking suture. Müller's muscle is easily separated since it is loosely attached to the levator aponeurosis but tightly adherent to the conjunctiva. A specially designed clamp is then used to grasp Müller's muscle and conjunctiva between the superior border of the tarsus and the 6-0 silk marking suture (11). As the Desmarres' retractor is released, the clamp is closed. The clamp then includes 7–9 mm of conjunctiva and Müller's muscle. The clamp is pulled downward while the skin is pulled upward to be sure that the levator aponeurosis has not been included within the jaws of the clamp. A 5-0 double-armed plain catgut mattress suture is run 1.5 mm below the clamp along its entire width in the temporal to nasal direction through the upper margin of the tarsus and through conjunctiva and Müller's muscle. The sutures are placed 2 mm apart traveling through conjunctiva and tarsus on one side and emerging from Müller's muscle and conjunctiva on the other side and vice versa. The tissue within the clamp is then excised with a surgical blade being placed between the clamp and the suture. After the tissue has been excised, the wound is closed in a manner very similar to that described for the Fasanella-Servat operation as modified by Beard (see preceding section). Putterman (5) has had a 10-year experience with this operation and feels that the results are excellent.

GAVARIS PROCEDURE

For acquired ptosis of 1–3 mm with good levator function or segmental ptosis of 1–3 mm, Gavaris (12) uses the following operation. He excises tarsus, Müller's muscle, and conjunctiva. He then advances the residual Müller's muscle and conjunctiva to the remaining upper border of the tarsus and uses three equally spaced double-armed 6-0 Prolene sutures, which are passed in mattress fashion from the conjunctiva through the skin and tied over sponge bolsters on the eyelid. The tarsus with its attached Müller's muscle and conjunctiva are resected in a manner similar to a modified Hughes' procedure. For 1 mm of ptosis, 4 mm of tarsus and 4 mm of Müller's muscle are excised. For 2 mm of ptosis, 5 mm of tarsus and 5 mm of Müller's muscle are excised. For 3 mm of ptosis, 5 mm of tarsus and 7 mm of Müller's muscle are excised. Gavaris notes that this procedure reduces the possibility of corneal abrasion either from exposed sutures or from a tarsal edge, and it permits segmental adjustment of lid level and contour during the immediate postoperative period. This is done by removing any one of the sutures after 48 hours without endangering the remaining correction.

SMALL'S A-FRAME METHOD

Small (13) has devised a procedure for resecting levator aponeurosis, Müller's muscle, and conjunctiva via the skin approach. He makes an incision in the lid crease area, and then reflects orbicularis muscle, orbital septum, and preaponeurotic fat out of the way. He places three temporary traction sutures through aponeurosis, Müller's muscle, and conjunctiva about 4–5 mm above the tarsal border. With traction on these sutures, the layers are elevated in the form of an A-frame, hence the name of the procedure. The posterior layers are elevated about 8–10 mm. This tissue is clamped, and the excess is excised. The clamped tissues are sutured together, and then the skin is closed. This procedure is done if the levator aponeurosis is intact and there is good levator function.

McCORD'S FULL-THICKNESS LID RESECTION

This procedure devised by McCord (14) can be used for congenital or acquired ptosis. When there is 11–16 mm of levator function in acquired ptosis, the resection equals the amount of ptosis plus 3 mm. For the acquired ptosis of Horner's syndrome in patients with 20 mm of levator function, the amount resected equals the amount of the ptosis. In this procedure, a lid crease incision is made, and the skin above it is undermined. An appropriate amount of skin is excised. The pretarsal and preseptal muscles are then partially excised along with tarsus, aponeurosis, Müller's muscle, and conjunctiva. Approximately 5 mm of tarsus are removed, and the rest of the measurement is made up of aponeurosis, Müller's muscle, and conjunctiva. The conjunctiva, Müller's muscle, and levator aponeurosis are sutured to the upper tarsal edge, and the skin is closed.

MUSTARDÉ'S SPLIT-LEVEL LID RESECTION

Mustardé (15) described a ptosis procedure that can be used for congenital or acquired ptosis. In this procedure, an ellipse of skin and underlying orbicularis muscle is removed. The lower part of the incision is at the intended lid crease. After the skin and muscle have been removed, the orbicularis muscle inferior to the resected area is dissected away from the anterior surface of the tarsal plate almost down to the lash line. The lid is then everted, and a section of tarsus with attached conjunctiva is removed. The upper 7 mm of tarsus are excised. The layer of aponeurosis, Müller's muscle, and conjunctiva is then sutured to the remainder of the conjunctival tarsal plate using 6-0 chromic catgut sutures with the knots buried. The skin is closed with four or five 6-0 chromic catgut sutures that also pick up the underlying fused layer of levator aponeurosis and orbital septum, thereby creating a lid crease. This technique is used with 7–9 mm of levator function. If there are 9 or more millimeters of levator function, the resection should be less extensive: 5–6 mm of skin and orbicularis are removed and only 4–5 mm of tarsal plate and attached conjunctiva should be removed.

TARSOFRONTALIS SUSPENSION

When there is poor levator function, 3 mm or less, a tarsofrontalis suspension is usually necessary to correct the ptosis. With poor levator function, there is usually a large amount of ptosis, 4 mm or more. As indicated in the chapter on congenital ptosis, there are many materials available for a tarsofrontalis suspension. Autogenous fascia lata is the best material for a permanent result. Children adapt quite well to the lagophthalmos and usually have no problem with the corneas after the postoperative period.

In adults with severe ptosis and poor levator function, the cause is often neuromuscular in origin. There may be an associated poor Bell's phenomenon or the older individual may have poor tear function. The corneas in the older individual will not fare as well with constant partial exposure. The material that has given consistent success with tarsofrontalis suspensions in acquired ptosis is silicone (16, 17). This silicone rod has the advantage of elasticity and allows the patient to close the eyes against the tarsofrontalis sling, assuming a moderate degree of orbicularis function. It also has the advantage of adjustability with a minor surgical procedure.

In the author's experience, this operation along with levator aponeurosis surgery will treat essentially all of the patients with acquired ptosis.

TECHNIQUE

The operation can be performed under local or general anesthesia, but all operations that were done thus far have been done with local anesthesia. Approximately 2 ml of 2% lidocaine with epinephrine are injected into each upper eyelid. The injection is given in the path to be followed by the silicone rod.

Two stab incisions are placed through the skin to the tarsus about 2 mm above the lash line. Three additional stab incisions are placed above the brow, and the central one is about 10 mm above the brow, with the lateral and medial ones being just above the brow hairs. Using the Wright needle to form tunnels between the stab incisions, the surgeon passes the silicone rod from one lid incision to the other, and then passes each end of the silicone rod to the respective brow incision (Fig. 37.7). The ends of the rod are then passed from the lateral or medial brow incision to the central incision (Fig. 37.8).

The depth of placement of the silicone rods is related to

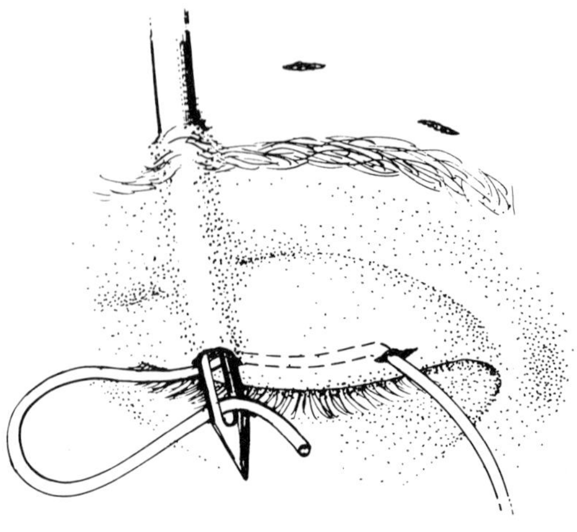

Figure 37.7. Passage of silicone rod through the epitarsal tissues using the Wright needle.

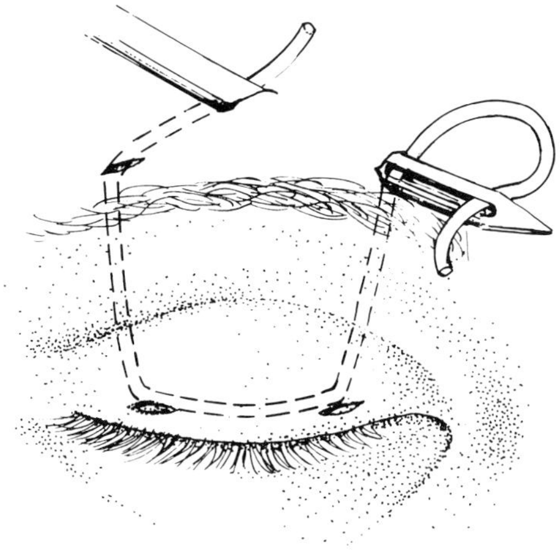

Figure 37.8. Formation of the pentagon by pulling the silicone rod deep to the tissues just above the brow.

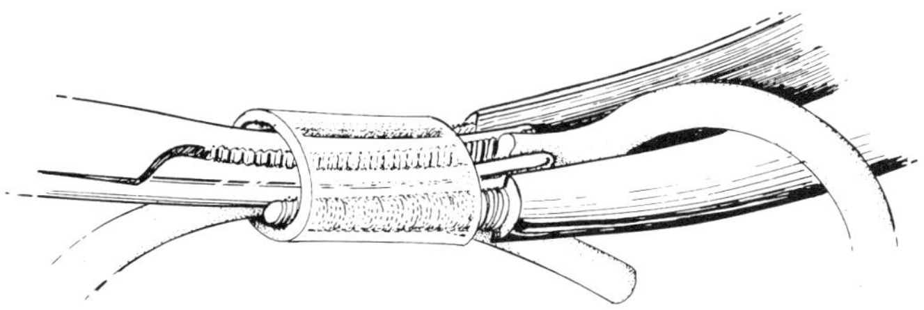

Figure 37.9. Use of the Watzke spreader to facilitate attachment of the silicone rod ends within the silicone sleeve.

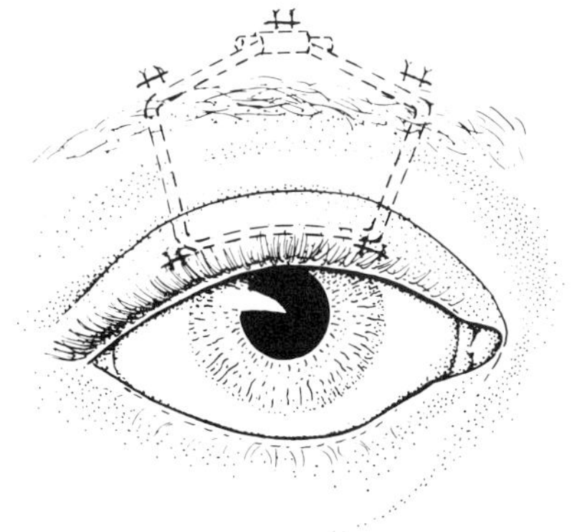

Figure 37.10. Final formation of the silicone sling.

function and cosmesis. The author attempts to place the rods within the epitarsal tissues between the medial lid and the lateral lid incisions. The placement between the brow incisions and lid incisions should be posterior to the orbital septum. To do this, the point of the Wright needle is slid over the orbital rim and then passed between the orbital septum and the levator muscle until it reaches the superior border of the tarsus. At that point, the needle is passed just anterior to the tarsus and brought out the lid incision. When the Wright needle is passed from the central brow incision to the lateral or medial brow incision, it should be deep to the subcutaneous tissue and fat.

When the silicone rods have been placed in both upper lids, the ends of each rod are attached through a silicone tube (Dow Corning Silastic No. 602-205). Use of the Watzke spreader will facilitate attachment of the rod ends (Fig. 37.9). Shortening the loops of the silicone rods will elevate the eyelids (Fig. 37.10). The brow incisions are closed with interrupted 6-0 nylon sutures, but the lid incisions are not sutured.

If awake, the patient can look in the appropriate direction and also attempt to close the eyes. Closure will be limited because of the previous injection with lidocaine. If the lid level is approximately 3 mm below the upper limbus looking straight ahead, the final position of the upper lid will be approximately 4 mm below the upper limbus in the primary position. This will allow a full range of vision, and the eyes can be kept open with normal effort.

During follow-up, the amount of closure, as well as the amount of eyelid opening, is evaluated. Each cornea is stained with fluorescein as an objective evaluation of the amount of keratopathy. The amount of punctate staining with fluorescein combined with the subjective complaint of burning or irritation is the parameter by which exposure keratopathy can be measured.

Antibiotic ointment to the wounds, systemic antibiotics, and frequent applications of artificial tears and lubricating ointments to the eyes are used during the first postoperative week. Use of artificial tears or lubricating ointment can then be gradually tapered during the ensuing weeks as determined by the amount of exposure keratopathy that exists.

COMPLICATIONS

One of the significant complications of tarsofrontalis suspension in adults is exposure keratopathy secondary to lagophthalmos. Care must be taken when performing this procedure in adults since their corneas do not seem to adapt as well as those of children who undergo tarsofrontalis suspensions. One of the advantages of a silicone rod is its elasticity, which allows the upper lid to drop down over the cornea with orbicularis contraction. In patients with neurological ptosis, a poor Bell's phenomenon or poor orbicularis function may be present, giving an increased risk of corneal exposure.

Formation of the lid crease may be asymmetrical, and in some cases, a double lid crease is formed. In some patients, the silicone rods can be seen through the skin (17). If a unilateral tarsofrontalis suspension is done, there will be asymmetry of the palpebral fissures in downgaze and upgaze and, perhaps, in primary gaze.

TYPES OF ACQUIRED PTOSIS

INVOLUTIONAL (SENILE PTOSIS)

The most common type of acquired ptosis is involutional, in which there is a weakness in the levator aponeurosis. The aponeurosis is either thin, infiltrated with fat, laced with actual holes, or disinserted from the anterior border of the tarsus. It may rest 3–10 mm above the upper border of the tarsus (2, 6). When the levator aponeurosis is disinserted, Müller's muscle can be seen attached to the conjunctiva in the space between the lower border of the aponeurosis and the upper border of the tarsus. In these cases, histopathological studies have shown Müller's muscle to be normal (2). In studies using light and electron microscopes, severe acquired ptosis was shown to have muscle fibers replaced by collagen and adipose tissues (18).

The clinical picture of aponeurosis weakness is that of an elderly persons (6th, 7th, or 8th decade) with a high lid crease (12–15 mm above the lash line) and ptosis of 1–5 mm. This is usually a bilateral condition (Figs. 37.11 and 37.12). However, in some patients, there is significant asymmetry, and it appears that only one lid is ptotic (Figs. 37.13 and 37.14). The levator function in these patients is usually 10 mm or more of excursion from downgaze to upgaze. This condition responds very well to levator aponeurosis surgery. Levator aponeurosis surgery has the advantage of correcting the anatomical defect and also of repairing up to 5 mm of ptosis. The Fasanella-Servat operation will usually correct only 2–3 mm of ptosis. If the ptotic lid responds to 10% phenylephrine hydrochloride, the procedure described by Putterman and Urist (5) gives a high rate of success.

PTOSIS FOLLOWING OCULAR SURGERY

Mild to moderate ptosis is a well-recognized sequela to cataract and other ocular surgery in a small percentage of cases. It may resolve spontaneously in 1–3 months. The cause has not been found. However, one usually finds a thinned or a disinserted aponeurosis (19).

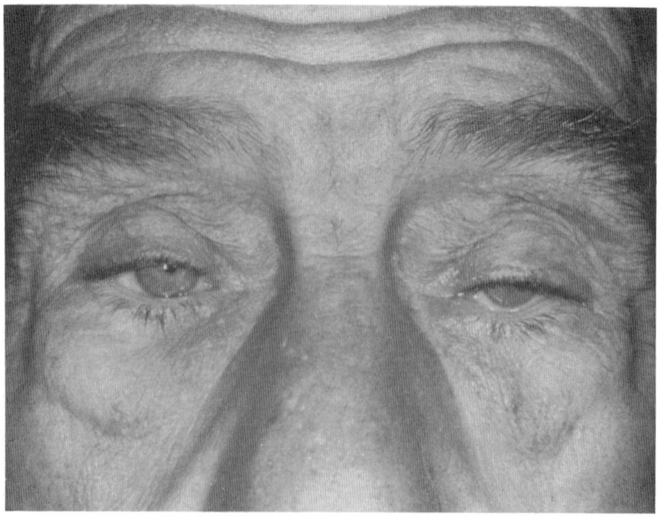

Figure 37.11. Man, age 70, with involutional ptosis.

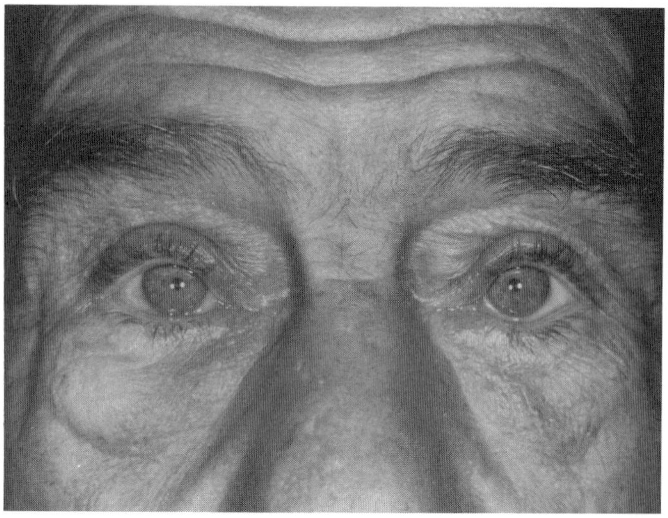

Figure 37.12. Same patient as Figure 37.11 three months after levator aponeurosis surgery.

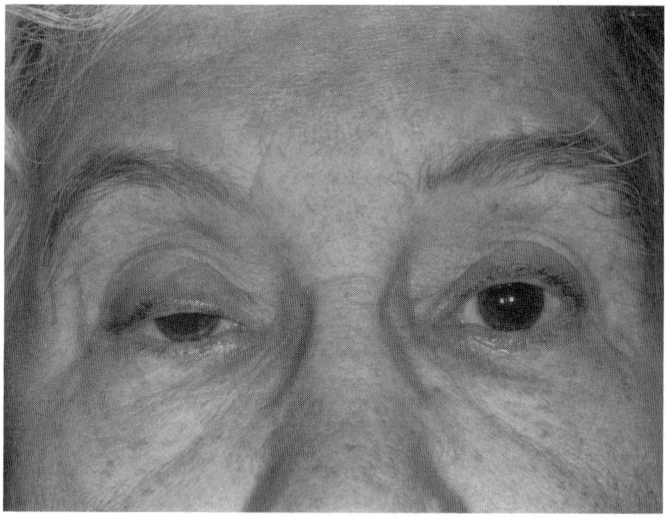

Figure 37.13. Woman, age 74, with involutional ptosis greater on the right than on the left.

This type of postsurgical ptosis is most likely an exacerbation of the tendency toward involutional ptosis, and it responds well to aponeurotic surgery (Figs. 37.15 and 37.16). It also responds well to the other procedures designed to correct 1–3 mm of ptosis, which are discussed elsewhere in this volume.

POSTENUCLEATION PTOSIS

If ptosis following enucleation cannot be corrected with the appropriate prosthesis, then ptosis repair is indicated. If there are 8 mm of levator function or greater, levator aponeurosis surgery should give appropriate correction (Figs. 37.17 and 37.18). For small amounts of ptosis, the Fasanella-Servat procedure or its modifications could be used. A small levator resection, as described in the chapter "Congenital Ptosis," would also yield good results. For

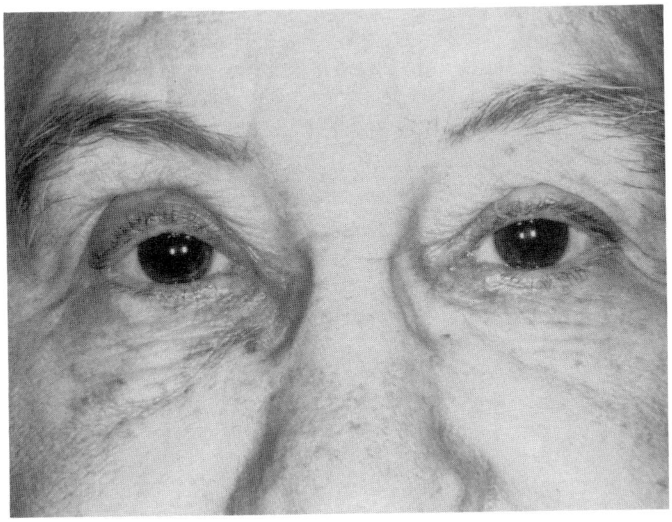

Figure 37.14. Same patient as Figure 37.13 after unilateral levator aponeurosis advancement in the right upper lid.

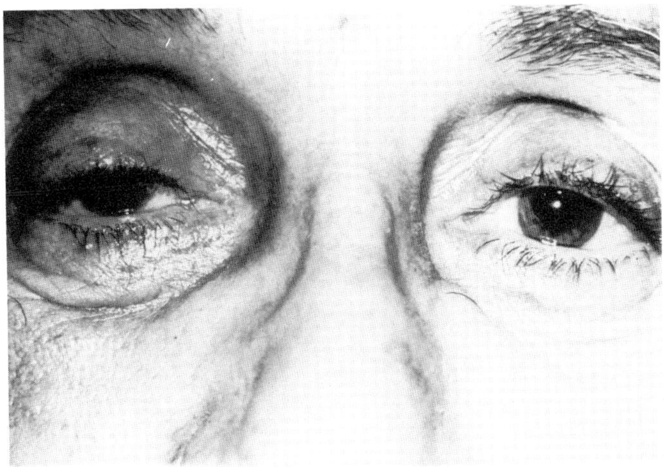

Figure 37.16. Woman, age 66, with ptotic right upper lid covering the pupil 6 months following cataract surgery on the right side. Note the high lid crease in both eyes indicating involutional ptosis of both upper lids.

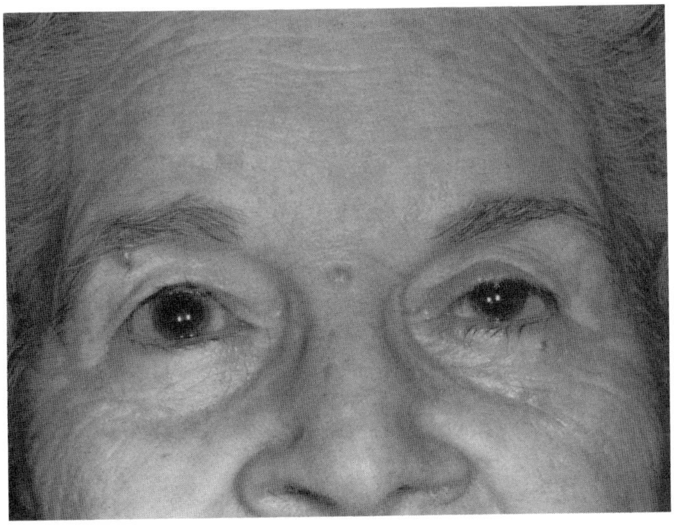

Figure 37.15. Woman, age 68, with left upper lid ptosis following cataract surgery on the left eye.

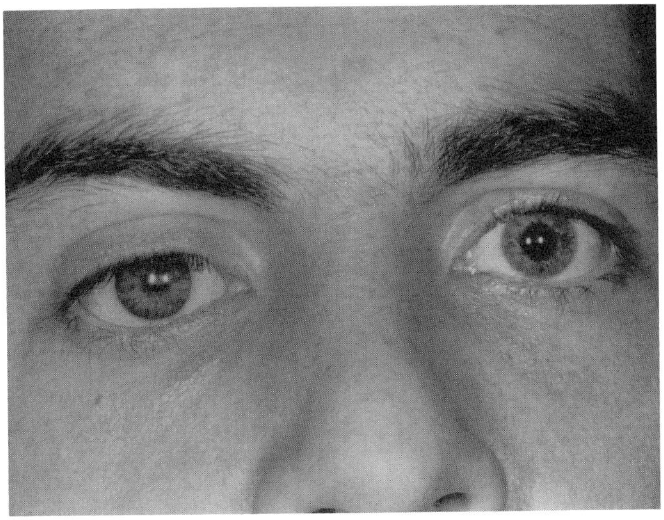

Figure 37.17. Man, age 32, with ptosis of the right upper lid twenty years after enucleation surgery of the right eye.

severe postenucleation ptosis in which the third nerve might be injured or the levator muscle severely compromised, a tarsofrontalis suspension would be indicated.

LATE ACQUIRED HEREDITARY PTOSIS

Some patients develop what appears to be an aponeurosis weakening in the 4th or 5th decade. In these patients, there is also a family history of a similar problem. Levator function is usually good, and levator aponeurosis surgery meets with excellent results.

BLEPHAROCHALASIS

Blepharochalasis is a rare condition in which frequent bouts of allergic edema occur in the eyelids. After multiple attacks, the eyelid tissues, including the levator aponeurosis, become thinned and weak. The orbital septum breaks down, and protruding orbital fat is often present. If there is good levator function, aponeurosis surgery is indicated for repair of this condition. However, if the allergic condition persists, ptosis may recur at a later date and additional procedures might be necessary.

CHRONIC PROGRESSIVE EXTERNAL OPHTHALMOPLEGIA

Chronic progressive external ophthalmoplegia is a muscular dystrophy affecting the extraocular muscles. The condition begins in childhood or adolescence and gradually develops over 20 to 40 years. Ptosis associated with limitation of extraocular movement and a poor Bell's phenomenon ensues.

Involvement of other organ systems may be present in association with extraocular movement disorders. Ptosis and dysphasis are the cardinal features of the oculopharyngeal syndrome, but there may be associated weakness of the facial, extraocular, and laryngeal muscles (20, 21). This disorder is usually found in members of a large

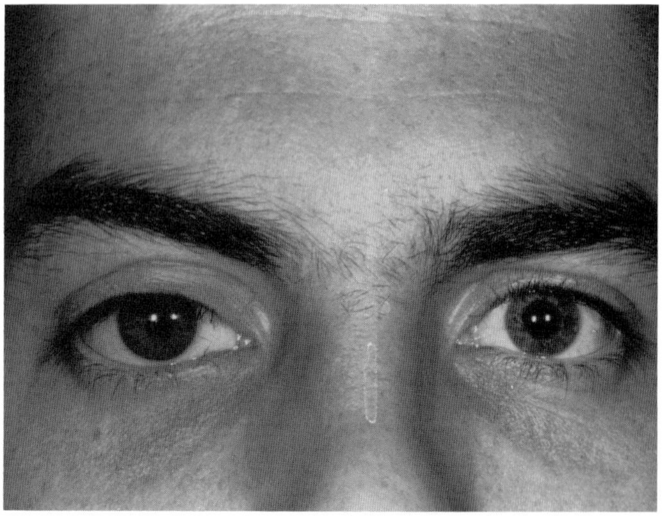

Figure 37.18. Same patient as Figure 37.17 one year following levator aponeurosis advancement of the right upper lid.

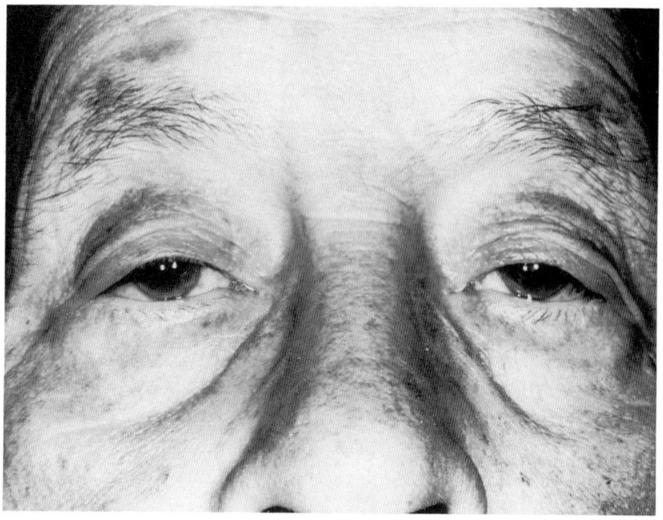

Figure 37.19. Man, age 67, with progressive external ophthalmoplegia.

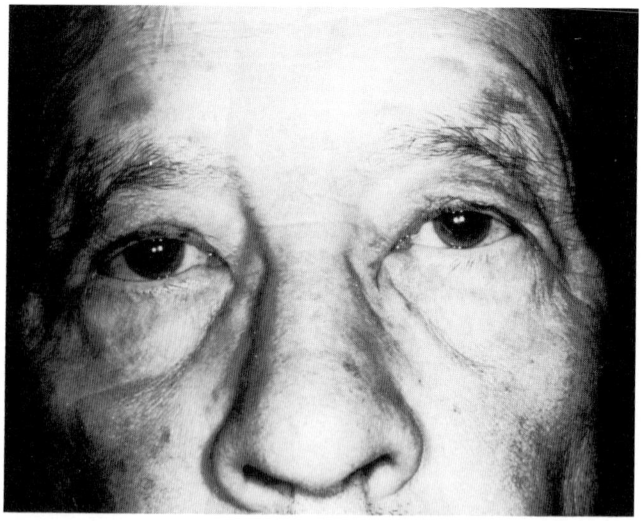

Figure 37.20. Same patient as Figure 37.19 three months following tarsofrontalis suspensions using silicone rods.

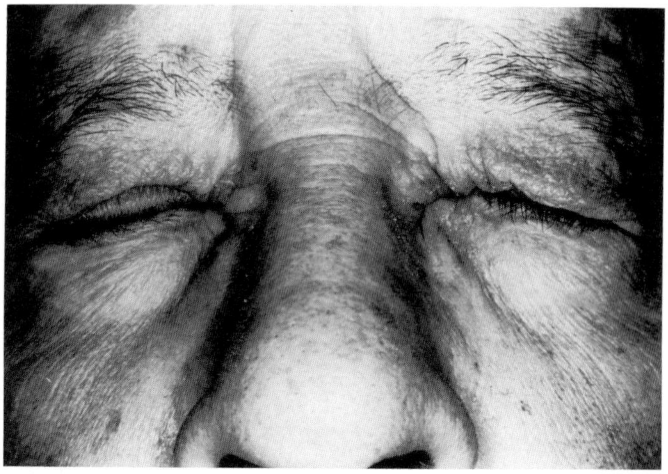

Figure 37.21. Same patient as Figures 37.19 and 37.20 three months following placement of silicone rods. Note the ability to close the eyes with the silicone rods in place.

French-Canadian family. The combination of external ophthalmoplegia, retinal pigmentary degeneration, and heart block is referred to as "Kearns-Sayre syndrome." Other organ systems such as the skeletal muscles and the endocrine glands may also be involved. Some cases of chronic progressive ophthalmoplegia associated with retinal pigmentary disturbances may have a hereditary component, and therefore, family members should be evaluated (22, 23).

When seen by the ophthalmologist, the ptosis may be moderate to severe, and the levator function is usually moderate to poor. If the levator function is moderate to good and the ptosis is moderate to mild, levator aponeurosis surgery or surgery on the tarsus-levator complex can be performed. However, since this is a progressive disease, the surgical results will only be temporary. A more permanent result can be obtained with a tarsofrontalis suspension. Because of the poor Bell's phenomenon, a tarsofrontalis suspension with fascia lata may result in significant corneal exposure. Use of silicone slings to elevate the eyelids above the pupils so that the patient can see properly and yet not have the cornea significantly exposed has been an effective treatment for these patients (17). The orbicularis function usually remains fairly good and the patient is able to close the eyes against the elasticity of the silicone slings. Use of artificial tears and/or ocular lubricants to combat the possibility of exposure keratitis is needed in the postoperative period, but the frequency of instillation of these medications can be significantly reduced 4–6 months after the surgical procedure (Figs. 37.19–37.21).

MYASTHENIA GRAVIS

Myasthenia gravis is an immunological disorder that often presents with ocular motility disturbances. In this condition the muscle and nerve are intact, but the receptor sites for neuromuscular transmission via acetylcholine are blocked by immunologic complexes. It has been estimated that approximately one-half of all patients with myasthenia gravis present initially with ocular signs. It is therefore necessary to consider this condition when viewing a patient with acquired ptosis. If myasthenia gravis is suspected, a test with edrophonium chloride (Tensilon) can be done. This is best done in a double-blind fashion. Two syringes are prepared, one with sterile saline and one with 10 mg of edrophonium chloride. The vial with edrophonium chloride can be mixed with 0.1 mg of atropine in order to decrease the parasympathetic signs that might occur with the injection of the Tensilon. The double-blind nature of the test is negated if the patient begins to sweat or feel light-headed after one of the injections. Two-tenths of 1 ml of one of the vials is injected into the intravenous catheter and 1 minute is allowed to elapse. If there is no reaction, the remaining 0.8 ml are injected, and the patient is observed to see if there is an improvement in the ptosis. The same test is then repeated with the second vial. A positive response would be an obvious improvement in the ptosis. Most patients with myasthenia gravis will give a positive Tensilon test. However, some patients with myasthenia gravis will not show any improvement with the Tensilon test.

Although side effects are rare, respiratory arrest, syncopal episodes or cholinergic crisis may be precipitated by intravenous Tensilon. Because of these risks, Tensilon should be given after a clinical evaluation of the patient rather than as a routine part of the evaluation for adult onset of ptosis.

If the diagnosis of myasthenia gravis is made, the treatment is usually best handled by a neurologist. There are some people who are refractory to medical treatment. In those cases, the author has had moderate success with surgical repair of the ptsosis using silicone slings for tarsofrontalis suspensions (Figs. 37.22–37.24).

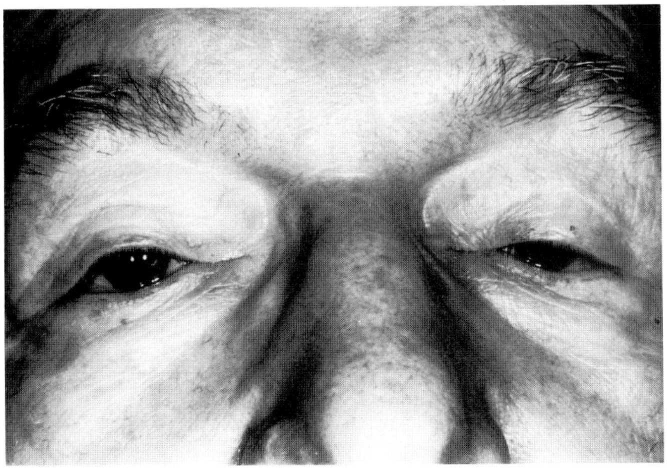

Figure 37.22. Man, age 72, with ptosis associated with myasthenia gravis.

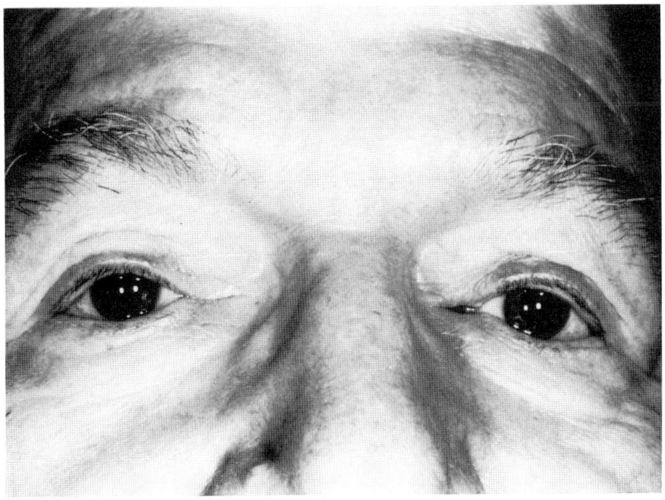

Figure 37.23. Same patient as Figure 37.22 three months following placement of silicone rods for tarsofrontalis suspensions.

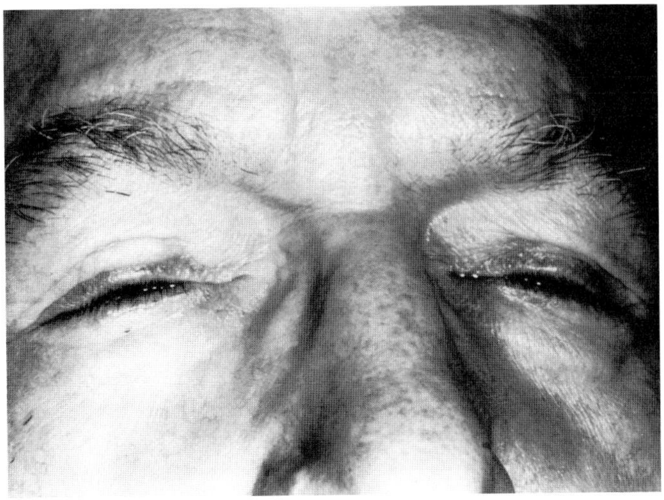

Figure 37.24. Same patient as Figures 37.22 and 37.23. Note the ability to close the eyes with the silicone slings in place.

PTOSIS ASSOCIATED WITH CONTACT LENS USE

Epstein and Putterman (24) reported five patients with acquired blepharoptosis after contact lens use. The patients were ages 25–55 years. All patients were found to have disinsertions or recessions of the levator aponeurosis, and ptosis improved in each case after reattachment of the aponeurosis to the superior tarsal border. The authors hypothesized that excessive eyelid manipulation disinserted the aponeurosis from the tarsus. Ptosis associated with contact lens were can also resolve spontaneously with elimination of the contact lens or replacement with a different kind of lens (Fig. 37.25).

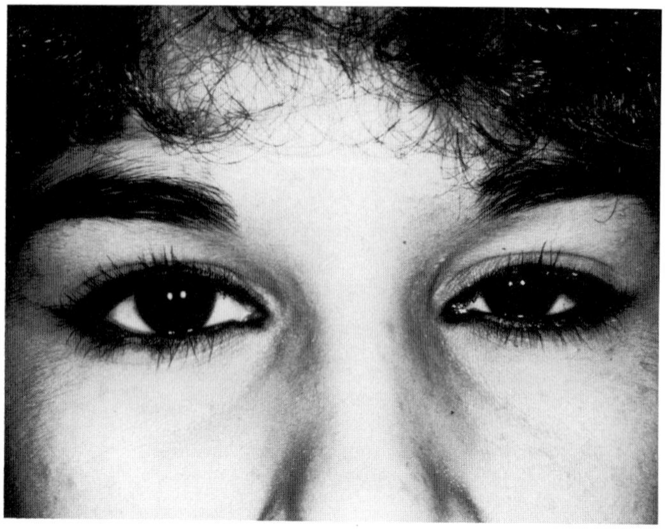

Figure 37.25. Girl, age 17, with ptosis of the left upper lid following soft contact lens wear. The ptosis resolved spontaneously after the lens was removed for 1 month.

HORNER'S SYNDROME

Horner's syndrome is caused by an interruption of the sympathetic innervation to the eye. Slight elevation of the lower eye and miosis is also associated with the ptosis. In some cases, there is anhidrosis of the affected side of the face and neck. The most common causes of Horner's syndrome are inflammatory processes, aneurysms, injuries, and surgical intervention. If the Horner's syndrome is permanent and the ptosis is cosmetically unacceptable or it affects vision, surgery can be considered. Levator aponeurosis surgery that also tucks Müller's muscle may yield good results. Anesthetic without epinephrine should be used for levator aponeurosis advancement when correcting ptosis associated with Horner's syndrome. The Fasanella-Servat procedure or one of its modifications can also be effective.

PTOSIS AND NORMAL PREGNANCY

Ptosis has been reported in association with normal pregnancy. Hypotheses for the cause include levator aponeurosis disinsertions associated with increased eyelid swelling and infiltration of water molecules into the collagen ground substance of the levator muscle and its tendon (25, 26). This type of ptosis is reported to respond well to the various operations to correct small amounts of acquired ptosis.

TRAUMATIC PTOSIS

Trauma to the eyelid, orbit, or brain may result in ptosis. Brain trauma usually involves the third nerve and gives a complete ptosis associated with a third nerve palsy. Orbital trauma, which could include foreign bodies, may give a complete ptosis if the superior branch of the third nerve is injured or a partial ptosis if the levator muscle is injured. Trauma to the eyelid itself may result in lacerations to the aponeurosis or aponeurotic disinsertion secondary to increased swelling (27).

For complete ptosis with poor levator function, a tarsofrontalis suspension is indicated. However, if the ptosis repair will result in diplopia and poor cosmesis secondary to strabismus, then ptosis correction may not be indicated. With unilateral complete ptosis in an adult, the decision must be made as to whether or not bilateral tarsofrontalis suspensions are indicated. In the author's experience, unilateral tarsofrontalis suspensions performed in awake adults have yielded acceptable results.

Exploration for a lacerated aponeurosis can be done after eyelid trauma. The exploration can be done immediately after trauma or at a later date. If exploration is done and the anticipated laceration is not found, levator aponeurosis advancement can be performed to correct the ptosis in an awake, cooperative patient with good to moderate levator function.

Traumatic ptosis will often resolve partially or completely within several days or several months. It may be prudent to wait 3–6 months before surgical intervention is undertaken.

NEUROLOGICAL PTOSIS

Nontraumatic involvement of the third nerve can occur in many disease states, including vascular malformation, tumors, and inflammatory and infectious processes. *Ophthalmoplegic migraine* is a condition characterized by severe unilateral migrainous headaches followed by ipsilateral oculomotor nerve paralysis. In most cases, the ophthalmoplegia resolves along with the migraine, but in some cases it becomes permanent. Multiple sclerosis has also been associated with ptosis. If surgical correction seems to be indicated in the occasional neurological ptosis, then the principles already described apply. That is, severe ptosis with poor levator function needs to be corrected by a tarsofrontalis suspension. Mild to moderate ptosis with moderate or good levator function will usually respond to levator aponeurosis surgery or one of the other techniques mentioned in this chapter.

REFERENCES

1. Beard C: *Ptosis*, ed 3. St. Louis, CV Mosby, 1981, p 41.
2. Dortzbach RK, Sutula FC: Involutional blepharoptosis. *Arch Ophthalmol* 98: 2045–2049, 1980.
3. Frueh BR: The mechanistic classification of ptosis. *Ophthalmology* 87: 1019–1021, 1980.
4. Duke-Elder S, MacFaul PA (eds): *System of Ophthalmology*. St. Louis, CV Mosby, 1974, vol 13, p 544.
5. Putterman AM, Urist MJ: Müller muscle-conjunctiva resection—technique for treatment of blepharoptosis. *Arch. Ophthalmol* 93: 619–623, 1975.
6. Jones LT, Quickert MH, Wobig JL: The cure of ptosis by aponeurotic repair. *Arch Ophthalmol* 93: 629–634, 1975
7. Older JJ: Levator aponeurosis tuck: a treatment for ptosis. *Ophthal Surg* 9: 102–110, 1978.
8. Older JJ: Levator aponeurosis surgery for the correction of acquired ptosis—analysis of 113 procedures. *Ophthalmology* 90: 1056–1059, 1983.
9. Harris WA, Dortzbach RK: Levator tuck: a simplified blepharoptosis procedure. *Ann Ophthalmol* 7: 873–878, 1975.
10. Beard C: *Ptosis*, ed 3. St. Louis, CV Mosby, 1981, p 151–153.
11. Putterman AM: A clamp for strengthening Müller's muscle in the treatment of ptosis. *Arch Ophthalmol* 87: 665–667, 1972.
12. Gavaris PT: Minimal ptosis surgery—a new technique. In Guibor P (ed): *Oculoplastic Surgery and Trauma*. Miami, Symposia Specialists, 1976, p 254.
13. Small RG: The A-frame operation for acquired blepharoptosis. *Arch Ophthalmol* 98: 516–519, 1980.
14. McCord CD Jr: An external minimal ptosis procedure—external

tarsoaponeurectomy. *Trans Am Acad Ophthalmol Otolaryngol* 79: 683–686, 1975.
15. Mustardé JC: *Repair and Reconstruction in the Orbital Region*, ed 2. Edinburgh, Churchill Livingstone, 1980, p 316–324.
16. Leone Jr, CR, Shore JW, Van Gemert JV: Silicone rod frontalis sling for the correction of blepharoptosis. *Ophthal Surg* 12: 881–887, 1981.
17. Older JJ, Dunne PB: Silicone slings for the correction of ptosis associated with progressive external ophthalmoplegia. *Ophthal Surg* 15: 379–381, 1984.
18. Hornblass A, Masazumi A, Wolintz A, Smith B: Clinical and ultrastructural correlation in congenital and acquired ptosis. *Ophthal Surg* 7: 69–76, 1976.
19. Paris GL, Quickert MH: Disinsertion of the levator aponeurosis of the levator palpebrae superioris muscle after cataract extraction. *Am J Ophthalmol* 81: 337–340, 1976.
20. Murphy SF, Drachman DB: The oculopharyngeal syndrome. *JAMA* 203: 1003–1008, 1968.
21. Johnson CC, Kuwabara T: Oculopharyngeal muscle dystrophy. *Am J Ophthalmol* 77: 872–879, 1974.
22. Leveille AS, Newell FW: Autosomal dominant Kearns-Sayre syndrome. *Ophthalmology* 87: 99–108, 1980.
23. Koerner F, Schlote W: Chronic progressive external ophthalmoplegia: association with retinal pigmentary changes and evidence in favor of ocular myopathy. *Arch Ophthalmol* 88: 155–166, 1972.
24. Epstein G, Putterman AM: Acquired blepharoptosis secondary to contact-lens wear. *Am J Ophthalmol* 91: 634–639, 1981.
25. Beard C. *Ptosis*, ed 3. St. Louis, CV Mosby, 1981, p 60
26. Sanke RF: Blepharoptosis as a complication of pregnancy. *Ann Ophthalmol* 16: 720–722, 1984.
27. Baylis HI, Sutcliffe T, Fett DR: Levator injury during blepharoplasty. *Arch Ophthalmol* 102: 570–571, 1984.

CHAPTER 38

Neuromuscular Ptosis Syndromes

GIL A. EPSTEIN, M.D.

Neurologic and muscular disease that affect the upper lid are frequently overlooked by the clinician. An understanding of the disease as well as the patient's degree of disability is imperative in choosing the proper treatment modality. Furthermore, the neuromuscular ptosis syndromes often vary in severity and change with time. This aspect makes these patients most challenging from a therapeutic standpoint.

As with all ptosis patients, an accurate history will guide the physician in making the proper diagnosis as well as assessing the severity of the disease. With many of the neuromuscular ptosis syndromes, other organ systems may be involved that often deserve medical attention. Similarly these syndromes may affect other components of the eye and need to be carefully assessed. Since surgical treatment is often risky, the patient and physician need a full understanding of the risks and benefits. Specific emphasis on ocular examination is given to extraocular motility, presence of diplopia, Bell's phenomenon, and corneal status.

It is the purpose of this chapter to give the clinician an understanding of neuromuscular syndromes causing ptosis as well as a rational therapeutic approach. Classification of neuromuscular syndromes causing ptosis are seen in Table 38.1. It is noteworthy that syndromes may fall into more than one category.

Table 38.1.
Neuromuscular Syndromes That Cause Ptosis

Congential
Marcus-Gunn jaw winking ptosis
Misdirected third nerve
Congenital fibrosis of the extraocular muscles
Acquired
Primarily Neurogenic
Disease of the third cranial nerve
Disease of the sympathetic pathways (Horner's syndrome)
Disease of interneuronal pathways (multiple sclerosis)
Primarily Muscular
Chronic progressive external ophthalmoplegia
Oculopharyngeal muscular dystrophy
Myotonic dystrophy
Myasthenia gravis
Thyroid disease
Corticosteroid induced
Pregnancy induced
Senile ptosis

CONGENITAL NEUROGENIC PTOSIS

MARCUS-GUNN JAW WINKING PTOSIS

Marcus-Gunn jaw winking ptosis is a well-recognized entity that has been reported to occur in from 4–6% of congenital ptosis. It is a form of synkinetic ptosis in which fibers of the fifth cranial nerve are misdirected into those third cranial nerve fibers that innervate the levator. The syndrome varies both in the degree of ptosis as well as the degree of jaw wink. It is most commonly unilateral and involves the left side predominantly. The ptosis can be seen to vary with the patient opening and closing the mouth, moving the jaw from side to side, and chewing (Figs. 38.1 and 38.2).

Sano (1) classified trigeminal oculomotor synkinesis into two groups. The more common is the *external pterygoid levator synkinetic group* in which the lid elevates with jaw thrusting to the opposite side (homolateral exter-

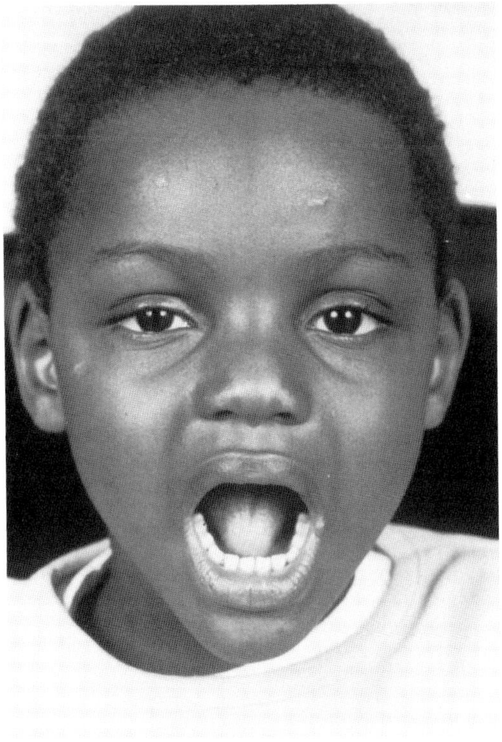

Figure 38.1. Patient with right upper lid ptosis with Marcus Gunn jaw winking syndrome.

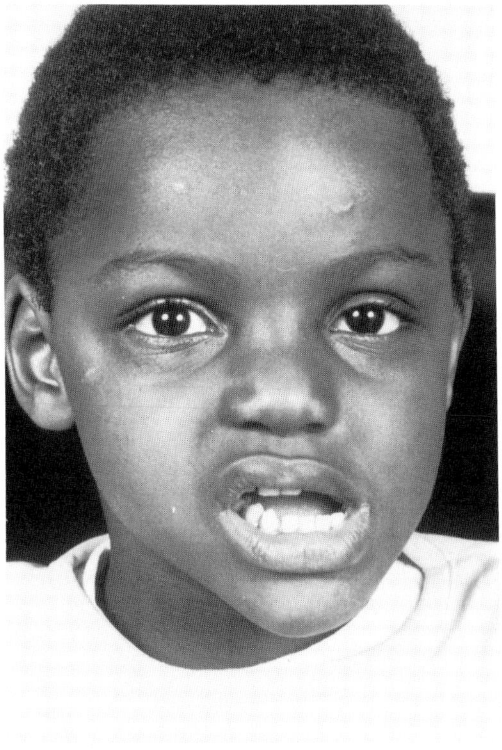

Figure 38.2. With jaw thrust to left, ptosis is resolved.

nal pterygoid), with the jaw projecting forward or the mouth opening (bilateral external pterygoids). The less common variety is the *internal pterygoid levator synkinetic group* in which the lid elevates with the mouth closing or teeth clenching. Pathoclinically, Sano (1) showed electromyographic evidence of co-contraction.

There is no genetic pattern identified with the disease, although familial cases have been reported. The superior rectus is involved in 75% of cases, and a double-elevator palsy is found in 25% of cases. Amblyopia is found in 50% of cases. Some feel the syndrome improves with age, although in 1883 Marcus-Gunn's first report of the syndrome was an adult patient (2). Pratt (3) studied 71 cases and found little change in jaw wink or ptosis over a 20-year follow-up.

Ptosis is classified as mild, moderate, or severe. The jaw wink is considered mild if it is 2 mm or less, moderate if 2–5 mm, and severe if greater than 5 mm. Two-thirds of cases have moderate to severe jaw wink and/or ptosis. If the jaw wink is minimal, then the patient should be considered as a simple congenital ptosis. Putterman (4) has advocated a Müllers muscle conjunctival resection for mild ptosis, which is similar to a Fasanella-Servat procedure (5). A levator resection is advocated for moderate and some severe cases of ptosis. Beard (6) advocates doing 4–5 mm more resection than usual, and he still finds undercorrection to be the rule. For severe ptosis, a supermaximum (greater than 30 mm) levator resection described by Epstein (7), or excision of the normal levator with bilateral autogenous fascia lata slings can be considered. The supermaximum levator resection is a logical procedure for severe ptosis since surgery is on one eyelid.

The supermaximum levator resection may be performed under local or general anesthesia. A 4-0 silk suture is placed through the superior rectus. The levator is isolated within a ptosis clamp and externalized.The conjunctiva is dissected from the Müllers muscle and attached to the tarsus with 6-0 plain catgut (Fig. 38.3*A*). A bone eyelid plate is placed between conjunctiva and the levator Müller complex. The medial horn is cut with the scissor directed superiorly so as to avoid the superior oblique tendon (Fig. 38.3*B*). The lateral horn is cut similarly, avoiding damage to the lacrimal gland while protecting the conjunctiva (Fig. 38.*C*).

The loose attachments between the levator and superior rectus are released optimally by applying countertraction (Fig. 38.3*D*). Meticulous dissection is necessary to avoid damage to the superior rectus. If the attachments are not severed, hypotropia may be encountered. Three 6-0 polyglycolic (Vicryl) sutures are placed 8 mm apart to connect the resected levator back to the tarsus (Fig. 38.3*E*, *F*). The lid is optimally placed at the superior limbus. A 4-0 double-armed silk suture is passed through the central superior fornix to prevent conjunctival prolapse (Fig. 38.3*G*). This suture is removed 7–10 days postoperatively, and an upper lid traction suture is taped to the cheek for usually 1 day but may remain if overcorrection or severe lagophthalmos is encountered (Fig. 38.3*H*). Advantages of the supermaximum levator are good cosmetic surgery on one eye and avoidance of brow scars. The disadvantage of the procedure is asymmetry of lid fissure width in downgaze.

If the jaw wink is severe or must be eliminated, excision of the levator as described by Beard (8) is necessary. Since a unilateral brow suspension is cosmetically unacceptable,

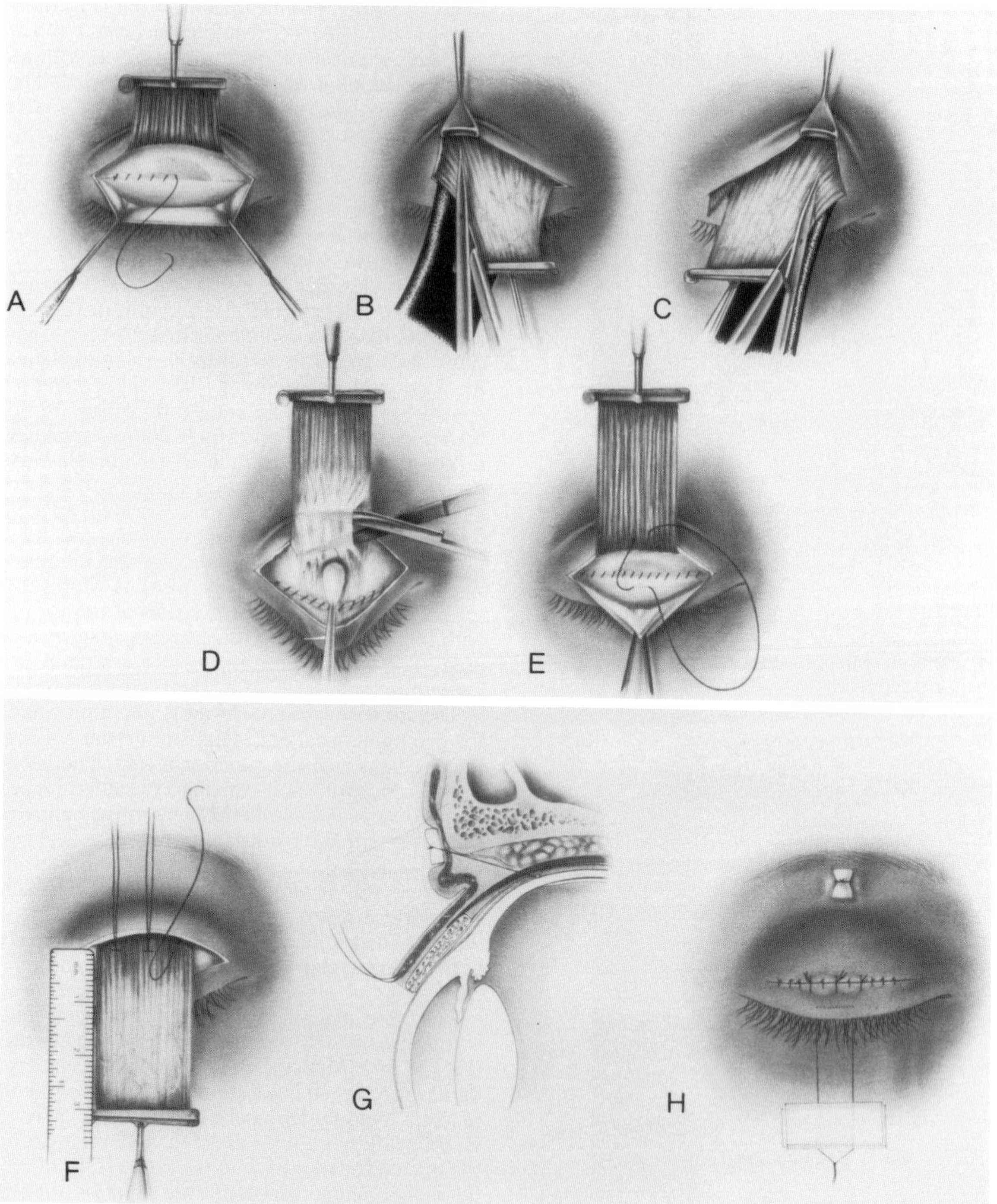

Figure 38.3. *A,* Levator has been isolated and is in external position. Conjunctiva is reattached to tarsus. *B,* Medial horn is cut in a straight upward fashion to avoid damage to the superior oblique tendon. *C,* Lateral horn is cut in a straight upward fashion to avoid damage to the lacrimal galand. *D,* The attachments between levator and superior rectus are released. *E,* A double-armed 6-0 polyglycolic (Vicryl) suture is placed 2 mm below the superior tarsal border. Each arm is passed through the levator. *F,* Verification of amount of levator resection is made with a sterile ruler. Care is taken not to stretch the levator. *G,* A double-armed 4-0 black silk suture is passed through the superior fornix to exit through skin to prevent conjunctival prolapse. The suture is tied over a cotton pledget. *H,* Lid is pulled downward with traction suture to allow high reattachment of septum to levator muscle to prevent postoperative lagophthalmos. (From Epstein GA, Putterman AM: Supermaximum levator resection for severe unilateral congenital blepharoptosis. *Ophthal Surg* 15: 971–979, 1984.)

both lids must be done. Attempts have been made unsuccessfully to treat the jaw-wink component by injecting alcohol into the pterygoid branches of the fifth cranial nerve (9). Recurrence and the inability to localize the specific branches were the reasons for failure.

Variations of the jaw winking have been described. The

inverted jaw-winking syndrome is associated with lid closure upon chewing. It is felt there is a synkinesis between the fifth and seventh cranial nerve (10). Osterle and associates (11) described ocular bobbing associated with jaw movement, which was felt due to synkinesis of the fifth cranial nerve to the superior rectus.

MISDIRECTED THIRD NERVE

Misdirected third nerve is a rare neuromuscular condition that is a synkinesis of branches of the oculomotor nerve. This is usually congenital, but may be seen following third nerve paresis (injury, tumor, inflammation, aneurysm). Surgery for this condition, if severe, is by dissociating the lid from the extraocular muscles in the form of a brow suspension with levator excision (9). Duane's retraction syndrome is probably a similar condition.

Patients have varying degrees of misdirection and usually present with anomalous lid position in different fields of gaze. The pupil may or may not be involved. A pseudo-Graefe's sign—elevation of the lid in downgaze as opposed to Graefe's sign in which the lid fails to descend—is commonly seen.

CONGENITAL FIBROSIS OF THE EXTRAOCULAR MUSCLES

Congenital fibrosis of the extraocular muscles, a rare condition that is often autosomal dominant, causes a severe bilateral ptosis. Patients typically have a backward head tilt and the eyes converge in upgaze. Frequently the forced duction test is positive. Leone and Weinstein (12) described unilateral nonfamilial congenital fibrosis associated with enophthalmos.

Surgery is indicated early if amblyopia threatens. This usually consists of a levator resection or brow suspension.

ACQUIRED, PRIMARILY NEUROGENIC PTOSIS

DISEASES OF THE THIRD CRANIAL NERVE

There are many etiologies causing third cranial nerve diseases. Location varies as to supranuclear, nuclear, or peripheral. Supranuclear lesions are primarily vascular or tumor in origin and often produce gaze palsies. Nuclear lesions have associated extraocular muscle palsies, and the ptosis is invariably bilateral. Vascular infarction, demyelination, and metastatic disease are the most common etiologies of nuclear oculomotor lesions. Infranuclear lesions may occur in the brainstem, cavernous sinus, superior orbital fissure, or orbit (Fig. 38.4). Causes include congenital, tumor (nasopharyngeal carcinoma, meningioma, pseudotumor, metastatic), vascular (aneurysm, carotid cavernous fistula, diabetes, migraine, arteritis), infectious (meningitis, herpes zoster), and traumatic (birth trauma, head injury) (13).

Treatment must be fashioned to the patient's degree of functional and cosmetic disability. Since many of the oculomotor lesions may resolve in varying degrees, surgical treatment should be delayed for 6–12 months or until the condition stabilizes. Frequent measurements and photographs are necessary to accurately assess the stability. If amblyopia is of concern, early treatment may be indicated. Crutch glasses are beneficial for some ptosis patients (Fig. 38.5).

It is frequently difficult to achieve good long-term results with surgery. Usually a brow suspension is needed. A bilateral procedure must be done to achieve optimal symmetry. A synthetic material (silicone, Supramyd) should

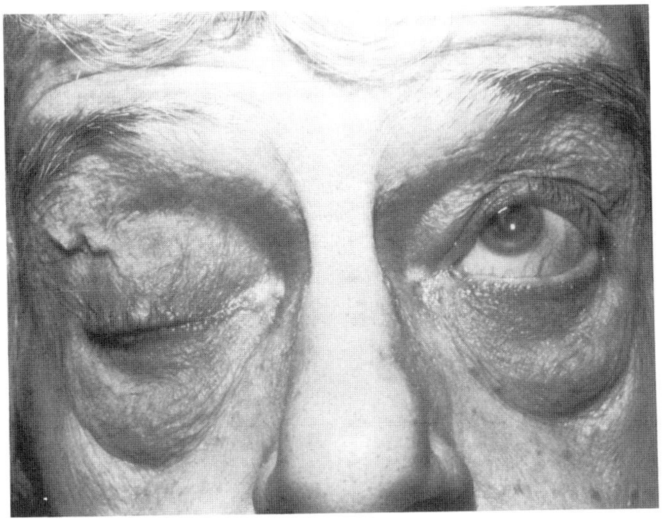

Figure 38.4. Woman, age 80, with right third cranial nerve paralysis from CVA.

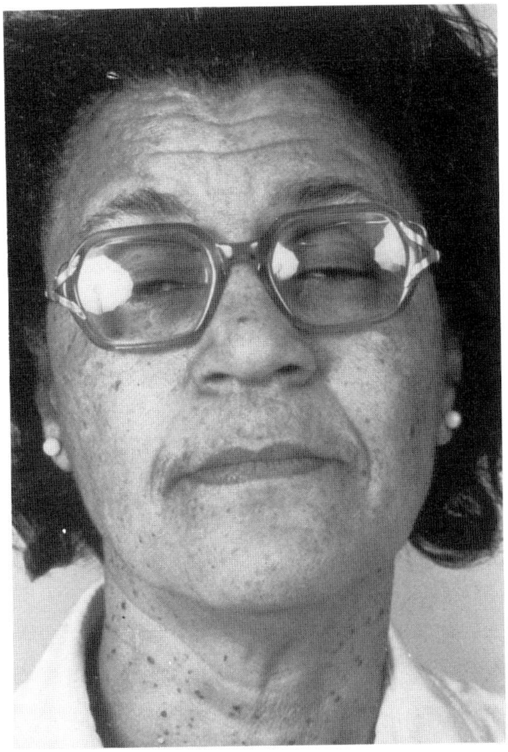

Figure 38.5. Crutch glasses attempting to lift upper lids.

be initially used to assess the postoperative adaptability of the eye. Silicone is the preferred material due to its elasticity, which allows the lid to snap back. If the eye cannot adjust to exposure, the sling may be easily reversed. If the eye adapts to the sling, fascia lata may be used later to replace the synthetic material should the ptosis recur.

Frequent lubrication is necessary postoperatively. Putterman (14) has described a temporary-suture tarsorrhaphy system to allow gradual adaptation to the environment (Fig. 38.6). Double-armed 4-0 silk Frost sutures are placed at the temporal and nasal aspect of the lower lid and fixated to the brow. A 4-0 silk suture is placed centrally in the lower lid, which can be utilized to close the eye at night. Lubrication may be gradually reduced prior to removing a suture; the upper lid suture is the last to be excised.

DISEASE OF THE SYMPATHETIC PATHWAYS

Horner's syndrome is a well-recognized syndrome that is characterized by minimal ptosis, miosis, anhydrosis, and pseudoenophthalmos (Fig. 38.7). Heterochromia may be present if the syndrome is congenital (Fig. 38.8). Pharmacologic agents such as cocaine and hydroxyamphetamine 1% (Paredrine) have been employed to distinguish central (brainstem or cervical spinal cord) preganglionic (chest or neck), or postganglionic (above the superior cervical ganglion) locations of the lesions (Fig. 38.9) (15). Etiologies of Horner's syndrome vary according to the location of the damage to the sympathetic pathway; the clinician should rule out bronchogenic carcinoma involving the apex of the lung and previous neck surgery (thyroid, carotid disease).

Stability of the condition is essential prior to surgery. Since the ptosis is minimal it can be usually corrected with either a Fasanella type procedure or a small levator resection. Attempts have been made to correct the pseudoenophthalmos (illusion of enophthalmos) due to a higher lower lid position secondary to paretic lower lid Müllers muscle. A lower lid Fasanella type procedure and/or lid retractor resection has been used with varying success (16).

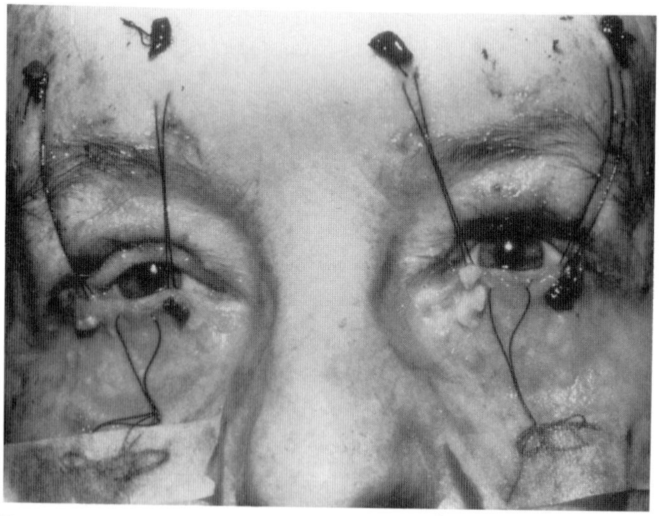

Figure 38.6. Suture tarsorrhaphy system used after silicone frontalis sling.

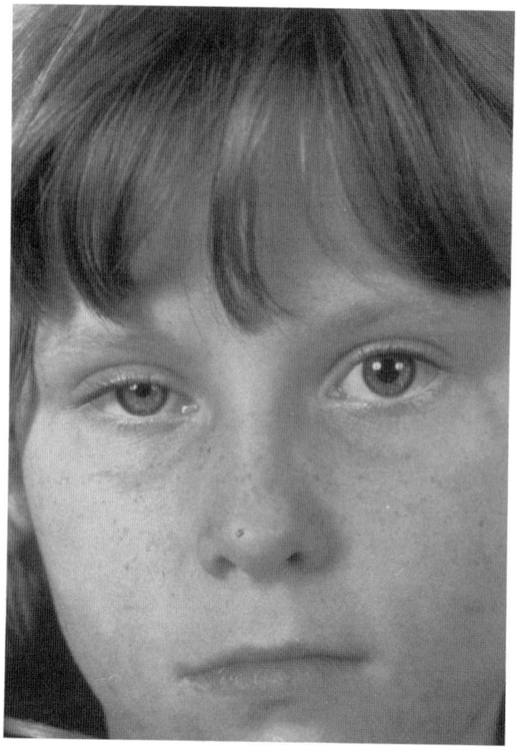

Figure 38.7. Horner's syndrome following head injury.

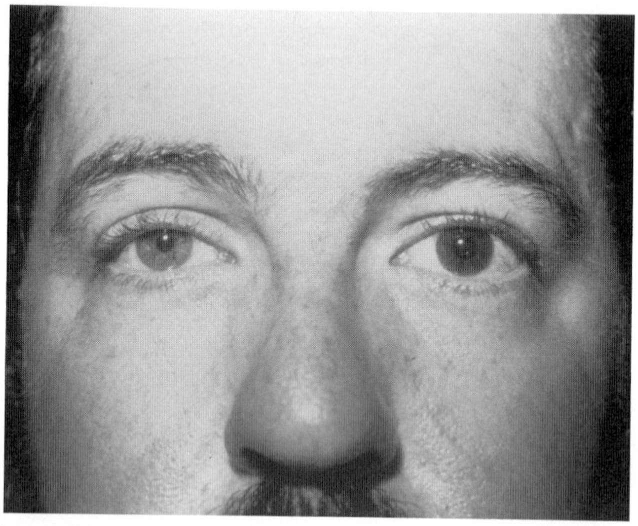

Figure 38.8. Congenital Horner's syndrome with heterochromia. Note lighter iris ipsilateral to ptosis.

DISEASE OF THE INTERNEURONAL PATHWAYS

Multiple sclerosis uncommonly causes ptosis that may resolve spontaneously. No therapy is advocated.

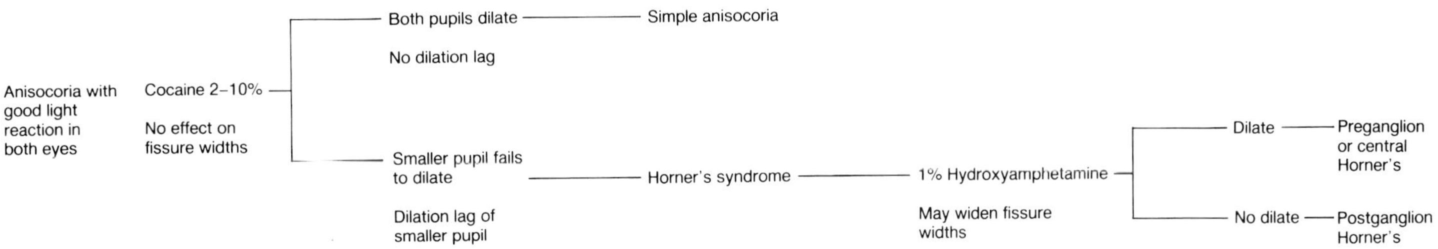

Figure 38.9. Flowchart for diagnosing Horner's syndrome.

ACQUIRED, PRIMARILY MUSCULAR PTOSIS

PROGRESSIVE EXTERNAL OPHTHALMOPLEGIA

Chronic progressive external ophthalmoplegia (CPEO) is a well-recognized neuromuscular syndrome that causes ptosis. It is slowly progressive and involves primarily the eyelids and extraocular muscles; however, other organ system abnormalities have been associated. Familial CPEO is present in half the cases and often begins in childhood or early adolescence; males and females are equally affected. The levator and extraocular muscles are first affected by CPEO, and the disease is slowly progressive and symmetrical (Fig. 38.10). The pupils are spared. Usually the forced duction test is negative, but may rarely become positive after long-standing fixation with secondary fibrosis. The edrophonium (Tensilon) test is negative. Other facial muscles including the orbicularis oculi may later be involved. Duchenne's muscular dystrophy differs in that the orbicularis oculi is the first lid muscle affected and the levator is usually spared.

Controversy arises as to the cause of CPEO. Traditionally CPEO is felt to be myopathic. Daroff (17) raised the issue as to a neurological origin by citing histologic evidence of neural atrophic changes. Further studies are necessary, and perhaps CPEO has a combined neuropathic and myopathic etiology.

Other syndromes corresponding to various organ system involvement have been described with CPEO. Kearns and Sayre (18) associate CPEO with cardiac conduction defects, elevated cerebrospinal fluid protein, spongiosis–encephalopathy, and retinal pigmentary degeneration. "Ophthalmoplegia plus" is another term coined by Drachman for this condition (19). The fundus picture resembles retinitis pigmentosa but usually visual function is not disturbed. Visual fields and electroretinographic studies may be normal.

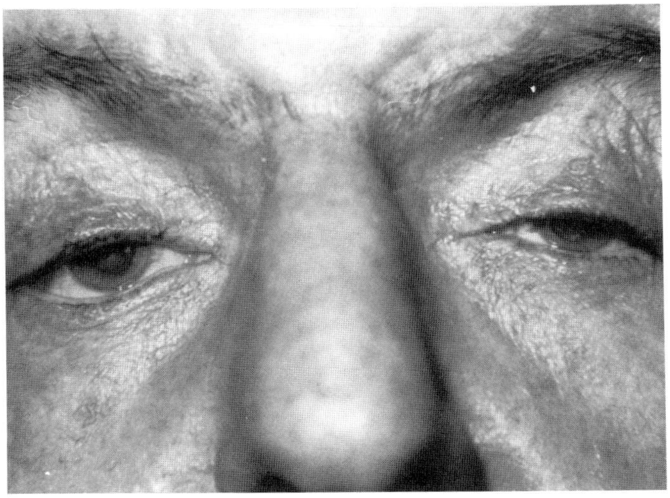

Figure 38.10. Chronic progressive external ophthalmoplegia with early fibrosis.

There is no systemic treatment for CPEO. Systemic corticosteroids have been tried unsuccessfully. Although diplopia rarely occurs with CPEO, extraocular muscle surgery may be necessary. In view of the poor superior rectus function, absent Bell's phenomenon, and the progressive nature of the disease, surgical correction may be unsuccessful. Crutch glasses are an initial alternative to surgery. Standard levator resection or Fasanella-type ptosis surgery provide transient relief. Anderson and Dixon (20) described success with levator advancement in correcting cases of CPEO. The patients were operated under local anesthesia, and the mean lid elevation was greater than 3 mm in a 1–2 year follow-up. In their series, the patients were intentionally undercorrected, and further aponeurotic surgery could be done as indicated. Bilateral brow suspension is the usual definitive treatment for CPEO. However, corneal exposure may be a problem in view of poor sursumduction and absent Bell's phenomenon. Use of synthetic materials should be utilized initially in the event that reversal is necessary. The suture tarsorrhaphy system should be employed postoperatively. Beard (6) advocates repeated skin excisions as the safest surgical treatment.

OCULOPHARYNGEAL MUSCULAR DYSTROPHY

This syndrome may represent a variant of chronic progressive external ophthalmoplegia. It is found in patients of French-Canadian descent and is characterized by ptosis and dysphagia beginning usually in the fourth to fifth decade of life. The extraocular muscles and Bell's phenomenon are usually unaffected. Levator function often is better than patients with CPEO. Electron microscopy reveals a decrease of striated muscle fibers and the disease is felt to be primarily a myopathy. Johnson and Kuwabara (21) recommend a levator resection if levator function is 9 mm or more and a brow suspension when it is 8 mm or less.

MYOTONIC DYSTROPHY

Myotonic dystrophy is a rare condition that produces multiple ocular and systemic abnormalities. The ptosis is usually mild and symmetrical. Other ocular findings include ophthalmoplegia, polychromatic cataract, retinal pigmentary changes, sluggish pupils with poor mydriasis, weak orbicularis oculi, and occasional low intraocular pressure. The disease begins in childhood or adolescence and often facial, neck and limb muscles are atrophied. There may be early frontal baldness. Due to the weakened orbicularis oculi associated with myotonic dystrophy, a more conservative approach is indicated. Usually a Fasanella-type procedure or levator resection is sufficient (22).

MYASTHENIA GRAVIS

Myasthenia gravis is often overlooked as a cause for acquired blepharoptosis and is a well-recognized neuromuscular ptosis syndrome. Although classified as a myopathic process, it is really a neuromuscular transmission defect characterized by a deficiency of acetylcholine. The disease can occur at any age; it rarely has a familial pattern. Ocular involvement occurs in 90% of myasthenia patients and is the initial complaint in 75% of cases. It is reported that 80% with ocular findings progress to involve other muscle groups (23). The disease is characterized by fatigue with remission. The clinician should seek the presence of general fatigue, diplopia, or varying degrees of facial asymmetry in all patients with ptosis.

The ocular findings are usually asymmetrical, and the ptosis may change from side to side. If unilateral ptosis is present, there may be contralateral lid retraction (24). Cogan (25) has described a lid twitch sign in myasthenia patients. As the patient looks from downgaze to primary position, the upper lid retracts only to resume the ptotic appearance. The extraocular muscles are variably affected; most often it is the medial rectus. The pupil and accommodation are invariably spared. With historical clues, the ocular examination can further demonstrate the signs of the myasthenic patient. Asking the patient to look upwards for a sustained period of time can fatigue the levator and the ptosis may worsen (Figs. 38.11 and 38.12). Osher and Glaser (26) demonstrated ocular gaze fatigue with prolonged lateral gaze. As mentioned previously, the lid twitch sign may be elicited.

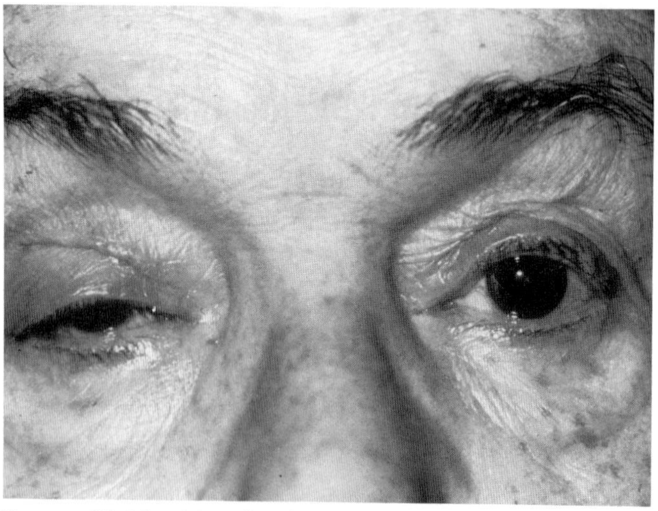

Figure 38.11. Myasthenia gravis before edrophonium test.

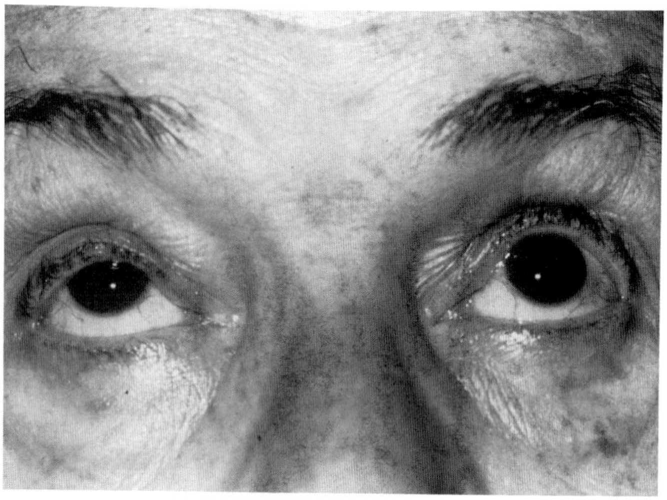

Figure 38.12. Myasthenia gravis upgaze before edrophonium test.

Edrophonium Test

The edrophonium (Tensilon) test is one of the most dramatic examinations in medicine. The test is performed by inserting a butterfly needle into an antecubital or hand vein. Initially 0.1 ml (1 mg) of Tensilon is given and the patient is observed for 1 minute for signs of systemic effect. After 1 minute, the remaining 0.9 ml (9 mg) is then given and the fissure width and/or the strabismus is measured frequently for 3 minutes. Atrophic sulfate (0.4 mg) should be readily available if too great a parasympathetic response is obtained. Rarely, false-positive results are seen, but false-negative occur more often due to infrequent or cursory measuring. Neostigmine (prostigmine) may alternatively be used diagnostically.

If the Tensilon test is positive, the patient should be referred to an internist or neurologist for therapy (Fig. 38.13). Treatment usually consists of Mestinon (pyridostigmine), although systemic corticosteroids have been used for resistant cases. A thyroid evaluation should be obtained due to an association of thyroid disease with approximately 5% of myasthenic patients. There is also a high incidence of thymoma with myasthenia. The Lambert-Eaton syndrome is a myasthenic-like disease associated with neoplasms, most prominently bronchogenic carcinoma. Systemic antibiotics such as streptomycin, neomycin, kanamycin, polymixin, bacitracin, and colistin have been implicated in causing a myasthenic-like syndrome.

Surgical treatment for ptosis secondary to myasthenia gravis can only be considered after medical therapy has stabilized the disease. Due to the varying involvement, surgical treatment may be unsuccessful. If the patient is functionally and cosmetically disturbed, a similar approach to the patient with CPEO may be employed. Crutch glasses may be tried initially. A Fasanella-Servat or levator aponeurosis surgery may be tried but definitive treatment is from brow suspension.

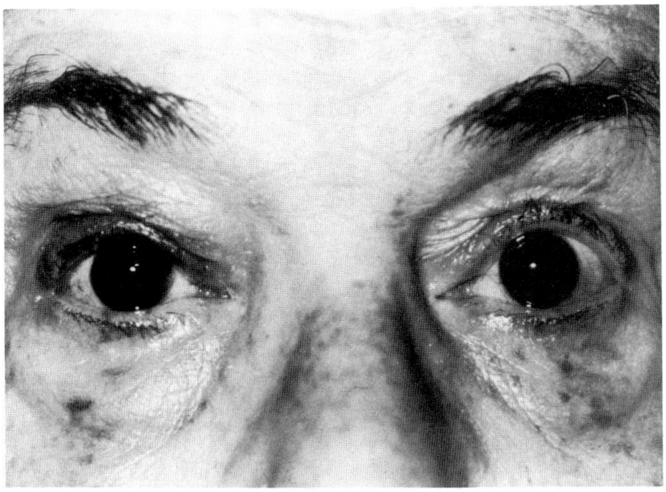

Figure 38.13. Myasthenia gravis after edrophonium test.

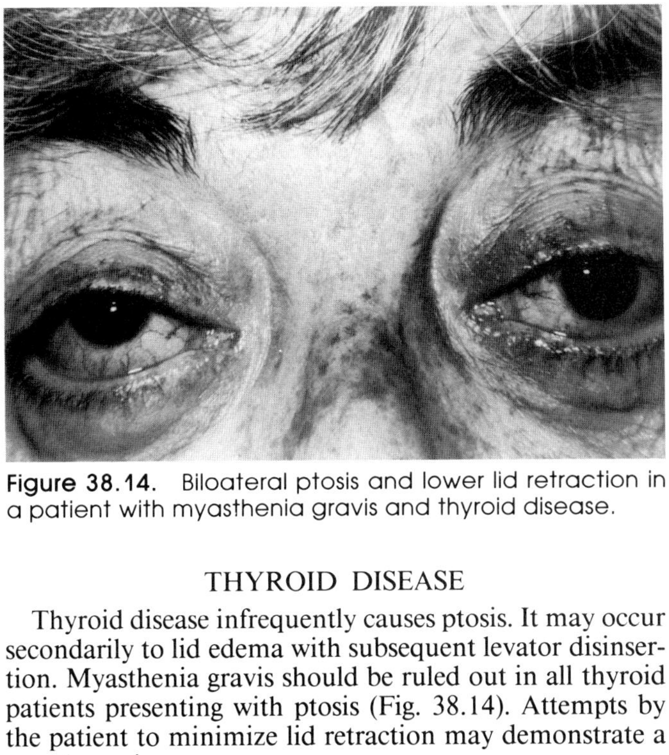

Figure 38.14. Biloateral ptosis and lower lid retraction in a patient with myasthenia gravis and thyroid disease.

THYROID DISEASE

Thyroid disease infrequently causes ptosis. It may occur secondarily to lid edema with subsequent levator disinsertion. Myasthenia gravis should be ruled out in all thyroid patients presenting with ptosis (Fig. 38.14). Attempts by the patient to minimize lid retraction may demonstrate a pseudoptosis.

Surgical correction of ptosis can be considered when lid measurement and photographs remain stable for at least 6 months. A levator advancement with or without a resection usually corrects the minimal to moderate ptosis seen with thyroid disease (27). A Fasanella-type operation can also be used successfully but frequently can cause overcorrection. Smaller excisions of tarsus, conjunctiva, and Müller's muscle, or conjunctiva and Müller's muscle alone are indicated.

CORTICOSTEROID INDUCED PTOSIS

There are reports of long-term use of topical corticosteroids being a causative factor in producing acquired ptosis. The ptosis is usually mild and may be secondary to the underlying disease (uveitis, chronic conjunctivitis, keratitis) or to excessive manipulation of the lids when instilling the medication. No histopathologic studies have been done, but levator disinsertion or dehiscence may be the cause. A Fasanella-type procedure or levator repair is usually corrective.

PTOSIS FROM PREGNANCY

Beard (6) has demonstrated cases of ptosis occurring shortly after delivery in pregnant women. He speculated the cause as being levator disinsertion, possibly due to increased interstitial lid fluid, high progesterone levels, or physical stress from delivery. A levator advancement with possible tuck or a Fasanella procedure is sufficient to correct the ptosis.

SENILE PTOSIS

This common form of ptosis is seen most commonly in the elderly patient (past the 6th decade of life). It is due to progressive thinning of the levator or disinsertion from the tarsus. The condition is characterized by ptosis, high lid crease (representing disinsertion of the aponeurosis), and normal levator function. A similar clinical picture is seen in patients with typically bilateral ptosis occurring in the fourth to sixth decade of life with a familial predisposition; this is termed "late acquired hereditary ptosis." These syndromes and their management will be discussed in another chapter.

REFERENCES

1. Sano K: Trigemino-oculomotor synkinesis. *Neurologia* 1: 29, 1959.
2. Gunn MR: Congenital ptosis with peculiar associated movements of the affected lid. *Trans Ophthalmol Soc UK* 3: 283, 1883.
3. Pratt S: Marcus Gunn phenomenon study said to find unexpected results. *Ophthalmol Times* July 15, 1984, pg. 28.
4. Putterman AM, Urist MS: Müllers muscle-conjunctival resection. *Arch Ophthalmol* 93: 619, 1973.
5. Fasanella RM, Servat J: Levator resection for minimal ptosis. Another simplified operation. *Am J Ophthalmol* 65: 493, 1961.
6. Beard C: *Ptosis,* ed 3. St. Louis, CV Mosby, 1981.
7. Epstein GA, Putterman AM: Super maximum levator resection for severe unilateral congenital blepharoptosis. *Ophthal Surg* 15: 971–979, 1984.
8. Beard CA: New treatment for severe unilateral congenital ptosis and for ptosis with jaw winking. *Am J Ophthalmol* 59: 252, 1965.
9. Walsh FS, Hoyt WF: *Clinical Neuro-Ophthalmology,* ed 3. Baltimore, Williams & Wilkins Co. 1969.
10. Frueh BR: Associated facial contractions after seventh nerve palsy mimicking jaw winking. *Ophthalmology* 90: 1105, 1983.
11. Oesterle CS, Faudkiner WJ, Clay R, Fold ER, Lucchese N, Putterman AM: Eye bobbing associated with jaw movement. *Ophthalmology* 89: 63, 1982.
12. Leone CR, Weinstein GW: Orbital fibrosis with enophthalmos. *Ophthal Surg* 3: 71, 1972.
13. Glaser JS: Infranuclear disorders of eye movements. In Duane TD: *Clinical Ophthalmology.* Philadelphia, Harper & Row, vol 2, 1983.
14. Putterman AM: Suture tarsorrhaphy system to control keratopathy after ptosis surgery. *Ophthal Surg* 11: 577, 1980.
15. Thompson HS, Monsher JH: Adrenergic mydriasis in Horner's syndrome. *Am J Ophthalmol* 72: 472, 1971.
16. Stasior OG, Roen JL: The anophthalmic socket and enophthalmos. In Stewart WB: *Ophthalmic Plastic and Reconstructive Surgery.* San Francisco, American Academy of Ophthalmology, 1984.
17. Daroff RB: Chronic progressive external ophthalmoplegia: A critical review. *Arch Ophthalmol* 82: 845, 1969.
18. Kearns TP, Sayre GP: Retinitis pigmentosa, external ophthalmoplegia and complete heart block: Unusual syndrome with histologic study in one of two cases. *Arch Ophthalmol* 60: 28, 1958.

19. Drachman DA: Ophthalmoplegia plus the neurodegenerative disorders associated with progressive external ophthalmoplegia. *Arch Neurol* 18: 654, 1968.
20. Johnson CC, Kuwabara T: Oculopharyngeal muscular dystrophy. *Am J Ophthalmol* 77: 872, 1974.
21. Anderson RL, Dixon RS: Neuromyopathic ptosis: a new surgical approach. *Arch Ophthalmol* 97: 1129, 1979.
22. Walker RR: Management of myogenic (Myopathic) Ptosis. *Trans Am Acad Ophthalmol Otolaryngol* 79: 697, 1975.
23. Rosenberg MA: in Principles and Practice of Ophthalmology ed. by Peyman GA, Saunders DR, Goldberg MF. Philadelphia, WB Saunders, 1980.
24. Burian HM, Burns CA: Ocular changes in myasthenic dystrophy. *Am J Ophthalmol* 63: 22, 1967.
25. Cogan DG: Myasthenia gravis: a review of the disease and a description of lid twitch as a characteristic sign. *Arch Ophthalmol* 74: 217, 1965.
26. Osher RH, Glaser JS: Myasthenic sustained gaze fatigue. *Am J Ophthalmol* 89: 473, 1980.
27. Waller RR: Evaluation and management of the ptosis patient. In McCord CD (ed): *Oculoplastic Surgery.* New York, Raven Press 1981.

CHAPTER 39

Lagophthalmos

EUGENE O. WIGGS, M.D.

Lagophthalmos means "incomplete closure of the eyelids," and the term is derived from the Greek word for hare. The Greeks believed that the hare slept with its eyes open. Lagophthalmos, which has varied causes, can be classified as follows:

1. Postsurgical: large levator resection and frontalis sling, upper blepharoplasty, lower eyelid and upper eyelid reconstruction, large inferior rectus recession;
2. In association with seventh nerve palsies: Bell's palsy, following resection of tumors from the cerebellar-pontine angle (usually acoustic neuromas), following parotid surgery (permanent facial nerve palsy existing if there is malignancy present, and frequently transiently for benign tumors);
3. Thyroid ophthalmopathy with upper and/or lower lid retraction;
4. Ectropion of the lower lid;
5. Anophthalmos with a sagging lower lid and increased curvature or scarred fornices, which prevents closing movements of the upper and/or lower lid;
6. Nocturnal lagophthalmos: a rare entity, which Duke Elder (1) notes is more common in Chinese;
7. Mechanical factors: high myopia, buphthalmos, proptosis;
8. Inflammatory and systemic cicatrizations such as scleroderma or mycosis fungoides;
9. Euryblepharon.

MANAGEMENT

Lagophthalmos, which is thought to be temporary as in an acute Bell's palsy, should be managed with emollient drops and ointments. Taping the eyelids shut at night also greatly benefits these patients, though they do incur problems with skin erosion from the tape over a prolonged period of time. If the patient develops exposure keratopathy in spite of drops, ointment and taping, and the cause of the lagophthalmos is thought to be temporary, a tarsorrhaphy which is temporary should be performed. I prefer the technique described by Scott and Johnson (2) because it does not involve the use of the eyelid margins; this use can predispose the patient to lid margin deformities and trichiasis. In this technique a flap of palpebral conjunctiva is mobilized from just below the inferior tarsus laterally and sewn into a slot just below the top of the superior tarsus. Any patient who has sustained both a fifth and seventh nerve palsy should have a permanent tarsorrhaphy performed as soon as is feasible to prevent corneal ulceration.

A flush-fitting scleral lens can be useful in the management of patients with a fifth and seventh nerve palsy. Soft lenses are not feasible because the patient is unable to blink and if the lens comes off the eye, the patient is unaware of it due to lack of sensation. A convenient moist chamber involves the use of swimming goggles, which the patient wears at night while sleeping.

POSTSURGICALLY INDUCED

Almost all children adapt to the lagophthalmos induced by larger levator resections or frontalis suspension operations. A combination of drops, ointments, moist chambers and/or Frost sutures is usually employed during the first several weeks postoperatively. Exposure keratopathy not relieved by drops and ointment is more easily managed by a Frost suture than a moist chamber on a short-term basis. Other physicians, however, have had excellent success with a moist chamber. If the patient has a corneal exposure problem postoperatively that has not been relieved by drops or ointment, it is a simple matter to gently pull the lower lid upward and tape the suture to the forehead. When not in use, the Frost suture is taped to the cheek. A monofilament suture is used to minimize postoperative reaction in the eyelid. Adults do not adapt as well and some may require drops and ointment indefinitely. Smaller levator resections used in the typical acquired adult-onset or senile ptosis and milder degrees of congenital ptosis do not generally induce lagophthalmos. Obviously, if a patient has a poor Bell's phenomenon, decreased tearing, a compromised orbicularis, or any combination of these, a more conservative lid-elevating procedure should be done if ptosis surgery is necessary.

The minimal lagophthalmos induced by a properly executed upper blepharoplasty frequently disappears within the first few postoperative weeks. The lagophthalmos disappears or is minimized because of a reactivation of the orbicularis, the effect of gravity, the disappearance of postoperative pain, and a probable slight stretch of the tissue. Exposure keratopathy develops in those patients who have had an unduly large amount of skin taken from the upper lid and/or who have a poor Bell's phenomenon and/or decreased tears. The presence of a good Bell's phenomenon does not mean that in deep sleep the patient will not have exposure keratopathy; some patients will and others will not. What is significant is that those who have an absent or poor Bell's phenomenon, decreased tears, or both will invariably have an exposure problem if lagophthalmos is present at the end of the operation. If drops or ointment do not alleviate the patient's postoperative exposure keratopathy, a full-thickness skin graft should be grafted to the upper eyelid. A skin graft is done only if exposure keratopathy is severe. The combination of lagophthalmos and severe lid lag following upper blepharoplasty (without obvious skin shortage) indicates that there has been incarceration of the orbital septum into the wound closure or the septum itself has been sewn closed. These patients need lysis of the septal adhesions and may or may not require a skin graft; intermarginal sutures are frequently helpful postoperatively. Kamin (3) has described the use of a conjunctival flap over the inferior aspect of the cornea as an alternative therapeutic modality for exposure keratopathy secondary to lagophthalmos.

Lagophthalmos after major eyelid reconstruction usually results from lower eyelid retraction. If corrective surgery is necessary, a technique that I have described for treating lower lid retraction may be of use (4). The technique consists of skin muscle and tarsal conjunctival transposition flaps from the upper to the lower eyelid. Large resections of the upper lid, which may be necessary for tumor ablation, can produce lagophthalmos due to a tight levator or full-thickness shortening of the upper lid. Both conditions also produce upper eyelid retraction. A taut levator is treated by a controlled levator recession as in an overcorrected levator resection. Full-thickness vertical shortening of the upper eyelid can be treated by skin and deeper laminar grafts placed at staggered levels in the eyelid so that each graft obtains a blood supply. A biopsy of any "excess scarring" at the time of stage 2 reconstruction or following a stage 2 reconstruction of the eyelid should be done to be sure recurrent tumor is not present.

Lagophthalmos due to surgery on the inferior rectus results from a recession of this muscle in excess of 4–5 mm without severing the capsulopalpebral fascial connections to the tarsus. These patients need to have an intermarginal lid suture placed after the connections between the capsulopalpebral fascia and the inferior tarsus have been severed. It is usually possible to relieve the lagophthalmos and lower lid retraction by a total severing of the fascial connections between the inferior rectus and the eyelid or a resection of the fascial band may be done. In either case an intermarginal suture should be left in place for approximately 5–7 days. In some instances a filler is inserted between the bottom of the tarsus and the recessed or resected capsulopalpebral fascia; a convenient tissue for this is ear cartilage from the scaphoid fossa, which helps to push the lower lid upward.

SECONDARY TO SEVENTH NERVE PALSY

ARION CERCLAGE TECHNIQUE

The problem of facial nerve palsy has intrigued and frustrated surgeons from a variety of disciplines. The numerous operations that have been described indicate that we are still searching for an ideal solution. Among the surgical remedies that have been tried for lagophthalmos secondary to facial nerve palsy are gold weights in the upper eyelid, eyelid magnets, and metallic springs. All of these attempts have been plagued by problems of extrusion. Probably the most ingenious solution has been proposed by Arion (5), who developed the use of a silicone rod for eyelid closure. Description of the technique is as follows: The medial and lateral canthus as well as both eyelids are infiltrated with local anesthetic containing epinephrine. The medial canthal tendon is isolated by a curved vertical incision over the tendon. A horizontal incision is made over the lateral orbital rim at the lateral canthus. Level with the lateral commissure, a hole is drilled through the orbital rim and a 4-0 nonabsorbable monofilament suture is passed through this hole. A 1-mm solid silicone rod is then passed under the medial canthal tendon, and this can be done using either a wire suture or a small curved surgical needle with a large eye. A special threader is then passed from a lateral to a medial plane in the lower eyelid between the tarsus and orbicularis while hugging the lid margin. One end of the silastic rod is inserted into the eye of the instrument, the instrument is drawn laterally, and the end is brought out through the lateral canthal wound. It is important to hug the margin in this maneuver because if the rod is placed lower in the lower lid it can cause ectropion. In the upper lid the threader is also passed from lateral to medial between the orbicularis and tarsus, but one can stay several millimeters from the lid margin as ectropion is not a problem and it is important not to injure the lash follicles. The other end of the silicone rod is then drawn medially and laterally. The ends of the silastic rod are then passed through the hole in the lateral orbital rim. Slight tension if placed on the silastic rod, and the patient is asked to open the eyes. The ideal tension is reached when the patient is able to readily open the eyes but with relaxation of the levator the lids close. Generally the amount of tension needed corresponds to the weight of a mosquito hemostat. When proper tension has been achieved the suture, that has been previously placed through the lateral orbital rim hole is tied securing the silastic rod. The ends of the silastic rod can be placed through a silicone sleeve such as is used in retinal detachment surgery; the silicone is sewn to the periosteum or the ends are pointed in opposite directions in the same plane as the skin. Make sure that the ends of the silastic do not stick upward toward the skin, as this predisposes to extrusion. The wounds are closed in layers (Fig. 39.1).

Erosion of the silastic through the tissue and a loosening of the silastic are the main complications of this operation. The operation has been more successful in theory than in practice, but it has benefited a few patients. In cases of prolonged seventh nerve palsy it may be necessary to perform a horizontal shortening operation on the lower eyelid to bring the eyelid into proper apposition to the globe.

ANASTOMOSES

Anastomoses have also been carried out between the facial nerve and the spinal accessory and hypoglossal nerves. At the present time the 12-7 anastomosis is more commonly done. This operation has the significant advantage of restoring facial tone, but it really does not provide much in the way of facial dynamics or significant lid closure. A great disadvantage of the 12-7 anastomosis is that the patient develops a hemiatrophy of the tongue with some subsequent slurring of speech which, though not great, in many of these patients is somewhat troublesome. A Z-plasty performed on the tongue has resulted in reneurotization of the atrophic side (6). This procedure has not stood the test of time but hopefully it will, as it could represent a remarkable advance in rehabilitation of the patient with a seventh nerve palsy. Patients also can develop mass facial movements with a 12-7 anastomosis and many patients find this aspect of the procedure also undesirable. Another attempt to produce dynamic lid closure has been with the temporalis transfer but great enthusiasm has not developed for this procedure, as it does not seem to produce the desired result in a majority of patients. Levator recession can also be helpful in some patients with a facial nerve palsy; this procedure reduces lagophthalmos and upper lid retraction.

TARSORRHAPHY

Among the more static procedures that have been developed are lateral tarsorrhaphy; the tarsorrhaphy technique that I use is described next: Local anesthetic containing epinephrine is infiltrated into the upper and lower eyelid. The upper lid margin is split over the lateral 4–6 mm of lid and a flap of tarsus conjunctiva is developed by making vertical-relaxing incisions. The lid margin on the posterior flap is sacrificed. A corresponding tarsal conjunctival defect including lid margin is made in the lower lid. The tarsal conjunctival flap from the upper lid is advanced into the lower lid defect and secured with horizontal mattress sutures tied over a bolster on the skin of the lower lid. Skin from the lower lid is advanced upward and sewn to the skin of the upper lid to complete the closure. With this technique one may sacrifice the hair-bearing portion of the lid margin from both eyelids or the lower eyelid only (Fig. 39.2). A generally superior cosmetic result is obtained in women by sparing the lashes of the upper lid laterally.

Patients with lagophthalmos due to facial nerve palsy usually need more than eyelid surgery. They require facial suspension as well. These patients invariably have a ptosis of the eyebrow, a partial collapse of the nostril on the side of the facial nerve palsy, and a drooping of the face that is accentuated by a downward-turning angle of the mouth. Ideally these patients can be treated by a brow lift, an upper blepharoplasty if necessary, a horizontal-shortening operation on the lower eyelid and a fascia lata sling to the lower eyelid and face. After a horizontal-shortening operation on the eyelid a thin strip of fascia is sewn to the medial canthal tendon, drawn through the lower lid just beneath the margin in the space between orbicularis and

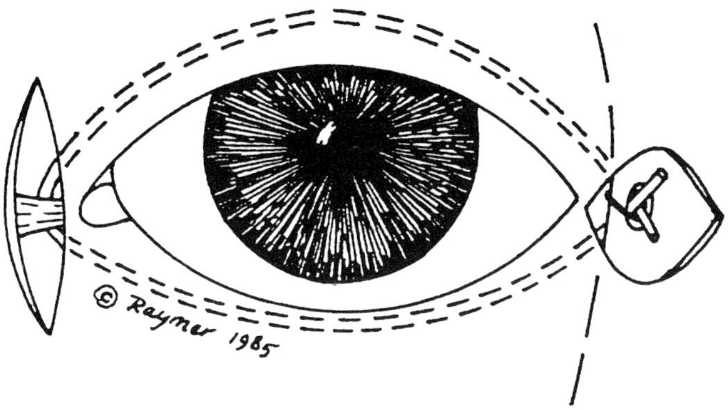

Figure 39.1. Arion rod before tightening.

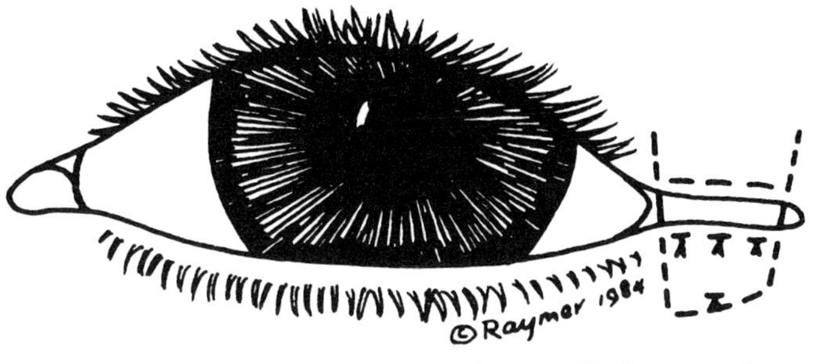

Figure 39.2. Tarsorrhaphy technique with tarsoconjunctival flap from upper lid advanced into lower lid defect. Spared lashes (frequently left on upper lid laterally) not shown for purposes of illustration. Skin wound not closed in illustration.

tarsus, and then sewn to the lateral orbital rim. I like to place several sutures in the tarsus to secure the fascia to the lower lid to prevent downward migration and ectropion induction. The fascia is brought through a periosteal tunnel in the lateral orbital rim. Skin wounds are closed in the usual fashion (7).

FASCIA LATA SLING TECHNIQUE

The fascia lata sling technique is as follows: A strip of fascia lata 1 by 20 cm is harvested from the lateral thigh. A temporal incision is made in front of the hairline on the side of the facial nerve palsy and dissection is carried down to the temporalis fascia. Three or four horizontal cuts are made in the temporalis fascia. Vertical incisions are made just lateral to the nasal ala, just lateral to the angle of the mouth, just past the philtrum on the upper lip on the uninvolved side, and in a corresponding position in the lower lip. Scissors then create subcutaneous tunnels between the temporal incision and the incision lateral to the nasal ala and the incision lateral to the angle of the mouth. Subcutaneous tunnels also connect the incision at the lateral angle of the mouth to the two lip incisions. The fascia lata is cut into two strips, the strip going to the nasal ala is about 3–4 mm wide. The two fascia lata strips are woven through the cuts in the temporalis fascia and secured with a hemostat. The fascial strip to the nasal alar area is then passed subcutaneously to the wound lateral to the nasal ala and sewn to the dermis with nonabsorbable sutures. The other wider piece of fascia is passed subcutaneously to the wound just lateral to the angle of the mouth and divided into three strips here. The fascia is then sewn under slight tension to the dermis at the lateral angle of the mouth after looping it around the orbicularis oris. The other two ends of the fascia are passed subcutaneously to the lip wounds and sewn to the dermis under slight tension. In the four lower facial incisions the fascia is sewn to the dermis on the side of the wound away from the temporal wound so as to facilitate tension-free wound closure. The four lower facial wounds are closed with monofilament skin sutures. The two fascial strips are then pulled upward and laterally and woven through the cuts in the temporalis fascia so as to slightly overcorrect the drooping at the lateral angle of the mouth and to slightly widen the nostril. When this has been accomplished, the fascia lata is sewn to the temporalis fascia with nonabsorbable sutures. The wound is then closed in layers. Though this operation is not a dynamic one, it is permanent and

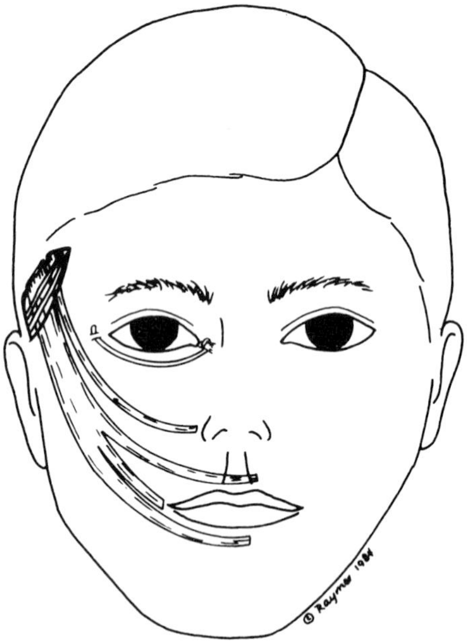

Figure 39.3. Placement of fascia lata strips for facial sling and fascia lata sling to the lower eyelid.

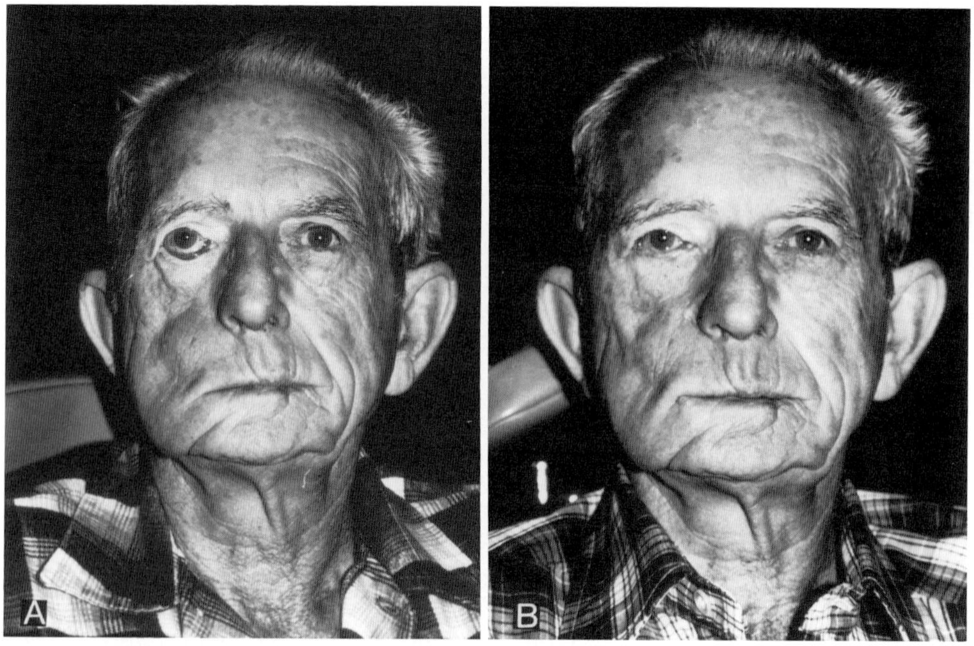

Figure 39.4. Patient with longstanding right facial nerve palsy before (*A*) and after (*B*) undergoing fascia lata sling to the right lower lid and right side of the face, as well as brow lift and horizontal shortening of the right lower lid.

produces reasonable facial symmetry. It is important that excess facial skin be resected by pulling the excess skin upward and temporally, and it will sometimes be necessary to extend the incision down in front of the ear. A nasolabial crease is created as necessary by resecting skin in this area and closing the wound so as to produce some inversion of the edges. A diagram of the operation is seen in Figure 39.3. A preoperative and postoperative picture of a patient with a longstanding facial nerve palsy is seen in Figure 39.4. This patient underwent a brow lift, a horizontal-shortening operation of the left lower eyelid, a fascia lata sling to the lower lid, and a facial sling.

SECONDARY TO THYROID OPHTHALMOPATHY

Lagophthalmos secondary to thyroid ophthalmopathy can result from inflammatory sequelae involving the levator muscle and/or lower eyelid retractors. The treatment of these conditions is described in detail elsewhere in this volume. The surgical procedure involves excising up to 2 mm from the superior tarsal muscle for upper lid retraction; for greater retraction, one carries out a controlled levator recession under local anesthesia. For most patients it is not necessary to use a "filler" between the recessed levator and the top of the tarsus. In the lower lid one may also use various types of fillers, including ear cartilage, between the recessed or resected lower lid retractors and the lower border of the tarsus. I think that the ear cartilage helps to push the lower lid upward and this is supplemented by severing the connections between the lower border of the tarsus and the lower lid retractors. An intermarginal suture is invaluable in these procedures, particularly in the lower lid operations. Figure 39.5 shows a patient with thyroid ophthalmopathy before and following ear cartilage grafts to the lower eyelids.

Lagophthalmos with resultant exposure keratopathy that is severe and cannot be controlled by more conservative measures can be an indication for orbital decompression. In general if the proptosis is severe, it is better to

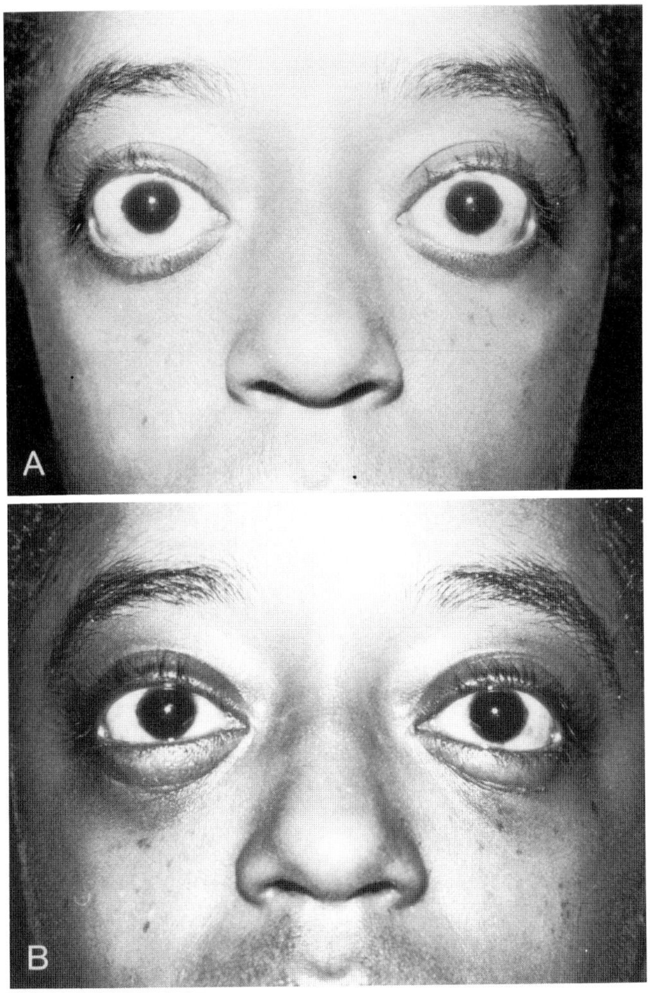

Figure 39.5. Preoperative (*A*) and postoperative (*B*) photographs of thyroid ophthalmopathy patient with severe lower eyelid retraction, who underwent retractor weakening and ear cartilage graft to the lower lids. No surgery was carried out on the upper lids even though they are lower postoperatively.

perform the decompression prior to eyelid surgery but in some milder instances I think it is preferable to proceed with eyelid surgery in an attempt to avoid a decompression. Ideally, the thyroid disease should be quiescent before eyelid surgery.

SECONDARY TO ECTROPION OF THE LOWER EYELID

Lagophthalmos resulting from ectropion of the lower lid is treated by a horizontal-shortening operation on the eyelid and lengthening of the anterior lamina of the lid if cicatricial ectropion exists. The lengthening of the skin lamina of the eyelid is best accomplished by a transposition flap of skin muscle from the ipsilateral upper eyelid or one may use a full thickness skin graft (Fig. 39.6). Generally the skin muscle flap is superior to a skin graft because of the blood supply present in the flap and better color match. For paralytic ectropion a horizontal-shortening operation combined with a fascia lata sling (7) or a lateral tarsal strip operation (8) may be used.

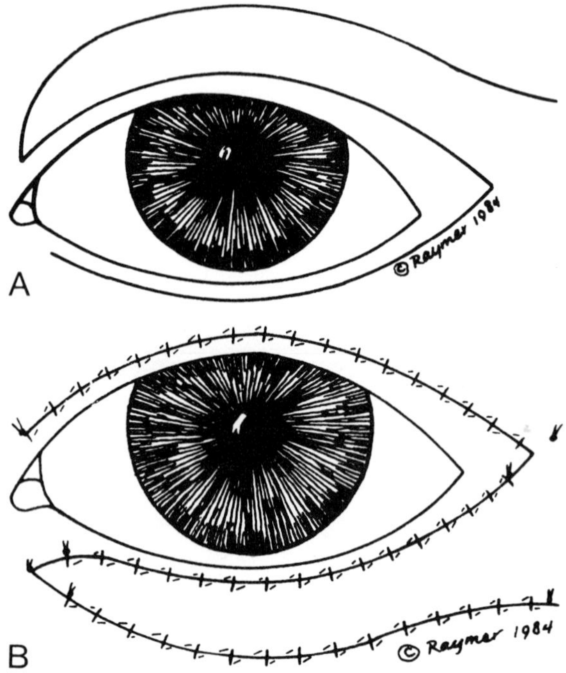

Figure 39.6. *A,* Outline of skin-muscle transposition flap on an upper eyelid and incision on the lower eyelid. *B,* Transposition of skin-muscle flap from upper to lower eyelid.

SECONDARY TO ANOPHTHALMOS

The lagophthalmos resulting from anophthalmos is frequently not amenable to surgery as one is often dealing with a contracted socket. The lagophthalmos in this situation results from scarring in the fornices and dome of the socket with significantly reduced lid motility. Some improvement can be obtained by placing the patient on squeezing exercises to improve the elasticity of the eyelids, but the changes here are only minimal in most cases. One thing that can be done is to help the patient retain a luster to the prosthesis. This can be done with various types of oils but I prefer a silicone drop manufactured under the name of Sil-Ophtho. Patients with this problem should not be placed on any drop which can dry and form a dry crust on their prosthesis, which further reduces the luster of the prosthesis. These patients also need to have a buff and polish of their prosthesis once or twice a year. Scrupulous cleaning of the prosthesis is also frequently necessary on a daily basis or more for some of these patients.

NOCTURNAL AND SECONDARY TO MECHANICAL FACTORS

Nocturnal lagophthalmos is best treated by the use of lid taping or an ointment at bedtime. The lagophthalmos resulting from high myopia, buphthalmos, or proptosis has to be treated on an individual basis, and it is difficult to generalize regarding treatment modalities. A tarsorrhaphy can be enormously beneficial to these patients; swimming goggles can sometimes provide a satisfactory moist chamber while sleeping at night.

Euryblepharon is a condition characterized by an abnormally large palpebral fissure. Some patients with euryblepharon develop severe exposure problems and corneal ulcers. A lateral tarsorrhaphy provides a great relief for these patients.

SECONDARY TO INFLAMMATION OR SYSTEMIC DISEASES

Lagophthalmos resulting from inflammatory and systemic diseases, which cause lid retraction and ectropion, have to be individually considered. Generally these patients have chronic difficulties, and most surgical measures are frequently only temporizing in nature. Some of the problems and partial solutions are exemplified by the following patient:

A 65-year-old white female had mycosis fungoides for many years. The patient developed severe lagophthalmos secondary to lower lid retraction and ectropion secondary to involvement of the lower lid by the lymphoma. The exposure keratopathy that she experienced eventually resulted in ulceration of the cornea in spite of drops, ointments, and intermarginal sutures. The patient was finally given some temporary relief by means of a horizontal-shortening operation on the lower eyelid and lengthening of the anterior lamina of the lower lid by means of a skin muscle transposition flap from the upper lid to the lower lid (Figs. 39.6 and 39.7). The patient also required a lateral tarsorrhaphy at a later date. After the operations the patient has had less exposure problems than before the operation.

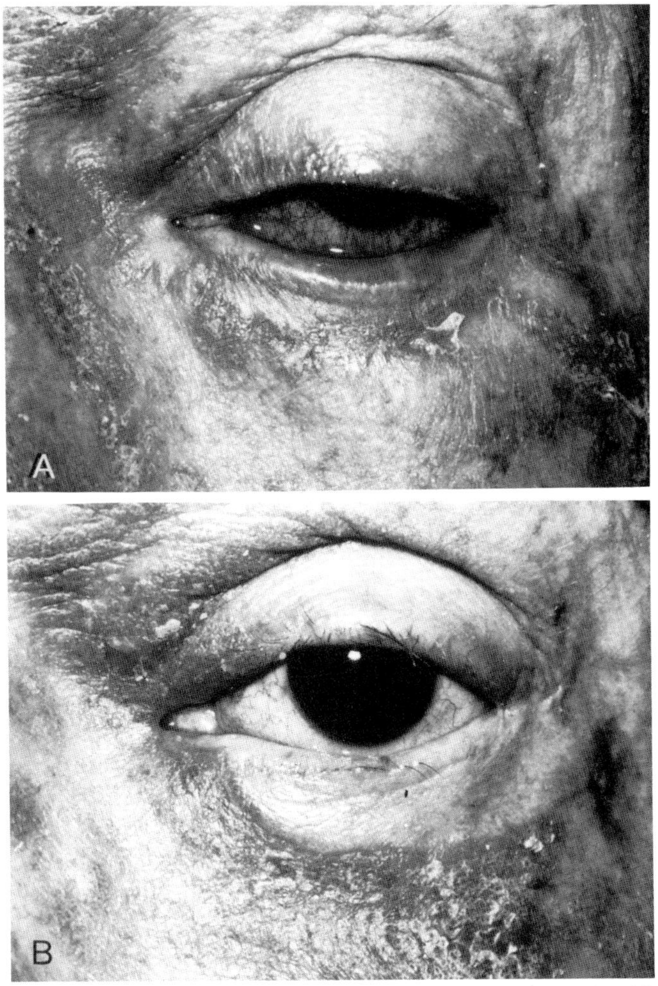

Figure 39.7. Patient with mycosis fungoides and cicatricial ectropion before (*A*) and after (*B*) undergoing horizontal shortening of the left lower eyelid and skin-muscle transposition flap from upper to lower eyelid.

REFERENCES

1. Duke-Elder S: *System of Ophthalmology.* London, Henry Kimpton, 1974, vol. 13, no. 1.
2. Scott AB, Johnson RC: A modified tarsorrhaphy technique. *Arch Ophthamol* 88: 530–531, 1972.
3. Kamin D: *Ophthalmol Times* 9: 32–33. 1984.
4. Wiggs EO: Treatment of lower lid retraction by tarso-conjunctival and skin muscle transposition flaps. *Ophthal Surg* 14: 663–665, 1983.
5. Arion HG: Dynamic closure of the lids and paralysis of the orbicularis muscle. *Int Surg* 57: 48–50, 1972.
6. Rubin LR et al: Reanimation of the hemiparalytic tongue. *Plast Reconstr Surg* 73: 184–192, 1984.
7. Wiggs EO et al: Surgical treatment of the denervated or sagging lower lid. *Ophthalmology* 89: 428–432, 1982.
8. Anderson RL, Gordy DD: The tarsal strip procedure. *Arch Ophthalmol* 97: 2192–2196, 1979.

CHAPTER 40

Ectropion of the Lower Eyelid

KENNETH V. CAHILL, M.D.
GEORGE F. BUERGER, JR., M.D.
JOHN D. SHEPPARD, JR., M.D.

Lower lid ectropion is a condition in which the lower lid margin is everted from the globe. Tears collect along the malpositioned lower lid, which leads to epiphora and cutaneous irritation. If palpebral conjunctiva is exposed, it becomes hyperemic, edematous, and uncomfortable. In advanced ectropion the exposed conjunctiva becomes keratotic, and corneal exposure can occur along with pain and possible visual loss.

CAUSES

Most causes of lower lid ectropion are acquired. Ectropion can occur on the basis of lower lid laxity or cicatricial changes of the lower lid. Laxity is usually the result of involutional stretching of the medial canthal tendon, lateral canthal tendon, or both. Although the tarsal plate may become less rigid as a result of inflammation of aging, it rarely stretches significantly. Laxity of the orbicularis oculi muscles can also contribute to the manifestation of an ectropion. This is frequently seen in patients with a seventh cranial nerve palsy. Enophthalmos resulting from orbital trauma or involutional fat atrophy can allow the lower lid to become lax and ectropic.

Cicatricial processes affecting lower lid skin, subcutaneous tissue, orbicularis oculi muscles, or the orbital septum can produce lower lid ectropion. This can be the result of trauma or skin diseases. Vertical lid lacerations that heal with cicatricial shortening are an obvious cause. Lower lid blepharoplasties in which excessive skin is removed, or if there is unrecognized preexisting lid laxity, can also cause ectropion. Burns may lead to tissue contraction and ectropion. These can be acute thermal injuries, chronic exposure to infrared radiation, or high-dose ionizing radiation. Some localized dermatologic conditions and diffuse scleroderma may also be responsible for ectropion. These cicatricial processes can occur alone or in combination with canthal tendon laxity.

Cicatricial ectropion should be differentiated from lower lid retraction. Inferior scleral show is frequently seen in patients with proptosis. In these cases the lower lid margin is not everted. Anterior displacement of the globe creates an appearance of lid retraction. Thyroid ophthalmopathy can also produce lower lid retraction on the basis of cicatrization. Since the cicatrization preferentially involves lid retractors, the lower lid margin is pulled down without eversion. Lower lid retraction requires different techniques for evaluation and management than does an ectropion.

Ectropion can also occur as a congenital defect. This is usually due to insufficient anterior lamellar lower lid tissue, resembling cicatricial ectropion. However, it may be complicated by concurrent maxillary hypoplasia, decreased tarsal rigidity, poorly developed canthal tendons, and low attachment of the lateral canthal tendon. Type II blepharophimosis syndrome and Treacher Collins' syndrome are examples of congenital ectropion with associated periocular anomalies.

EVALUATION OF PATIENT

The portion of the ocular examination to evaluate ectropion should begin with careful facial observation. Skin lines and wrinkles should be noted. Patients who have sustained burns, spent a career in proximity to industrial furnaces, or been affected by scleroderma will show an absence of normal skin lines. Scars from injuries or previous surgeries should be searched for. Lid inflammation and signs suggestive of occult lid carcinoma should not be overlooked. Exophthalmometry is helpful to rule out proptosis that might be responsible for lid retraction but not for ectropion. In congenital cases, maxillary hypoplasia and low lateral canthal tendon position may be present. Lid tension can be judged by gently pulling the lid margin away from the globe, paying attention to the amount of tension present and how quickly the lid returns to its previous position. The lid margin is then gently pulled laterally. The lower puntum is observed. If there is no medial canthal laxity, the punctum will not be displaced. If the punctum can be displaced past the medial limbus, significant canthal laxity is present. The lateral canthal tendon is evaluated in a similar fashion. Orbicularis oculi muscle strength is tested by asking the patient to close the eyes as the examiner provides digital resistance. Manually pushing the lower lid margin superiorly when the patient is relaxing is a test for cicatricial restriction. Ordinarily, the lid margin should elevate easily to obscure the pupil while the patient is in primary gaze. Finally, the upper lids and retroauricular regions should be inspected for the suitability of obtaining skin grafts if cicatricial signs are present.

MEDICAL THERAPY

Initially a bland or antibiotic ophthalmic ointment should be used to help protect exposed conjunctiva and corneal epithelium. This will often result in significant improvement in conjunctival engorgement, lid swelling, and lid margin position. Maximal improvement from this medical therapy is usually seen within 3 weeks. An ointment containing a corticosteroid may produce more rapid relief than a plain petrolatum ointment or an antibiotic preparation, but should not be used if the corneal epithelium is not intact, if the patient is a steroid responder, or it the patient has had Herpes simplex keratitis.

Corticosteroid creams (hydrocortisone valerate, 0.2%) may be used on the eyelid skin during active cicatricial stages of dermatologic conditions to try to limit cutaneous shrinkage. Scars due to eyelid surgery or trauma may go through hypertrophic and contractive stages. These complications can often be minimized by early subcutaneous injections of small volumes (0.1–0.5 ml) of corticosteroids (triamcinolone acetonide, 10 mg/ml). These injections may cause skin depigmentation, skin atrophy, and transient (weeks to months) white subcutaneous deposits. Two or three injections at 2-week intervals may be necessary for a maximal effect.

SURGICAL TECHNIQUES FOR INVOLUTIONAL ECTROPION

Conjunctivoplasty for Punctal Ectropion

In early or very mild ectropion, outward displacement of the lower punctum may be the only apparent abnormality. A vertically directed punctum will generally not result in epiphora. But if it everts and becomes stenotic due to chronic drying of its mucous membrane surface, epiphora is likely.

Punctal ectropion can be alleviated by a conjunctivoplasty, which is performed with local anesthesia. The lower canaliculus is identified by placing a lacrimal probe. A diamond of conjunctival and subconjunctival tissue 4 mm high and 8 mm wide is excised inferior to the punctum (Fig. 40.1). This diamond-shaped defect is then closed using three interrupted sutures of 6-0 polyglactin (Vicryl, Dexon) with buried knots. The sutures incorporate a bite of deep lid tissue in the depth of the diamond-shaped site and the conjunctival edges to maximize the inward rotation of the punctum.

Punctoplasty for Punctal Stenosis

A stenotic punctum can be permanently enlarged using a Jones "two snip" punctoplasty. If this is performed as an isolated procedure, topical 4% cocaine or 4% Xylocaine (lidocaine HCl) solution applied for 1 minute with a cotton pledget will provide sufficient anesthesia. The two snips can be used to create a 2-mm-high "V" opening, which enlarges the punctum posteriorly (Fig. 40.2*A*). Alternatively, the first cut can be 2 mm high vertically through the posterior wall of the vertical canaliculus (Fig. 40.2*B*). The second cut is then directed medially through 2 mm of the horizontal canaliculus. Sharp-pointed iris or Westcott scissors and toothed 0.5 mm forceps work well for this procedure. The patient should be seen twice at weekly intervals following the punctoplasty. At these visits a punctal dilator should be used if the punctum shows signs of reclosure.

Experience has shown that the "one snip" punctoplasty is of no lasting value and should not be done. A "three snip" procedure (Fig. 40.2*C*), which removes a square of tissue from the posterior wall of the vertical canaliculus, should be avoided because a visible lid margin deformity may result.

Smith Lazy-T for Medial Ectropion

If the lower lid shows laxity and medial palpebral conjunctiva is exposed due to ectropion, a simple conjunctivoplasty will not be sufficient. The Smith Lazy-T (1) works well in these cases. A standard pentagonal wedge is resected 4 mm lateral to the lower punctum (Fig. 40.3). The horizontal width of the pentagon is 5–8 mm, depending on the laxity of the lid. A conjunctivoplasty is then performed inferior to the punctum. In this procedure it is easiest to excise an isosceles triangle of tissue, whose base is 4 mm high, along the medial edge of the pentagonal

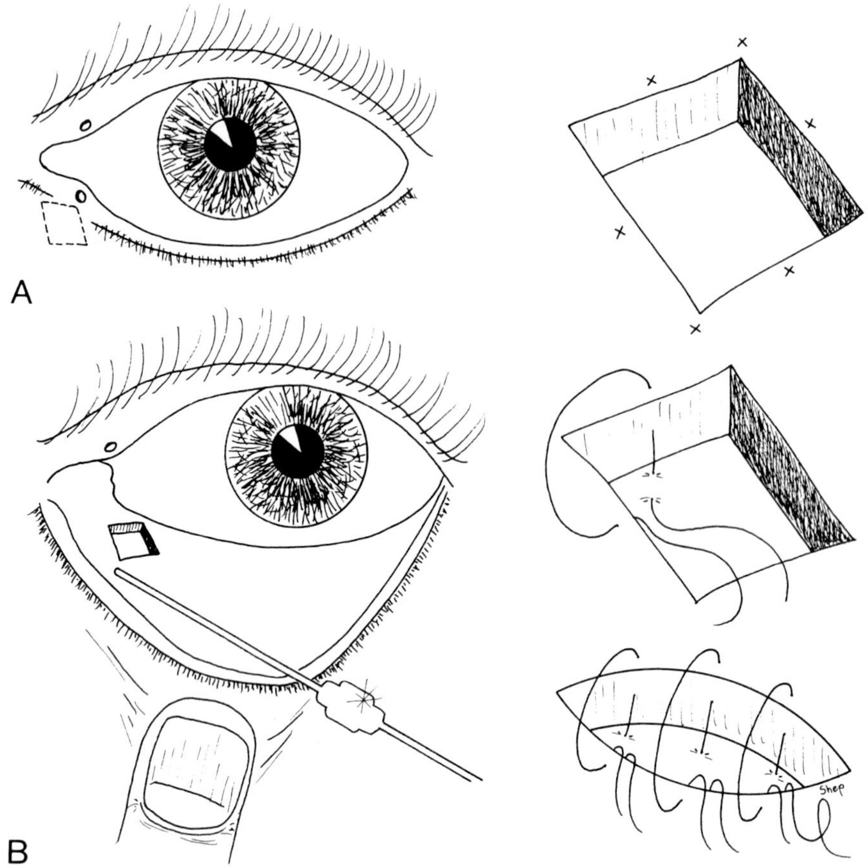

Figure 40.1. Conjunctivoplasty for repair of mild medial lower lid ectropion involving the punctum. *A*, A diamond conjunctival and subconjunctival tissue is excised. *B*, A lacrimal probe identifies the location of the lower canaliculus so that it can be avoided. Vertical closure of the diamond draws the ectropic punctum toward the globe.

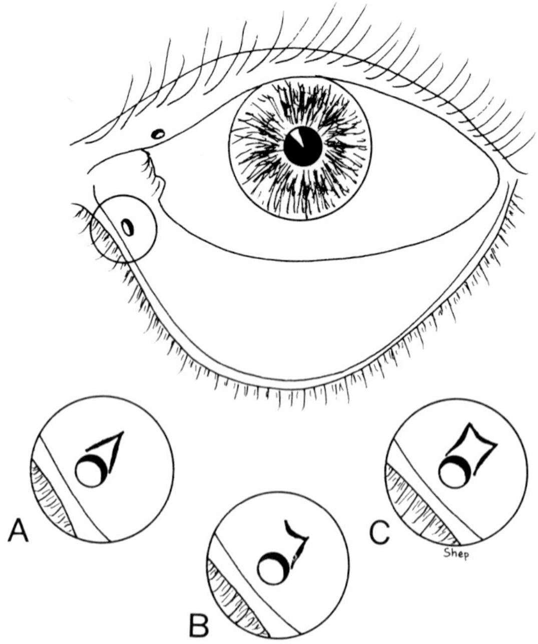

Figure 40.2. Jones punctoplasty. *A*, Two snips excise a "V" from the posterior wall of the vertical canaliculus. *B*, Two snips can be used to open the posterior wall of the vertical and 2 mm of the horizontal canaliculus. *C*, Three snips to excise a square of tissue are rarely indicated. This may result in excessive tissue removal and a visible lid margin deformity.

resection. The legs of this triangle extend 8 mm medially. The triangle is closed in the same way as described for the diamond-shaped conjunctivoplasty. The pentagonal lid resection is closed using two partial-thickness 5-0 polyglactin tarsal sutures and a standard lid margin and skin closure using 6-0 black silk. Skin sutures can be removed in 6 days. An alternative is to use 6-0 catgut (Ethicon G-1916) for skin closure. This eliminates the need for removing skin sutures. The lid margin silk sutures are removed in 10–14 days.

Bick Lid Shortening for Lateral Canthal Laxity and Ectropion

If lower lid lateral canthal laxity has caused a lower lid ectropion, lateral lid shortening with canthal reattachment is an effective therapy. The procedure described by Bick (2) works very well. Tissue scissors are used to cut inferolaterally from the lateral canthal angle through the full thickness of the lower lid (Fig. 40.4). This cut follows the direction of the lateral upper lid curvature and extends 12 mm. The medial edge of this incision can then be drawn laterally to determine how much excess lid tissue should be excised. There is no need to create a pentagonal wedge in this site. The excess tissue is excised as a "V" with tissue scissors. The horizontal distance of lid margin excised will generally be between 6 and 10 mm. When there has been involutional stretching and laxity of the lateral canthal tendon, this excised wedge contains very little tarsal tissue.

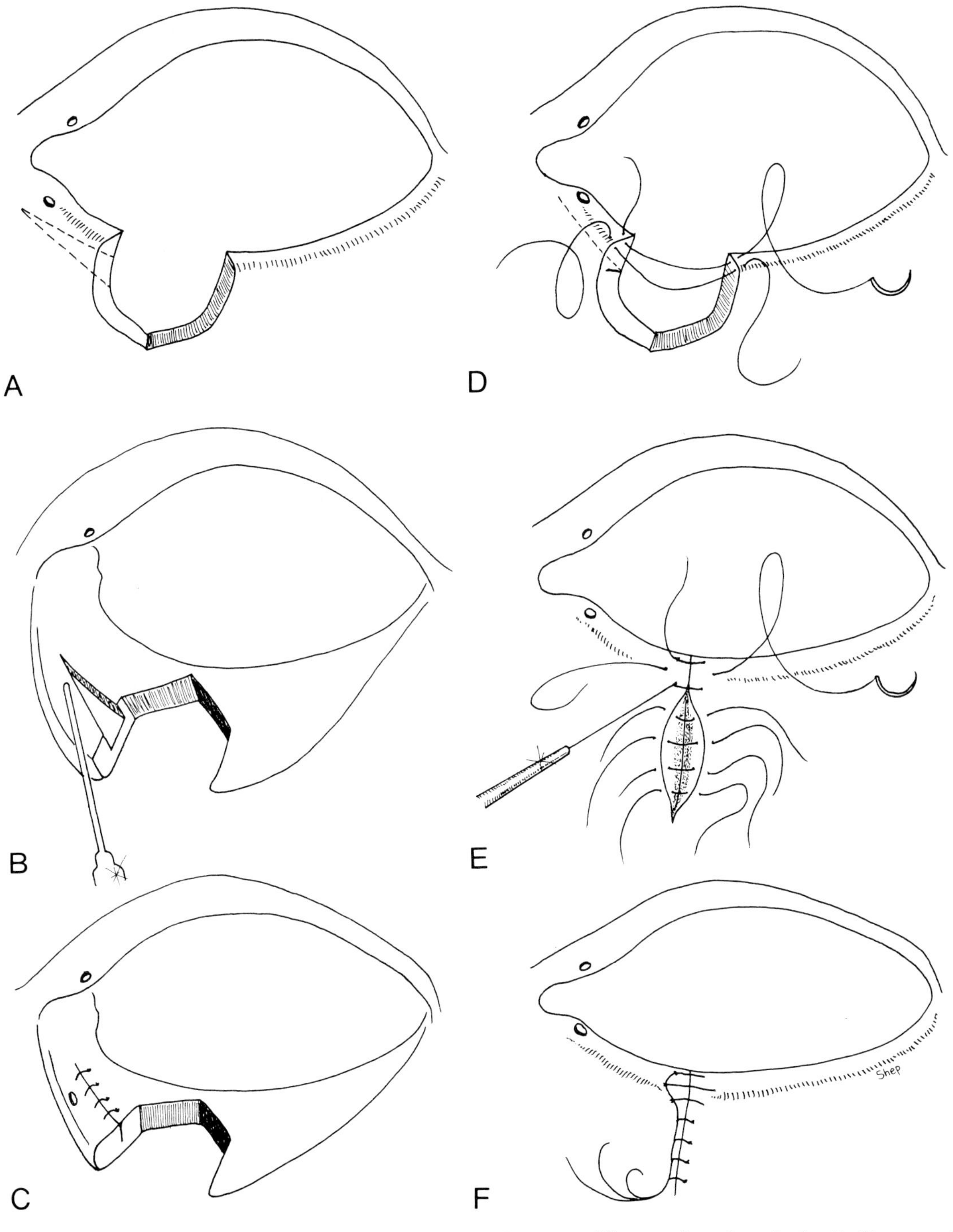

Figure 40.3. Smith Lazy-T procedure for correction of moderate medial lower lid ectropion. *A*, Pentagonal wedge resection temporal to the lower punctum. *B*, Excision of tissue wedge from conjunctival surface of lid inferior to the punctum. A Bowman probe is used to identify the location of the canaliculus so that it can be avoided. *C*, Closure of the conjunctivoplasty. *D*, Closure of the pentagonal wedge resection site with lid margin sutures. *E*, Closure of skin with interrupted sutures. *F*, Final appearance. The ends of the lid margin sutures are held away from the globe by tying them under one of the skin sutures.

The tarsal tissue that is exposed is then sutured to remaining lateral canthal tissue along the lateral orbital tubercle with a 5-0 polyglactin suture. Accurate placement of this suture is facilitated by use of the firm, half-round P-2 needle. Before this suture is tied, the bites of tarsus and lateral canthal tendon should be checked to make certain they are secure. Another 5-0 polyglactin suture is used to unite the gray lines of the upper and lower lid at the lateral canthal angle. An additional suture can be placed from the lower tarsal border, laterally to deep tissue. Interrupted skin sutures complete the closure.

Tarsal Strip Procedure

The tarsal strip procedure (3, 4) is a modified method of shortening the lower lid and reattaching it to the lateral canthus. This provides a stronger lateral canthal tendon

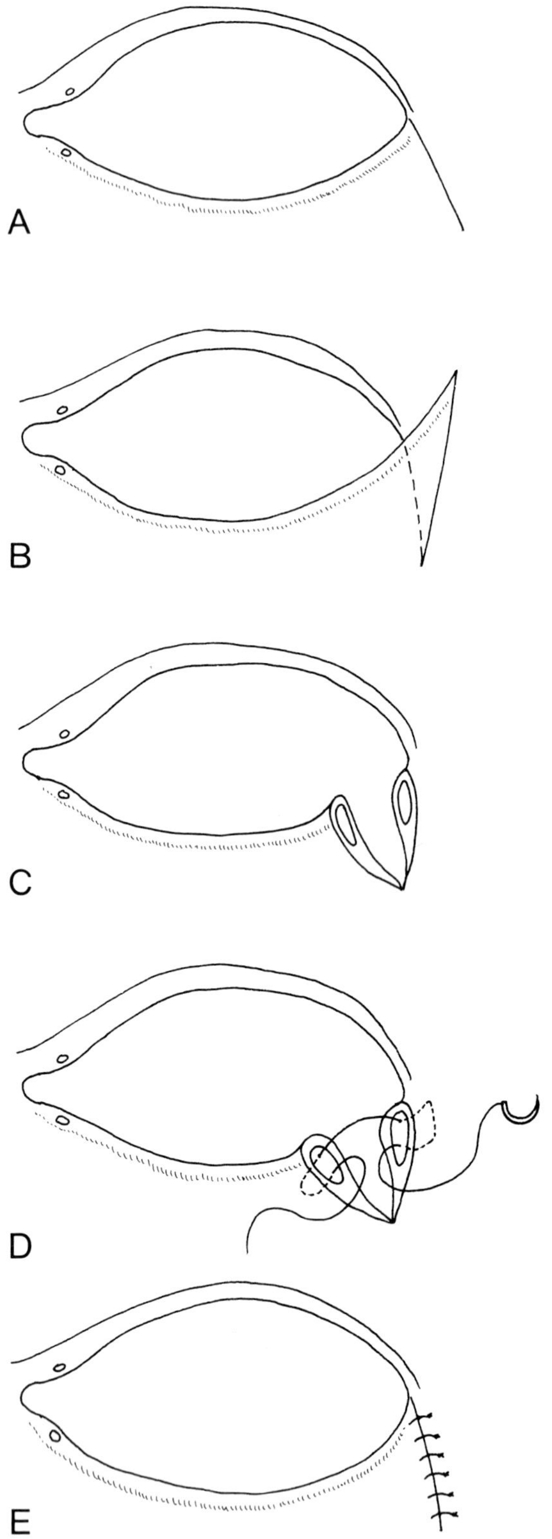

Figure 40.4. Bick lateral lid shortening for correction of ectropion due to lower lid laxity. *A*, A full-thickness incision is made at the lateral canthus following the curvature of the upper lid. *B*, Traction is used to determine the amount of lid tissue to be excised. *C*, The cut end of the tarsal plate is identified so that it can be attached to the lower arm of the lateral canthal tendon. *D*, A suture is used to unite the cut end of the lower tarsus to the lateral canthal tendon at the lateral orbital tubercle. *E*, Final appearance after skin closure.

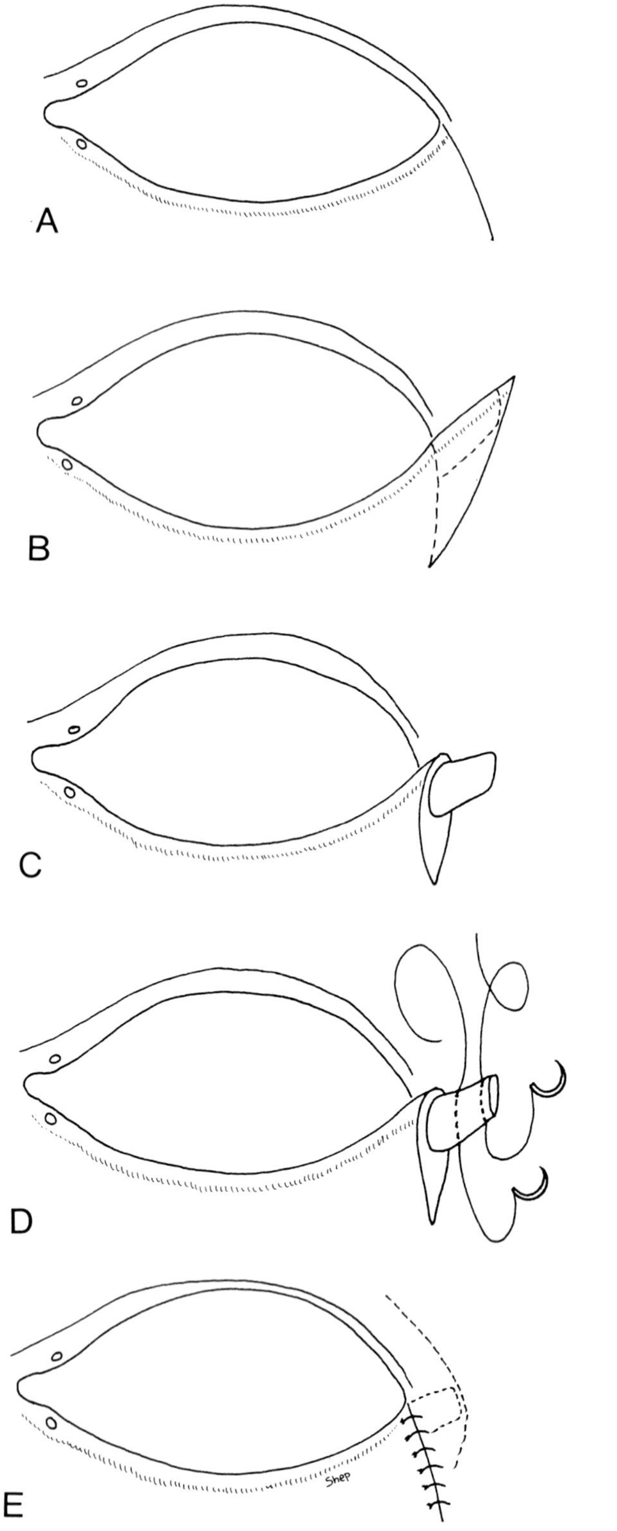

Figure 40.5. Lateral tarsal strip procedure. *A*, A full-thickness lid incision is made at the lateral canthus following the curvature of the upper lid. *B*, The amount of lid laxity is determined by gentle traction of the free edge of the lower lid over the lateral canthal region. *C*, Excess lid tissue is excised, preserving the remaining tarsus. All epithelium must be removed from the tarsus. *D*, Sutures are used to attach the remaining strip of tarsus to the periorbita of the lateral orbital tubercle. *E*, Final appearance after skin sutures have been placed.

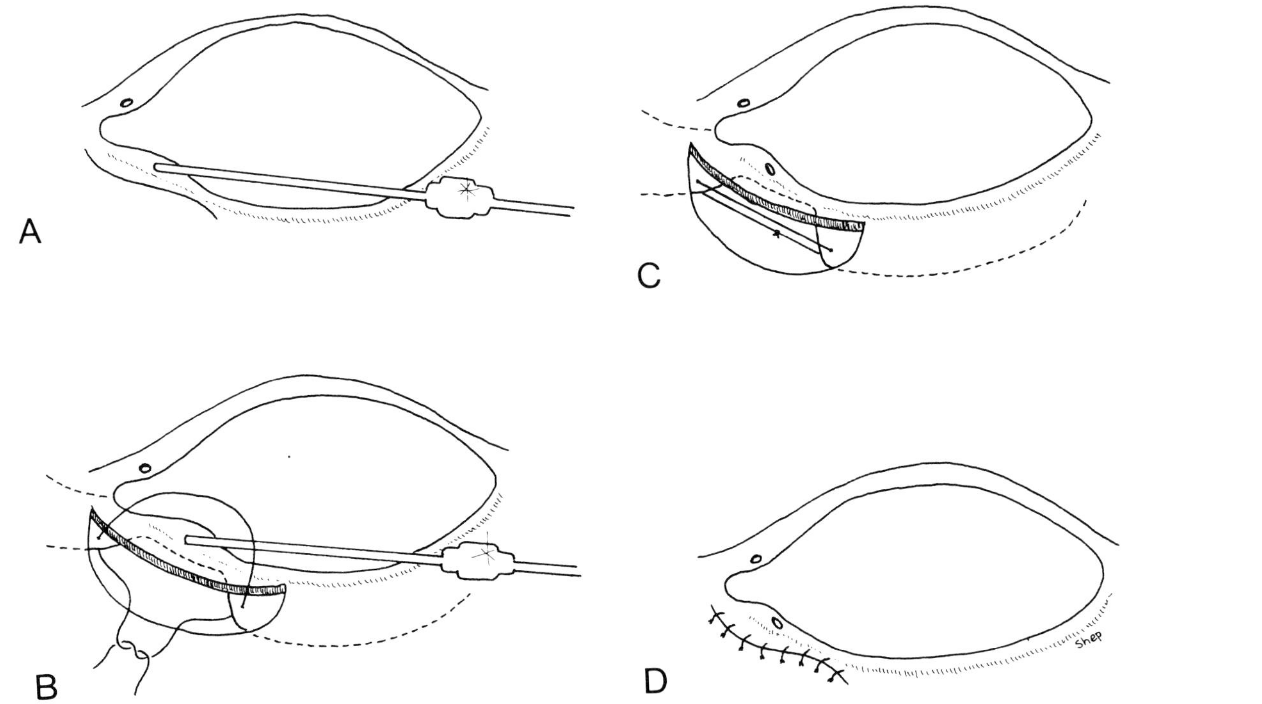

Figure 40.6. Plication of the inferior arm of the medial canthal tendon. *A*, The inferior canaliculus is identified and avoided with a lacrimal probe. *B*, A horizontal incision through skin and muscle allows exposure of the lower arm of the medial canthal tendon. *C*, A suture is placed between the medial canthal tendon and the lower tarsus stabilizes the medial aspect of the lower lid. *D*, Skin closure.

and is particularly helpful in the anophthalmic socket, where the lower lid must help support a prosthesis. This differs from the Bick procedure in two respects. First, instead of excising a full-thickness wedge of eyelid tissue, tarsus is retained (Fig. 40.5). All epithelium must be removed from this exposed tarsus. Second, the tarsal strip is drawn across the intact upper limb of the lateral canthal tendon. Two points of suture fixation can be made, one to the lateral canthal tendon and one to the periosteum of the lateral orbital rim. A 5-0 polyglactin suture with the P-2 needle works very well for this. The remaining closure is performed in the same fashion as the Bick procedure.

Medial Plication for Extreme Medial Canthal Laxity

Occasionally the lower lid's medial canthal attachments will be found to be quite lax. In some cases the lower punctum can be pulled over as far as the pupil when the lower lid is stretched laterally. Usually, lateral punctal displacement does not compromise lacrimal drainage postoperatively and involutional ectropion repair should be performed as just discussed. Because the medial canthal tendon has both superficial and deep attachments, successful tightening of this structure is difficult. The deep tissue attaches to the posterior lacrimal crest. Surgery in this area may damage the lacrimal drainage system. The superficial tissue attaches to the anterior lacrimal crest. When the superficial portion alone is tightened, the deep attachment remains lax. This can allow anterior displacement of the medial aspect of the lower eyelid, resulting in a gap between the posterior lid margin and the globe.

If the medial attachment of the inferior tarsus is so lax that the Smith Lazy-T or the Bick technique alone will not provide adequate lid tension, a medial plication should be used along with a lid-shortening technique. A lacrimal probe is placed in the lower canaliculus, a skin incision is made inferior to the canaliculus extending from just lateral to the punctum to just medial to the canthal angle (Fig. 40.6). Either a nonabsorbable or a polyglactin 5-0 suture is placed to attach the medial end of the inferior tarsal plate to the anterior portion of the medial canthal tendon. The suture placement in the medial canthal tendon should be at the level of the medial canthal angle just lateral to the anterior lacrimal crest. After the lacrimal probe is removed, the suture should be tightened so that the position of the punctum is stabilized. The goal should be to prevent further lateral displacement of the lower punctum. Attempting to draw the punctum more medially may result in canalicular kinking and loss of lacrimal pump function. The skin incision is then closed.

MANAGEMENT OF PARALYTIC ECTROPION

Elderly patients with facial palsy or patients with longstanding facial palsies are likely to exhibit lower lid laxity and ectropion. The lid protractor weakness and complications of corneal exposure make this condition a more difficult management problem than involutional ectropion due only to lid laxity. Ophthalmic ointments, moisture chambers, and night-time occlusion therapy are all helpful modalities. Temporary suture tarsorrhaphies may be indicated acutely. An ectropion that persists after spontaneous improvement of the facial palsy has ceased can be evaluated and treated with the same techniques as involutional ectropion. However, if significant lagophthalmos persists despite any spontaneous orbicularis recovery, then ectropion surgery will not be sufficient. In these cases, reanimation surgery should be considered for repositioning the lids. This can include the placement of a gold weight or spring into the upper lid. Silicone rods and facial reanimation surgery are covered elsewhere in this volume.

In some cases of severe permanent facial palsy, a permanent tarsorrhaphy may be indicated if other medical and surgical treatments fail. When performed properly the cosmetic impairment of a tarsorrhaphy can be minimal. If medial ectropion is not severe, a lateral tarsorrhapy alone will suffice. If there is prominent exposure of the cornea or medial palpebral conjunctiva, a medial tarsorrhaphy will also be necessary. The epithelial surface of the upper and lower lids is excised from the eyelid margin with a sharp-pointed microsurgical blade for approximately 10 mm adjacent to the canthal angle (Fig. 40.7). A large chalazion clamp positioned with the flat plate on the posterior side of the lid protects the globe, provides hemostasis, and stabilizes the lid margin for this step. The excision should not involve cilia. In a medial tarsorrhaphy the excision may extend laterally past the puncta, since the puncta are posterior to the normal lid margin. A medial tarsorrhaphy does not seem to change tear drainage in these patients, who already have impaired lacrimal pump function. Medial to the puncta the tarsorrhaphy is closed with interrupted 6-0 polyglactin subcutaneous sutures and also skin sutures. It is helpful to have lacrimal probes in the canaliculi while placing these sutures to avoid canalicular damage. Transmarginal 4-0 silk sutures passed through pieces of a large sterile rubberband are all that is necessary to approximate lateral tarsorrhaphies. They are also placed lateral to the puncta to help support medial tarsorrhaphies. The sutures are tied so that the rubberband "bumpers" lightly indent the skin and approximate the tarsorrhaphies sites without causing pressure necrosis. These sutures should be left in place for 3 weeks. Tarsorrhaphies should always be made wider than required because some separation and stretching is likely. It is very easy to open this type of tarsorrhaphy if there is an overcorrection or if orbicularis function improves.

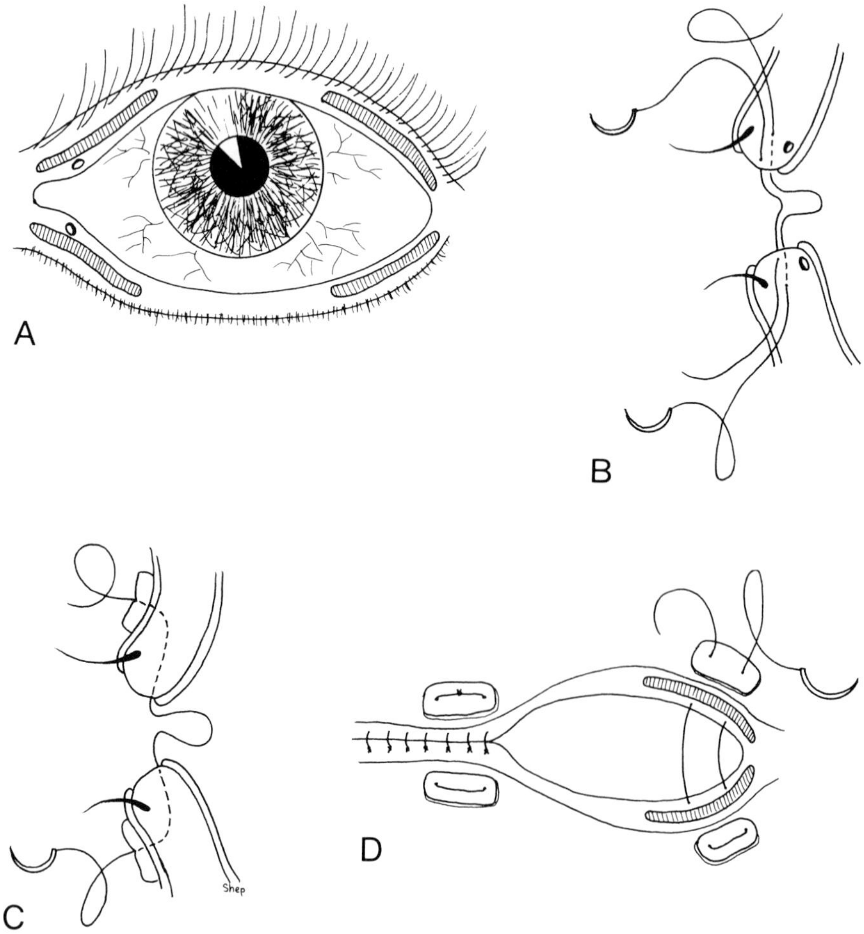

Figure 40.7. Tarsorrhaphies can be formed laterally and medially. These may be indicated in some cases of permanent paralytic ectropion. *A*, Excision of epithelium from the lid margin. *B*, Side view of suture placement anterior to the puncta and canaliculi. These sutures pass through the gray line in areas of the lid where there is tarsus. *C*, Pieces of sterile rubber band spread the force of the suture over a wider area of skin. *D*, Medially the skin edges should be sutured. This is not necessary temporally.

MANAGEMENT OF CICATRICIAL ECTROPION

Repair of cicatricial ectropion should be deferred until active scar contraction has ceased. If there is concurrent lower lid laxity, this can be corrected at the same time as the cicatricial ectropion repair.

Occasionally there will be a tight narrow scar resulting from trauma or prior excision of a skin lesion. In these cases the linear scar can be excised and a cutaneous Z-plasty can be used to eliminate recurrent traction along this line. If the scar involves the lid margin, it may be necessary to perform a full-thickness pentagonal resection and closure to create a normal lid-margin contour.

If the cicatricial process is not limited to a narrow band, skin grafting is necessary to augment the deficient lower lid skin. Full-thickness grafts are preferrable. Retroauricular or upper lid skin produces the best results, although supraclavicular, medial upper arm, and preauricular skin grafts provide a reasonable graft. If necessary, 0.018 inch thick split-thickness grafts can be used. The graft bed is prepared by making a skin incision 3 mm inferior to the lid margin (Fig. 40.8). A 4-0 black-silk, gray-line suture can be placed centrally in the lower lid to provide gentle superior traction. Subcutaneous cicatricial tissue should be excised until the lower lid margin can be easily elevated to a position higher than the pupil when the globe is in primary position. This excision may need to include tissue down to and including the orbital septum. Orbital fat need not be excised. Careful hemostasis is necessary. The skin graft should cover the defect completely while the lower lid margin is held at the level of the pupil. The graft is sewn in place with 6-0 black silk sutures. One end of these sutures should be left long. A piece of Telfa gauze cut to match the skin graft is placed over the graft. Then a firm roll of cotton saturated with ophthalmic antibiotic ointment is placed on the Telfa. Long arms of the silk sutures from the upper and lower graft edge are tied over the cotton to produce a pressure dressing. The 4-0 lid traction suture is removed and is replaced with intermarginal 6-0 polypropylene (Prolene) sutures placed through the gray line of both the upper and lower lids. There should be three intermarginal sutures placed medially, centrally, and laterally. If this is the patient's only visually useful eye, the central suture can be omitted to provide a small visual aperture. The pressure dressing and skin sutures are removed in 1 week. Telfa covered with an eye patch should be taped firmly over the eyelids during the 2nd postoperative week. The intermarginal sutures should be left in place for 2 weeks. The skin graft will initially show a sunken contour, but this disappears after 1–2 months.

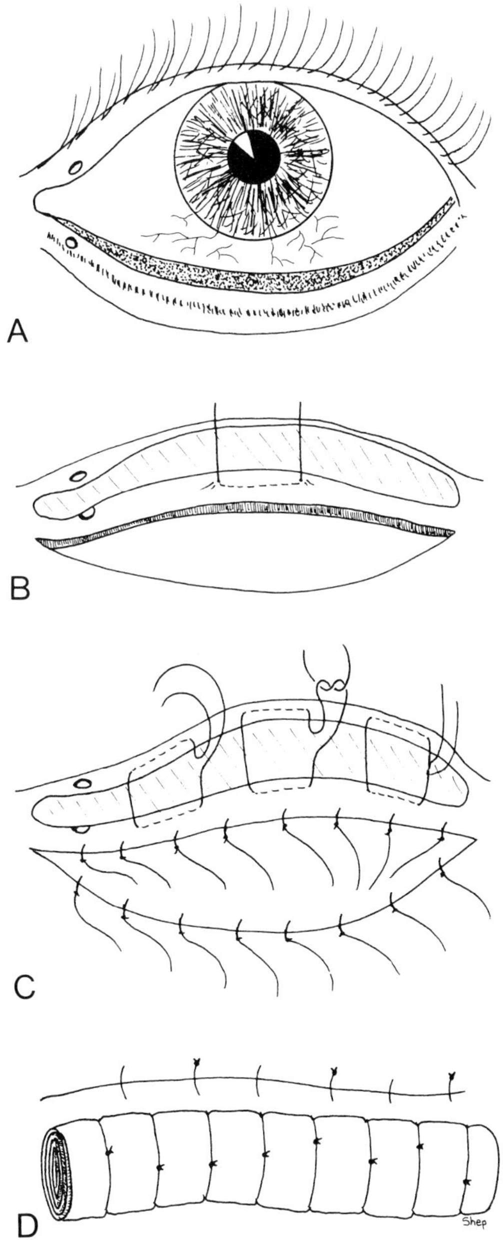

Figure 40.8. Skin grafts to the lower lid are utilized in the repair of cicatricial lower lid ectropion. *A*, The incision is made in a subciliary position. *B*, All subcutaneous cicatricial tissue is excised. *C*, Placement of a free skin graft and of gray line intermarginal sutures. *D*, A bolster is secured over the free skin graft. The intermarginal sutures are tied so that the lid margins are held in apposition.

MANAGEMENT OF CONGENITAL ECTROPION

Congential ectropion generally involves a deficiency of tissue in the anterior lamella of the lower lid. This can be corrected using the technique described for acquired cicatricial ectropion. In these patients, subcutaneous lower lid tissue is incised, but there is no cicatricial tissue to excise. If coexisting maxillary hypoplasia requires correction, this should be carried out before ectropion repair is performed. If there is lateral canthal dystopia, this can be managed at the same time as the ectropion.

REFERENCES

1. Smith B: The "lazy-T" correction of ectropion of the lower punctum. *Arch Ophthalmol* 94: 1149, 1976
2. Bick MW: Surgical management of orbital tarsal disparity. *Arch Ophthalmol* 75: 386, 1966
3. Tenzel RR: Treatment of lagophthalmos of the lower lid. *Arch Ophthalmol* 81: 366–368, 1969.
4. Tenzel RR, Buffam FV, Miller GR: The use of the "lateral canthal sling" in ectropion repair. *Can J Ophthalmol* 12: 199–202, 1977.

CHAPTER 41

Telecanthus

MICHAEL A. CALLAHAN, M.D., F.A.C.S.
ALSTON CALLAHAN, M.D., F.A.C.S.

Telecanthus has been defined by Mustardé (1) as increased intercanthal distance (ICD); when compared to the interpupillary distance (IPD) the normal distance between the two medial canthi should measure approximately half of the distance between the two pupils (interpupillary distance). Thus, telecanthus is present when the ICD/IPD fraction is greater than 0.5; there are primary and secondary types (Table 41.1).

Primary telecanthus results from attenuation of the medial canthal tendons (MCT) and is usually associated with other soft tissue abnormalities, such as epicanthus, the blepharophimosis syndrome, or after trauma. Secondary telecanthus is due to underlying bony abnormalities with an abnormal separation between the orbits because of an increased thickness of the interorbital bones (the nasofrontomaxilloethmoidal bony complex); examples are hypertelorism and the complex craniofacial syndromes. Surgical correction of primary telecanthus is achieved by shifting the soft tissues; secondary telecanthus, by midline resection of bones. If the MCT is sectioned traumatically and not rejoined, primary telecanthus will occur. Fractures of the nasoethmoidal complex lead to secondary telecanthus and typically a rounded appearance of the medial canthus.

The most commonly encountered form of epicanthus is epicanthus palpebralis, which is characterized by a vertical fold extending from the medial aspect of the upper lid to a corresponding point on the medial aspect of the lower lid, partially obscuring the caruncle. Other forms of epicanthus less commonly associated with telecanthus are epicanthus superciliaris, which is described as a vertical fold of skin extending from below the medial aspect of the eyebrow over the inferior orbital rim; epicanthus tarsalis, which is characterized by a horizontal fold of skin extending over the upper lid and medial canthus; and epicanthus inversus, which is similar to epicanthus tarsalis, except the horizontal fold of skin involves the lower lids.

Table 41.1
Types of Telecanthus

Primary telecanthus
Epicanthus
Blepharophimosis syndrome
Trauma
Secondary telecanthus
Primary hypertelorism
Craniofacial abnormalities (e.g., Crouzon's disease, Apert's syndrome)
Trauma

Epicanthus results from a horizontal maldistribution of skin and subcutaneous tissue between the medial canthus and the nose; also the orbital fibers of the orbicularis that normally tuck under the horizontal portion of the MCT instead course anterior to the tendon like a web.

If the loose skin over the dorsum of the nose is pinched up between the thumb and forefinger, the epicanthal fold can be temporarily reduced. This diagnostic maneuver was the idea behind the von Ammon procedure (1), in which an ellipse of skin was excised over the nasal dorsum. With this procedure, the epicanthus usually recurred as the rather conspicuous scar over the nose widened with the passage of time. The failure of this procedure taught that the skin must be rearranged within the canthus, which it will do when the proper procedure is performed.

TELECANTHUS CORRECTION

SURGICAL CORRECTION OF PRIMARY TELECANTHUS

Successful surgical correction of primary telecanthus must consist of reorganization of the three soft tissue elements within the medial canthus responsible for the abnormality: skin and underlying fascia, subcutaneous tissues and muscle, and MCT. Various procedures have been developed to correct these abnormalities (Table 41.2). Telecanthus and epicanthus usually coexist, and the severity of each is variable. Some patients exhibit more telecanthus than epicanthus and vice versa; when surgery is indicated, both problems must be corrected. Most cases of congenital primary telecanthus, except for the blepharophimosis syndrome, can be corrected by MCT tucking or resection combined with a Y-to-V or Roveda procedure for the epicanthus.

The Y-to-V flap and Roveda procedures involve incision, undermining, and movement of skin horizontally and vertically from the medial canthus toward the midline. The Y-to-V flap is preferred for surgical correction of blepharophimosis, because a great deal of subcutaneous soft tissue must be excised and the medial canthi has to be wired transnasally. The resultant skin scar is more even with this procedure than with Roveda's.

Y-to-V Surgical Technique

The Y-to-V surgical technique is described as follows (Fig. 41.1): With a marking pen or dye draw a horizontally oriented "Y" over the medial canthal area with the base of the stem near the nose at the desired new position of the canthus. Pinching the skin together over the nasal dorsum will help with this determination. Extend the arms of the "Y" to the supraorbital and infraorbital folds, with the apex being just nasal to the crest of the fold. Make the skin incision with a blade (Bard-Parker) and excise the subcutaneous tissues over the MCT. Advance the canthus toward the midline, trim the flaps, and then suture them in two layers with absorbable sutures (Vicryl 6-0) subcutaneously and nonabsorbable sutures (nylon 6-0) for the skin (Fig. 41.2).

Roveda Surgical Technique

Roveda's correction for epicanthus palpebralis is described as follows (Fig. 41.3): First, with dye draw a line parallel to and about 5–6 mm medial to the crest of the epicanthal fold. At the midpoint of the curve, level with the canthal angle, incise the skin an subcutaneous tissues in the form of a horizontal "Y." Extend the stem of the Y a distance of 5–7 mm toward the nose. When viewed directly from in front, the five-point junction between the curved line and the Y incision should lie 1–2 mm medial to the underlying canthal angle.

Table 41.2
Surgical Correction of Soft Tissue Elements Responsible for Primary Telecanthus

Soft Tissue	Surgical Procedure
Skin	Y to V
	Roveda
Soft tissue	Excision
Medial canthal tendon	Tucking
	Resection
	Two drill holes in the medial orbital wall
	Bone piton
	Bone screw
	Transnasal wiring

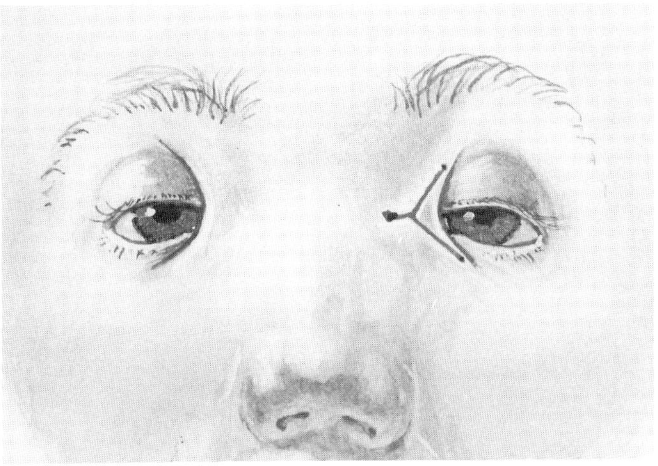

Figure 41.1. Y-to-V correction of epicanthus with base of stem at desired point of new canthus.

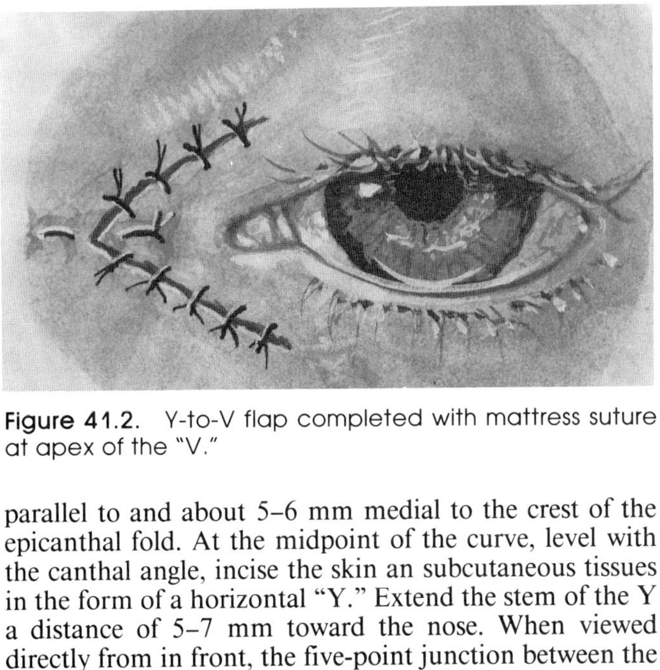

Figure 41.2. Y-to-V flap completed with mattress suture at apex of the "V."

Second, incise the long curved line that you have drawn, and undermine the skin in all directions from this incision. Excise the excessive subcutaneous tissue and orbicularis below the small flaps so the skin will lie flat.

Third, trim off the two small triangular flaps of skin medially (delimited above by the dotted line; below it is pulled inferiorly by a skin hook). Advance the two triangular flaps toward the midline to fill the spaces vacated by the triangular flaps just excised. Avoid grasping these flaps with forceps, which crush the tissue and lead to scarring. Handle the flaps carefully with small, single skin hooks.

Finally, meticulously close the now W-shaped incision with fine nonabsorbable sutures (nylon 6-0). Allow these sutures to remain approximately 5–7 days. Medial canthal skin is thicker than that of the lid and contains more

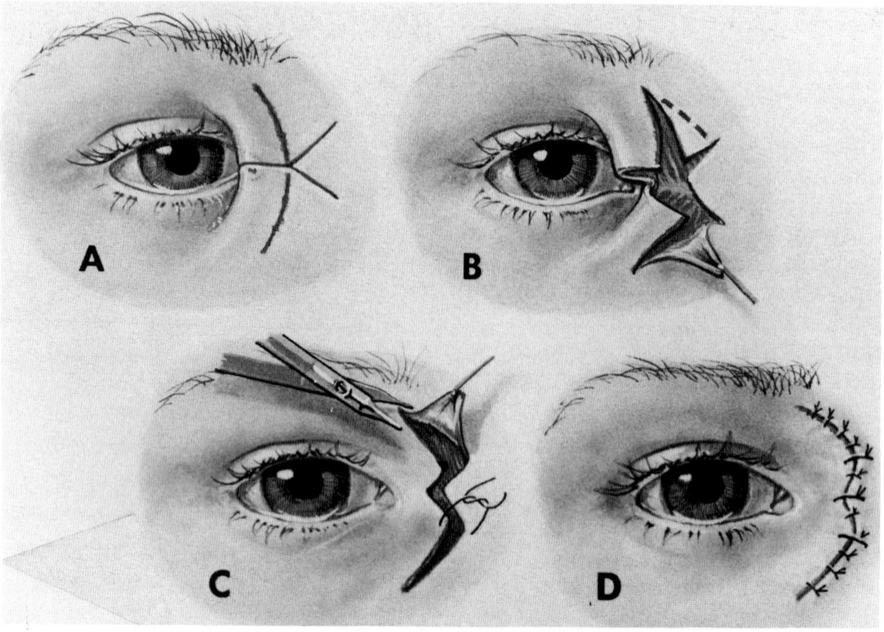

Figure 41.3. Roveda's correction of epicanthus palpebralis. *A,* Y incision is fashioned. *B,* Flaps are undermined. *C,* Flaps are trimmed and aligned. *D,* Closure with interrupted sutures of "W" flap.

glandular elements; consequently scarring is more likely, so suture carefully. Small "dog ears," or areas closed with excessive skin tension, will also promote unwanted scarring, so trim tissues with this complication in mind.

SOFT TISSUE EXCISION

The soft tissue lying between the dermis and periosteum of the medial canthal area, including subcutaneous tissue and skeletal muscle, should be excised under direct visualization. The primary caveat is to avoid canalicular damage by inserting lacrimal probes into the canaliculi prior to the dissection.

MEDIAL CANTHAL TENDON SHORTENING FOR REATTACHMENT PROCEDURES

The MCT is formed by the insertions of the three divisions of the orbicularis into the medial orbital wall. At the midpoint of the lid the pretarsal orbicularis is intimately associated with the tarsus; it splits into superficial and deep heads, which insert into the anterior and posterior lacrimal crests, respectively. The preseptal orbicularis also splits into superficial and deep heads, which join the pretarsal orbicularis to form these anterior and posterior crura; the deep head of the preseptal orbicularis inserts into the lacrimal diaphram. The orbicularis' third division (the orbital portion) inserts under the anterior crus of the MCT along the inferior and superior orbital rims. Zide (2) and Anderson (3) have recently described a third branch of the MCT's insertion that bifurcates superiorly from the anterior crus as the latter inserts into the anterior lacrimal crest. It ascends 4-5 mm along the anterior lacrimal crest and then inserts in the orbital portion of the frontal bone. Zide (2) believes the anterior and superior crura of the MCT are stronger than the posterior crus.

The presence of this superior branch helps to explain two clinical phenomena: (*a*) the failure of the medial canthus to migrate inferiorly following sectioning of the MCT's anterior crus directly in front of the lacrimal sac, as is sometimes done during a DCR; (*b*) the disturbing tendency of an avulsed canthus to migrate inferiorly as healing occurs unless it is anchored posterior and superior to the insertion of the anterior crus. If these relationships of the MCT are kept in mind, the reconstructive surgeon can more accurately resect or reattach it.

MCT tucking and resection is indicated only in mild cases of telecanthus associated with epicanthus. For blepharophimosis repair or the traumatic telecanthus that may accompany severe nasoethmoidal fractures, it is inadequate. It is possible to tuck an elongated MCT with a Burch tendon tucker. A nonabsorbable suture (Prolene 5-0) is wrapped around the base of the tuck, much as is done in superior oblique strengthening procedures, and the loop is folded over the MCT medially or laterally and sutured with absorbable suture (Vicryl 6-0). Better correction can be obtained by sectioning 4–5 mm of the MCT and suturing the cut ends with nonabsorbable suture (Prolene 6-0). A large enough stump should be left attached to the periosteum so that secure fixation will be obtained. If the proximal portion of the canthal tendon is sectioned too close to the periosteum, there is a possibility that the suture might pull through the remaining tissue, permitting the telecanthus to recur. Severe degrees of telecanthus must be corrected with transnasal wiring to effectively and permanently shorten the distance between the two canthi.

Transnasal Wiring for Telecanthus

After the skin incision (usually Y to V) and subcutaneous tissue resection, the surgical objective of pulling both canthi toward the midline with a transnasal wire is accomplished by dividing the anterior and superior crura of the medial canthal tendons near their attachment to the bone. The stumps are used as landmarks for the osteotomies, which should be 5–7 mm in diameter and located just anterior to the lacrimal sac fossa on the anterior lacrimal crest (Fig. 41.4). After the osteotomies, the nasal mucosa is exposed and incised to accommodate transnasal wiring. [In preparation for this, the nasal cavity should be packed with cocaine hydrochloride (10% solution) and phenylephrine hydrochloride ophthalmic solution USP (Neosynephrine hydrochloride, 0.25% solution) to minimize bleeding as the wire is drawn through the mucosa and septum.] The osteotomies can be made with either a Hall drill, a chisel, a mallet, or a Stryker saw.

Wire the canthi with 24-gauge stainless steel wire (0.51 mm) attached to a ski needle (Fig. 41.5). (Conventional needles are suitable for obtaining bites of the canthal structures, and a Wright needle or Mustardé awl can be used to pass the wire across the nasal cavity.) First take a bite of the MCT near the medial end of the two right tarsi; then direct the needle into the lower part of the bony opening, penetrating the mucosa, the nasal septum, and mucosa on the left side. Draw the needle and wire across the nasal cavity and insert the needle and wire through the conjoined MCT near the medial aspect of the two left tarsi. Direct the wire back across the nasal cavity of the upper part of the opening; detach the needle and twist the ends together so that the canthal structures are drawn into the bony openings. Cut the ends that have been twisted together short and "knuckle" them backward toward the mucosa.

The patient's face should be viewed from each side of the operating table and also from above and below. The spacing of the canthi should be verified with a ruler to be certain they are equidistant from the midline of the nose.

To achieve these goals, the surgeon may need to repass the wire transnasally through a slightly different route; also the bites of the subcutaneous tissues must sometimes be adjusted. If one canthus will not advance far enough medially to be symmetrical with the other side, a transconjunctival lateral canthotomy on the involved side will usually release it satisfactorily.

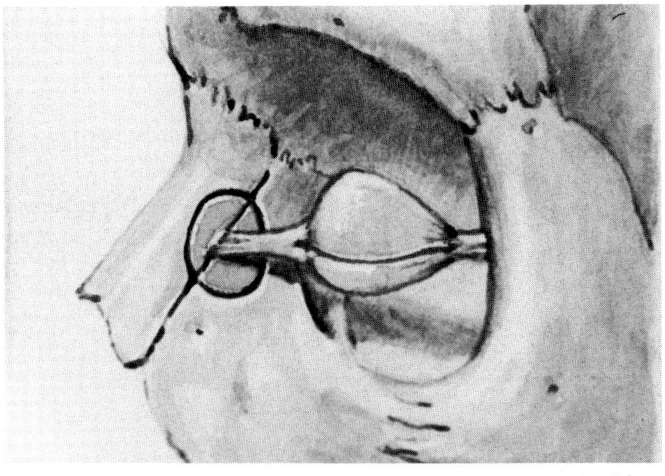

Figure 41.4. Outline of osteotomy for transnasal wiring. Medial canthal tendon is sectioned, and its insertion is used as a landmark for the bony opening.

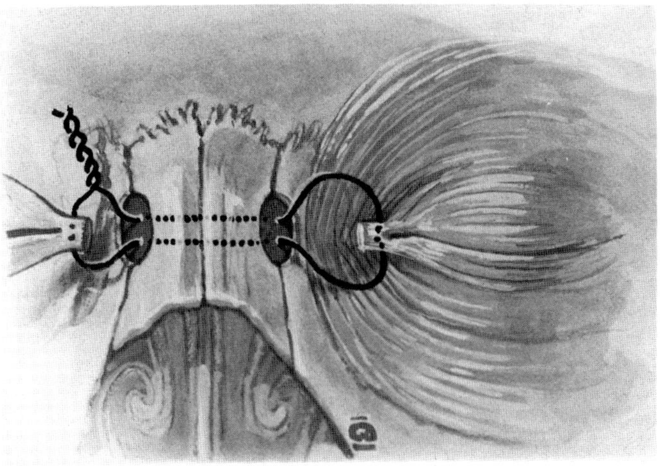

Figure 41.5. Transnasal wiring of both medial canthal tendons. Wire started on the right passing transnasally to catch the left medial canthal tendon, and then back through the nasal septum to the right side.

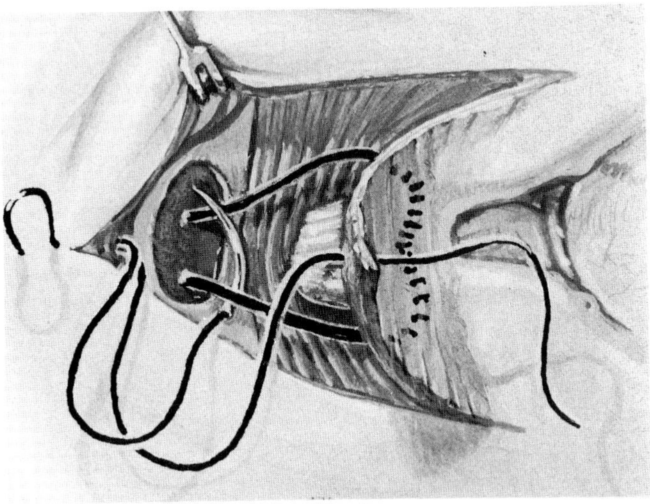

Figure 41.6. Just prior to twisting the wire, which brings the canthi toward the midline, a mattress suture is placed through the wire's loop. This forces the skin and soft tissues back against the medial orbital wall imparting concavity to the medial canthus.

Any remaining excessive muscle and subcutaneous tissue can be removed to permit the medial canthal skin to flatten. The mattress suture in the apex of the "V" should be looped under the transnasal wire loop (Fig. 41.6). Place the other skin sutures individually (nylon 6-0).

TRAUMATIC TELECANTHUS

We present four ways to reattach a traumatically detached medial canthus. These methods have evolved over the past 35 years. We have found that the MCT must be attached to the bone of the medial orbital wall for permanent correction and that periosteum is of insufficient strength.

The first method of bony fixation of a MCT is to drill two holes: one above the other along the posterior lacrimal crest. Do not make them in the ethmoidal bone for these delicate bones will simply crumble. Insert a stainless steel wire (25-gauge) into one opening (Fig. 41.7), and draw it out the other with an Iris hook. Bring the ends of the wire through the MCT and twist them to fixate the canthal structures. Knuckle the twisted ends under and turn them posteriorly. This procedure replaces the canthal structures satisfactorily, but is technically difficult because sometimes an inordinate amount of time is spent locating and pulling the wire out of the second hole; occasionally, bleeding from the ethmoidal arteries is significant.

A time-tested and still useful method of medial canthal reattachment was suggested by Mustardé in 1966; it is especially useful when one medial orbital wall has been demolished. After a skin incision 5-7 mm is made along the normal medial orbital wall (just anterior to the attachment of the MCT's anterior crus) drill a hole, insert an awl and penetrate the nasal septum to surface on the abnormal side either through a drill hole or traumatic bony window (Fig. 41.8). Thread a stainless steel wire through the detached canthal tendon and then through the awl's eye and draw it back across the nasal cavity to the normal side. Complete fixation by twisting the wire's ends over a stainless steel modified Kirschner pin[a] (Fig. 41.9). Excise any hypertropic scarred soft tissue and bone that prevents the canthus from properly advancing to the midline. This method is still applicable and is effective, but has the undesirable feature of invading the normal orbit. This adds more risk, especially when the orbit contains the patient's only eye.

Wilkins (6) suggested a perforated stainless steel bar[b] to be used in certain situations as the one cited above of a monocular patient or when there is a large traumatic bony window with relatively normal surrounding bone. Insert this 15–25 mm steel bar through the bony opening lengthwise, and then once the bar is inside the medial orbital wall, rotate it 90° to span the bony opening (Fig. 41.10). This sets the tendon in place without upsetting the nasal

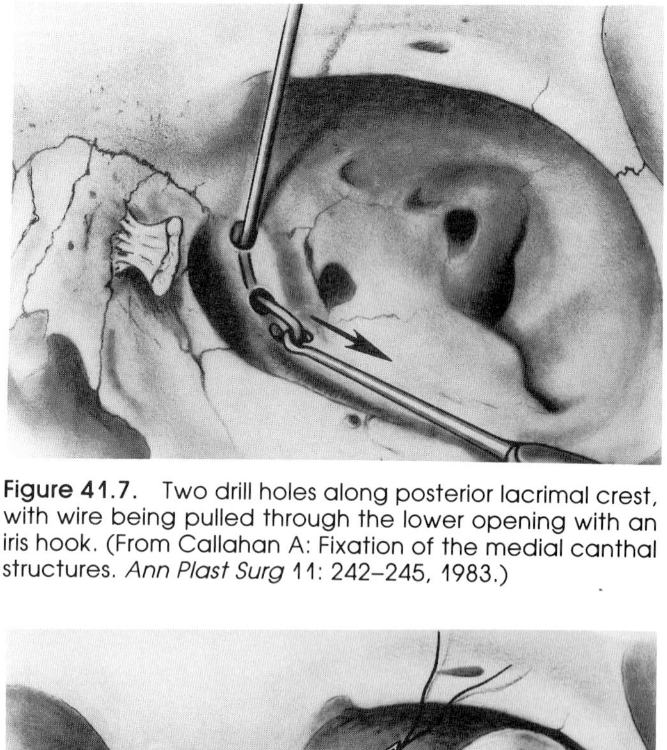

Figure 41.7. Two drill holes along posterior lacrimal crest, with wire being pulled through the lower opening with an iris hook. (From Callahan A: Fixation of the medial canthal structures. *Ann Plast Surg* 11: 242–245, 1983.)

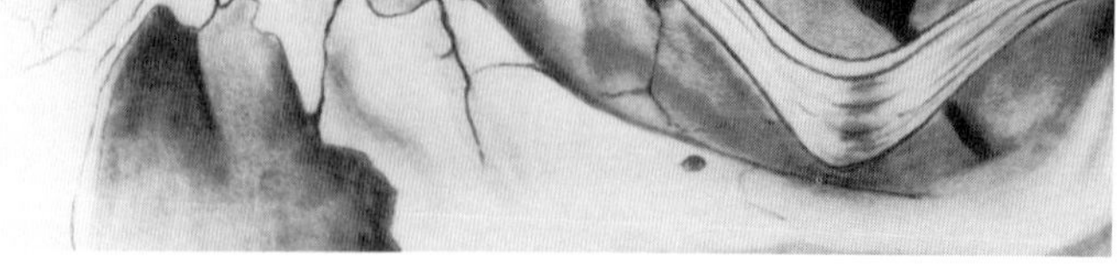

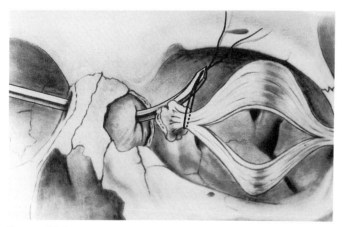

Figure 41.8. Mustarde's transnasal wiring of a unilaterally detached medial canthal tendon. (From Callahan A: Fixation of the medial canthal structures. *Ann Plast Surg.* 11: 242–245, 1983.)

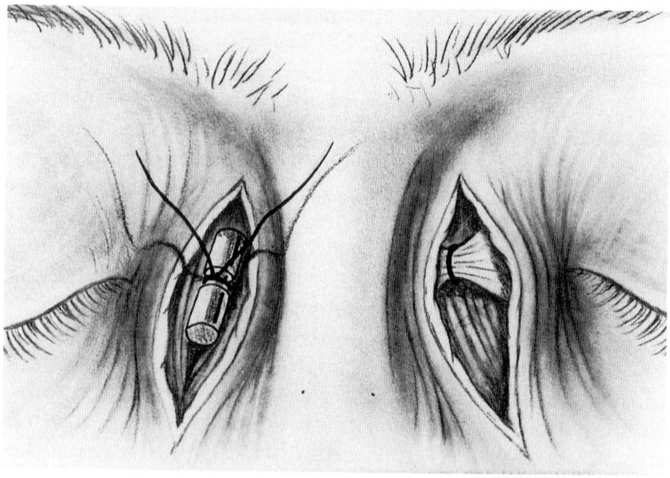

Figure 41.9. Twisting the wire over a Kirschner pin on the normal side. (From Callahan A: Fixation of the medial canthal structures. *Ann Plast Surg* 11: 242–245, 1983.)

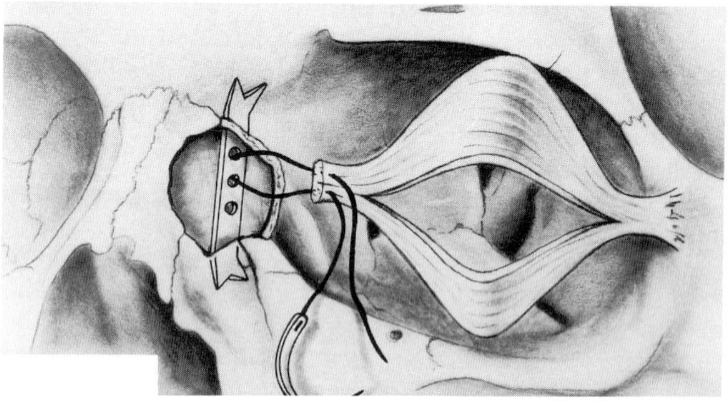

Figure 41.10. Wilkins' bar for refixation of a medial canthal tendon when a large bony defect has been created in the medial orbital wall. (From Callahan A: Fixation of the medial canthal structures. *Ann Plast Surg* 11: 242–245, 1983.)

[a] C. W. Cox, Jr., Eye Foundation Hospital, 1720 University Boulevard, Birmingham, AL 35233

[b] Jedmed Instrument Co., 1430 Hanley Industrial Court, St. Louis, MO 63144

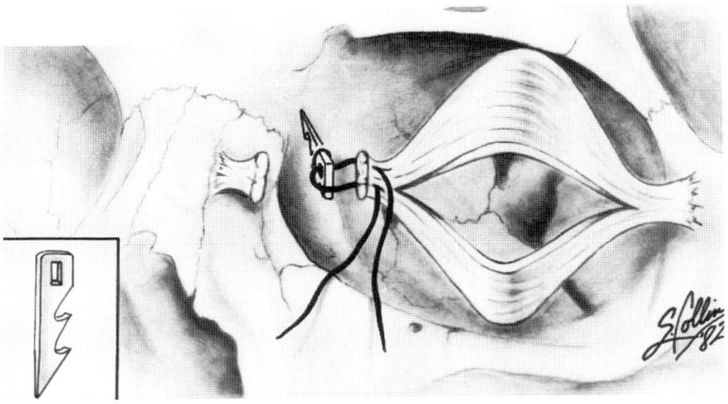

Figure 41.11. Bone piton refixation of medial canthal tendon. Piton (*inset*) is driven into thick bone of the posterior lacrimal crest. (From Callahan A: Fixation of the medial canthal structures. *Ann Plast Surg.* 11: 242–245, 1983.)

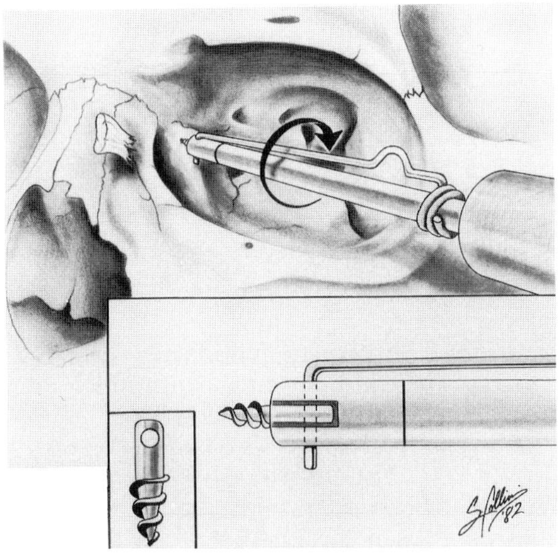

Figure 41.12. Nelson bone screw fixation of medial canthal tendon. *Inset,* Screw is attached to special screwdriver shaft by a pin that passes through holes in the tip of the shaft and bone screw. (From Callahan A: Fixation of the medial canthal structures. *Ann Plast Surg.* 11: 242–245, 1983.)

cavity or normal contralateral orbit. The tendon may be sutured to this strut without damage to the nasal cavity.

To streamline canthal fixation, our innovative Eye Foundation Hospital instrument makers, C. W. Cox, Jr. and Terrell Nelson, suggested a stainless steel piton[c]. With this device the canthal tendon can be secured to the bone, much like a tent pole rope is tethered to a piton driver into the ground. With the aid of a special stainless steel holder, drive the piton into the bone (Fig. 41.11), disconnect the holder, and attach the canthal structures to the piton's eye. In some cases where the bone is thin or trauma has been sufficient to fracture or weaken the bone, the piton will pull out, which will necessitate the Wilkins' bar or transnasal wiring. Another unique problem is that sometimes the bone is fractured as the piton is driven in.

[c] Jedmed Instrument Co., 1430 Hanley Industrial Court, St. Louis, MO 63144

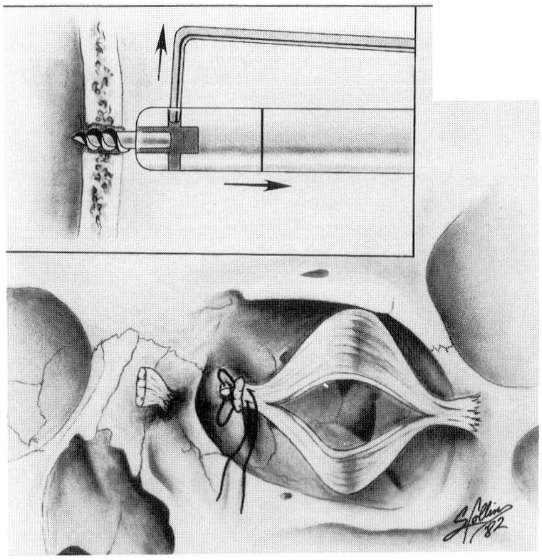

Figure 41.13. After the screw is in place (*inset*), the pin is removed and the canthus is wired to the screw's eye. (From Callahan A: Fixation of the medial canthal structures. *Ann Plast Surg* 11: 242–245, 1983.)

This problem led, in 1982, to Nelson's development of a stainless steel screw[c] that could be screwed into a small drill hole in the medial orbital wall (Fig. 41.12). The diameter of the threaded part of this screw at its widest point is 2.2 mm; thus drill a 1.3-mm-diameter pilot hole at the desired point of fixation and twist the screw in with a special screwdriver. Once the screw is in place detach the screwdriver from the screw and wire the canthal tendon to the screw's eye (Fig. 41.13).

The medial canthus must be replaced three-dimensionally; not only must the canthal tendon be drawn towards the nose on a horizontal level so that it is even with the contralateral side without telecanthus, but it must also be fixated posteriorly to hold the medial end of the lids against the globe so lacrimal fluid will not pool in front of the eye.

REFERENCES

1. Mustardé JC: *Repair and Reconstruction in the Orbital Region.* London, Livingstone, 1966, pp 340 and 349.
2. Zide BM, McCarthy J: The medial canthus revisited: anatomical basis for canthopexy. *Ann Plast Surg* 11: 1–9, 1983.
3. Anderson RL: Medial canthal tendon branches out. *Arch Ophthalmol* 95: 2051, 1977.
4. Callahan MA, Callahan A: *Ophthalmic Plastic and Orbital Surgery.* Aesculapius, Birmingham, AL, 1979.
5. Jones LT, Reeh MJ, Wirtschafter JD: *Ophthalmic Anatomy: A Manual With Some Clinical Applications.* American Academy of Ophthalmology and Otolaryngology, Rochester, MN, 1970.
6. Wilkins RL: Personal communications, 1969.

CHAPTER 42

Management of Lagophthalmos with the Palpebral Spring and Silastic Elastic Prosthesis

ROBERT E. LEVINE, M.D.

In the normal eyelid, the function of the orbicularis oculis is opposed by the levator palpebrae superioris. In the presence of facial paralysis, the levator is working against a markedly weakened or completely denervated orbicularis. The eye opens but cannot be closed, resulting in potentially severe corneal complications.

Two implantable prosthetic devices have been designed to simulate orbicularis function and oppose the levator. In 1965, Morel-Fatio and Lalardrie (1) reported on a design of a palpebral spring made of stainless steel wire. In 1972, Arion (2) described the use of a silastic band to help close the eye. Subsequent reports have been published by others (3–12; N. Chin, personal communication, 1969) of their experience with these devices.

During the past 15 years, I have had the opportunity to implant over 100 silastic prostheses (Figs. 42.1 and 42.2) and over 200 palpebral springs (Figs. 42.3–42.5). Both techniques have been modified through the years from their original descriptions. The information contained in this chapter is based on my personal experience with these devices.

GENERAL CONSIDERATIONS

SELECTION OF PATIENTS

Patients who are considered candidates for implantation of a dynamic lid closure device are those who are not expected to recover facial nerve function, or those who are expected to require at least 6 months for significant improvement in lid closure to occur. Very few patients with idiopathic Bell's palsy require any surgical procedure. Most of the patients who have come to surgery have had acoustic neuromas, facial nerve neuromas, meningiomas, cholesteatomas, glomus jugulare tumors, or severe injuries of the facial nerve. Patients who expect to have the prostheses for the rest of their lives are made to understand the possibility that the prosthesis may need to be repositioned or replaced sometime in the future. Those who can reasonably expect return of function in the future, either because the facial nerve will recover or because a nerve graft will begin to function, are advised that the prosthesis may need to be adjusted or removed when function of the nerve or nerve graft occurs. Patients who do not have access to medical follow-up are not candidates for prosthesis implantation.

Most patients with long-term facial paralysis who can be adequately managed by medical means do not require prosthesis implantation. However, young, active patients who require a regimen of frequent drops and lid taping may find that such a regimen interferes with their lifestyle. With a prosthesis in place, such patients often lead more nearly normal lives, with a markedly reduced medical regimen.

Among those patients who have been most enthusiastic about the implanted prosthesis are those who have lived

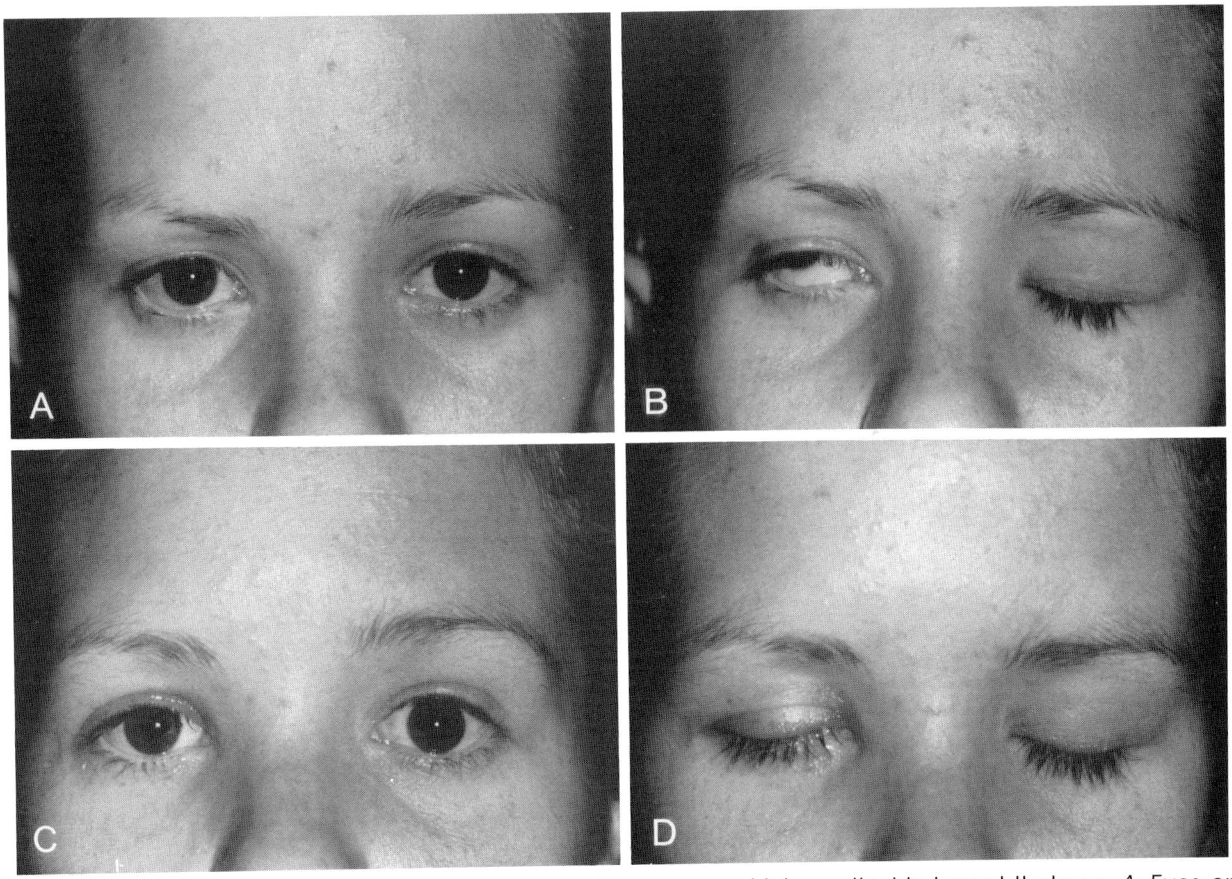

Figure 42.1. This 23-year-old patient underwent removal of a CPA meningioma that impinged on the facial nerve and required resection and direct nerve grafting of that nerve, which resulted in lagophthalmos. *A*, Eyes open. *B*, Attempted closure. *C* and *D*, A silastic elastic prosthesis was placed for improvement in her lid function.

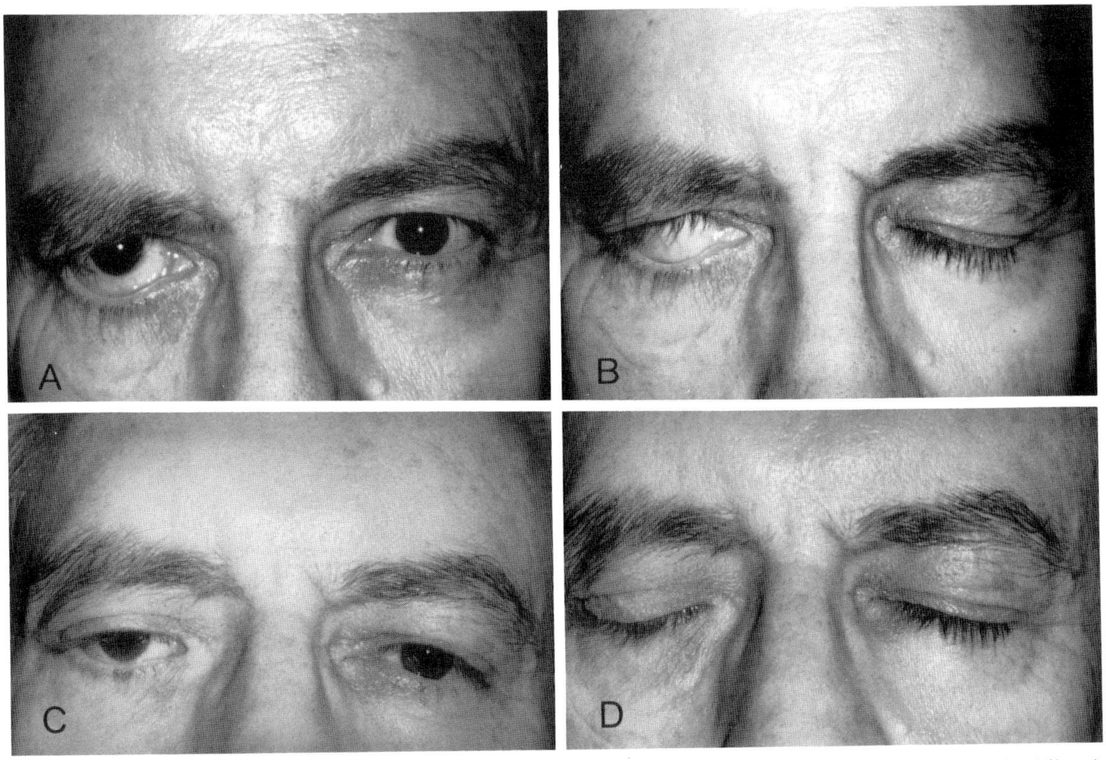

Figure 42.2. This 62-year-old male underwent acoustic neuroma surgery with subsequent marked right lower lid lagophthalmos and moderate right upper lid lagophthalmos. *A* and *B*, Preoperative. *C* and *D*, After implantation of silastic elastic prosthesis and medial canthoplasty.

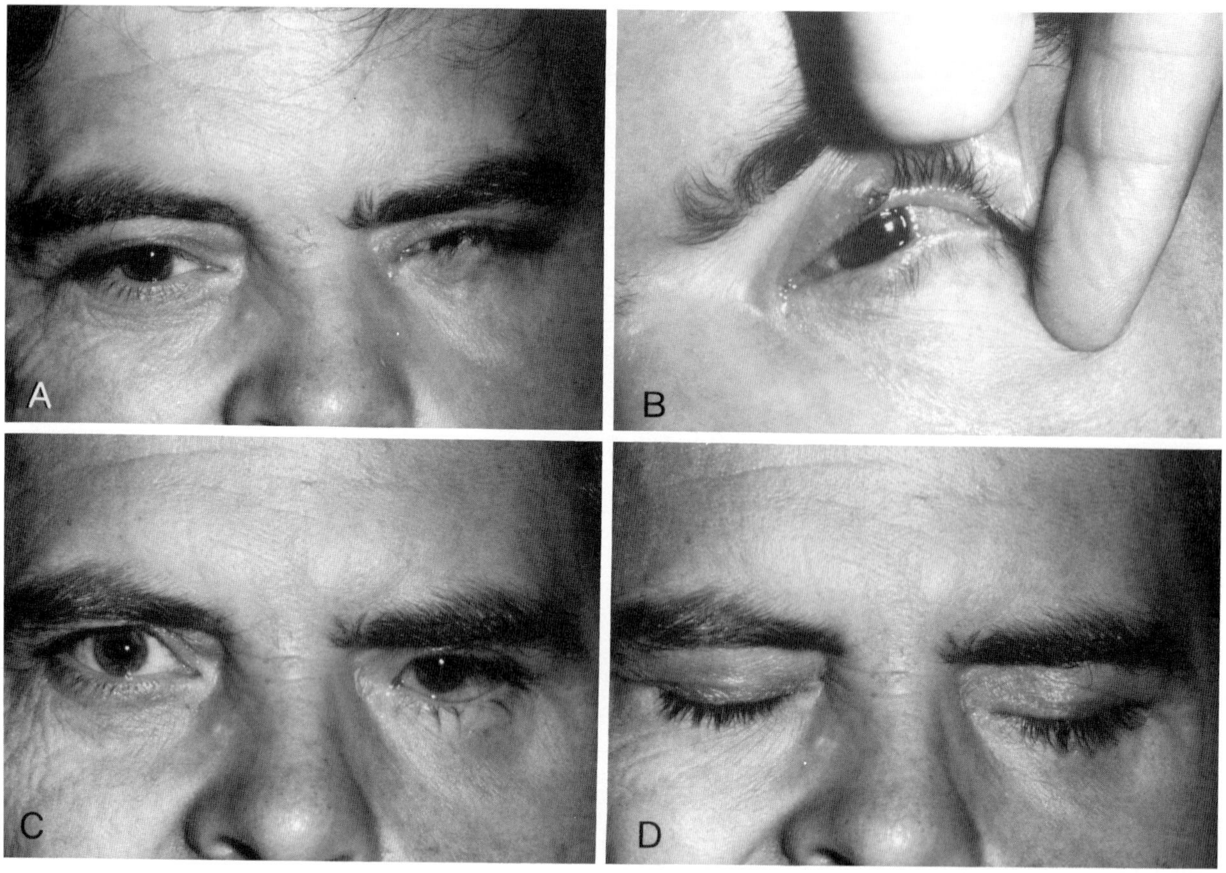

Figure 42.3. This 40-year-old patient underwent removal of a large acoustic neuroma in 1978, resulting in total loss of corneal sensation and facial movement. A tarsorrhaphy was performed on the involved eye shortly after the original surgery and was opened 2 years later. During the following year he had multiple corneal ulcerations and attempts at additional tarsorrhaphies, which did not hold. *A* and *B*, Permanent tarsorrhaphy was placed in 1981 in which the levator was brought through the upper lid and secured to the lower lid. The eye was functionally useless and a cosmetic liability, which he kept covered with a black patch when I first saw him in 1982. The lids were opened and the upper eyelid reconstructed. *C* and *D*, Subsequently a palpebral spring was placed in the upper lid, allowing him to use the eye and providing good closure.

for some period of time with a tarsorrhaphy. With the prosthesis in place, they are relieved of the limited field of vision and the marked disfigurement that accompanies all but minimal tarsorrhaphies. Several patients had their lids sewn completely closed or nearly completely closed by other physicians prior to having spring implantation (Fig. 42.3).

OPHTHALMIC CONSIDERATIONS

The palpebral spring can provide complete closure of the upper lid. It does not weaken significantly with time. Since it is placed only in the upper lid, it does not affect lower lid position or function. It is easily adjustable in the office through a simple skin incision.

By contrast, although the Arion prosthesis can close a lid securely (Fig. 42.3), it should not be relied upon to do so for more than several months, since it stretches and becomes weaker at any time from 2 months to 1 year after surgery. Patients who require secure lid closure, such as those with coexistent fifth nerve involvement and/or poor Bell's phenomenon, are therefore better served with a spring than a silastic prosthesis. Although medial canthoplasty is frequently combined with spring implantation to elevate the lower lid, patients with significant lower lid droop (Fig. 42.2) and/or ectropion who could tolerate some degree of lagophthalmos of the upper lid are good candidates for silastic prosthesis implantation. Because the upper lid is under the constant pull of the levator whereas the lower lid is not, the lower lid stretching of the prosthesis is significantly less than that of the upper lid. The improvement of lower lid position that can be achieved therefore can be maintained for many years.

A patient with only moderate upper and lower lid lagophthalmos who is expected to recover significantly in 6 months to 1 year and is not at high risk for corneal problems may do very well with a silastic prosthesis. If the prognosis is correct, the weakening of the prosthesis will parallel the return of normal function. By the time normal function has completely returned, the prosthesis will have functionally self-destructed and will not need to be removed.

In summary, then, those patients with severe or long-

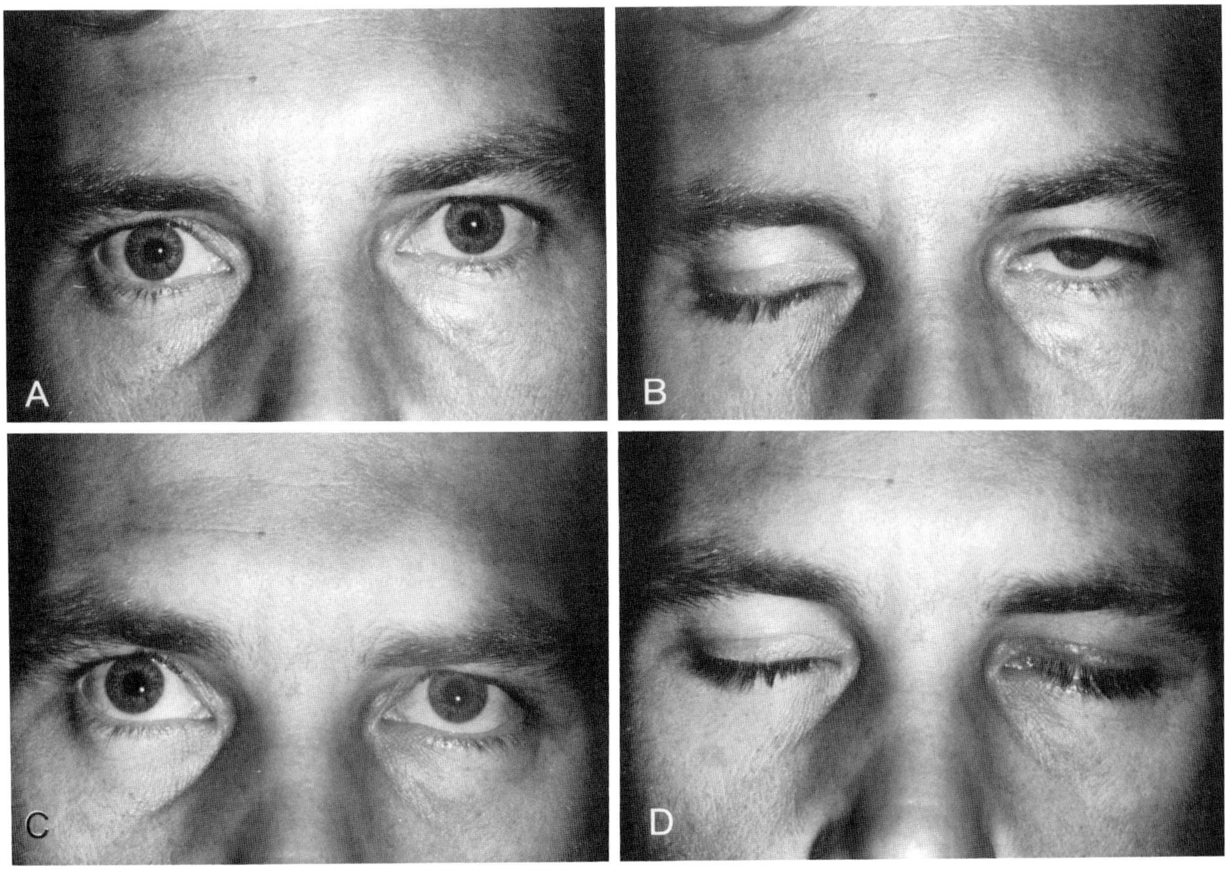

Figure 42.4. This 30-year-old patient sustained an iatrogenic injury to his facial nerve in the course of an otologic procedure, resulting in inability to close the eye on the affected side. *A*, Eyes open. *B*, Attempted closure. *C* and *D*, A palpebral spring was placed with enough tension to adequately close the eye so that the residual lagophthalmos did not result in discomfort. By not placing enough tension on the spring to achieve full closure, no pseudoptosis was created in the primary position. One year after a nerve graft, closure and facial nerve tone were better as compared to the photographs shown. Function is not yet good enough, however, to permit removal of the spring.

term upper lid closure problems and/or factors placing them at high risk for corneal damage are best served with the spring. Those with a lesser degree of upper lid problem but who have significantly lower lid droop are good candidates for the silastic prosthesis.

PALPEBRAL SPRING

PRINCIPLE OF OPERATION

The spring, which is individually made for each patient prior to surgery, is formed from 0.008-0.010 inch stainless steel orthodontic wire. It is shaped like an open safety pin (Fig. 42.6). The fulcrum and upper arm of the spring are secured to the orbital rim periosteum. The lower arm, which is free to move, is placed in the upper lid between orbicularis and tarsus. When the patient opens the eye, the levator pulls the lower arm of the spring superiorly, allowing the lid to open. When the levator tone is relaxed on attempted lid closure, the spring overcomes the levator and pushes the lid shut.

TECHNIQUE OF SPRING IMPLANTATION

The spring should be fashioned prior to surgery by first making a loop of 0.008-0.010-inch stainless steel orthodontic wire. With one round-nosed pliers to bend and a second pair of pliers to fixate the wire, a loop at the fulcrum should be formed approximately 5 mm in diameter. The loop should be as flat as possible. The posterior portion of the loop will be the arm of the spring and will rest on the periosteum of the orbital rim. The anterior extension will be the lower arm and will be positioned in the upper eyelid overlying the tarsal plate. Curves should be placed in the arms of the spring, which conform to the contour of the lid. One curve should be in the frontal plane, allowing the upper arm of the spring to conform to the curvature of the orbital rim and the lower arm to conform to the contour of the upper eyelid. A second curve should be made anteroposteriorly for the upper arm of the spring to fit the orbital rim and for the lower spring arm to fit the curvature of the globe below.

With ocular protection from a scleral shell, local anesthetic with epinephrine should be injected overlying the

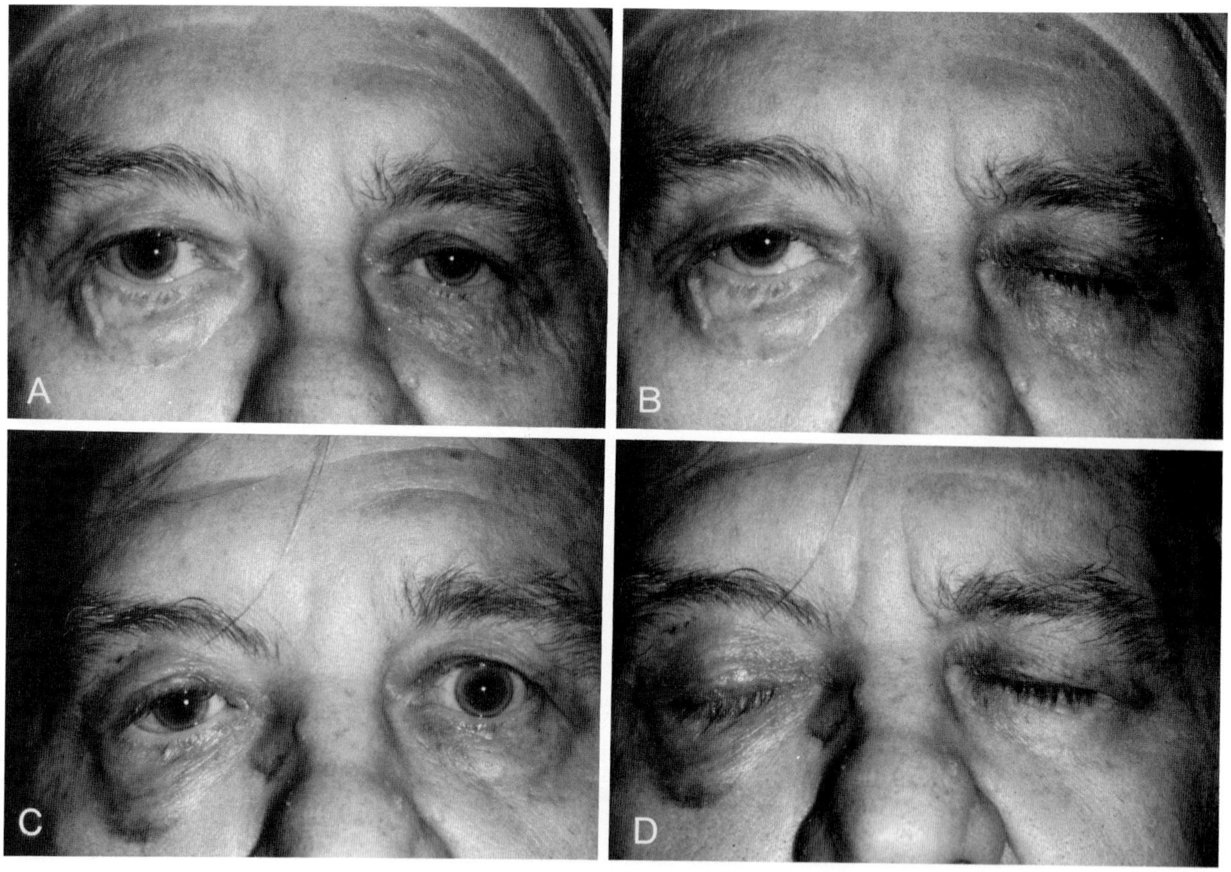

Figure 42.5. A 69-year-old patient with facial weakness following acoustic neuroma surgery. *A* and *B*, Eyes open and closed. *C* and *D*, One week following implantation of palpebral spring and medial canthoplasty.

midtarsus of the upper lid and at the lateral orbital rim. Only the minimum amount of infiltration anesthesia should be used, so as to prevent lid akinesia that might interfere with evaluation of lid function.

The separation of the arms of the spring in the closed position should be approximately one and a half times the separation when the lids are opened. With severe lagophthalmos, the ratio can be increased to two. Intraoperatively, reducing the tension of the spring is easier than increasing the tension. Consequently, the arms should initially be too far apart rather than too close together.

To insert the spring, the surgeon makes a 1-cm incision slightly superior to the midtarsus, about 5 mm medial to the center of the upper lid, lying parallel to the lid margin. Dissection is carried to the anterior surface of the tarsus. A 2-cm incision should be made over the lateral orbital rim, with dissection carried to the periosteum.

A blunted 22-gauge spinal needle should be passed in a slightly inferior direction from the medial incision at the midtarsus in a plane between the anterior surface of the tarsus and the orbicularis oculi. The needle is directed to pass 2 mm superior to the lashes at the lateral extent of the upper lid, emerging at the lateral orbital rim incision.

The undersurface of the upper lid should be checked to ensure that the tarsus has not been inadvertently penetrated. The stylet should be removed and the end of the previously prepared spring passed into the needle. The needle is withdrawn and the spring is brought into position (Fig. 42.6).

A permanent suture, such as 4-0 mersilene, should be placed through the fulcrum of the spring and secured to the periosteum of the orbital rim. An extra bite of periosteum should be taken prior to tying the stitch. The spring should be made so that the fulcrum is placed as far laterally as practical on the orbital rim.

With the scleral shell removed, the spring contour should be checked with the eye opened and closed. Ideally, the spring should be positioned so the lower arm moves slightly posteriorly on opening the lid; this is to accommodate normal lid movement in that direction. Two additional 4-0 mersilene sutures are used to secure the fulcrum, and an additional bite of periosteum is taken with each stitch.

Loops should be formed in the upper and lower ends of the wire with the orthodontic pliers. The superior loop should lie at the upper end of the lateral incision, and the inferior loop should lie about 5 mm medial to the center of the upper lid. To allow for smooth contour, the loop in the lower arm should be directed superiorly and the excess wire cut (Fig. 42.6). Each loop should be closed so that no sharp free end could possibly perforate the tissues.

With precise placement, pressure on adjacent tissues is minimal; this prevents any point from extruding or migrating. To secure the arm in the lower lid, a piece of 0.2-

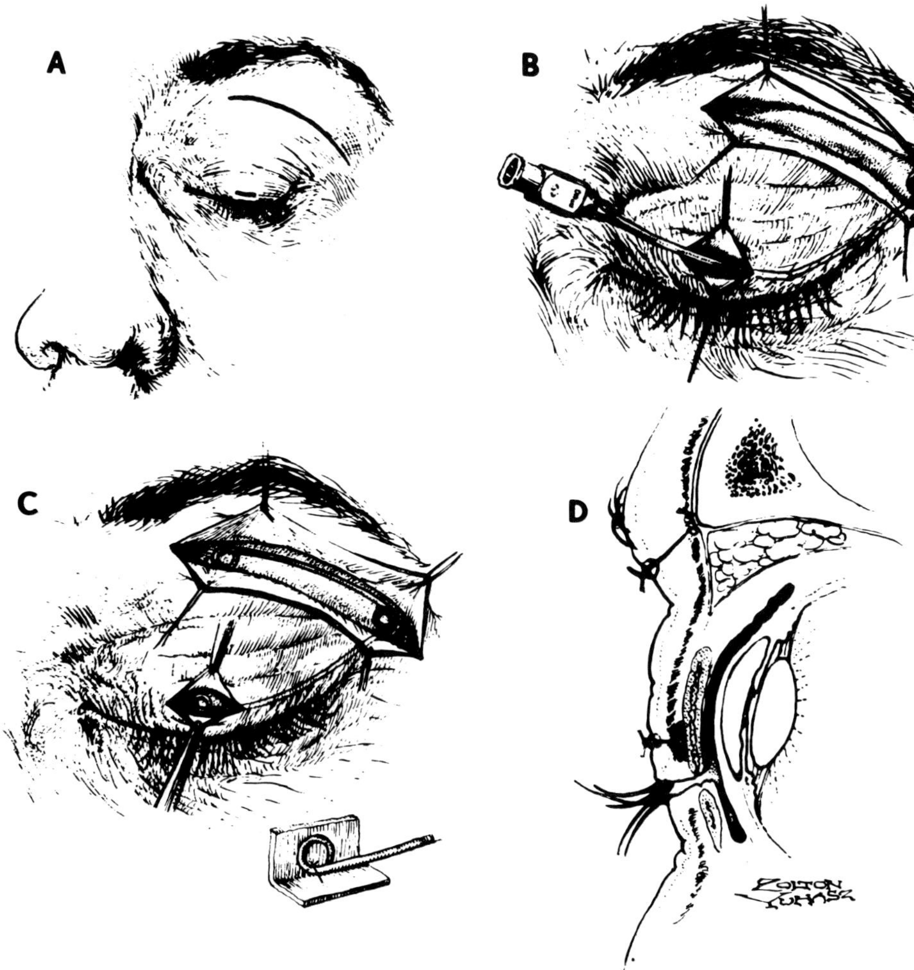

Figure 42.6. Technique of implantation of palpebral spring. *A*, Lid incisions. *B*, Spring is threaded through needle and brought into position as needle is withdrawn. *C*, Spring is adjusted to conform to lid contours and secured at its fulcrum to periosteum. Lower end of spring is encased in pressed 0.2 mm Dacron patch material to which it is secured with an 8.0 nylon suture tied internally. (From Levine RE: Management of the eye after acoustic tumor surgery. In House WF, Luetje CM (eds): *Acoustic Tumors*. Baltimore, MD, University Park Press, 1979, vol 2, chap 6.)

mm-thick Dacron patch, which has been folded in a Gelfoam press and placed in a steam autoclave, is cut and placed around the wire. The crease is directed toward the lid margin. The piece should be approximately 5 mm wide and 10 mm long (Fig. 42.6). The Dacron is secured to the loop of the spring by a nylon 8-0 suture tied internally. The Dacron patch can be held in position in the upper lid by closing overlying tissues meticulously with vertical mattress sutures and interrupted skin sutures of 6-0 Ticron.

Final tension in the spring can be accomplished by varying the position of the upper arm or bending the wire with two instruments. The upper arm should be secured to the periosteum with three 4-0 mersilene sutures; again an extra bite of periosteum is taken with each stitch.

A final inspection of the spring should be made with the patient seated and supine and tension adjusted as needed. Slight overcorrection is preferred.

The lateral wound can be closed with 5-0 plain sutures deeply, and interrupted or running 6-0 Ticron sutures for the skin. Ophthalmic antimicrobial ointment and a moderate-pressure dressing should be placed and removed the next day. Swelling should resolve over the following week, at which time skin sutures can be removed.

Spring adjustments can be made by injecting a local anesthetic and making an incision above the lower arm of the spring adjacent to the fulcrum to expose 0.5 cm of wire. Tension on the wire can be adjusted with two pliers, and the wound can be closed with one or two sutures.

Adjustments may be required to fine-tune the spring or to reduce tension as facial nerve function returns. In patients with satisfactory return of facial function, the spring can be removed. Patients with permanent facial paralysis generally tolerate the spring well for many years. The key to success is meticulous attention to detail at surgery.

Problems with the spring can include extrusion, migration, breakage, infection, and requirement for postoperative adjustment. Therefore, patients selected for this procedure must be followed carefully while the spring is in. The secure closure, simulated blink, and relief of exposure keratitis that can be provided with this technique make the results gratifying.

SILASTIC ELASTIC PROSTHESIS

PRINCIPLE OF OPERATION

The prosthesis consists of a 1-mm silastic rod that is anchored medially by being sewn through the medial tendon and laterally by being sutured to orbital rim periosteum. The upper arm opposes the levator in the same manner as the spring. The lower arm supports the lower lid like a hammock.

TECHNIQUE OF SILASTIC PROSTHESIS IMPLANTATION

Local anesthesia is infiltrated over the origin of the medial canthal tendon and over the lateral orbital rim. The eye is protected with a scleral shell. A curvilinear incision is made medially through skin and the tendon exposed by blunt dissection (Fig. 42.7*A–D*). Laterally, the dissection is carried down to expose the periosteum at the inner aspect of the lateral orbital rim. Hemostasis is achieved with bipolar cautery. The prosthesis, which has been soaked in gentamycin (the parenteral solution is used), is then threaded on a number 14 Ferguson needle and sewn through the medial canthal tendon as a figure-of-8 suture.

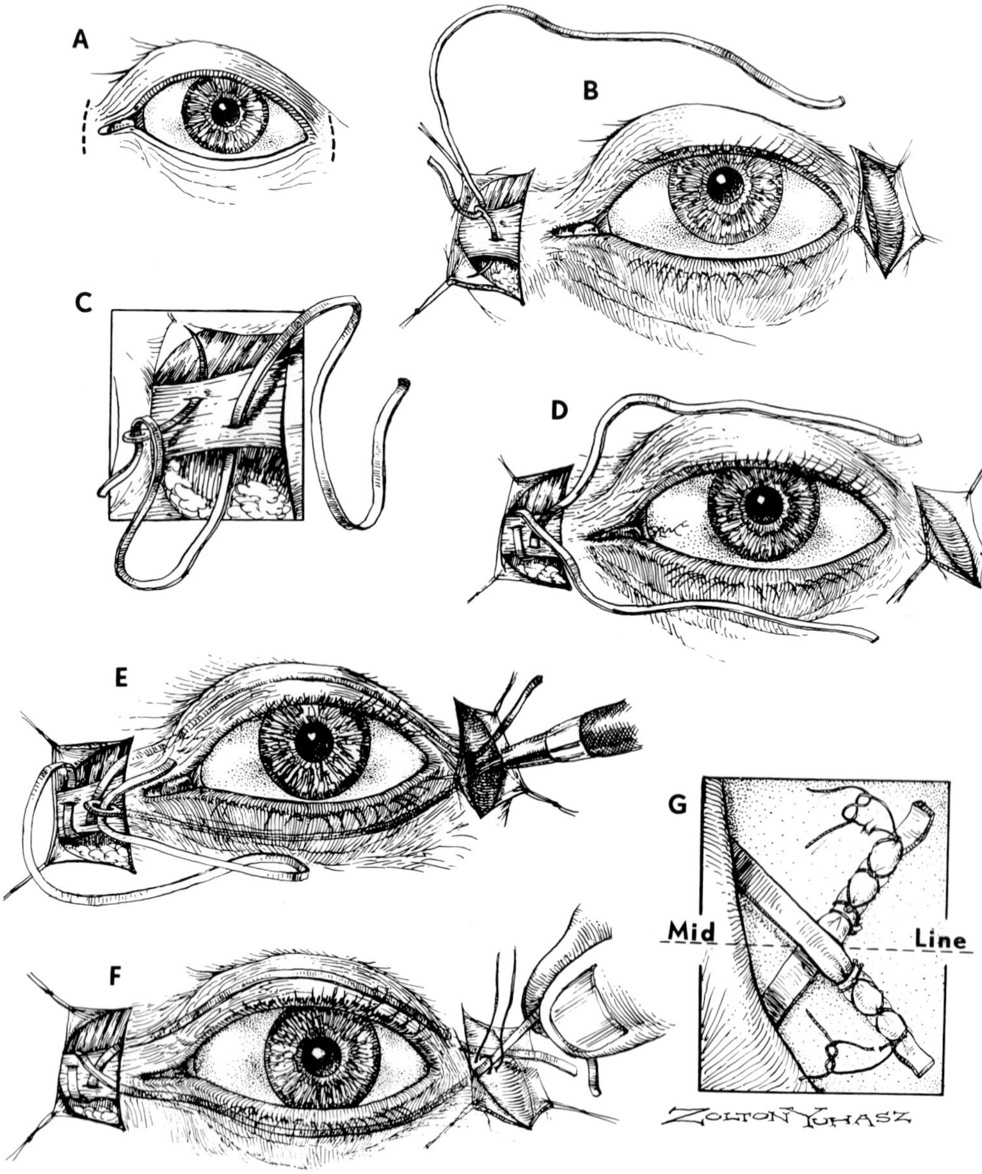

Figure 42.7. Technique of implantation of silastic elastic prosthesis. *A*, Incision sites. *B*, Medial canthal tendon is exposed and prosthesis is sutured through tendon. *C*, Detail of suturing of prosthesis. *D*, Figure-of-8 suture is completed. *E*, Introducer is passed through lateral incision to emerge medially and lower arm of prosthesis is threaded into introducer. *F*, Lower arm of prosthesis is brought through lower lid, and upper arm is brought through in similar manner. Suture is placed to secure lower arm of prosthesis to orbital rim periosteum. *G*, Detail of suturing of prosthesis to periosteum (see description in text). (From Levine RE: Management of the eye after acoustic tumor surgery. In House WF, Luetje CM (eds): *Acoustic Tumors*. Baltimore, MD, University Park Press, 1979, vol 2, chap 6.)

It is important that the inferior arm of the prosthesis leave the tendon at a point that is maximally superior, medial, and posterior. Similarly, the superior arm must come from an anchoring that is as inferior, medial, and posterior as possible. Gentle tension is then placed on both arms of the prosthesis so no slack remains in the figure-of-8 suture. Laterally, the cleavage plane between orbicularis and the anterior aspect of tarsus is entered in the upper and lower lids. A special introducer (Fig. 42.7*E*) is then passed along this cleavage plane in the lower lid just below the lashes to emerge at the medial wound. The lower arm of the prosthesis is threaded into the introducer, which is then withdrawn laterally, thereby placing the prosthesis in the lid. In a similar manner, the upper arm is brought laterally, except that the passage is carried out at the level of mid-tarsus rather than adjacent to the lashes. Gentle tension is again placed on the arms of the prosthesis. It is important not to manipulate the prosthesis with instruments except close to the ends (which will eventually be cut off) since such manipulation will weaken or break the silastic.

A 2-0 Ethoflex suture is placed slightly above the medial raphe at the inner aspect of lateral orbital rim periosteum. A second suture bite is taken through periosteum. A similar stitch is placed just below the medial raphe. The superior stitch is the lateral anchor for the lower arm of the prosthesis. The silastic is then pulled through the loop and the suture loosely tied. Lower lid position is then inspected, with the patient both supine and in an upright position.

Tension on the lower arm of the prosthesis is adjusted to bring the lid against the globe at a point on the cornea that is symmetrical to the opposite eye. A slight additional tension (overcorrection) is then employed to allow for future stretching of the prosthesis, and the Ethoflex suture is tied. In a similar manner, adequate tension is placed on the upper arm of the prosthesis to close the eye. Slight overcorrection again is made and the suture tied. The ends of each suture are then looped over and under the prosthesis, resulting in a slight bend with each tie. This is repeated several times to prevent the prosthesis from slipping. The prosthesis is cut and further secured to periosteum with the same suture, thereby causing each end to be held firmly against the orbital bone. Laterally, deeper layers are closed with interrupted 5-0 plain sutures and skin with running 6-0 Tevdek. Medially, closure is achieved with vertical mattress sutures and interrupted sutures of 6-0 Tevdek. Twenty milligrams of gentamycin parenteral solution are injected subcutaneously at each wound site while taking care not to place the needle deep enough to damage the prosthesis.

The eye is dressed with antimicrobial ointment and a moderate pressure dressing, which is removed the next day. Moderate lid swelling usually subsides within the first postoperative week at which time the skin sutures are removed. However, especially in patients who undergo prosthesis implantation shortly after tumor removal and whose postoperative course included swelling at the original surgical site (e.g., patients with meningitis), some degree of lid swelling may persist for a month or more.

In some patients, placing adequate tension on the lower arm of the prosthesis results in a lateral ectropion. If this occurs, the position of the prosthesis in the lid should be checked, since one major cause of ectropion is placement of the prosthesis too far from the lid margin. In that case, the lower arm of the prosthesis should be removed from the lid, the introducer placed closer to the lashes, and the prosthesis rethreaded into the lid. If the prosthesis is found to be in the proper position, but there is, nevertheless, ectropion, it is due to the additional unequal tension on the lid from its lateral attachments. In that case, the suture should be loosened and lateral attachments should be dissected free, allowing the lid to assume the position dictated by the placement of the prosthesis. The upper lid attachments to the orbital rim may also need to be dissected free to bring that lid into its proper position.

EXPERIENCE WITH THE IMPLANTED PROSTHESIS

Some of the difficulties encountered at the outset with the use of the spring and silastic rod have been overcome by modifications of technique. An initial problem with the spring was the difficulty of fixating the lower arm to tarsus by a direct suturing technique. If the sutures were not secure, the lower arm could dislocate. With the current method, there is no direct suturing to tarsus. Rather, the spring is secured to a piece of Dacron, which in turn becomes firmly adherent to tarsus by the ingrowth of granulation tissue into the Dacron. Moving the fulcrum of the spring as far laterally as possible has increased the mechanical advantage of the spring, thereby allowing less residual ptosis in the primary position. Because there still is closing tension even in the primary position with both devices, the operated eye may have a narrower palpebral fissure than the unoperated eye if enough tension is placed on the device to assure full closure. In those patients with good Bell's phenomenon and no associated fifth nerve problems, a mild degree of residual lagophthalmos may be traded for improved cosmesis in the open position. In some patients the narrow fissure provides additional corneal protection that is helpful to them.

Arion originally described anchoring the prosthesis to a hole drilled in the orbital rim. I have found suturing the prosthesis to periosteum to be an equally secure method of fixation though it is much simpler than drilling. In some patients, placing a medial canthoplasty at the time of silastic implantation enhances the effect of the procedure and allows for desired results with less tension on the prosthesis. A medial canthoplasty is often used with a spring to deal with the coexistent lower lid problem.

Critics of alloplastic devices have pointed out that these devices may extrude, break, or malfunction, and indeed they may. The same criticism can be applied with equal validity to other implanted devices used elsewhere in the body ranging in complexity from hip pins to programmable pacemakers. The merit of implanted devices should not stand or fall on those criticisms however, but rather on how well they carry out their tasks compared with other available modalities. In my experience during the last 17 years with many hundreds of facial paralysis patients, I have come to rely heavily on the spring and silastic implants in those patients requiring surgical management of ocular problems. Unless facial nerve function returns or there is sufficient reinnervation of the lid by a nerve graft procedure, no other available procedure provides the degree of reanimation afforded by the dynamic prostheses. Even functioning temporalis transfer procedures provide lid movement only in association with nonphysiologic associated movements of the face. From a practical standpoint, therefore, the lid is often static.

In the appropriate patient, a dynamic prosthesis, placed with meticulous attention to surgical detail, can move a patient an important step away from disability and toward normality.

REFERENCES

1. Morel-Fatio D, Lalardrie JP: Le ressort palpebral: Contribution a l'etude de la chirurgie plastique de la paralysie faciale. *Neuro-chir* 11: 303, 1965.
2. Arion HG: Dynamic closure of the lids in paralysis of the orbicularis muscle. *Int Surg* 57: 48, 1972.
3. Guy CL, Ransohoff J: The palpebral spring for paralysis of the upper eyelid in facial nerve paralysis. *J Neurosurg* 29: 431, 1968.
4. Levine RE, House WF, Hitselberger WE: Ocular complications of seventh nerve paralysis and management with the palpebral spring. *Am J Ophthalmol* 73: 219, 1972.
5. English FP, English KP: The palpebral spring in facial palsy. *Med J Aust* 1: 223–225, 1972.
6. English FP, Apel JVT: Cerclage technique for dynamic eyelid closure in facial paralysis. *Br J Ophthalmol* 57: 750, 1973.
7. Morgan LR, Rich AM: Four years' experience with the Morel-Fatio palpebral spring. *Plast Reconstr Surg* 53: 405–409, 1974.
8. Wood-Smith D: Experience with the Arion prosthesis. In Tessier P (ed): *Symposium on Plastic Surgery in the Orbital Region.* St. Louis, CV Mosby, 1976.
9. Marrone AC, Soll D: Modification of the Arion encircling silicone spring. Thesis for membership in the American Society of Ophthalmic Plastic and Reconstructive Surgery, Inc, 1977.
10. Lessa S, Carreirao S: Use of an encircling silicone rubber string for the correction of lagophthalmos. *Plast Reconstr Surg* 61: 719–723, 1978.
11. Levine RE: Management of the eye after acoustic tumor surgery. In House WF, Luetje CM (eds): *Acoustic Tumors.* Baltimore, University Park Press, 1979, vol 2, chap 6.
12. Jelks GW, Ransohoff J: Early correction of orbicularis oculi paralysis with an encircling silicone prosthesis. *Neurosurgery* 12: 1983.

CHAPTER 43

BLEPHAROSPASM: DIAGNOSIS AND TREATMENT

GARY S. WEINSTEIN, M.D.
RICHARD L. ANDERSON, M.D.

Blepharospasm is defined as bilateral involuntary, spasmodic closure of the eyelids. It may occur in isolation or as a component of a group of dystonias involving other muscles innervated by the facial nerve. When intermittent lower facial movements accompany the eyelid spasms, the disorder is known as Meige's syndrome, idiopathic orofacial dystonia, or spasm facial median. With more extensive mandibular involvement, Brueghel's syndrome or oromandibular dystonia is diagnosed.

Patients with these disorders are most disabled by the eyelid spasms that render them functionally blind. This chapter discusses the etiology, signs and symptoms, differential diagnosis, and current treatment of blepharospasm. Emphasis will be placed on extirpation of the squeezing eyelid muscles (Anderson myectomy) and the use of botulinum A toxin. These treatments are the best presently available for eliminating the eyelid spasms and allowing a normal life-style.

ANATOMY AND PHYSIOLOGY

The seventh cranial nerve supplies the muscles of facial expression including the orbicularis oculi. A neuroanatomical description of its course is necessary to understand the sites of action of the different treatment modalities. Neurons originating in the motor cortex pass down the rostral brainstem to synapse in the seventh nerve nucleus located in the reticular formation of the lateral pons. The nerve exits the brainstem at the caudal border of the pons just lateral to the recess between the olive and the inferior cerebellar peduncle. It has a long course in the petrous portion of the temporal bone and exits from the stylomastoid foramen. After first giving off a postauricular branch, the location of the main trunk varies from directly below the external auditory meatus to the lower tip of the ear. The nerve usually enters the parotid gland at two-thirds of the distance between the angle of the mandible and the temporomandibular joint or slightly lower. Within the substance of the gland, the nerve divides into two branches. The temporofacial branch, which transmits motor fibers to the orbicularis oculi muscles, divides into two temporal branches and a zygomatic branch. The cervicofacial division supplies the lower face and divides into buccal, supramandibular, and inframandibular branches. The buccal, or middle branch, which originates from the temporofacial division in 24% of patients, the bifurcation in 12%, and the cervicofacial division in 64%, frequently anastamoses with the zygomatic branch to supply the lower medial portion of the orbicularis oculi muscle (1). Therefore, sectioning the temporofacial division alone with not eliminate the buccal branches in 76% (12% and 64%) of cases, and contractions of the lower medial orbicularis oculi fibers will persist.

The orbicularis oculi muscles are thinnest and broadest inferotemporally, and thickest and strongest inferomedially. Their full extent is often unrecognized, so that incomplete extirpations are performed. The pretarsal muscle fibers are responsible for involuntary reflex blinking while the preseptal and preorbital fibers are used for voluntary forceful eyelid closure (2). During a normal blink, the orbicularis oculi contract and the levator muscles relax to allow the upper eyelids to move downward. Blinking increases in chronic schizophrenia and in the Gilles de la Tourette syndrome because of central dopaminergic hyperactivity in the midbrain and basal ganglia (3). An increased blink rate is also an early sign of blepharospasm and Meige's syndrome.

ETIOLOGY

In the past, essential blepharospasm was thought to be a functional disorder and patients were often referred to psychiatrists. The current belief that essential blepharospasm and Meige's syndrome are organic diseases is supported by a high correlation with essential tremor (4) and a positive family history in some patients (4–7).

The bilaterality of these syndromes suggests a pathologic focus rostral to the facial nucleus. Postulated sites include a lesion between the bulbar reticular formation and the 4S area of the motor cortex (8), a rostral brainstem infarct with denervation sensitivity of the facial nuclei (9), or a basal ganglia disorder because patients with Parkinson's disease (10) may have eyelid fluttering and an increased blink reflex with glabellar tap (11–13). Histopathologic studies of the muscle fibers reveal only areas of hypertrophy and atrophy (14).

SIGNS AND SYMPTOMS

The mean age at onset of essential blepharospasm is 56 years (8) and females predominate (8, 10, 15). Henderson (8) estimated that 1 of every 10,000 patients seeking medical care at the Mayo Clinic had blepharospasm, although one would predict a lower incidence in the general population. Patients usually present to an ophthalmologist, neurologist, or psychiatrist.

The onset is heralded by variable episodes of increased blinking lasting from seconds to as long as 20 minutes (10). Subjective complaints include burning eyes and a drawing or clamping sensation around the eyelids. The blinking may be unilateral at first, but becomes bilateral with time. Within 6 months to 3 years (15, 16), progression to episodic involuntary spasms of eyelid closure occurs. Precipitants include bright sunlight, air pollution, wind, noise, eye movement, head movement (8), stress, television, and reading (10). Patients are usually asymptomatic in the morning or after resting (8). They may develop "tics" or mannerisms that involve using other muscles innervated by the facial nerve or acts of mental concentration to decrease the frequency and intensity of the spasms (8). Examples include humming, whistling, yawning, coughing, mouth opening, chewing gum, using a toothpick, eating, extending the neck, rubbing ones eyelids or other areas of the face, covering one eye, playing the piano, or solving puzzles or mathematical problems. Although remissions have been described following major life crises such as fighting with a spouse, being accosted, or having a myocardial infarction, relentless progression is the rule (8). In the advanced stages, patients develop severe spasms that render them functionally blind, socially reclusive, and unable to work or care for themselves.

The sine qua non of this disease is true blepharospasm with the eyes clamped tightly shut (Fig. 43.1), and not just increased blinking or twitching. Periocular whitening can be observed during a spasm because the arterial inflow is constricted and blood is expressed from the venous system. Attempts to manually pry the eyelids open to oppose the spasms lead to stretching and excoriation of the skin (8, 17), attentuation of its attachments to the underlying orbicularis oculi, and eventual dermatochalasis (14). The excess eyelid skin, in turn, can touch the eyelashes and trigger additional spasms (18).

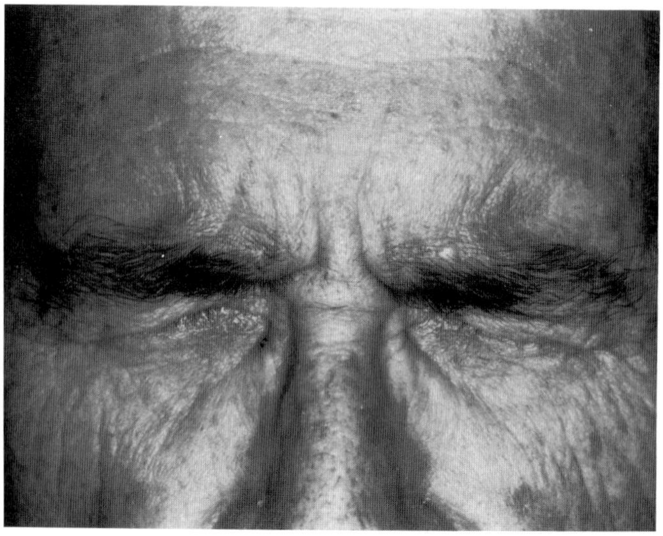

Figure 43.1. Patient with severe blepharospasm demonstrating secondary brow ptosis and dermatochalasis.

Examples of other periocular structures weakened by the opposing forces of blepharospasm and forced eyelid opening include brow ptosis from weakened brow attachments to the frontalis muscles and blepharoptosis secondary to attenuation or disinsertion of levator aponeurotic fibers (14). These problems, in combination with dermatochalasis, can block the patient's superior visual field even when not in spasm. Stretching of the medial and lateral canthal tendons as well as possible overaction of the orbicularis oculi lead to entropion or ectropion of the lower eyelid (8). Many patients with blepharospasm also have poor tear function, which should be evaluated preoperatively.

Associated ocular signs include impersistence of gaze, spasms of vertical gaze, and eyelid retraction (19). The nonocular signs reported, such as tongue thrusts, head jerks, and head tilts (19), are part of Meige's syndrome rather than essential blepharospasm.

DIFFERENTIAL DIAGNOSIS

A complete ophthalmologic and neurologic examination is required to establish the diagnosis. Corneal irritation from keratitis sicca, spastic entropion, eyelash abnormalities, or blepharitis may cause a blepharospastic response (14). If a drop of topical anesthetic decreases the spasms significantly, corneal irritation should be suspected and the primary problem treated. The eyelids of patients with photophobia secondary to anterior uveitis and posterior subcapsular cataracts may also be in a state of semicontraction or tonus even when not actually closed (8).

Reflex blepharospasm has been reported as a normal finding in premature infants (20), a hereditary disorder with onset in early childhood that improves after the first decade (6), a response to glabellar tap in patients with Parkinson's disease (13), and a release phenomenon in nondominant temporoparietal lesions where the spasms persist on the functioning side for several weeks (20).

Our experience indicates that blepharospasm more commonly exists as part of a spectrum of movement disorders. Meige's syndrome combines blepharospasm with abnormal lower facial movements such as involuntary chewing, trismus, lip pursing, jaw deviation, wide opening of the mouth, and tongue protrusion, retraction, and writhing (21). Patients may also demonstrate spasmodic dysphonia with grunting, platysmal contractions, torticollis, retrocollis, arm dystonia, or postural tremor. In patients with blepharospasm previously treated with seventh nerve avulsion, it may be difficult to differentiate Meige's syndrome from aberrent regeneration of the nerve (22). Brueghel's syndrome, which is also known as oromandibular dystonia, is a more severe form of Meige's syndrome that is characterized by continuous mandibular and cervical spasms (10). Although both syndromes may present with blepharospasm (4) and are treated with the same techniques, the success rate is decreased and the lower face and neck movements are only variably improved.

A careful drug history must be obtained because dopamine stimulators (23) and nasal decongestants containing antihistamines and sympathomimetics have been reported to cause blepharospasm (4, 24). These drugs should be discontinued for a trial period prior to establishing the diagnosis.

Several movement disorders involving the orbicularis oculi may mimic blepharospasm. Tardive dyskinesias with choreiform facial movements may develop in psychotic patients when phenothiazines are discontinued (25). Eyelid tremors and prolonged violent blepharospasms can be observed in patients with postencephalitic Parkinson's disease. Individual orbicularis muscle bundles may flicker and quiver in facial myokymia associated with brainstem disease (8). Myokymia can persist for 6 months, is generally absent during sleep, and is accompanied by narrowing of the palpebral fissure and elevation of the angle of the mouth (27). A benign, self-limited form involves the lower eyelids and is precipitated by stress, fatigue, or caffeine.

An apraxia of eyelid opening has been reported in progressive supranuclear palsy, Huntington's chorea, extrapyramidal syndromes, cerebral diplegia and Parkinsonoid-like syndromes (28). These patients are unable to voluntarily open their eyelids after closure, although true spasms are lacking.

Hemifacial spasm is characterized by unilateral tonic and clonic contractions of muscles innervated by the seventh nerve that continue during sleep (29). Rare bilateral cases have been reported, but the left and right sides of the face are not synchronized or involved to the same degree (29, 30). Some cases secondary to vascular or neoplastic lesions compressing the seventh nerve in the posterior fossa have been relieved with surgical decompression (31). A careful neurologic workup including a computer tomography scan is indicated to search for posterior fossa pathology such as an ectatic basilar artery stimulating the underlying facial nerve.

Habit spasms are stereotypical, repetitive mannerisms or facial tics of variable frequency. Rare patients with Gilles de la Tourette syndrome appear blepharospastic but they also grunt, sniff, clear their throats and exhibit coprolalia.

Functional or hysterical blepharospasm should be considered only as a diagnosis of exclusion. It may follow an emotional or traumatic event in younger patients (age 25–40 years) with no preceding history of increased blinking (32). In contrast with essential blepharospasm, the spasms are under volitional control and are not improved by rest or worsened with fatigue (8). Patients are also less disabled and may improve with psychotherapy (33), conditioning in a group setting (34), behavior modification (35), hypnosis, biofeedback techniques (36, 37) or no treatment.

MEDICAL TREATMENT

Psychotherapy (33), hypnosis, biofeedback (36, 37), relaxation therapy, acupuncture and the use of ptosis crutches have been tried. Reported successes may actually represent the treatment of hysterical rather than essential blepharospasm.

Medical treatment is undertaken initially in hopes of ameliorating the spasms and avoiding the need for surgical intervention. Centrally active medications decrease aberrant impulses impinging on facial nerve nuclei in the brainstem, while peripherally acting medications relax or inhibit contractions of the orbicularis oculi. Henderson (8) documents the early treatment of blepharospasm as well as the rationale for using certain medications. Patients with concomitant depressions were treated with stimulants, although sedative hypnotics were tried if patients were agitated.

The long list of usually ineffective centrally acting drugs includes antipsychotics (phenothiazines, butyrophenones, reserpine), affective disorder agents [lithium carbonate (4), tetrabenazine (38)], antianxiety agents (39) (meprobamate), stimulants (8) (amphetamine sulfate), sedative hypnotics (8, 16) (phenobarbitol), parasympathomimetics (8) (lecithin, choline, physostigmine), antimuscarinics (8) [tincture of belladona, scopolamine (40], catecholamine synthesis inhibitors (8) (α-methyl-p-tyrosine), antihistamines (diphenhydramine hydrochloride), and anticonvulsants (clonazepam) (4, 41). Treatment with antiparkinsonian drugs such as amantadine (39), mixtures of carbidopa and levodopa (4, 16), trihexyphenidyl (4), and anticholinergics (16) were tried because of the association of blepharospasm with Parkinson's disease. Centrally acting antispasmodics such as baclofen and orphenadrine citrate are currently under investigation. We prescribe the latter agent prior to surgery as well as postoperatively for persistent lower facial spasms, although tachyphylaxis frequently develops within 2 weeks.

SURGICAL TREATMENT

Functionally impaired patients with essential blepharospasm or Meige's syndrome who have not tolerated or responded to medication are candidates for injections or surgical therapy. Numerous procedures have been devised to interrupt the pathway from the motor cortex neurons to the orbicularis oculi muscles. At present, orbicularis extirpation appears to have the most long-lasting effect with a low recurrence rate and concomitant correction of the secondary anatomic defects (22).

FACIAL NERVE INTERRUPTION

Subcorticotomy of the facial area of the nondominant cortex has been reported (42), although an intracranial approach is associated with increased morbidity and mortality. Prior to the successful use of myectomy, most treatments attempted to destroy seventh nerve fibers. Alchohol injections 1 cm anterior to the ear, on a line drawn from the lateral canthus to the junction of the tragus and lobule of the ear, were used to chemically necrose the temporofacial division of the nerve (8). Stimulating electrodes facilitated accurate injection into the nerve sheaths (43), which was required for success. Although the injections caused only transient pain, few experienced any benefit for greater than 6 months, spasms tended to recur earlier after each subsequent injection, and cicatricial contraction of the overlying soft tissues was cosmetically unacceptable (4). Percutaneous thermolysis of the nerve minimized scarring, but the long-term results continued to be unsatisfactory (44).

More permanent results were sought by stretching, sectioning, or avulsing the nerve (8). When performed at the brainstem or stylomastoid foramen, the cervicofacial branches of the nerve were unnecessarily damaged and regeneration was common. Reynolds (17) popularized selective facial nerve avulsion to prevent lower facial paralysis. Patients who improved after 1% xylocaine was injected in the region of the facial nerve and were willing to accept the associated paralysis were candidates for the procedure. General anesthesia, with the tracheal tube positioned to observe the angle of the mouth for drooping, was utilized. The incisions were placed 2 cm anterior to the external auditory meatus at the inferior border of the zygoma, and then extended downward for 5 cm. The branches to be avulsed on each side were placed on a hemostat and rotated several times. After 24 hours, the procedure was repeated if no improvement was evident. Some surgeons applied silver radioopaque clips to the coagulated ends of the proximal nerve stumps for later localization with x-rays to facilitate retreatments for recurrences (45).

Blepharospasm recurred within 6 months after facial nerve avulsion in 30–50% of cases (17, 39, 46). One study found no significant effect in over 100 patients (15). The iatrogenic facial nerve palsy often exacerbated preexisting brow ptosis, dermatochalasis, and lower eyelid ectropion and laxity and caused epiphora secondary to "lacrimal pump" dysfunction and corneal exposure from lagophthalmos (39, 46, 47). When cervicofacial fibers were also damaged, upper lip paresis resulted in eating problems, drooling, mouth droop, and absent facial expression (46, 47). Other complications included prominent surgical scars, ectopic parotid secretion, and transcutaneous parotid fistulas, although the latter two problems were usually transient (47).

BOTULINUM TOXIN

More recently, the spasms have been treated with injections of botulinum A toxin that interfere with acetylcholine release from nerve terminals (48, 49). Early treatments consisted of injecting 2.5 mg (units) subcutaneously in each side. The toxin was placed in all four eyelids several millimeters from the lash margin and the zygomatic regions (to block the lateral orbicular fibers). The central portion of the upper eyelid was avoided to spare the levator aponeurosis from blockade by the toxin. Currently, doses of up to 55 mg (units) are injected in each side and the toxin is placed in the brow regions and lower face in addition to the areas described above. Most patients respond within 2–3 days, but an early overcorrection is possible. Patients are clinically improved for an average of 10 weeks before repeat injections of higher dosages are required (49). Although no cumulative or permanent effect has been observed, it has been postulated that antibody formation may lead to tachyphylaxis (49). Early complications that have been reported include exposure keratopathy, blepharoptosis, and diplopia. The optimal dosage, number of injections, and long-term complications have not yet been established.

The unacceptable recurrence and complication rates, exacerbation of preexisting tissue defects, and theory that muscles are less likely to regenerate than nerves reoriented the therapeutic approach toward impairment or removal of the orbicularis muscles. Periobicular alchohol injections were tried early on but they resulted in stiffness and cicatricial contraction of the overlying skin (4).

ORBICULARIS EXTIRPATION

Surgical myectomies have been performed for many years but recent refinements have increased the success rate (50). The procedure is indicated in patients who fail to respond to other forms of therapy. Early operations are unsuccessful because insufficient muscle was removed and the anatomic defects were not fully corrected. Fox (51) advocated surgical excision of the orbicularis fibers in the upper eyelid through a blepharoplasty incision, but the pretarsal fibers were spared and the blepharospasms persisted. Callahan (52) reported a 75% recurrence rate with excision of a 10 × 40- to 50-mm section of orbicularis muscle at the lateral raphe. The corrugator muscles were excised if the frontalis muscles participated in the spasms, and levator tucks were performed when involutional blepharoptosis was present. Other techniques, such as upper eyelid blepharoplasties (18) and bilateral fascia late slings (53) were added to partial myectomies in an attempt to improve the success rate.

With the above techniques, many patients still required reoperations or were not significantly improved. This suggested the need for more aggressive extirpation of the eyelid protractors including the orbicularis oculi, procerus, corrugator superciliaris, and facial nerve fibers in the postorbicular fascia. The myectomy operation that was developed is performed through a browplasty and sometimes also a blepharoplasty incision that enables full correction of the anatomic changes (14, 50). The browplasties correct brow ptosis, which improves cosmesis, increases the superior visual field, and facilitates use of the frontalis muscles to break the spasms. Blepharoplasties are only added if excess skin is present and there is no lagophthalmos after the browplasty incision has been closed. Although the additional lid crease incision facilitates removal of pretarsal orbicularis fibers, hemostasis, and lid crease formation, it compromises the eyelid's vascular supply, increases the operative time, and can result in lagophthalmos and corneal irritation. Lateral canthal tendon plications are added when lower eyelid laxity is present. The levator aponeurosis is reapproximated to tarsus if blepharoptosis was present before or if iatrogenic disinsertion occurs during surgery.

Preoperatively, patients are asked to estimate the percentage of time the spasms impair their reading, driving, watching television, or working. A history of prior bleeding problems or medications that interfere with hemostasis such as acetylsalicylic acid should be elicited. Patients are made aware of the presence of any lower facial spasms preoperatively because these dystonias may become more bothersome and progressive following surgery. They are informed that numbness of the forehead from cutting the supraorbital nerve and some lagophthalmos from removal of orbicularis muscle fibers can be expected; although both problems are usually transient. They are also told that lower facial movements may not be improved by surgery and that approximately 45% of patients with Meige's syndrome require additional extirpation of lower eyelid orbicularis muscles.

General anesthesia is more comfortable than local for both the patient and surgeon because the operation is lengthy and multiple injections are required. Intraoperative hemostasis can be facilitated by injecting 1% lidocaine hydrochloride with epinephrine 1:100,000 subcutaneously in the region of the brow, upper eyelid, temple, zygoma, and lateral one-third of the lower eyelid. Local anesthesia offers the advantages of greater safety in high-risk patients, better intraoperative hemostasis, and the ability to quantitate dermatochalasis and eyelid height. When local anesthesia is being used alone, equal amounts of 2% lidocaine hydrochloride with epinephrine 1:100,000 solution and 0.5% bupivacaine are injected in the areas described above as well as through the brow to the periosteum. Gentle pressure facilitates diffusion of the anesthetic.

Gentian violet is used to outline a browplasty incision. A smaller browplasty is planned in males because of the differences between the sexes in natural brow height and contour. A No. 15 scalpel blade is used to completely incise the brow to periosteum (Fig. 43.2). Full-thickness brow is then removed with a Steven's scissors and Paufique forceps (Fig. 43.3). The supraorbital arteries and nerves are usually included in the brow excision because residual muscle remains when an attempt is made to spare them.

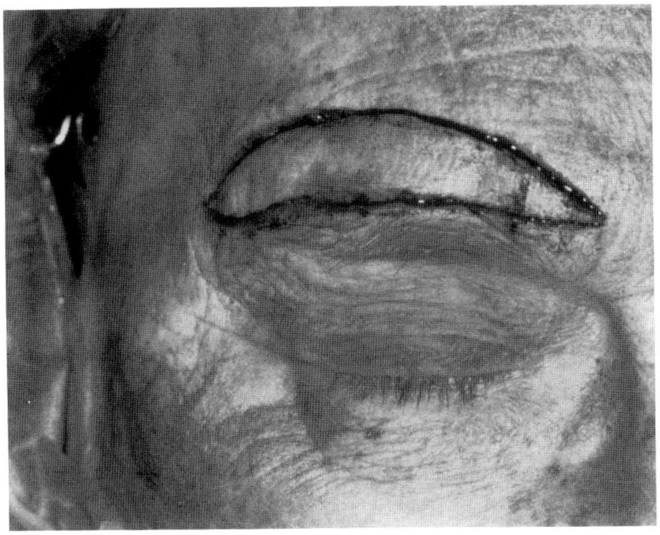

Figure 43.2. Incisions for full-thickness browplasty have been completed. Vertical gentian violet line indicates location of supraorbital artery and nerve.

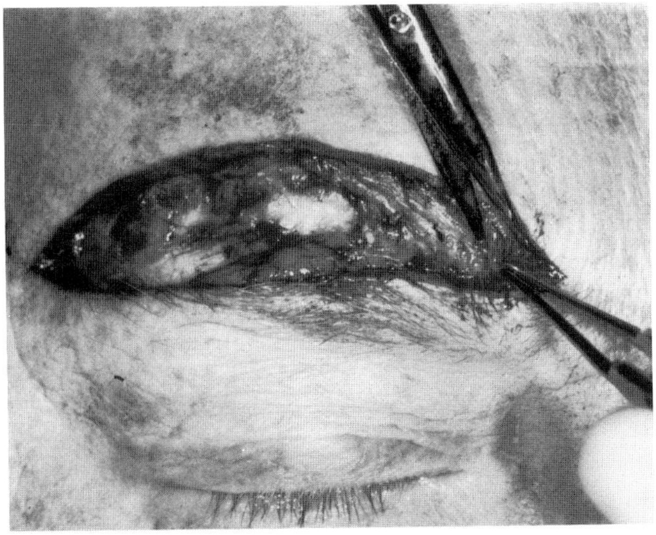

Figure 43.3. Brow has been excised to periosteum.

The resection of the lower portion of the frontalis muscle helps to permanently elevate the brow and allows the patient to counteract residual spasms. Bipolar cautery is used throughout the operation to achieve hemostasis.

Large skin hooks are placed at the lower border of the incision beneath the brow hairs, which are preserved by not injuring the underlying hair follicles, muscle fibers, or dermal tissues. While traction on the orbital orbicularis muscle fibers is applied below the brow with a Paufique forceps, a Stevens scissors is used to develop a dissection plane between skin and muscle. Skin necrosis and injury are avoided if the small subcutaneous vessels are not cauterized and if the assistant properly manipulates the skin hooks to allow observation of both the surgical plane and the scissors' blades through the thin overlying skin. Visualization of all dissection planes through the browplasty incision is further enhanced with a fiber optic headlight.

The superficial surgical plane is continued inferiorly to just above the upper eyelid margin, medially across the midline to include the corrugator and procerus muscles (Fig. 43.4), temporally to include the entire lateral raphe, and inferiorly around the orbital rim to include the lateral one-third of the lower eyelid orbicularis oculi (Fig. 43.5).

After all except the medial two-thirds of the lower eyelid orbicularis fibers have been dissected from overlying skin and before muscle is removed, a deep plane is created underlying the same muscles. This allows excision of the protracting muscles en bloc, which reduces bleeding, facilitates more complete muscle removal, and reduces operating time. The superior orbicularis muscle is grasped with a forceps and the upper eyelid orbicularis muscle is bisected with a Stevens scissors. The medial stump is carefully dissected from the orbital septum and tarsus to avoid cutting orbital fat and the levator aponeurosis. This plane is extended medially to remove muscle from the periosteum overlying the frontal and nasal bones in the glabellar region. The medial orbicularis, corrugator superciliaris, and procerus muscles are amputated as one piece because bleeding from the supraorbital, infraorbital, and angular veins can be copious.

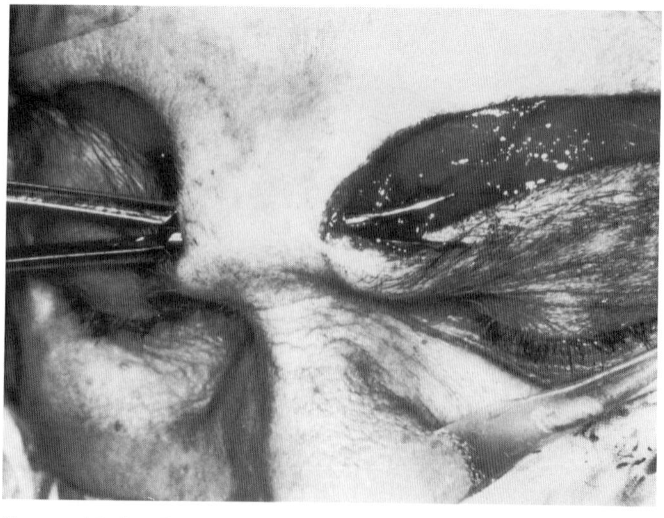

Figure 43.4. Elevation of glabellar region with a hemostat shows dissection plane between skin and corrugator and procerus muscles.

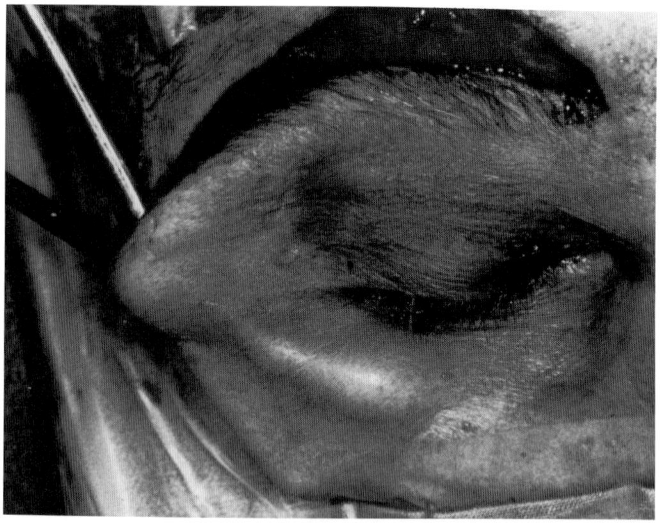

Figure 43.5. A scissors placed through the temporal portion of the browplasty incision demonstrates how the lateral third of the lower eyelid orbicularis can be undermined and removed.

The lateral orbicularis fibers are dissected from the septum and tarsus in a similar manner. This plane is continued laterally and inferiorly for several centimeters beyond the orbital rim to separate orbicularis oculi and peripheral facial nerve fibers from the underlying temporalis fascia and zygoma. The large temporal block of orbicularis muscle is amputated at the junction of the lateral one-third and medial two-thirds of the lower eyelid. A Metzenbaum scissors and Addison forceps are used because of the long distance between the brow incision and the inferior extent of muscle removal. Prior to closure (Figs. 43.6 and 43.7) all bleeding points and vessels in spasm are meticulously cauterized with a bipolar unit to prevent hematoma formation.

Rarely, a very conservative blepharoplasty is needed if considerable excess skin is still present after the brow is sutured into position. Additional preseptal and pretarsal fibers can be excised through the incision, although a small strip of orbicularis muscle should be left over the eyelash follicles and margin to facilitate eyelid closure. A blepharoplasty may compromise the blood supply to the upper eyelid skin and brow flap, increase the operative time, and possibly induce postoperative lagophthalmos and skin contracture. In cases where a blepharoplasty is not indicated, a deep eyelid crease still forms because the removal of orbicularis fibers allows the skin to adhere directly to the underlying levator aponeurosis.

Prior to closure, the levator aponeurosis is reapproximated to tarsus with several interrupted 5-0 polygalactin 910 sutures if disinsertion (iatrogenic or involutional) has occurred. If lower eyelid laxity is noted after resecting orbicularis and seventh nerve fibers in the lateral portion of the lower eyelid, the lateral canthal tendon is plicated by passing a 4-0 polygalactin 910 suture on a half-circle needle between the tendon and the periosteum of the lateral orbital rim. In patients with marked lower eyelid

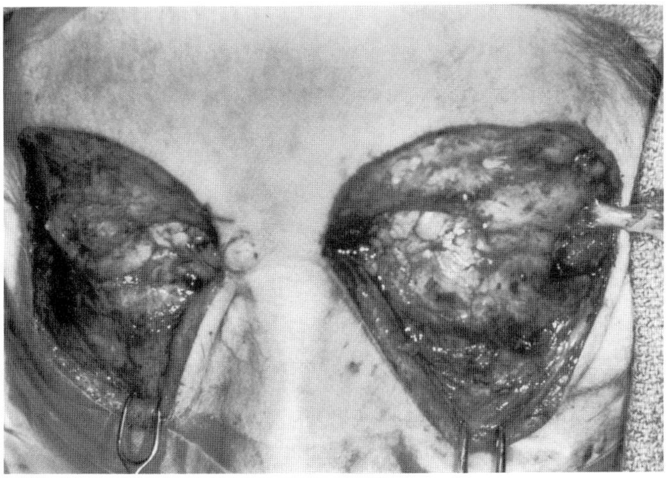

Figure 43.6. A plane was developed between skin and muscle and then between muscle and periosteum, orbital septum, and tarsus. The muscle was excised en bloc, and the brow and upper eyelid flaps were reflected downward to demonstrate subtotal orbicularis extirpation.

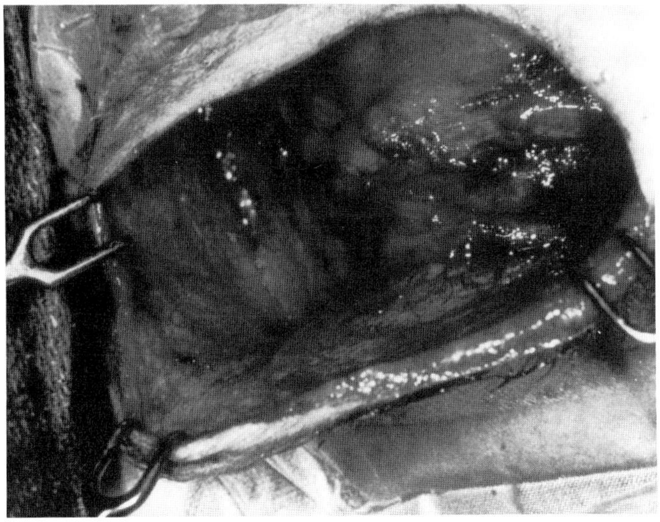

Figure 43.7. The brow and upper eyelid are reflected inferolaterally to demonstrate the temporal extent of myectomy, which includes the entire lateral raphe of the orbicularis.

spasms, the lower eyelid orbicularis fibers are extirpated at this time (see below).

Hematomas can be prevented by suction drains in the early postoperative period (Fig. 43.8). Collections of blood can prevent lid crease formation if the skin is unable to adhere to the underlying levator aponeurosis. A trocar with drain attached is passed through the brow incision and out through the skin overlying the most dependent (inferolateral) portion of the dissection plane on each side. The fenestrated tubes are placed just inside the superior orbital rim with the ends positioned medially along the nose. The drains are attached to a suction apparatus, placed on low continuous suction, and secured to the skin with 4-0 silk sutures.

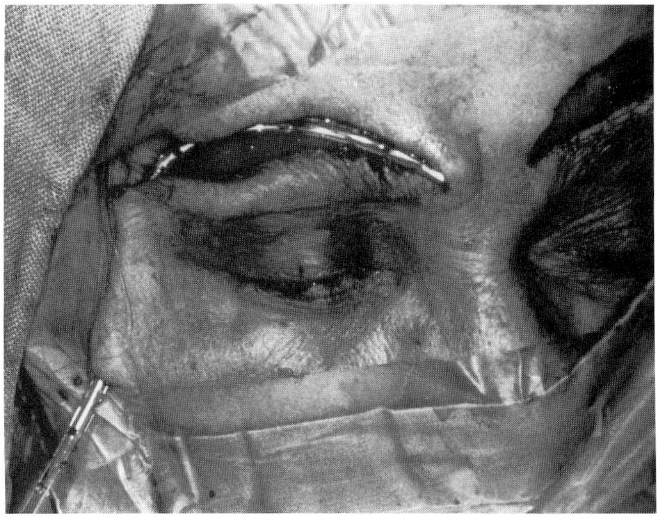

Figure 43.8. A hemovac drain has been placed by using a trochar to make a stab incision through the most inferior portion of the myectomy. The drain is trimmed and adjusted so that the superior portion lies under the supraorbital rim in the upper eyelid. It is sutured to skin with 4-0 silk sutures to prevent migration during the day of surgery, attached to low continuous suction, and removed the morning following surgery.

The brow is closed in three layers. Deep brow tissues are attached to the resected edge of the frontalis muscle with 4-0 polygalactin 910 sutures to achieve brow motility. The subcutaneous tissues and skin are then reapproximated with 5-0 chromic catgut interrupted and 6-0 nylon vertical mattress sutures, respectively. If a blepharoplasty has been performed, a running 7-0 nylon suture is used to close the incision. After antibiotic ointment is placed on both eyes and along the wounds, a moderate-pressure dressing and ice bags are used to minimize postoperative swelling.

The myectomy operation can also be performed via a bicoronal or hairline incision combined with an eyelid incision (54). We have utilized this in female patients with minimal brow ptosis but have avoided its use in patients with thin hair, male pattern baldness, or large amounts of brow ptosis. This method risks vascular compromise because the blood supply to the coronal flap comes from the area in which the myectomy is performed and the brow may not function as well as with a standard browplasty incision.

In the immediate postoperative period, superficial pain is uncommon because most sensory nerves in the operative areas have been excised. Patients with intense retrobulbar pain are seen on an emergent basis to exclude hematoma formation with increased orbital tension and decreased optic nerve perfusion. The dressings are promptly removed to assess orbital tension, visual acuity, pupillary reactions, and central retinal artery perfusion. Hematomas should be treated with suture removal, expression of the clots, and cauterization of residual bleeding points.

On the first postoperative morning, pressure dressings and drains are removed and any collections of edema or blood are gently milked out through the drainage sites. The patients are reexamined several hours later for delayed hematomas, which should be drained if present. Patients are discharged on the second morning after surgery and instructed to use artificial tears and nightly ointment for several weeks to prevent exposure keratopathy secondary to lagophthalmos.

Complete healing occurs between 3 months and 1 year after surgery. Blepharospasm patients treated with this technique average an 80–90% functional improvement after a follow-up period of 2 years (50). This level decreases to 50–80% improvement when marked lower facial movements are prominent. In general, the more extensive the lower facial squeezing, the poorer the response to any form of therapy. In patients presenting with marked squeezing of the lower eyelids or in those approximately 20% of patients with immediate or delayed functionally debilitating lower eyelid spasms after surgery on the upper eyelids, extirpation of the medial two-thirds of the lower eyelid orbicularis fibers is performed. If there is a question about whether or not the lower eyelids will require surgery and the patient lives within a reasonable distance, waiting is preferred since some patients may be less bothered with lower eyelid spasms following myectomy.

An infraciliary blepharoplasty incision is marked with gentian violet. The lower lids are injected subcutaneously with the same anesthetic solution described above, and incised with a No. 15 scalpel blade (Fig. 43.9). A plane between the muscle fibers and orbital septum is developed laterally with a Stevens scissors, and extended medially to the nose and inferiorly to the orbital rim. Care is taken not to cut the lower eyelid retractors, inferior oblique muscle, or pretarsal muscle fibers at the eyelash margin needed to avoid ectropion and tearing.

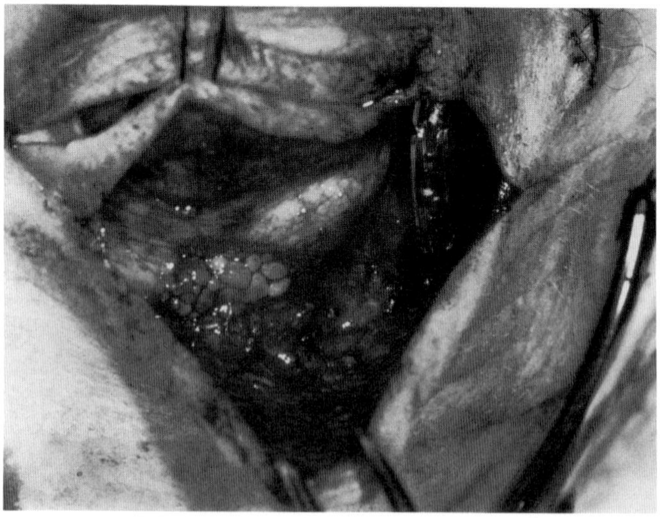

Figure 43.9. Lower lid orbicularis fibers are removed through a blepharoplasty incision. Fibers were dissected from orbital septum and fat and then from skin prior to excision. A suction drain is visible laterally.

The orbicularis fibers are separated from skin and deep tissues (as described for upper eyelids) and are excised inferiorly to the orbital rim and medially to the nose with a Stevens or Metzenbaum scissors (Fig. 43.9). The skin incision is closed with a running 7-0 nylon suture after hemostasis has been achieved. Drain placement is rarely required for lower eyelid surgery alone and postoperative care is similar to the upper eyelid procedure.

The myectomy operation is also utilized in patients with hemifacial spasm who have not responded to the neurosurgical placement of a sponge between an enlarged basilar artery and the facial nerve or who prefer myectomy to neurosurgical intervention. Because the operation is performed unilaterally, less brow elevation is planned to avoid asymmetry. A lower eyelid myectomy is performed in all cases because lid and cheek spasms are frequent. The improvement in the lower lid region appears to be much greater and more predictable than with blepharospasm. In addition, myectomy poses fewer major risks and complications than craniotomy and should be considered in more cases.

Serious postoperative complications are rarely a problem when the technique is properly performed. Postoperative hematomas should be drained to avoid necrosis of overlying tissues, secondary infection, and optic nerve damage. Supraorbital nerve damage frequently causes forehead anesthesia, which resolves within 6 months in approximately 50% of patients and in nearly all cases by 2 years. Patients frequently also note a tight forehead sensation. Transient mild superficial keratitis, which commonly results from lagophthalmos or "dry eyes," is treated with artificial tears and ointment. Excess skin removal occurred in several early cases when skin was removed from the upper eyelids. These patients required skin grafts to cure the lagophthalmos and secondary corneal irritation. This problem has not occurred since eliminating blepharoplasty from the standard procedure.

Less common complications include chronic lymphedema lasting up to 3–4 months and partial loss of brow hairs. The latter problem most likely results from direct injury to the brow hair follicles at the time of surgery or vascular ischemia. The operation can also be complicated by lateral canthal deformity from inadvertent cantholysis or unrecognized tendon laxity, and blepharoptosis secondary to inadvertent levator aponeurotic disinsertions. Both problems can be corrected by minor surgical procedures.

Patients may have residual eyelid twitching postoperatively, but true spasms with functional visual problems are rare. Because muscle does not regenerate, recurrences should not occur if the myectomy is meticulously performed. Postoperative lower facial spasms, which are only variably improved with these procedures, may respond to orphenadrine citrate or other antispasmodics.

CONCLUSION

At present, there is no cure for essential blepharospasm, Meige's syndrome, or Brueghel's syndrome. Systemic medications ameliorate the spasms in some patients, but many develop debilitating blepharospasms that render them functionally blind. The use of botulinum A toxin appears to work well for up to 2–3 months before repeat

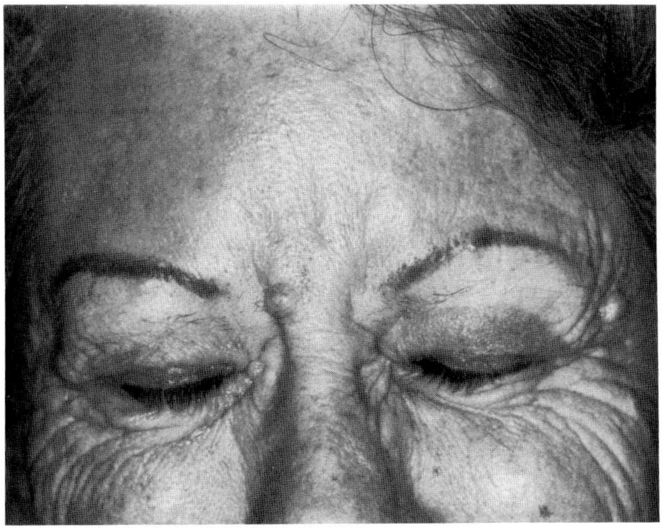

Figure 43.10. Patient with Meige's syndrome, brow ptosis, dermatochalasis, and phimosis. Note alopecia of brows and how patient has used a marker to try to make brows appear at a higher level.

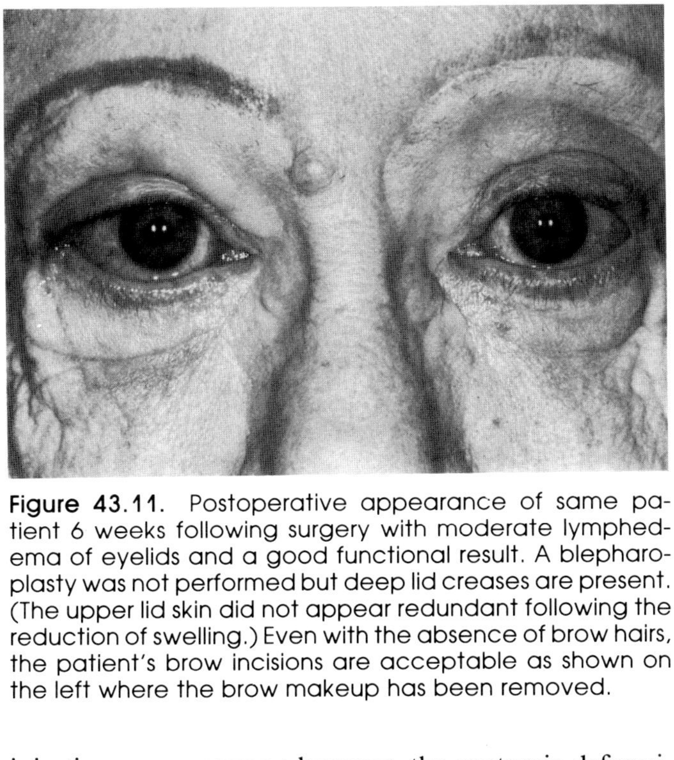

Figure 43.11. Postoperative appearance of same patient 6 weeks following surgery with moderate lymphedema of eyelids and a good functional result. A blepharoplasty was not performed but deep lid creases are present. (The upper lid skin did not appear redundant following the reduction of swelling.) Even with the absence of brow hairs, the patient's brow incisions are acceptable as shown on the left where the brow makeup has been removed.

injections are necessary; however, the anatomic deformities caused by years of spasm are left uncorrected. In patients who are willing to have repeated injections, it is a useful alternative to surgical intervention and may eliminate residual spasms following surgery.

Surgery is indicated in patients who do not respond well to systemic medications or botulinum A toxin injections. In the past, facial nerve avulsions were performed, which paralyzed the face, exacerbated preexisting brow and eyelid problems, and had a high recurrence rate. In contrast, orbicularis extirpation corrects the concomitant functional and cosmetic deformities with a lower recurrence rate, a 4.5 times less need for additional surgical procedures, and better patient acceptance [Figs. 43.10 and 43.11 (22)]. Recent advances in the diagnosis and treatment of blepharospasm have dramatically improved the lives of patients with debilitating eyelid spasms.

REFERENCES

1. McCormack LJ, Cauldwell EW, Anson BJ: The surgical anatomy of the facial nerve—With special reference to the parotid gland. *Surg Gynecol Obstet* 80: 620, 1945.
2. Gordon G: Observations upon the movements of the eyelids. *Br J Ophthalmol* 35: 339, 1951.
3. Stevens JR: Disturbances of ocular movements and blinking in schizophrenia. *J Neurol Neurosurg Psychiatr* 41: 1024, 1978.
4. Jankovic J, Ford J: Blepharospasm and orofacial-cervical dystonia: Clinical and pharmacological findings in 100 patients. *Ann Neurol* 13: 402, 1983.
5. Tolosa ES: Clinical features of Meige's disease (Idiopathic orofacial dystonial), A report of 17 cases. *Arch Neurol* 38: 147, 1981.
6. Irvine AR et al: Familial reflex blepharospasm. *Am J Ophthalmol* 65: 889, 1968.
7. Nutt BG, Hammerstad JP: Blepharospasm and oromandibular dystonia (Meige's syndrome) in sisters. *Ann Neurol* 9: 189, 1981.
8. Henderson JW: Essential blepharospasm. *Trans Am Ophthalmol Soc* 54: 453, 1956.
9. Jankovic J, Havins WE, Wilkins RB: Blinking and blepharospasm. *JAMA* 248: 3160, 1982.
10. Marsden CD: Blepharospasm-oromandibular dystonia syndrome (Brueghel's syndrome): A variant of adult-onset torsion dystonia? *J Neurol Neurosurg Psychiatr* 59: 1204, 1976.
11. Boiardi A, et al: Electrophysiological evidence for a neurohumoral dependence in the changes of the late glabellar response in man. *Eur Neurol* 13: 513, 1975.
12. Rushworth G: Observations on blink reflexes. *J Neurol Neurosurg Psychiatr* 25: 93, 1962.
13. Loeffler JD, Slatt B, Hoyt WF: Motor abnormalities of the eyelids in Parkinson's disease. *Arch Ophthalmol* 76: 178, 1966.
14. Gillum WN, Anderson RL: Blepharospasm surgery—An anatomical approach. *Arch Ophthalmol* 99: 1056, 1981.
15. Frueh BR, et al: A profile of patients with intractable blepharospasm. *Trans Am Acad Ophthalmol Otolaryngol* 81: 591, 1976.
16. Coles WH: Essential blepharospasm. *South Med J* 66: 1407, 1973.
17. Reynolds DH, Smith JL, Walsh TJ: Differential section of the facial nerve for blepharospasm. *Trans Am Acad Ophthalmol Otolarygol* 71: 656, 1967.
18. Castanares S: Blepharospasm: A new approach to treatment. *Plast Reconstr Surg* 51: 248, 1973.
19. Coles WH: Signs of essential blepharospasm. *Arch Ophthalmol* 95: 1006, 1977.
20. Fisher CM: Reflex blepharospasm. *Neurology* 13: 77, 1963.
21. Tolosa ES, Klawans HL: Meige's disease: A clincial form of facial convulsion, bilateral and medial. *Arch Neurol* 36: 635, 1979.
22. McCord CD Jr, et al: Treatment of essential blepharospasm I. Comparison of facial nerve avulsion and eyebrow-eyelid muscle stripping procedure. *Arch Ophthalmol* 102: 266, 1984.
23. Weiner WJ, Nausieda PA: Meige's syndrome during long-term dopaminergic therapy in Parkinson's disease. *Arch Neurol* 39: 451, 1982.
24. Powers JM: Decongestant-induced blepharospasm and orofacial dystonia. *JAMA* 247: 3244, 1982.
25. Jankovic J: Drug induced and other orofacial-cervical dyskinesias. *Ann Intern Med* 94: 788, 1981.
26. Metz LN, Magee KR: Postencephalytic blepharospasm. *Arch Ophthalmol* 63: 692, 1960.
27. Harrison MS: The facial tics. *J Laryngol Otol* 90: 561, 1976.
28. Goldstein JE, Cogan DG: Apraxia of lid opening. *Arch Ophthalmol* 73: 155, 1965.
29. Eckman PB, Kramer RA, Altrocchi PH: Hemifacial spasm. *Arch Neurol* 25: 81, 1971.
30. Ehni G, Woltman HW: Hemifacial spasm: A review of one-hundred and six cases. *Arch Neurol Psychiatr* 53: 205, 1945.
31. Janetta PJ, et al: Etiology and definitive microsurgical treatment of hemifacial spasm: Operative techniques and results in 47 patients. *J*

Neurosurg 47: 321, 1977.
32. Assael M: Hysterical blepharospasm. *Dis Nerv Syst* 28: 256, 1967.
33. Cavenar JO Jr, Brantley IJ, Braasch E: Blepharospasm: Organic or functional? *Psychosomatics* 19: 623, 1978.
34. Reckless JB: Hysterical blepharospasm treated by psychotherapy and conditioning procedures in a group setting. *Psychosomatics* 13: 263, 1972.
35. Sharpe R: Behaviour therapy in a case of blepharospasm. *Br J Psychiatr* 124: 603, 1974.
36. Peck DF: The use of EMG feedback in the treatment of a severe case of blepharospasm. *Biofeed Self Regul* 2: 273, 1977.
37. Roxanas MR, Thomas MR, Rapp MS: Biofeedback treatment of blepharospasm with spastic torticollis. *Can Med Assoc J* 119: 48, 1978.
38. Jankovic J: Treatment of hyperkinetic movement disorders with tetrabenazine: A double-blind crossover study. *Ann Neurol* 11: 41, 1982.
39. Weingarten CZ, Putterman AM: Management of patients with essential blepharospasm. *EENT* 55: 8, 1976.
40. Tanner CM, Glantz RH, Klawans HL: Meige disease: Acute and chronic cholinergic effects. *Neurology* 32: 783, 1982.
41. Merikangas JR, Reynolds CF III: Blepharospasm: Successful treatment with clonazepam. *Ann Neurol* 5: 401, 1979.
42. Dvorak M, Nemec J: Beitrag zur neurochirurgischen therapie des hartnackingen blepharospasmus. *Ophthalmologica* 148: 130, 1964.
43. Greenwood J Jr: The surgical treatment of hemifacial spasm. *J Neurosurg* 3: 506, 1946.
44. Battista AF: Hemifacial spasm and blepharospasm: Percutaneous fractional thermolysis of branches of facial nerve. *NY J Med* 77: 2234, 1977.
45. Fisch U, Esslen E: The surgical treatment of facial hyperkinesia. *Arch Otolaryngol* 95: 400, 1972.
46. Dortzback RK: Complications in surgery for blepharospasm. *Am J Ophthalmol* 75: 142, 1973.
47. Frueh BR et al: The effects of differential section of the seventh nerve on patients with intractable blepharospasm. *Trans Am Acad Ophthalmol Otolaryngol* 81: OP595, 1976.
48. Scott AB: Botulinum toxin treatment of eyelid disorders and of thyroid myopathy. Presented at The American Society of Ophthalmic Plastic and Reconstructive Surgery, Chicago, Illinois, November 4, 1983.
49. Frueh BR, Felt DP, Wojno TH, Musch DC: Treatment of blepharospasm with botulinum toxin. *Arch Ophthalmol* 102: 1464, 1984.
50. Anderson RL, Weinstein GS: The long-term results of myectomy for blepharospasm. Presented at The American Society of Ophthalmic Plastic and Reconstructive Surgery, Atlanta, Georgia, November, 1984.
51. Fox SA: Relief of intractable blepharospasm. *Am J Ophthalmol* 34: 1351, 1951.
52. Callahan A: Surgical correction of intractable blepharospasm. *Am J Ophthalmol* 60: 788, 1965.
53. Callahan A: Blepharospasm with resection of part of orbicularis nerve supply. *Arch Ophthalmol* 70: 508, 1963.
54. McCord CD Jr, et al: Treatment of essential blepharospasm II. A modification of exposure for the muscle stripping technique. *Arch Ophthalmol* 102: 269, 1984.

CHAPTER 44

Treatment of Involuntary Facial Spastic Disease with Botulinum Toxin

DANIEL TOWNSEND, M.D.
GARY BORODIC, M.D.

Since 1978, Scott and associates at the University of California at San Francisco have been studying the role of botulinum toxin (Oculinum) in a variety of ophthalmologic disorders (1). Initially used in the treatment of strabismus, the toxin in recent years has been under intense studies by research collaborators throughout the United States for its use in the control of involuntary movement disorders of the facial muscles such as essential blepharospasm, Meige's syndrome, hemifacial spasm, spastic entropion, facial dystonia associated with basal ganglion disease, and aberrant regeneration of the seventh nerve with a reverse Marcus-Gunn phenomenon. Further applications in the fields of ophthalmology and neuroophthalmology are currently being investigated.

PHARMACOLOGY

The toxin is produced by the Gram-positive bacteria *Clostridium botulinum*. Six antigenically distinct toxins are produced, but only toxin type A has been used in human research so far. The mechanism of action is thought to be to prevent the release of the neurotransmitter acetylcholine from the nerve terminal at the neuromuscular junction; the electrical excitability and the conductivity of acetylcholine do not appear to be affected by botulinum.

Using data extrapolated from monkey research, researchers have established the lethal dose for 50% survival of the group (LD_{50}) to be 2.0 μg for humans. The usual range needed for facial movement disorders range from 8 ng to 40 ng. The drug has also been quantitated in biologic units. One biologic unit represents the LD_{50} for a mouse. Hence, the doses used in the therapy of facial movement disorders range from 0.4–2% of the estimated LD_{50} for a human.

METHOD OF TREATMENT

The techniques used for hemifacial spasm, a unilateral problem, and benign essential blepharospasm, a bilateral disorder, are similar. The freeze-dried toxin is available from the Smith-Kettlewell Eye Research Institute in San Francisco. This toxin is reconstituted in normal saline and small nanogram doses are drawn up into syringes for therapeutic use. Prior to the injection of the Oculinum, local lid blocks using Xylocaine are usually performed. Toxin is given in approximately four to five sites in appropriately spaced subcutaneous tissues in the upper

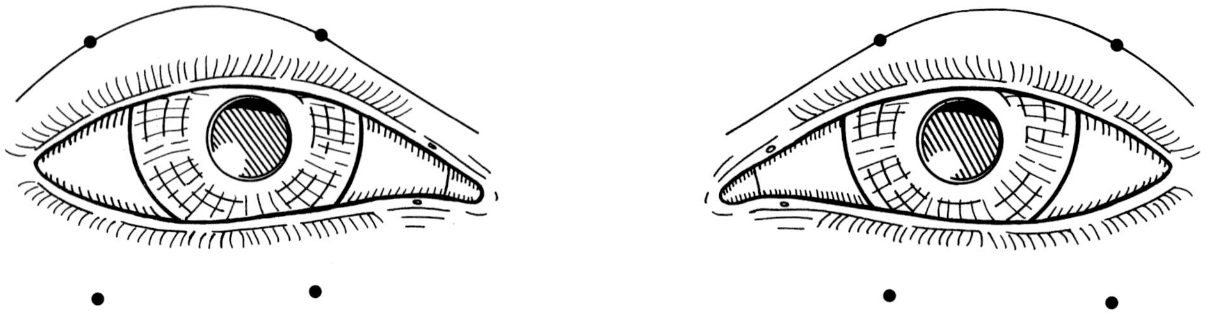

Figure 44.1. Injection points (*dots*) for toxin.

and lower eyelids. The toxin is injected on top of or into the orbicularis muscle (Fig. 44.1).

Caution must be observed when the injection is given near the levator muscle, as ptosis can result, and when the injection is given near the lower punctum, where medial ectropion with secondary epiphora can be produced. Preoperative baseline ophthalmologic examinations (including videotaping of spasms and measurements of forced eyelid closure) are often important. Other organic causes of facial spasm and blepharospasm, including bacterial induced blepharitis, chronic uveitis, "dry eye" syndrome, and contact lens intolerance must be ruled out or treated first.

RESULTS

Botulinum toxin has been used in more than 500 patients treated by 50 investigators in the United States to provide effective although transient relief of facial spasms (2). Studies have revealed that treatment will last an average of 8–12 weeks before symptoms fully return and retreatment is necessary. Initial relief has been seen within 2–4 days of treatment with the maximal effect usually noted within 7–14 days. Patients with residual blepharospasm following surgical intervention can also be effectively treated with this drug.

Frueh and coworkers (3) have shown via studies of mechanical measurements of forced lid closure that the initial force of the eyelid is reduced 10–20% after initial injections with botulinum toxin, via weakening of the orbicularis oculi muscles. Those same authors have also reported that 10 of 14 patients with benign essential blepharospasm required a second treatment with botulinum. Other investigators (4) have reported that 17 of 28 patients required two or more injections over a period of 1–2 years. The authors of this chapter have also found that 50–60% of their current research subjects have needed retreatment within 2–4 months. Most investigators have also observed that the majority of patients had gradual return of their spasms to baseline levels; this usually took several months on the average.

SIDE EFFECTS

So far, no serious sustained systemic side effects have been seen with this form of therapy. Local side effects, including ectropion, epiphora, diplopia, transient blurring of vision, ptosis, lagophthalmos, and exposure keratitis are possible. All these effects appear to be short-lived and only local therapy (i.e., topical lubricants) seem to be required. The symptoms can sometimes last from 1–6 weeks. With graduated doses given, the authors have found prolonged exposure keratitis and lagophthalmos to be quite rare. Consecutive injections appear to have no cumulative effect. Generally, according to the protocol defined by Scott (2), doses can be doubled with each retreatment. It is unknown how permanent the effects of retreatment may be or if retreatment may result in orbicularis atrophy, which may have lasting effects.

SUMMARY

Botulinum toxin injection appears to be a relatively safe albeit temporary therapy for outpatient treatment of hemifacial spasms and other forms of involuntary facial movement disorders. Patient acceptance is high and morbidity appears to be low. It provides a promising and simple alternative and adjunct to the much more extensive surgical procedures previously advocated for these forms of neuroophthalmic disease. The injections are not a cure—relief of symptoms generally last from 2 to 3 months, with approximately 70% of the patients requiring more than one injection. It can be especially effective in patients with residual spasm following surgical interventions, or it could be used as a primary mode of therapy.

Questions surrounding proper doses, number of times injections can be repeated with effectiveness, future developments of toxin antibodies, and the role of the drug in other neuromuscular diseases where local paresis is desired have not yet been answered. The long-term effectiveness of the therapy also remains to be determined.

REFERENCES

1. Scott AB: Botulinum injection of eye muscles to correct strabismus. *Trans Am Ophthalmol Soc* 79: 734–771, 1982.
2. Scott AB: Blepharospasm—treatment by botulinum toxin. Research to Prevent Blindness, Science Writers Seminar, October 1984.
3. Frueh BR, Douglas PF, Wojno TH, Musch D: Treatment of blepharospasm with botulinum toxin. *Arch Ophthalmol* 102: 1464–1469, 1984.
4. Perman KI, Baylis HI, Rosenbaum AL, Kirschen DG: The use of botulinum toxin in the treatment of benign essential blepharospasm. Presented at the American Academy of Ophthalmology Annual Meeting, Atlanta, Georgia, November 1984.

SECTION VII

TRAUMA

CHAPTER 45

Management of Eyelid Trauma

RICHARD P. CARROLL, M.D., F.A.C.S.

A systematic approach to the patient sustaining eyelid trauma involves both a general and specific evaluation. Associated systemic injuries may require consultation, and treatment of such injuries often take priority over the eyelid problem. Once serious systemic injury has been controlled, attention may be directed to evaluation of the eye, and finally to evaluation of the lids.

HISTORY

Circumstances surrounding the injury are important not only because they often influence and dictate the course of treatment but also because they may prove essential in resolving later compensation claims and medical legal disputes. Often the initial history proves to be the most accurate account; it is untainted by extraneous factors relating to financial rewards and time off work. The time and place of injury, how the trauma was sustained, whether safety glasses were worn at the time of injury, whether others were involved, the possibility of foreign-body or chemical injury, and whether the patient received any prior treatment should be recorded in every case. The patient should also be questioned with regard to previous injuries as well as preexisting conditions such as eyelid asymmetry. Preinjury photographs are invaluable in documenting preexisting abnormalities.

EVALUATION

Injury to the eyelids can be conveniently divided into *blunt* and *penetrating trauma.* If possible, visual acuity should be recorded for each eye before administering drops or treating the patient in any way. Without a pretreatment acuity, a completely unrelated vision problem such as amblyopia may later be attributed to the treatment given by an unsuspecting physician. In all cases, a thorough but careful examination of the eye should be performed. The extent of the initial examination of the globe will be tempered by associated ocular injuries. It may sometimes be prudent, as with the patient with massively swollen lids who is suspected of having a lacerated globe, to delay all or part of the examination until the patient is in the controlled atmosphere of the operating room. Timely recognition of associated injuries such as hyphema, angle recession, lens dislocation, and retinal edema or detachment will only be possible if a search for them is made routinely in every patient presenting with eyelid trauma. Preservation of vision obviously takes priority over the management of injury to the eyelids and other extraocular structures.

Once associated systemic and ocular involvement have been ruled out, repair of the eyelid can usually be carried out on an elective basis within 24 hours. Indeed it may be preferable to delay repair either because of the nature of the injury or because of practical circumstances such as the availability of experienced operating room personnel. Waiting 12–24 hours until the initial edema subsides will sometimes facilitate repair of the lacrimal drainage apparatus, while delays of several days are preferable in many orbital fractures to allow for accurate assessment of ocular motility and visual acuity. On the other hand, there is no merit in treating "dirty" wounds such as dog bites of the lid any differently than other eyelid injuries. Contrary to classic teaching on the management of contaminated wounds, these injuries can be cleaned up and repaired primarily with no greater risk of infection and considerably less risk of deformity than would be expected if the wound were allowed to heal by secondary intention (1).

Peripheral nerve function and extraocular motility should be carefully assessed in both blunt and penetrating trauma. Impaired motility or suspicion of an intraorbital foreign body should encourage obtaining appropriate radiologic studies. The Caldwell and Waters views of the orbit will be sufficient to detect most orbital fractures, but when these are equivocal, computerized tomography study is worthwhile.

PENETRATING EYELID INJURIES

A precise knowledge of eyelid and orbital anatomy is essential if one is to obtain consistently good results following repair of eyelid injuries. Anatomy may be considered in terms of superficial structures (skin, subcutaneous tissue, and orbicularis muscle), deep structures (orbital septum, fat, levator complex, and conjunctiva), lid margin, and adjacent structures. Postoperative lagophthalmos secondary to vertical shortening of the lid should come as no surprise to the surgeon who repairs a lid injury with only a vague idea of the intimate relationship between the orbital septum and the levator aponeurosis. Similarly, involvement of adjacent structures such as the lacrimal drainage apparatus and the canthal tendons must be searched for, recognized, and managed at the time of the primary repair to minimize the need for secondary reconstructions. Regardless of the individual circumstances of the injury, the surgeon must be committed to taking the time necessary to ensure the best possible primary repair.

SUPERFICIAL EYELID LACERATIONS

The management of eyelid lacerations depends on both the location and the depth of the injury. Even with relatively superficial injuries to the eyelid not involving the margin, certain general principles of surgical repair must be kept in mind (2). The wound should be thoroughly cleaned and debrided of all foreign material to avoid postoperative tatooing of the tissue, but conservative debridement of the eyelid tissue is advocated. Fortunately, the excellent vascular supply permits even completely avulsed fragments of eyelid tissue to heal well as free grafts. Surgeons often have an opportunity to instruct paramedical personnel on the management of trauma, and it is worthwhile to point out that avulsed lid tissue should be looked for at the site of the injury, kept moist, and brought with the patient to the surgeon.

The smallest-caliber suture that will accomplish the repair should be used. Less important is the surgeon's individual preference for natural versus synthetic suture material or the preference for running versus interrupted placement. Regardless of these variables, wound edges should be slightly everted once the sutures have been placed and tied. A technique for proper suture placement is illustrated in Figure 45.1. The needle is introduced approximately 1 mm from the wound edge in a vertical direction so that, once placed, the suture assumes a trapezoid configuration. This configuration encourages subcutaneous tissue to push the skin edges slightly outward, allowing for the natural flattening of the wound that occurs as wound healing proceeds over the next 6–12 months. Such suture placement will help avoid depressed scars once the wound-healing process is complete. Sutures are usually removed in 3–5 days to minimize scarring and prevent "hatch" marks.

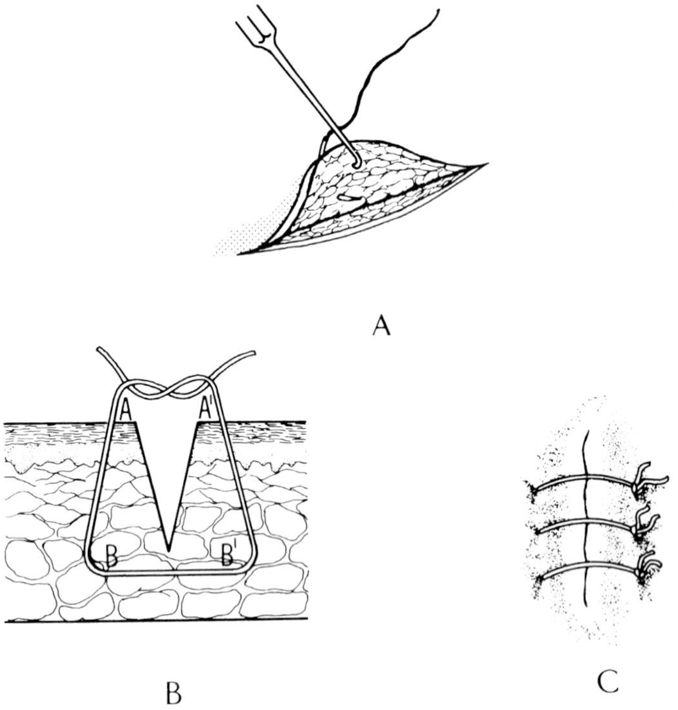

Figure 45.1. *A*, Needle is introduced approximately 1 mm from the wound edge in a vertical direction. *B*, Desired trapezoid configuration. *C*, Slightly everted wound edges after sutures have been tied.

DEEP EYELID LACERATIONS

A meticulous search for foreign bodies and an evaluation of levator muscle and the orbital septum should be carried out before repairing deeper eyelid lacerations. Because some foreign material such as glass is sometimes missed on x-ray, radiologic examination of the orbit does not eliminate the need to carefully examine the wound for foreign bodies at the time of surgery. The danger of removing intraorbital foreign bodies that are not affecting the eye must be weighed against the risk of leaving them in place. Both the nature and the size of the foreign material will influence this decision.

Posttraumatic eyelid edema often makes it difficult to clinically assess the levator function in the immediate postinjury period; this again highlights the need to be familiar with eyelid anatomy so that the levator complex can be properly evaluated during surgery. A lacerated levator aponeurosis or muscle should be isolated and carefully sutured at the time of the initial repair to reduce the possibility of secondary ptosis surgery. It is customary to observe a traumatic ptosis for 9–12 months until all spontaneous return of function has occurred. After this time, exploration of the lid is undertaken with revision and resection of scar tissue and repair of the ptosis. The patient in Figure 45.2 is an example of a patient with a complete traumatic ptosis; he had an almost complete spontaneous resolution of the ptosis 12 months following penetrating injury to the eyelid.

Should fat be noted in the wound, one can be reasonably certain that the orbital septum has been violated. This is not to say that the orbital septum must always be repaired. In fact, if one is unsure of the anatomy, suturing of the septum should probably not be done to avoid incorporating these sutures into adjacent superficial or deep lid structures that may result in postoperative vertical shortening of the lid (Fig. 45.3).

If scarring involves only the superficial structures of the eyelid, simple fusiform excision with primary closure or more complex rearrangements of tissues using single or multiple Z-plasties, W-plasties, or broken-line closures may be effective. Which of these techniques or combination of techniques will best deal with a particular scar will depend upon the relationship of the scar to the relaxed

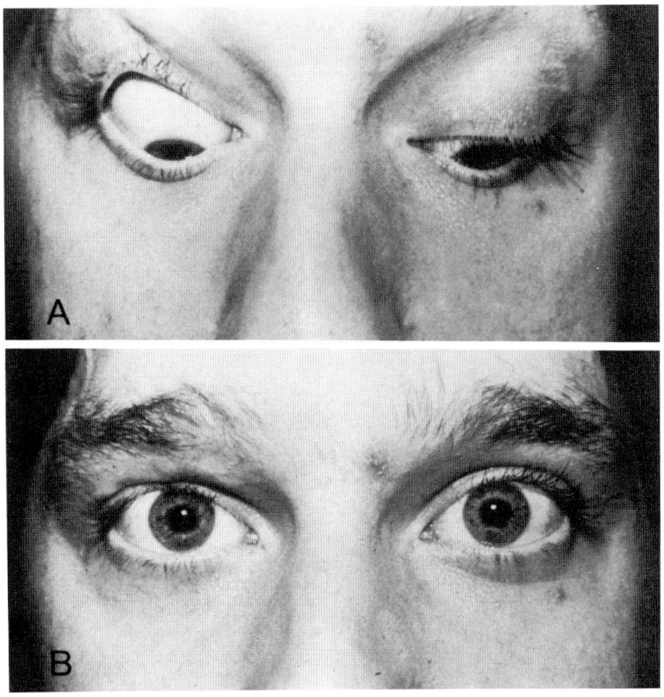

Figure 45.3. *A*, Patient with previously traumatized right upper lid in primary gaze. *B*, Patient in panel *A* showing severe lagophthalmos in downgaze due to incorporation of the orbital septum in the superficial sutures during the primary repair.

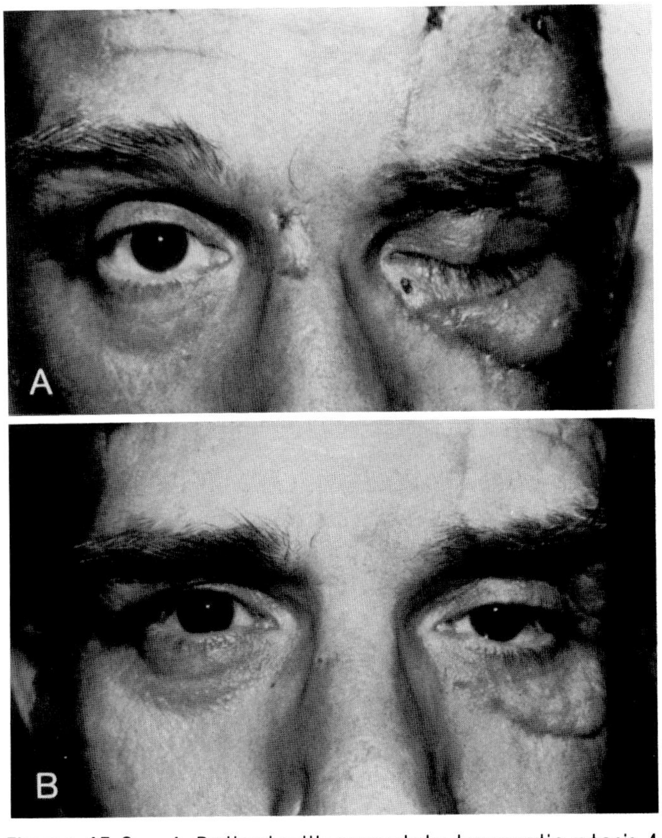

Figure 45.2. *A*, Patient with complete traumatic ptosis 1 wk after injury. *B*, Patient in panel *A* showing spontaneous resolution of complete traumatic ptosis one year after injury.

skin-tension lines that run horizontally in the eyelids and periorbital area. In general, the fusiform excision is most useful for revision of scars that closely follow the relaxed skin tension lines. The W-plasty and the broken-line closure will camouflage a variety of antitension line scars of the eyebrows and forehead. Usually single or multiple Z-plasties are preferred for all other periorbital antitension line scars.

When cicatricial changes involve the deeper structures of the eyelid, resulting in retraction or ectropion of the lid, more involved reconstructive procedures are necessary. Retraction of the upper eyelid can be satisfactorily treated with a two-step procedure involving an incision and revision of the cicatrix, which is combined with vertical lengthening of the lid using a full-thickness postauricular skin graft. Traumatic retraction of the lower eyelid usually requires a three-step procedure with the addition of a full-thickness horizontal shortening of the stretched lid to the above two steps.

EYELID MARGIN LACERATION

The success of eyelid margin repair will depend on proper suture placement and satisfactory suture tension. Historically, many methods of repair, such as halving procedures or figure-of-8 sutures, have been advocated; however, none of these methods seem to offer any advantage over direct repair of the laceration (Fig. 45.4). Postoperative notching of the eyelid margin is undesirable because of the cosmetic deformity that results and, just as importantly, because the notch may functionally impair proper tear drainage.

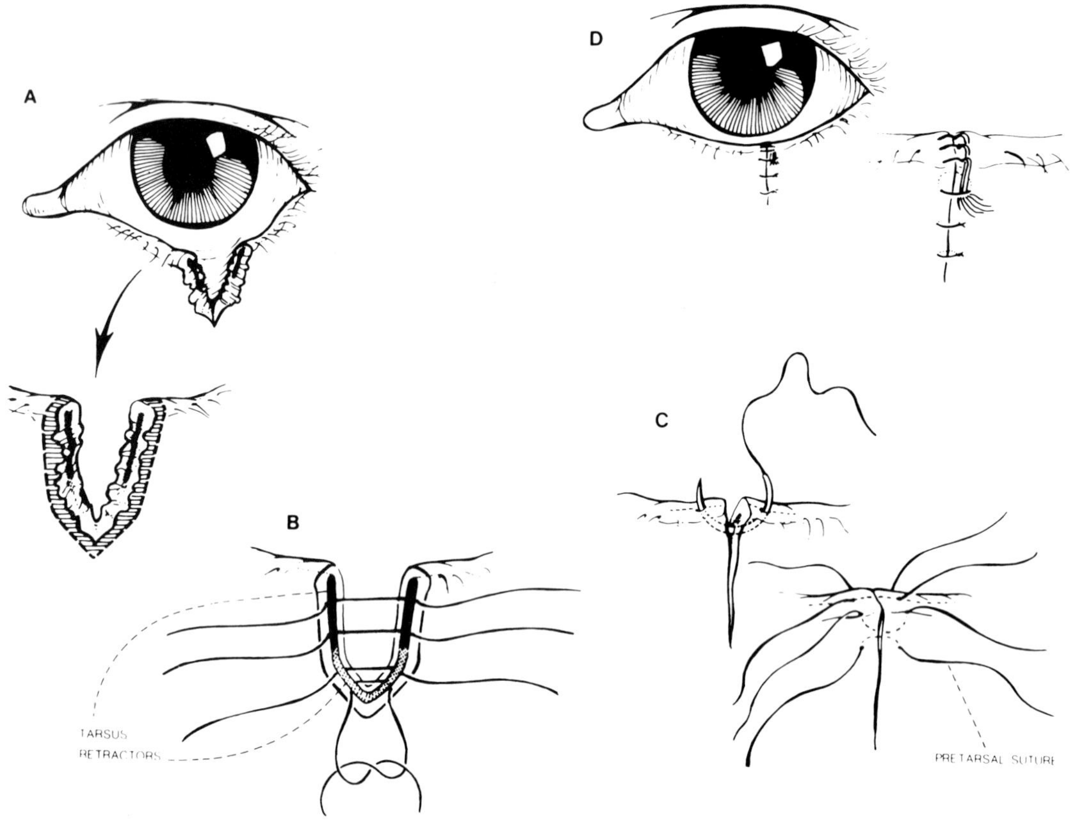

Figure 45.4. Repair of the eyelid margin. *A*, If the laceration is ragged, it is sometimes useful to create a pentagonal defect by freshening the wound edges. *B*, Absorbable sutures are used to close the cut edges of the tarsus and the lower lid retractors. Knots are tied anteriorly to avoid erosion through the conjunctiva. *C*, Nonabsorbable sutures are used to close the eyelid margin and skin edges. Three sutures are placed in the margin: one in the lash line, a second in the posterior edge of the margin, and a third in the gray line. These sutures as well as the pretarsal suture are taken into the tarsus. *D*, The three-margin sutures are tied under the pretarsal sutures to avoid corneal irritation.

If the edges of the laceration are ragged, it is sometimes preferable to freshen the edges with razor-blade fragment or one of the "supersharp" blades. Unlike the V-shaped incision advocated in the past, a pentagonal defect will ensure parallel tarsal edges for suturing and eliminate one of the iatrogenic causes of a postoperative notch. Two skin hoods are then used to pull the edges of the defect together to asess potential wound tension. Should any undue tension exist, either because of a shortage of tissue or because of edema, a cantholysis of the appropriate limb of the lateral canthal tendon of the involved eyelid is performed. Multiple interrupted absorbable sutures are then used to bring the cut edges of the tarsus and the eyelid retractors together. Special care is taken in the upper eyelid not to involve the conjunctiva in these sutures to avoid postoperative corneal abrasion and irritation.

Once the absorbable sutures are tied, the eyelid margin is sutured. Three 6-0 silk sutures are placed: one of these sutures is placed in the lash line; a second, in the posterior edges of the margin; and a third, in the gray line. These sutures are introduced 1 mm from the edges of the laceration and are placed about 1 mm into the tarsus, thereby reinforcing the absorbable sutures. The margin sutures are tied with just enough tension to slightly evert the edges of the wound. A postoperative notch can result from either tying the margin sutures too tightly or too loosely. If tied too loosely, the wound will separate and the edge will contract as healing occurs; if tied too tightly, the tissue within the suture may necrose.

The three margin sutures are left approximately ½ inch long to be tied anteriorly under the fourth skin suture placed in the pretarsal area. This suture is placed into the anterior half of the tarsus to ensure good apposition between the pretarsal orbicularis and the anterior tarsal surface. The margin sutures are secured under this pretarsal suture to keep them away from the cornea. Finally, skin suturing is completed with multiple nonabsorbable sutures through the skin and orbicularis muscle. It is helpful to have an assistant place a single-pronged skin hook in the apex of the pentagon for traction to ensure accurate placement of these interrupted sutures.

Should a portion of the full-thickness eyelid be missing, the eyelid may be reconstructed using the techniques traditionally used when reconstructing the eyelid following tumor removal. One of the most useful techniques in this regard is the Tenzel myocutaneous semicircular advancement flap that can be used to repair defects in both the upper and lower eyelids. This technique is illustrated in the chapter on congenital coloboma of the eyelid.

Few patients sustaining eyelid margin trauma in the

nasal portion of the eyelid margin escape without disruption of the lacrimal drainage apparatus. Repair or rerouting of the lacrimal drainage system should be carried out at the time of the primary repair if at all possible. Specific techniques will be discussed elsewhere, but in general, lacrimal reconstruction is usually carried out using a silicone stent around which the lacerated canaliculi are sutured.

CANTHAL ANGLE INJURIES

A three-dimensional perspective (Fig. 45.5) as well as familiarity with the configuration of the canthal angles are essential to ensure an optimum functional and cosmetic result. Tendon involvement may be diagnosed using the simple lash-traction test in which the lacerated or avulsed eyelid is grasped with a toothed forcep and pulled in a direction opposite the injury. Resistance will be absent if the tendon is involved in the injury. Precise diagnosis of canthal tendon injury will permit appropriate repair during the initial reconstruction and will often eliminate the need for complex secondary reconstruction.

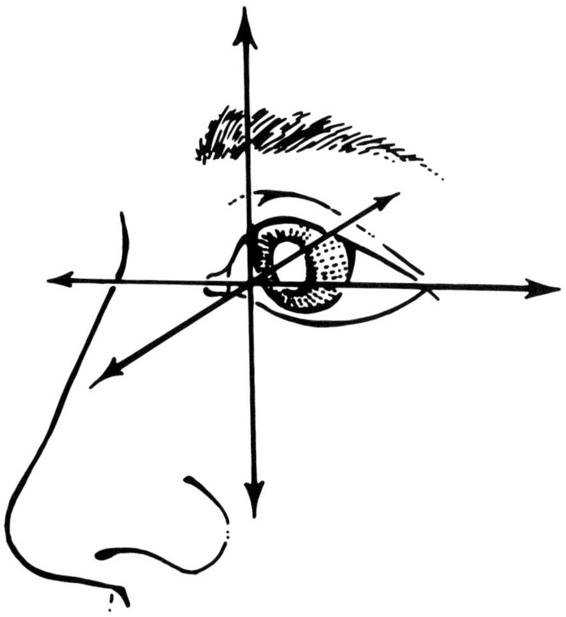

Figure 45.5. Injury may displace a medial canthus horizontally, vertically, and/or in the anterior-posterior plane. A three-dimensional perspective is useful in approaching reconstruction of this area.

The three-dimensional perspective mentioned previously emphasizes that injury may displace the canthal angle horizontally, vertically, and/or anteroposteriorly. Proper reconstruction requires careful assessment of the preoperative canthal position and its relationship to the rest of the face. Photographs of the patient taken before the injury can be most useful in this evaluation. It is also important to keep in mind that the medial canthal angle has a rounded configuration, whereas the lateral canthal angle is sharp. Failure to take these anatomical details into consideration will result in unnecessary postoperative deformity, which will have cosmetic and functional implications.

Knowledge of the anatomy of the canthal tendons (Fig. 45.6) is crucial to their proper repair. The medial canthal tendon originates from two bony prominences: the anterior lacrimal crest and the posterior lacrimal crest. While the anterior origin is broad based, it is the posterior limb of the medial canthal tendon that primarily influences the position of the medial canthal angle. It is therefore critical to determine whether or not the posterior limb of the tendon is involved in the injury. If only the anterior limb of the tendon is involved, direct suturing of the cut edges

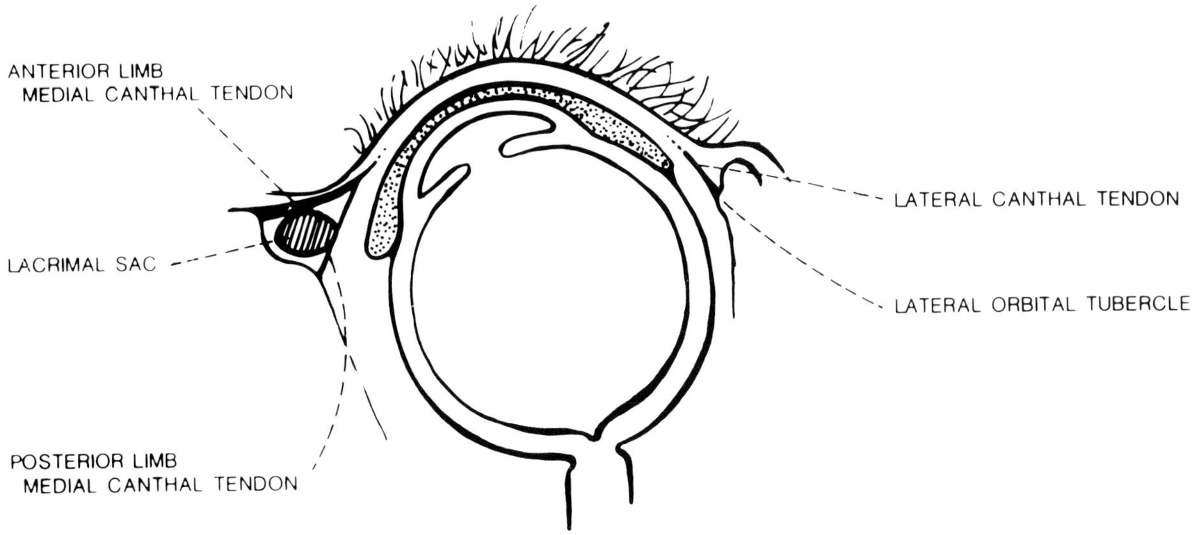

Figure 45.6. The medial canthal tendon originates from both the anterior lacrimal crest and the posterior lacrimal crest. The lateral canthal tendon originates inside the lateral orbital rim from the lateral orbital tubercle.

of the tendon is all that is required. If the posterior limb of the tendon is involved, there will be anterior displacement of the medial canthal angle, and the unsuspecting surgeon who simply reattaches the avulsed tendon to the anterior lacrimal crest will later find it necessary to deal with a deformity like the one shown in Figure 45.7.

In patients with complete avulsion of the medial canthal tendon, that is, injury to both the anterior and posterior limbs, one must determine whether or not a fracture of the nasal or lacrimal bones is also present. If there is no fracture, the avulsed tendon may be wired to the ipsilateral posterior lacrimal crest by threading a 28-gauge wire through two small burr holes placed at the posterior lacrimal crest. If a fracture is present, the fracture first must be reduced, after which a transnasal wire is used to stabilize the fracture and to maintain the correct medial canthal tendon position. The transnasal wires are placed at the posterior lacrimal crest. Depending on the extent of the injury, associated damage to the lacrimal drainage apparatus can sometimes be treated at the time of the medial canthal tendon repair. In other patients it is preferable to reconstruct the lacrimal apparatus as a secondary procedure.

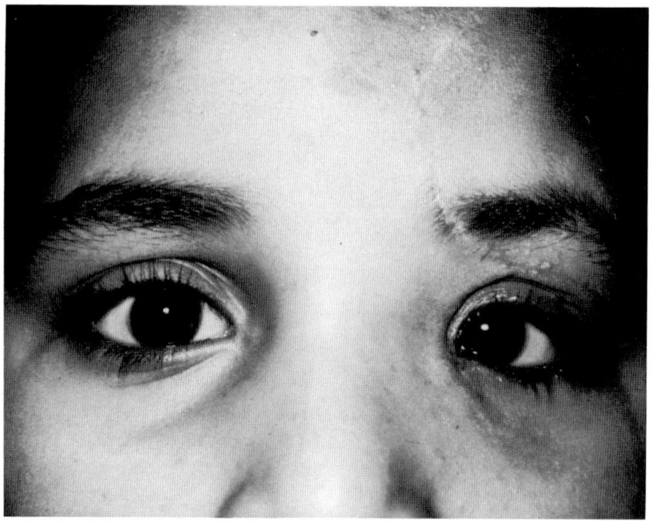

Figure 45.7. Two months following a primary repair, this patient illustrates traumatic displacement of the left medial canthus. The injured canthus is displaced laterally, inferiorly, and anteriorly.

The lateral canthal tendon originates from the orbital tubercle just inside the lateral orbital rim. The avulsed lateral canthal tendon is therefore wired inside the rim through burr holes at the tubercle.

BURNS

The management of surface injury to the lids caused by thermal or chemical burns will depend on the degree of injury. Prior to treatment of the lids, underlying ocular injury must be treated and foreign material (e.g., soot, ashes, debris, chemicals) must be meticulously removed. First- and second-degree burns will usually respond well to meticulous hygiene accompanied by wet dressings and antibiotic ointment. Third-degree burns on the other hand destroy all the epidermal elements of the lids, which gives rise to contraction manifested by cicatricial retraction or ectropion of the lids. The globe is placed at risk for ulceration and secondary infection.

Moist chambers and ocular lubricants are useful as temporizing measures to protect the eye, but aggressive surgical management is often required in severely burned eyelids. While intramarginal lateral tarsorrhaphy and medial canthoplasty may successfully offer the desired protection in mild retraction, more severe cases require vertical lengthening of the lid with full-thickness skin grafts. When available, full-thickness postauricular skin has been found to be the most satisfactory donor tissue for both upper and lower lid reconstruction in most of these patients; the supraclavicular site is an alternate choice. In the upper lid the vertical lengthening is combined with revision of the cicatrix; in the lower lid horizontal tightening of the lid is also usually necessary because of stretching of the lids by the cicatrix. In anticipation of further retraction postoperatively, more surgery than might ordinarily be done; i.e., a more extensive tarsorrhaphy or a larger graft should be carried out in these patients.

SUMMARY

The key to the responsible management of eyelid trauma is accurate diagnosis. Accurate diagnosis combined with complete familiarity with eyelid anatomy and reasonable technical skill will permit an optimum primary repair and will eliminate the need for many secondary reconstructions.

REFERENCES

1. Shannon GM: The treatment of dog bite injuries of the eyelids and adnexa. *Ophthal Surg* 6: 41–44, 1975
2. Carroll RP, Wilkins RB: General principles and basic techniques. In Stewart WB (ed): *Ophthalmic Plastic and Reconstructive Surgery. American Academy Ophthalmology Manual.* San Francisco, American Academy Ophthalmology, 1984, pp 11–31.

CHAPTER 46

Skin Wound Repair in Orbital and Periorbital Trauma

CHARLES K. BEYER-MACHULE, M.D., F.A.C.S.
AMIRAM SHAPIRO, M.D.

Skin wound repair is superseded by the priority placed on a patient's general status. These conditions include an adequate airway, control of hemorrhage, treatment of shock, evaluation and treatment of neurological problems, evaluation of the extent of other injuries, and the evaluation of ocular and lid trauma.

An early history and physical evaluation of a patient aids in the assessment of subspecialty services that may be required. A subsequent complete physical examination, x-ray, and laboratory studies provide further insight into the severity of the injury. Axial and coronal computerized tomograms aid in visualizing and localizing foreign bodies, including nonmetallic ones, as well as provide succinct information about bony alignments.

Extensive lid lacerations or avulsions often signify ocular involvement and require especially careful examinations. Undue manipulations of such tissues in an emergency room setting must be avoided, but is better reserved for scrutiny and repair in a fully equipped operating room with a stable patient. Nothing is worse than a hasty wound repair in an emergency room on an unable or uncooperative patient. Well-timed primary repairs under suitable operative conditions will avoid secondary procedures in most instances.

Full ocular and adnexal examinations include complete assessment of visual acuity, anterior segment biomicroscopy, tonometry, gonioscopy (if indicated), indirect ophthalmoscopy and visualization of the peripheral retina, diplopia testing, exophthalmometry, measurement of levator function, documentation of the degree of ptosis (if present), forced duction tests (if entrapment of extraocular muscles is suspected), and visual field testing, if suitable. Photographic documentation of all injuried patients is mandatory (1–9).

SURGICAL REPAIR

GENERAL PRINCIPLES

Primary emphasis in the ophthalmologist's approach is placed on saving the eye. Next, the lacrimal excretory continuity is established by suitable and accepted methods. A surgeon must be adaptable and master a series of different methods of canalicular realignment and intubation. Obviously, the location and severity dictate the required treatment. A versatile treatment will create better results (8). (The reader is referred to the appropriate chapters in this volume that address treatment of lacrimal injuries.)

Lacerations in the canthal region frequently create rounding of the canthal angles. The latter is brought on by the orbicularis function pulling the canthus away from its tendinous attachment. Reinsertion of the canthus is essential prior to repair of skin or lid lacerations. This is best accomplished with nonabsorbable sutures of proper caliber, e.g., 3-0 or 4-0 material.

Seemingly superficial upper lid lacerations may cover separations of the levator underneath it. The realignment of such a damaged levator muscle avoids a secondary ptosis as a complication.

Complete and thorough knowledge of the anatomy of

the tissues involved is a prerequisite towards a good repair (10, 11).

FIRST AID FOR SKIN WOUNDS

All contaminated materials and debris should be removed by sterile methods. A wound is irrigated with sterile saline. Alcoholic solutions should be avoided. Infection and scar formation are enhanced by devitalized tissues, blood clots, or foreign material. Debridement of lids is kept to obviously devitalized tissues. In general, the blood supply of lids assures a better healing potential (4, 12–17).

SUTURES IN SKIN LACERATION

As a general rule, suture materials in the orbital and periorbital areas should be fine, flexible, provide good tensile strength, be of suitable material to be easily tied to a flat knot, and should not interfere with the blood supply (18).

Synthetic absorbable sutures are used for repair of deep tissue layers of the lid and for closure of skin wounds in patients in whom suture removal may necessitate general anesthesia, e.g., children. Catgut sutures absorb in approximately 1 week. They are rigid when dry. Newer synthetic materials, e.g., Vicryl[a] or Dexon,[b] absorb after about 3 weeks. All the listed sutures are known to cause some inflammatory reaction. We favor Vicryl sutures for deep and superficial wound closure; we have experienced only minimal inflammatory reactions with the use of these sutures.

Removal of sutures should be carried out at the earliest possible time to prevent scarring secondary to fibrosis in the area of the suture repair. As lid skin heals quite rapidly, suture removal can be accomplished after 4–5 days in the area of the lids. Periorbital skin sutures should be removed after approximately 7–10 days (10, 18–20).

BASIC PRINCIPLES IN LID WOUND REPAIR

In view of the good blood supply in the lids, the danger of infection is reduced and a primary closure can be accomplished without risks (13, 17).

For purpose of reapproximation a lid may be anatomically divided into three layers: (*a*) the innermost tarsoconjunctival layer, (*b*) the intermediate muscular layer, (*c*) the superficial skin layer. The optimal goal is to repair all of the listed tissue layers or realign at least two of them (6, 12, 17, 18, 21, 22).

The only exceptions to this rule are superficial lid lacerations parallel to the lid margin, especially if these injuries lie within the area of the lid crease. These lacerations may not require suture repair if they are superficial (5, 6, 17).

If the laceration extends beyond the eyelid into the periorbital area, deep subcutaneous tissue realignment is required to avoid depressed scars and to relieve tension on skin margins and sutures. When a lid laceration reaches into the region of the eyebrow, attention is focused on the realignment of the hairy margins. An eyebrow should not be shaved in an effort to avoid potential loss of cilia of the brow (8, 23, 24).

[a] Ethicon Company, Somerville, NJ 08876.
[b] Davis and Geck, Danbury, CT 06810.

Deep upper lid trauma involves the aponeurosis of the levator muscle until proven otherwise! If the levator aponeurosis is not realigned a secondary ptosis may ensue. A cooperative patient under local anesthesia may demonstrate a dehiscence of the levator aponeurosis by being asked to look upwardly while the surgeon can inspect the movement of the levator aponeurosis. The lower border of the aponeurosis must be realigned to the anterior surface of the tarsus approximately 2–3 mm. From its upper border with three double-armed sutures. We prefer the use of 6-0 Vicryl material for this purpose (6, 12, 16, 25).

Nonabsorbable sutures such as silk, nylon, and Dacron may be applied to realign the lid skin. Silk sutures are soft, flexible, and easy to manipulate but are the most irritating among the three types of listed sutures. Nylon monofilament is a popular skin closure material, because it causes the least skin reactions. Dacron sutures are even more flexible than nylon and likewise, cause less skin reaction than silk. We favor nylon material in its monofilament variety for the ease of the removal of the material postoperatively.

If the tarsoconjunctival lid layer is severed in an injury, it must be repaired first before realigning the levator aponeurosis to the anterior tarsal tissue as described before.

In canthal lacerations, as noted before, we prefer nonabsorbable material as Prolene[a] or 28- or 30-gauge wire, which is passed through burr holes drilled into the posterior lacrimal crest for realignment. In these type of patients the nasolacrimal system must be thoroughly evaluated as many of the described lacerations involve the lacrimal excretory structures (8).

Injury to the lateral canthus only rarely causes a disfiguring problem; the lateral border of the tarsus can be reattached to the lateral palpebral raphe or to the adjacent periosteum through a tunnel made by blunt dissection with blunt curved scissors through the covering orbicularis muscle. Fixation of the lateral canthus is accomplished with either a 5-0 absorbable Vicryl or similar quality material (6, 8, 10, 21) (Fig. 46.1).

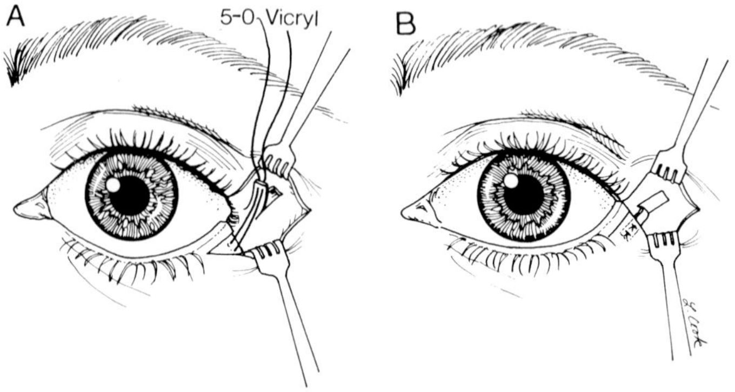

Figure 46.1. Periosteal flap. *A*, The flap is cut from the bone at the lateral orbital rim. A double-armed 5-0 Vicryl suture is passed through its upper border. *B*, Flap is sutured to the lateral upper border of the free tarsus of the involved lower lid. (From Beyer-Machule CK: *Plastic and Reconstructive Surgery of the Eyelid.* New York, Thieme-Stratton, 1983, pp 10–83.)

Whenever the lateral fixation of a canthus is imperiled by existing wound tension, a periosteal flap may be extended towards the free element of the lid in an effort to secure a good continuity of wound repair. Such a periosteal flap is prepared as a pedicle from the lateral orbital rim and is of approximately 5 mm width (6, 8, 10).

LID SKIN WOUND REPAIR WITHOUT LOSS OF TISSUE

If a laceration involves the lid margin, the first suture should be placed into the gray line from one free lid edge to the gray line of the other. For these purposes, we favor 6-0 Vicryl or an equivalent material. The arms of such a suture are left long for subsequent traction. If orbital fat protrudes into the wound, it can be easily reposited or removed; meticulous hemostasis is emphasized with this procedure. Application of electrocautery is kept to a minimum, but it affords the best suitable means of achieving such hemostasis. The next procedure is to realign the two adjoining lid marginal edges with at least one more suture, of a similar material as described before, at the lash line. Care is taken that the posterior lid marginal suture is tied into the central and anterior one to avoid its potential contact with the cornea.

Realignment of the tarsal edges can be accomplished with three interrupted 6-0 absorbable sutures of the material noted before. These sutures are deep enough for good reapproximation but do not penetrate the tarsal tissue. Conjunctiva is not included in these sutures. All buried sutures are tied with four knots, and the sutures are cut on the knots.

The repair of the muscle layer is next and this is done with the use of separate 6-0 absorbable sutures. The lid skin lacks subcutaneous tissue of any substance. Therefore, lid skin closure requires no subcutaneous sutures. It is aligned with 7-0 caliber sutures. We favor Vicryl material for the same reasons as discussed under "Sutures in Skin Lacerations."

To avoid depressions of scars, skin sutures should not include deeper tissues. There must be no tension on wound edges. Sutures are placed near the edges of the laceration to minimize formation of suture tunnels. The latter represent epithelialization tunnels along the suture lines (6, 8, 16, 18, 23) (Fig. 46.2).

Any remaining excessive skin after a continuous skin closure, a "dog ear", can be excised along dynamic skin lines for best functional and cosmetic repair.

The marginal sutures that were left long for traction purposes are fixed to the opposing firm surfaces with nonallergic tape. This traction affect everts the approximated lid margins slightly. These sutures are cut short near the lid edges in 24–48 hours. Ultimately, the everting effect will bring about the desired straight lid alignment with wound healing. It is emphasized that a straight margin at the time of the initial wound closure without traction sutures may ultimately result in an undesirable lid notch as a wound contracts and heals (17, 22, 26–29).

LID SKIN WOUND WITH LOSS OF TISSUE

As a general rule, it can be stated that a lid defect of less than 25% of the lid margin is easily reconstructed utilizing the described direct-closure technique. Lid defects encompassing 25–40% require usually a lateral cantholysis and subsequent lid realignment (1, 6, 16, 30, 31).

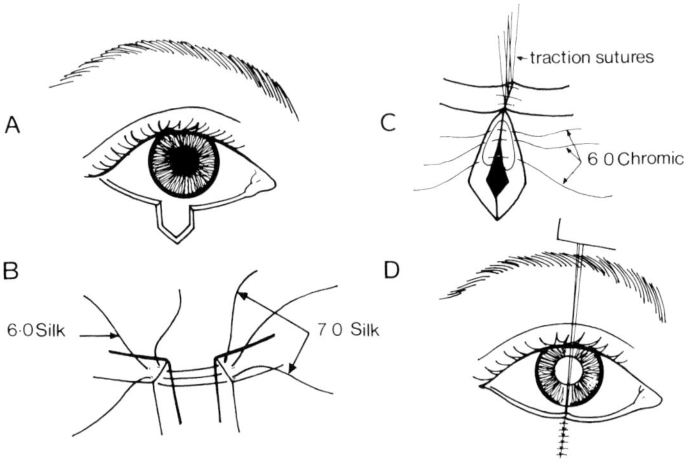

Figure 46.2. *A*, The defect is noted in the right lower lid. *B*, Three sutures are located into the lid margin, and the posterior suture is incorporated into the middle one to avoid contact with the cornea. Sutures are left long for traction; 7-0 silk or 6-0 silk or Vicryl are used. *C*, The slight everting effect of the realigned lid margin is emphasized. *D*, Skin has been sutured and the traction sutures are placed to the forehead. (From Beyer-Machule CK: *Plastic and Reconstructive Surgery of the Eyelid.* New York, Thieme-Stratton, 1983, pp 10–83.)

A lid defect between 40–75% may be reapproximated by advancement of the lateral free-lid component and with the aid of a semicircular skin flap. This lid repair technique applies to both upper and lower lids alike (6, 32).

Large lower lid defects may be reconstructed by use of the Landoldt-Hughes technique, a Mustardé rotation skin flap, or a Beyer-Bathrick tarsoconjunctival graft with advancement of a skin graft (6, 15, 33–37).

Large upper lid defects can be reestablished by the Cutler-Beard technique, a Wesley-McCord modification of the Cutler-Beard repair, or by a Mustardé repair principle. These methods require a two-staged approach and the involved eye is closed for a period of 6–12 weeks between the two surgical stages (6, 16, 33, 38, 39).

Lately we have favored the application of one or two composite grafts as a method for repair for large defects of both upper and lower lids. This method includes grafts taken from the opposite lids that are complemented with pedicle skin grafts and free skin graft to cover the defect created by the rotation of a pedicle graft (46).

REPAIR OF PERIORBITAL SKIN WOUNDS WITHOUT LOSS OF TISSUE

The periorbital skin is thicker than that of the adjacent lids and has a considerable depth of subcutaneous tissue. This difference between the structures increases with age. Like skin in most parts of the human body, periorbital skin becomes thicker. By the same token, lid skin becomes thinner with age.

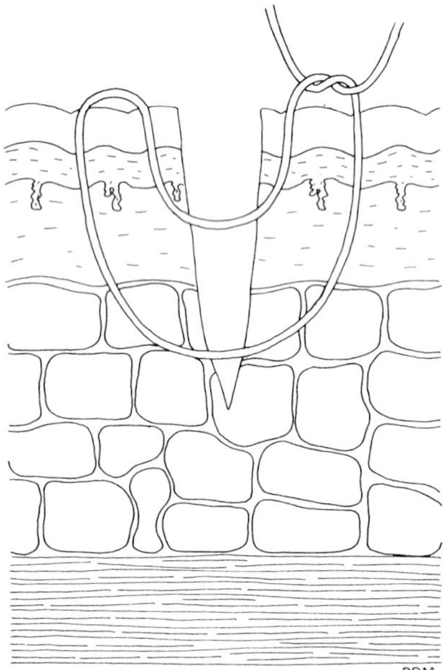

Figure 46.3. A shallow vertical mattress suture. (From Reeh MJ, Beyer CK, Shannon GM: *Practical Ophthalmic Plastic and Reconstructive Surgery*. Philadelphia, Lea & Febiger, 1976, pp 17–31.)

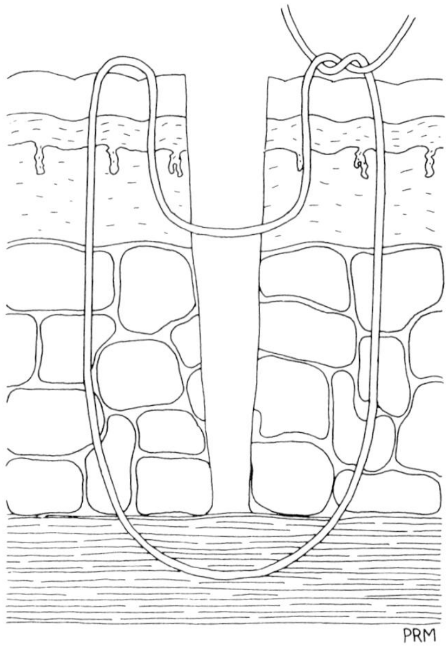

Figure 46.4. A deep vertical mattress suture. (From Reeh MJ, Beyer CK, Shannon GM: *Practical Ophthalmic Plastic and Reconstructive Surgery*. Philadelphia, Lea & Febiger, 1976, pp 17–31.)

In suturing thick skin, the surgeon must take care to avoid subcutaneous dead spaces. This can be done by subcuticular (subdermal) absorbable realigning sutures that are tied with buried knots facing inwardly. Sutures of 4-0 to 6-0 caliber are used according to the tension on the wound margins. Similar sutures are utilized to reapproximate the deeper muscle layers, if necessary. Running superficial dermal sutures can be applied in addition to the deeper interrupted ones to further reduce wound tension.

The epidermis is usually realigned with 6-0 interrupted or continuous sutures of absorbable or nonabsorbable quality, as previously advocated for lid wound repair.

Mattress sutures are useful for approximation of skin wounds with tension. Depending on the type and severity of the laceration, they may be placed more superficially or more deeply. The superficial sutures include the epidermis, dermis, and superficial cutaneous fat (Fig. 46.3). The deep sutures extend to the level of the fascia (Fig. 46.4). The near-fat/far-near suture, as described by Smith, relieves tension on the wound edges and can be easily combined with the interrupted supporting sutures (Fig. 46.5). Mattress and the near-far/far-near sutures are usually of 4-0 to 6-0 caliber. Steri-strips[c] are attached perpendicularly to the wound margin to further minimize wound tension. Moderate-pressure bandages help to reduce subcutaneous spaces and reduce edema and hematoma formation postoperatively (4, 19, 28, 41, 42).

PERIORBITAL SKIN WOUND WITH LOSS OF TISSUE

When tissue loss is minimal, skin next to the wound edges is undermined by blunt and sharp dissection with

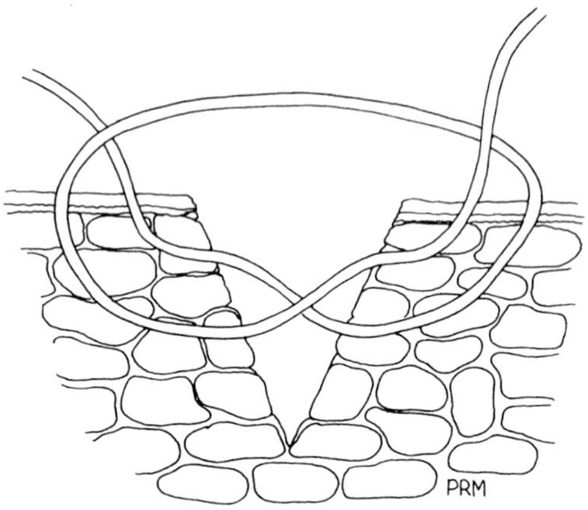

Figure 46.5. The near-far/far-near suture (Smith). (From Reeh MJ, Beyer CK, Shannon GM: *Practical Ophthalmic Plastic and Reconstructive Surgery*. Philadelphia, Thieme-Stratton, 1976, pp 17–31.)

blunt curved scissors. Residual wound tension can be overcome by deeper buried absorbable interrupted sutures or by a running subcutaneous dermal nylon suture. The superficial skin is realigned primarily with 6-0 suture. In elderly patients with more profound lid laxity, larger wound defects can be reapproximated by direct closure (21).

When a more profound tissue loss if encountered, skin or skin muscle flaps are helpful in such wound repairs. Such flaps may be of sliding, transpositional, or rotational type. In order to assure a proper blood supply to the skin flaps the length of the flap should not be more than twice the width of its base. A practical test for evaluating the circulation of the graft is to look for blanching at the distal end of a graft on applying mild digital pressure over the

[c] 3M Co., Surgical Products Division, St. Paul, MN 55144.

graft and then noting the rate of capillary-filling color within 4 seconds after removal of the pressure. A layer by layer realignment of a pedicle is advised (18, 43–47).

When a lid defect involves the skin surface only, a free skin graft can be chosen for coverage of the defect. The graft color and texture should be matched as much as possible to the recipient area. In lid defects the opposite lid provides the best donor material for a graft. For periorbital defects, skin can be obtained from the retroauricular area, the supraclavicular or infraclavicular region, or from the undersurface of an upper arm. A free graft may be of split-thickness type to include epidermis and partial dermis or of full-thickness type to a depth of the subcutaneous fat. Full-thickness grafts contract less than split-thickness ones and provide better skin color and texture. In general, however, a split-thickness skin graft has better viability. Grafts are secured to the surrounding skin with 6-0 or 7-0 silk or Vicryl suture and are subsequently covered with a Telfa[d] dressing soaked in garamycin ophthalmic solution and covered with a pressure dressing. This method provides a uniform pressure over a graft and minimizes edema and hematoma formation and soaks the graft in an antibiotic medium during its initial phase of transfer and healing. Thus, it increases its chances for survival and viability (4, 6, 17, 18, 21, 42, 46).

[d] Kendall Company Hospital Products, Boston, MA 02101.

COMPLICATIONS

A skin laceration may result in scarring and discoloration. With the passage of time, scars diminish and discolorations fade. Softening of a scar may be accelerated by gentle massage of the scar with the tip of a finger for 10 minutes two to three times a day. We advocate massage of scars with a topical hydrocortisone ointment, commencing 10 days after surgery when the fibrosis is still in an early stage. This principle may reduce or minimize some of the wound deformities of scarring. If a scar persists after 6 months, it can be removed surgically with a subsequent W-plasty or Z-plasty. Some surgeons favor performing a Z-plasty as part of the primary wound repair to reduce or divert wound tension for better cosmetic and functional effects. A Z-plasty creates triangular flaps adjacent to the incision in the skin, with the angles of the "Z" being about 60° from the main incision. The flaps are then undermined and transposed to create a "Z" out of the original straight scar or laceration (Fig. 46.6). Small irregular raised scar tissues at the border or peripheral to the lids may be removed by dermabrasion (8, 16, 23, 48–51) (Fig. 46.7–46.9).

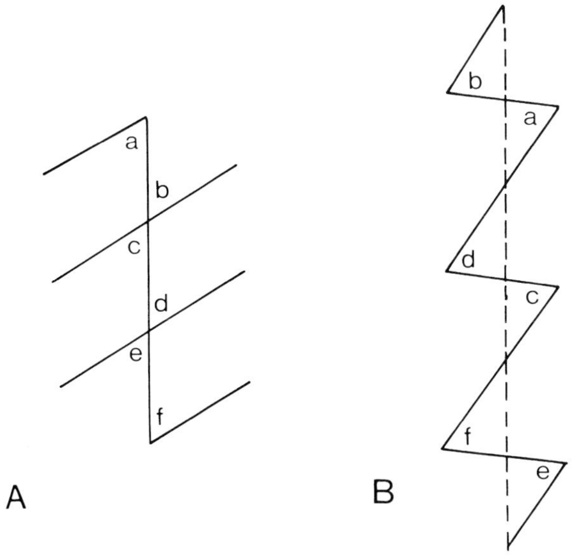

Figure 46.6. Z-plasty. *A,* The original vertical cut along the *line a–f* and the oblique parallel lines for the Z-plasties are cut. *B,* After transposing the flaps the Z-plasty is created. *Dotted line,* the line of the original scar, which has been diverted from a vertical to a Z-line. (From Beyer-Machule CK: *Plastic and Reconstructive Surgery of the Eyelid.* New York, Thieme-Stratton, 1983, pp 10–83.)

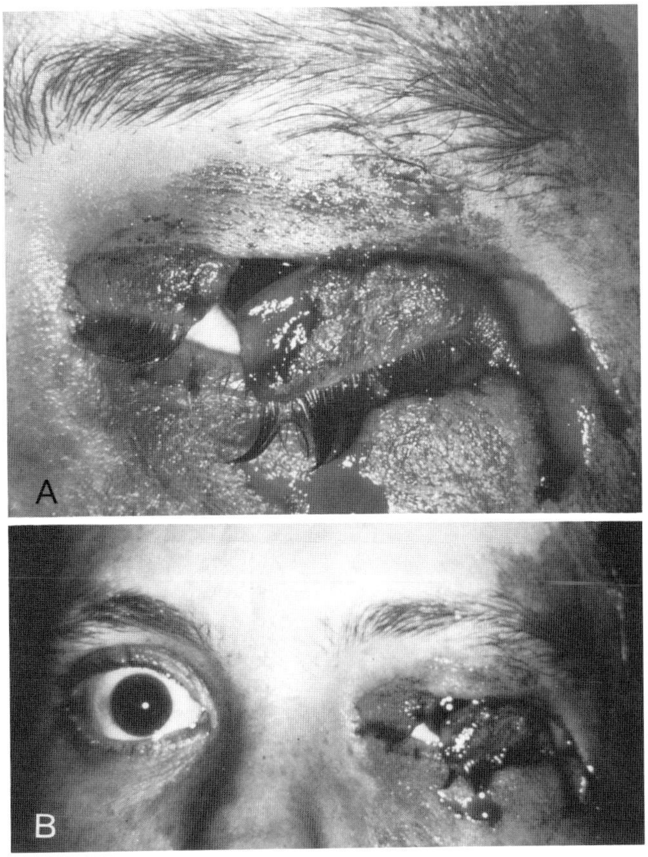

Figure 46.7. The appearance of an acute dog-bite injury involving the entire left upper lid, lateral canthus, and outer lower lid. The canthus is severed, the upper lid nearly evulsed and deep as well as superficial structures are severely injured.

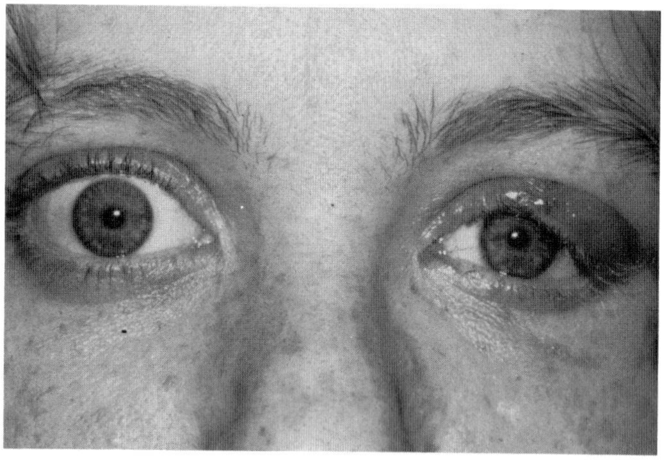

Figure 46.8. The appearance of the patient after a meticulous layer-by-layer realignment of all anatomical structures.

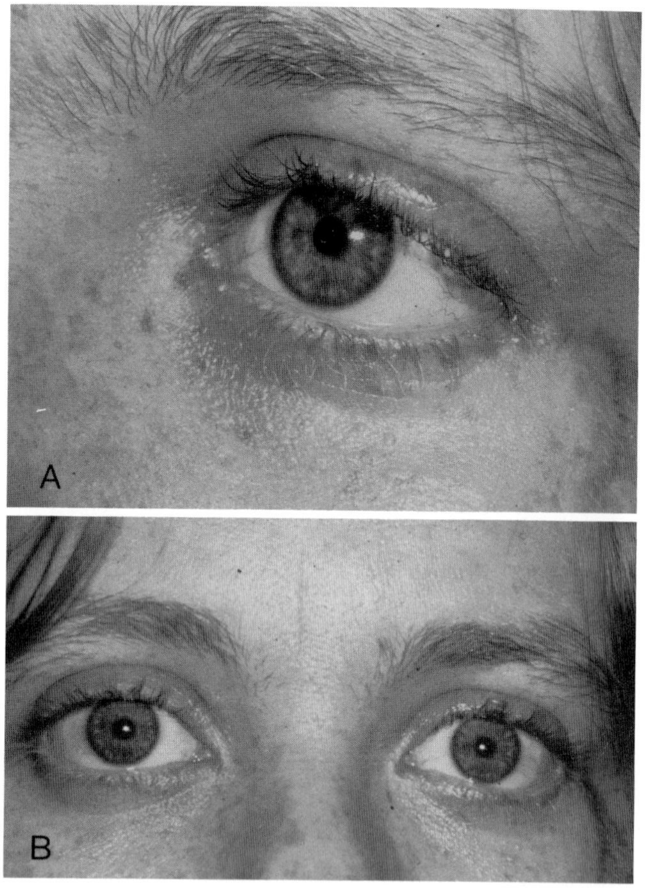

Figure 46.9. *A–C*, The appearance of the same patient 3 months after the initial repair.

SUMMARY

Orbital and periorbital skin lacerations may involve trauma to vital organ systems, mainly the ocular globe. A complete physical and ocular examination is required before any ocular or lid repair. Surgery should be performed under optimal conditions on a stable patient. The laceration is best closed by a layer-by-layer technique with emphasis on realigning anatomical structures accurately and precisely. Lid skin that is virtually devoid of subcutaneous tissue rarely requires subcutaneous sutures. The repair of lid skin lacerations includes suturing of the tarsoconjunctival layer, the realignment of the levator aponeurosis in the upper lid, reapproximation of the orbicularis muscle, and closure of the skin. Canthal tendon realignment may require placement of nonabsorbable or wire material for best functional repair. Emphasis is placed on intubation of canalicular laceration and their realignment. Applicable suture materials and methods of wound repair are listed.

REFERENCES

1. Barton Jr FE, Berry WL: Evaluation of the acutely injured orbit. In Aston SJ, Hornblass A, Meltzer MA, Rees TD (eds): *Third International Symposium on Plastic and Reconstructive Surgery of the Eye and Adnexa.* Baltimore, Williams & Wilkins, 1982, p 41.
2. Callahan MA, Callahan A: *Ophthalmic Plastic and Orbital Surgery*, Birmingham, AL, Aesculapius, 1979, pp 156–167.
3. Doucet TW, Harper D, Rogers J: Penetrating orbital foreign body with intracranial involvement. *Ann Ophthalmol* 15: 325–327, 1983.
4. Fox SA: *Ophthalmic Plastic Surgery*, ed 5. New York, Grune and Stratton, 1976, pp 82–91, 633–643.
5. Grove Jr AS: Computed tomography in the management of orbital trauma. *Ophthalmology* 89: 433–440, 1982.
6. Beyer-Machule, C. K.: Lid trauma. In C. K. Beyer-Machule and G. K. von Noorden (eds): *Atlas of Ophthalmic Surgery, Vol. 1: Lids, Orbits, Extraocular Muscles.* Thieme, Thieme-Stratton, Stuttgart, New York, 1985.
7. Mathog RH: Reconstruction of the orbit following trauma. *Otolaryngol Clin North Am* 16: 585–607, 1983.
8. Reeh MJ, Beyer CK: Mismanaged trauma. In Soll DB (ed): *Management of Complication in Ophthalmic Plastic Surgery.* Birmingham, AL, Aesculapius, 1976, pp 78–92.
9. Weisman RA, Savino PJ, Schut L, Schatz N: Computed tomography in penetrating wound of the orbit with retained foreign bodies. *Arch Otolaryngol* 109: 265–268, 1983.
10. Hughes WL: *Reconstructive Surgery of the Eyelids*, ed 2. St. Louis, CV Mosby, 1954, pp 162–170.
11. Ruedemann AD: Immediate treatment of lid lacerations. *Trans Am Ophthalmol Otolaryngol* 61: 629–630, 1957.
12. Callahan A: *Surgery of the Eye.* Springfield, IL, Charles C Thomas, 1950, pp 71–73.
13. Cole JG: Primary treatment of eyelid lacerations. In Tessier P, Callahan A, Mustardé JC, Salyer KE (eds): *Symposium on Plastic Surgery in the Orbital Region.* St. Louis, CV Mosby, 1976, vol 12, pp 39–41.

14. Gabarro P: Late management of the eyelid scars and retractions from burns and lacerations. In Troutman RL, Converse JM, Smith B (eds): *Plastic and Reconstructive Surgery of the Eye and Adnexa.* Washington, Butterworth, 1962, pp 203–207.
15. Hübner H: Zur Wiederhestellung des inneren Lidwinkels. *Klin Mbl Augenheilk* 169: 207–211, 1976.
16. Mustardé JC: *Repair and Reconstruction in the Orbital Region.* Baltimore, Williams & Wilkins, 1966, pp 2–26, 135–175.
17. Scheie HG: Lacerations of the eyelid. In Troutman RC, Converse JM, Smith B (eds.): *Plastic and Reconstructive Surgery of the Eye and Adnexa.* Washington, Butterworth, 1962, pp 208–212.
18. Reeh MJ, Beyer CK, Shannon GM: *Practical Ophthalmic and Plastic Surgery,* Philadelphia, Lea & Febiger, 1976, pp 17–31.
19. Converse JM: Introduction to plastic surgery. In Converse JM (ed): *Reconstructive Plastic Surgery,* ed 2. Philadelphia, WB Saunders, 1977, vol 1, pp 3–68.
20. Wilkins RB, Carroll RP: General principles and techniques. In *Ophthalmic Plastic Surgery.* American Academy of Ophthalmology and Otolaryngology, 1977, pp 11–13.
21. Beyer-Machule CK: *Plastic and Reconstructive Surgery of the Eyelids.* New York, Thieme-Stratton, 1983, pp 10–83.
22. Callahan A: Repair of eyelid laceration. In Smith B, Converse JM, Wood-Smith D, Obear M (eds): *Proceeding of the Second International Symposium on Plastic and Reconstructive Surgery of the Eye and Adnexa.* St. Louis, CV Mosby, 1967, pp 215–219.
23. Lipshutz H: Principles of skin and mucous membrane scar correction. In Soll DB (ed): *Management of Complications in Ophthalmic Plastic Surgery.* Birmingham, AL, 1976, pp 66–70.
24. Wang MH, Macomber WB, Elliott RA: Deformities of the eyebrow. In Converse JM (ed): *Reconstructive Plastic Surgery,* ed 2. Philadelphia, WB Saunders, 1977, vol 2, pp 956–957.
25. Hartman DC: Treatment of the late results of lid lacerations. *Trans Am Acad Ophthalmol Otolaryngol* 61: 631–634, 1957.
26. Smith B: Primary repair with loss of tissue of the eyelids. In Tessier P, Callahan A, Mustardé JC, Salyer KE (eds): *Symposium on Plastic Surgery in the Orbital Region.* St. Louis, CV Mosby, 1976, vol 12, pp 42–45.
27. Smith B: Eyelid reconstruction. In Soll DB (ed): *Management of Complications in Ophthalmic Plastic Surgery.* Birmingham, AL, Aesculapius, 1976, pp 221–223.
28. Smith B, Nesi FA: *Practical Techniques in Ophthalmic Plastic Surgery.* St. Louis, CV Mosby, 1981, pp 16–17, 43–45.
29. Wheeler JM: Halving wounds in facial plastic surgery. In *Proceedings of the Second Congress Pan-American Surgical Association.* Honolulu, Pan-Pacific Surgical Association, 1936, pp 228–1930.
30. Hughes WL: A new method for rebuilding a lower lid. *Arch Ophthalmol* 17: 1008–1017, 1937.
31. Tenzel RR: Reconstruction of the central one half of an eyelid. *Arch Ophthalmol* 93: 125–126, 1975.
32. Beyer CK, Bathrick ME: One-stage lower eyelid reconstruction. *Ophthal Surg* 13: 551–554, 1982.
33. Cutler NL, Beard C: A method for partial and total upper lid reconstruction. *Am J Ophthalmol* 39: 1–7, 1955.
34. Hübner H: KolobomverschluB mittels freiez Tarsus-Lidrandüberpflanzung. *Klin Mbl Augenheilk* 168: 677–682, 1976.
35. Hübner H: Totalersatz des Oberlides. *Klin Mbl Augenheilk* 169: 6–9, 1976.
36. McCord CD, Nunery WR: Reconstruction procedure of the lower eyelid and outer canthus. In McCord CD (ed): *Oculoplastic Surgery.* New York, Raven Press, 1982, pp 194–198.
37. Putterman AM: Viable composite grafting in eyelid reconstruction. *Am J Ophthalmol* 85: 237–241, 1978.
38. McCord CD, Wesley R: Reconstruction of the upper eyelid and medial canthus. In McCord CD (ed): *Oculoplastic Surgery.* New York, Raven Press, 1982, pp 178–180.
39. McLean JM: Plastic reconstruction of the upper lid. *Am J Ophthalmol* 24: 46–48, 1941.
40. Beyer-Machule CK, Shapiro A, Smith B: Double composite lid reconstruction. *J Ophthalmol Plast Reconstr Surg* 1:97, 1985.
41. Dingman RO, Converse JM: The clinical management of facial injuries and fractures of the facial bones. In Converse JM (ed): *Reconstructive Plastic Surgery,* ed 2. Philadelphia, WB Saunders, 1977, vol 2, pp 625–646.
42. Wilkins RB, Berris CE: Diagnosis and treatment of lacrimal drainage insufficiency. In McCord CD (ed): *Oculoplastic Surgery.* New York, Raven Press, 1982, pp 1–11.
43. Burian F: Use of tubed pedicle flap. In Troutman RC, Converse JM, Smith B (eds): *Plastic and Reconstructive Surgery of the Eye and Adnexa.* Washington, Butterworths, 1962, pp 40–41.
44. Converse JM, McCarthy JG, Braver RO, Ballantyne DL: Transplantation of skin: grafts and flaps. In Converse JM (ed): *Reconstructive Plastic Surgery,* ed 2. Philadelphia, WB Saunders, 1977, vol 1, pp 195–209.
45. Crikelaiz GF: Closure of defects by advancement and rotation flaps. In Troutman RC, Converse JM, Smith B (eds): *Plastic and Reconstructive Surgery of the Eye and Adnexa.* Washington, Butterworths, 1962, pp 37–40.
46. Iliff CE, Iliff WJ, Iliff N: *Oculoplastic Surgery.* Philadelphia, WB Saunders, 1979, pp 5–17, 329–334.
47. Smith B: Basic principles in ophthalmic plastic surgery. In DeVoe AG, Fox SA, Naquin H, Sanders TE, Smith B, Veizs ER, Wadsworth JAC (eds): *Symposium on Surgery of the Ocular Adnexa.* St. Louis, CV Mosby, 1966, pp 1–5.
48. PF Garber, D MacDonald, CK Beyer-Machule: Ophthalmic plastic and reconstructive surgery, BC Smith, RC Della Rocca, FA Nesi, RD Lisman (eds) vol 1, CV Mosby Co., St Louis, 1987.
49. Holmes EM: Closure of defects by z-plasty technique. In Troutman RC, Converse JM, Smith B (eds): *Plastic and Reconstructive Surgery of the Eye and Adnexa.* Washington, Butterworths, 1962, pp 35–37.
50. Smith B, Beard C: Abrasion treatment for skin scars; corneal tattooing. In *Ophthalmic Plastic Surgery.* American Academy of Ophthalmology and Otolaryngology, 1961, p 208.
51. Stallard HB: *Eye Surgery,* (ed 3). Baltimore, Williams & Wilkins, 1958, pp 155, 232–245.

CHAPTER 47

Chemical Injuries of the Eye

JOEL CONFINO, M.D.
JOHN F. MEAGHER, M.D.
STUART I. BROWN, M.D.

Chemical injuries to the eye present the clinician with a range from the most minor of problems, requiring little or no treatment, to the most complex ophthalmologic and oculoplastic reconstructive challenges. They can occur in a wide variety of situations, as oculotoxic chemical substances are ubiquitous in our environment. The most common occurrences are household injuries with cleaning substances containing ammonia, lye, or other strong alkalies; industrial and occupational accidents; and criminal assaults.

PATHOPHYSIOLOGY

The severity of the injury is related to the type of chemical, its concentration, and duration of contact (1). The epidermal, conjunctival, and corneal epithelium provide the main barrier to penetration. In general, acid burns are less severe as they precipitate tissue proteins upon contact, creating insoluble complexes and retarding further penetration. Studies on the penetration of acids showed that the epithelium is protective if the pH is greater than 2.5 (2). However, stronger acids may penetrate and cause severe stromal and intraocular damage.

Alkaline substances are potentially the most injurious to the eye. Alkali enters the eye through disruption of epithelial cell membranes, which allows access to deeper tissues. The hydroxyl ion reacts with tissue fats to form soaps, which is followed by a denaturation of proteins. As with acids, pH concentration, type of cation, and duration of contact determine the severity of injury (2). Grant (3) found that alkaline compounds with pH greater than 11 caused the most damage, and that lipid solubility determines the rate of penetration. Ammonium hydroxide penetrates most rapidly because of high lipid solubility; sodium hydroxide (lye) is the secondmost injurious. Calcium hydroxide (lime) generally causes more superficial injury, because of the low solubility of calcium soaps. Damage from all the alkalies is rapid, and destruction is probably complete within seconds after the exposure.

The poor buffering capacity of ocular tissue allows for rapid entry of alkali into the anterior chamber where extensive damage may occur to the iris, ciliary body, trabecular meshwork, and lens (4). Lysis of cells in the anterior chamber destroys the blood-aqueous barrier, which leads to large amounts of inflammatory and necrotic debris. This, in addition to tissue shrinkage and prostaglandin release, can cause a rise in intraocular pressure. All of the above changes occur within seconds after exposure. The aqueous pH may remain elevated for a long period of time; this activity could result in further damage of the intraocular contents (5).

CLINICAL COURSE

CLASSIFICATION

Hughes (6) provided the first classification of chemical injuries to the eye based on corneal clarity and degree of vascular compromise of surrounding conjunctiva and sclera:

1. Mild:

Erosion of corneal epithelium;
Faint haziness of cornea;
No ischemic necrosis of conjuctiva or sclera.
2. Moderately severe:
Corneal opacity blurs iris details;
Minimal ischemic necrosis of conjunctiva and sclera.
3. Very severe:
Blurring of pupillary outline;
Blanching of conjunctival and scleral vessels.

Various modifications of this system have been proposed in an attempt to define an early prognosis based on initial appearance (7–9). The key to prognosis is the degree of limbal and corneal exposure. If the limbus and cornea are partially burned, the cornea generally heals. If the limbus and cornea are totally burned, healing is prolonged and the eyes are in danger of perforation.

If the cornea and conjunctival surfaces are burned, the eyes heal and the degree of corneal opacity will depend on the length of time without epithelium function. Essential to the uninterrupted healing of the eye is the absence of symblepharon. Symblepharon results in the inability of the lid to close completely or creates a juxtalimbal mass that interrupts spread of tears over the cornea. Final healing will be delayed and the cornea will usually become densely opacified or ulcerated.

POSTTRAUMATIC COURSE

Many of the severe long-term effects of chemical injuries develop later in the clinical course. Lid and conjunctival scarring leading to ectropion, entropion, trichiasis, lagophthalmos, and symblepharon develop over the ensuing days and weeks. Two raw surfaces are required for symblepharon formation (10), and diffuse damage to bulbar and palpebral conjunctiva may lead to symblepharon formation and fornix shortening. Exposure of the globe, and/or reduction or absence of tears resulting from scarring of the lacrimal tubules, can lead to severe drying of the ocular surface.

The corneal and conjunctival epithelium will attempt to regenerate, but persistent epithelial defects will often develop, which lead to opacification, vascularization, or ulceration.

Corneal ulceration and perforation are the most dangerous long-term complications. Slow epithelial healing due to tear film insufficiency, corneal denervation, and lack of a reservoir of regenerative epithelium predispose to ulceration, probably as a result of collagenolytic enzymes. The major source of collagenase appears to be the invading polymorphonuclear leukocytes (PMNs), and the corneal epithelium is a minor contributor (11–18).

TREATMENT

Treatment of ocular chemical injuries is directed toward minimizing the initial injury, maintaining and preserving physiologic function, and restoring vision.

Intensive and immediate irrigation of the eye is the first treatment. Various solutions and methods of delivery have been used with equal effect. The nearest water source should be used to irrigate the eyes as quickly as possible for at least 30 minutes. Irrigation with saline, Ringer's solution, and other buffered solutions may also be used. Irrigation should continue until the pH of the conjunctival cul-de-sac returns to 10. This can be verified with pH paper. The fornices must be carefully inspected and cleaned of residual solid chemical material. Because the aqueous pH may be abnormal due to intraocular penetration, some studied have advocated paracentesis of the anterior chamber with the removal of 0.1–0.2 ml of aqueous and replacement by buffered solution (19–21). All the above must be questioned in the light of experimental evidence showing corneal and lens damage occurring within 10 seconds after exposure. No study has yet shown the value of irrigation, let alone anterior chamber paracentesis.

Once irrigation is completed, supportive and preventive therapy for the potential complications may be instituted. Topical antibiotic drops providing broad-spectrum coverage against secondary bacterial infection should be used until reepithelialization is complete. Cycloplegics should also be used to prevent posterior synechia early in the postburn course and later if hypopyon or hyphemia occur. Topical cycloplegics are suggested.

If the pressure is elevated, those drugs that inhibit aqueous formation, such as topical timolol maleate 0.5% or systemic carbonic anhydrase inhibitors, should be used first.

The use of corticosteroid therapy in the treatment of chemical eye injuries has been controversial. In our experience corticosteroids do not have a beneficial effect on the postinjury inflammatory response, and it may be harmful to the alkali burned cornea by potentiating collagenase activity (22, 23). They definitely do not prevent or alter the hypopyon or hyphema that can accompany chemical burns in approximately 25% of the severe burns. We feel that corticosteroids play no useful role early in the rehabilitative course, but should be used as an adjunct to conjuctival or corneal surgery if required.

Topical ascorbate therapy has been shown in animal studies to have moderate protection against corneal ulceration and perforation (24–26). The premise is based on the association of low ascorbate levels and defective collagen synthesis seen in alkali injuries. One animal study showed that if ascorbate concentration in the aqueous is maintained at a sufficient level via supplementation, then the incidence of corneal ulceration is markedly decreased (27). A clinical study evaluating the use of supplemental topical and oral ascorbate in humans is currently being conducted.

Failure to reepithelialize may be due to several factors: Extensive damage to corneal, limbal, and conjunctival epithelium may lead to chronic, slowly healing epithelial defects due to alteration in the basement membrane and conjunctival metabolism. Scarring of the lids and conjunctiva may lead to symblepharon, ectropion, and exposure due to improper lid closure. Trichiasis may further aggravate the corneal epithelium, and loss of conjunctival goblet cells and lid abnormalities may lead to instability of the tear film.

The first and foremost goal of therapy is to promote reepithelialization. To promote epithelial healing, the surgeon's initial treatment is to close the lids by patching. Once the conjunctival swelling is reduced, a bandage soft lens may be applied. The progress of reepithelialization must be carefully monitored since our experience is that the major cause for the failure of epithelialization (which leads to ulceration) is lagophthalmos caused by symblepharon. If symblepharon is determined to be the cause of a halt in the progress of epithelialization, reconstructive conjunctival surgery should be immediate (28). We prefer using flaps of conjunctiva instituted adjacent to the symblepharon for the initial treatment. This is possible if the conjunctiva is epithelialized. Important to the success of this approach is the separation of the subconjunctival inflamed connective tissue from the surface layer, which prevents postoperative shrinkage.

Additionally, it is essential to recess the flap from the limbus, which in effect reduces the amount of conjunctival mucous epithelium needed to interrupt the lid from the globe. Finally, it is not necessary to have both the scleral and lid surface covered; i.e., covering the sclera is sufficient. This will prevent the lid from adhering to the globe, and in time the lid will be surfaced with epithelium.

Swelling of the crystalline lens and obliteration of the anterior chamber may occur; this must be treated by lens extraction regardless of the stage of healing of the surface.

Various substances, based on in vitro and animal studies, have been used in the attempt to inhibit collagenase-mediated corneal ulceration (29–34). Disodium EDTA, calcium EDTA, L-cysteine, penicillamine, and acetylcysteine have been shown experimentally to inhibit collagenase activity by chelation of calcium required for enzyme activity and by reduction of disulfide bonds. They have been very effective in preventing perforation of the alkali burned rabbit cornea. Efficacy in humans has been difficult to prove; L-cysteine has demonstrated a positive effect (30–34). Recently, citrate has been shown to decrease the risk of ulceration in severe experimental alkali burns (35). The mechanism of action is thought to be inhibition of PMN-related collagenase activity through calcium chelation. Topical medroxyprogesterone has also been shown experimentally to lessen collagenase activity via inhibition of enzyme synthesis (36, 37). We have found in our treatment of human burns that collagenase inhibitors are only rarely needed if the above approach to therapy is carried out. We only use inhibitors if epithelialization halts despite good lid approximation.

CORNEAL TRANSPLANTATION

Rehabilitative surgery in the alkali-burned vascularized cornea, with abnormal conjunctiva and lid function, is problematic. Marked tear reduction is a contraindication to corneal transplant. In most cases surgery involves, in addition to a penetrating keratoplasty, lid and fornix reconstruction, cataract extraction and excision of fibrous tissue from the anterior chamber, and glaucoma surgery. However, with meticulous surgery and proper follow-up, a successful result can be obtained in many cases (28, 38–40).

The donor cornea must be carefully selected. The epithelium should be intact, and care must be taken during transplantation not to disrupt it. Alkali-burned eyes have abnormal epithelium that will only slowly heal over a stromal defect, if at all; this leads to stromal opacification and an optically unsuccessful result. Healthy donor epithelium is needed to recover the surface.

The procedure begins with a conjunctivoplasty and lid repair, to remove the conjunctival overgrowth, repair shortened fornices, and correct symblepharon. Inadequate lid closure may lead to graft failure due to exposure and epithelial erosions and must be corrected at or before the time of keratoplasty. A horizontal incision is made through the conjunctival overgrowth, which is then undermined and, using scissors, dissected free of the subconjunctival tissue over the sclera. Bleeding is usually extensive and must be controlled with cautery to facilitate proper dissection. The subconjunctival tissue is then mobilized, freed fro the sclera, and excised en bloc. The conjunctiva is then recessed, which leaves a smooth corneal and scleral surface. Next the fornices must be reestablished and deepened to allow for proper lid closure. When symblepharon is present, the lids are cut free from the globe and the conjunctiva is cut into flaps and mobilized to cover raw sclera areas where the lids are not lined by conjunctiva, particularly in the fornix. The flaps must be positioned so that at least one side of all opposing surfaces is lined with conjuctiva. The conjunctiva is then sutured to the sclera with 7-0 silk mattress sutures to help maintain its new configuration. If additional tissue is needed, conjunctiva from the other eye, if available, or mucous membrane grafts may be used. The superotemporal conjunctiva should be avoided so as not to interfere with the lacrimal gland ductules. In most cases, recession and rearrangement of the conjunctiva in itself is sufficient for reestablishing the fornices. A trephine is then used to excise the donor button from the donor cornea.

The host cornea is then partially incised with a trephine. A razor-blade knife is then used to deepen the incision to the level of the Descemets-retrocorneal membrane complex. The host cornea is then removed, and the retrocorneal membrane is gently freed from the iris and excised with a knife and spatula. The dissection is carried peripherally into the angle that is opened with a spatula or blunt scissors. If the membrane cannot be freed from the iris then the iris-membrane structure must be excised. Cataract extraction is then performed if necessary. If the vitreous face is broken, an anterior vitrectomy is performed until the iris plane is free of vitreous. The graft is then placed over the host bed and sutured in place, and care is given to avoid inflicting trauma to the epithelial surface.

The most important postoperative management problem relates to the maintenance of the donor epithelium on the graft and the progressive resurfacing of the *host* cornea with donor epithelium. The eye is kept patched until reepithelialization is complete. Fluorescein is used to stain the cornea and scleral surface to aid detection of defect. If patching is not sufficient, a bandage soft contact lens is used to protect the corneal epithelium. The fit must be carefully assessed so that the lens is neither too loose and irritating to the epithelium, nor too tight.

If the fit becomes inadequate, or erosions reoccur, the lens must be changed. Meticulous management of reepithelialization cannot be overemphasized, as failure can cause an otherwise successful graft to opacify. If epithelialization fails, the graft will melt and may fail.

Presently, the authors' experience with corneal transplantation indicates that approximately two-thirds of the grafts remain transparent. However, in order to have long-term success, the patient must be under direct observation for the first 6 months.

REFERENCES

1. Hughes WF, Jr: Alkali burns of the eye: I. Review of the literature and summary of present knowledge. *Arch Ophthalmol* 35: 423–449, 1946.
2. Lemp MA: Cornea and sclera. *Arch Ophthalmol* 92: 158–170, 1974.
3. Grant WM: *Toxicology of the Eye*, (ed 2). Springfield, IL, Thomas, pp 88–101.
4. Pfister RR: Chemical injuries of the eye. *Ophthalmology* 90: 1246–1253, 1983.
5. Paterson CA, Pfister RR, Levinson RA: Aqueous humor pH changes after experimental alkali burns. *Am J Ophthalmol* 79: 414–419, 1975.
6. Hughes WF, Jr: Alkali burns of the eye. II. Clinical and pathologic course. *Arch Ophthalmol* 36: 189–214, 1946.
7. Ballen PH: Treatment of chemical burns of the eye. *Eye Ear Nose Throat Mon* 43: 57–60, 1964.
8. Roper-Hall T: Thermal and chemical burns. *Trans Ophthalmol Soc UK* 85: 631–653, 1965.
9. Pfister RR: Chemical corneal burns. *Int Ophthalmol Clin* 24: 157–167, Summer, 1984.
10. Kaufman HE, Thomas EL: Prevention and treatment of symblepharon. *Am J Ophthalmol* 88: 419–423, 1979.
11. Brown SI, Weller CA, Wasserman HE: Collagenolytic activity of alkali-burned corneas. *Arch Ophthalmol* 81: 370–373, 1969.
12. Brown WI, Weller CA, Akiya S: The pathogenesis of ulcers of the alkali-burned cornea. *Arch Ophthalmol* 83: 205–208, 1970.
13. Gnadinger MD, Itoi M, Slansky JJ, Dohlman CH: The role of collagenase in the alkali-burned cornea. *Am J Ophthalmol* 68: 478–483, 1969.
14. Brown SI, Wasserman HE, Dunn MW: Alkali burns of the cornea. *Arch Ophthalmol* 82: 91–94, 1969.
15. Brown SI, Weller CA: The pathogenesis and treatment of collagenase-induced diseases of the cornea. *Trans Am Acad Ophthalmol Otolaryngol* 74: 375–383, 1970.
16. Brown SI, Weller CA: The cell origin of collagenase in the normal and wounded cornea. *Arch Ophthalmol* 83: 74–77, 1970.
17. Pfister RR, McCulley JP, Friend J, Dohlman CH: Collagenase activity intact corneal epithelium in peripheral alkali burns. *Arch Ophthalmol* 308–313, 1971.
18. Kenyon KR, Berman M, Rose J, Gage J: Prevention of stromal ulceration in the alkali-burned cornea by glued on contact lens: evidence for the role of polymorphonuclear leukocytes in collagen degradation. *Invest Ophthalmol Vis Sci* 18: 570–587, 1979.
19. Bennett TO, Peyman GA, Rutgard J: Intracameral phosphate buffer in alkali burns. *Can J Ophthalmol* 13: 93–95, 1978.
20. Paterson CA, Pfister RR, Levinson RA: Aqueous humor pH changes after experimental alkali burns. *Am J Ophthalmol* 79: 414–419, 1975.
21. Grant WM: Experimental investigation of paracentesis in the treatment of ammonia burns. *Arch Ophthalmol* 44: 399–404, 1950.
22. Brown SI, Weller CA, Vidreh AM: Effect of corticosteroids on corneal collagenase of rabbits. *Am J Ophthalmol* 70: 744–747, 1970.
23. Donshik PC, Berman MB, Dohlman CH, Gage J, Rose J: Effect of topical steroids on ulceration in alkali-burned corneas. *Arch Ophthalmol* 96: 2117–2120, 1977.
24. Levinson RA, Paterson CA, Pfister RR: Ascorbic acid prevents corneal ulceration and perforation following experimental alkali burns. *Invest Ophthalmol* 15: 986–993, 1976.
25. Pfister RR, Paterson CA: Additional clinical and morphological observations on the favorable effect of ascorbate in experimental ocular alkali burns. *Invest Ophthalmol Vis Sci* 16: 478–487, 1977.
26. Pfister RR, Paterson CA, Hayes SA: Topical ascorbate decreases the incidence of corneal ulceration after experimental alkali burns. *Invest Ophthalmol Vis Sci* 17: 1019–1024, 1978.
27. Pfister RR, Paterson CA, Spiers JW, Hayes SA: The efficiency of ascorbate treatment after severe experimental alkali burns depends on the route of administration. *Invest Ophthalmol Vis Sci* 19: 1525–1529, 1982.
28. Brown SI: Transplantation of the severely alkali-burned cornea. In Shimizo K, Oosterhuis JA (eds): *XXIII Concilium Ophthalmologicum, Kyoto, Japan, 1978.* Amsterdam-Oxford, Excerpta Medica, 1979, vol 1 p 285–286.
29. Brown SI, Akiya S, Weller CA: Prevention of the ulcers of the alkali-burned cornea. *Arch Ophthalmol* 82: 95–97, 1969.
30. Brown SI, Weller CA: Collagenase inhibitors in prevention of ulcers of alkali-burned corneas. *Arch Ophthalmol* 83: 352–353, 1970.
31. Brown SI, Hook CW: Treatment of corneal destruction with collagenase inhibitors. *Trans Am Acad Ophthalmol Otolaryngol* 75: 1199–1207, 1971.
32. Brown SI, Tragakis MP, Pearce DB: Treatment of the alkali-burned cornea. *Am J Ophthalmol* 74: 316–320, 1972.
33. Slansky HH, Berman MB, Dohlman CH, Rose J: Cysteine and acetylcysteine in the prevention of corneal ulceration. *Am Ophthalmol* 2: 488–491, 1970.
34. Francois J, Cambie Feher J, Vanden Eeckhout E: Collagenase inhibitors (penicillamine). *Am Ophthalmol* 5: 391–408, 1973.
35. Pfister RR, Nicolari ML, Paterson CA: Sodium citrate reduces the incidence of corneal ulcerations and perforation in extreme alkali-burned eyes, acetylcysteine and ascorbate have no favorable effect. *Invest Ophthalmol Vis Sci* 21: 486–490, 1980.
36. Newsome DA, Gross J: Prevention by medroxyprogesterone of perforation in the alkali-burned rabbit cornea: inhibition of collagerolytic activity. *Invest Ophthalmol Vis Sci* 16: 21–31, 1977.
37. Lass JH, Campbell RC, Rose J, Foster CS, Dohlman CH: Medroxyprogesterone in corneal ulceration; its effects after alkali burns in rabbits. *Arch Ophthalmol* 99: 673–676, 1981.
38. Brown SI, Tragakis MD, Pearce DB: Corneal transplantation for severe alkali burns. *Trans Am Acad Ophthalmol Otolaryngol* 76: 1266–1274, 1972.
39. Brown SI, Bloomfield SE, Pearce DB: A follow-up report on transplantation of the alkali-burned cornea. *Am J Ophthalmol* 77: 538–542, 1974.
40. Brown SI: Techniques and problems associated with transplantation of the alkali-burned cornea. *Ophthalmol Dig* August, 1974, pp 27–32.

CHAPTER 48

Microsurgical Repair of Lacrimal Canaliculus in Medial Canthal Trauma

CHRISTINE L. ZOLLI, M.D., F.A.C.S.

Trauma to the soft tissues of the face resulting in eyelid avulsions and in the severance of the lacrimal canaliculi is not rare. It is especially common in children (1) (e.g., from dog bites, bike falls, sticks) and in young adults (e.g., from fistfights, sport activities). In a survey of eye trauma admissions to Wills Eye Hospital over a 3-year period (1980–1982), 84 cases of canalicular lacerations were reviewed (2). Five of these involved avulsion of both the upper and lower canaliculi. In this survey, eyelid avulsion was second only to hyphema in requiring hospitalization and ahead of ruptured globe, other facial lacerations involving the orbit, fractures, intraocular or orbital foreign body, commotio retinae, vitreous hemorrhage, and possible neurologic injury. The largest group of injured canaliculi was in young adults between the ages of 10 and 40. Forty-seven cases were in this group, or 56% of all canalicular lacerations. The next largest group was children under 10 years old (23 cases, or 28%), and in half of these (46%), the cause of injury was a dog bite. Only 14 cases (16%) occurred in people over 40, with even distribution among the decades.

Three types of avulsion patterns are seen clinically: (*a*) the abrupt canalicular, (*b*) the abrupt total disinsertion of the eyelid from the medial canthal plane, and (*c*) the biplane avulsion. The midcanalicular laceration is usually caused by sharp objects, fingernails, or glass (Fig. 48.1). Total eyelid disinsertion occurs infrequently because large forces are required to produce it (Figs. 48.2–48.5).

The biplane avulsion is the most common (Fig. 48.6). It may present as a small cut on the skin, yet an extensive canalicular laceration is found internally, in a posterior and medial direction. In this biplane type of avulsion, the skin-orbicularis tear is more lateral to where the canaliculus and the posterior crus of the medial canthal tendon are severed. The latter tissues are torn under the anteromedial aspect of the caruncle, about 2 mm in front of the junction with the lacrimal sac.

Traumatic medial canthal eyelid avulsions, because of the complex anatomy, form, and function of the medial canthal area, require special care and meticulousness in their surgical repair. The laterally retracted eyelid has to be reattached very accurately to the severed portion of the medial canthus, to reconstruct the lacrimal drainage system and to restore the proper angle of the lid to prevent epiphora and midfacial disfigurement, which is readily noticeable. A definitive repair at the time of the primary procedure will reduce the need for additional surgeries.

Precise microsurgical repair of the canaliculus is the mainstay of a good medial canthal avulsion repair. Once the tissues surrounding the canaliculus are brought together, the eyelid is automatically brought to its original angle and assumes its preinjury contour. Reuniting the canaliculus means reuniting the posteriorly directed lid tissues (Horner's muscle and the posterior crus of the medial canthal tendon), and that reestablishes the correct tissue relationships and makes the remainder of the repair a straightforward plastic surgery.

Routine use of the operating microscope is advocated for all lacrimal canalicular surgery. A standard ophthalmic objective lens (Zeiss f-175, Weck f-150) gives a good

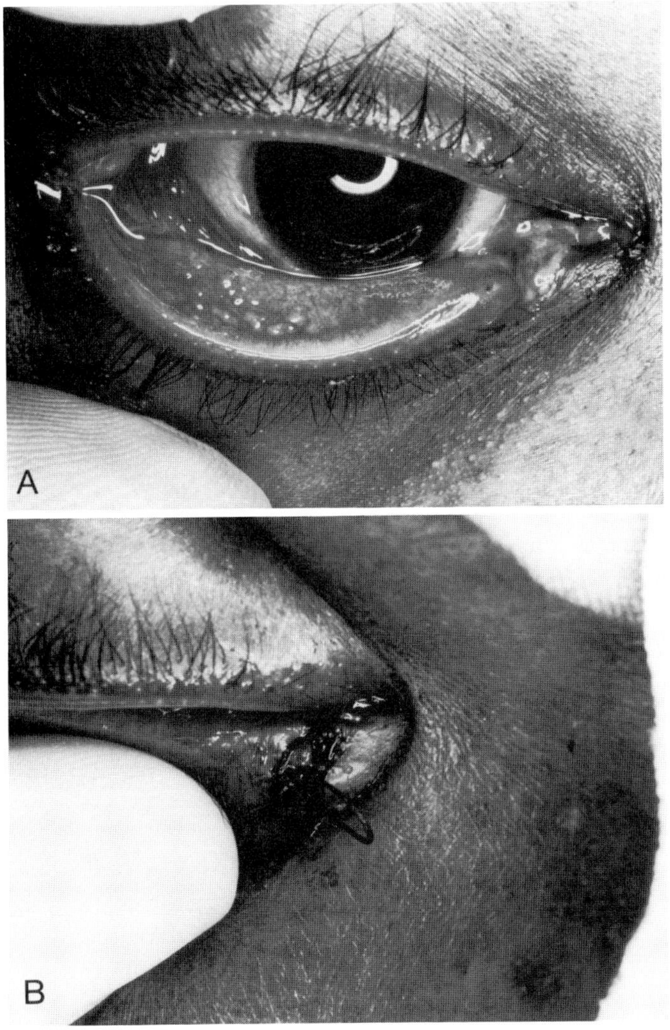

Figure 48.1. Midcanalicular eyelid laceration before (*A*) and after (*B*) repair. Veirs rod was employed as a stent.

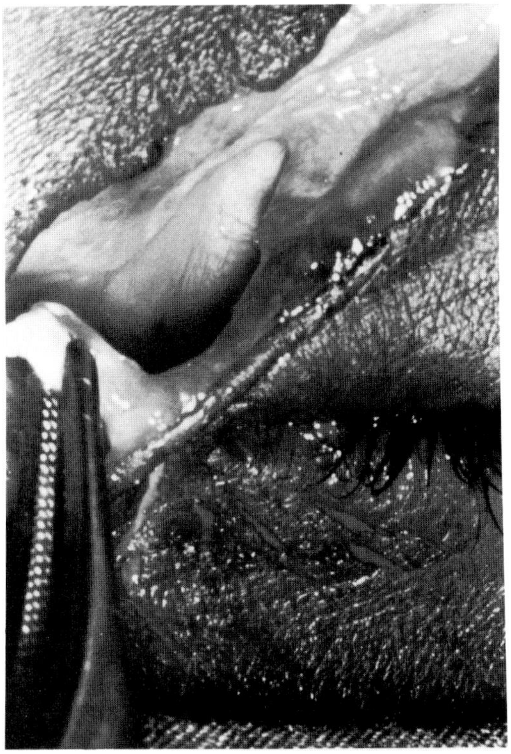

Figure 48.2. Total avulsion of eyelids from medial canthus with avulsion of medial canthal tendon. Patient hit her face against the corner of a piece of furniture.

working range. It provides magnification and the excellent necessary illumination to locate the harder-to-find medial cut end of the canaliculus. With it, the use of pigtail probes (3) and other devices put through the fellow canaliculus is usually unnecessary. The surgical technique that is described next involves working only with the torn canaliculus.

MATERIALS

ANESTHESIA

Though children and apprehensive adults may require general anesthesia, the majority of avulsion repair surgery can be done with local anesthetic agents.

A local anesthesia of Xylocaine 2% plain or with 1:100,000 epinephrine, alone or mixed in equal amounts with 0.5% Marcaine, works well. Related anesthetic agents, such as Nescaine or Carbacaine, may also be employed. The anesthetic solution is infiltrated directly into the thorn tissues, that is, into both sides of the wound, and to the medial canthus area and under the caruncle. The unused solution should be kept for booster injections, as the brisk circulation in the region causes rapid absorption of the anesthesia and early return of pain sensation.

SURGICAL INSTRUMENTS

A lid repair tray and lacrimal instruments are required. The lid repair instruments should include several different sizes of toothed forceps, such as Adson, Bonnacolto or Castroviejo; a medium-strength needle holder, such as Castroviejo curved, Westcox and suture scissors, and a few hemostats. A pair of tying forceps, such as a Harms or Barraquer type, is also useful.

Lacrimal instruments should include these items:

1. Punctum dilator (such as Nettleship);
2. Bowman probes;
3. Worst pigtail probe;
4. Lacrimal canula;
5. Canalicular stent.

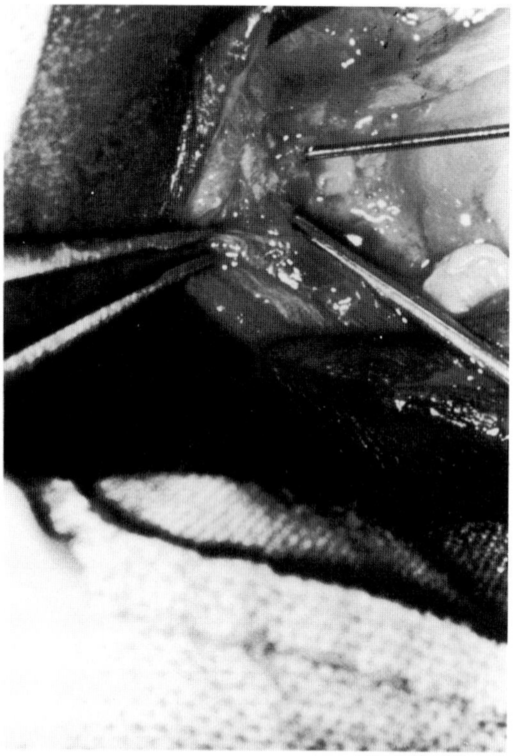

Figure 48.3. Upper and lower canaliculus were severed. Probes identify the medial cut ends of the canaliculi. (Same patient as in Fig. 48.2.)

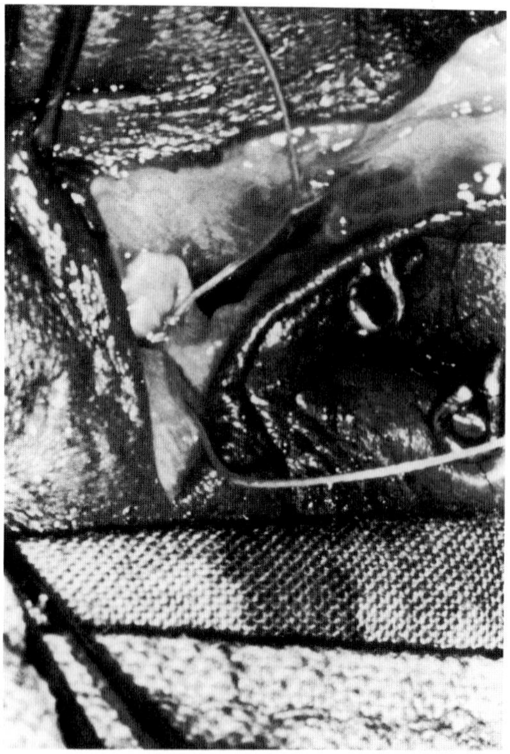

Figure 48.4. After repair of canaliculi over two Johnson wires, the medial canthal tendon is shortened and affixed to the point of severance with a double-armed 4-0 Mersilene suture.

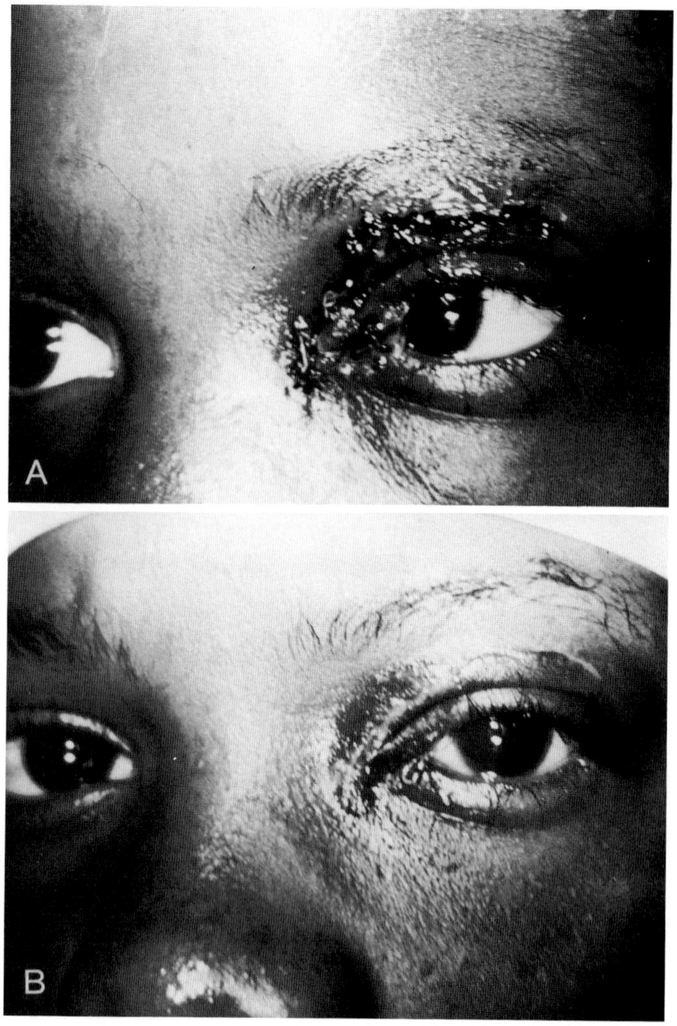

Figure 48.5. Same patient as in Figs. 48.2–48.4, 1 (*A*) and 3 (*B*) weeks after repair. Medial canthus is apposed well; however, the scar is thick.

Bowman probes should be available in a few assorted sizes; sizes 0, 1, 2, 3, are the most useful. The probes in sizes 00 and 000 are generally very thin and wire-sharp, easily perforate the canalicular lumen, and often get maneuvered into false passages. Therefore, the thicker probes are better. Once past the punctum, these thicker probes slide smoothly within the lumen, outlining its course, and will not exit through a wrong opening if, for instance, there is a partial cut in the wall of the canaliculus. Probes larger than size 3 are apt to rupture the punctum when pushed into the canaliculus.

Worst pigtail probe (3) is helpful in locating the medial cut end of the canaliculus and for passing certain stent materials, e.g., sutures or silicone tubing.

When lacrimal instruments are not available, a surgeon can fashion makeshift lacrimal devices. A sterile safety pin makes an excellent punctum dilator; heavy-grade surgical steel wire, doubled on itself, makes a good probe; and a 25-gauge needle with the tip cut off with the scissors can serve as a lacrimal canula.

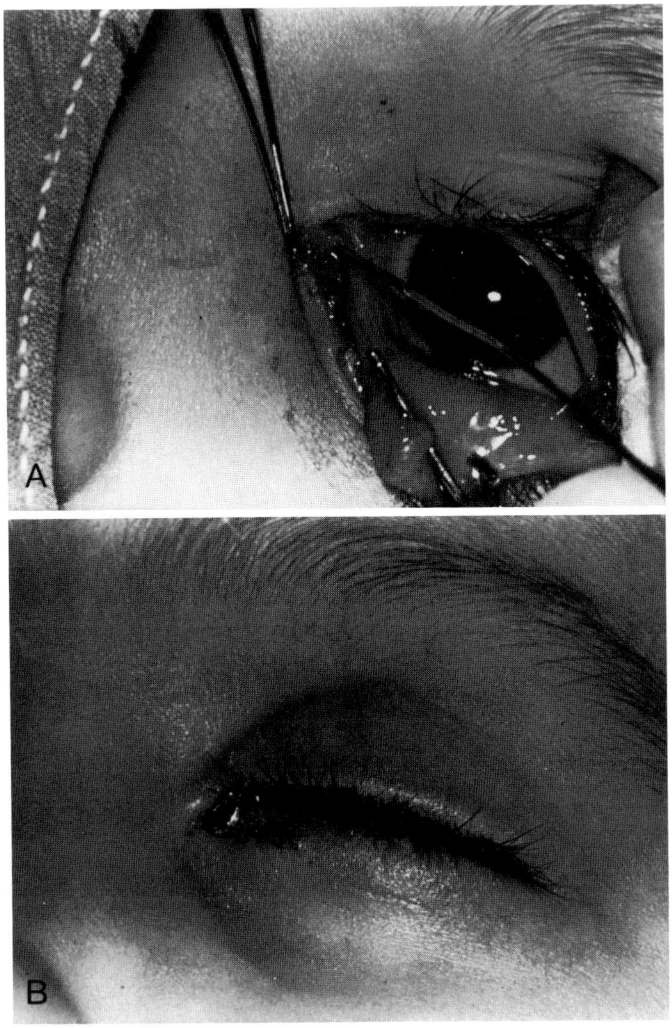

Figure 48.6. A biplane eyelid avulsion before (*A*) and after (*B*) repair. A Johnson wire remains in the reanastomosed canalicular lumen.

Canalicular Stents

An indwelling canalicular stent serves to align the cut sides of the canaliculus during the repair and to maintain an open lumen after the repair and to maintain an open lumen after the repair while the eyelid is healing. The length of time the stent should be kept in the canaliculus varies; 3 weeks is the usual time, as the mucosa of the canalicular lumen unites quickly.

Varied and ingenious devices have been developed and utilized as canalicular stents, for example, 22-0 and 3-0 silk or nylon and Mersilene sutures, Teflon rods, polyethylene tubing, silicone tubing, Veirs, Quickert, and Johnson metal rods (4–8).

If surgeons find themselves with emergency repair in situations where no premade stents are available, fashioning a small-diameter rod from materials readily available in the operating room is easy to do. Some ways are as follows:

Smith (8) suggests taking a doubly armed 4-0 silk suture, straightening one of the needles between two hemostats, cutting the sharp point off with a wire cutter, and thus fashioning a Viers rod-like device.

Another stent material can be the cut end of a Bowman's lacrimal probe. A portion of the probe, 20–25 mm in length, is cut off with a wire cutter or strong scissors; then, with a hemostat, one end is twisted into a closed loop and a Johnson-like wire is thus fashioned. The straight end of the metal is guided to bridge the canaliculus, and the loop is affixed with a suture to the skin side of the lid margin. A rod made of size 0 or 00 surgical steel wire may be similarly constructed and used as a canalicular stent.

SURGICAL TECHNIQUE

Repair of the eyelid avulsion begins with microsurgical lacrimal canalicular reanastomosis, which is done with the use of a microscope or loupe.

If infiltration anesthesia is used, gentle compression and massage will reduce the bulging of tissues and restore the suppleness of wound edges.

The first step is to dilate the punctum of the injured canaliculus with a punctum dilator or with the tip of a safety pin and to pass a Bowman's probe and thereby identify the cut distal end of the canaliculus. Next the medial cut end of the canaliculus is identified.

IDENTIFYING THE MEDIAL CUT END OF THE CANALICULUS

When a microscope is used, finding the medial cut end of the canaliculus is generally very straightforward. The microscope is lowered to illuminate and to focus over the nasal portion of the lacus lacrimalis and of the caruncle. The caruncle may be grasped with toothed forceps and lifted up and laterally. The cut canaliculus should appear deep under the anteromedial aspect of the caruncle. The medial cut end of the canaliculus can be differentiated from the silvery cut strands of the medial canthal tendon (MCT) by its mucosa-cuffed orifice, which retains an oval shape, whereas the cut ends of the MCT elongate and stretch with tissue manipulation.

Another way of identifying the cut inner canalicular lumen is to march up hand-over-hand with two toothed forceps along the medial cut skin wound over the lid margin into the conjunctival border and then explore fascial folds along the cut conjunctiva.

These two maneuvers, and good illumination, succeed almost always in locating the canalicular ends. If difficulty is still encountered, Morrison's technique of submerging the medial canthal angle under saline and injecting air through the opposite canaliculus may be tried. Also, injecting diluted methylene blue while compressing the area of the sac may bring results. If excess of methylene blue is covering all the tissues, immediate brisk irrigation with saline will clear it out sufficiently to permit the surgeon to continue with the surgery.

Employing a Worst Pigtail Probe

A Worst pigtail probe affords rapid and effective canalicular identification in experienced hands. With a little practice and gentleness most surgeons learn to be proficient with this instrument. Many in fact use it—after they have identified the canalicular cut ends by direct visualization—to thread certain types of canalicular stents; i.e., suture materials or silicone tubing through the lumen of both canaliculi, over which the tissue repair is then made (Fig. 48.7).

Once the tip of the pigtail probe, curving in the proper direction, passes the punctum and enters the lumen of the uninvolved opposite canaliculus, the shaft is straightened out to keep the curved portion flat in the plane of the canaliculi. The tip of the probe is then gently wiggled with a snake-like motion through that canaliculus. With a twisting motion of the fingers holding the probe, the tip is made to execute a sharp turn into the involved canaliculus and out of its cut medial end where it then can be visualized.

A suture or a silicone tubing (silastic 0.6 mm outside diameter, Dow Corning) is affixed to the pigtail probe. The probe is withdrawn and the material is pulled out through the punctum of the uninvolved canaliculus. The probe is then reintroduced through the punctum of the

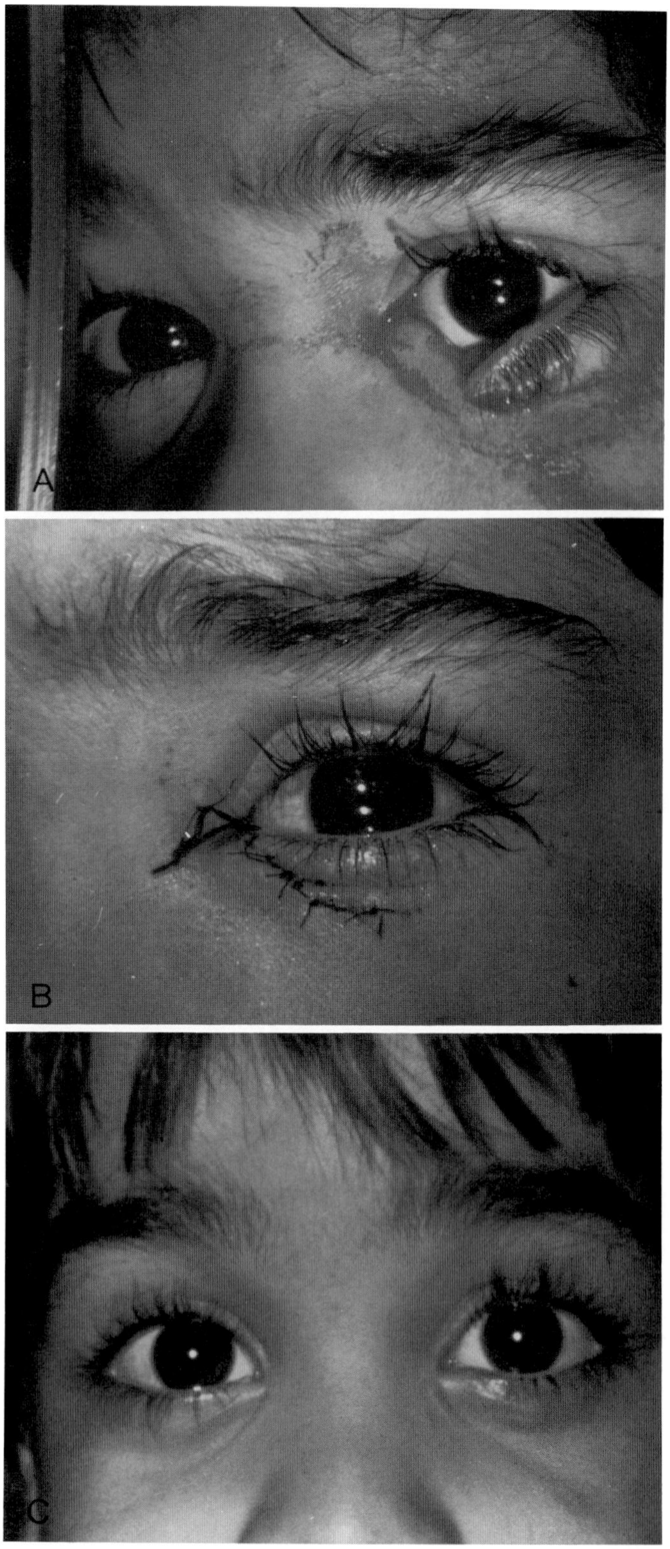

Figure 48.7. *A*, Patient was injured after falling on a fence. *B*, A Worst pigtail probe and a canalicular stent 4-0 silk suture were used in repairing this canalicular laceration. Suture was tied between the canaliculi and affixed to the skin of the nose away from the globe for 4 weeks. *C*, Four weeks after repair.

cut canaliculus to come out at its distal cut end. The silicone tubing protruding from the medial cut end is affixed to its tip again and drawn out through the involved punctum, thus completing the loop inside both canaliculi. The completed loop can then be tied and affixed away from the eye to the skin of the angle.

REPAIRING THE CANALICULUS

Before any sutures are placed to repair the canaliculus, the avulsed tip of the eyelid is grasped with toothed forceps and approximated to the medial canthus as a test of whether it will stay there with a relatively little tension. If excessive amounts of tension are felt, a lateral canthotomy or canthotomy and cantholysis may be required; this is to make sure that the pericanalicular tissue wound will not pull apart, notch, or otherwise deform after the repair from extensive tension on the wound.

When the involved canaliculus is repaired alone, without involving the opposite one, a rigid stent such as Veirs rod, a cut piece of the Bowman's probe, or a Johnson wire is very suitable. A Johnson wire, or a stent of surgeon's choice, is inserted through the punctum of the involved canaliculus, guided to bridge the cut sides of the wound, and pushed to stay in as far as the lacrimal sac. Then the tissue next to the canalicular lumen is united with strong sutures (e.g., 5-0 absorbable sutures).

REPAIRING THE JUXTACANALICULAR TISSUE

Juxtacanalicular tissue repair involves placing two deep sutures vertically into the muscle layer surrounding the canaliculus in close proximity to the canalicular walls, one anterior (Fig. 48.8) and the other posteriorly. When these two sutures are tied, the canaliculus is brought into align-

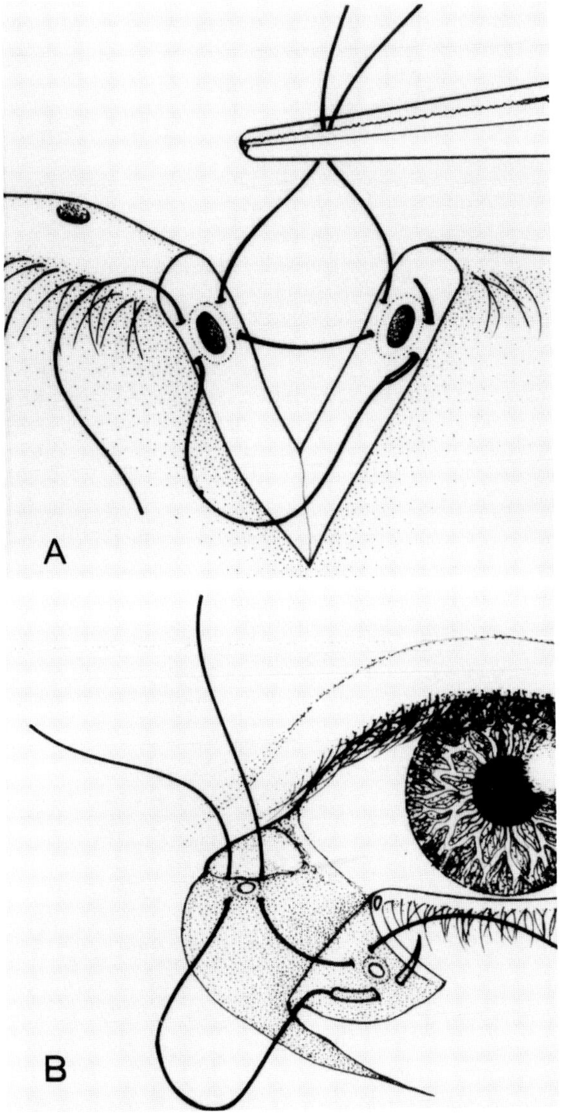

Figure 48.8. Juxtacanalicular suture placement. *A*, In midcanalicular laceration. *B*, In avulsion situation.

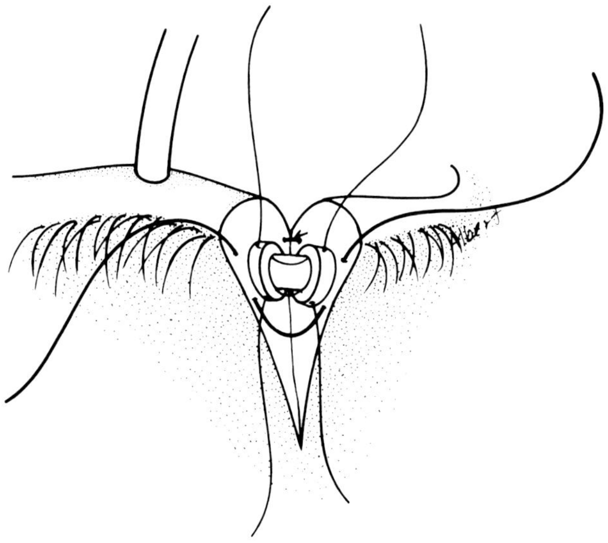

Figure 48.9. Canalicular mucosa may be anastomosed directly with two 9-0 nylon sutures placed superiorly and inferiorly.

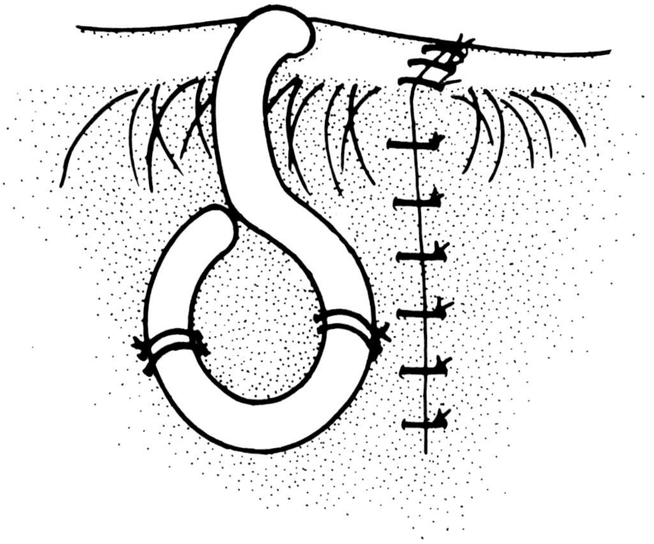

Figure 48.10. Remainder of the repair is to coapt the lid margin and the skin. Johnson wire is affixed securely to the skin.

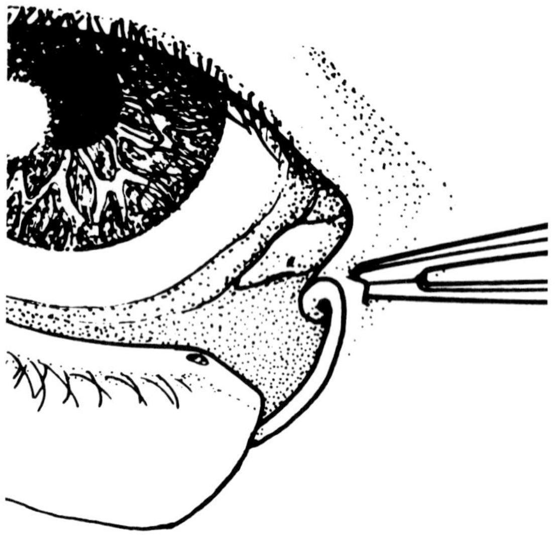

Figure 48.11. Lid margin continuity is achieved by unrolling the skin at the medial edge of the wound and searching for a skin-mucosal junction in which to place the suture.

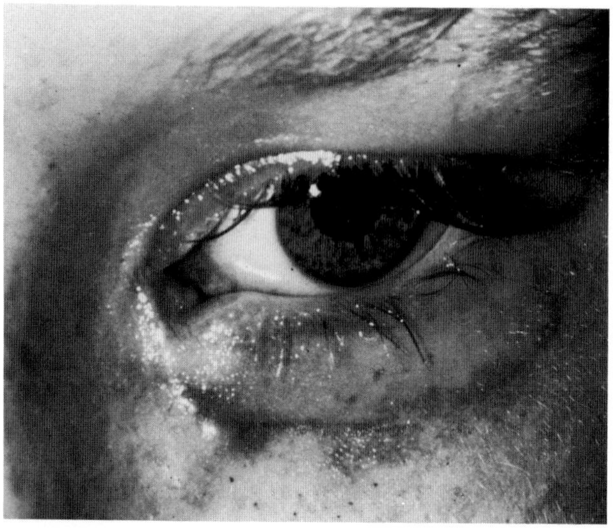

Figure 48.12. A deformity produced by downward misdirection of eyelid skin.

ment with the cut ends touching. When the canalicular stent is in place, generally, these sutures alone will suffice to achieve the repair of the canaliculus. When the microscope is used, it is easy to place end-to-end anastomotic mucosal sutures of 9-0 nylon (one superiorly and one inferiorly) to further guarantee a canalicular wall continuity.

Suture placement is easier when a long Bowman's probe is kept in the lumen; then, once the sutures are ready to be tied, the Bowman probe is withdrawn and a permanent stent, e.g., a Johnson wire, is put in its place.

The posterior juxta canalicular suture is tied first; the two mucosal sutures, superior and inferior, are tied second; and finally the anterior juxta canalicular suture is tied (Fig. 48.9), which completes the repair of the canaliculus.

The twisted loop of Johnson wire is affixed securely to the skin of the lid with 4-0 silk suture (Fig.48.10). This indwelling stent will remain in the canaliculus for 3 weeks.

COMPLETING THE REPAIR OF THE WOUND OF THE MEDIAL CANTHAL AVULSION

Since the avulsion in general is located beyond the nasal end of the tarsal plate, the lid margin at the point of the laceration no longer has a three-dimensional shape. In the medial canthal avulsion, the medial upper border of the skin wound is generally drawn up and coiled inward. The medial upper border has to be unrolled and everted out (Fig. 48.11) before uniting it with the corresponding lateral margin to avoid pull-down deformity (Fig. 48.12).

It is best to find the skin-conjunctiva junction on the lateral and on the medial side of the avulsion wound, and place a suture (6-0 silk or the like) exactly at that point on both sides.

The remainder of the repair involves closing the external skin wound with 6-0 silk or nylon sutures if the laceration lines do not extend far; if they do, one or two absorbable (5-0 Vicryl, 5-0 Dexon, or 6-0 plain) sutures are placed subcutaneously approximating the orbicularis muscle before the overlying skin is closed.

EDITOR'S COMMENT

Repairing the canaliculus comprises 90% of the medial canthal eyelid avulsion repair. The importance of a good microsurgical lacrimal canalicular repair is appreciated not only for the restoration of lacrimal drainage function, but also in terms of achieving correct anatomical lid reanastomosis (9, 11).

The use of the operating microscope is advocated (10, 12). With it, the two cut ends of the canaliculus can be readily identified and the sutures more accurately placed.

Most repaired canalicular lacerations heal promptly and without late lumen stenosis. The incidence of eyelid deformities and related complications (hypertrophic scars, keloids, granulomas) can be reduced by careful microsurgical repair; though, the avulsions involving the upper eyelid, often complicated by ptosis, require reoperations more frequently (13, 14) than those in the lower eyelid.

REFERENCES

1. Billson A, et al: Traumata to lacrimal system in children. *Ophthalmology* 36: 828, 1978.
2. Saxon A, Zolli C, data to be published.
3. Worst JG: Method for reconstructing torn lacrimal canaliculus. *Am J Ophthalmol* 53: 520, 1962.
4. Henderson JW: Management of obstructions of lacrimal canaliculi with polyethylene tubes. *Arch Ophthalmol* 49: 182, 1953.
5. Lauring L: Silicone intubation of the lacrimal system: pitfalls, problems and complications. *Ann Ophthalmol* 8: 489, 1976.
6. Veirs ER: Treatment of frequent disorders of the lacrimal drainage system. *Am J Ophthalmol* 53: 39, 1962.
7. Johnson CC: A canaliculus wire. *Am J Ophthalmol* 78: 854, 1974.
8. Smith B, Dodick JM: Repair of lid lacerations involving the lower lacrimal canaliculus. *Can J Ophthalmol* 3: 263, 1968.
9. Callahan A: *Reconstructive Surgery of the Eyelids and Ocular Adnexae.* Aesculapius, Birmingham, AL 1966.
10. Heinze J: Microsurgery and the lacrimal system. *Adv Ophthalmol* 37: 87, 1978.
11. Mustarde JC: *Repair and Reconstruction in the Orbital Region.* New York, Churchill-Livingstone, 1980.
12. Baylis HI, Axelrod R: Repair of the lacerated canaliculus. *Ophthalmology* 85: 1271, 1978.
13. Walter C: Problems in the reconstruction of the inner canthus and the lacrimal duct. *J Maxillofac Surg* 4: 34, 1976.
14. Tessier P: Eyelid lacerations. The emergency in eyelid surgery. *Bull Mem Soc Fr Ophthalmol* 85: 423–32, 1972.

CHAPTER 49

Thermal Eyelid Burns

ALFRED C. MARRONE, M.D.

Serious eyelid burns and ocular injuries occur in a small but significant number of all burn patients. They occur in a much higher percentage of patients with extensive burns. Most patients with serious lid burns also have extensive and life-threatening burns elsewhere. Consequently, a vast majority of eyelid burn patients are managed for long periods of time in burn centers by a team of physicians necessary to handle these most complex medical and surgical problems.

The depth of thermal skin injuries is dependent on the temperature of the external source of the burn and particularly on the length of time of the exposure.

Before discussing the treatment of eyelid burns, it is necessary to understand the natural course of the stages of these injuries. The depth of cellular injury extends from the most superficial first-degree burn to a deeper destruction within the dermis in the second-degree burn and full-thickness dermal necrosis in a third-degree burn. Because the eyelid is thin, if it is exposed to the full thermal injury, it is not uncommon to find the eyelid deeply burned, whereas the surrounding skin may be less burned. The next section further describes this factor.

NATURAL HISTORY

The natural course of an eyelid burn depends on many factors, particularly the depth of the burn and the extent of the burn in the surrounding facial tissues.

A first-degree burn presents no significant permanent threat to the eyelid. It should heal well without compromise of lid function in several days. Edema of the lid may impair opening, but this is only transient.

Superficial second-degree burns with bullae formation will usually create more edema; the edema reaches a maximum in 8–48 hours and will usually subside within several days. The bullae usually rupture early. Contracture of lid skin or permanent compromise of lid function is also not expected in such a burn unless it becomes infected, in which case the depth of tissue destruction and inflammation will result in a clinical course more similar to a deep second- to third-degree burn.

Deep second-degree burns can vary in their clinical course, depending on their depth and damage to surrounding tissues. The spectrum can range from minimal tissue shrinkage and good skin healing within 1–3 weeks to significant contracture necessitating a release and grafting procedure later in the course. A deep second-degree burn should epithelialize itself in about 14–28 days although the skin will be red for several months and not be of completely normal appearance. Further contracture can occur even after epithelialization occurs although the rate of progression usually slows down considerably. Deep second-degree burns can convert to third-degree burns if there is an extension of avascularity in the transition zone between viable and nonviable tissue.

Third-degree eyelid burns initially present with a devascularized, usually greyish skin (or blackened by smoke or char). Massive edema sets in during the first few hours and usually results in complete closure of the lids in 8–24 hours. The extent of this edema varies considerably with each burn because of the massive fluid and electrolyte imbalances that occur in the first few hours following the injury of a patient who has considerable burn damage elsewhere in the body (Fig. 49.1).

About 20% of patients with deeply burned eyelids will develop spontaneous eversion of the upper lids. This is a result of the edema, which develops in the deeper lid

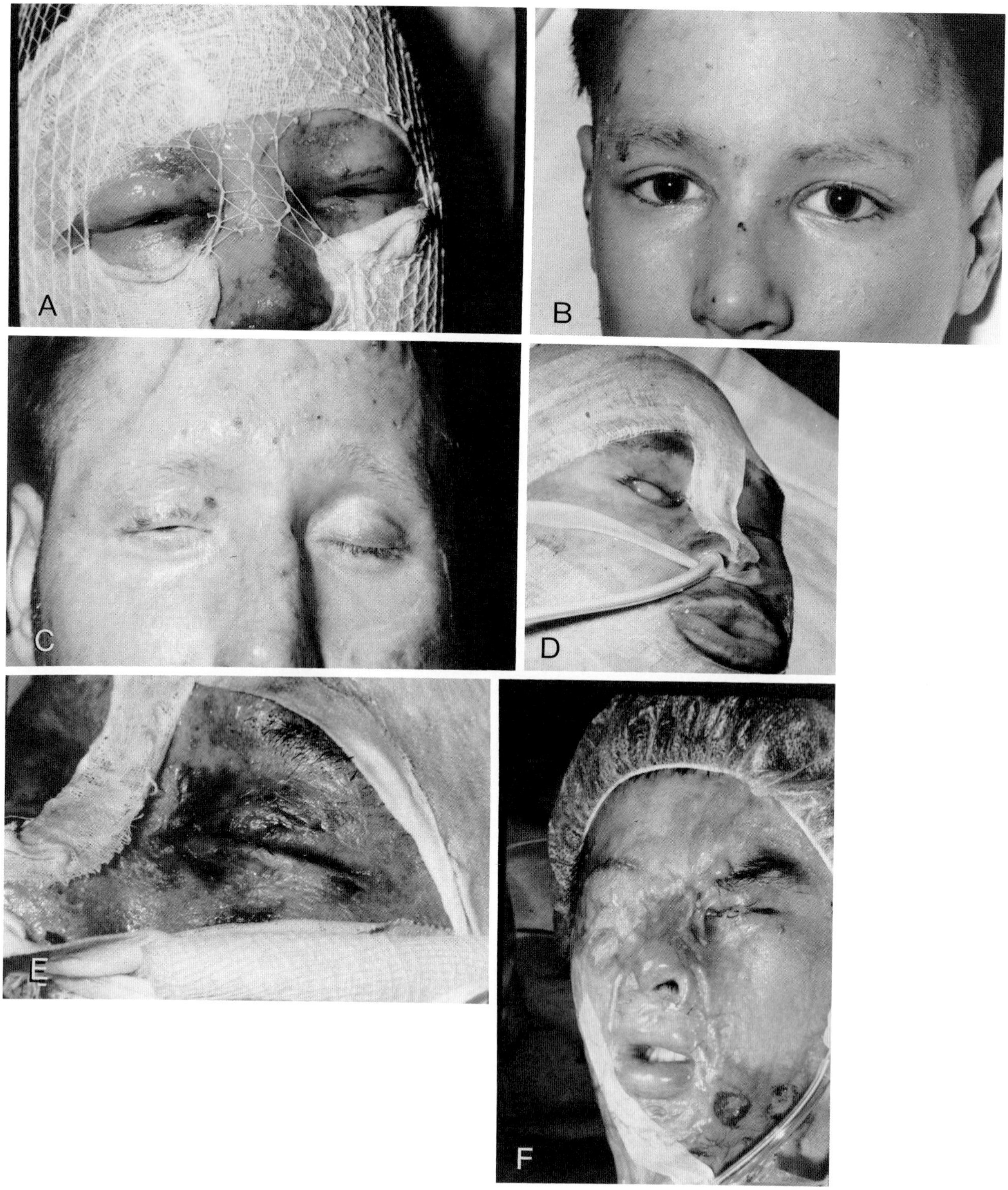

Figure 49.1. Degree of burns. *A*, Superficial second-degree burns following flash-injury burn. Note vascularity of skin along with edema. *B*, Same patient as in panel *A* 1 week later with good healing. *C*, Another patient 1 month following second-degree burns, deeper on the right side than on the left. No surgery has been performed on the lids. Note retraction of right upper lid but little retraction of the left. *D*, Typical facial appearance of severe third-degree burns from motorcycle fire. Note massive edema, avascular skin, and spontaneous eversion of right upper lid. *E*, Same patient as in panel *D* 3 weeks later, with sloughing of necrotic skin and some viable skin present on the left side. *F*, Same patient as in panel *D* 8 months later after split-thickness grafting. Note the degree of contracture and spontaneous fusing of burned lid margins on the right side.

tissues (conjunctiva and perhaps levator), pushing the inner layers of the upper lid inferiorly around the stiff and relatively immobile burned and charred skin.

During the first 1–2 weeks, the burned skin will become a necrotic eschar and will slough. This occurs spontaneously: However, the sloughing is usually hastened by cleansing and gentle debridement by the nursing staff. After the slough of necrotic tissue, granulation tissue can be seen to develop. Along with the excellent blood supply in this tissue, there is development of myofibroblasts that contribute to the massive contracture of deeply burned tissue. This contracture will continue even after skin grafting, but it is minimized by successful and early grafting. The contracture continues for at least 6 and as long as 18 months following injury. Naturally, the ability of the lids to cover the eye during relaxed closure and even forced closure will be compromised by the contracture, which will cause lagophthalmos and ectropion. This is the major oculoplastic problem facing the surgeon in the immediate and later stages of healing.

INITIAL EXAMINATION AND TREATMENT

There are several aspects of the initial examination of the patient with eyelid burns that affect the further course of treatment. It is of course necessary to establish whether any ocular injury is present. In badly burned lids, especially from flash-type injuries, it is common to see corneal epithelial burns that often present as a grey, opaque coagulum, which is easily debrided with a cotton-tipped applicator under topical anesthesia. Usually the underlying stroma is quite clear, but occasionally it is edematous. It usually clears in just a few days. Stromal scarring from thermal (nonchemical, nonelectrical) burns rarely occurs (less than 2% in my experience) and usually only causes minimal or no visual defects. Hot grease or oil more frequently causes corneal scarring. Superficial corneal burns are best treated by instilling antibiotic ointment after evaluation and repeating this several times a day until the cornea is well epithelialized. I prefer a pseudomonas-effective antibiotic such as polymixin-bacitracin combination. It is best to avoid neomycin because its superficial toxicity may provide a route for infection into the cornea. I also avoid prophylactic use of gentamycin or tobramycin because such treatment may potentially select resistant organisms. In nearly 200 burn cases in 9 years, with significant ocular involvement, we have not had any infectious ulcers with this therapy. Antibiotic ointment is discontinued when the cornea is well epithelialized. If the patient has a significant epithelial burn and if the anterior chamber is deep, then initial cycloplegia with 0.25% scopolamine drops is indicated in most cases (unless pupillary neurologic signs are monitored). The edema present in the eyelid functions very well to keep the lids closed, which makes patching unnecessary.

In treating exposure of the eyes prior to surgical repair, it is best to use bland ointment with antibiotics. Ointments without irritating preservatives (such as Duolube) are best.

Conjunctival edema along with mild to moderate erythema often occurs, even in the absence of any corneal injury. This subsides in a few days when the initial edematous phase resolves.

Careful evaluation for superficial foreign bodies should be done. Singed lashes are usually present in a thermal burn and should be cleansed to eliminate the possibility of char falling into the eye.

Pupil responses should be noted especially if an objective visual acuity cannot be done. A fundus examination should be performed if possible. This is particularly important in electrical burns, where electrical damage can often cause optic nerve and retinal injury and late cataract formation.

In the initial examination, it is often difficult to be fully accurate about the depth or extent of eyelid and surrounding burns. Although many cases are very obvious, others are less so. Because of the protective blepharospasm that occurs during many injuries and because the upper eyelid skin is often protected by its redundancy, it is not uncommon for the physician to make an initial assessment of third-degree burns only to find that there is considerable viable skin intermixed with necrotic skin. This skin may often be enough to eliminate a surgery or at least to postpone surgery until the patient is more stable. Similarly, the surrounding thicker facial skin may represent deep second- rather than third-degree burns in some areas. For this reason, we usually do not surgically debride eyelid skin as early as other areas. Rather, cleansing with saline-soaked fine gauze or wet-to-dry dressings is likely to preserve what cellular elements are present.

Part of the initial assessment should include potential donor sites. For example, if the ears are badly burned (as they frequently are if the eyelids and face are also burned), then retroauricular skin may be either burned or might need to be preserved for ear reconstruction. Other donor sites should be evaluated. The patient with much good skin in the supraclavicular or infraaxillary area might benefit from a full-thickness graft earlier rather than temporizing with a split-thickness.

If spontaneous eversion of the lids develops, it is almost always necessary to place a temporary tarsorrhaphy suture. I prefer to use two horizontal mattress 4-0 monofilament nylon or Prolene suture to pull the margin areas together and to bolster the suture with small pieces of catheter material that have rounded edges. These sutures are usually necessary for only a few days until the edema subsides. Failure to correct the eversion usually results in further conjunctival edema and exposure damage. I have occasionally been able to reinvert the tarsus with a Desmarres retractor or a bent paper clip. Then by holding the lid in position for 10 minutes with digital pressure, the cycle of edema leading to eversion and more edema can be broken. If this can be done, the need for early tarsorrhaphy may be eliminated.

During the first days, the burned skin should be gently cleaned and debrided with saline or fine-mesh gauze.

Saline-soaked wet-to-dry dressings are occasionally useful if thick eschar is present. Facial burns are usually coated with silver sulfadiazine or sulfamyalon, but these are somewhat irritating and best not used on eyelid skin.

TARSORRHAPHIES

Following the initial therapy of corneal and conjunctival burns, the first and probably most controversial decision to make is whether to perform a tarsorrhaphy, with or without intermarginal adhesions. Various authors have taken differing approaches to this. In general, it is best to make this decision depending on the individual characteristics of the case.

Usually I prefer not to use tarsorrhaphies if they can be avoided, especially with intermarginal adhesions. If the patient does not become comatose, ocular lubrication, eye movement, and a normal Bell's reflex are adequate to protect the globe. If minimal exposure is present during sleep, the use of bland ointment is usually more than adequate, especially with an alert and conscientious nursing staff. However, if the patient becomes comatose and the eyes remain in a relatively fixed position without good lid closure, then lubricants are usually not satisfactory. At this point, tarsorrhaphies are more reasonable especially if the patient is nonresponsive.

It should be noted, however, that a tarsorrhaphy will not overcome the relentless contracture and separation of the lids. They simply keep the lids better opposed and minimize exposure until definitive therapy can be initiated.

My personal preference is never to use tongue-in-groove-type tarsorrhaphies because they are destructive to the lid margin. The greater strength of such an adhesion is of little use in preventing severe contracture.

SURGICAL PROCEDURE

The surgical procedure for a tarsorrhaphy includes the following:

1. The patient is injected with Xylocaine with epinephrine subcutaneously.
2. Careful examination of cornea is done before closing lid.

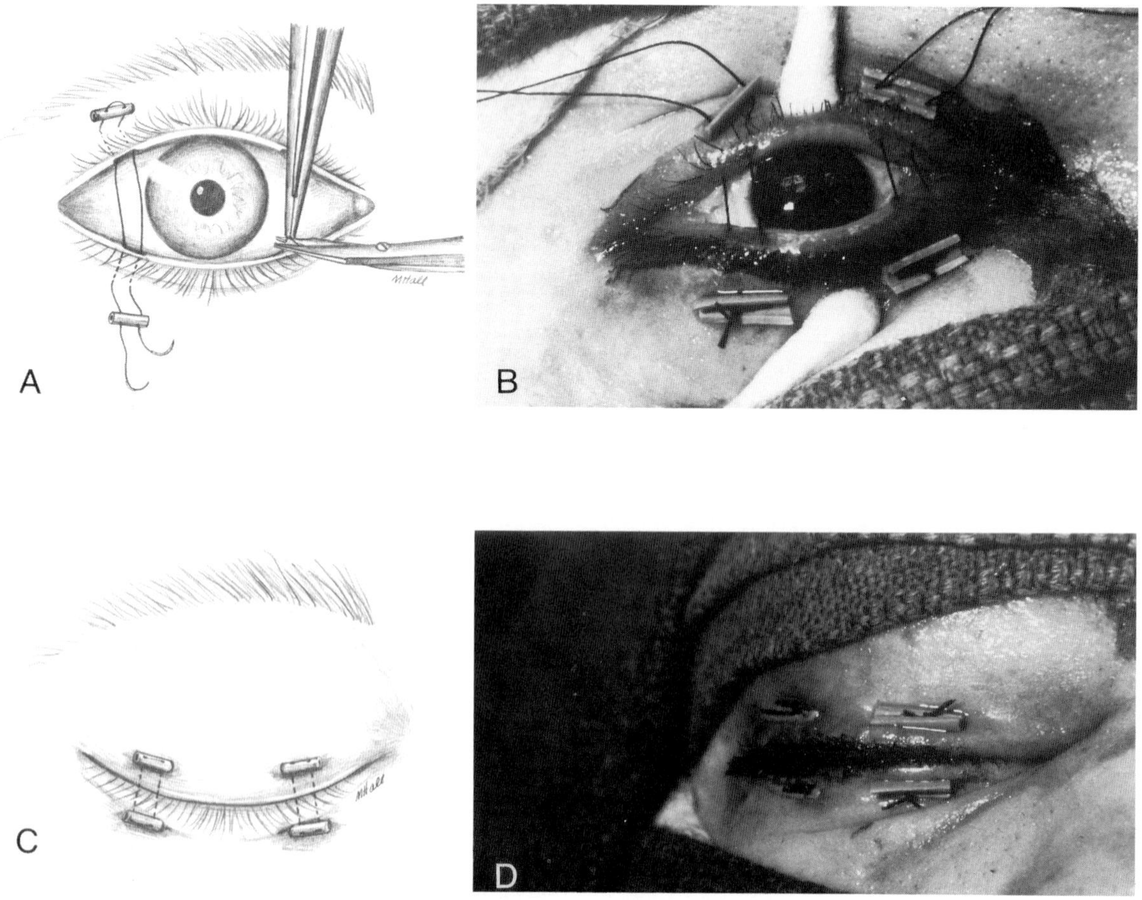

Figure 49.2. Tarsorrhaphies with intermarginal adhesion. *A*, Method of excising skin of margin over tarsus without excising lashes. *B*, Patient with tarsorrhaphies with intermarginal adhesions being performed. Note tissue excision. *C*, Placement of sutures with intermarginal adhesions. *D*, Same patient after sutures are tied.

3. If intramarginal adhesions are to be performed, the margin skin at the junction of the horizontal thirds of the eyelid covering the tarsus is removed with a fine Wescott scissors. The tarsus should be exposed but not excised.

4. Whether or not intermarginal adhesions are performed, a horizontal mattress 4-0 nylon or Prolene suture, which has been passed over a bolster (6 mm-long pieces of Robinson catheter with the edges rounded), is then placed through the lower lid skin about 6 mm below the margin and into the tarsus. The sutures should then pass intratarsally and exit through the margin. In the case of an intermarginal adhesion, the sutures should exit through the cut tarsal edge on the margin. The sutures then pass through the upper margin and pass intratarsally for about 6–7 mm and out through the skin; they are then tied through another bolster. These sutures should not contact the eye at any point. Usually two such horizontal mattress sutures are placed per eyelid, which divides the lid into thirds.

5. Polysporin ointment is instilled onto the sutures and through the lids to the surface of the lid.

6. If intermarginal adhesions are preferred, the suture can be removed about 10–12 days with adequate adhesion.

In general, I prefer tarsorrhaphies with intermarginal adhesion in the more severely burned patient who is comatose and whose lid and facial burns are so extensive that more than one surgical procedure will probably be necessary. In this case I prefer to do the tarsorrhaphies early, after 4–7 days, so the adhesion develops before contracture becomes a problem.

If the patient remains alert, tarsorrhaphies can usually be avoided and grafts can proceed one eye at a time. This allows patients to maintain visual contact with their surroundings. If the burns are less extensive, then tarsorrhaphies are rarely necessary and often a definitive one-stage release and full-thickness graft can be performed later in the course of the patient's healing.

SKIN GRAFTING WITHOUT SURGICAL RELEASE OF CONTRACTURE

If a patient has extensive skin loss of one or both eyelids on each side, it is usually advisable to perform a graft as soon as the necrotic tissue sloughs (with daily cleansings) and granulation tissue begins to form. At this point if it is clear that there is little or no viable skin remaining, it does little good to wait further. Contraction in such a case is relentless and lid distortion will be greater if grafting is delayed. It is also unlikely that a single procedure will suffice in such a case because contracture usually continues to advance in the eyelids and the surrounding facial tissues. If subsequent release and grafting is likely to be necessary, the primary graft should be done early before a release is necessary so that the depth of surgical incision can be kept as superficial as possible. Successful grafting also seems to minimize contracture.

If thin but full-thickness skin is plentifully available from appropriate areas—retroauricular; supraclavicular; infraaxillary; or even groin, foreskin, or scrotal skin—then this is the preferred donor site. Full-thickness grafts contract much less than split-thickness grafts, and if properly done, the success of the graft is better. However, in the more advanced burn cases, the full-thickness skin that is meagerly available must usually be saved for later reconstruction.

The second best alternative is a relatively thick, split-thickness graft that is taken from a donor site where the skin is not thick. It is best to use a split-thickness graft and to obtain the greatest percentage of skin thickness from an area where the skin is naturally thin. Areas of the arms, lower leg, and dorsum of the foot are often good sites.

SURGICAL PROCEDURE

The surgical procedure for skin grafting without release of cicatricial tissue is as follows (Fig. 49.3):

1. The lids that are to be grafted are carefully debrided of any necrotic tissue or superficial granulation tissue by scraping with a scalpel. Actual excision of tissue should be avoided or done very carefully because any viable underlying orbicularis should be preserved to obtain the optimal amount of lid closure. Usually if the upper and lower lids are to be grafted simultaneously (usually split-thickness skin), intramarginal-type tarsorrhaphy has already been done. If it has not, the lid edges can be sutured together with a running nylon subcuticular-type suture to hold the edges together without interfering with the graft.

2. For a split-thickness graft, the donor skin is harvested with a dermatome, which is set at 0.014 to 0.018 inches in thickness. Meticulous hemostasis with a bipolar cautery is performed in the recipient bed prior to suturing the graft. The skin is then placed over the upper lid and lower lid, usually separately, and any surrounding tissues to be grafted. Several small perforations should be made in the graft for drainage. It is sutured into position to any viable skin along the margins with interrupted 6-0 nylon or braided nylon sutures. It is also sutured in interrupted fashion around the edges of the graft so that the grafted skin is kept taut against the recipient bed.

3. The grafts are covered with a dressing, such as Interface or Vaseline gauze, that can be more easily removed later. A stent is then molded of cotton balls soaked in saline with gentamycin added. The stents are placed over the grafts and are molded into position and then sutured into position, with pressure placed by several horizontal mattress nylon sutures passed into the tissue surrounding the graft. It is preferable not to pass the stenting sutures through the grafted tissue to prevent bleeding when they are tied. The pressure caused by the stent minimizes the accumulation of blood or serum under the graft. It also acts as a splint to immobilize the lids.

4. The dressing can be kept moist with saline every 4–6 hours. The dressing can be removed in about 7 days for split-thickness grafts although it can be left longer if the wounds are clean. If full-thickness skin is used, 5–7 days is sufficient.

5. If full-thickness skin is used, it is usually best to do either upper or lower lids one at a time. In this way the

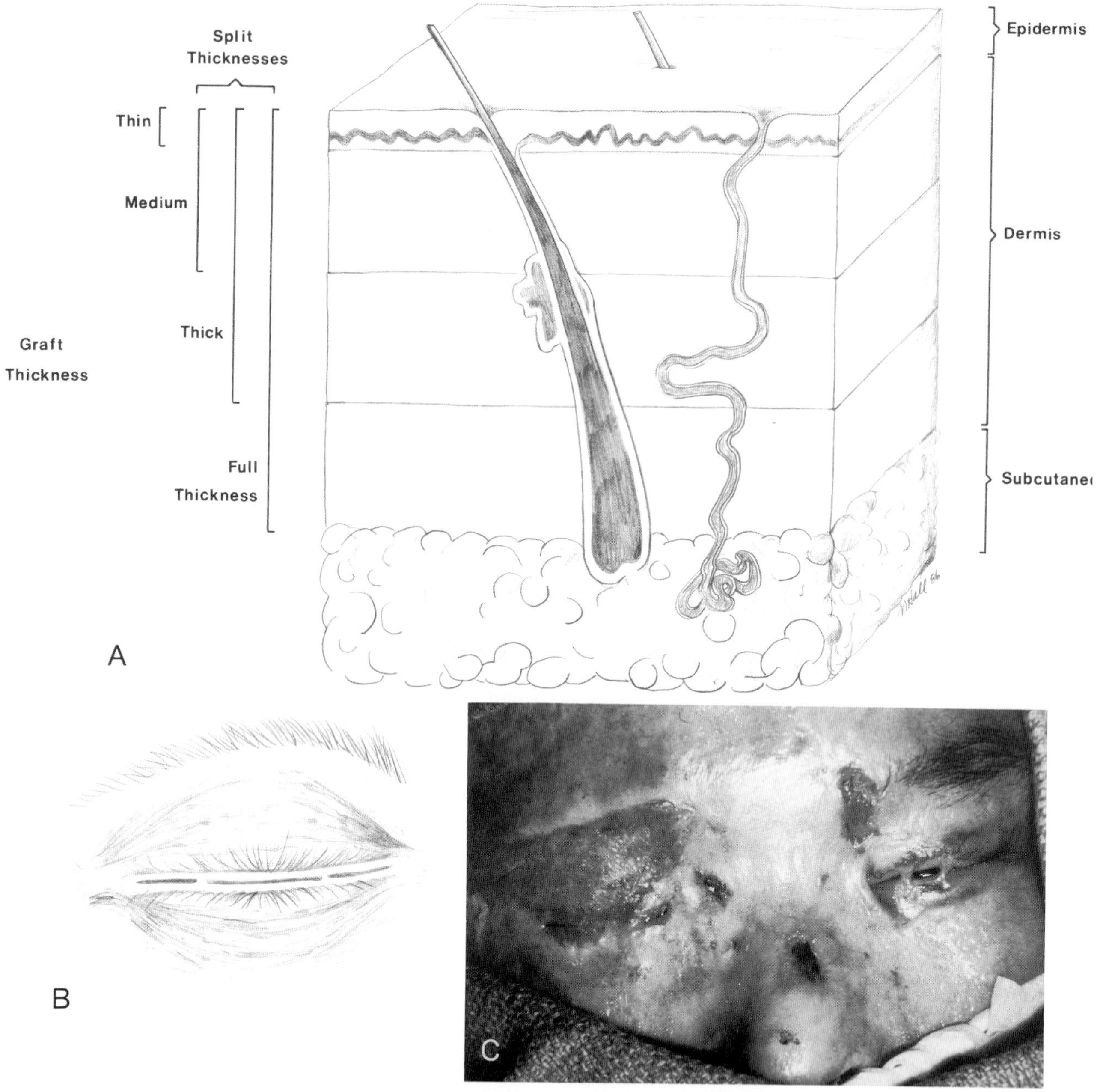

Figure 49.3. Early split-thickness grafting without contracture release. *A*, Cross-section of skin showing relative depth of skin structure and types of skin grafts. *B*, Recipient bed after necrotic tissue and superficial granulation have been debrided. *C*, Patient seen in panels *D–F*, with granulation tissue ready for grafting. (Other facial areas have already been grafted.) *D*, Split-thickness graft sutured into position. *E*, Split thickness graft sutured into position. Note position of tie-over sutures for stenting. They do not pass through the recipient bed or the graft. *F*, Wet-cotton stent in position. *G*, Appearance of graft 10 days postoperatively.

lid to be grafted can be stretched with a Frost-type suture, which lengthens the recipient bed. The graft should be trimmed to match the size of the recipient bed. Leaving excess full-thickness skin only adds to the thickness of the graft without enhancing the eventual outcome. It is important to stretch the recipient bed as far as possible rather than to add excess donor skin. Full-thickness skin should be sutured very carefully to existing skin; this usually done with running and locking sutures. Edge-to-edge suturing enhances the final appearance. Drainage incisions and a stent dressing should be done in a similar fashion to a split-thickness graft.

6. It is preferable to avoid using the sutures between the graft and the recipient bed to tie over the bolster. This creates an elevated ridge that often remains unsightly. This also creates tension in the recipient bed by the sutures, which can cause bleeding under the graft. By placing separate tie-over sutures a few millimeters beyond the graft for tension, the recipient bed is less likely to bleed, as the stent presses flatly against the graft. I also reinject the recipient bed and surrounding tissue with the epinephrine-containing anesthetic just prior to suturing to enhance hemostasis during the suturing and postoperative period.

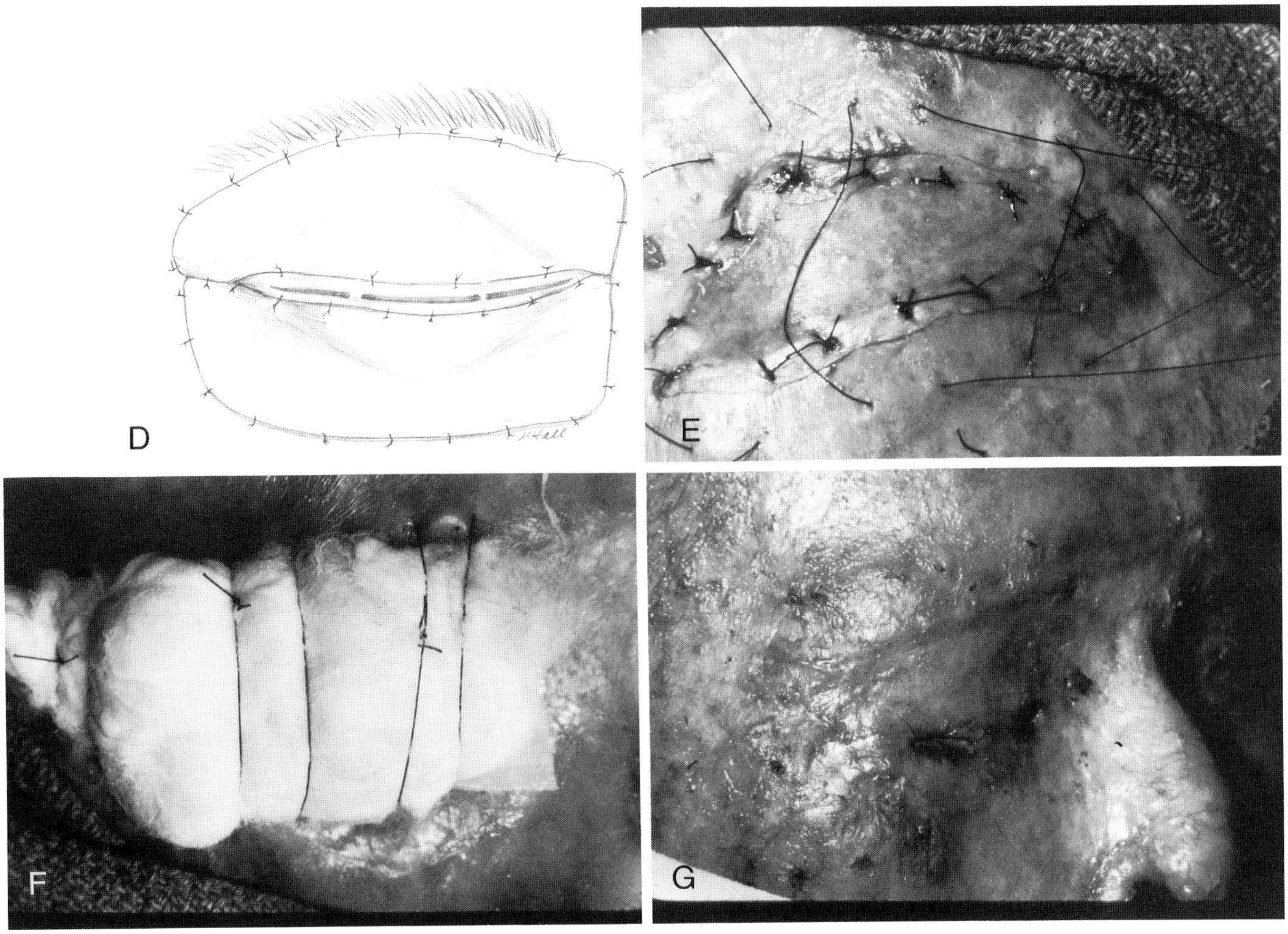

Figure 49.3. *D–G.*

SKIN GRAFTING WITH RELEASE OF CICATRICIAL CONTRACTURE

When a contracture has progressed to a point where the lid will no longer adequately protect the globe, then a release of the contracture must be performed.

The principle for releasing is the same as for the upper and lower lids. An incision must be made through the contracted skin and the anterior tissues. The contracture often involves the orbicularis and can even extend deep into the septum and preaponeurotic fat in severe burns in the late healing phase. The incision must be brought deep to the contracture until the eyelid is mobilized enough to lie in its normal closed position. To enhance the surgical results, the release should actually allow the lid to be pulled into overcorrection.

Care must be taken to preserve the pretarsal orbicularis and the nerve supply to this muscle in order to retain as much function as possible. For this reason the incisions should be planned not to cross the nerve supply in the lateral canthal area.

Because it is advisable to overcorrect the eyelids when performing a release to allow further contracture in the operative site and in the surrounding burn tissues, it is usually necessary to operate on one lid per side at a time. The opposing lid can then be operated when the first graft is healed.

Because full-thickness grafts contract much less than split thickness grafts, they are the superior donor material. If the availability of appropriately thin full thickness skin is limited, then the skin should be used when the release and grafting is expected to be the final procedure.

SURGICAL PROCEDURE

The surgical procedure for release of cicatricial contracture and graft of eyelid is as follows:

1. Local anesthetic with epinephrine is injected subcutaneously and subconjunctivally. Injection should also be placed in the opposing lid because traction sutures will be placed.
2. For the upper eyelid, a marking pen is used to draw a line in the desired lid-crease area. Care should be taken to preserve the pretarsal orbicularis. The incision usually extends beyond the lateral commissure of the lids, but this extension can be performed later as the lid is released so that it is not overextended. Usually I prefer a pointed Westcott or Iris scissors to make the incision, so that the

inner blade easily slides just beneath the contracture. The mobilized lid can then be grasped with a toothed forceps and pulled downward. The cicatricial tissue should be further incised in a superior and deep direction until the tarsal portion of the eyelid can be pulled downward further than the normal resting position. The resting position of the eyelid should be normal at this time. Care should be taken not to damage the levator unless it is involved in the contracture. In that case it may have to be incised down to the conjunctiva in order to adequately mobilize the lid. If the contracture is very deep, the plane of the incision usually extends through the septum and is brought onto the surface of the levator aponeurosis. This nearly always will mobilize the lid entirely and preserve both levator function and pretarsal orbicularis function (Figs. 49.4 and 49.5).

3. For a lower lid release, the incision is usually made just below the lash line and is extended laterally and in the direction of a normal "crow's foot." This prevents the incision from cutting across the nerve fibers and damaging orbicularis function. If the cicatricial tissue is only skin deep, the lid will release very well without incising the orbicularis. If the contracture extends deeper, then the plane of dissection should be brought inferiorly as well as deeply so the pretarsal orbicularis is preserved against the tarsus. As in the upper lids, the release should be extensive

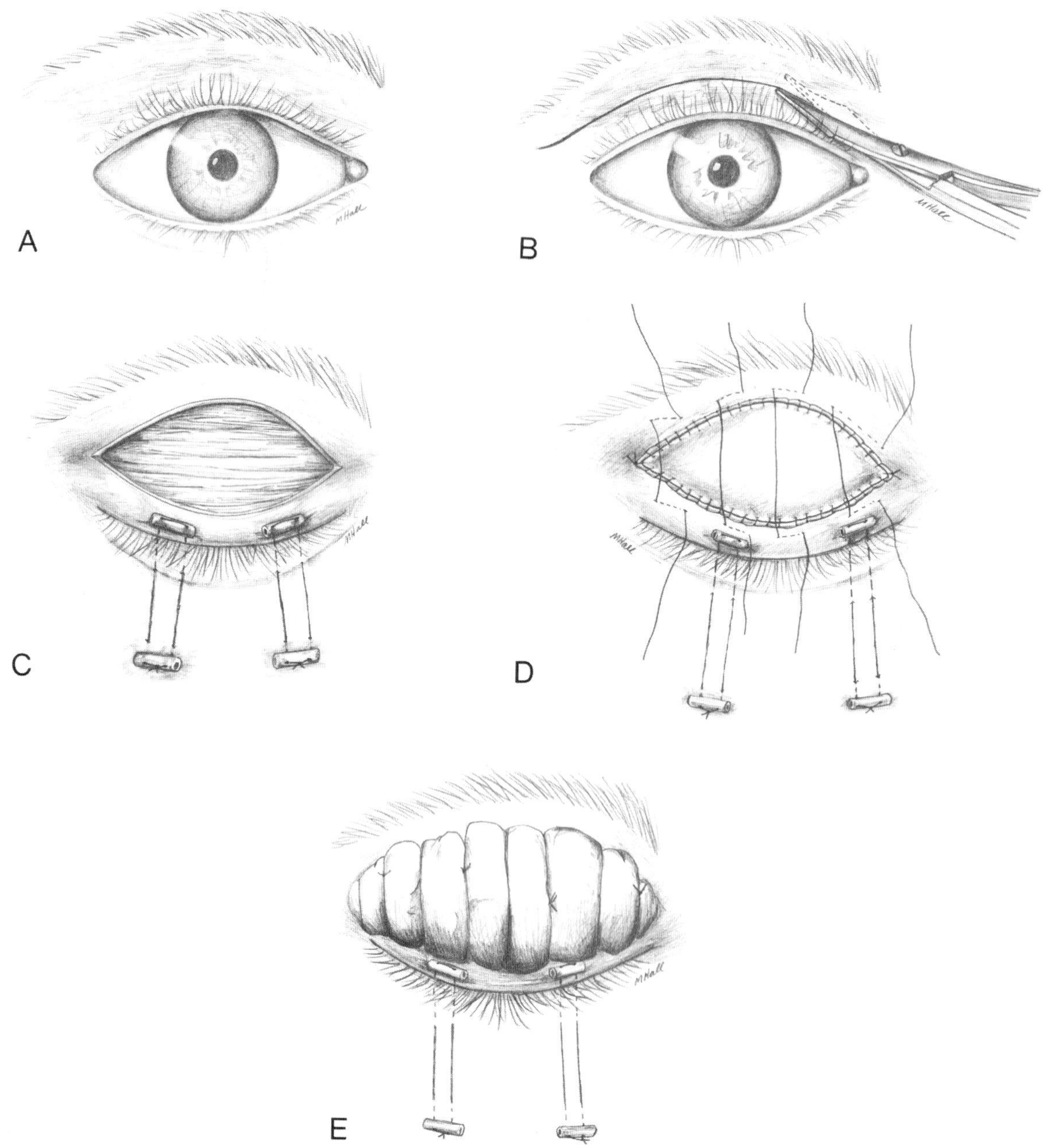

Figure 49.4. Upper lid release and grafting. *A*, Retraction of upper lid from cicatrization. *B*, Position of incision and release of cicatrization with scissors. *C*, After release of contracture. Lid is pulled down with traction sutures. *D*, Graft sutured into position and tie-over horizontal mattress sutures in position. *E*, Wet-cotton stent in position.

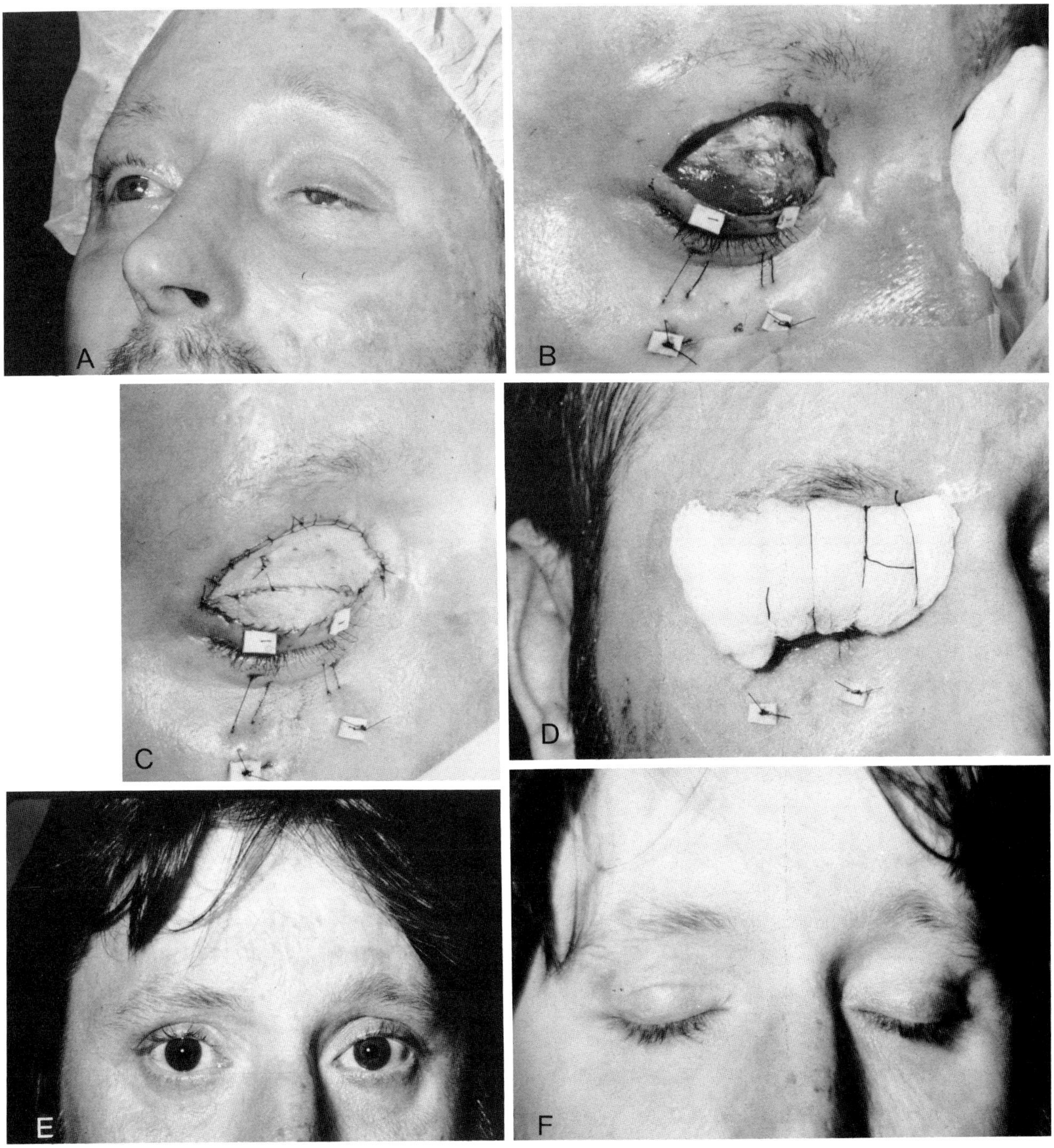

Figure 49.5. Upper lid release and grafting. *A*, Exposure of right eye from upper lid contracture while patient is under anesthesia. *B*, Cicatrix is released and traction sutures are placed. Note blanching of skin from epinephrine in the anesthetic injection. *C*, Full-thickness retroauricular skin graft (in two pieces) sutured into position. *D*, Stent in position as it immobilizes the lid. *E*, The patient several years later with eyes open; *F*, With eyes closed. Function and cosmesis are excellent.

enough to allow the lid to rest in the normal position and to allow it to be pulled upward with minimal traction to a hyperelevated position.

4. At this point, traction sutures are placed from the released lid through the lid margins, out through the opposing lid skin, and then sutured to the brow or cheek skin to stretch the released lid and recipient grafting site. This immobilizes the lid and increases the area of the vascular bed for a given area of graft.

5. Meticulous hemostasis of the recipient bed with a bipolar cautery is obtained with as little cauterization as possible. Reinjection of the bed with epinephrine and local anesthesia enhances this hemostasis.

6. The graft, preferably of full thickness, is sutured into

position. If full-thickness skin is used, the graft should be spread out so that there is no excess, but at the same time it should not be sutured under tension. Edge-to-edge suturing of graft to host skin results in the best cosmesis. If the graft is of split thickness, I prefer to use interrupted sutures and to leave the edges slightly overlapped.

7. The graft site is covered with Interface or Vaseline-coated gauze.

8. The stenting method using horizontal mattress sutures placed around but not through the graft, as previously described, is utilized. Wet cotton is molded into position over the graft. The cotton can be soaked with antibiotics. The stent sutures are tied tightly, which creates a pressure dressing against the graft.

9. The stent is left in place for about 5–7 days for full-thickness grafts and about 7–9 days for split-thickness grafts if no infection is evident. The traction suture may be left in position for a few days more for immobilization and to ensure good coverage of the eye before the opposing lid is released and grafted (Figs. 49.6 and 49.7).

10. Along with removal of the stents, it is preferable to keep the grafts moist for a few weeks with ointment. Steroid ointment should be avoided.

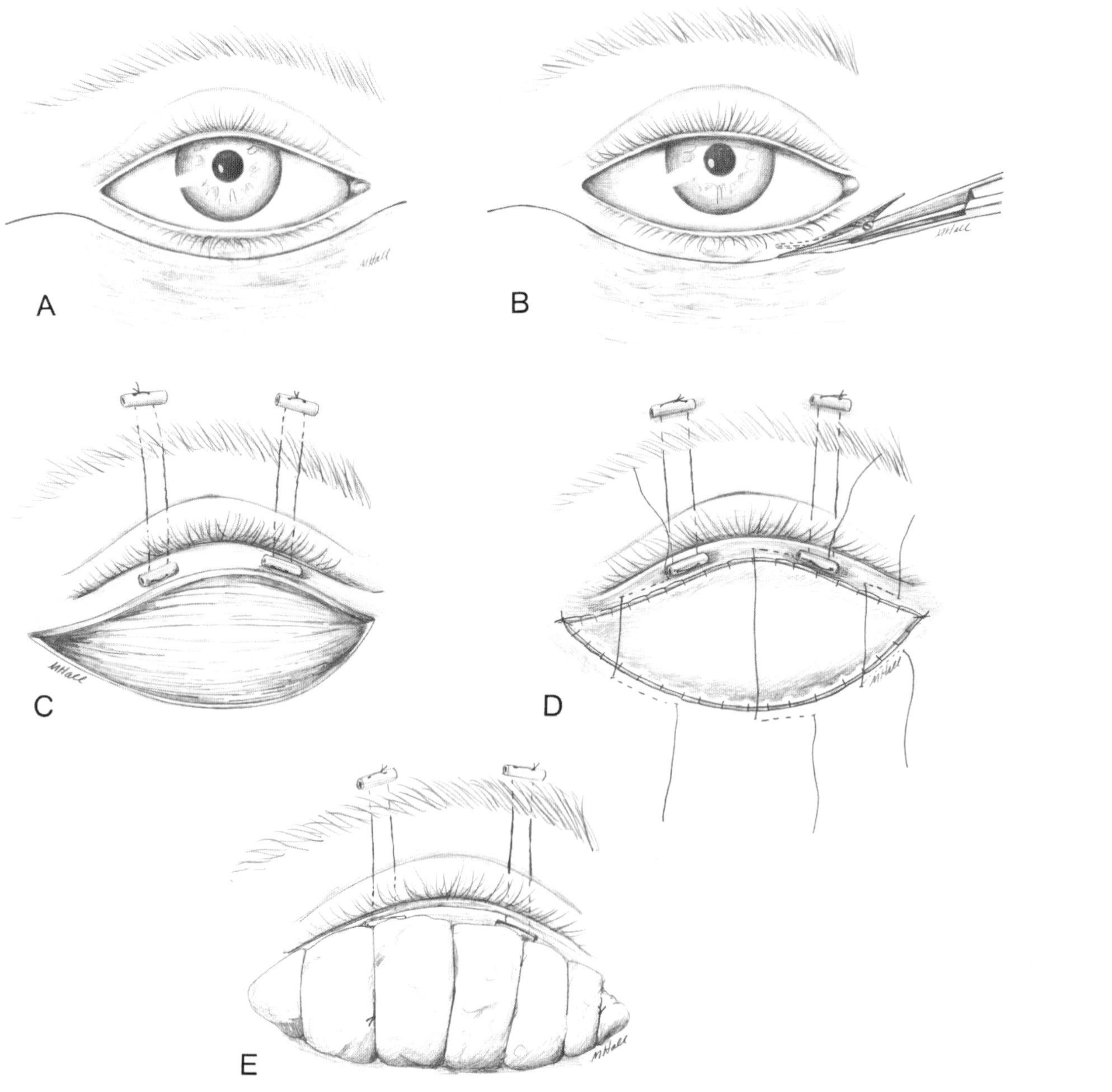

Figure 49.6. Lower lid release and grafting. *A*, Proper position of incision through retracted skin. *B*, Scissor incising and releasing cicatrix while sparing the orbicularis. *C*, Release completed and traction sutures in position expanding the recipient bed. *D*, Graft sutured into position and horizontal mattress tie-over sutures placed. *E*, Wet cotton stent in position at conclusion of surgery.

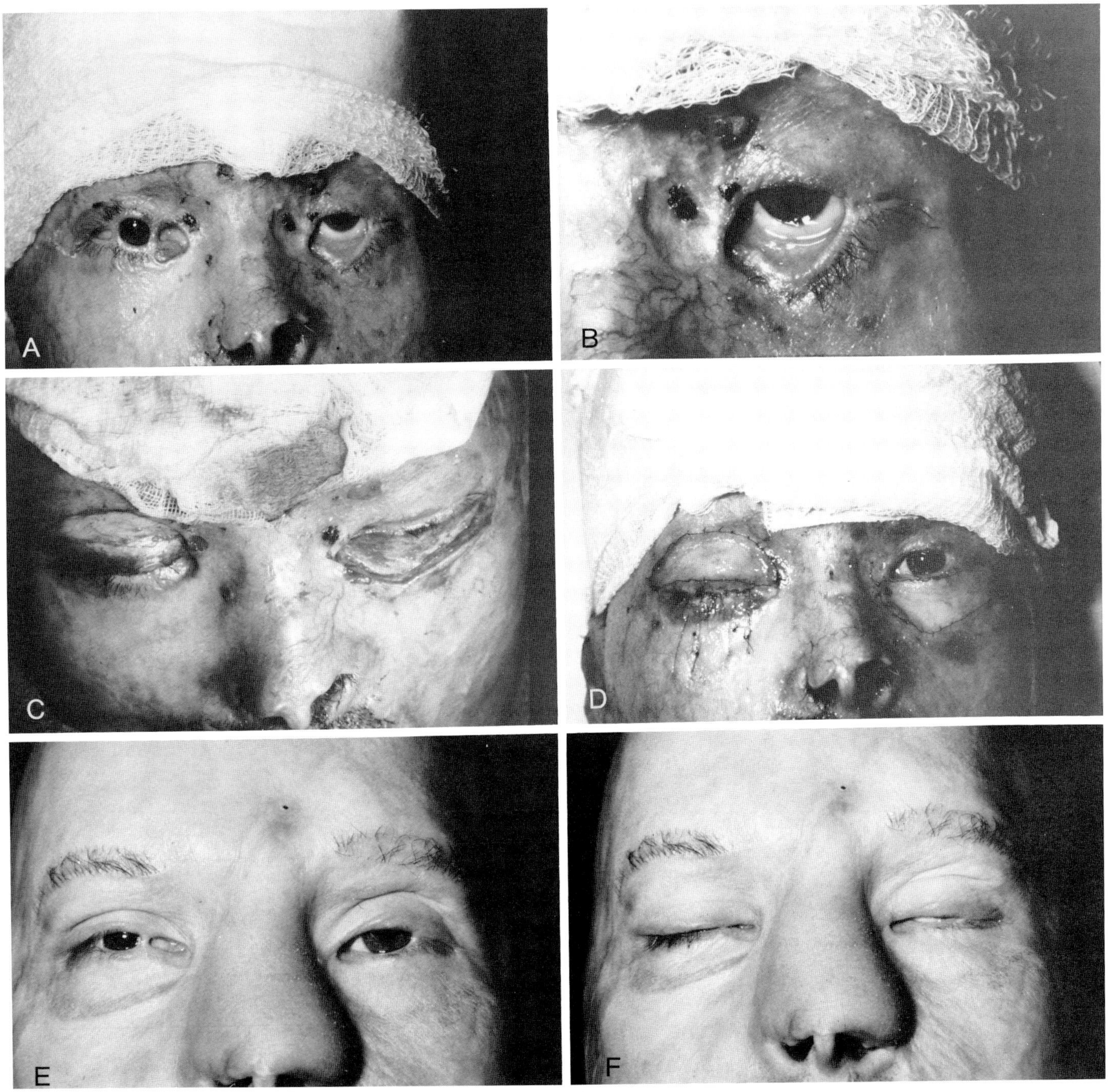

Figure 49.7. Lower lid release and grafting. *A*, Patient pictured 2 months after third-degree burns. Split grafting and intermarginal adhesions have previously been performed. *B*, Note the greater exposure on the nasal side of the left lower lid where the intermarginal adhesion failed to adhere. *C*, The right upper and left lower lids have been released. *D*, Patient pictured 1 week after full-thickness grafts were placed. Note position of left lower lid. Right upper lid traction sutures are still in position. *E* and *F*, Patient shown 2 years postoperative. Lid position and closure are good. (Note nasal half of left lower lid.) Patient did not have intermarginal adhesions released because he was transiently lost to follow-up. Also note the brow grafts performed by another surgeon.

SLOUGH OF FULL-THICKNESS EYELID

If an entire full-thickness eyelid sloughs—that is, not just the skin, but the tarsal elements as well—then the reconstructive problems are quite difficult. Virtually all of the reconstructive procedures used in oculoplastic surgery depend on local flaps, but these are unlikely to be possible because there are deep burns surrounding the full-thickness slough. The standard and probably most viable way of repairing the slough of an eyelid with surrounding third-

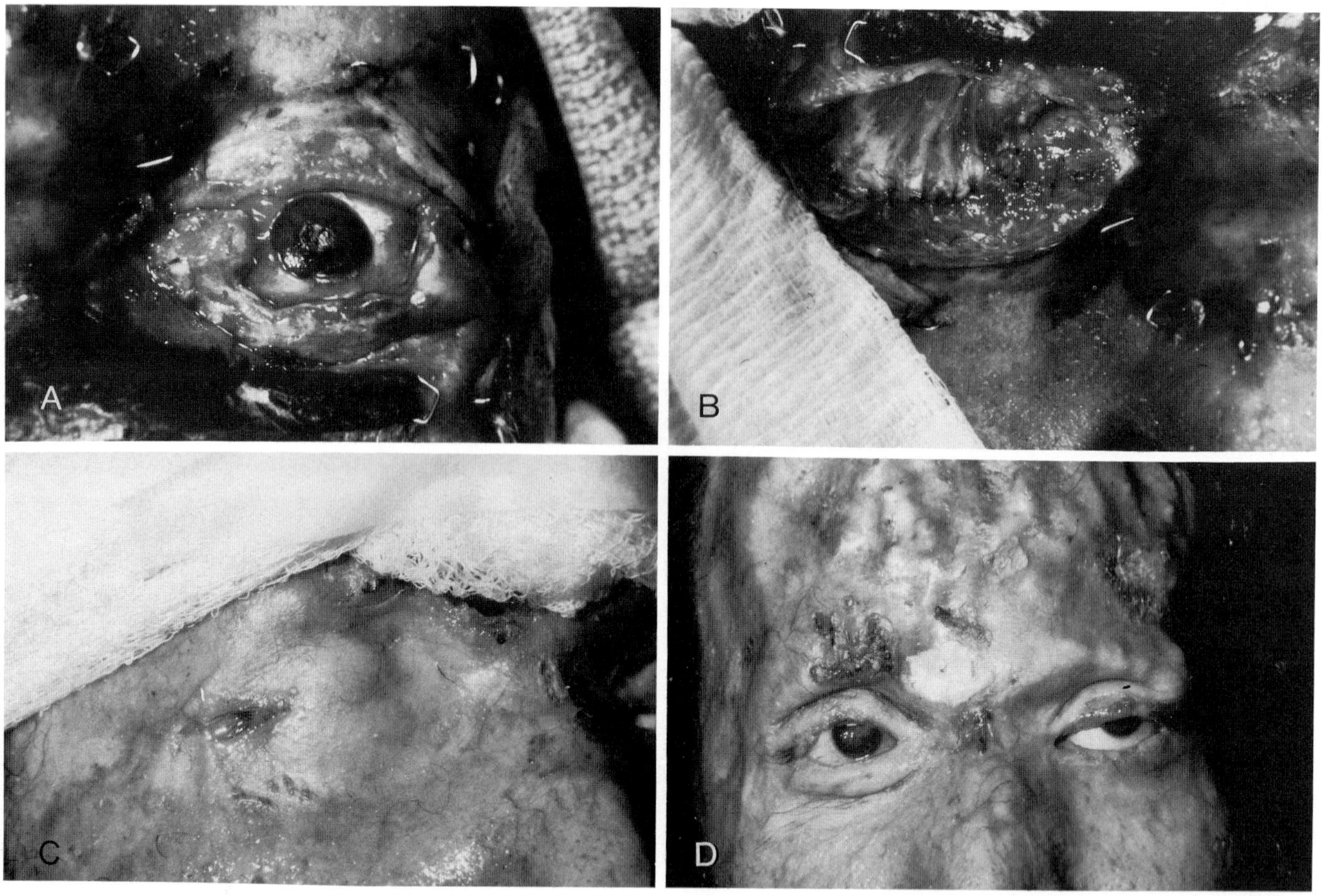

Figure 49.8. Slough of full-thickness upper lid and portion of lower lid. *A*, Loss of majority of upper lid tissue following high voltage electrical burn. Lower lid margin is also necrotic. *B*, Advancement of levator as a conjunctivally lined flap. *C*, Full-thickness skin graft over reconstructed upper lid and lower lid. Globe is now protected. *D*, Appearance after separation. Further reconstruction will be necessary.

degree burns is to use some form of conjunctival flap from the fornices or perhaps a tarsoconjunctival flap such as a modified Hughes' flap if it is the lower lid that sloughs. This will create a vascular bed, and a full-thickness graft can be placed over the vascular bed and then left for a period of time before separation. Loss of the upper lid is a greater problem because there is less tissue in the lower fornices to utilize and the opening and closing functions of the upper lid are impaired. The use of conjunctival flaps covered by skin grafts is a viable method of protecting the eye until further reconstruction can be accomplished.

Distant, tubed pedical flaps such as a deltopectoral flap can also be utilized to protect an eye, but these are very difficult to accomplish in a patient who is likely to have multiple burns in other areas of the body. These flaps are occasionally useful in late reconstruction, but the thickness of the skin in these areas makes the result less than satisfactory for eyelid reconstruction. The flaps must be lined with mucous membrane grafts and are more useful for the lower lid.

I have recently repaired the slough of virtually an entire upper lid and a portion of the lower lid by advancing the levator muscle. This was done after incising the horns in a fashion similar to levator resection surgery, but with an advancement rather than a resection. This provided an excellent vascular bed and good coverage along with the ability to open the lid. This was covered with a full-thickness graft. The lids now have been separated and appear to be functioning quite well, but a longer follow-up is necessary before recommending this procedure. All of these procedures to replace the loss of the entire upper lid with surrounding tissue suffer from the lack of orbicularis, which is necessary for lid closure. Obviously if coverage of the eye is not obtained by one of these procedures, the resultant exposure keratopathy will surely result in a corneal ulcer before long (Fig. 49.8).

LATE RECONSTRUCTION

After lid closure has been restored and the lids are protected and comfortable, it is then preferable, if possible, to wait until all inflammation and contracture is complete and the tissue is as supple as possible before any final surgery is performed. At times the cicatrization will continue, and it may be necessary to do an additional release

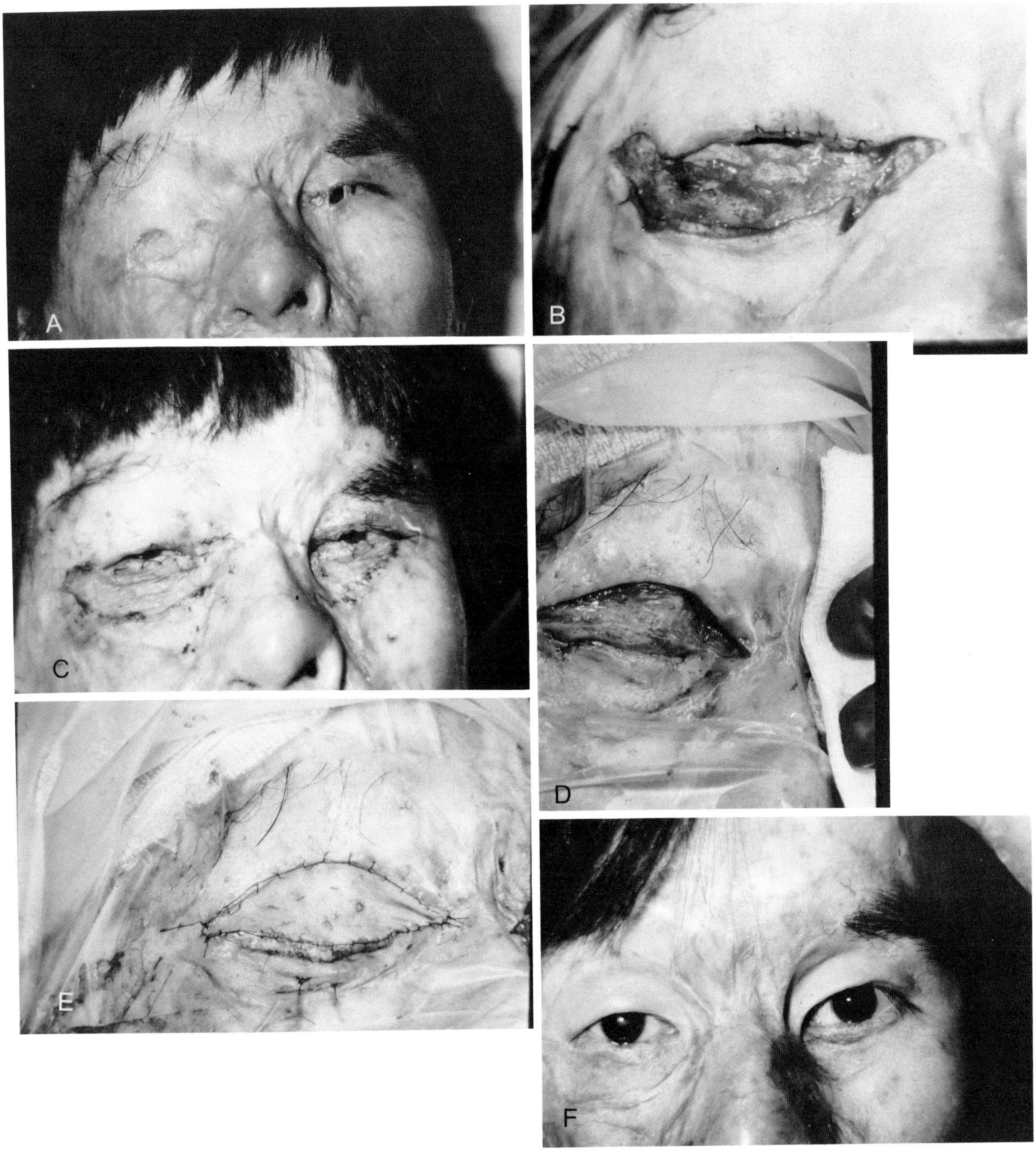

Figure 49.9. Late reconstruction. *A*, Same patient as in Figs. 49.1*D–F* and 49.3*C–F*. He is now 16 months after injury. Note the spontaneous fusion of the right lids and massive contracture. *B*, Release of right lower lid and excision of some thickened scars. *C*, Ten days following released lower lids and split-thickness grafts. Full-thickness graft was not done because very little donor skin was available. *D*, Release of left upper lid 1 month later. *E*, Full-thickness graft in position in left upper lid. Right side was done simultaneously. *F*, Result 18 months later. Note difference between full-thickness upper lid grafts and split-thickness lower lid grafts. Only one procedure per eyelid was done between panels *A* and *F*.

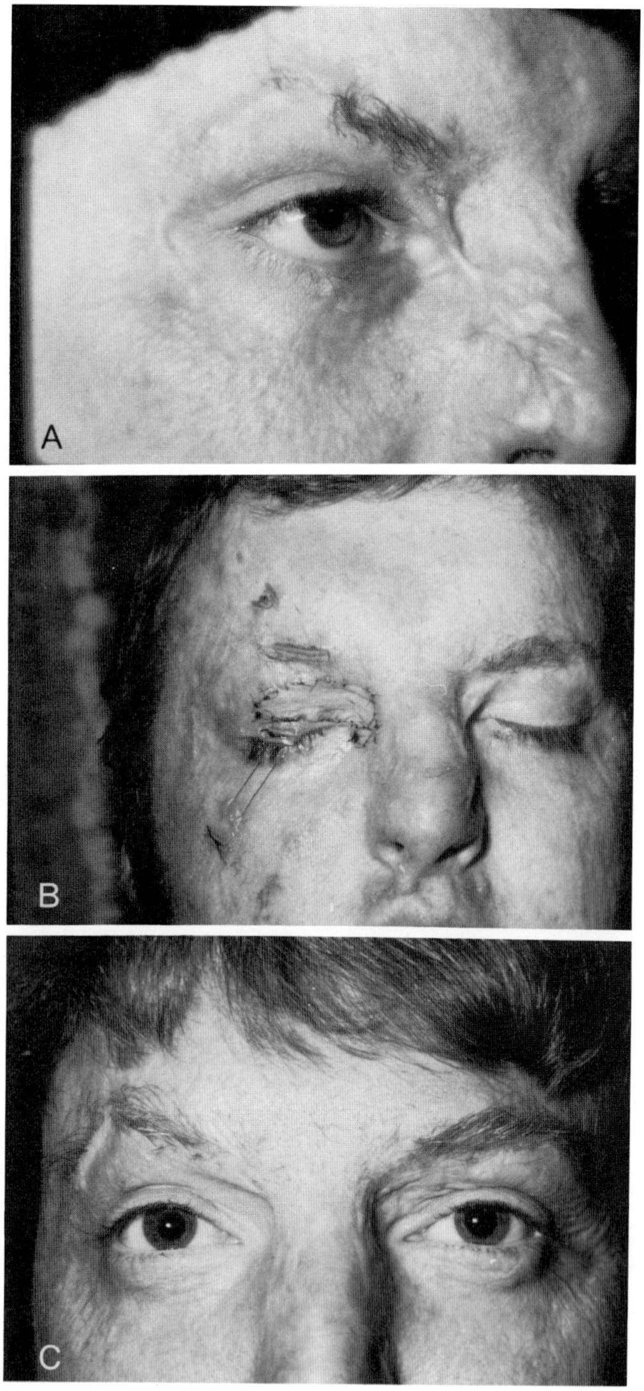

Figure 49.10. Canthal web repair. *A*, Patient 5 months after flash burn with lower lid graft already performed. Note nasal burns, which contribute to the densely scarred canthal web. *B*, Same patient 1 week following excision of web and full-thickness graft. Note unoperated web on left side. *C*, Patient several years later. Note the absence of webbing and the good cosmetic result of full-thickness grafts in both lower lids.

and graft before the inflammation has subsided. Although this is not the ideal time, a good result at this stage may eliminate further surgery.

Late reconstructive principles are the same as those for early reconstruction except that results are much more predictable because the underlying and surrounding tissue is not inflamed. It is important to remember that any further surgery in the paraorbital region, such as the nose or cheek, may have an effect on the lid. This surgery may add to or lessen the lid contraction and could consequently have a significant effect on the lid condition (Fig. 49.9).

A frequent occurrence in patients with deep nasal burns is webbing of the canthal tissues with pseudoepicanthal folds. If these folds are supple and caused by contracture on the nose, then multiple Z-plasties often work well. I have found that if the webs are densely scarred themselves,

Z-plasties are ineffective; I have obtained much better results by excising the entire scarred web and replacing it with a full-thickness graft (Fig. 49.10).

In late reconstructions as in the earlier phases, if thickened scar tissue or bands of tissue between grafts would result in an unsightly result, it is advisable to excise these areas if this will not compromise function. However, excision of wide areas of scars in the eyelid area is risky because of the potential destruction of underlying orbicularis. Also, excising scar tissue that has matured creates a wider area of fibrosis and contracture than would result by simply releasing the contracture. This should be done only if necessary and with caution.

SUMMARY

The proper treatment for severe eyelid burns is enhanced by early accurate assessment of the future course of the injury. Proper and careful planning of early skin grafting; tarsorrhaphies, if necessary; and later release and grafting will enhance the functional and cosmetic results. Attention to detail to ensure successful skin grafting is probably the single most important aspect of eyelid burn care that is under the surgeon's control. Eliminating future visual problems or chronic eye discomfort is a significant part of the rehabilitation of the severely burned patient.

SUGGESTED READINGS

Artz CP, Moncrief JA, Pruitt BA, Jr, et al: *Burns: A Team Approach.* WB Saunders, 1979.

Asch MJ, Moylan JA, Bruck HM, et al: Ocular complications associated with burns. Review of a five-year experience including 104 patients. *J Trauma* 11: 857–861, 1971.

Asch MJ, Pilger IS: Ophthalmological problems related to burn injury. *Eye Ear Nose Throat Mon* 54: 114–116, 1975.

Boswick JA, Jr: Burns of the head and neck. *Surg Clin North Am* 53: 97–104, 1973.

Burns CL, Chylack LT, Jr: Thermal burns: The Management of Thermal Burns of the Lids and Globes. *Ann Ophthalmol* 11: 1358–1368, 1979.

Chih-chun Y, Wei-shia H, Tsi-siang S, et al (eds): *Treatment of Burns.* Berlin, Shanghai Scientific and Technical Publishers and Springer-Verlag, 1982.

Constable JD, Carroll JM: The emergency treatment of the exposed cornea in thermal burns. *Plast Reconstr Surg* 48: 309–311, 1970.

Converse JM: Burn deformities of the face and neck. *Surg Clin North Am* 47: 323–354, 1967.

Converse JM, McCarthy JG, Dobrkovsky M, et al: Facial Burns, In Converse JM (ed): *Reconstructive Plastic Surgery.* Philadelphia, WB Saunders Company, 1957.

Converse JM, Smith B: Repair of severe burn ectropion of the eyelids. *Plast Reconstr Surg* 23: 21–26, 1959.

Ecker HA: Reconstruction of the eye socket and eyelids following deep burn. *Plast Reconstr Surg* 41: 278–279, 1968.

Edlich RF, Nichter LS, et al: Burns of the head and neck. *Otolaryngo Clin North Am* 17: 1984.

Falvey MP: Secondary correction of the burned eyelid deformity. *Plast Reconstr Surg* 62: 564–570, 1978.

Feller I, Grabb WC, et al (eds): *Reconstruction and Rehabilitation of the Burned Patient.* National Institute for Burn Medicine, 1979.

Goodwin CW: Current burn treatment. *Adv Surg* 18: 145–176, 1984.

Grabb WC, Smith JW, et al (eds): *Plastic Surgery, A Concise Guide to Clinical Practice.* 1973.

Guy RJ, Baldwin J, Kwedar S, et al: Three-years' experience in a regional burn center with burns of the eyes and eyelids. *Ophthal Surg* 13: 383–386, 1982.

Huang TT, Blackwell SJ, et al: Burn injuries of the eyelids. *Clin Plast Surg* 5: 571–581, 1978.

Hummel RP, et al (eds): *Clinical Burn Therapy.* Bristol, UI Wright & Sons, 1982.

Jackson DM, Roper-Hall MJ: Preservation of sight after complete destruction of the eyelids by burning. *Burns* 7: 221–226, 1983.

Khitrov FM: Clinical features and treatment of bilateral cicatricial deformities of the eyelids. *Acta Chir Plast* 26: 84–93, 1984.

Linhart RW: Burns of the eyes and eyelids. *Ann Ophthalmol* 10: 999–1001, 1978.

Luce EA, Hoopes JE: Electrical burn of the scalp and skull. *Plast Reconstr Surg* 54: 359–363, 1974.

Majno G, Gabbiani MG, Hirschel BS, Ryan GB, Statkov PR: Contraction of granulation tissue in vitro: similarity to smooth muscle. *Science* 173: 548–550, 1971.

Petajan JH, Voorhees KJ, et al: Extreme toxicity from combustion products of a fire-retarded polyurethan foam. *Science* 187: 742–744, 1975.

Records RE: Primary care of ocular emergencies. 2. Thermal, chemical and nontraumatic eye injuries. *Postgrad Med* 65: 157–163, 1979.

Rodeheaver GT, Hiebert JM, et al: Initial treatment of chemical skin and eye burns. *Compr Ther* 8: 37–43, 1982.

Rodeheaver GT, Kurtz L, et al: A promising new skin wound cleanser. *An Emerg Med* 9: 572–576, 1980.

Roper-Hall MJ: Thermal and chemical burns. *Trans Ophthalmol Soc UK* 85: 631–653, 1965.

Silverstein P, Peterson HD, Col MC: Treatment of eyelid deformities due to burns. *Plast Reconstr Surg* 51: 38–43, 1973.

Sloan DF, Huang TT: Reconstruction of eyelids and eyebrow in burned patients. *Plast Reconstr Surg* 58: 340–346, 1976.

Smith BC, Nesi FA: Upper lid loss due to formalin injection: Surgical reconstruction. *Ophthalmology* 86: 1951–1955, 14.

Soll DB, et al: *Management of Complications in Ophthalmic Plastic Surgery.* Birmingham, AL, Aesculapius, 1976.

Zaikova MV, Koroleva EV: A blepharoplasty indicated by consequences of thermomechanical injuries of eyelids. *Acta Chir Plast* 22: 232–240, 1980.

CHAPTER 50

Eyelid Burns: A General Plastic Surgeon's Approach

HAGAI TSUR, M.D.

The eyelids will be involved in most facial burns (1, 2). The globe itself, however, is infrequently involved, because of the reflex closing of the eyes during the occurrence of the injury. Most cases of corneal ulceration in burns are secondary to the development of eyelid deformities due to the burn injury and are therefore preventable; they are secondary to exposure keratitis and infection.

The eyelids are especially vulnerable in the acute stage because of the extremely thin and delicate skin and during the healing phase which is associated with the phenomenon of wound contraction. The tarsal plates that compose the "skeleton" on the eyelid are only loosely attached to the bony skeleton by the palpebral ligaments on both sides and by means of the relatively weak layer of the orbital septum to the periphery of the orbit. This is the reason why burns of the eyelids that are not watched and treated properly can often cause ocular damage and even loss of vision.

ETIOLOGICAL FACTORS AND CLASSIFICATION

As in all other burns there are three major etiological factors: thermal, chemical, and electrical (2–6).

Thermal burns can be caused by several mechanisms; flame and flash are the most common causes of eyelid burns; flame as a direct cause of ocular burn is uncommon. These burns are most commonly caused by house fires, that is to say they are flame burns, and only seldom are they caused by scalding or by electricity. Outdoor burns are usually caused by fires; a common factor is gasoline ignition. In industry most burns are chemically induced and are caused by chemical splashes of either acid or alkaline sources. Electrical burns of the eye are extremely rare.

In thermal injuries the degree of the injury is a function of two factors: temperature and exposure time. In flash burns, for instance, there is intense heat that acts momentarily, and therefore the degree of the injury is usually slight and superficial. In flame burns, however, the damage is usually deep since the time of exposure to the heat is prolonged and causes relatively massive destruction of tissues.

Skin burns are usually divided into three groups according to the depth of the damage to the skin: The first degree is the most superficial; the damage is confined to the epidermal layer only. Clinically a first-degree burn is manifested by erythema alone. In the second-degree burn there is partial dermal loss, and clinically it is characterized by vesication. In the third-degree burn there is destruction of the full-thickness of the skin, and clinically it appears as a dry pale surface.

In chemical burns, the extent of the injury varies according to the inocuous agent; it may vary from simple conjunctival irritation to massive destruction of the cornea, conjunctiva, and eyelids. Acid burns are usually self-limiting and the damage is usually superficial, unless the contact was prolonged. Alkali burns, on the other hand, cause much more extensive tissue destruction.

In electrical burns the damage is caused as a result of

the heat and the electrical current itself. The amount of damage is related to the intensity of the current, to its voltage, and to the resistance of the areas through which the current travels (7). The characteristic feature of electrical burns is that the damage is progressive. The electrical burn usually damages the skin of the face and eyelids, and only seldom is there direct damage to the globe itself. In cases where the globe is damaged, the pathological changes are usually very extensive and severe; most of the global structures are affected and usually exontheration of the globe and orbit is necessary.

EARLY EVALUATION AND TREATMENT

The early treatment depends on the etiological factor, therefore, a careful history is important. For example, a chemical burn should be treated by continuous copious irrigation and a thermal injury should be treated by application of cold compresses.

A careful initial examination of the eye should be performed at the time of the patient's arrival to the hospital, regardless of the severity of the patient's general condition. This is extremely important since in 24 hours a thorough eye examination is much more difficult to perform because of the severe swelling that develops, necessitating the use of lid retractors. Usually it is very hard to determine initially the degree of involvement of the eyelids. Parameters that usually serve to determine the depth of a burn are not always clear because of the rapidly developing edema in this region. Analgesia to pin prick for instance, which helps in diagnosing third-degree burns in other parts of the body, is unreliable in the eyelids. The appearance of the burn surface is not helpful in diagnosis either: it might look red, pale, or even black and yet be of partial thickness only.

The degree of visual impairment, if present, is examined by checking visual acuity using a simple eye chart or finger-counting. The conjunctiva and cornea are examined directly and also be fluorescein staining with ultraviolet light for detection of any corneal injury.

Chemosis or diffuse conjunctival swelling, which usually indicate conjunctival injury, are not reliable in a case of burn injury since such physical signs can be produced by overhydration during the first stage of burn resuscitation.

EARLY TREATMENT OF THE OCULAR BURN

In chemical burns, copious continuous irrigation with water, saline, or any other bland solution has to be performed for 24–48 hours to achieve efficient corneal lavage. We do not recommend the use of neutralizing solutions since these can cause additional damage (see Chapter 47).

In thermal burns, it is very important to perform close monitoring of the conjunctiva and cornea, by frequent inspection, especially in a patient who is partially alert or obtunded and cannot report the early signs of corneal involvement, which are pain and blurred vision. Conjunctivitis, which is associated with swelling and suppuration, should be treated by repeated irrigations of the eye and instillation of antibiotic eye solutions and ointments three to four times daily. Usually the conjunctivitis will subside within a few days.

Thermal injury of the cornea is diagnosed by the finding of proteinaceous coagulation on the corneal surface (3). Treatment is by topical antibiotics and close inspection by fluorescein stainings for prevention of corneal ulceration. If corneal abrasion or ulceration develops, it should be treated by antibiotics, cycloplegics, and patching. A culture should be taken and frequent slitlamp examinations should be performed to determine efficacy of the treatment. If a deep ulcer develops, it should be treated surgically by a conjunctival flap. As stated earlier, a true flame burn of the cornea is rare; the injury to the cornea associated with the burn injury is caused usually not by the flame itself but by foreign bodies in an explosion.

The initial corneal treatment is preventive; its aim is to protect and moisten the corneal epithelium by instillation of the ophthalmic drops and ointments. The patient's head should be kept elevated in order to decrease the amount of conjunctival and palpebral edema.

EARLY TREATMENT OF THE PALPEBRAL BURN

As mentioned previously, it is difficult or impossible to determine initially the depth of the eyelid burn; the diagnosis is actually made retrospectively by the progress of the healing process and the response to treatment. Burns that do not heal spontaneously within 3 weeks are defined as third-degree burns of full-thickness dermal damage. These burns will cause permanent deformities during the postburn course.

An experienced clinician can make a gross distinction in distinguishing between the most superficial burns from the deep ones, which include those with partial dermal damage and those with total dermal burns. Superficial burns heal spontaneously within a relatively short period of about 1 week and do not leave any permanent deformity. This type of burn is usually caused by scalding or flash explosions. The treatment is minimal. In the immediate postburn period, ice saline soaks should be employed in order to prevent progressive damage and decrease the palpebral edema. In order to prevent wound sepsis, topical antibacterial agents like sulfamylon are used; these may cause burning and stinging sensations but are not toxic to the eye.

The superficial burns will heal within 5–7 days, and the deep ones will form within this period a black eschar. At this stage, loose wet soaks are applied to facilitate separation of the eschar and cleansing of the sloughing wound. If infection does not develop in the deep burn, one can expect that those burns in which the dermal damage was partial will heal spontaneously by epithelialization without necessitating resurfacing by skin grafts. This process takes place between the tenth and fourteenth postburn day.

In the full-thickness burn, the eschar is usually thick and its separation is slower—between 14 and 21 days. A layer of granulation tissue will appear underneath the separating eschar, which will have to be resurfaced by skin grafting. It has to be stressed that the method of treating the facial and palpebral burn wound described above is relatively conservative compared with the rather aggressive approach to the burn wound in other parts of the body. There I usually recommend early excision and grafting of the burn wound, whereas in the face, I firmly believe that the method described gives better results and in many cases saves unnecessary surgery.

THE TARSORRHAPHY ISSUE

Review of the medical literature reveals that a few authors still recommend the use of tarsorrhaphy in the early stages of treatment of palpebral burns for the purpose of preventing corneal exposure (8).

I feel, and so do other authors (1, 6), very strongly against this approach. My experience has shown that the tarsorrhaphy cannot prevent the development of ectropion in a later postburn stage. A tarsorrhaphy is very difficult to perform in an eyelid that is extremely edematous and with friable lid margins, and in most cases the chances of its holding successfully are poor. In those cases where the tarsorrhaphy does hold, the patient ends up with severe permanent deformity of the lid margin (Fig. 50.1). Only in extremely severe cases of corneal exposure that cannot be overcome by conservative means is there justification for performing a tarsorrhaphy single-thickness on both lids that can allow separation in a later stage (6).

In the early edema phase, there is actually no need for a tarsorrhaphy: the eyelids are closed by the swelling, thus protecting the cornea, which is even difficult to get at for examination (Fig. 50.2). Following the absorption of the edema, but before the separation of the eschar from the eyelids, usually the normal protective function of the eyelids is maintained; it is only after spontaneous healing by epithelialization or skin grafting, that the wound contraction forces start to act. These forces, however, are too powerful for the tarsorrhaphy to overcome.

Instead of performing a tarsorrhaphy, I prefer to watch the eye closely in order to prevent exposure keratitis and chronic conjunctivitis and infection, which are the potential hazardous complications of a developing ectropion. This is done by protecting the eye with ointments; if this proves ineffective, an early reconstruction of the eyelids is performed. This will also be performed in cases where the rest of the patient's burn wound is not completely covered.

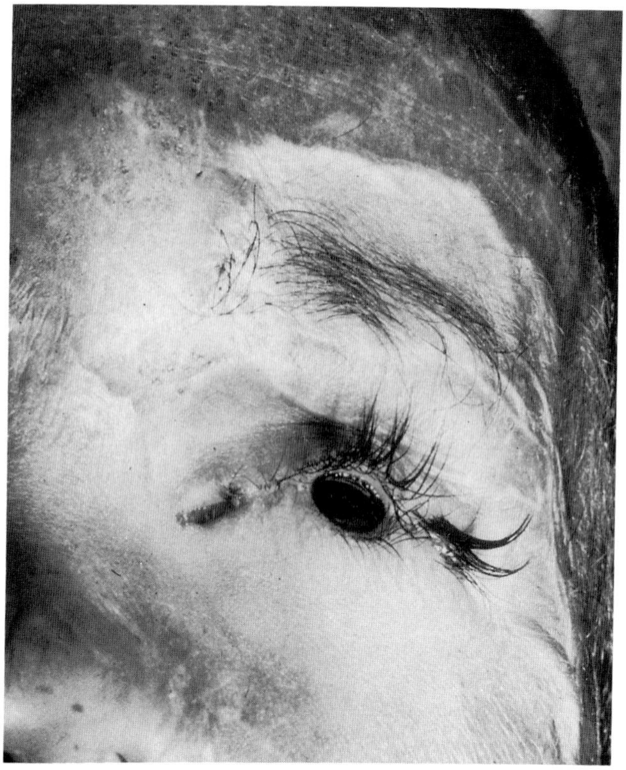

Figure 50.1. Tarsorrhaphy that caused severe deformity of the eyelids.

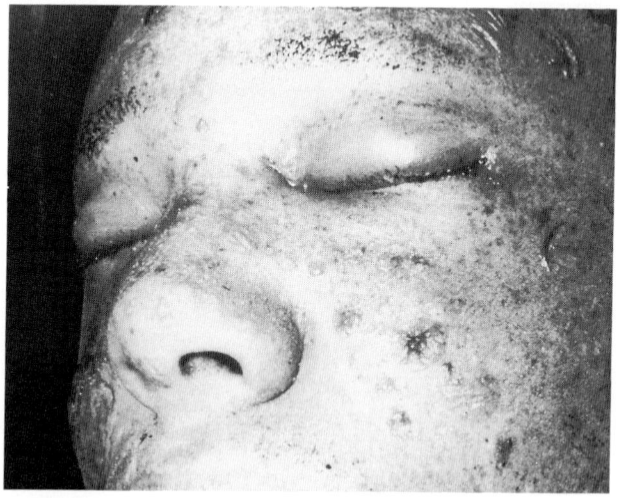

Figure 50.2. Acute facial burn involving the eyelids. Severe palpebral edema prevents opening of the eye, thus providing corneal protection.

SURGICAL TREATMENT DURING THE SUBACUTE AND CHRONIC STAGES

All palpebral burns are resurfaced within a few weeks from the time of injury, either spontaneously or by a skin graft. If the palpebral burn was relatively superficial and the surrounding facial skin was not injured, then the situation will remain static. In cases where the burn was deep and had to be grafted, or even if it was spontaneously resurfaced by epithelialization, a progressive process of wound contracture and scar hypertrophy will take place.

This process will cause severe deformities that will have to be either prevented or surgically corrected.

This postburn wound contraction process in the eyelid is similar to that which takes place after a healing burn wound in any other part of the body, but here the scar contracture affects the eyelid more severely, causing a special clinical manifestation because of the eyelid's loose skeletal connections.

The most common deformity in the eyelid is the ectropion, which results in vertical shortening of the eyelid (Fig. 50.3). If the skin surrounding the eye region was affected as well, the deformities will be more severe; in fact, a deformity of the eyelid can develop even in cases where the eyelid was spared and only the surrounding tissues were burnt. Skin contracture of the cheeks, nose, or forehead and temporal regions will exert tension on the eyelids and the canthi. The lower eyelid is more affected by the process of scar contracture since it has less loose skin available than the upper lid.

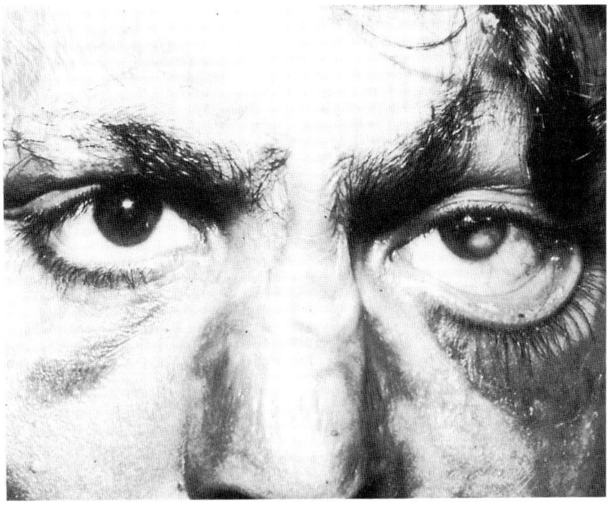

Figure 50.3. Cicatricial ectropion of the lower eyelid.

SURGICAL TREATMENT DURING THE ACUTE STAGE

Soon after the separation of the eschar, the raw surface should be resurfaced with a skin graft, both in full-thickness and in deep dermal burns. It is true that in deep dermal burns, one can expect spontaneous epithelialization but this will result in more severe contracture than with skin grafting.

A relatively thick split-thickness skin graft of 14-18/1000 inch is being employed. This type of skin graft revascularizes well and provides resurfacing of better quality than the thin split-thickness skin grafts.

In cases where surgery has to be postponed because of the patient's general condition, the granulation tissue might become hypertrophic. In such an event the soft superficial layer should be scraped mechanically from the firm, well-vascularized base underneath, prior to the skin grafting, or this soft hypertrophic layer can be flattened by 0.25–0.5% hydrocortisone solution soaks for 24–48 hours prior to surgery. Systemic antibiotic treatment should commence prior to surgery.

LATE COMPLICATIONS

These complications develop as a result of intrinsic factors due to the process of wound contracture in the eyelids themselves, as well as a result of extrinsic factors, such as contracture of scarred or grafted tissues in areas adjacent to the eyelids. When both of these factors exist, the extrinsic causes should be resolved first, and only then should the intrinsic factors be dealt with.

The process of wound contracture takes place in burnt areas that have healed spontaneously, as well as in grafted areas; it is more severe in thin grafts than in thick ones.

This active process of wound contracture continues for about a year postburn, and then the situation becomes static. During this year deformities may occur, the most common of which is lid ectropion. If it is at all possible, corneal exposure that develops during this period should be dealt with conservatively; the definitive surgical repair should be postponed to the static phase because then the changes of recurrence are minimized (34). Conservative treatment includes artificial tears, eye ointments, and blinking exercises. I do not recommend performing tarsorrhaphy for the reasons mentioned earlier. If corneal exposure cannot be controlled conservatively, my choice is to operate, knowing that an additional operation will probably be required for recurrent ectropion, rather than to perform a tarsorrhaphy that will result in a deformity.

Definitive reconstructive surgery starts approximately 1 year after the burn; by that time the hypertrophic scars become paler and softer and, most importantly, there is a slight degree of mobility of the scars or grafted areas on the underlying tissues due to the development of loose connective tissue underneath the scars.

Lower Lid Ectropion

Lower lid ectropion is the most common eyelid burn complication (Fig. 50.4) (8, 9). It usually appears a few weeks to a few months following the burn injury. The treatment during the acute and convalescent period is nonsurgical and only after about 1 year is a surgical release indicated. The indications for surgical intervention are corneal exposure and epiphora, as well as cosmetic considerations.

An opening incision is performed immediately under the ciliary margin from canthus to canthus and is extended laterally and slightly superiorly for about 1.5 cm beyond the lateral canthus. All cicatricial tissues are removed, and the skin is released as much as possible. The lid is pulled toward the superior orbital rim by traction sutures placed in the lid margin, overlapping the upper lid in order to create the largest possible defect, to account for future graft contracture.

A full-thickness skin graft is preferred here. Its main advantage is its minimal postoperative contracture. The best donor site regarding texture and color match is of course the face itself; theoretically the upper eyelid should be preferred, but in the vast majority of cases it is also

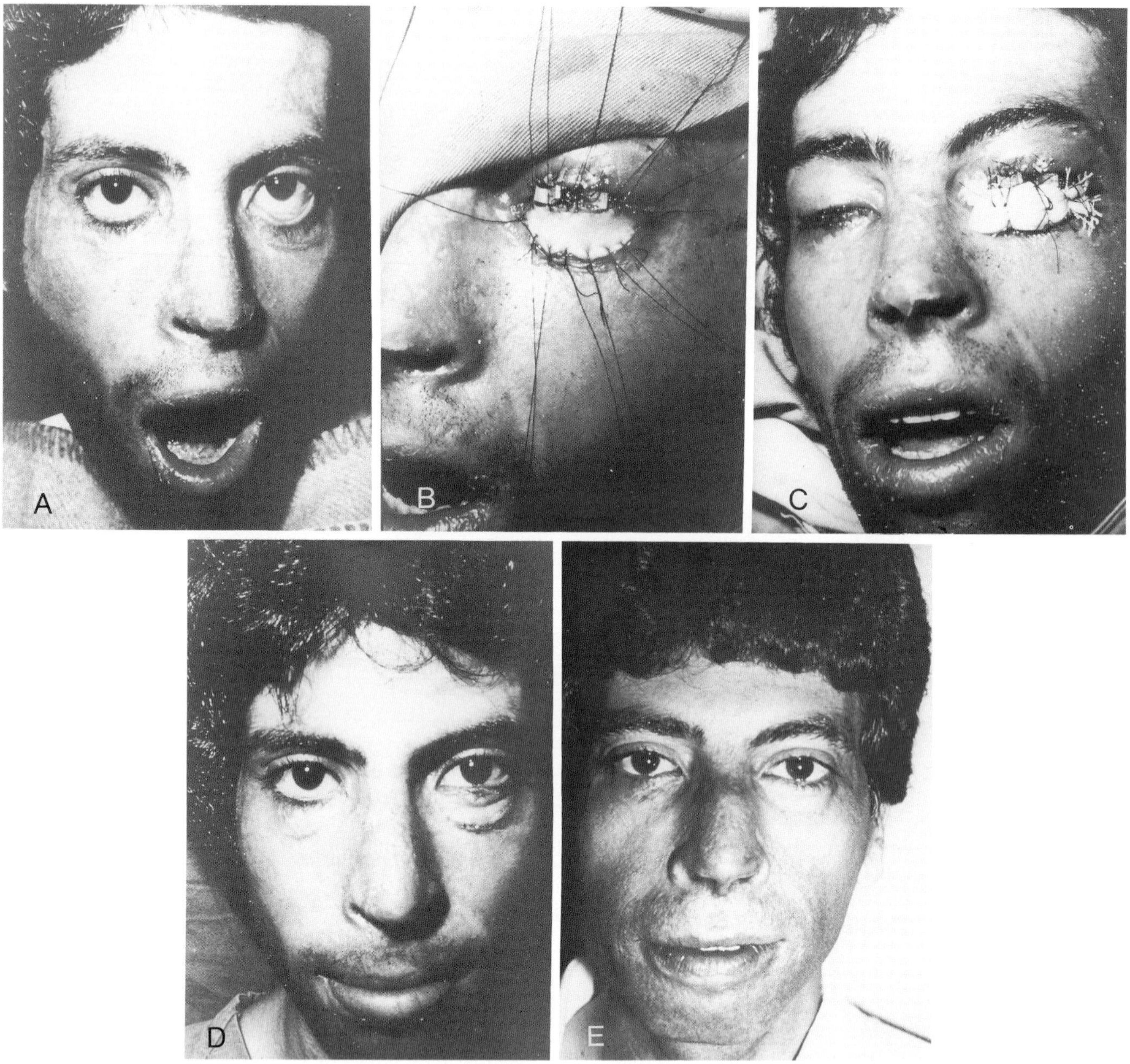

Figure 50.4. Surgical release of lower lid ectropion achieved through use of postauricular full-thickness skin graft. *A*, Lower lid ectropion, most pronounced when facial skin stretches while the patient fully opens the mouth. *B*, Full-thickness graft applied. Note overcorrection. *C*, Tie-over dressing applied. *D*, Two weeks postoperative. *E*, Five years postoperative.

involved and its quantity is limited. For this reason, retroauricular skin is most frequently used. The retroauricular skin is relatively thin and its take is good. If this area is involved as well in the burn injury and is not available, the supraclavicular skin or the upper inner arm skin is used, despite the fact that their color match is inferior to the postauricular skin. The graft is fixed in position by a tie-over dressing for about 5 days.

Upper Lid Ectropion

The upper eyelid is the one that normally protects the cornea. Marked retraction will cause drying of the cornea with resulting corneal damage (Fig. 50.5). In most cases, in spite of upper lid retraction or erosion, patients are still capable of protecting their corneas effectively, mainly because of Bell's phenomenon, which is the upward rotation of the eyeball during sleep or attempted lid closure. An additional indication for surgical correction is obviously the cosmetic consideration.

The upper lid requires a thinner skin graft in order to retain mobility, in contrast to the less mobile lower lid, where a thicker graft will provide support and stability.

Here it is also extremely important to put the skin graft in excess in order to counteract subsequent contracture.

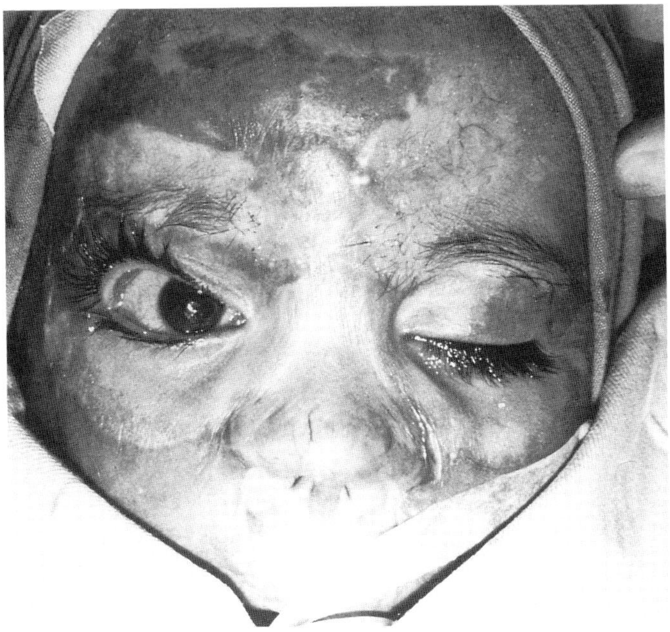

Figure 50.5. Severe ectropion of upper eyelid. (Photograph taken while patient attempts to close the eye.)

A similar transverse incision across the whole lid is performed; this incision extends laterally into the temporal region. All scar tissue is carefully removed, and the lid is pulled down by traction sutures and released until it is overlapping the lower lid. The raw surface is covered with the skin graft, which is secured and fixed with a tie-over dressing for about 5 days. If both eyelids of the same eye require surgical repair, one lid is repaired and the other one is left to a subsequent session. However, if two upper eyelids or two lower lids necessitate surgery, they can be corrected at the same operating session. This is in spite of the fact that the patient's vision will be obscured for a few days.

Medial Canthal Deformities

Prominent medial canthal scarring occurs usually when there is a deep palpebral burn with burns in the adjacent nasal bridge area. It can also be an outcome of palpebral and nasal resurfacing (10).

The medial canthal scarring takes the form of a hood or an epicanthal hypertrophic fold. There is in some cases a forward displacement of the medial canthus with forward displacement of the lacrimal puncta, which causes epiphora.

The repair of this pericanthal scarring is accomplished by excising the scar, releasing the canthus and replacing it to its normal position, and resurfacing the raw area thus created with a skin graft. In the cases where the scarring takes the form of a band rather than a hood or a hypertrophic mass, a regular Z-plasty or a double interlocking Z-plasty can correct the deformity.

Symblepharon

Symblepharon is a rare complication of burns of the eye region, since a burn that will injure the palpebral and bulbar conjunctiva will usually destroy the globe and will necessitate enucleation in an early stage. Surgical correction is by release of the adhesions between the eyelid and the eyeball and resurfacing by a conjunctival flap or a free mucosal graft.

Eyebrow Deformities

The degree of the cicatricial damage to the brow varies from partial to complete alopecia, depending on the severity and depth of the burn injury. The reconstruction can be performed either by a composite graft of hair-bearing scalp or by a scalp island flap. The method of repair depends on the amount of damage, and the vascular condition of the region.

The composite hair-bearing scalp grafts require almost ideal conditions for complete take. They are limited in size, and in order for them to undergo satisfactory vascularization, they should be narrow and not exceed a width of 5 mm. Therefore, in many cases there is partial failure, which results in hairless spaces between the grafts because of the poor vascularity of the recipient site that is in the midst of heavy scar tissue.

Better results are achieved by using an island scalp flap based on a branch of the superficial temporal artery. In both techniques, attention should be given to the design of the flap in reference to the direction of the hair growth. Usually if the graft is taken from the vicinity of the ipsilateral mastoid area, there is good match of the transferred tissue in texture, density, and direction of growth of the hair as compared with a normal brow (Fig. 50.6).

The patient's gender also influences the choice of the procedure: Because women can camouflage a missing eyebrow deformity nicely, especially if it is partial, by using makeup and an eyebrow pencil, a free composite graft can be used satisfactorily in them; in males, who require a thick, bushy eyebrow, a flap procedure is preferable.

SUMMARY

In most facial burns there is some involvement of the eyelids. The initial treatment of eyelid and adnexal structures must be aimed at protecting the corneal surface and maintaining a clean wound that is free of sepsis.

Ocular complications do not endanger life, but do cause high morbidity rate and may cause loss of vision if not treated early and properly.

There are complications in the globe, mainly conjunctivitis and corneal exposure and ocular adnexal complications, mostly lid ectropion. Very often the ocular problems are neglected because of the patient's severe general condition, and these non-life-saving problems seem to be secondary. However, an early diagnosis should be achieved by conducting a thorough examination regardless of the

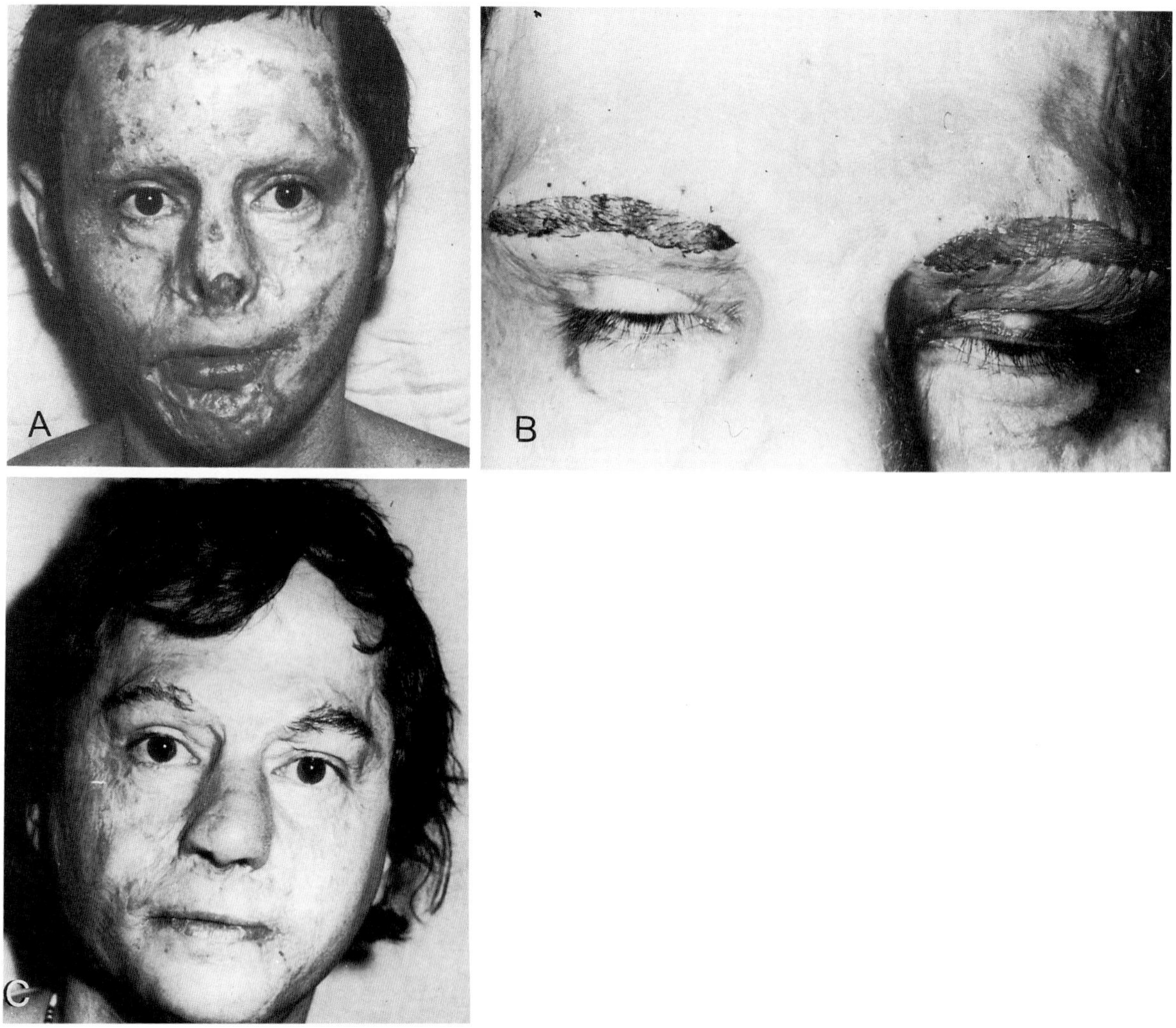

Figure 50.6. Reconstruction of eyebrows with a free composite hair-bearing scalp flap. *A*, Preoperative. *B*, Immediately postoperative. *C*, Two years postoperative. (Patient also had reconstruction of nose, lips, and chin.)

patient's discomfort. An aggressive and effective conservative treatment should be started prophylactically, or for curative purposes if complications have appeared already.

The initial treatment of eyelid burns should include efforts for protecting the corneal surface. Corneal exposure is encountered in the early recovery period because of damage to the eyelid either by the burn itself or by secondary infection; in the subacute and chronic postburn recovery stage corneal exposure due to lid contracture because of wound contracture in the eyelid itself or as a result of traction of adjacent scarred areas.

REFERENCES

1. Frank DH, Wachtel T, Frank HA: The early treatment and reconstruction of eyelid burns. *J Trauma* 23: 874–877, 1983.
2. Huang TT, Blackwell SJ, Lewis SR: Burn injuries of the eyelids. *Clin Plast Surg* 5: 571–581, 1978.
3. Asch MJ, Moylan JM, Bruck HM, Pruitt BA: Ocular complications associated with burns: review of a 5-year experience including 104 patients. *J Trauma* 11: 857–861, 1971.
4. Burns CL, Chylack LT: Thermal burns: the management of thermal burns of the lids and globes. *Ann Ophthalmol* 11: 1358–1368, 1979.
5. Linhart RW: Burns of the eyes and eyelids. *Ann Ophthalmol* 10: 999–1001, 1978.
6. Schofield AL: A review of burns of the eyelids and their treatment. *Br J Plast Surg* 7: 67–91, 1954.
7. Bienfang DC, Zakov ZN, Albert DM: Severe electrical burn of the eye. *Graefes Arch Ophthalmol* 214: 147–153, 1980.
8. Silverstein P, Peterson HD: Treatment of eyelid deformities due to burns. *Plast Reconstr Surg* 51: 38–43, 1973.
9. Sloan DF, Huang TT, Larson D, Lewis SR: Reconstruction of eyelids and eyebrows in burned patients. *Plast Reconstr Surg* 58: 340–346, 1976.
10. Converse JM, Smith B: Repair of severe burn ectropion of the eyelids. *Plast Reconstr Surg* 23: 21–26, 1959.

SECTION VIII

COSMETIC OPHTHALMIC PLASTIC SURGERY

CHAPTER 51

Evaluation of the Cosmetic Surgery Patient

MICHAEL PATIPA, M.D., F.A.C.S.

The preoperative evaluation of patients considering cosmetic eyelid surgery should assess the physical conditions to be improved and the psychological motives for the desired cosmetic change; it should also determine whether the patient's expectations are realistic and attainable. Careful consideration of these details will help prevent postoperative complications and dissatisfaction.

The preoperative evaluation may commence by inquiry into what type of cosmetic surgery the patient desires. Some surgical candidates have spent many hours studying their eyes and eyelids in the mirror while anticipating and planning for cosmetic surgery. They may quickly and succinctly outline their goals and expectations. Individuals who can describe their surgical goals and express realistic expectations are generally good candidates for cosmetic surgery.

An impulsive decision to undergo cosmetic surgery is frequently inspired in the hope that a changed physical appearance will convert an unpleasant situation in one's life. Such individuals frequently have unrealistic expectations of the results they can secure from cosmetic surgery. Thus, an individual in the midst of a midlife crisis who expects a cosmetic blepharoplasty to turn the clock back 20 years will be dissatisfied following surgery, when he or she neither feels nor looks 20 years younger.

Recently widowed individuals who intend cosmetic surgery to serve as a means for reentry into the social world will still be burdened by grief and insecurity following surgery if they have not resolved their personal emotions prior to undergoing surgery.

It should be clear that cosmetic surgery candidates require careful, detailed discussion and evaluation prior to surgery (1). Surgery should be postponed or even denied to individuals with severe personal and emotional problems until they have had the opportunity to resolve those conditions that inappropriately motivate their quest for cosmetic improvement. This will help the surgeon from failing to provide those patients with satisfactory results (2).

An excellent method for patients to explain their surgical goals is by providing a small hand mirror and asking them to demonstrate which features they would like changed or corrected (Fig. 51.1). This also provides the surgeon an opportunity to separate those individuals with realistic expectations from those with unrealistic or unattainable surgical goals (3). Individuals requesting removal of all the fine wrinkles and laugh lines, those pulling their canthi laterally in an attempt to obtain almond-shaped oriental eyelids, and those who desire their deep nasolabial folds to be smoothed via a blepharoplasty must be informed that conventional cosmetic eyelid surgery will not succeed in accomplishing these goals.

An additional benefit of providing patients the opportunity to describe and exhibit their surgical goals is that this period provides the surgeon an opportunity to carefully observe the patients under relaxed conditions while they are preoccupied with their discussion. It is important to take this opportunity for observation as the patient will inevitably become tense as the surgeon approaches and begins the physical examination.

A common chief complaint among patients requesting cosmetic upper eyelid surgery is a sensation of heaviness of the upper eyelids. This may be accompanied by complaints of excessive upper eyelid skin, functional visual complaints including aesthenopia (i.e., eye fatigue) late in the day, obstruction of the superior field of vision due to

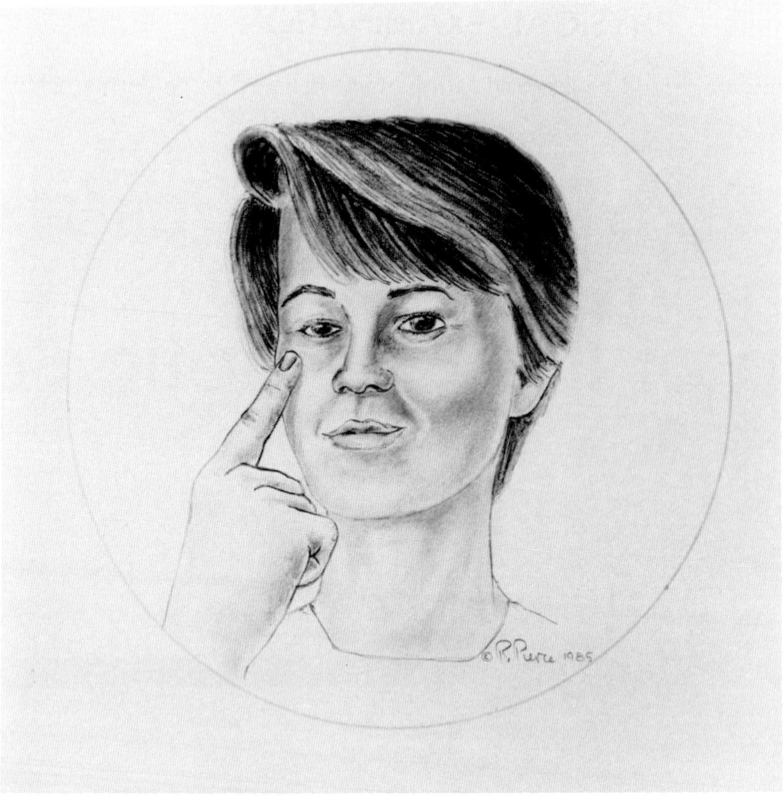

Figure 51.1. Cosmetic surgery candidates should be given the opportunity to exhibit the features they would like changed or cosmetically improved.

the overhanging eyelid skin, or the sensation of peering through their eyelashes in upgaze. Listening to and recording such complaints is important in order to direct the physical examination toward recognition of the true etiology of the symptoms. The differential diagnosis of complaints such as difficulty in keeping one's eyelids open should include belpharoptosis, eyebrow ptosis, severe dermatochalasis, blepharospasm, or myasthenia gravis. In addition, documenting visual symptoms and complaints may be important for proper completion of insurance forms many months following surgery.

MEDICAL HISTORY

The history should include questions regarding both the ocular and medical history. A history of strabismus, amblyopia, eye patching as a child, or previous ocular surgery or ocular trauma should be obtained. If the patient has undergone previous strabismus, eyelid, orbital, or retinal surgery, they may be at increased risk of orbital hemorrhage due to orbital neovascularization.

A history of previous cosmetic eyelid surgery forewarns the surgeon to expect scar tissue and more bleeding than usual. It also serves to caution the surgeon toward conservative excision of skin and orbicularis muscle in order to prevent overcorrection and the possible complications of ectropion or lagophthalmos.

On occasion, the patient may not be aware of a monocular decrease in vision. The recognition of poor vision prior to surgery avoids the possibility of having the visual impairment discovered following the procedure and blamed on the surgery. In addition, a decision to perform elective cosmetic surgery on a monocular individual must be carefully considered in determining the type of procedure such a patient may safely undergo (4–6).

Systemic disorders such as diabetes mellitus, sickle cell disease, or other conditions that might cause visual impairment should be addressed. Patients with thyroid orbitopathy, uncontrolled hypertension, or bleeding diathesis may be predisposed to orbital hemorrhage and risk of visual loss.

A history of current medications should specifically include questions regarding the use of anticoagulants, aspirin, or aspirin-containing compounds. These medications alter normal platelet function and normal blood clotting. Following consultation with the patient's medical physician and obtaining medical clearance, the patient should discontinue anticoagulants or aspirin 2 weeks prior to surgery.

PHYSICAL EXAMINATION

The patient's general facial features should be assessed. A round- or moon-faced individual may have orbital fullness. Attempts to surgically eliminate the prominent fat pockets and provide tight eyelid skin and deep eyelid creases may result in an unnatural appearance of exophthalmic eyes.

EYEBROW EXAMINATION

The eyebrows require careful attention during the examination of a patient for upper eyelid surgery (7). As the surgeon sits facing the patient, the patient is asked to close the eyes and relax the forehead in order to reduce any elevation of the eyelids and eyebrows by the frontalis muscle. The eyebrow is palpated with one or two fingers and the location relative to the supraorbital rim is noted. The eyebrow normally inserts at or above the level of the supraorbital rim. In insertion is below the supraorbital rim, the ptotic eyebrow may push the underlying eyelid tissue down, over the visual axis or field of vision. This is frequently the etiology of the heaviness or fatigued eyelid sensation of which patients complain.

Segmental eyebrow ptosis may occur nasally or temporally or the entire eyebrow may be ptotic. The surgeon should lift the eyebrow with two fingers to a position just above the supraorbital rim. This frequently results in a dramatic reduction of the excessive upper eyelid tissue that was believed to be dermatochalasis but was actually due to the ptotic eyebrows. Usually, correction of the eyebrow ptosis alone provides satisfactory cosmetic and functional results. Those patients who undergo eyebrow ptosis repair combined with upper eyelid blepharoplasty will require significantly less upper eyelid skin excision following the eyebrow elevation.

Failure to recognize the presence of eyebrow ptosis may result in excessive upper eyelid skin excision during the blepharoplasty and increased eyebrow ptosis, because of the eyebrows having been pulled further down by the upper eyelid skin excision.

If a coronal eyebrow elevation procedure is considered for the correction of eyebrow ptosis, one must look for the presence of a high forehead, receding hairline, or thinning hair. These findings, particularly in a male, may contraindicate a coronal brow elevation and indicate a midforehead or suprabrow elevating procedure. The presence of glabellar wrinkles and forehead rhytides should be noted as these may also be corrected at the time of a coronal brow elevation.

Suprabrow tissue excision for eyebrow elevation, when properly performed, provides excellent functional and cosmetic improvement. It is important to carefully measure the amount of tissue to be excised preoperatively (Fig. 51.2). Place a dot with a felt-tip pen within the top row of

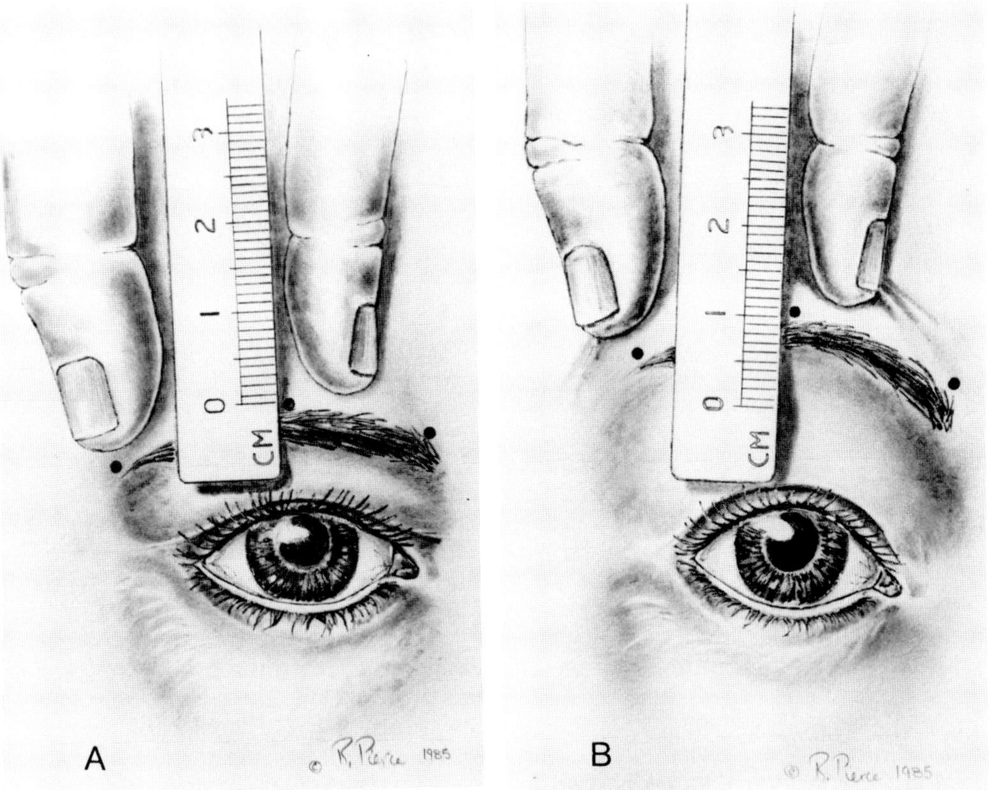

Figure 51.2. *A*, Ink dots are placed at the medial, central, and lateral third of the ptotic eyebrow. The dots are aligned with a millimeter ruler. *B*, The eyebrow is elevated to the intended postsurgical height and the number of millimeters traversed is recorded.

cilia of the eyebrow at the medial, central, and lateral thirds of each eyebrow. A millimeter ruler is oriented perpendicular to the eyebrow and the ink dot aligned with a point on the ruler. The eyebrow is elevated to the intended postsurgical height and the number of millimeters the dot has traversed is recorded. This is the amount of tissue to be excised. Measurements are performed in each third of the eyebrow. The eyebrow elevation generally measures approximately 10 mm.

UPPER EYELID EXAMINATION

As mentioned earlier, careful evaluation and detailed surgical planning are necessary in order to attain satisfactory results from cosmetic eyelid surgery. Men and women undergoing upper eyelid blepharoplasty surgery generally expect elimination of their excessive upper eyelid skin and bulging fatty pockets. Women additionally may request a deep supratarsal sulcus and high lid-crease appearance, as well as a smoothed pretarsal surface as a bed for their makeup application.

Skin Fat Examination

With the patient seated and looking straight ahead, the excessive upper eyelid skin is gently lifted up and away from the pretarsal surface of the upper eyelid. Having already assessed the extent the eyebrow contributes to the patient's dermatochalasis, the surgeon can estimate the amount of excessive upper eyelid skin to be excised. The wooden end of a cotton-tipped applicator can be used to roll the excessive upper eyelid skin backward and off the pretarsal eyelid surface, thereby allowing the patient to preview the surgical result. This simulates the eyelid's appearance following supratarsal fixation or other type of procedure for lid crease formation (8). The effect attained by eyelid-crease formation should be demonstrated to the patient because some individuals may not want the deep supratarsal sulcus. This is particularly true in men, although women who have had prominent eyelid folds all their lives may also reject this change in their appearance.

Lateral rhytides, or crow's feet, as they are commonly called, generally cannot be completely eliminated by a blepharoplasty. The patient should be forewarned that, although some of the wrinkles will be smoothed or reduced, the fine periorbital laugh lines are dynamic facial features that will remain after surgery.

Large bulging unsightly fat pockets are more common in the nasal upper eyelid. The longer, narrower central fat pocket of the upper eyelid may require excision in order to expose a levator aponeurosis defect or permit lid-crease formation.

To assess the fatty pockets, the surgeon instructs the patient to close the eyes lightly and the surgeon applies gentle pressure to the globe and orbital contents by pressing on the eyes through the closed eyelids. Excessive fat will bulge foreward and the location and degree of fat herniation should be recorded in the patient's chart for reference at the time of surgery. Some surgeons find it helpful to evaluate the fat pockets with the patient supine, as well as seated, as this previews the appearance of the fat at the time of surgery.

Blepharoptosis Evaluation

The patient population undergoing blepharoplasty surgery is frequently the same group that has levator aponeurosis dehiscences or disinsertions that result in acquired blephoaroptosis. Recognizing the presence of blepharoptosis allows the surgeon to correct it at the time of blepharoplasty surgery, which may be the procedure actually required rather than a cosmetic blepharoplasty (9, 10).

The vertical palpebral fissure height normally measures 9–10 mm. The signs of acquired blepharoptosis include a diminished vertical palpebral fissure height and good-to-excellent levator function on eyelid excursion from downgaze to upgaze (i.e., 8 mm or more). The upper eyelid crease, which is normally located 10 mm from the upper eyelid margin or eyelashes, may be displaced backwards into the orbit. A superiorly displaced upper eyelid crease indicates the presence of a dehiscence or disinsertion of the levator aponeurosis.

The eyelid tissues may be thinned due to a levator aponeurosis disinsertion, even to the extent of permitting the underlying ocular structures to be visible through the closed eyelids.

The vertical palpebral fissure height is measured with the eyes in straight-ahead primary gaze. In order to block any elevating influence of the frontalis muscle, the surgeon immobilizes the eyebrows by applying pressure, in a posterior direction, against the suprabrow frontalis muscle. Measurements of the palpebral fissure heights are recorded, and the difference between the recorded height and a 10-mm standard is considered to be the amount of ptosis. Figure 51.3 illustrates 4 mm of ptosis of the left upper eyelid. It is important to determine whether the ptosis is congenital or acquired in order to plan the appropriate procedure. This is best determined by ascertaining the age of onset of the ptosis and by careful measurements of levator excursion.

Levator excursion is measured by asking the patient to look in extreme downgaze. The millimeter ruler is aligned with the upper eyelid. Pressure is applied against the eyebrow with the examiners finger. This immobilizes the frontalis muscle. The patient then looks in extreme upgaze and the number of millimeters traversed by the upper eyelid is the levator excursion (Fig. 51.4).

Upper Eyelid Crease

It is important to note the location of the upper eyelid crease. While the examiner elevates the eyebrow with the hand, the patient is instructed to look down and then slowly up until the upper eyelid skin begins to retract backward into the orbit. The eyelid crease represents the fibrous attachment of the levator aponeurosis to the overlying orbicularis muscle and skin. The distance from the upper eyelid margin to the upper eyelid crease normally measures 10 mm. This location serves as the lower edge of the skin ellipse excision during a blepharoplasty.

A lid crease measurement of less than 8 mm indicates the need to reform the lid crease during the blepharoplasty. A superiorly displaced eyelid crease may indicate the presence of acquired ptosis due to a levator aponeurosis

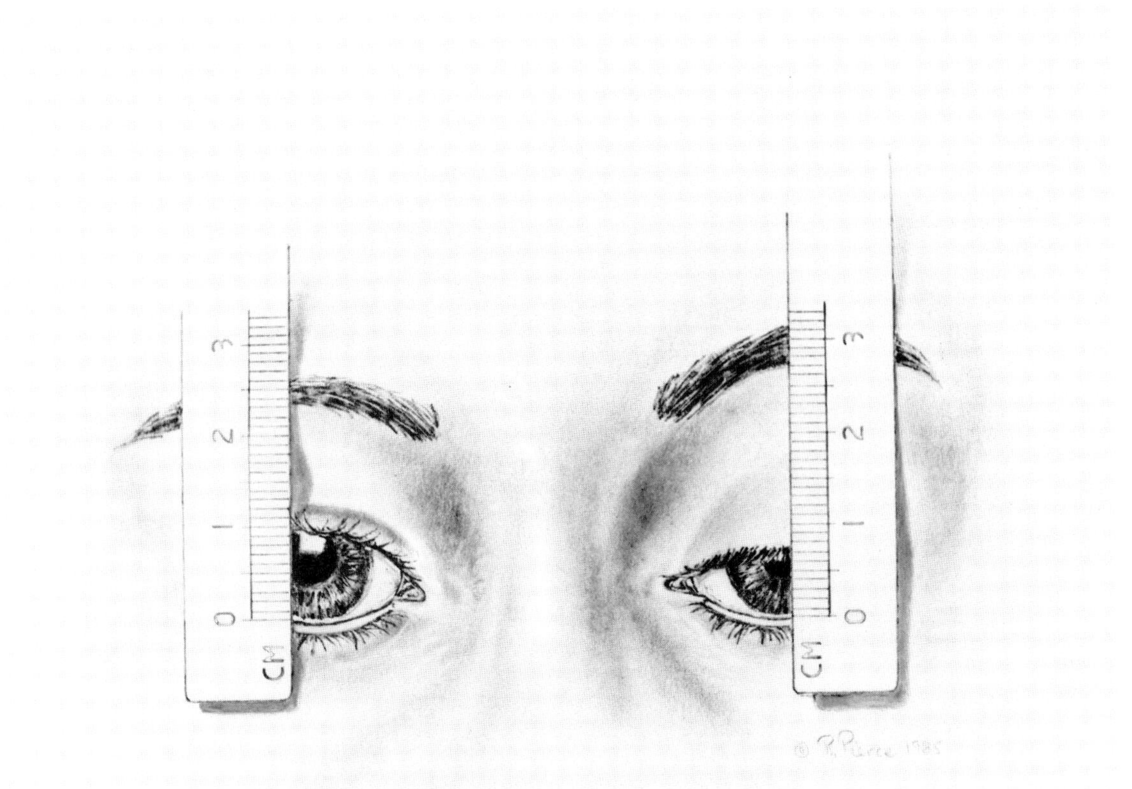

Figure 51.3. The vertical palpebral fissure height normally measures 10 mm. The left eyelid exhibits 4 mm of ptosis. Note the superiorly displaced left upper eyelid crease suggestive of a levator aponeurosis defect. The left eyebrow is elevated as a compensatory attempt to elevate the ptotic eyelid.

defect. Failure to recognize a superiorly displaced eyelid crease may result in postoperative asymmetry of the eyelid creases, which is quite difficult to correct.

LACRIMAL GLAND PROLAPSE

Prolapse of the lacrimal gland may be misdiagnosed as bulging orbital fat in the superior lateral orbit (11). Preoperative recognition of lacrimal gland prolapse permits planning for the correction of this abnormality at the time of blepharoplasty. Recognition of a prolapsed lacrimal gland will also prevent the inadvertent excision of lacrimal gland tissue while removing orbital fat.

OPHTHALMOLOGIC EXAMINATION

The most important fact to document during the preoperative evaluation is the visual acuity in each eye. The vision should be measured with glasses or contact lenses. If the visual acuity is not 20/20 in each eye, a refraction and ocular examination should be performed to determine the best corrected vision and to rule out any undiagnosed ocular pathology. Surgeons have performed uneventful cosmetic surgery and then have been confronted with charges of visual loss, presumably due to the elective blepharoplasty. Preoperative documentation of prior existing amblyopia, traumatic visual loss, or other causes of visual defects immediately avoids a potentially serious legal problem. In addition, a patient with undiagnosed visual loss may not be a candidate for a cosmetic blepharoplasty with fat removal because of the risk of orbital hemorrhage.

Normal ocular motility with absence of diplopia or strabismus should be documented. Following a hand light in the cardinal fields of gaze and an alternate cover test will reveal any ocular motility problem (12).

Fundoscopy should be performed to document normal optic nerves and absence of any retinal vascular disease.

VISUAL FIELDS

A peripheral visual-field examination documenting preoperative field loss, which is restored by the elimination of excessive upper eyelid skin, is often required by insurance companies if a blepharoplasty is intended for functional visual improvement.

A confrontation visual field is performed by sitting face to face, 2–3 feet from the patient. The patient occludes one eye with one hand and fixes gaze on the examiner's eye facing the patient's unoccluded eye. As the examiner's hand moves towards the visual axis from the periphery, the patient responds when the hand is first seen. This is performed in the superior temporal and inferior temporal quadrants. Comparison of the visual field with that obtained with the eyelids or eyebrows elevated commonly reveals suppression of the superior temporal field when there is extensive dermatochalasis. In a similar manner, a comparison of the peripheral visual field with and without

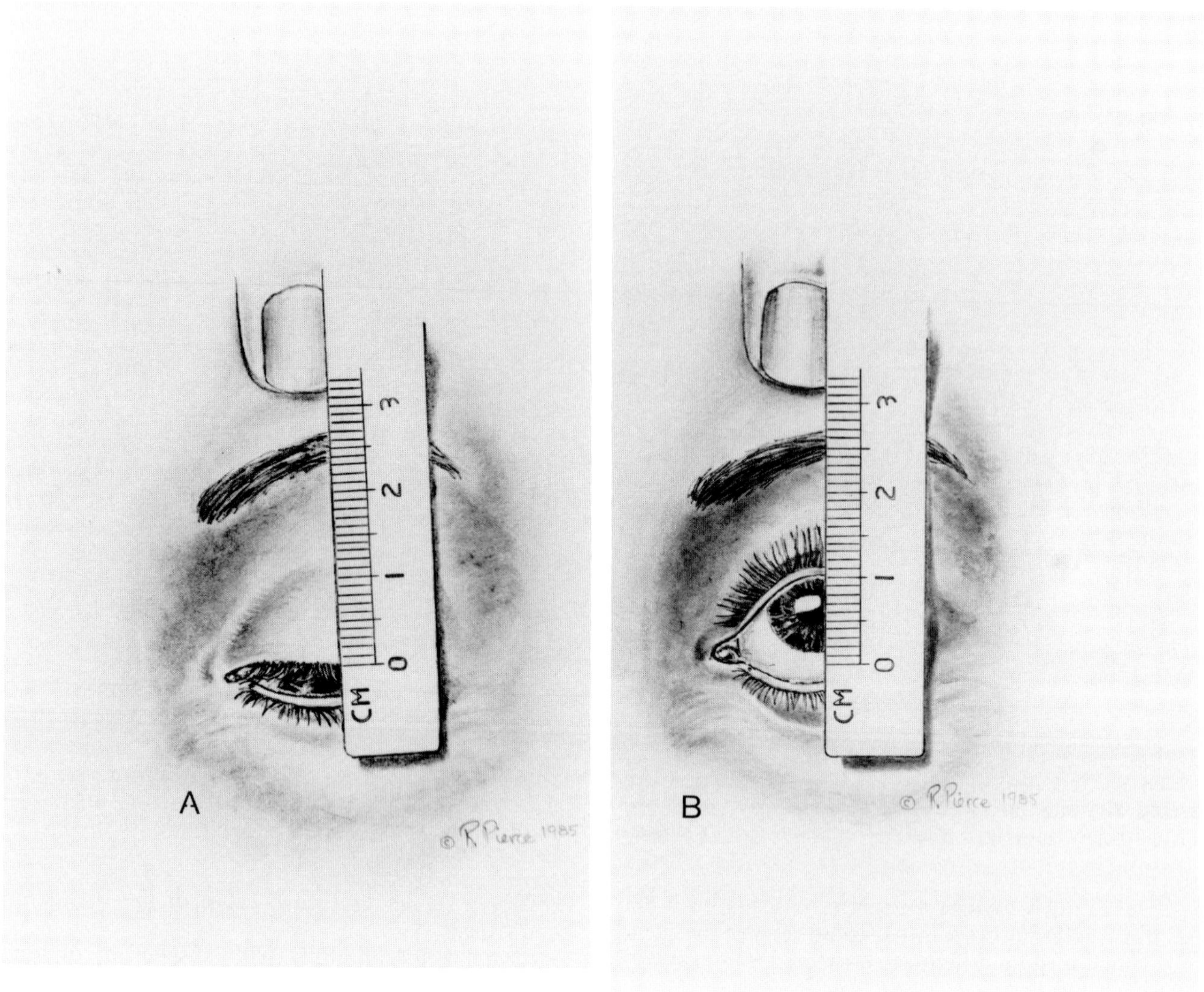

Figure 51.4. *A*, In downgaze, the upper eyelid margin is aligned with the millimeter ruler. *B*, In extreme upgaze, the eyelid excursion measures 11 mm.

elevating the excessive eyelid skin may be obtained with a tangent screen or perimetry examination.

LACRIMAL FUNCTION

Base line lacrimal secretion should be assessed preoperatively by Schirmer testing or clinical examination using the slitlamp. Patients with borderline lacrimal secretion who are asymptomatic may develop frank keratitis sicca with all of the associated symptoms of dry eyes following excessive excision of upper eyelid skin. The presence of dry eyes preoperatively suggests the need for conservative skin excision at the time of the blepharoplasty. A method for supratarsal fixation or other types of eyelid crease formation also permits an aesthetically acceptable cosmetic result without the need for excessive upper eyelid skin excision (13).

PHOTOGRAPHS

Preoperative photographs in straight-ahead and lateral gaze provide documentation of the patient's appearance prior to surgery and permits comparison with postoperative results. Thirty-five millimeter slides are used for clinical records. A preoperative Polaroid photo is an excellent reference source and memory refresher at the time of surgery. Photographic documentation has been valuable in preventing medical and legal problems when the photographs simply remind the patient of their preoperative appearance. The surgeon may be exonerated of charges by an unhappy patient when the latter is confronted with photographs exhibiting the preoperative appearance or condition.

LOWER EYELID EXAMINATION

The lower eyelids have traditionally posed a significant risk for postoperative complications following blepharoplasty surgery. An ectropion, following an elective cosmetic blepharoplasty, that requires secondary reconstructive surgery will remain an unpleasant memory and experience for both the surgeon and the patient. As previously stated, the preoperative evaluation is the best opportunity to recognize and avert postoperative complications by permitting proper surgical planning.

The lower eyelids should be evaluated for the degree of excessive skin, excessive orbicularis muscle, bulging fatty pockets, presence of "bags on bags," and the lower eyelid tone or degree of eyelid laxity. Young patients, most commonly women, request lower eyelid cosmetic surgery when they notice bulging fatty pockets, which cause an appearance of chronic fatigue or premature aging. These patients may require fat excision without removal of lower eyelid skin. They are candidates for an infraciliary skin incision or behind the eyelid blepharoplasty without a skin incision and scar. This condition requires preoperative recognition in order to prevent an unnecessary lateral canthal surgical scar.

More commonly encountered are the patients with obviously protruding fatty pockets and a moderate-to-severe degree of excessive lower eyelid skin. These patients require careful evaluation of their lower eyelid tone to determine whether an incipient lower eyelid ectropion may become a frank ectropion following a blepharoplasty. The term "bags on bags" describes a condition of excessive lower eyelid skin, orbicularis muscle festoons, lower eyelid laxity, and protruberant fatty pockets (14). Patients with this condition frequently require a lower eyelid horizontal tightening procedure to correct their eyelid laxity and provide additional eyelid support.

Consultation and Discussion

As in upper eyelid surgery, a satisfactory understanding by the surgeon and the patient of the goals attainable by a lower eyelid blepharoplasty should be clearly understood prior to undertaking cosmetic surgery. Providing patients with a mirror, as previously described, and asking them to show what they would like to attain, helps summarize the expected goals. As mentioned earlier, patients who wish to have their crow's feet eliminated or nasolabial folds flattened should be warned that these goals are unattainable and complications may arise if such procedures are attempted.

A cotton-tipped applicator may be rolled over the lower eyelid skin in the lateral direction, thereby roughly duplicating the effect of a blepharoplasty following removal of excessive fat and skin.

Bags on bags of the lower eyelids may be due to a longstanding dermatochalasis or may be secondary to a systemic medical disorder. Renal function and abnormal thyroid status are two conditions that may cause chronic lower eyelid edema. Further questioning in order to rule out these disorders is mandatory.

Lower Eyelid Tone

The lower eyelids are supported against the globe by the medial and lateral canthal tendons, the suspensory ligament, lower eyelid retractors, the tarsus, and the orbicularis muscle. Lower eyelid laxity, which is most commonly due to stretching of the canthal tendons, may be converted from an asymptomatic incipient or borderline ectropion into a frank ectropion following blepharoplasty. Preoperative evaluation of the lower eyelid tone allows the surgeon to recognize the possible need for a horizontal eyelid shortening, thereby preventing an ectropion.

The two simplest, yet most effective tests for evaluation of lower eyelid laxity, are the "snap-back test" and the eyelid distraction test. The snap-back test, as the name implies, is a subjective evaluation of the rate and force with which the lower eyelid is passively returned to the globe by the lower eyelid–supporting structures. The examiner should become adept at evaluating snap back; with experience, the examiner can acquire a sense of what should be considered normal.

The examiner should instruct the patient not to blink during the snap-back test. Otherwise, the orbicularis muscle will contribute to the eyelid's return to the globe. The

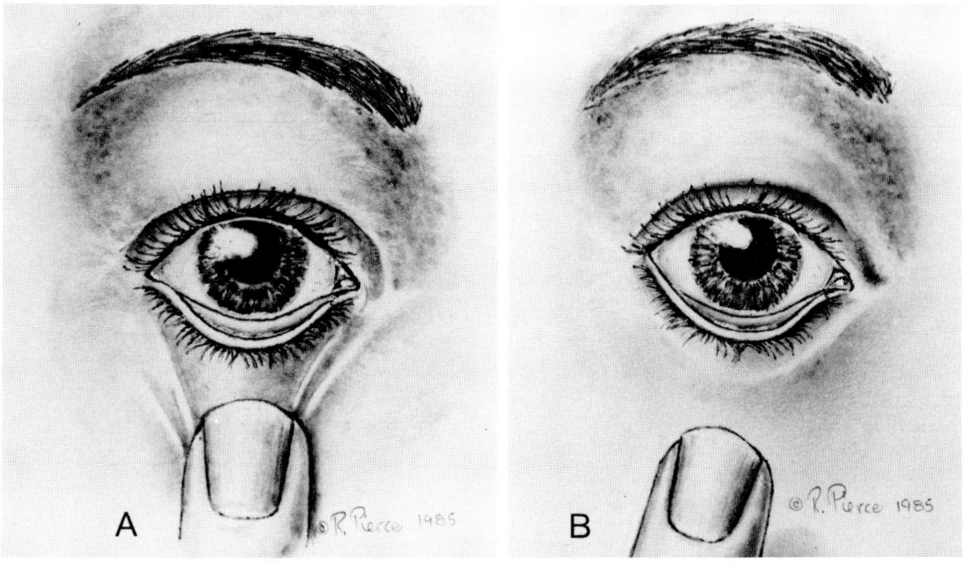

Figure 51.5. *A*, The snap-back test assesses lower eyelid laxity. The examiner pulls the lower eyelid away from the globe and instructs the patient not to blink while the lower eyelid is gently released. *B*, If the lower eyelid remains suspended away from the globe or only slowly returns, there is eyelid laxity, which requires correction.

examiner's index finger pulls the lower eyelid away from the eye. The eyelid is then released, and the force with which the eyelid returns to the globe is assessed. The eyelid should briskly snap back without the patient blinking. If there is a slow return to the globe or if the eyelid remains suspended away from the globe, lower eyelid laxity is present. This finding indicates the need for horizontal eyelid shortening to prevent an ectropion (Fig. 51.5).

The eyelid distraction test measures the distance the lower eyelid can be retracted from the eyeball. A distance greater than 6–8 mm is considered an indication of lower eyelid laxity, which requires lower eyelid tightening (Fig. 51.6).

Skin Evaluation

The amount of skin to be excised at the time of surgery may be estimated preoperatively by having the patient widely open the mouth and look in extreme upgaze. This places the lower eyelid skin on stretch and ensures that a patient is not predisposed to a cicatricial ectropion due to tight malar or lower eyelid skin. In addition, performing this maneuver during the preoperative examination, helps patients to understand when they are instructed to repeat the maneuver at the time of surgery.

Fatty Pockets

Evaluation of the lower eyelid fatty pockets is performed in a manner similar to that described for the upper eyelid fat evaluation. The patient is instructed to close the eyes, and with slight pressure applied to the globe by the surgeon's fingers, the presence and degree of pouching orbital fat pockets is assessed. Attention should always be given to the lateral fat pocket as it may not protrude as conspicuously while the patient is supine during surgery. Failure to recognize and remove the lateral fat pocket at the time of surgery is a commonly encountered complication following lower eyelid blepharoplasty.

Lateral Canthal Tendon Laxity

Detachment or stretching of the lateral canthal tendon results in lower eyelid laxity. In addition, a phimotic-appearing eye with a rounded lateral canthal angle may occur due to a lateral canthal tendon detachment. Under normal circumstances, the distance between the lateral orbital rim and lateral end of the eyelid is negligible. If the examiner finds a finger-width distance between the lateral orbital rim and lateral canthus, this is evidence of a lax lateral canthal tendon (Fig. 51.7). The lateral tarsus may require repositioning against the lateral orbital rim at the time of surgery (15, 16).

Medial Canthal Tendon Laxity

Medial canthal tendon laxity must also be recognized preoperatively (Fig. 51.8). The lower eyelid is pulled laterally, and this should result in minimal lateral punctal movement. If the punctum can be pulled laterally to the medial limbus, this suggests a medial canthal tendon

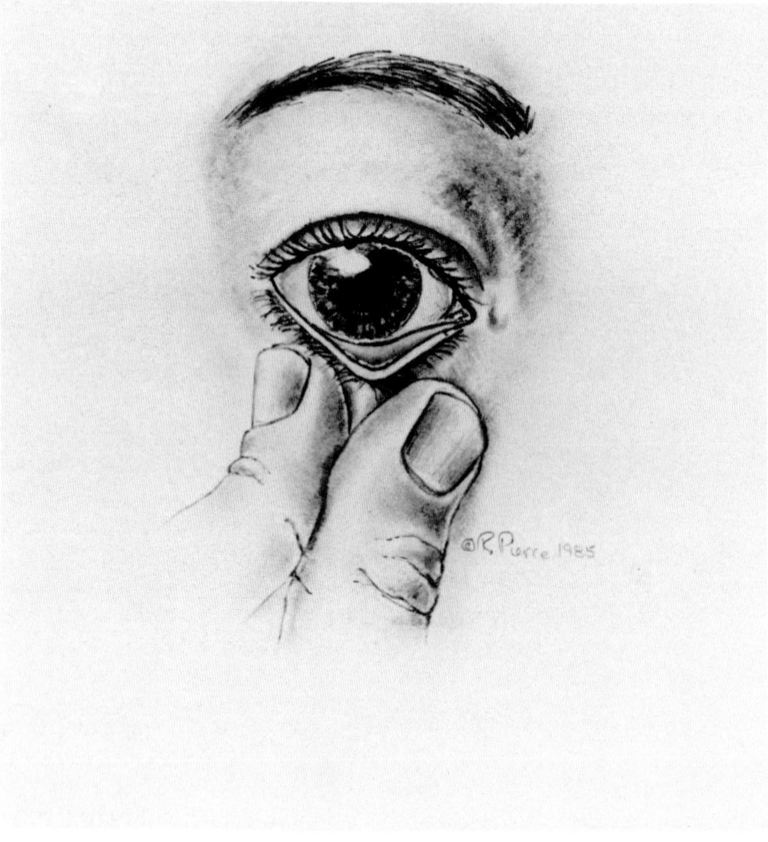

Figure 51.6. As the lower eyelid is pulled from the globe, a distance greater than 6–8 mm suggests lower eyelid laxity.

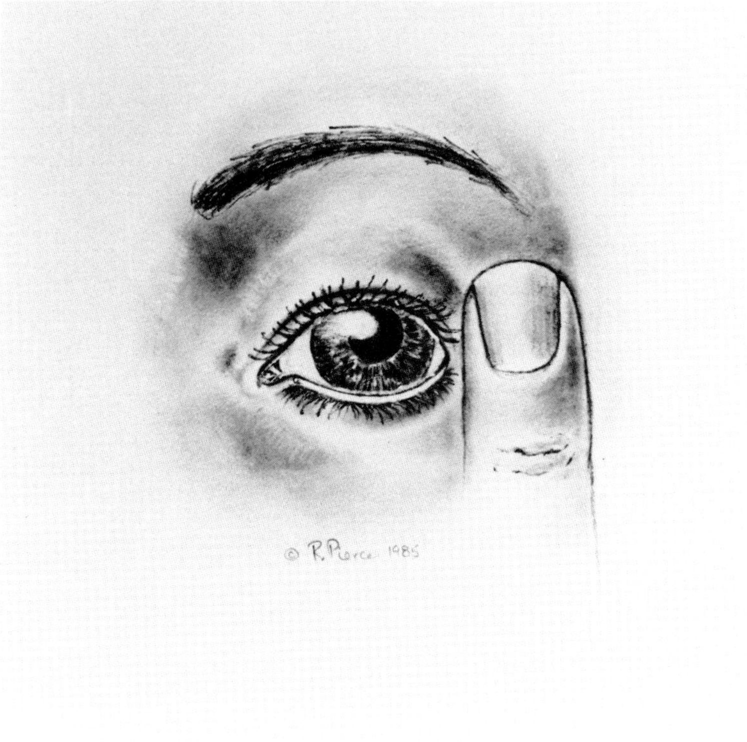

Figure 51.7. A lateral canthal tendon defect exists if there is a finger-width distance between the lateral canthal angle and the orbital rim.

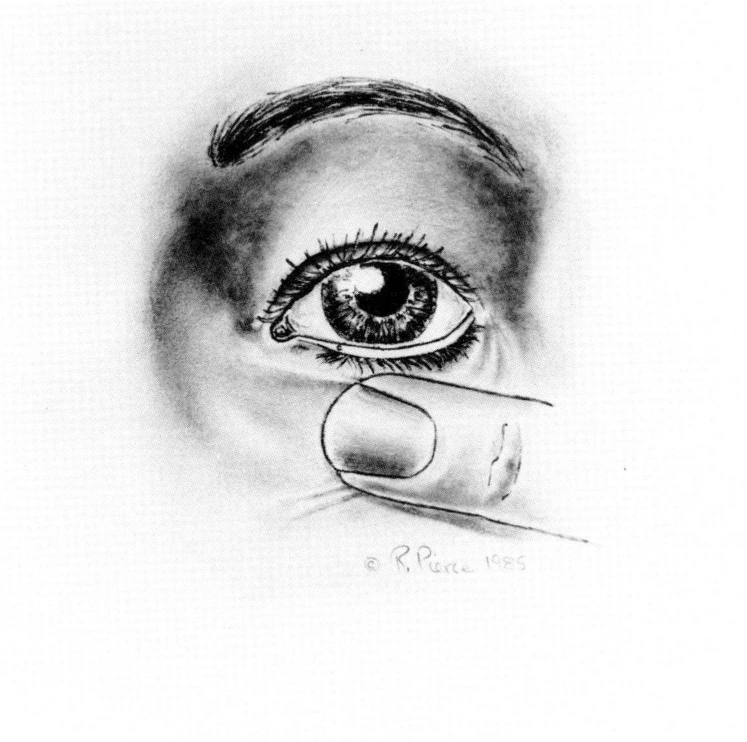

Figure 51.8. Medial canthal tendon laxity may be demonstrated if the lower punctum can be easily pulled laterally to the medial limbus.

dehiscence or detachment, which may require surgical correction by a medial canthal tendon plication (17).

"Bags on Bags"

When a "bags on bags" condition is due to involutional skin changes, a significant reduction of excessive skin and fatty tissue can be attained with surgery. Most patients will be satisfied with the significant reduction of the excessive tissues following a conventional blepharoplasty, which may be enhanced by a horizontal shortening and plication of the orbicularis muscle. Others, however, may require a direct secondary excision of the bags with a subtle but visible facial scar. The patient should be preoperatively instructed of this possibility.

CONCLUSION

A step-by-step preoperative evaluation of the cosmetic surgery patient prepares surgical candidates for their postoperative result and provides the surgeon many details and facts that will assist in surgery and in providing the patient with a satisfactory result.

REFERENCES

1. Rees TD: Selection of patients. In Rees TD (ed): *Aesthetic Plastic Surgery.* Philadelphia, WB Saunders, 1980, p 19–28.
2. Knorr NJ, et al: Psychiatric surgical approach to adolescent disturbance in self-image. *Plast Reconstr Surg* 41: 248–253, 1968.
3. Putterman AM (ed): *Cosmetic Oculoplastic Surgery.* New York, Grune-Stratton, 1982, p 13, 28–30.
4. Waller RR: Is blindness a realistic complication in blepharoplasty procedures? *Trans Am Acad Ophthalmol* 85: 730–735, 1978.
5. Wiggs EO: Blepharoplasty complications. *Trans Am Acad Ophthalmol* 81: 583–586, 1976.
6. Moser MH, et al: Sudden blindness following blepharoplasty: report of seven cases. *Plast Reconstr Surg* 51: 364–370, 1973.
7. Dingman RO, et al: Forehead and brow lifts and their relationship to blepharoplasty. *Ann Plast Surg* 2: 32–36, 1979.
8. Sheen JH: Supratarsal fixation in upper blepharoplasty. *Plast Reconstr Surg* 54: 424–431, 1974.
9. Wilkins RB, Patipa M: The recognition of acquired ptosis in patients considered for upper eyelid blepharoplasty. *Plast Reconstr Surg* 70: 431–4343, 1982.
10. Hornblass A: Ptosis and pseudoptosis and blepharoplasty. In Rees TD (ed): *Modern Trends in Blepharoplasty.* Philadelphia, WB Saunders, 1981, p 811–830.
11. Horton CD, et al: Treatment of a lacrimal bulge in blepharoplasty by repositioning the gland. *Plast Reconstr Surg* 61: 701–702, 1978.
12. Hayworth RS, et al: Diplopia following blepharoplasty. *Ann Ophthalmol* 16: 448–451, 1984.
13. Tenzel RR: Cosmetic blepharoplasty. *Int Ophthalmol Clin* 18: 9, 1978.
14. Furnas DW: Festoons of orbicularis muscle as a cause of baggy eyelids. *Plast Reconstr Surg* 54: 424–431, 1974.
15. Bick MW: Surgical management of orbital tarsal disparity. *Arch Ophthalmol* 75: 386–389, 1966.
16. Schaefer, AJ: Lateral canthal tendon tuck. *Ophthalmology* 86: 1879–1882, 1979.
17. Furnas DW, Bircell MS: Eyelash traction test to determine if the medial canthal ligament is detached. *Plast Reconstr Surg* 52: 315–317, 1973.

CHAPTER 52

Evaluation of the Blepharoplasty Patient

ALBERT HORNBLASS, M.D., F.A.C.S.
NEIL D. GROSS, M.D.

Cosmetic eyelid procedures are an important part of the oculoplastic surgeon's armamentarium. This chapter will focus upon the specific psychological and medical concerns that need to be addressed in blepharoplasty candidates. Selected oculoplastic conditions related to this procedure will be highlighted (Table 52.1). Surgical approaches designed to treat these problems will be discussed.

PREOPERATIVE EVALUATION

In evaluating patients for cosmetic eyelid surgery, the surgeon must determine several factors (1). First and foremost, patients' aims and goals must be ascertained. It must be determined whether their hopes are realistic, and whether they can be achieved with surgery.

These questions can be answered during the preoperative consultation. At this time, the patient's behavior should be noted and carefully evaluated. Occasionally, more than one session is necessary to determine the patient's true self-image and surgical goal. Psychiatric evaluation may be helpful (2).

All patients should be examined with the aid of a hand-held mirror, so that real and "imagined" flaws can be uncovered. During this time, the patient can be shown that certain facial characteristics, such as increased lower lid pigmentation or fine skin lines, cannot be eliminated with a blepharoplasty.

Cosmetic surgery can be a gratifying experience for both the patient and the doctor; however, frustration can develop when a patient with a "perfect result" remains dissatisfied. Certain patients exhibit particular characteristics that may help to identify them to the physician as potentially "difficult." Physicians with experience develop a sixth sense as to which patients will have unusual problems adjusting to a good postoperative result.

The surgeon should learn to be wary of patients who are overly anxious for an appointment, or who are extremely irritated by a delay in the schedule. These patients' responses are frequently out of proportion to the stimuli. Some underlying factor may be fueling their reaction.

Table 52.1.
Oculoplastic Conditions

Eyebrow ptosis
Dermatochalasis
Herniated orbital fat
Eyelid ptosis
Pseudoptosis
Prolapsed lacrimal gland
Hypertrophic orbicularis muscle
Horizontal lid laxity
Scleral show
Eyelid erythema
Crow's feet
Surgical implantation of pigment in the eyelid margin

Patients who are unkempt or who have poor hygiene should be viewed with suspicion. Patients who are undergoing surgery because of someone else's desire frequently become unhappy patients.

Patients who are "perfectionists," almost by definition, will never be totally satisfied. These patients may spend hours in front of a magnifying mirror, inspecting tiny scars. The surgeon also must be wary of patients who seem to ignore preoperative instructions, such as medication orders or requests for preoperative photographs.

Age (3) and social status may also affect a patient's assessment of the postoperative result. For example, middle age often plays an important role in the decision to undergo cosmetic eyelid surgery. Some individuals may seek to regain lost youth through surgery. Others are frustrated with their professional or social positions and seek a cosmetic improvement to lift their spirits. Unfortunately, a blepharoplasty cannot solve these underlying problems.

During the preoperative evaluation, all blepharoplasty candidates should be checked for dry eyes and thyroid disease. Patients who are keloid formers should be discouraged from having surgery. In some cases, the surgeon may consider superficial radiation preoperatively to lessen scar formation. Patients who complain of brow ache, fatigue, or superior visual field loss should be evaluated for ptosis. Visual field examination should also be performed for medical and insurance documentation.

The initial consultation should last for 20 or 30 minutes. If the interview is extended by the patient, another appointment should be scheduled. Uncertainty about the surgery will also necessitate a second visit. If possible, a relative or friend should accompany the patient to the consultation. Possible complications of the proposed surgery should be reviewed in the presence of the patient and the companion in appropriate detail (4). It is wise to give a patient a detailed letter concerning instructions and expectations. This information can be printed and given out routinely by the surgeon's secretary.

Finally, both the surgeon and the patient must "feel comfortable" with each other. Open and frank communication is of utmost importance. If the surgeon feels uncomfortable or hostile toward a particular patient, it would be prudent not to accept the patient for cosmetic surgery.

SURGICAL OBJECTIVES

The following objectives are sought in cosmetic *upper* eyelid blepharoplasty: removal of an appropriate amount of redundant eyelid skin; the production of an area of well-defined pretarsal skin, readily visible in the postoperative lid; symmetric, inconspicuous scars; a well-defined orbitopalpebral sulcus; and symmetry of the upper lids (5, 6). The *lower* lid should be free of notable pouchiness associated with herniation of the fat pads; there should also be no scleral show between the limbus and lower eyelid margin (7).

SPECIFIC CONDITIONS ASSOCIATED WITH BLEPHAROPLASTY

EYEBROW PTOSIS

Eyebrow ptosis may occur in patients with a facial nerve paralysis or a unilateral tumor. It may also accompany dermatochalasis or blepharochalasis (see the following sections) (Figs. 52.1 and 52.2). Brow ptosis occurs when there is inferior migration of the eyebrow. It is usually more prevalent laterally. Gentle elevation of the brow will determine whether or not the primary problem is a droopy brow.

This condition may be corrected by a suprabrow skin and muscle resection (8). However, the scar may be very conspicuous. In order to diminish the visible scar, the surgeon should place the incision above the brow, tangential to the cilia. If the eyebrows are surgically lifted, the skin should be minimally excised from the upper lids to avoid lagophthalmos. The patient should be warned that sensory nerves may be cut, resulting in forehead anesthesia.

To avoid supraciliary scarring, others have employed the transcoronal brow lift technique (9). This approach involves a radical dissection of the forehead and requires a low, thick hairline. Pronounced sensory loss, alopecia, and scalp necrosis have occurred.

Another surgical alternative for the treatment of eyebrow ptosis is the midforehead lift or "glabellaplasty" (10).

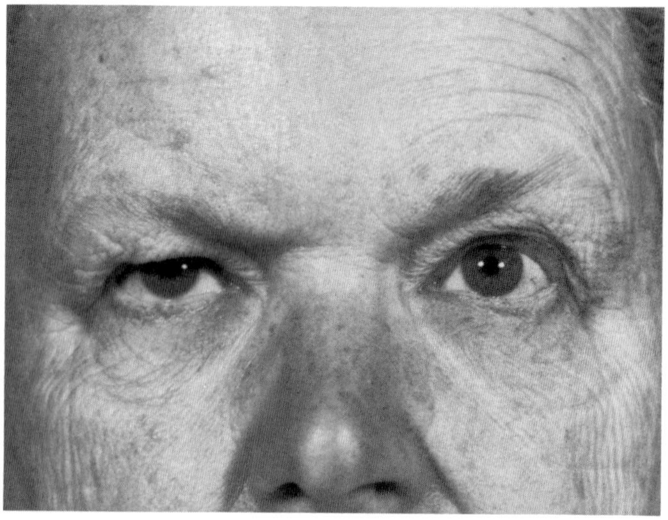

Figure 52.1. A 63-year-old female with right eyebrow ptosis. Her pseudoptosis is secondary to dermatochalasis. Hooding is accentuated by the brow ptosis.

This approach is recommended for patients who are not candidates for the transcoronal approach and have preexisting furrows in which to place the incision.

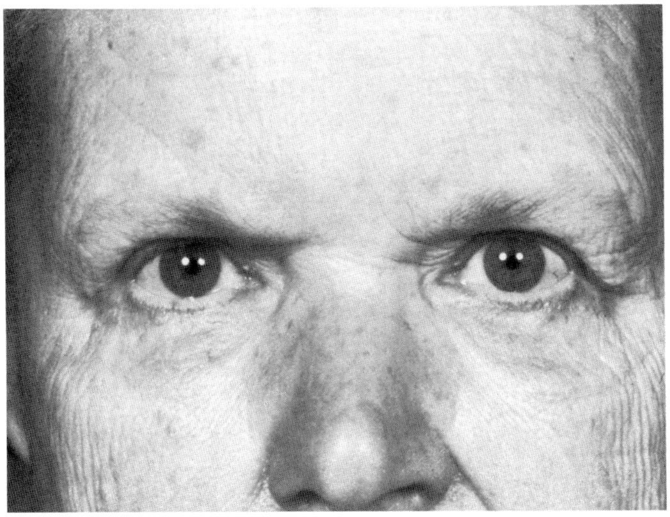

Figure 52.2. Improvement of the pseudoptosis with conservative excision of excess right upper lid skin is shown in this postoperative photo. Note that the position of the ptotic right eyebrow is unchanged. Patient refused brow surgery.

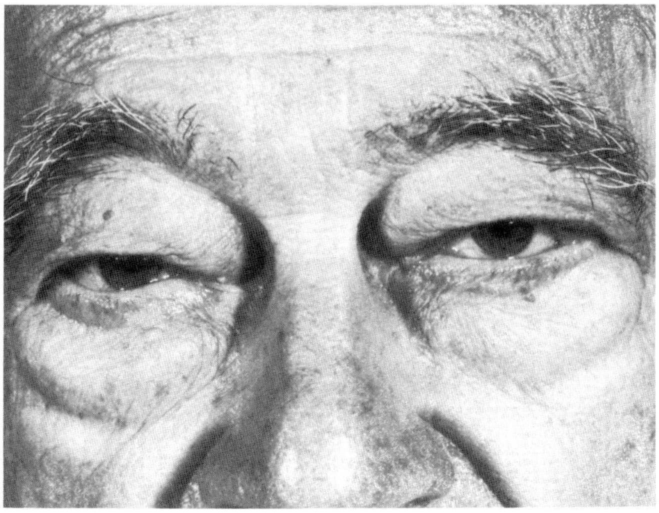

Figure 52.3. A 68-year-old male with pronounced upper lid dermatochalasis. Ptosis adiposa and herniated orbital fat with bilateral lower lid laxity are also depicted.

DERMATOCHALASIS

Dermatochalasis describes a redundancy or relaxation of the skin of the lids (Figs. 52.3 and 52.4). Patients can be evaluated for this condition by selectively pinching the skin of the upper eyelid and noting if there is any eversion of the eyelid margin (11, 12).

Abnormally crinkled, pigmented nasal lower eyelid skin is sometimes associated with dermatochalasis. Nasal excision of abnormal lid skin can be used to improve the cosmetic appearance of the lower lid (13).

BLEPHAROCHALASIS

Blepharochalasis is a rare condition that typically affects both upper eyelids. It is characterized by atrophy and relaxation of the lid tissues following intermittent lid edema. This condition usually occurs in young people, especially at puberty. Occasionally, it can be inherited as an autosomal dominant trait. It can be associated with allergy (15). Blepharochalasis has been associated with the floppy eyelid syndrome (16). Blepharochalasis was reported recently in an individual with unilateral agenesis of the kidney, multiple abnormalities of the vertebral column, and congenital heart disease (17). Treatment is directed at the etiology of the lid edema.

ORBITAL FAT HERNIATION

Herniation of orbital fat is a common condition afflicting people of all ages. Certain individuals may have herniated fat without excess eyelid skin or muscle. The condition may be familial (Figs. 52.5 and 52.6).

Careful preoperative evaluation will help to identify the orbital fat compartments (18). Patients with lower lid orbital fat festoons are difficult to treat (19). Frequently, the "bags on bags" situation will persist after blepharoplasty. Local excision of the festoons may be the only way to treat this condition, despite residual scars.

Fat excision must be undertaken carefully. Excessive traction, inadequate cauterization of the medial fat pad vessels, or insufficient cauterization after fat amputation can lead to retrobulbar hemorrhage and visual loss. Excision of fat in monocular patients is discouraged for this reason. An alternative method for treating herniated orbital fat includes tightening of the orbital septum (18). Techniques employing electrocautery (14, 20–23) or the carbon dioxide laser (24) have been advocated as alternative means for fat dissolution.

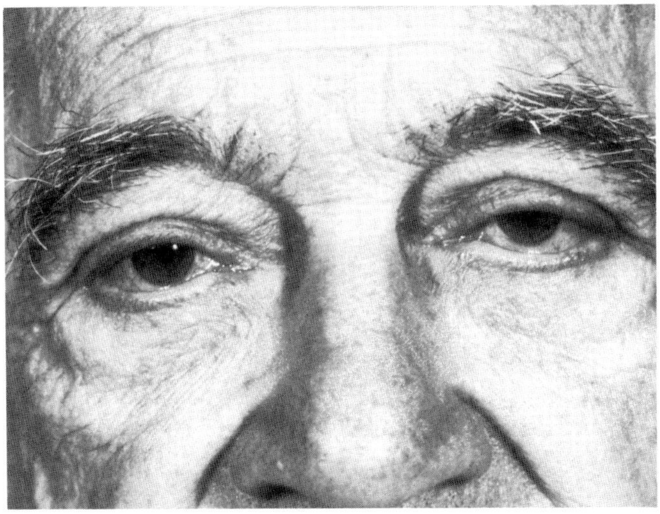

Figure 52.4. Bilateral excision of excess skin of the upper lids with removal of herniated orbital fat and bilateral lower lid horizontal shortening was performed.

Patients with Graves' eye disease frequently develop unsightly orbital fat herniation. These patients must first be carefully evaluated for exposure keratopathy, lagophthalmos, lid retraction, and compressive optic neuropathy before excision of fat is contemplated (Figs. 52.7 and 52.8).

Removal of the unsightly tissue can provide a dramatic improvement in the patient's appearance; however, it is

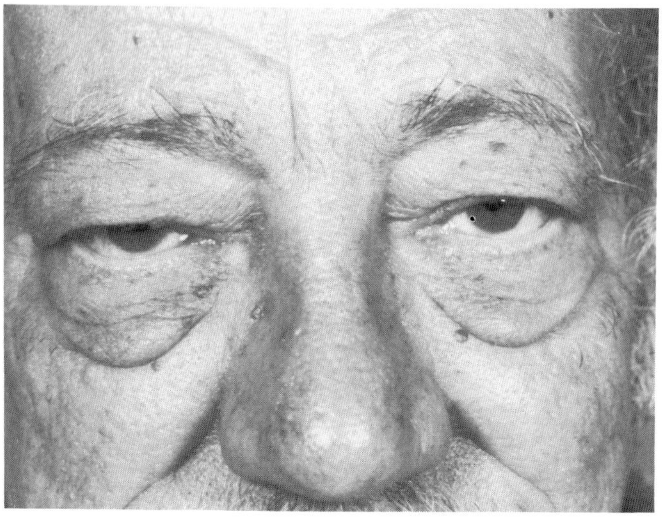

Figure 52.5. A 62-year-old male with herniated orbital fat and festoons of skin. A bilateral pseudoptosis secondary to hooding with bilateral lower lid laxity is also present.

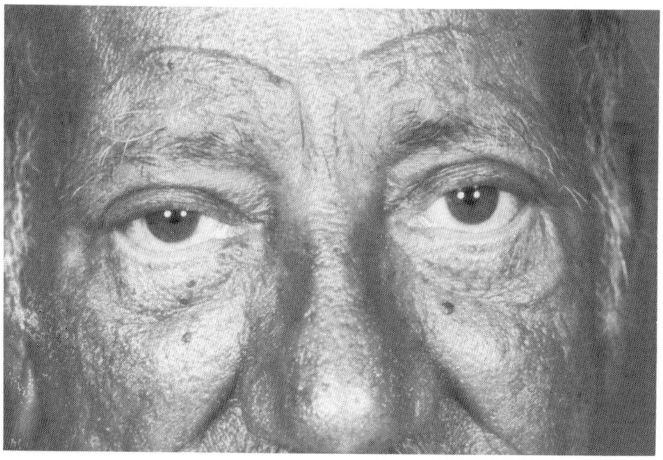

Figure 52.6. Surgical correction including a four-lid blepharoplasty with excess of orbital fat and bilateral lower lid horizontal shortening was performed. Mild festooning of the lower lid skin remains.

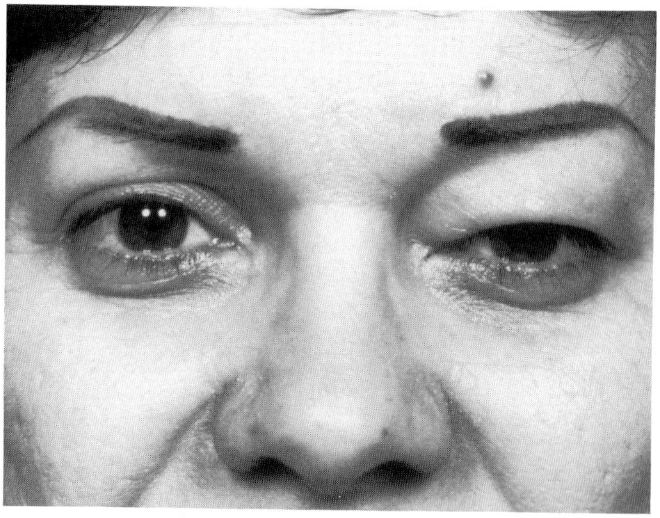

Figure 52.7. A 37-year-old female with thyroid ophthalmology with left exophthalmos and bilateral herniated fat of the orbits.

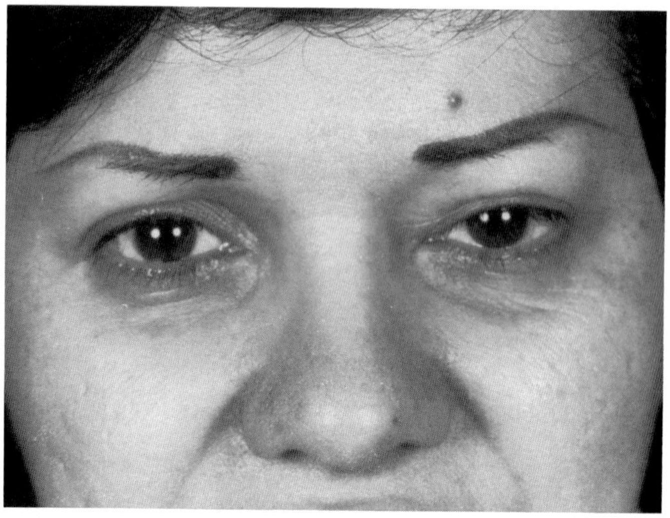

Figure 52.8. A bilateral blepharoplasty with excision of herniated orbital fat and reformation of the left upper lid crease was performed.

recommended that removal of skin be avoided in these cases. Scleral show, with subsequent keratopathy, can result, even if the most conservative skin resection is performed. Treatment of this complication may require a skin graft or a lateral tarsal strip (28).

EYELID PTOSIS

Ptosis may be a preexisting problem in the patient who is interested in a blepharoplasty (25). In these patients, etiology of the ptosis must be ascertained first. Patients with dermatochalasis and involutional ptosis generally do well with a blepharoplasty in combination with a Fasanella-Servat (tarsoconjunctivo-Muellerectomy) (26) or a blepharoplasty with a Putterman Muellerectomy (27). Some cases may require levator aponeurosis surgery, especially if there is a high lid fold and a thin lid.

PSEUDOPTOSIS

Pseudoptosis occurs in patients with microphthalmos, enophthalmos, phthisis, hypotropia, or dermatochalasis. The approach for the treatment of pseudoptosis in the blepharoplasty candidate is covered in detail in Chapter 63.

PROLAPSED LACRIMAL GLAND

Bulging at the temporal aspect of the upper lid or lateral canthus may be the result of a prolapsed lacrimal gland. Double eversion of the eyelid with the Desmarres retractor or digital pressure on the globe will verify the diagnosis. Occasionally, the lacrimal gland may be visible when the surgeon simply raises the upper lid and notes the position of the pink or yellow lacrimal gland tissue on the globe.

This condition may be repaired by replacement of the gland in the lacrimal fossa with a nonabsorbable suture. Several interrupted sutures are placed in the temporal portion of the superior cul-de-sac and anchored to periosteum (29). A Schirmer test should be performed preoperatively and postoperatively (30).

HYPERTROPHIC ORBICULARIS MUSCLE

Patients who have an exaggerated smile or squint frequently may have a hypertrophic orbicularis muscle (31). This deformity consists of a horizontal bulging of the lower lids immediately below the palpebral margin. This is very different from the irregular bulging caused by the herniation of the intraorbital fat. Treatment is directed towards excision of the orbicularis muscle, with excision of redundant skin (32).

ENTROPION AND LOWER LID LAXITY

All patients undergoing lower lid blepharoplasty should be checked for lower lid laxity. Some patients may not have overt ectropion but may actually have poor eyelid apposition. This can result in epiphora or a persistent conjunctival hyperemia.

Lid laxity is determined by the "snap test." The patient is instructed to tilt the head downward while the surgeon gently pulls the lower lid away from the globe. If there is good muscle tone, the lid should retract back to the globe. The longer it takes to retract, the more severe the laxity of the lid. This condition is common in patients who are 50 years of age and older.

Patients with lower laxity must have this corrected during the blepharoplasty, or lower lid ectropion can result. A full-thickness horizontal lid shortening (33, 34) or plication of the canthal tendons is recommended (32).

SCLERAL SHOW

Scleral show may be the result of a previous blepharoplasty procedure (35) (Figs. 52.9 and 52.10). It can also occur secondary to lid retraction in thyroid disease. Vertical skin shortening from cicatrization secondary to rosacea or sun exposure usually results in ectropion with scleral show.

Patients afflicted with scleral show may complain of its unsightliness and can experience discomfort from punctate keratopathy. Thyroid patients can be corrected by undergoing recession of the lid retractors with or without the insertion of a scleral (36) or a retroauricular cartilage (35) graft. A full-thickness skin graft or direct tissue expansion can be used to provide vertical length in cicatricized lids. Superior displacement of the lateral canthal tendon also has been advocated as a technique for reducing scleral show (37).

EYELID EDEMA

Some of the causes of eyelid edema include allergy, systemic hypertension, low-grade infections, thyroid disease, toxins, renal disease, long-standing blepharospasm, anemia, lymphedema, parasitic lid infestation, and angioneurotic edema. The laxity and distensibility of the subcutaneous connective tissue in the lids make them a ready site for the accumulation of fluid.

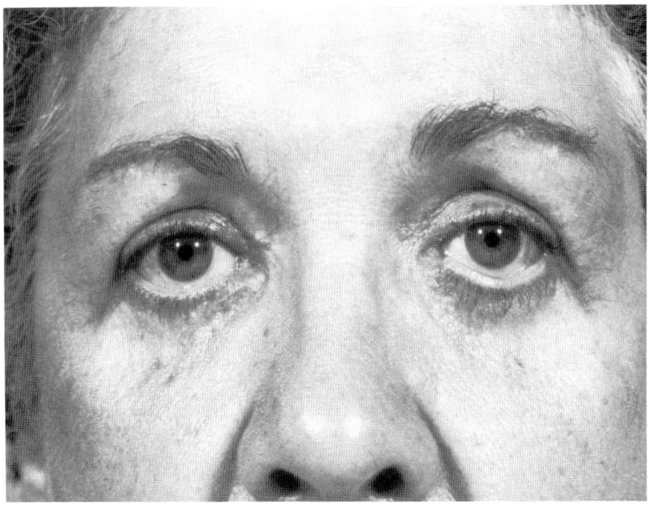

Figure 52.9. A 53-year-old female with horizontal lid laxity, scleral show, and mild ectropion following blepharoplasty surgery.

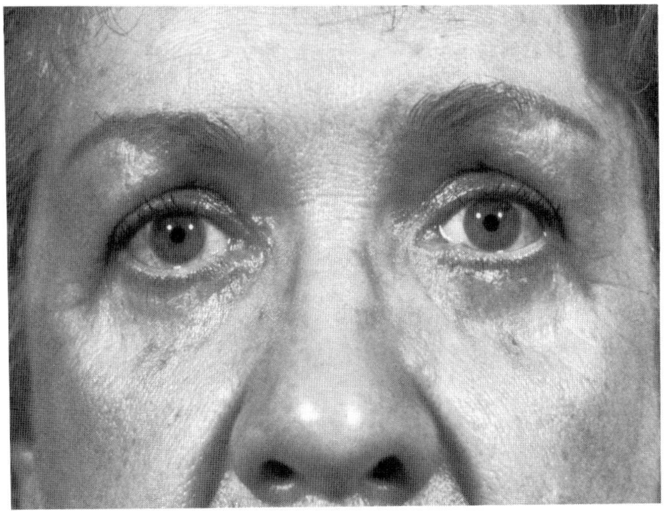

Figure 52.10. A bilateral horizontal lid shortening with lateral tarsal strip canthoplasty repaired the scleral show and ectropion.

Eyelid edema is a very difficult problem to treat. Patients who undergo blepharoplasty will frequently have residual postoperative edema. Patients with recurrent edema of the eyelids would not benefit from eyelid surgery. Treatment of the edema should be directed at the underlying pathologic cause.

EYELID ERYTHEMA

Eyelid erythema may be due to the overfilling of the arterial and capillary circulation. This can be caused by fever, local irritation, or vasomotor blepharitis.

Again, treatment should be directed at the cause of the irritation. Surgery should be avoided. Cosmetic makeup, vasoconstrictors, and steroids can be used (38). Recently,

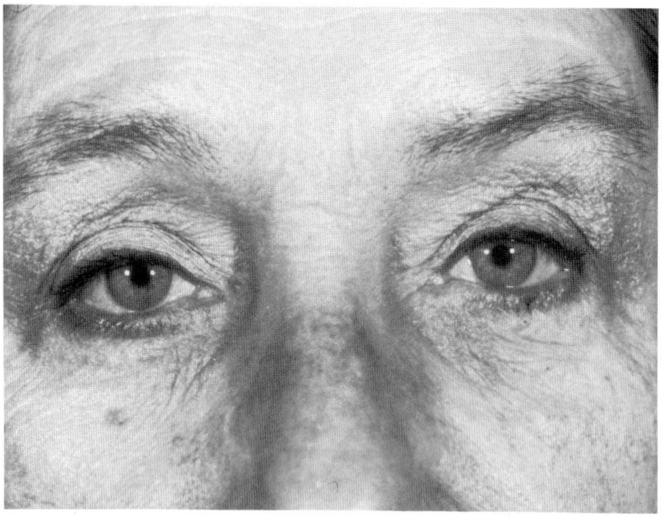

Figure 52.11. Preoperative photograph of blepharopigmentation candidate.

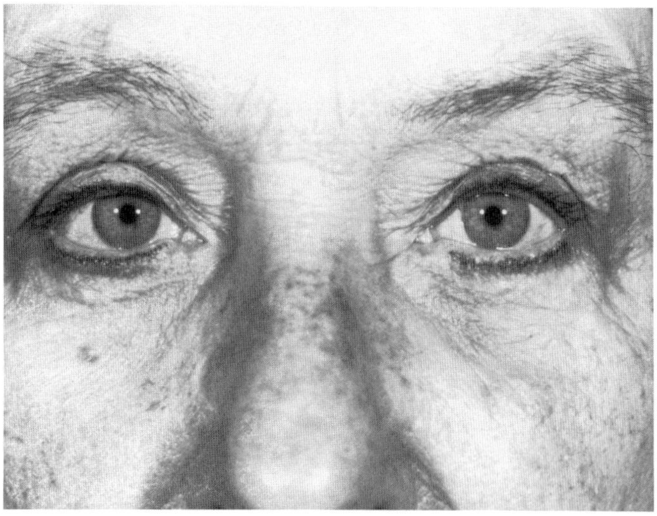

Figure 52.12. Postoperative photograph of patient who has undergone bilateral upper and lower lid blepharopigmentation.

the argon laser has been employed selectively to treat small vessels on the eyelids.

CROW'S FEET

Skin folds and wrinkles in the lateral canthal area are difficult to improve. The orbicularis oculi muscle flap seems to permit a predictable correction in selected cases (39).

SURGICAL IMPLANTATION OF PIGMENT TO THE EYELID MARGIN

Many women and physicians who do cosmetic lid surgery have become interested in the surgical application of pigment to the eyelid margin. This technique is known as the "Permalid Liner" method. Advocates claim that it enhances the effects of blepharoplasty and frees the individual from the daily chore of applying eyeliner (7).

The procedure of pigmentation implantation is analogous to tattooing. The Accent pigment contains 98% iron and 2% titanium (41). It is implanted in the eyelid margin with a needle (Figs. 52.11 and 52.12).

A histopathologic study of the pigment reveals rapid and deep migration of the substance into the dermis and lymphatic drainage system of the eyelid. Systemic exposure to the pigment may occur via the lymphatics (40). Long-term effects from exposure to the pigment are not known. Permanent lash loss has been reported as a side effect (41).

REFERENCES

1. Rees TD: Selection of patients. In Rees TD (ed): *Aesthetic Plastic Surgery*. Philadelphia, WB Saunders, 1980, p 1928.
2. Knorr NJ, Hoopes JA, Edgerton ND: Psychiatric surgical approach to adolescent disturbance in self-image. *Plast Reconstr Surg* 41: 248–253, 1968.
3. Abrahamson IA, Jr: Eye changes after forty. *Am Fam Physician* 29: 171–181, 1984.
4. Courtiss AH: Selection of alternatives in aesthetic blepharoplasty. In Rees TD (ed): *Modern Trends in Blepharoplasty*. Philadelphia, WB Saunders, 1981, p 739–754.
5. Baker DJ: Upper blepharoplasty. *Clin Plast Surg* 8: 635–662, 1981.
6. Sheen JH: Supratarsal fixation in upper blepharoplasty. *Plast Reconstr Surg* 54: 424–431, 1974.
7. Angres GG: The Angres Permalid-Liner method to enhance the result of cosmetic blepharoplasty. *Ann Ophthalmol* 17: 176–177, 1985.
8. Lewis JR, Jr: A method of direct brow lift. *Ann Plast Surg* 10: 115–119, 1983.
9. Ellenbogen R: Transcoronal eyebrow lift with concomitant upper blepharoplasty. *Plast Reconstr Surg* 71: 490–499, 1983.
10. Brennan HG, Rafaty MD: Midforehead incisions in the treatment of the aging face. *Arch Otolaryngol* 108: 732–734, 1982.
11. Gonzalez VM: An update on blepharoplasty. *Aesthet Plast Surg* 7: 1–11, 1983.
12. Beekhus GJ: Blepharoplasty. *Otolaryngol Clin North Am* 15: 179–193, 1982.
13. Putterman AM: Simultaneous treatment of lower eyelid dermatochalasis and abnormal-appearing skin. *Am J Ophthalmol* 96: 6–9, 1983.
14. Custer PL, Tenzel RR, Kowal Czyk AP: Blepharochalasis syndrome. *Am J Ophthalmol* 99: 424–428, 1985.
15. Finney JL, Peterson HD: Blepharochalasis after a bee sting. *Plast Reconstr Surg* 73: 830–832, 1984.
16. Goldberg R, Seiff S, McFarland J, Simms K, Schorr N: Floppy eyelid syndrome and blepharochalasis. *Am J Ophthalmol* 102: 376–381, 1986.
17. Chose S, Kalra BR, Dayal Y: Blepharochalasis with multiple system involvement. *Br J Ophthalmol* 68: 529–532, 1984.
18. Cook TA, Dereburg J, Hurrah R: Reconsideration of fat pad management in lower lid blepharoplasty. *Arch Otolaryngol* 110: 521–524, 1984.
19. Furnas DW: Festoons of orbicularis muscle as a cause of baggy eyelids. *Plast Reconstr Surg* 61: 540–546, 1978.
20. Tobing HA: Electrosurgical blepharoplasty: A technique that questions the conventional concepts of fat compartmentalization. *Ann Plast Surg* 14: 59–63, 1985.
21. Kaye BL: The use of disposable cautery in blepharoplasty. *Plast Reconstr Surg* 75: 444–445, 1985.
22. Liv D: Reply: the use of disposable cautery in blepharoplasty. *Plast Reconstr Surg* 75: 445, 1985.
23. Liv D, Stassor O: Thermal orbital injuries resulting from disposable cauteries. *Plast Reconstr Surg* 74: 1, 1984.
24. Bater SS, Munezler WS, Small RG, Leonard JE: Carbon dioxide laser blepharoplasty. *Ophthalmology* 91: 233–244, 1984.
25. Hornblass A: Ptosis and pseudoptosis and blepharoplasty. In Rees TD (ed): *Modern Trends in Blepharoplasty*. Philadelphia, WB Saunders, 1981, p 811–830.
26. Fasanell RM, Servat J: Levator resection for minimal ptosis: Another simplified operation. *Arch Ophthalmol* 65: 493–496, 1961.

27. Putterman AM, Uris MJ: Muller muscle-conjunctiva resection. *Arch Ophthalmol* 93: 619–623, 1975.
28. Anderson RL, Gordy DD: The tarsal strip procedure. *Arch Ophthalmol* 97: 2192–2196, 1979.
29. Smith B, Petrelli R: Surgical repair of prolapsed lacrimal glands. *Arch Ophthalmol* 96: 113–114, 1978.
30. Hornblass A, Ingis JM: Lacrimal function tests. *Arch Ophthalmol* 97: 1654–1655, 1979.
31. Furnas DW: The orbicularis oculi muscle: Management in blepharoplasty. *Clin Plast Surg* 8: 687–706, 1981.
32. Soll DB (ed): *Management of Complications in Ophthalmic Plastic Surgery.* Birmingham, AL, Aesculapius, 1976, p 295–344.
33. Shagets FW, Shore JW: The management of eyelid laxity during lower eyelid blepharoplasty. *Arch Otolaryngol Head Neck Surg* 112: 729–732, 1986.
34. Rees TD: Prevention of ectropion by horizontal shortening of the lower lid during blepharoplasty. *Ann Plast Surg* 11(1): 17–23, 1983.
35. Tenzel RR: Complications of blepharoplasty. Orbital hematoma, ectropion and scleral show. *Clin Plast Surg* 8: 797–802, 1981.
36. Ortiz-Monasterio F, Rodriguez A: Lateral canthoplasty to change the eye slant. *Plast Reconstr Surg* 75: 1–10, 1985.
37. Victor WH, Hurwitz JJ: Cicatricial ectropion following blepharoplasty: Treatment by tissue expansion. *Can J Ophthalmol* 19: 317–319, 1984.
38. Duke-Elder S: The ocular adnexae. In *System of Ophthalmology.* St. Louis, CV Mosby, 1974, vol 18, p. 8–19.
39. Aston SJ: Orbicularis oculi muscle flaps: a technique to reduce crow's feet and lateral canthal skin folds. *Plast Reconstr Surg* 64: 206–216, 1980.
40. Tse DT, Folberg R, Moore K: Clinicopathologic correlate of a fresh eyelid pigment implantation. *Arch Ophthalmol* 103: 1515–1517, 1985.
41. Hornblass A: Patient selection for cosmetic oculoplastic surgery. In Putterman A: *Cosmetic Oculoplastic Surgery.* New York, Grune & Stratton, 1982, p 28–44.

CHAPTER 53

Upper Eyelid Blepharoplasty

ALLEN M. PUTTERMAN, M.D.

Dermatochalasis (excessive skin) and herniated orbital fat are the most common cosmetic problems of the upper eyelid. The excessive skin is usually located over the temporal two-thirds of the lid, and the herniated orbital fat commonly occurs over the nasal one-third. At times the skin is so excessive that it drapes over the lid margin and obscures vision. (In this situation, many insurance companies will consider patient reimbursement for cost of the surgery if the functional problem can be documented with photographs and visual fields.)

If the upper eyelid crease is close to normal (usually about 10 mm above the eyelid margin), the excessive skin and herniated fat can be removed without excision of the orbicularis muscle and without reconstruction of the upper eyelid crease. However, if the upper eyelid crease is low (0–8 mm) or is duplicated or asymmetric, then reconstruction of the eyelid crease along with excision of skin, orbicularis muscle, and orbital fat is indicated. When the crease is reconstructed, less of the upper eyelid skin needs to be excised. This is advantageous in patients with keratitis sicca because it avoids the postoperative complications of lagophthalmos and exposure keratopathy.

Eyebrow ptosis also can lead to a redundant upper eyelid fold. It is important to assess the position of the eyebrow; if it is found to be a significant contributing factor to the fullness to the upper lid fold, then elevation of the brow must be considered (1). This is usually accomplished by excising an ellipse of skin above the brow or by means of the popular coronal brow lift (1).

Prolapse of the lacrimal gland is another problem that can lead to upper eyelid fullness. In this situation, a subcutaneous bulge appears over the temporal eyelid. Since there is no temporal upper lid fat to herniate, the surgeon must recognize that fullness in this area is caused by a prolapsed lacrimal gland (1). The treatment is fixation of the gland to the lacrimal fossa periosteum. Mistaking the gland for fat could lead to excision of the gland and severe keratitis sicca.

Blepharochalasis is a rare problem that produces redundant tissue of the upper eyelid (2). It is usually caused by allergic edema and leads not only to dermatochalasis, herniated orbital fat, and a low lid crease, but also upper eyelid ptosis and horizontal laxity. Treatment of blepharochalasis usually consists not only of excising excess skin, orbicularis muscle, and herniated orbital fat but also of reconstructing the lid crease, performing a levator aponeurosis advancement and tuck ptosis procedure, and horizontally tightening the upper lid by removing a full-thickness section of the lid at its temporal end.

SURGICAL TREATMENT OF UPPER EYELID DERMATOCHALASIS AND HERNIATED ORBITAL FAT

SKIN MARKING

The surgeon uses a marking pen to outline excessive upper eyelid skin. If the lower eyelid also is being treated surgically, a lateral canthal line is drawn on the lower eyelid first to ensure at least 5 mm of skin between the upper and lower lateral canthal incisions (Fig. 53.1*A* and *B*). This line starts about 2–3 mm temporal to the lateral canthus and travels in a horizontal and slightly downward direction for a total of 1–1.5 cm. The upper lid fold is elevated with the surgeon's finger, and the patient is instructed to gaze slightly upward. A line is drawn where the lid creases with this maneuver (Fig. 53.1*C* and *D*). The line begins nasally above the upper punctum, extends

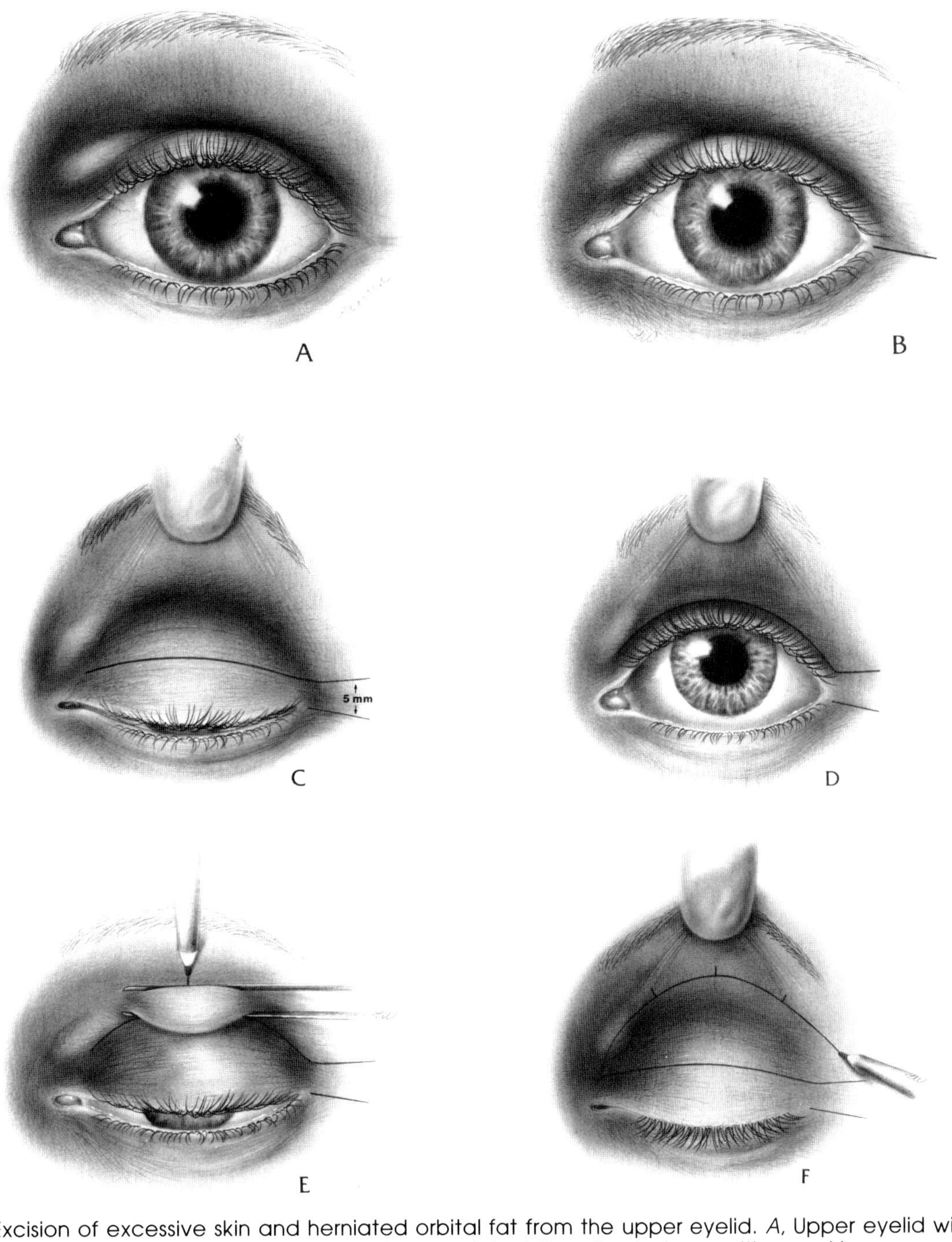

Figure 53.1. Excision of excessive skin and herniated orbital fat from the upper eyelid. *A*, Upper eyelid with dermatochalasis (excessive skin) and nasal herniated orbital fat. *B*, A 1- to 1.5-cm line is drawn with a marking pen over the lateral canthal lower lid incision site. The line begins 2–3 mm temporal to the lateral canthus and extends 1–1.5 cm in a horizontal but slightly downward direction. *C*, Upper lid skin fold is elevated by the surgeon raising the eyebrow so that a marking pen can indicate the upper eyelid crease site. This begins above the punctum and extends 1–1.5 cm beyond the lateral canthus in one of the natural canthal creases. The distance from the lower eyelid lateral canthal mark to the upper eyelid mark should be at least 5 mm. *D*, When the patient looks slightly upward, the marked line in the upper lid should fall into the upper eyelid crease that forms on slight upgaze. *E*, A smooth forceps grasps the center marked line with one blade and the other blade grasps the skin superiorly. The forceps is reapplied until all redundant upper lid skin is eliminated and the upper lid is elevated slightly from its closed position with the forceps blades meet. A mark is made centrally at the site of the upper forceps blade in this position. *F*, The central, temporal, and nasal superior marks are connected together and extended to the nasal and temporal extremes of the lid crease line.

to the lateral canthus, and then slopes slightly upward in one of the lateral canthal creases, about 1–1.5 cm beyond the lateral canthus.

A smooth forceps is placed horizontally to grasp the skin at the central aspect of the marked line and is applied to the skin superiorly. The forceps is closed at various levels until the amount of skin pinched together eliminates all excessive eyelid skin and minimally elevates the upper lid from its apposition to the lower lid (Fig. 53.1*E*). A mark is made at the superior site. The procedure is repeated nasally and temporally. The surgeon uses a marking pen to connect these three lines with the nasal and temporal ends of the eyelid crease line (Fig. 53.1*F*).

The contralateral upper eyelid is marked in a similar manner, and the amount of excessive skin outlined is compared with that of the first upper lid. Measurements are made from the upper lid margins to the lid crease lines and between the upper and lower marked lines. These

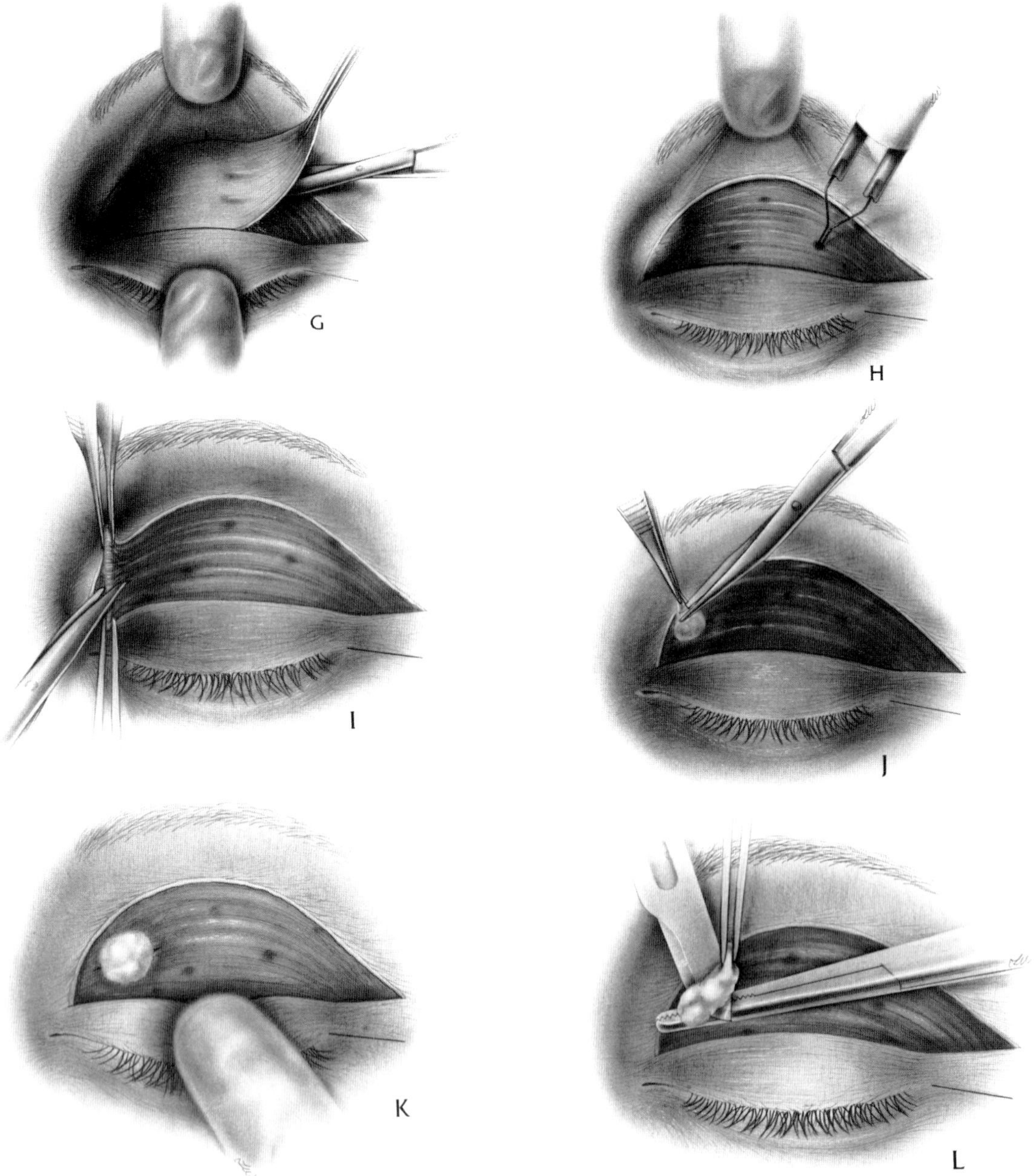

Figure 53.1. *G*, The outlined area of excessive skin is undermined and severed from underlying orbicularis muscle. *H*, Disposable cautery establishes hemostasis. *I*, A forceps grasps nasal orbicularis. As one forceps pulls the orbicularis directly downward, the superior forceps pulls upward and outward. The orbicularis tended with this maneuver is cut with a Westcott scissors that is directed inward and slightly upward. This should allow entrance into the space beneath the orbicularis where herniated orbital fat is located. *J*, The nasal herniated orbital fat capsule is grasped with forceps and severed. *K*, Pressure is applied to the globe through the upper eyelid to determine the amount of fat that herniates with gentle pressure. *L*, Nasal orbital fat that prolapses with gentle pressure is clamped with a hemostat and excised by running a No. 15 Bard-Parker blade along the edge of the hemostat.

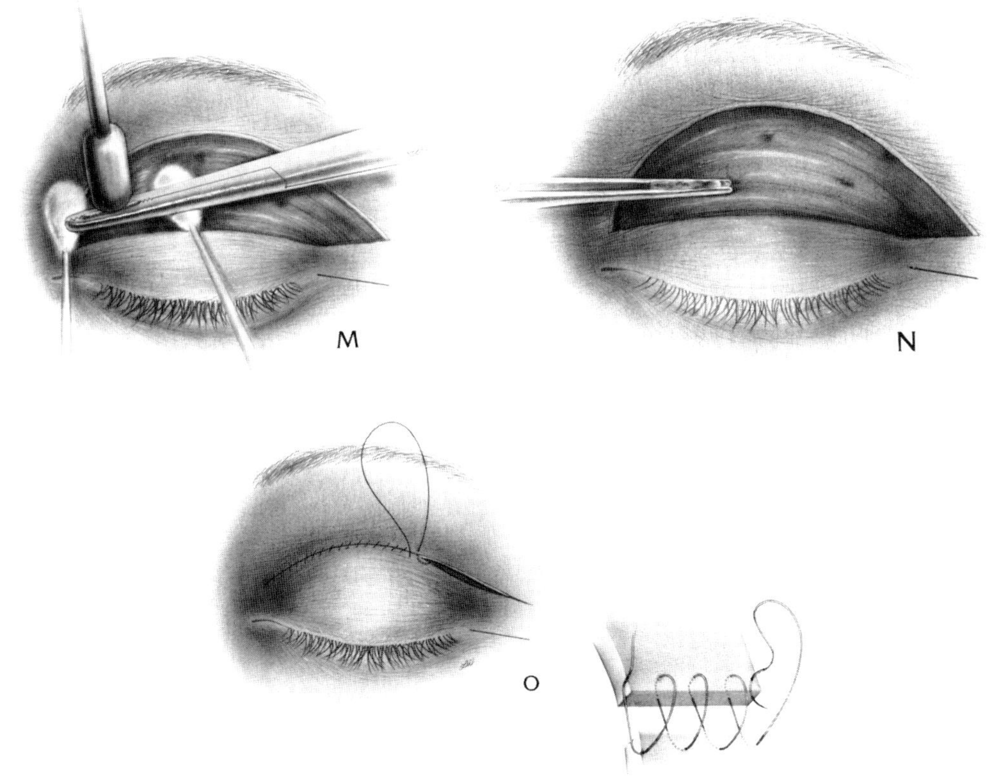

Figure 53.1. *M*, Cotton-tipped applicators separate the hemostat from underlying lid tissue, and Bovie cautery is applied to the hemostat to cauterize the excised nasal orbital fat stump. *N*, A forceps holds the nasal herniated orbital fat stump after the release of the hemostat, while the surgeon checks that hemostasis has been achieved before allowing the fat to slip back into the orbit. *O*, A continuous 6-0 black silk suture runs nasally to temporally to unite the skin edges. (From Putterman AM (ed): *Cosmetic Oculoplastic Surgery*. New York, Grune & Stratton, 1982.)

measurements should be similar if the amount of skin fold noted preoperatively is the same. Otherwise, differences in measurement should correspond to the preoperative asymmetry. (For example, if the left upper lid fold is more redundant or the left eyebrow is more ptotic than the right, a slightly greater outlined ellipse of skin is expected on the left upper lid compared with the right.)

SKIN EXCISION

Two-percent lidocaine with epinephrine is injected subcutaneously over the outlined upper eyelid and lateral canthus for anesthesia, hemostasis, and hydraulic dissection of skin from orbicularis muscle. A No. 15 Bard-Parker blade is used to incise along the upper eyelid marks in a nasal to temporal direction, first over the lower line and then on the upper line. Next, the skin is severed from orbicularis muscle with Westcott scissors (Fig. 53.1*G*). The assistant stretches the upper lid skin by pulling upward on the brow and downward on the upper lid margins. The surgeon finds the plane between skin and orbicularis by observing the points of the scissors beneath the translucent skin. (The upper lid skin is the thinnest in the body and the scissors blades should be easily seen beneath it. Also, while observing the undersurface of the skin, the surgeon should readily see the operating light shining through the thin skin; this should also facilitate the skin-orbicularis dissection.) An Accu-temp disposable cautery (No. 4300, Concept Medical Division, South Clearwater, FL) is used to control all bleeding (Fig. 53.1*H*).

EXCISION OF ORBITAL FAT

Any herniated fat noted preoperatively is removed next. Usually, nasal orbital fat (white) is herniated, but at times, the middle fat (yellow) is also displaced. [There is no temporal fat in the upper lid; a protrusion in this area is usually caused by a prolapsed lacrimal gland and should be handled by the replacement of the gland in the lacrimal fossa (1).]

Slight pressure is applied to the eyelids and globe, and the nasal orbicularis is observed for tenting by the herniated fat. The orbicularis at this site is picked up with forceps and pulled upward and outward, away from the globe. The assistant grasps the orbicularis close to the crease incision and pulls the lid downward. (This maneuver pulls the orbicularis away from the levator aponeurosis.) The surgeon severs the orbicularis between these two forceps with a Westcott scissors that is directed slightly upward and inward (Fig. 53.1*I*). (Severing the orbicularis in this manner creates a space between orbicularis and levator aponeurosis that should be easily seen at this time. Herniated orbital fat should be observed in this potential space.)

Pressure is applied to the globe, and fat protruding through the opening of the orbicularis is noted; the fat capsule is grasped with forceps and severed (Fig. 53.1*J*). Pressure again is applied to the globe, and fat should now flow through the orbicularis opening (Fig. 53.1*K*). The fat that protrudes easily with gentle pressure on the globe is grasped with forceps and pulled outward from the wound. (It is important not to pull too vigorously on the fat, because the anterior nasal orbital fat communicates with the posterior orbital fat, through which the ophthalmic and ciliary arteries may pass. Undue tension on these vessels could theoretically rupture them, and could lead to permanent blindness.) The fat that protrudes with this maneuver is clamped with a straight hemostat and severed by slicing with a Bard-Parker blade against the hemostat (Fig. 53.1*L*). [The surgeon should inspect the hemostat before applying it to make sure that the jaws meet completely when closed. If they do not, the fat can slip out of the hemostat and lead to serious bleeding that is difficult to control and has the potential to cause blindness (3).] Hemostasis is achieved with a Bovie cautery applied to the hemostat. A setting on the Bovie is chosen to cauterize adequately without charring the tissue. The hemostat is held away from other lid tissues with cotton-tipped applicators (Fig. 53.1*M*).

The fat beneath the hemostat is grasped with a forceps, and the hemostat is released. The surgeon inspects the severed fat for bleeding before allowing it to retract into the orbit (Fig. 53.1*N*). Any bleeding is treated with a disposable Concept cautery applied to the severed end of the orbital fat until the bleeding is controlled.

Any herniated midorbital fat noted preoperatively is removed in a similar fashion through the same orbicularis opening. Occasionally, an orbicularis incision slightly temporal to the nasal site is necessary to isolate midorbital fat.

Care must be taken to avoid pulling the levator aponeurosis into the hemostat clamped with the orbital fat. The tissue beneath the hemostat should be inspected carefully to make sure that it is fat and not levator aponeurosis before it is severed.

The surgeon covers the orbicularis muscle with a 4 × 4 inch pad that is soaked in lidocaine with epinephrine and wrung out. The same procedure then is followed for the contralateral upper eyelid.

SKIN CLOSURE

The skin incisions are sutured closed with continuous 6-0 black silk in multiple close bites that are pulled snugly during closure (Fig. 53.1*O*). I prefer to use running continuous 6-0 black silk through the upper eyelid wound. This suture is easier to work with than the stiffer nylon or polypropylene (Prolene) sutures. However, suture cysts are a common complication that require hydroylsis at a later date.

Alternative sutures to the 6-0 running black silk include the continuous 6-0 Prolene or a subcuticular suture of 6-0 nylon. (I have found that the nylon is difficult to remove and have caused wound dehiscences in doing so, even though it is removed 10–14 days postoperatively.) A 6-0 catgut suture can be used to eliminate the discomfort of suture removal. The dissolving of this suture, however, is not always predictable, and I believe that it can cause more scarring than the nonabsorbable suture. Polyglactin 910 (Vicryl) and 6-0 polyglycolic (Dexon) sutures also dissolve with minimum reaction; however, the process takes 4–6 weeks, and a good deal of scarring can be created in that time. Another alternative is to use interrupted 6-0 black silk or nylon sutures and remove them by pulling them out rather than by cutting them from the skin. This procedure prevents suture cysts and tunnels because the outer surface of any cyst or tunnel is pulled off with this technique. I find that this maneuver is surgically displeasing and prefer to contend with hyphercation of the cysts postoperatively.

W-PLASTY AND TRIANGULAR EXCISION FOR MEDIAL DERMATOCHALASIS

If there is a moderate amount of medial canthal skin, a W-plasty is performed medially. Instead of the upper and lower lines ending in a point medially, they are connected together as a "W" (Fig. 53.2*A*). On closing the central triangle of the W, it is pulled temporally to eliminate nasal dermatochalasis (Fig. 53.2*B*, *C*). Another technique to accomplish elimination of redundant medial canthal skin is to remove a triangle of tissue above the nasal skin resection site. A superior nasal cut is made about 8–10 mm from the nasal skin resection ellipse (Fig. 53.3*A*). The skin nasal to this cut is undermined, and the flap is pulled temporally to create slight tension (Fig. 53.3*B*). The place where the overlapped flap meets the underlying skin edge determines the site at which this triangular skin flap is excised. Suturing this area together reduces the excess medial canthal skin (Fig. 53.3*C*). (It is unwise to create incisions nasal to the punctum to eliminate excessive nasal skin, because webs at the canthal folds and excessive scarring may be produced. I prefer the W-plasty rather than the triangular skin resection to reduce medial canthal skin.)

RECONSTRUCTION OF THE UPPER EYELID CREASE

A line is drawn at the site of the proposed lid crease. This is usually 10–12 mm above the upper lid margin centrally (Fig. 53.4*A*). The line begins at a point vertical with the punctum and extends 1–1.5 cm temporal to the lateral canthus. The measurement from the lid margin to the crease line over the temporal third of the lid is the same as at the central distance; it is usually 2 mm less over the nasal one-third of the lid.

A smooth forceps is placed horizontally to grasp the skin at the central aspect of the marked line and is applied to the skin superiorly. The forceps is closed at various levels until the amount of skin pinched together eliminates all excessive eyelid skin without lash eversion (Fig. 53.4*A*). (This varies from removal of the skin without crease formation, for which lash eversion and slight lifting of the upper lid margin from the lower lid margin are the end points.) A mark is made at the superior site. The procedure

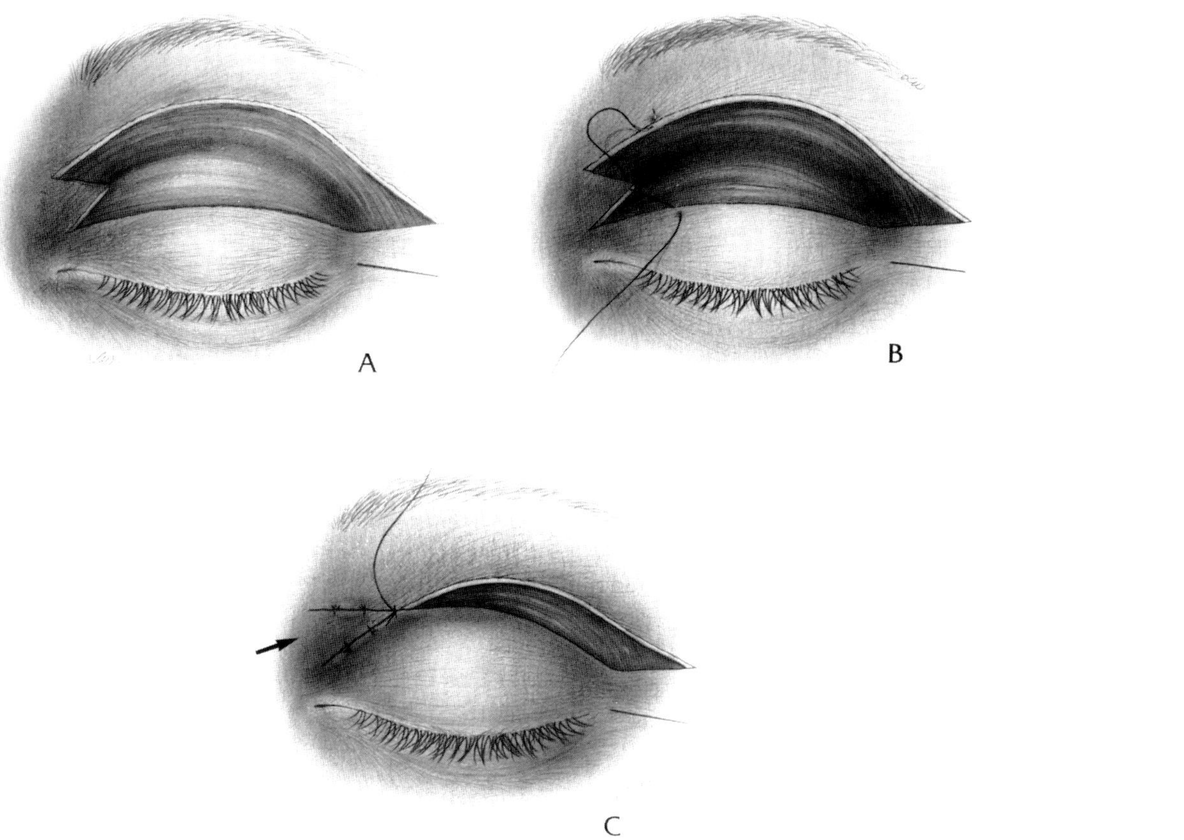

Figure 53.2. Treatment of nasal upper lid excessive skin with W-plasty. *A*, A W-incision is made at the nasal aspect of the upper eyelid skin resection site. *B*, A 6-0 black silk suture passes through skin edges approximately 5–8 mm temporal to passage through the subcutaneous apex of the W-incision. *C*, The 6-0 black silk depicted in *panel B* is tied so that the apex of the "W" is drawn temporally to reduce medial canthal skin. Several interrupted 6-0 black silk sutures are used to close upper and lower limbs of the triangular incision sites. (From Putterman AM (ed): *Cosmetic Oculoplastic Surgery*. New York, Grune & Stratton, 1982).

is repeated nasally and temporally. The surgeon uses the marking pen to connect these dots with the nasal and temporal ends of the upper crease line (Fig. 53.4*B*).

The contralateral upper lid is marked in a similar manner, the amount of excessive skin is outlined, and measurements of the lid crease position are compared until symmetry is achieved.

Two-percent lidocaine with epinephrine is then injected subcutaneously over the outlined skin ellipse. A skin incision is made with a No. 15 Bard-Park blade and the outlined skin ellipse is undetermined from orbicularis muscle and excised (Fig. 53.4*C*).

An 8–10 mm strip of orbicularis muscle is then excised from underlying levator aponeurosis across the eyelid just above the crease incision site (Fig. 53.4*D*). Picking up the orbicularis muscle with forceps during this excision minimizes injury to the levator aponeurosis.

If there is herniated orbital fat, it is excised next. Commonly, orbital fat will prolapse when gentle pressure is applied to the eye, since removal of the orbicularis muscle exposes the orbital septum (Fig. 53.4*E* and *F*). If orbital fat does not prolapse with this maneuver it is isolated as previously outlined for removal of the nasal orbital fat under excision of orbital fat. The orbital fat that flows forward with gentle pressure applied to the eye is clamped with a hemostat and excised, and then Bovie cautery is applied to the fat stump as previously outlined.

The upper eyelid crease is then reconstructed. This is accomplished by attaching four or five 6-0 white polyester (Mersilene) sutures from levator aponeurosis or superior tarsal border to the orbicularis of the lower skin flap, in a mattress fashion (Fig. 53.4*G–I*). The superior aspect of the lower skin muscle flap is grasped with forceps and is pulled over tarsus and levator aponeurosis to the position that the eyelashes are properly everted. The distance from the lid margin to this area is the desired lid crease position site. The needle of the Mersilene suture is then passed from right to left through levator aponeurosis or tarsus at this level, engaging approximately 3 mm of tissue. The needle is then passed through orbicularis through adjacent orbicularis muscle of the upper aspect of the lower skin flap from left to right, engaging approximately 3 mm of tissue. The suture ends are then drawn up and tied with approximately four knots, and the suture ends are cut close to the knot. One of the key sutures is at the temporal end of the lid, several millimeters nasal to the lateral canthus.

The skin is then closed with a continuous 6-0 black silk

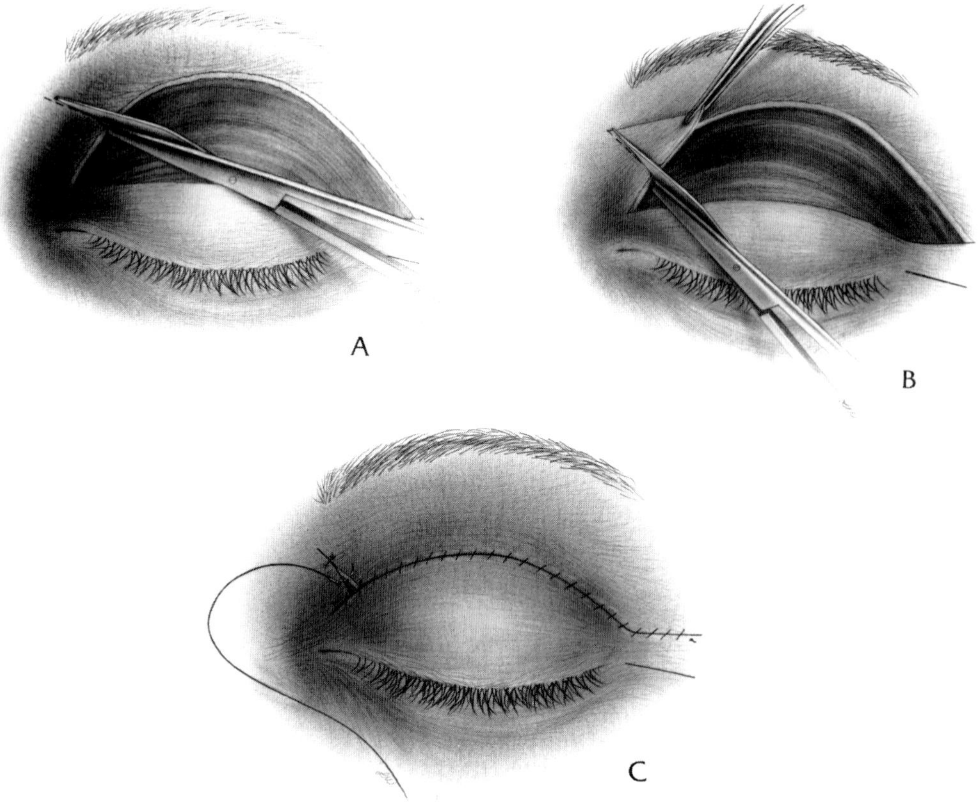

Figure 53.3. Nasal triangular technique to treat upper eyelid nasal dermatochalasis. *A*, Scissors severs skin in a superonasal direction, approximately 8–10 mm from the nasal end of the upper eyelid skin resection site for a distance of approximately 10 mm. *B*, The skin flap is drawn temporally and superiorly in the area of excessive skin to the degree needed to reduce medial canthal dermatochalasis. The triangle overlapping the underlying skin incision site is excised. *C*, Closure of the superonasal incision pulls the excessive medial canthal skin temporally and eliminates it. (From Putterman AM (ed): *Cosmetic Oculoplastic Surgery*. New York, Grune & Stratton, 1982.)

suture run nasally to temporally (Fig. 53.4*J*). (Care must be taken to avoid severing or removing the Mersilene suture during the running of the 6-0 black silk suture. Other suture material can be used as outlined under "Skin Closure".) The other lid is then treated similarly. (It is important that the eyelash and lid crease positions are symmetric.)

An alternative technique to reconstruct the upper eyelid crease is to excise an ellipse of skin and underlying orbicularis together. Then 6-0 Vicryl interupted sutures unite the tarsus or levator aponeurosis to each edge of skin. I prefer the described procedure rather than the alternative technique, since the crease is less evident on downgaze or with lid closure when the described technique is used. Also, postoperative ptosis and tightness of the lid on upgaze seems less with the described procedure.

POSTOPERATIVE CARE

No dressings are used after surgery so that the eyelids and eyes are visible for inspection. The patient is instructed to apply ice-cold compresses on the eyelids: 4 × 4-inch pads are soaked in a bucket of saline and ice and are applied with slight pressure to the lids. When the pads become warm, they are dipped again into the saline and ice and reapplied. The process is repeated for about 24 hours. The applications should be fairly constant for the first few postoperative hours. After that, the compresses are applied for about 20 minutes, with 15-minute rest periods in between until bedtime. The applications are resumed on awakening.

To reduce edema postoperatively, the patient lies in bed with the head about 45° higher than the rest of the body. Nurses should check for bleeding associated with proptosis, pain, or loss of vision; this is checked by counting fingers with each eye every 15 minutes for the first 2 hours postoperatively. If loss of vision occurs secondary to retrobulbar hemorrhage, it can be detected quickly and treated by opening the incision involved (2).

The 6-0 black silk sutures are removed 4 days postoperatively. The incision is supported with ¼ inch Steri-strips applied over weak areas, usually the lateral upper and lower canthal incision sites, for 3 more days.

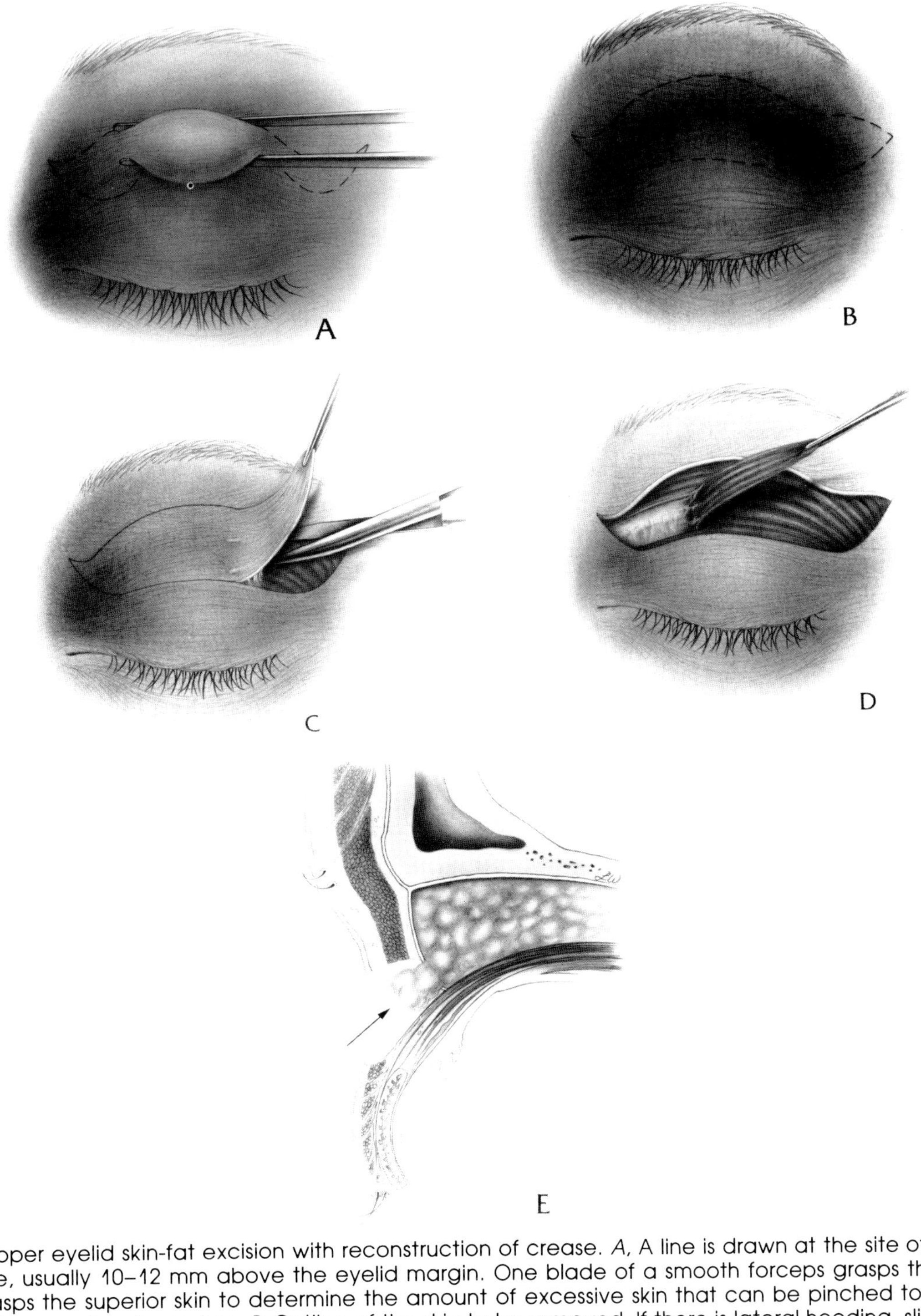

Figure 53.4. Upper eyelid skin-fat excision with reconstruction of crease. *A*, A line is drawn at the site of the proposed upper lid crease, usually 10–12 mm above the eyelid margin. One blade of a smooth forceps grasps this line and the other blade grasps the superior skin to determine the amount of excessive skin that can be pinched together without elevating the lid or everting the lashes. *B*, Outline of the skin to be removed. If there is lateral hooding, slightly more skin is removed in this area. *C*, Skin is removed from the orbicularis muscle after the premarked lines are incised with a No. 15 Barde-Parker blade. *D*, Eight- to 10-mm strip of orbicularis muscle is excised from underlying levator aponeurosis just above the lid crease site. *E*, The orbital septum is opened across the wound, and the fat is removed as previously described.

RESULTS

Over 600 lids have been treated by excising excessive skin and herniated orbital fat without lid crease reconstruction (Fig. 53.5). Patients have been followed from 3 months to 15 years postoperatively. Suture cysts have occurred in over 75% of these patients and have been successfully treated with light hydrolysis. It has been nec-

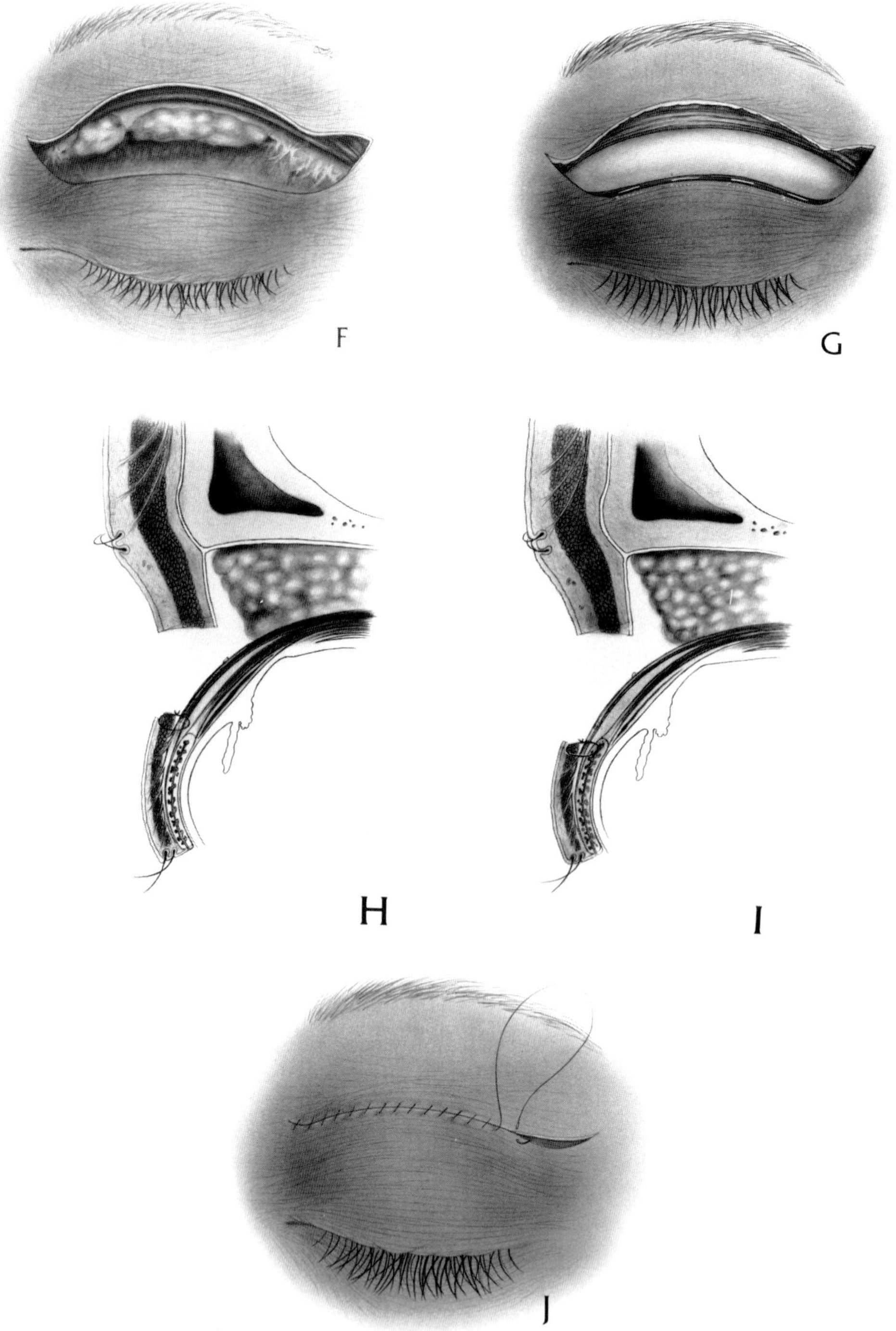

Figure 53.4. *F*, Demonstration of two orbital fat pads. *G*, Four fixation sutures of 6-0 white braided (Mersilene) polyester fibers go from the upper edge of the inferior orbicularis to the levator aponeurosis or to the aponeurosis and tarsus. *H*, Fixation of the orbicularis muscle from the lower skin flap to the levator aponeurosis. *I*, Fixation of the orbicularis muscle to levator aponeurosis and superior tarsus. *J*, Closure of skin wound with 6-0 continuous black silk suture. (From Tenzel RR: Upper eyelid crease formation. In Putterman AM (ed): *Cosmetic Oculoplastic Surgery*. New York, Grune & Stratton, 1982, pp 179–186.)

essary to remove more skin in three patients. None of the patients has developed secondary ptosis or lagophthalmos.

Over 100 eyelids have been treated by reconstruction of the upper eyelid crease along with skin-fat excision with at least a 3-month postoperative follow-up (Fig. 53.6). There have been more complications in this group of patients compared with those undergoing skin fat excision without crease formation. These include multiple incidences of asymmetrical lid-crease formation and eyelash eversion. A temporary ptosis occurred in several patients and resolved spontaneously several months postoperatively. Some patients also had noted a tight sensation and

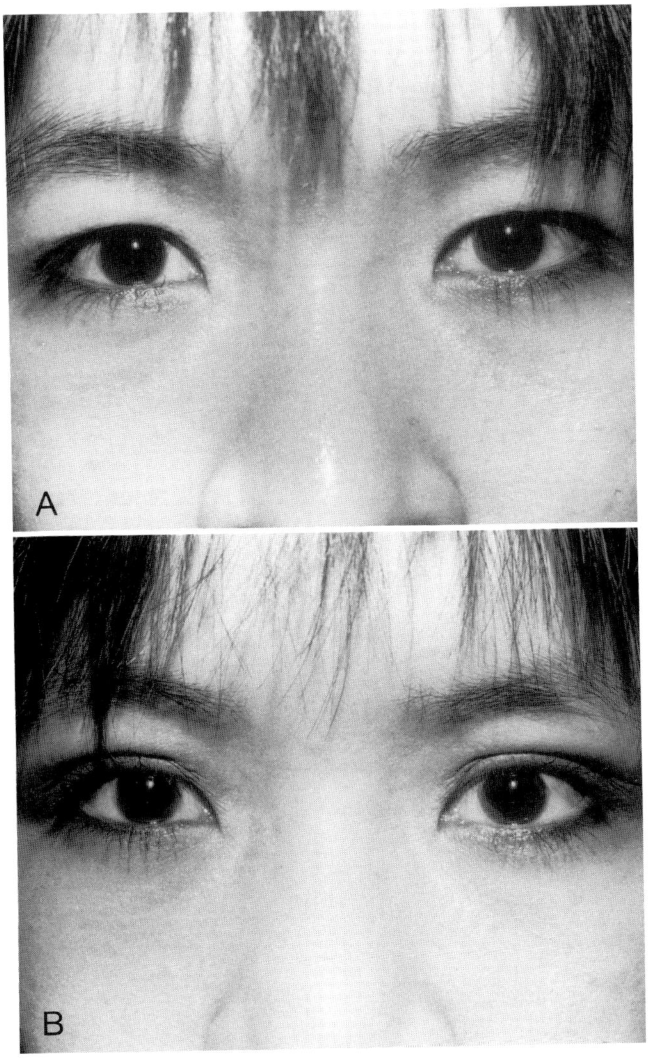

Figure 53.5. *A*, Preoperative photograph of patient with dermatochalasis and herniated orbital fat of upper eyelids. *B*, Postoperative photograph of same patient after excision of excessive skin and herniated orbital fat.

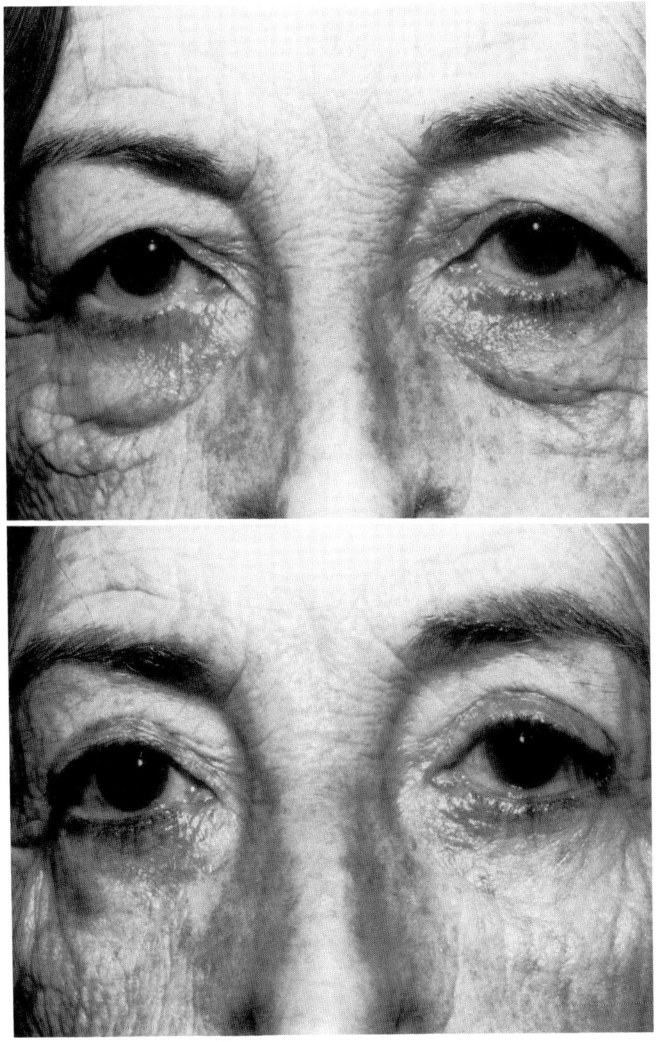

Figure 53.6. Preoperative (*A*) and postoperative (*B*) appearance in patient following skin fat excision with reconstruction of upper eyelid crease.

difficulty in elevating their eyelids on upgaze. This too resolved spontaneously several months postoperatively. Suture cysts occurred in approximately 75% of these patients and responded to light hydrolysis 2 months postoperatively. Several patients had a late suture abcess secondary to the Mersilene suture that resolved after removal of these sutures.

SUMMARY

Cosmetic oculoplastic surgery of the upper eyelid can lead to pleasing results. This is most frequently accomplished by excising excessive skin and nasal herniated orbital fat without reconstructing the upper eyelid crease. In many of these cases a functional improvement, including an increase of the superior visual field, is also accomplished. A W-plasty or triangular excision carried out over the nasal third of the lid can resolve redundant nasal upper eyelid skin without creating unsightly webs.

Reconstruction of the upper eyelid crease along with excision of the excessive skin, herniated orbital fat, and orbicularis muscle is desirable in patients who have low, duplicated, or asymmetric lid creases or in patients with the potential for keratitis sicca.

EDITOR'S COMMENT

I have found that when excising orbital fat with a Bard-Parker blade flush against the hemostat, the orbital fat may retract and sometimes the fat may not cauterize sufficiently. I prefer to excise the skin with a scissor and leave a small edge of the fat above the hemostat. I can then put my cautery directly onto the fat and thus visualize the actual cauterization of the fat. Dr. Putterman has stressed correctly that one should only amputate the amount of fat that easily protrudes under digital pressure and that one should not go into the orbit to seek orbital fat. My own preference for skin closure of the upper lid is either a 6-0 or a 5-0 subcuticular nylon suture. This helps avoid some of the suture cysts that Dr. Putterman has suggested is a common complication.

Early removal of sutures is critical, and I remove almost all sutures in 72 hours, including the subcuticular suture. Dr. Putterman's experience is particularly helpful in his discussion of the reconstruction of the upper eyelid crease, which is critical when one is looking for symmetry in a cosmetic blepharoplasty.

ACKNOWLEDGMENT

I would like to acknowledge Linda Warren for creating the illustrations.

This chapter was supported in part by Core Grant EY 1792 from the National Eye Institute, National Institutes of Health, Bethesda, Maryland.

REFERENCES

1. Putterman AM: *Cosmetic Oculoplastic Surgery.* New York, Grune & Stratton, 1982, pp 99–116, 148–186, 210–219.
2. Collin JRO, Beard C, Stern WH, Schoengarth: Blepharochalasis. *Br J Ophthalmol* 63: 542–546, 1979.
3. Putterman AM: Temporary blindness after cosmetic blepharoplasty. *Am J Ophthalmol* 80: 1081–1083, 1975.

CHAPTER 54

Lower Eyelid Blepharoplasty: The Cutaneous Approach

THOMAS D. REES, M.D., F.A.C.S.
WILLIAM B. NOLAN, M.D.

Good, bad, and indifferent results following blepharoplasty are often measured in millimeters. Marking the incisions with dye can determine these extremes. Despite the small tolerance for error, accurate assessment of the lower eyelid deformity is as essential as the actual surgical procedure. This chapter is concerned only with the lower eyelid and with the transcutaneous approach to lower lid blepharoplasty in particular, as contrasted to the transconjunctival incision. In many ways the upper eyelid operation is as critical, if not more so, than the lower lid, since the upper lids are essential to cover the cornea and provide protection and lubrication of the globe during sleep, whilst it is entirely possible to have severe ectropion of the lower lids and still not endanger the cornea.

This chapter discusses the evaluation and treatment of lower eyelid deformities including dermatocholasis, pseudoherniation of orbital fat, various deformities of the orbicularis muscle, and some aspects of the prevention and treatment of loss of tone of the lower lids, commonly referred to as "senile ectropion," which is actually a misnomer since it can occur in a host of orbital irregularities quite apart from senility. Preoperative evaluation with emphasis on applied anatomy, physical examination, and preoperative photographs is clearly of critical importance; however it will not be detailed here since examination and diagnosis is detailed elsewhere in this volume. Instead, the surgical indications and methods of the transcutaneous lower eyelid blepharoplasty are described in some detail with emphasis on the avoidance of complications. It will be repeatedly stressed that a thorough evaluation of the deformity is the key to obtaining an optimal result.

PREOPERATIVE EVALUATION

The preoperative evaluation includes a thorough examination of the orbital region and its contents as well as an analysis of the preoperative photographs. The operative plan is designed on the basis of the information gleaned from the evaluation. The general plan of the surgery evolves from the evaluation, but hard and fast surgical decisions cannot be made until the actual surgery. Room must be left for variations in the surgical plan based on findings at surgery. Photographs are important, and these should be of a standardized and professional quality. They are used in the operating room for continued monitoring of the patient's normal preoperative visage. A supine patient on an operating table loses many of the anatomical characteristics that guide the surgeon in devising a surgical plan. If, during the preoperative evaluation, information is obtained that indicates ophthalmic disease or associated systemic problems, the consultation of the appropriate specialist should be obtained. The plastic surgeon frequently requires the advice and guidance of an ophthalmologist in such matters. In our experience there are very few conditions of the eye that prohibit plastic surgery of the lids, but all problems should be recognized and evaluated preoperatively, including such obvious steps as a general visual acuity test.

Physical evaluation of the lower lid should consist of a systematic exercise in applied anatomy. The components of the lid that are routinely evaluated (in addition to the eye) are the skin, muscle, fat, bony orbital rims, conjunctiva, and the lacrimal system. The elasticity of the lid is also an important factor. When examining the skin, the surgeon notes the general appearance and degree of redundancy as well as the size and number of rhytides. The amount of excess of the orbicularis muscle and any special characteristics of this muscle such as unusual muscle folds, bands, or abnormalities that may occur during animation of this structure are also noted. Almost all patients have some degree of excess of the orbicularis muscle that requires consideration during surgery, a fact only recently appreciated by most surgeons (2, 4). We routinely resect muscle, along with skin, in our patients. The amount of excision ranges from only 1 or 2 mm to much more along the cut edge of the skin muscle flap. Marked excess of muscle ("festoons") require quite separate attention (2). The amount of excess muscle can be approximately determined preoperatively by pinching the palpebral bag between the thumb and index finger and rolling the excess tissue. Muscle can be recognized tactilely by the sense of bulk in most patients. Another test of muscle bulk is the

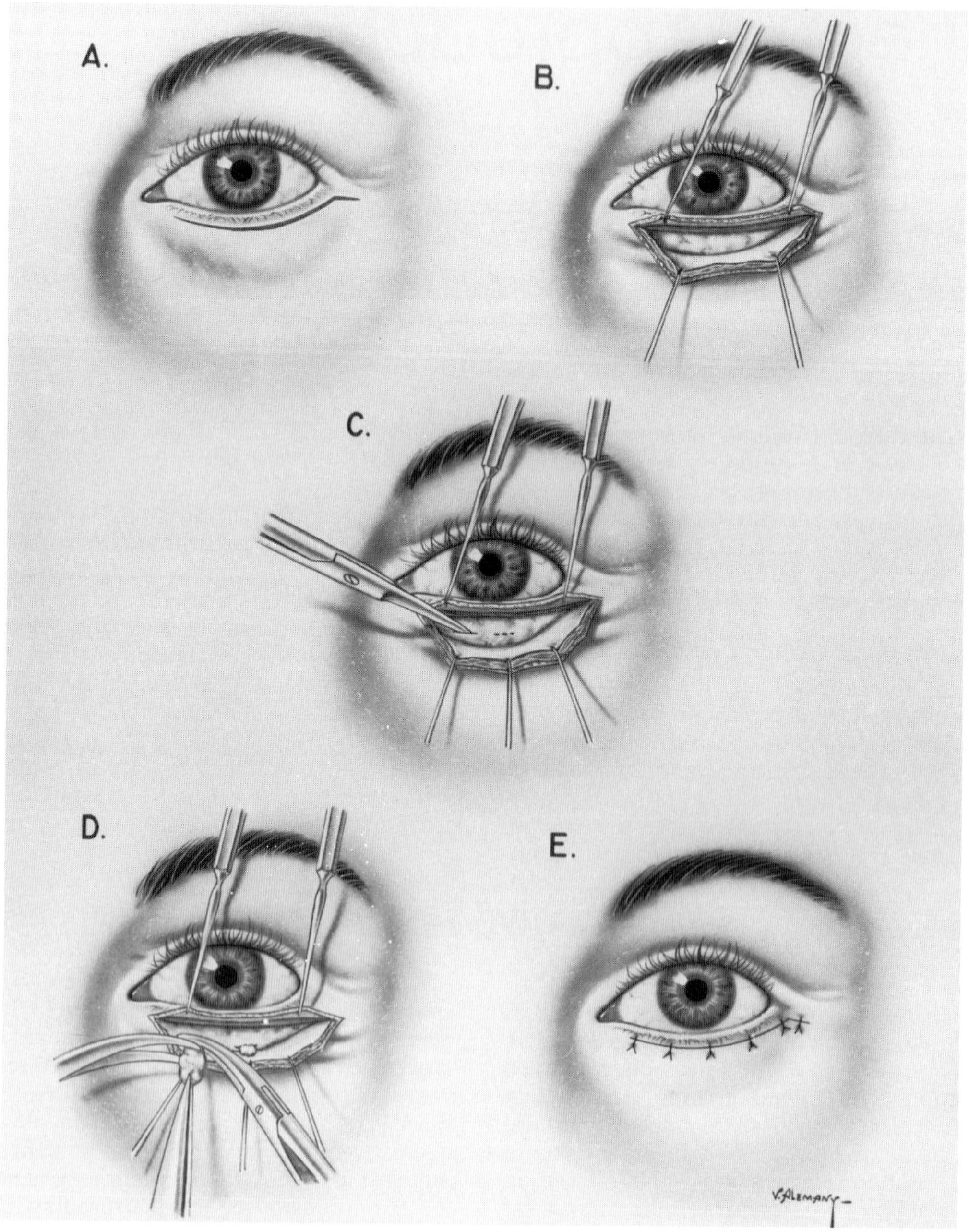

Figure 54.1. *A–E,* Simple skin muscle flap blepharoplasty in the young adult with familial fat bags. The dissection is limited, and the lateral extension of the wound can be ended just lateral to the lateral canthus. The fat can be removed through stab wounds in the orbital septum.

"squinch" test. The appearance and location of the bags and folds are observed during forceful orbicularis contraction. Ruggae and fold of excess muscle along with skin come into prominence during such animation if muscle is redundant, otherwise the muscle tightens and the skin folds become effaced, but relatively less than the muscle.

The orbital fat is assessed by first visualizing the location of the medial, middle, and lateral components. Especially in younger patients with minimal excess skin and/or muscle, the fat bulges are obvious and located where expected. The fat bulges are accentuated by gentle pressure on the globe and by having the patient gaze upwards.

It is exceedingly important to assess the configuration of the bony orbital rims and the relationship of the palpebral bags to the rims before blepharoplasty. The degree of prominence of the infraorbital margins are especially critical. Excessive prominence of the infraorbital rims can result in relative enophthalmos postoperatively if too much fat is resected (3). Hypoplasia of the maxilla with recessed rims in the presence of aggressive excision of fat or skin can result in tight eyelid margins that accentuate the forward projection of the globes and a "bug-eyed" look postoperatively, which at times results in marked scleral show and apparent ectropion.

Lower eyelid elasticity is determined by the traction and snap-back test. The lid is pulled away from the globe, pinched between the thumb and forefinger. The distance from the globe in millimeters is noted. Any distance over 6 mm arouses suspicion of laxity. Next, the lid is released and the degree of snap back onto the globe noted. If the recoil is slow and sluggish, insufficient elastic force must be suspected to overcome the downward pull of the healing flap. Ectropion can be the ultimate result of surgery in such cases. A variation in the procedure to include horizontal shortening or slinging of the lower lid should be included in the operative plan if such hypoelasticity is present (5).

Scleral show is an important clinical observation. Scleral show is normal in some patients, or can be a signal of exophthalmos or loss of lower lid tone. Scleral show constitutes a warning that excision of tissue must be undertaken cautiously and conservatively to avoid worsening the condition, or that horizontal shortening of the lid may be in order during the blepharoplasty procedure.

The lacrimal system is evaluated by checking for Bell's phenomenon and performing a Schirmer's test. Temporary lagophthalmos after blepharoplasty is the rule rather than the exception, and the lacrimal system is stressed to

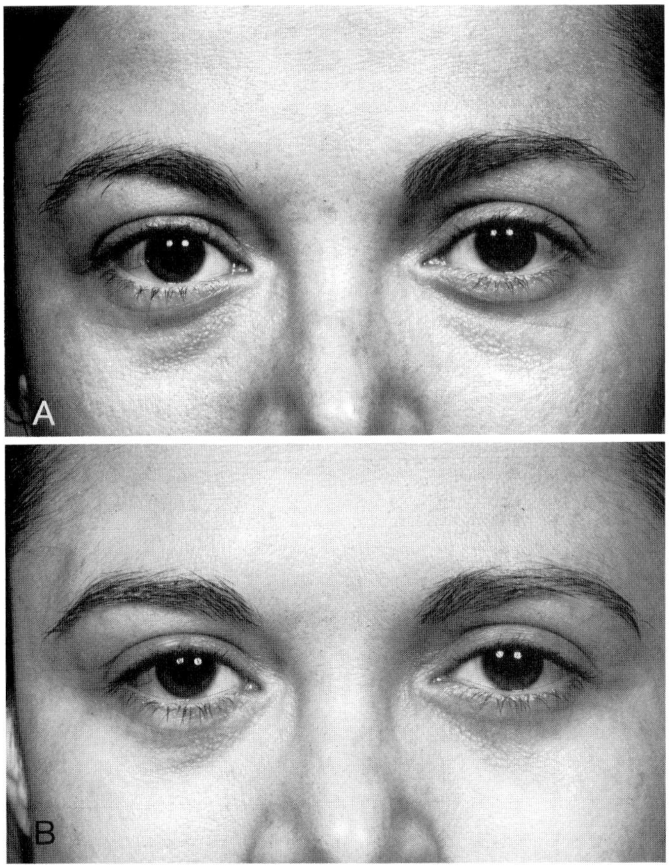

Figure 54.2. *A,* Typical palpebral fat bags in a young patient with a familial predisposition. *B,* Such a problem is easily cured according to the technique in Figure 54.1.

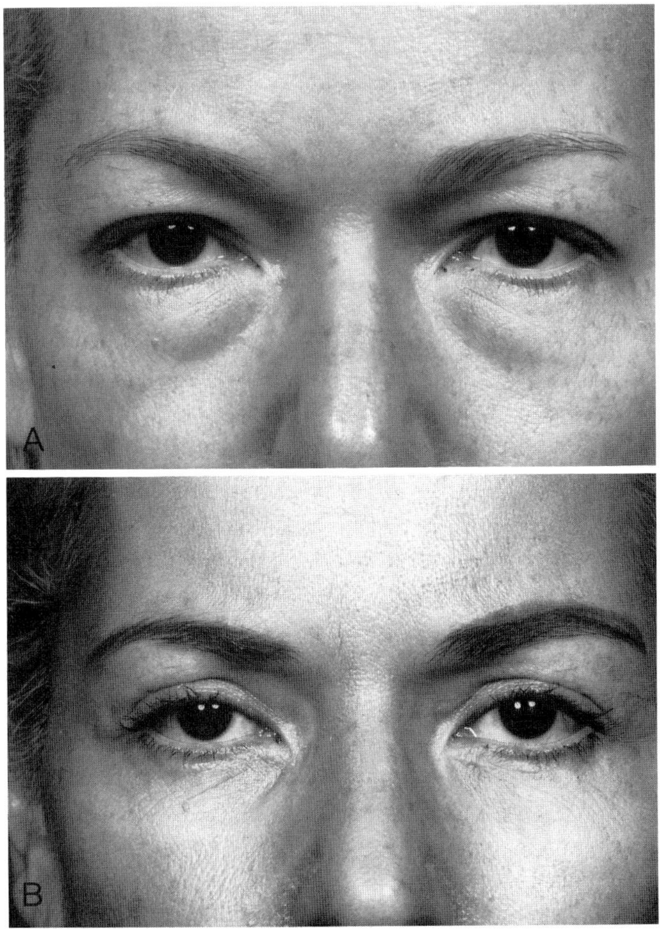

Figure 54.3. *A,* Marked redundancy of the periorbital fat in a 30-year-old woman also with a strong family history of this physical feature. *B,* Such a patient is also operated according to the technique in Figure 54.1.

maintain lubrication of the cornea. Deficient tearing must be suspected in a Schirmer's test of less than 10 mm. A positive Bell's test and normal blinking of the lids should also be present.

TRANSCUTANEOUS SURGICAL TECHNIQUE

The lower eyelid incision is marked in the first natural skin crease below the lash line. This crease is easily visualized in most patients at about 2–3 mm below the ciliary margin. The proposed incision is marked laterally into a natural rhytide of the "crow's foot." In young patients with minimal excess of skin and muscle, but only redundant fat, the incision can be ended at the lateral canthus to avoid lateral scars (Figs. 54.1 and 54.2).

When marked excess of skin and muscle is present the incision extends quite far laterally into the natural "laugh line" (Fig. 54.3). Marked caudal angulation of this incision as advocated in many early reports is not necessary and results in an obvious scar against natural facial lines.

After marking the incision, the surgeon infiltrates the tissues with the local anesthetic solution containing epinephrine to achieve vasoconstriction and hemostasis. It is

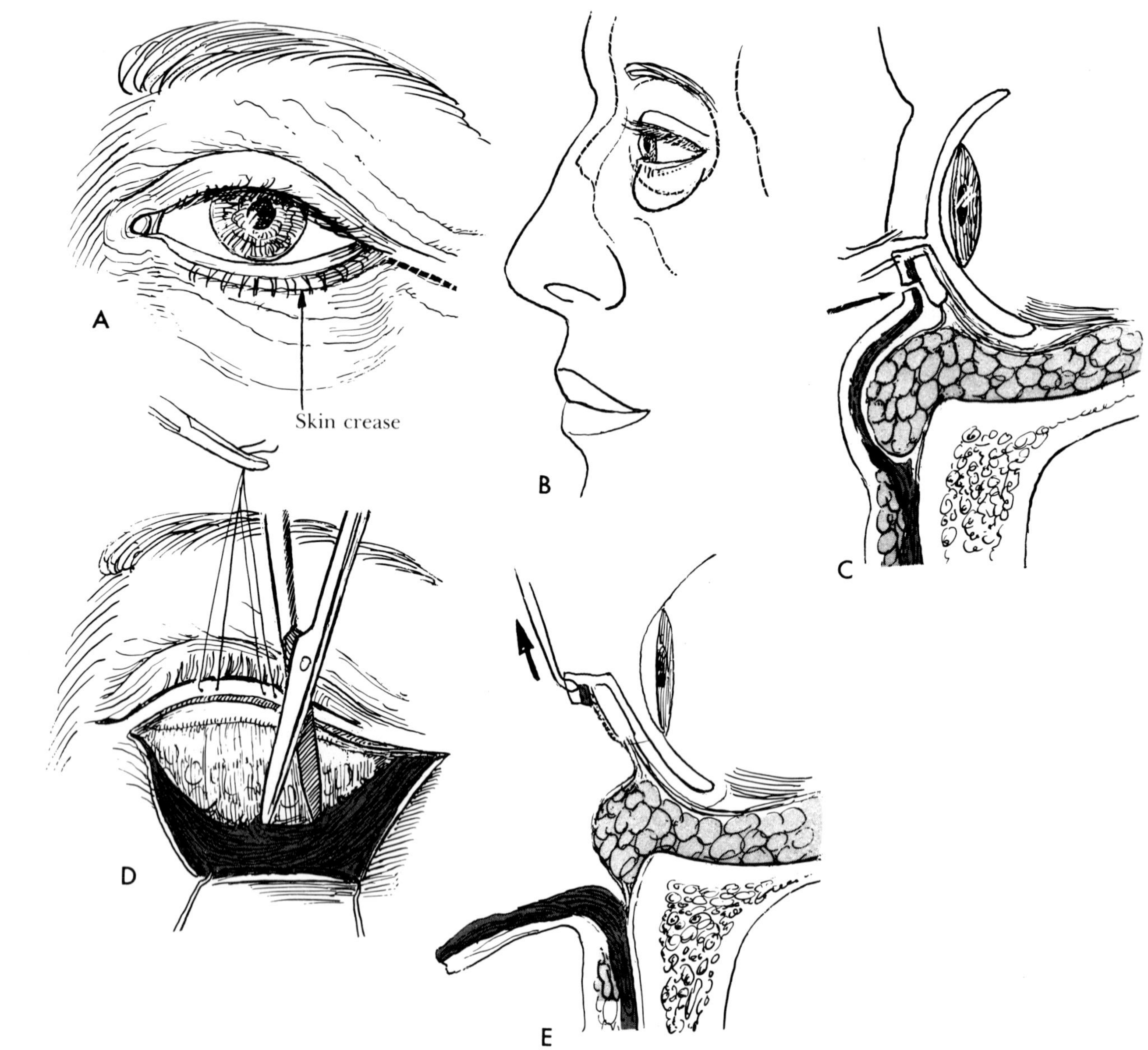

Figure 54.4. *A–O* The more extended skin muscle technique of blepharoplasty is shown (see text). This technique is useful for most blepharoplasty operations. The entire flap of skin muscle can be dissected down to and even beyond the orbital rim depending on the severity of the deformity. In more extensive problems, the orbital septum is opened throughout its length to gain full access to the three major fat pockets. From Rees TD: *Aesthetic Plastic Surgery*. Philadelphia, WB Saunders, 1981.)

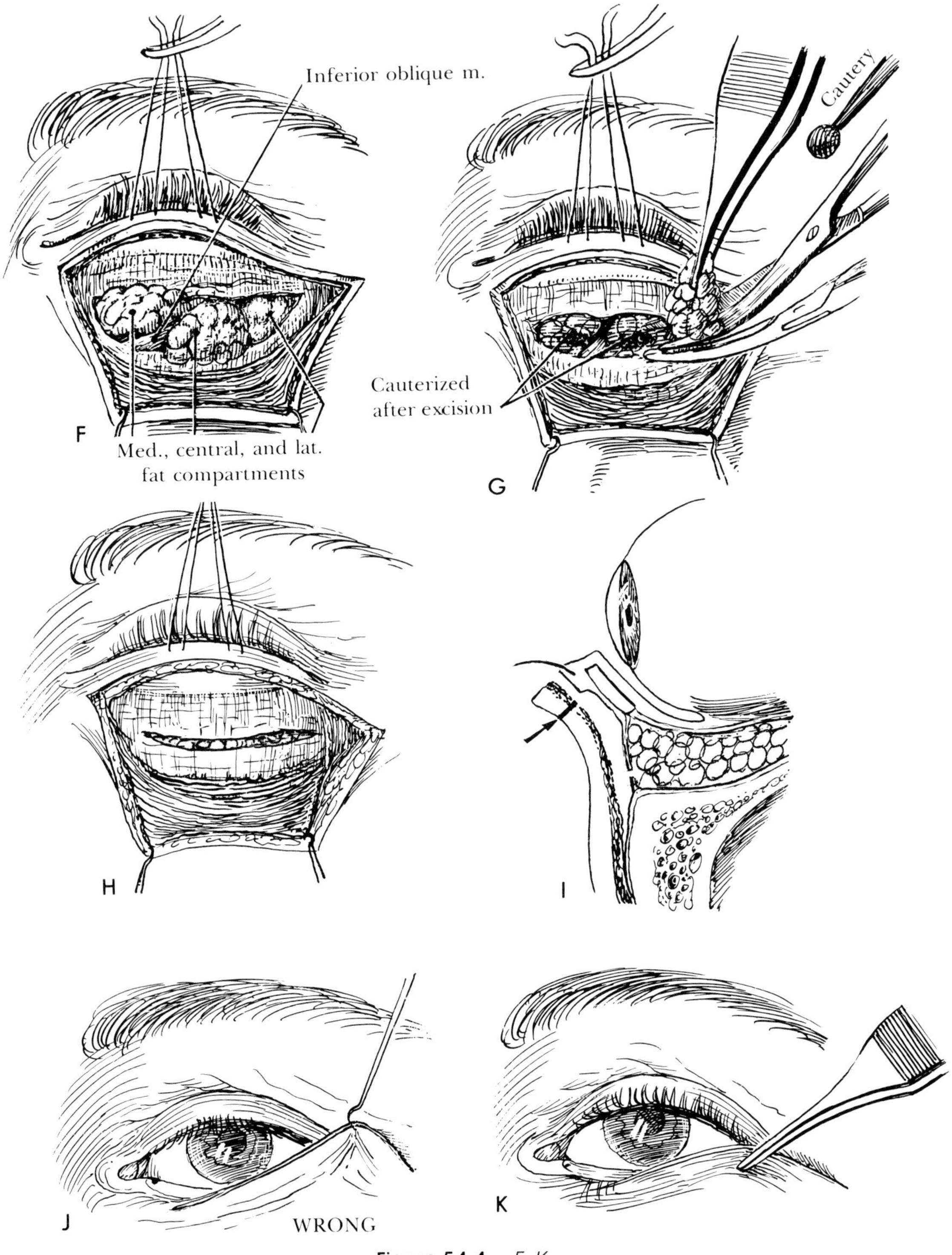

Figure 54.4. *F–K.*

wise to inject the tissues several minutes before surgery for maximum result.

The incision is begun with a lateral cut with a No. 15 blade, and the remainder of the incision developed medially with a pair of fine pointed scissors. Scissors are helpful in avoiding injury to the lashes. The depth of the incision varies depending on whether a skin flap or a skin muscle flap is planned. In approximately 95% of the authors' cases, a skin muscle flap is used. During development of a skin muscle flap, the incision is beveled slightly in a caudal direction so as to retain a strip of muscle horizontally across the lower lid overlying the tarsus (Fig. 54.4). This strip of pretarsal muscle is important to aid in tarsal function and strength as well as to provide a natural small fold postoperatively, which is cosmetically superior to a flat lid. Fixation of the skin flap to the tarsus, as advocated

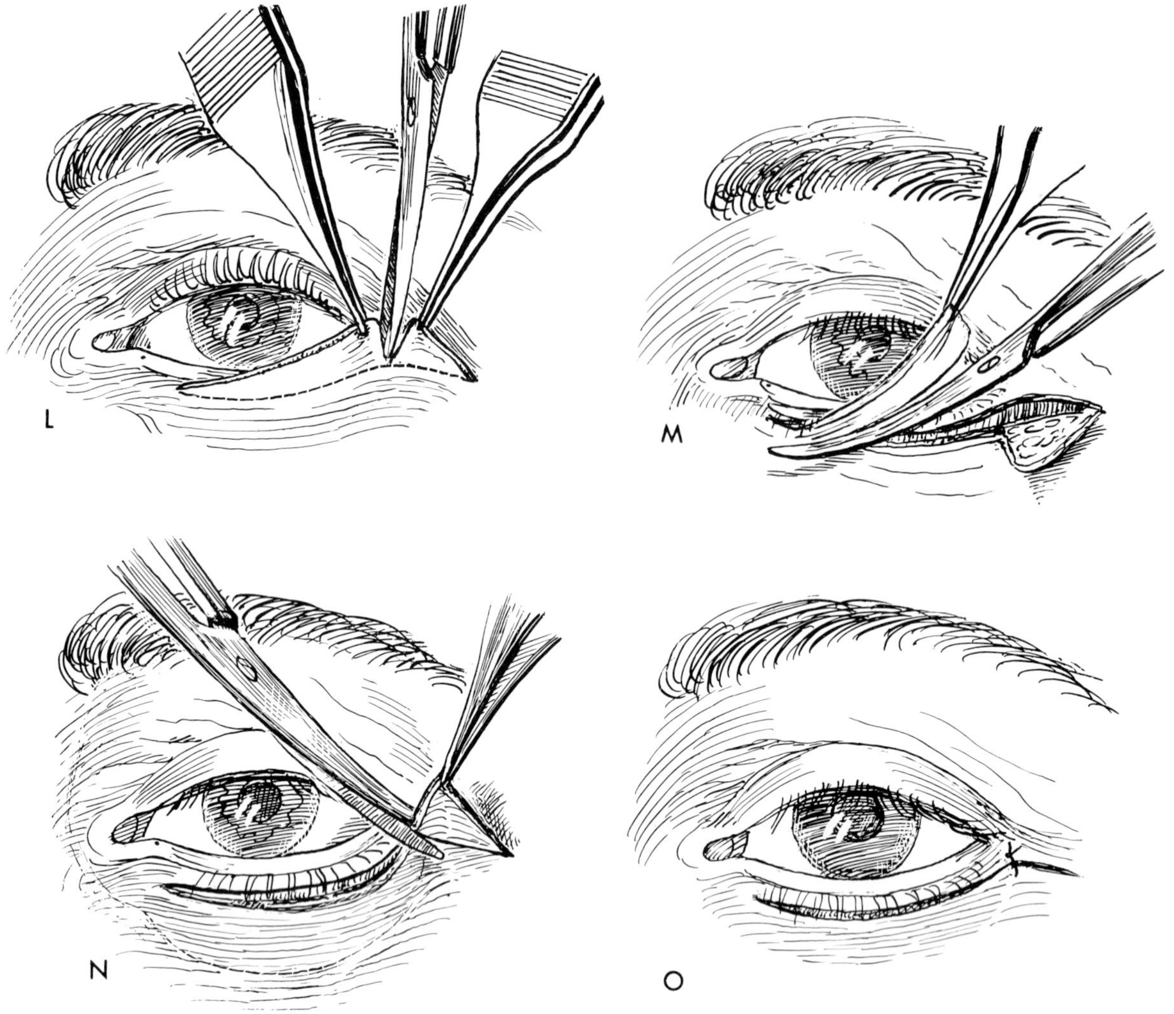

Figure 54.4. *L–O.*

by some surgeons, is not necessary to establish this small natural ridge of tissue.

The choice between a skin flap or a skin muscle flap is subjective and based on the surgeon's assessment of the amount of excess of skin as compared with muscle and to the extent of the skin involvement in the palpebral bags. In the past, the authors employed the skin flap much more frequently than in recent years. The limits of the effectiveness of the skin muscle flap have been extensively explored by the senior author (T.D.R.). We now believed that a skin flap is uncommonly necessary (less than 5%) and that a skin muscle flap can do the job in almost all instances. Occasionally, such as in those patients with unusual deformities such as excessive "festoons" of muscle, both a skin flap and a skin muscle flap may be necessary to achieve a natural drape of the tissues (Fig. 54.5) (3). Dissection of the skin muscle flap is far easier than a skin flap. The plane is relatively avascular and the plane exists without firm attachments. Blunt dissection may be all that is required.

If a skin flap is decided upon, the dissection between the skin and muscle is best carried out with blunt small scissors to avoid stab wounds through the skin. The cut-and-spread technique is used and the skin flap developed as far caudally as required to overcome the redundancy of the palpebral bag. Following completion of the remainder of the procedure, the excess skin is resected much as the redundant flap is trimmed during the skin muscle flap operation (Fig. 54.6).

The plane of the skin muscle is best located in the middle or medial portion of the wound since the dissection is facilitated here rather than laterally, where the plane blends with the tissues at the lateral extremity of the orbit. Lateral dissection of the flap may be required; this involves transection of the fibers of the orbicularis muscle, which results in bleeding and retraction of the divided muscle fibers. It is therefore easier to begin the dissection at about the midlash level and extend the plane both medially and laterally from this point. The flap is usually elevated to the infraorbital rim and sometimes caudal to this level, if the palbebral bags extend downward onto the cheeks. Meticulous hemostasis is obtained with fine-tipped jeweler's forceps and electrocautery. Bipolar cautery can also be used. Small sponges soaked in weak adrenaline solution are also helpful to obtain a dry wound.

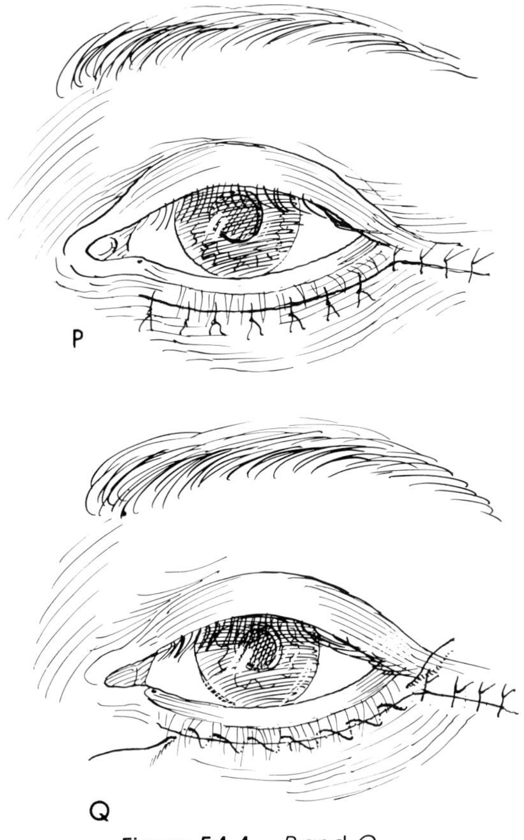

Figure 54.4. *P* and *Q*.

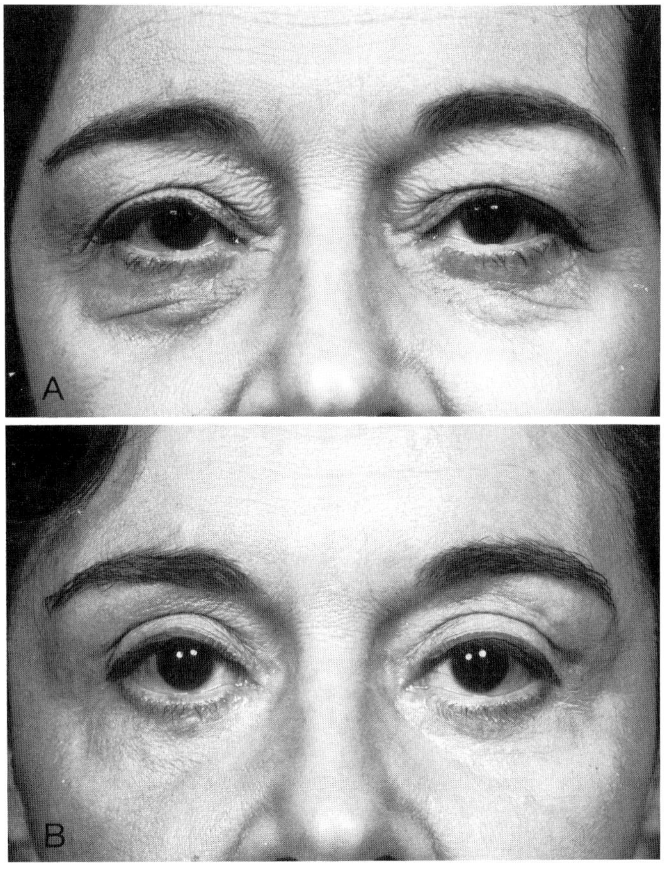

Figure 54.5. Example of the results of blepharoplasty by the skin muscle technique in an older patient with a more advanced degree of bulging of the orbital fat and attenuation of the septum.

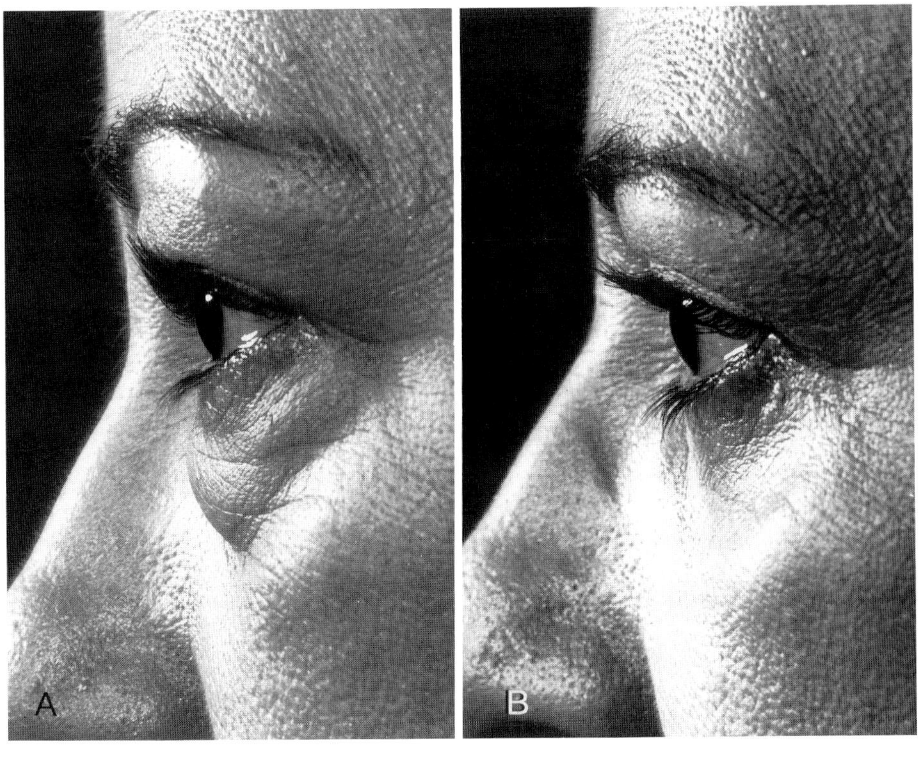

Figure 54.6. Results of skin muscle flap blepharoplasty with marked pseudoherniation of the orbital fat, lateral view.

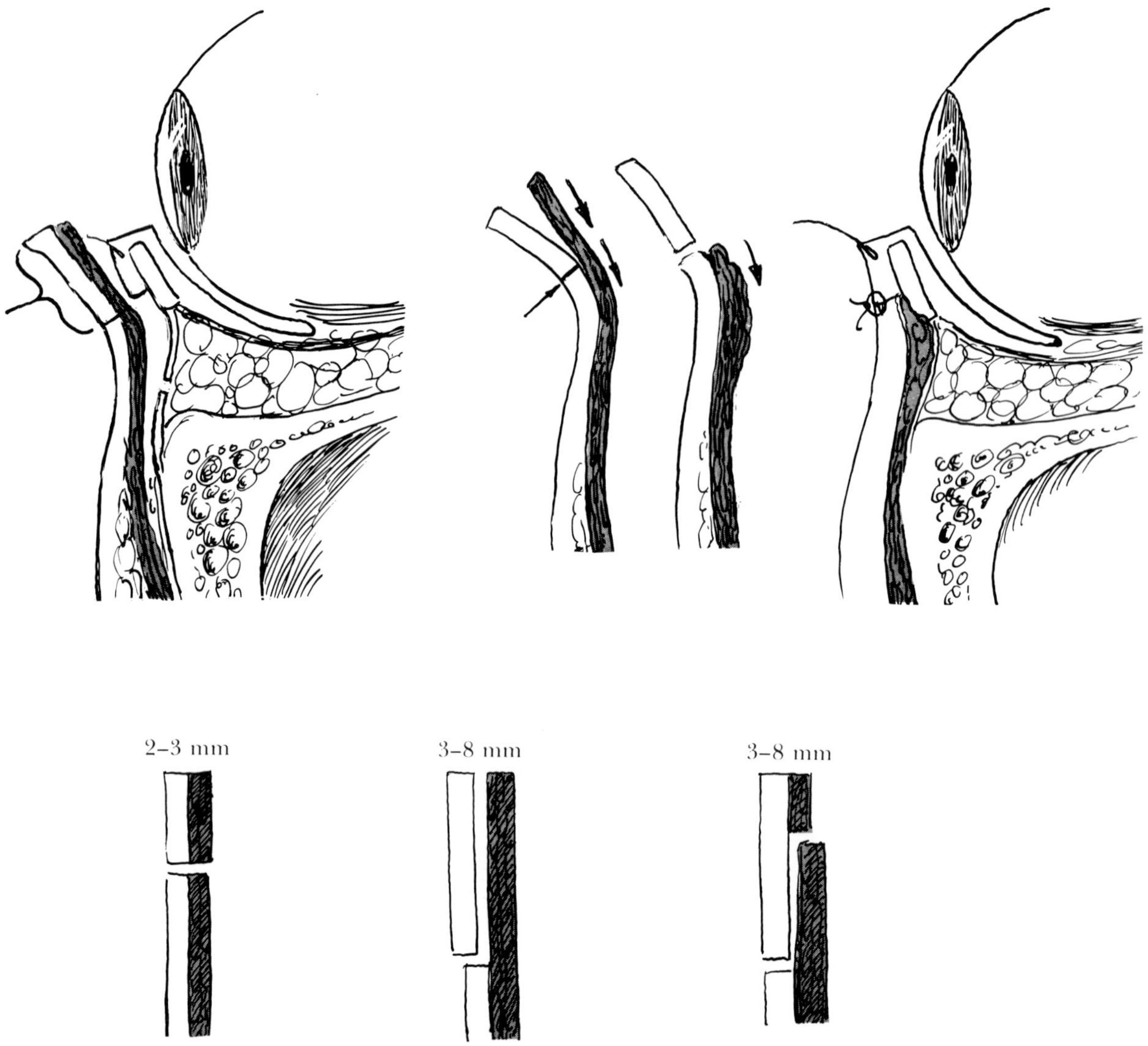

Figure 54.7. Care should be exercised in tailoring the flap so that a small strip of muscle remains over the tarsus (the pretarsal muscle), and so that there is not vertical drag on the lid margin, which can result in eversion of the lid margin. (From Rees TD: *Aesthetic Plastic Surgery*. Philadelphia, WB Saunders, 1981.)

Fat excision is estimated on the basis of the degree of protrusion of the fat after gentle pressure is applied on the globe. The three major compartments of the lower lid are usually apparent during this maneuver. The exact location of these compartments is very easy to visualize after elevation of a skin muscle flap. Attenuation of the orbital septum is often noted. The excess fat is delivered through an incision in the orbital septum that can be either extensive or simply local stab wounds over the individual fat pockets, depending on the nature of the deformity. Repair of the orbital septum is unnecessary. The excess fat is teased from the rent in the septum by gentle traction with forceps, the base is crushed with a hemostat, the excess is excised, and the stump is coagulated and sealed to avoid bleeding after retraction into the orbit, which can result in a deep orbital hematoma. The exact amount of fat to resect must be carefully evaluated and is largely a matter of judgment and experience. This evaluation simply cannot be learned except by hands-on experience. It depends on the amount and protuberance of the fat as well as on the prominence of the orbital rim, the size and protrusion of the eyeball, and other factors. Suffice it to say that it is obviously preferable to resect too little than too much. A second resection is preferable to trying to correct an enophthalmos—virtually an impossible task to perform in the seeing eye. In the presence of hypoplasia of the maxilla, considerable fat can be resected, while in the presence of strong orbital rims, the resection must be exceedingly conservative (3).

Following excision of the excess fat, the skin and/or skin muscle flap is carefully re-draped over the infraciliary wound edge (Fig. 54.7). It is important that the eyes be in a neutral position, and that the fat pads are tucked away beneath the rent in the orbital septum before this maneuver is undertaken in order to avoid distortion of the lid margin and excessive excision of the flap leading to a shortage of tissue and ectropion. The flap is simply draped over the wound edge without either lateral or cephalic traction.

A lateral key suture point is located by executing a small

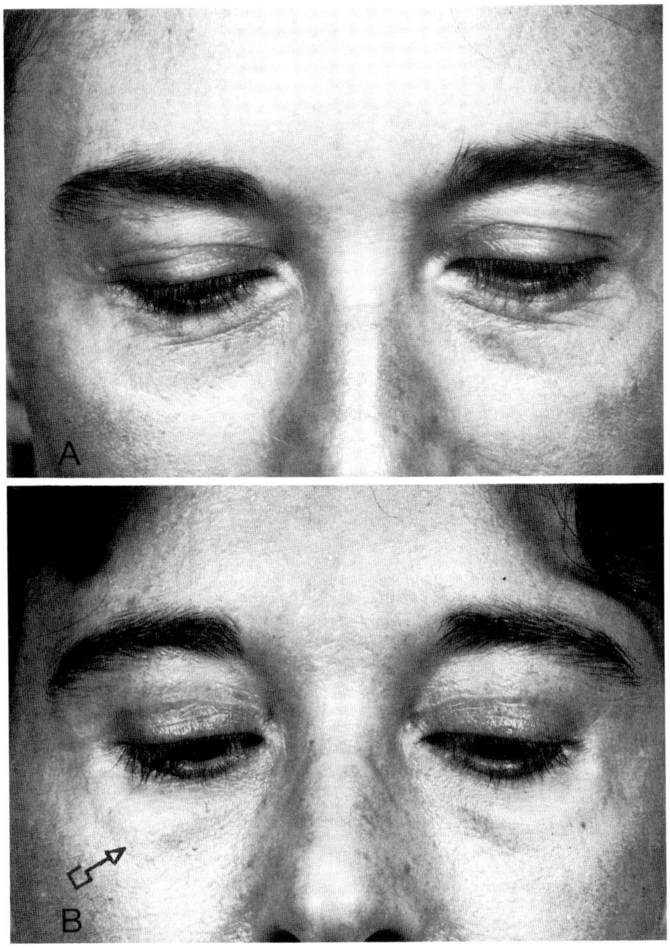

Figure 54.8. The unwary surgeon can be led into a trap if blepharoplasty is performed on the patient with a strong or protruding infraorbital margin without careful preoperative evaluation. In the patient shown, adequate fat removal was carried out at surgery; however, postoperatively a bulge was still present to her great distress. The bulge was caused by prominence of the bony margin that was not recognized preoperatively. Careful palpation of the bone is important to anticipate such a problem.

vertical cut in the flap just at the lateral canthus. A 6-0 nylon suture is placed at this point to serve as a reference. The remaining flap excess is carefully excised millimeter by millimeter with small sharp pointed scissors, first from the key suture medially and then from the key suture laterally. The classic maneuvers in the awake patient of opening the mouth or gazing upwards are helpful, but not at all mandatory in determining the amount of flap to excise. Making sure that the lid is in a neutral position and that there is no tension whatsoever on the flap is mandatory, however, for safe excision.

If this step is performed properly, the flap should lie in its new position with the wound edges in gentle and exact opposition with no gaps between the edges. The incision is then carefully closed with meticulous suturing of fine sutures such as 6-0 nylon or silk. Either running or interrupted sutures can be used, since all sutures from the lid must be removed within 4–5 days to prevent epithelial tunnel formation. Usually the sutures beneath the lash margin are removed in 48 hours after surgery, and the lateral sutures are left another 2 or 3 days.

ANCILLARY PROCEDURES

Special variations in the typical palpebral bag deformity requires special variations in the treatment technique, aside from the operative procedure just described. These include excessive muscle festoons (2), secondary bags or bulges of the malar eminences (Fig. 54.8) (3), hypotonia of the lids (senile ectropion) (4, 5), and marked wrinkling of the periorbital region (Fig. 54.9 and 54.10).

In those patients with a marked excess of muscle referred to by Furnas (2) so aptly as festoons, it is helpful to isolate the muscle flap separately from the skin flap, which results in two separate flaps: one of skin and one of muscle. The muscle problem can be dealt with separately from the skin. It can be tightened laterally as a sling, even suspended to the periosteum, or simply trimmed of all excess. Frequently a considerable block of muscle tissue can be excised, especially from the lateral wound element. The horizontal expanse of the muscle is thereby tightened, and the direction of muscle pull changed from horizontal to lateral.

Ridges of swelling or frank bags located beneath the eyelids on the malars are not related to the palpebral bags and are rarely corrected by blepharoplasty, although with

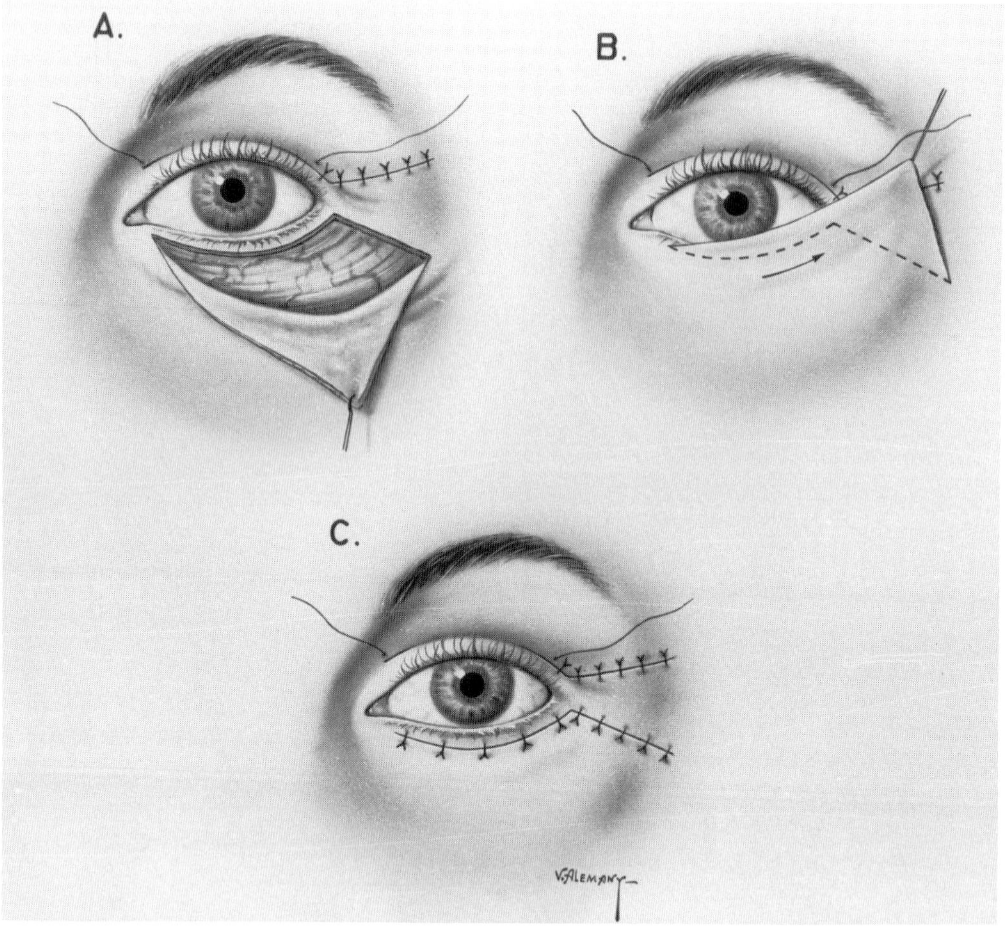

Figure 54.9. The skin flap operation without incorporation of the muscle in the flap is currently utilized only in very few and selected patients by the authors, only when there is marked excess and wrinkling of the skin with minimal fat protrusion. The skin flap operation is almost relegated to history. In this illustration the lateral triangle is exaggerated, and it should be noted that the lateral pull on the skin flap shown here must be curtailed.

extensive undermining some improvement can be achieved (Fig. 54.11). The deformity is often related to chronic and recurrent edema of unknown etiology (Fig. 54.12) (3).

Preoperative scleral show has been discussed previously. The treatment of this problem or the prevention of further show is based on the anatomical configuration of the lid and the globe as well as the maxilla. In the absence of exophthalmos, simple and mild hypotonicity of the lower lid with 1 or 2 mm of scleral show are treated with simultaneous wedge resection of full-thickness lower lid at the time of blepharoplasty (3, 5). Removal of a wedge of 5 to 7 mm can be accomplished without difficulty and with little or no deformity of the lid margin following surgery. Meticulous anatomical repair of all lid layers, and especially approximation of the tarsal plate and grey line of the lid margin, are keys to success. After elevation of the skin or skin muscle flap, the wedge is resected from the lateral one-third of the lower lid with small straight scissors. After resection of fat and flap, the flap is draped over the wedge resection repair and sutured as always.

When wrinkling of the skin is a prominent feature even after a thorough blepharoplasty, chemical peel should be considered in likely candidates (3). Deep peel is also useful in patients with excessive hyperpigmentation, especially of the superficial layers of the dermis. Deep chemical peel should not be carried out at the same time as blepharoplasty because of the possibility of necrosis of such thin skin. Usually an interval of about 6 weeks is considered best following surgery before a peel is done.

COMPLICATIONS

Most complications associated with lower lid blepharoplasty are avoidable. It is important to anticipate potential problems, and always when in doubt, one should err on the side of conservatism.

Increased postoperative scleral show or frank ectropion is usually the result of excessive skin resection or of failure to recognize conditions that predispose to this deformity. Preoperative careful assessment of tissue laxity and skin excess is essential. Simultaneous wedge resection to shorten the horizontal length of the lid was previously discussed. In more severe degrees of drooping lid or in the presence of exophthalmos, wedge resection may not suf-

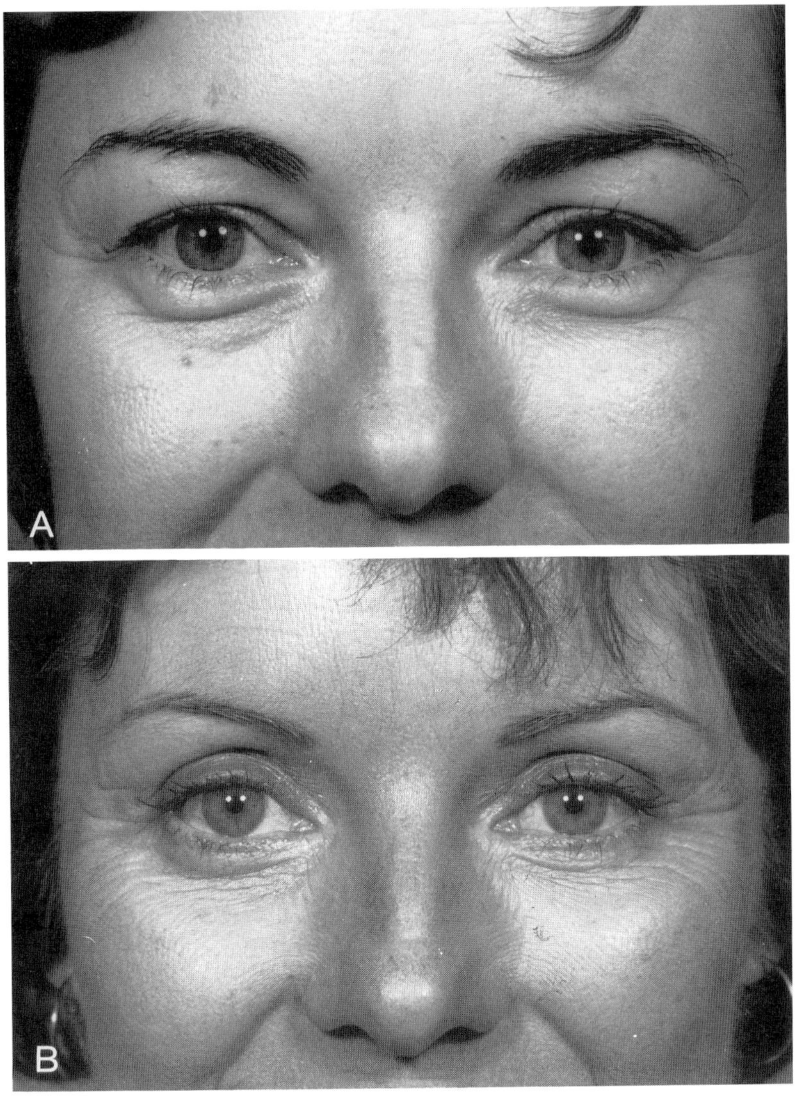

Figure 54.10. *A*, In some patients, the cephalic portion of the orbicularis muscle becomes excessively prominent during facial animation as demonstrated in this young woman. *B*, The postoperative smiling view shows the marked attenuation of the muscle roll that can be achieved. *C*, Correction of the problem is illustrated in the drawing. The muscle roll can either be cautiously excised, or in some instances imbricated with a fine 7-0 suture of nonabsorbable material. (From Rees TD: *Aesthetic Plastic Surgery*. Philadelphia, WB Saunders, 1981.)

fice and indeed can sometimes increase the scleral show. In such patients tarsal suspension to the lateral rim periosteum should be considered. This particular technique is especially helpful with secondary ectropion. In most patients postoperative ectropion is temporary and transient. It is related to edema, chemosis, and ordinary forces of wound healing. Such problems are best treated conservatively by providing lid support either by taping or suspension (Frost) suture. Protection of the cornea with artificial tears and lubrication is important until the process is resolved.

Great caution should be exercised in operating on patients with a combination of scleral show and a low Schirmer's test. The risk of a postoperative dry-eye syndrome is increased significantly in such patients. Of course, reduction in normal blinking response or ophthalmoplegia with inability to elevate the eyes only adds to the likelihood of problems.

Complications from excessive bleeding are primarily avoided by obtaining hemostasis. Patients with bleeding tendencies can often be screened by anemnesis or coagulation studies. All drugs, such as aspirin-containing compounds should not be consumed for at least 10 days before surgery, and the patients should be so instructed. During surgery it is especially important to coagulate every visible bleeding point and to sear the stumps of the fat pedicles to avoid deep orbital bleeding. Retrobulbar hematoma is a dreaded complication, but often surprisingly benign in its course. Injecting blindly deep into the orbit during blepharoplasty is ineffectual in blocking traction pain from the fat pockets and is potentially dangerous since most retrobulbar hematomas are the result of such deep injections.

Other complications can occur. The most serious of these is blindness, a very rare problem indeed when one considers the large number of blepharoplasties performed each year. A more detailed description of such an obscure complication is not within the scope of this chapter.

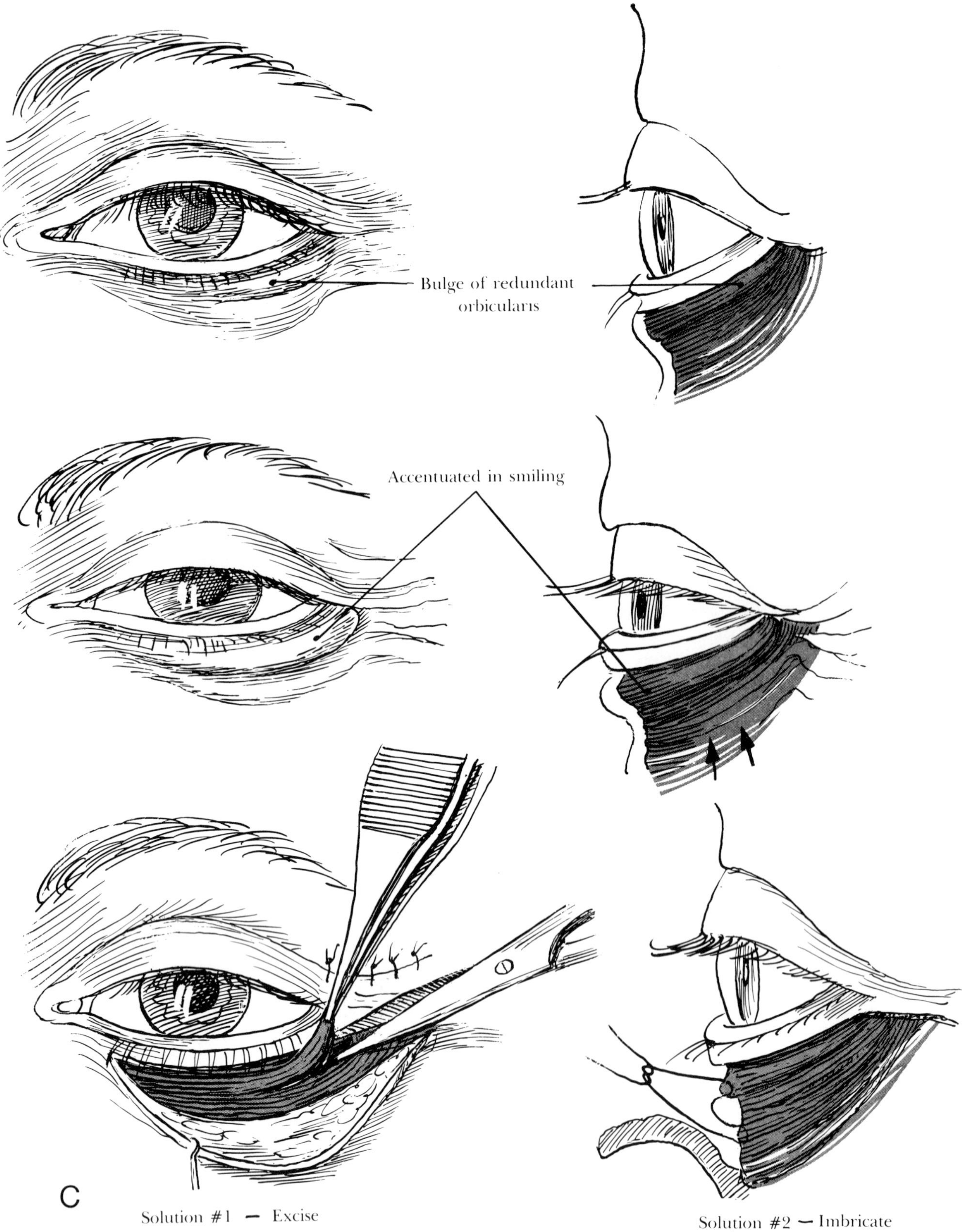

Figure 54.10. *C.*

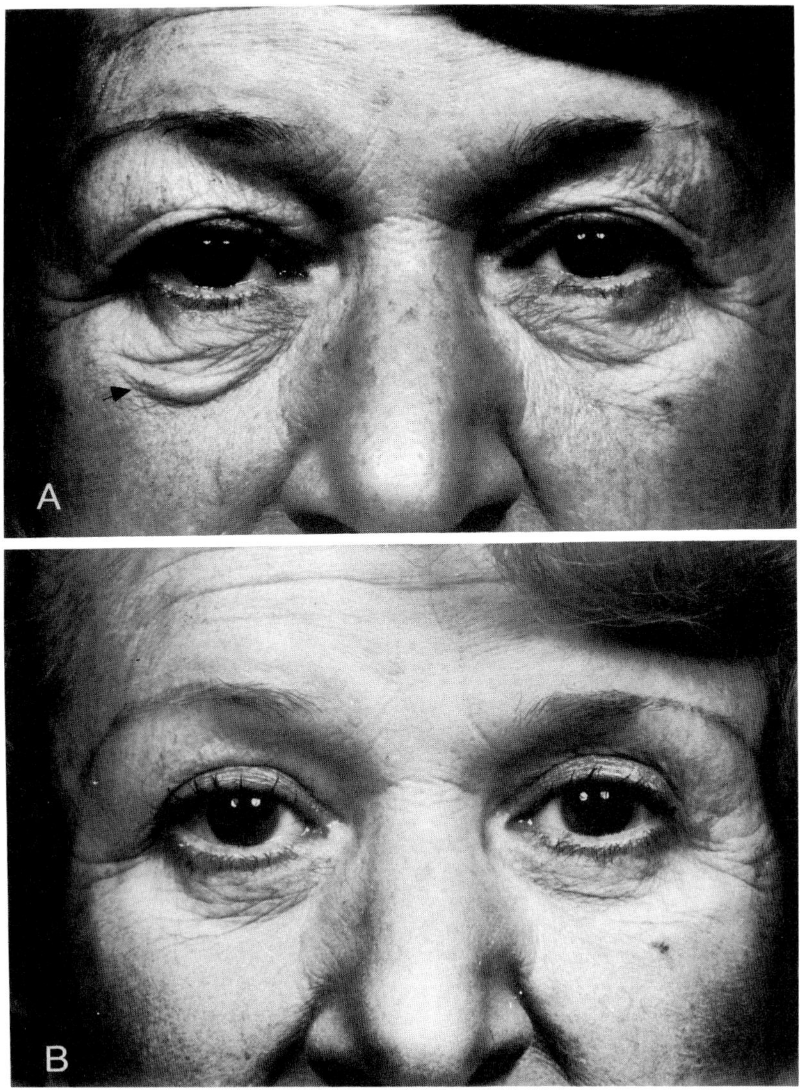

Figure 54.11. The so-called cheek bag can be a very difficult problem. The deformity is usually not removed by ordinary blepharoplasty since its cause is often obscure; the deformity is usually the result of chronic regional edema of unexplained etiology. When the deformity is severe, such as in this patient, a viable option is excision, provided the patient is willing to accept an external scar. *A*, The preoperative deformity. Note that the cheek swelling is partially camouflaged by the eyelid bag. *B*, Following blepharoplasty, the palpebral bags are gone, but the edema, causing the malar swelling is worsened. The prominence of the cheek bag is even more noticeable. *C–H*, Following direct excision of the area. (From Rees TD: *Aesthetic Plastic Surgery*. Philadelphia, WB Saunders, 1981.)

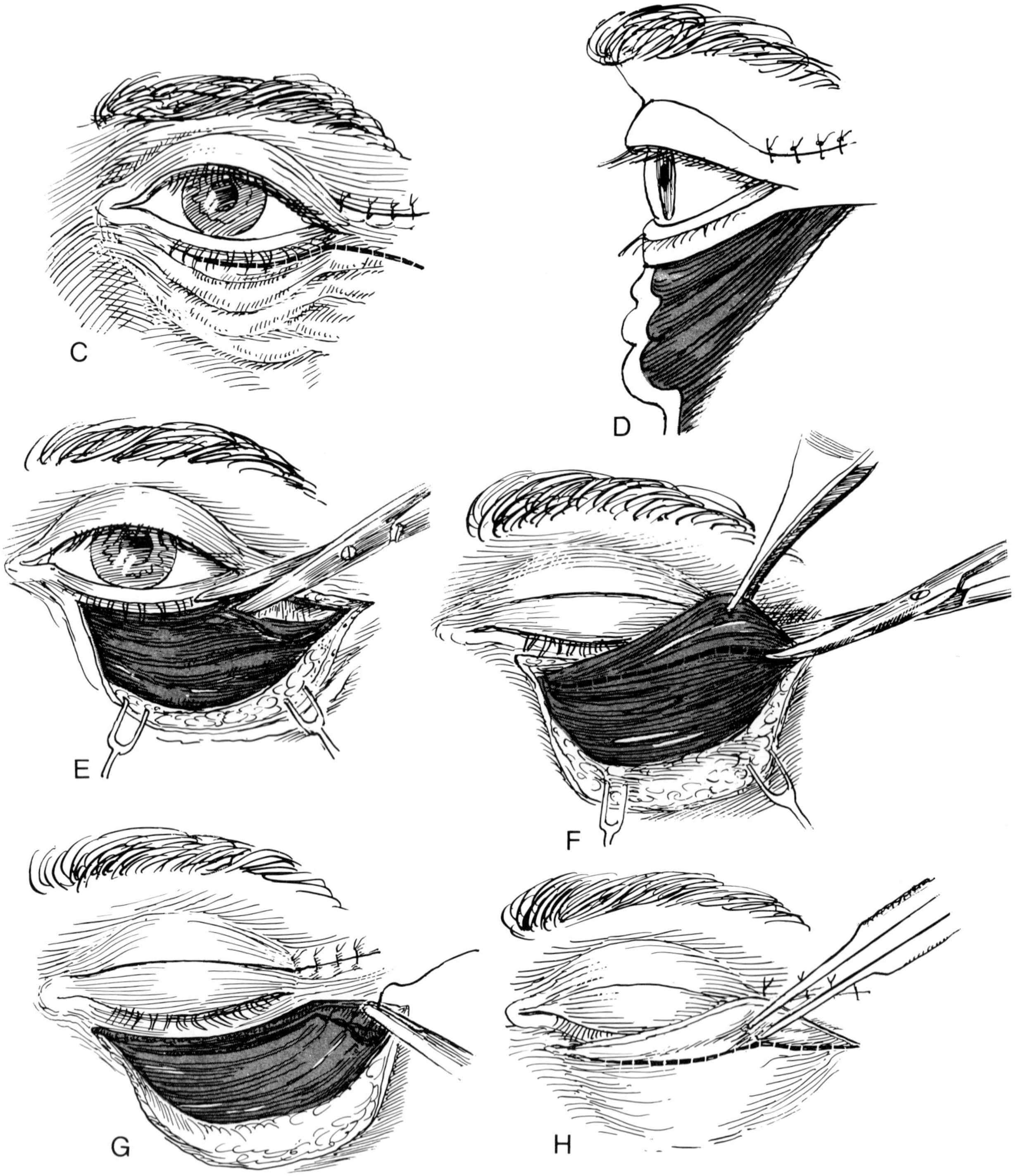

Figure 54.11. *C–H.*

SUMMARY

The benefits of lower lid blepharoplasty and the avoidance of problems in this procedure depend on careful preoperative evaluation of each patient and on careful, atraumatic operative technique. Systematic evaluation of the deformity allows the surgeon to plan an intelligent surgical approach and to vary the technique according to the problem at hand.

Although certainly one of the most satisfying operations in aesthetic surgery, blepharoplasty is also one of the most technically demanding. The margin of tolerance for a safe and successful result in lower lid blepharoplasty is small. Two to 3 mm can be the difference between good and bad

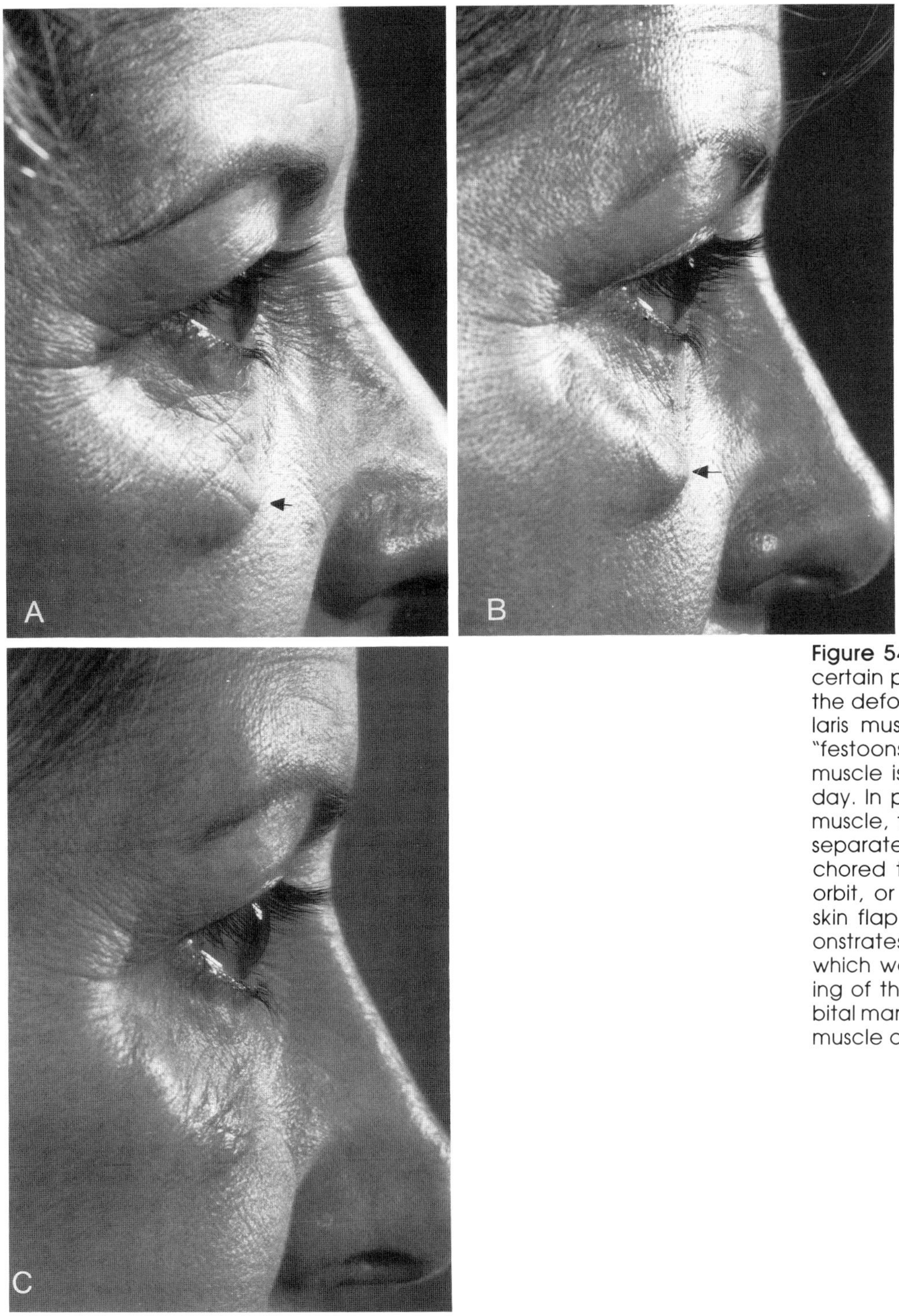

Figure 54.12. Furnas recognized that in certain patients the major component of the deformity is excessive folds of orbicularis muscle, which he so aptly named "festoons." Direct surgery to the orbicularis muscle is the rule in most operations today. In patients with marked festoons of muscle, the muscle can be treated as a separate layer. It can be trimmed, anchored to the periosteum of the lateral orbit, or simply shortened much like the skin flap is shortened. The patient demonstrates festooning of the right lower lid, which was corrected by wide undermining of the skin muscle flap below the orbital margin and separate trimming of the muscle as shown in the illustration.

results. With attention to these details and the development of a technical armamentarium that includes different variations in technique, the ophthalmic surgeon can perform blepharoplasty safely and effectively.

REFERENCES

1. Beare R: Surgical treatment of senile changes in the eyelids: the McIndoe-Beare technique. Proceedings of the Second International Symposium on Plastic and Reconstructive Surgery of the Eye and Adnexae. St. Louis, CV Mosby, 1967.
2. Furnas DW: Festoons of orbicularis muscle as a cause of baggy eyelids. *Plast Reconstr Surg* 61: 540, 1978.
3. Rees TD: Blepharoplasty. In Rees TD (ed): *Aesthetic Plastic Surgery*. Philadelphia, WB Saunders, 1981, vol 2, 459–525.
4. Rees TD, Tabbal N: Lower blepharoplasty, with emphasis on the orbicularis muscle. *Clin Plast Surg* 8: 643, 1981.
5. Rees TD: Prevention of ectropion by horizontal shortening of the lower lid during blepharoplasty. *Ann Plast Surg* 2: 17, 1983.

CHAPTER 55

Lower Eyelid Blepharoplasty: Transconjunctival Approach

KEVIN I. PERMAN, M.D.
HENRY I. BAYLIS, M.D.

The transconjunctival approach to lower eyelid blepharoplasty is rapidly gaining popularity. This is due to increasing sophistication of younger patients who are interested in aesthetic surgery and to a greater awareness of its potential benefits and complications. Historically, the majority of blepharoplasty candidates that have herniated orbital fat pads of the lower lids also have redundant lower eyelid skin; as a result, the surgical approach of choice has been the infraciliary incision, in which both redundant skin and herniated orbital fat could be removed. But what of the patient who exhibits herniated orbital fat without redundant eyelid skin? These patients would benefit from the transconjunctival approach, in which the orbicularis-septal complex is not compromised and, as a result there is decreased risk of postoperative lower eyelid retraction, which is the most common and dreaded complication of lower eyelid blepharoplastic surgery.

This approach is not new. In 1924, Bourquet (1) described the transconjunctival approach to herniated orbital fat in the lower lid. The procedure was further popularized by Tessier (2), who used the conjunctival approach to the inferior orbital rim in his surgeries for hypertelorism and craniofacial dysostoses.

Skin quality and muscle tone are the major criteria in the selection of this surgical approach. The authors do not consider age as a variable because, although the vast majority of the patients who are good candidates for the transconjunctival approach are young, we do encounter a few middle-aged and older patients who have good skin and muscle tone and would therefore also benefit from the transconjunctival approach. We also find this approach is more widely accepted by the patient who acknowledges the problem of herniated orbital fat but would avoid a cutaneous incision at all cost (3).

ANATOMY

As in all surgery, a brief review of the surgical anatomy facilitates discussion of the approach. The lower eyelid is divided into anterior and posterior lamellae. The skin and orbicularis make up the anterior lamella, while the tarsus and conjunctiva make up the posterior lamella. The inferior tarsal muscle and capsulopalpebral fascia insert into the inferior border of the tarsus. The anatomy is shown in cross section in Figure 55.1. From this illustration one can appreciate how herniated orbital fat can be approached by an incision through the conjunctiva and lower eyelid retractors. Entrance into the orbital fat is made posterior to the orbital septum, and as a result there is no violation of the anterior lamellae of the lower eyelids. The herniated orbital fat may be approached anterior to the septum, but the authors prefer a retroseptal approach.

TECHNIQUE

The conjunctiva of the lower eyelid is infiltrated with 2–3 ml of 2% lidocaine mixed with 1:100,000 epinephrine and hyaluronidase (Figs. 55.2). Fifteen to 20 minutes is allowed to elapse for maximum hemostasis. Until recently, we had favored the use of scissors to incise the conjunctiva, but in our current experience, we find that the needle-tipped cutting cautery offers an equally sharp incision and better hemostasis (Figs. 55.3); in addition, we have not encountered any postoperative scarring of the conjunctiva from this instrument. A plastic lid plate is used to protect the globe and to define the angle of the plane of the incision (Fig. 55.1), which is to be made just superior and posterior to the infraorbital rim. Another useful landmark is a stab incision made 5 mm below the lower tarsal border in the central part of the lower eyelid. The advantage of the cautery over scissors for the initial incision and dissection should now become evident. Gradually the tool is passed through the conjunctiva and lower eyelid retractors until a knuckle of bulging orbital fat is identified. Once this fat is allowed to protrude through the central incision, this plane is developed nasally toward the punctum and laterally to the end of the tarsus with the curved Stevens scissors (Figs. 55.4 and 55.5). Light digital pressure with retropulsion on the globe is applied by the assistant to ease the excision of orbital fat. The fat excision proceeds in a temporal to medial direction. This is because the temporal fat lies more posteriorly and tends to recede while the patient is lying in a supine position. Blood vessels are identified and pushed away prior to excision of fat. Actual excision may be carried out with either scissors or cautery (Fig. 55.6). Clamping is performed only if major blood vessels cannot be avoided. The middle and medial fat pads are resected in a similar fashion. Care should be taken to avoid injury to the inferior oblique muscle, which often can be identified as a "valley" between the middle and medial fat pads. Some surgeons use this as an indication that fat removal is in danger of becoming excessive.

As in all blepharoplasty surgery, the fat is retained in the surgical field to compare with the amount excised from the other eyelid. Closure of the eyelid is accomplished with two or three interrupted 6-0 plain or mild chromic sutures that approximate the lower eyelid retractors and conjunctiva (Fig. 55.7). Ice compresses are applied for 24 hours. This minimizes postoperative edema and bleeding. Pressure patching is not advised in blepharoplasty surgery. Hot compresses are then substituted, which aids in the healing and accelerates the resolution of the postoperative ecchymosis. Patients are advised to avoid direct exposure to the sunlight; this precludes tattooing secondary to hemoglobin pigment oxidation.

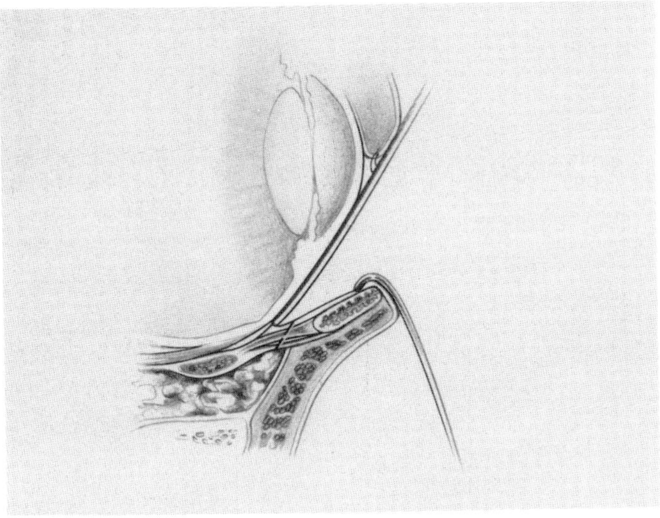

Figure 55.1. Sagittal section of lower eyelid depicts dotted line retroseptal plane of incision to be made.

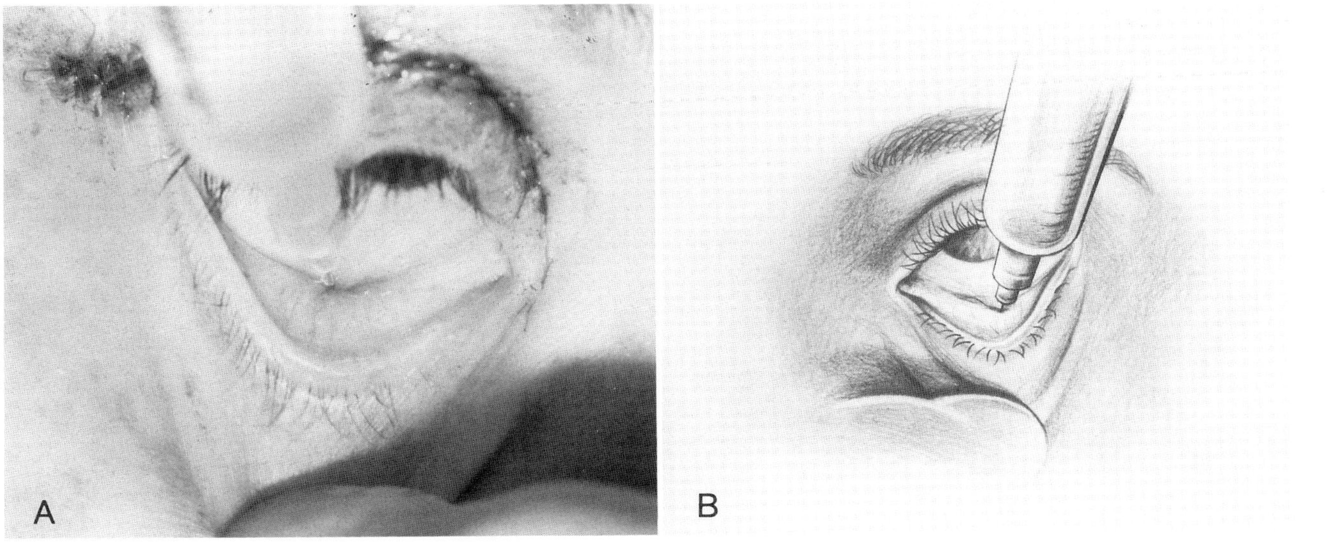

Figure 55.2. *A, B,* Anesthetic injection into lower fornix.

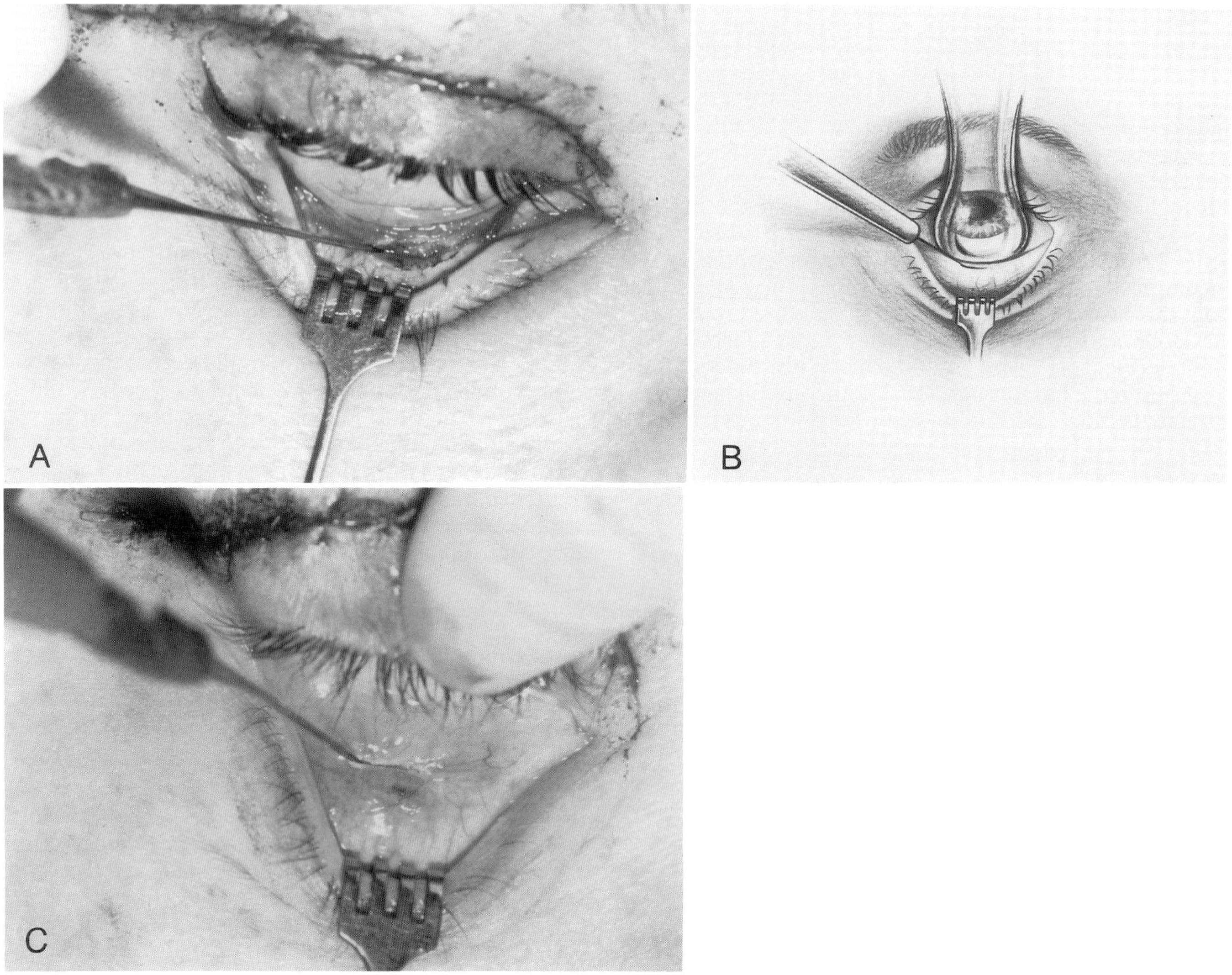

Figure 55.3. *A, B,* Needle tip cautery (cutting mode) to make incision. Plastic lid plate protects globe and provides retropulsion. *C,* Digital pressure is an alternative.

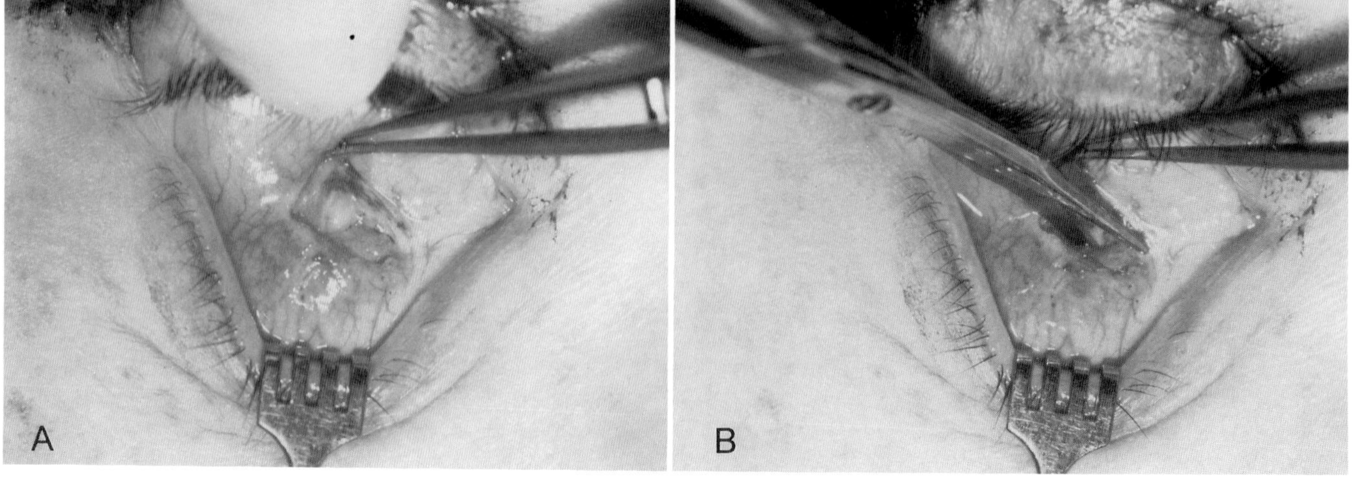

Figure 55.4. *A, B,* Once the fat is identified, the incision is extended with scissors.

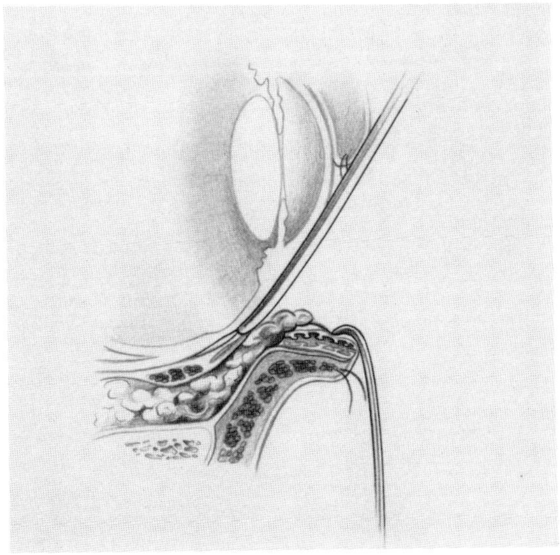

Figure 55.5. Illustration of protruding knuckle of orbital fat. The orbital septum is not violated.

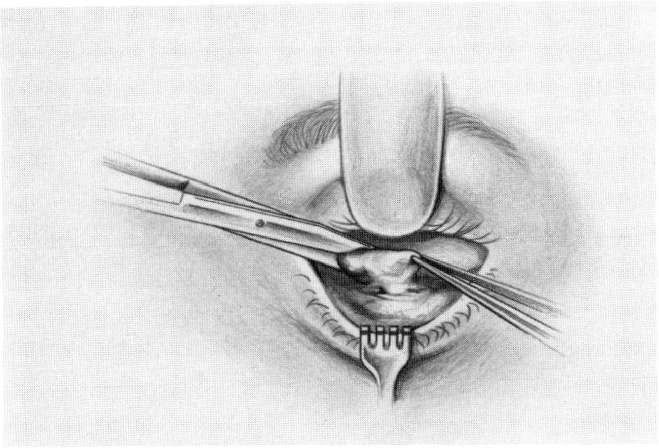

Figure 55.6. Excess orbital fat is resected.

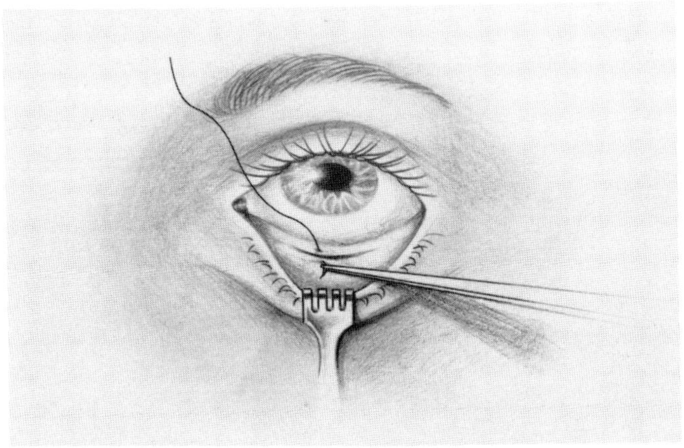

Figure 55.7. Closure is carried out with interrupted 6-0 plain suture.

RESULTS

Over the past 4 years, we have operated on 72 patients via the transconjunctival approach. There were 65 females and seven males. The ages ranged from 18 to 68 years, with a mean age of 42 years. In 15 patients the surgery was performed secondarily as a refinement of a need for greater fat excision. The only complication we encountered was in a particular patient who developed an S-configuration to the lower lid. This was felt to be due to a wound dehiscence between the conjunctiva and lid retractors. The problem was rectified by returning the patient to the operating room and advancing the lid retractors with interrupted 6-0 plain suture. Our mean follow-up for our transconjunctival series is 2.4 years.

DISCUSSION

Patients today are considering blepharoplasty surgery at a younger age. As a result the infraciliary approach may not be to the patient's or surgeon's advantage; cutaneous scars may be prominent and the risk of postoperative scleral show is increased. This is a common complication of lower eyelid blepharoplasty, resulting from an excessive shortening of the anterior lamella from the skin excision or a scarring of the orbicularis-septal complex, which is violated during the infraciliary incision (4–6). These two etiologies are avoided during the transconjunctival approach, and if the patient in question would benefit from fat excision alone, the transconjunctival route should be the approach of choice. We recommend the retroseptal approach as opposed to the preseptal approach. In our experience, avoiding compromise to the orbital septum will decrease the chances of postoperative lower eyelid retraction.

We recommend the transconjunctival approach not only as a primary procedure but also as a secondary procedure when residual fat is evident from the initial surgery, no matter what the initial approach was. If the initial surgery was via an infraciliary incision, a second skin incision may be avoided by repeating this approach.

REFERENCES

1. Bourquet: Les hernies graisseuses de l'orbite; notre traitment chirurgical. *Bull Acad Med Paris* 92, 1924. Quoted in Schwartz E, Randall P: Conjunctival incision for herniated orbital. *Ophthal Surg* 11: 276–279, 1980.
2. Tessier P: The conjunctival approach to the orbital floor and maxilla in congenital malformation and trauma. *J Maxillofac Surg* 1: 3, 1973.
3. Baylis HI, Sutcliff RT: Conjunctival approach in lower lid blepharoplasty. *Adv Ophthal Plast Reconstr Surg* II: 43–81, 1983.
4. McCord Jr CD: Techniques in blepharoplasty. *Ophthal Surg* 10: 40–55, 1979.
5. McCord Jr CD, Shore JW: Avoidance of complications in lower lid blepharoplasty. *Ophthalmology* 90: 1039–1046, 1983.
6. Levine MR, Boynton J, Tenzel RR, Miller GR: Complications of blepharoplasty. *Ophthal Surg* 6: 53–57, 1975.

CHAPTER 56

The Eyelid Crease

PAUL T. GAVARIS, M.D.

The ancient Greeks believed that symmetry was the essence of beauty. The eyes and their complementary structure, the eyelids, having such a prominent and focal position on the human face, epitomize this truism. Eyelid surgery, whether a blepharoplasty or blepharoptosis, should have as its goal the attainment of symmetry. Eyelid parameters such as horizontal and vertical dimensions, contour, direction of lashes, and position of the eyelid crease all play a significant role in creating this symmetry. Naturally there are degrees of variations from this so-called ideal—yet each can look natural and even quite beautiful. However, when there exists a slight uneveness or asymmetry between the two sides, the result can be a serious blemish.

As ophthalmic surgeons, we should be able to correctly predict and reconstruct the height and contour of the eyelid crease. It should function and look as natural as the original or opposite crease, and most of all it should be appropriate for that individual patient, whether he or she is Oriental or Occidental and has an average, a high, or a low crease.

ANATOMY

In recent years, the anatomy of the upper eyelid has been studied thoroughly and correlated more closely with respect to its function and its reconstruction (1). We know that the levator aponeurosis passes inferiorly and anteriorly towards its insertion onto the orbicularis fiber and dermis of the lid skin where it creates the primary lid crease. Immediately preceding this interdigitation, the aponeurosis also intercepts the orbital septum and forms a so-called conjoined fascial envelope wherein lies the preaponeurotic orbital fat. The position of this envelope or juncture is usually 2–3 mm above the primary lid crease, however, the height of the lid crease is different for each individual (Fig. 56.1). For example, in the average Occidental eyelid we find the primary lid crease 8–12 mm above the lid margin, when measured at the pupillary axis. Nasally, it slopes down 2 mm or more, whereas temporally it tapers off slightly less. In contrast, the Oriental lid usually has its primary crease much lower, i.e., 2–5 mm above the lid margin or even as low as the lash line (Fig. 56.2). Since the position and relationship of the primary lid crease and the septal aponeurotic junction (conjoined fascia) is constant, the preaponeurotic orbital fat extends much closer toward the lashes in the Oriental eyelid, thereby presenting the characteristic "thicker," "hooding," or "single" eyelid (Fig. 56.3). This orbital fat can be found anterior to the tarsus in many Orientals. Hooding is seen rarely in Occidentals except in the elderly or in patients with significant blepharochalasis. The difference, therefore, between the Caucasian and Asian eyelid is in the level of the attachment of the levator aponeurosis to the lid skin; i.e., the position of primary eyelid crease (compare Fig. 56.1 and Fig. 56.2). We can, therefore, conclude that the primary lid crease is a function and result of the action and direct insertion of *only* the levator aponeurosis upon the lid skin. Tarsus plays no role in the presence, position, height, or contour of the lid crease. Clinical and histologic studies confirm this, despite catch phrases such as "supratarsal fixation" found in the literature (2–7).

In the lower lid, analogous to the levator aponeurosis, there is the extension of the capsulopalpebral fascia, which likewise inserts onto the lower eyelid skin to create the crease (8) (Fig. 56.3) Its location below the lid margin likewise varies from 3–5 mm in Caucasians to 1–2 mm in Asians (compare Fig. 56.1 and Fig. 56.2).

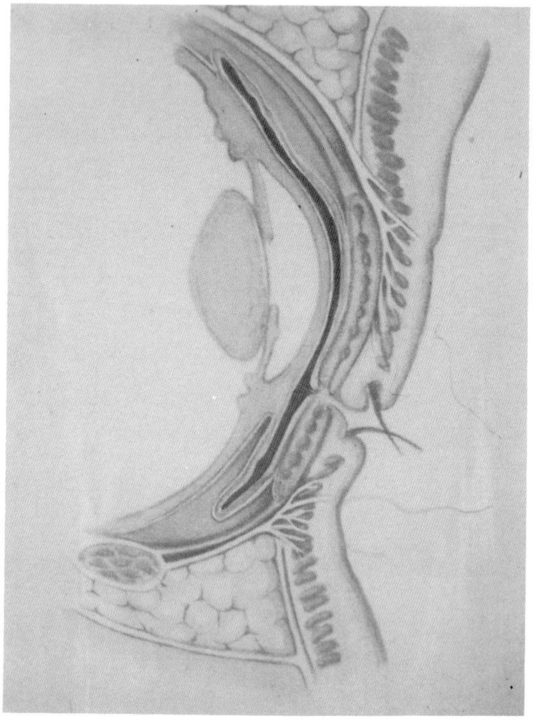

Figure 56.1. Typical Occidental upper and lower lid structures and their relationships.

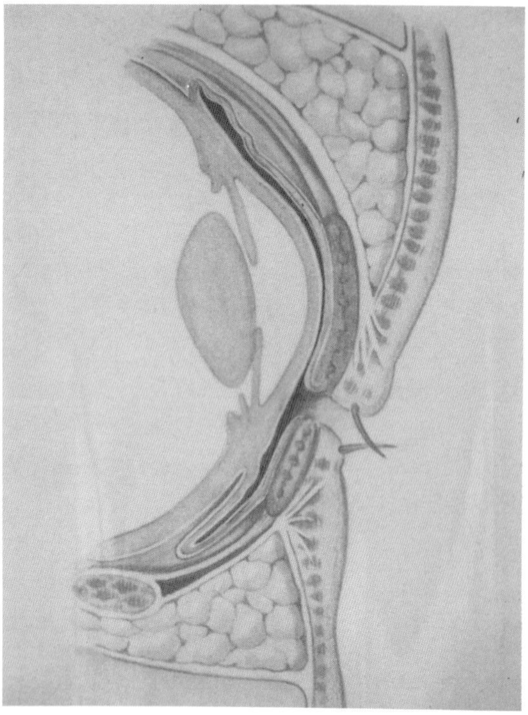

Figure 56.2. Oriental lid. The levator aponeurosis begins to insert quite low near the lashes in the upper lid as well as in the lower lid. Note the position of orbital fat anterior to the tarsus that gives the typical "hooding" characteristic to the Oriental lid.

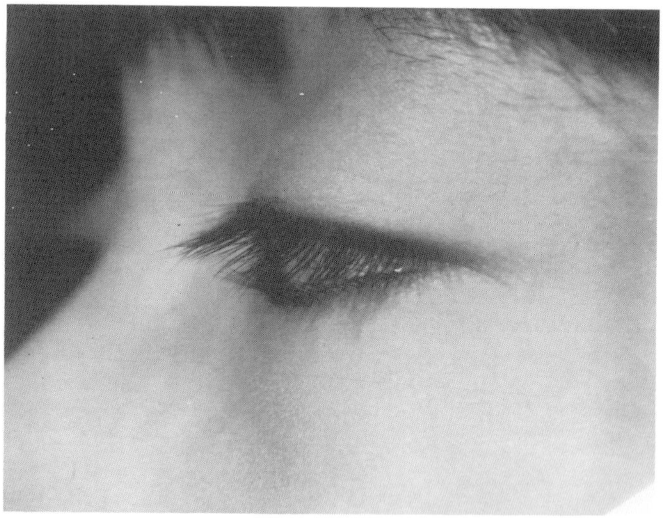

Figure 56.3. Note the low or lack of eyelid crease both in the upper and lower lid, which are the extremes often seen in Orientals.

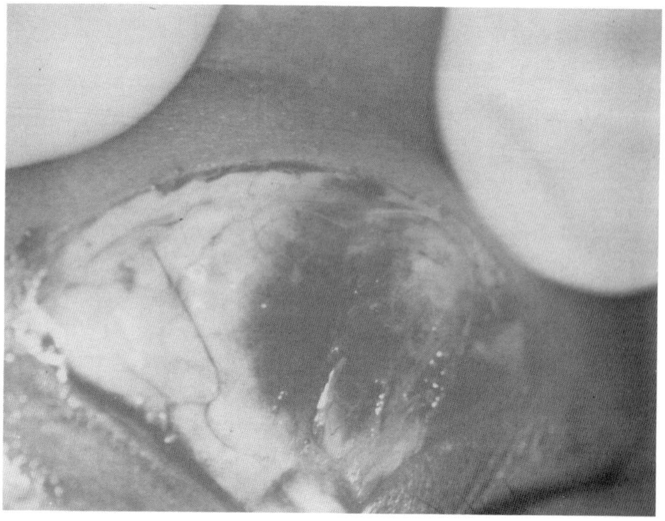

Figure 56.4. Retropulsion of the globe is necessary to prolapse the orbital fat within the septal aponeurotic fascial envelope, which will clearly delineate the septum from the aponeurosis. This preaponeurotic fat is a constant anatomical landmark sought during eyelid and ptosis surgery.

For purposes of clarification, the eyelid fold is a function of the presence of a lid crease, position of the lid, and degree of excess skin or dermatochalasis. In a young individual, a slight fold of skin overhangs the crease but is absent on downgaze as the action of the levator is minimized. In an elderly individual with excessive dermatochalasis, the lid fold overhands the crease significantly in primary gaze and can even persist on downgaze. In severe ptosis there might be a crease but rarely a lid fold (Fig. 56.17).

EYELID CREASE IN BLEPHAROPLASTY

The paticnt should have a thorough preoperative consultation and discussion especially regarding the desires of the patient and the capabilities of the surgeon. The patient is appropriately prepared and draped, open-faced, so that no inadvertent pull by the drapes of the forehead and brow above, or the cheek and lower lids tugged on inferiorly. If Betadine paint is used, it should be rinsed thoroughly so as not to camouflage fine rhytides of the lid and to accentuate the patient's natural crease. Using a fine-tipped marking pencil or toothpick with methylene blue dye, the surgeon outlines the primary lid crease position with single dots. Centrally, the crease should be from 8–10 mm above the lash margin, and the skin should be held slightly taut. Nasally, 6–8 mm is measured in a line above the punctum. Temporally, the mark is made 7–9 mm above the lateral canthus. If an excess of dermatochalasis is present, this incision can be made a bit longer or converted to a W-plasty. In Orientals, the crease is made 5–7 mm centrally or lower depending upon the desired endpoint, i.e., either "Occidentalizing" or retaining the original crease-fold characteristics. The upper incision line is similarly marked off. About 2 ml of 2% Xylocaine with 1:100,000 epinephrine is mixed in a 2:1 ratio with 0.5% Marcaine and injected subcutaneously along the outlined area. A No. 76 Beaver blade is grasped with a blade holder so that 0.75 mm of the blade is extending beyond the blade holder tip. The skin incision is then made perpendicular to the markings while keeping the lid skin on maximum stretch at the cutting site. This preset blade reduces the chances of cutting the levator aponeurosis inadvertently, such as might occur with a Bard-Parker blade in inexperienced hands. Skin and orbicularis are then dissected with a Bard-Parker blade using a "skinning technique over a finger" or with Wescott scissors. An additional strip of orbicularis is excised between the cut skin edges to expose the underlying orbital septum. The conjoined fascia, usually seen 2–3 mm above the primary lid crease position, can be difficult to delineate if there is little preaponeurotic fat present. Slight pressure superiorly on the globe will push the fat within the fascial envelope, delineating its location (Fig. 56.4). A horizontal-snip incision of the septum is then made, which allows the fat to herniate forth. This incision is extended nasally and temporally across the septum. The fat is teased gently from its septae and vessels, clamped, cut, and cauterized using a bipolar wet field unit. The levator aponeurosis fibers are now in full view. For closure, the surgeon approximates the nasal skin edges with two interrupted 6–0 Ethibond sutures, while being certain to include deep levator aponeurosis fibers (horn?) with each closure, otherwise a bulge or thick scar may ensue during healing. Then a continuous running lock stitch of 6–0 Ethibond is used to close the remaining incision. First the lower skin-dermis edge, with a few strands of orbicularis, is picked up with 0.5 mm forceps, then with the lid skin pulled flat against the

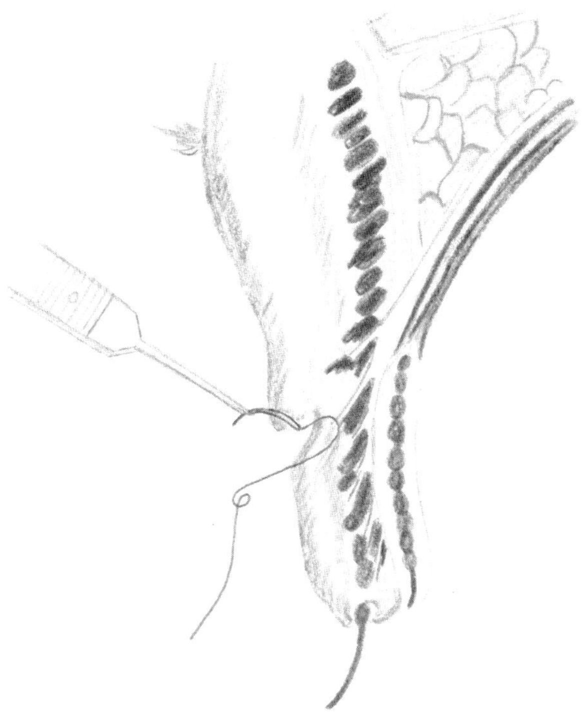

Figure 56.5. The suturing technique used in creating a natural eyelid crease anatomically; i.e., by suturing skin, orbicularis, levator aponeurosis, orbicularis, and skin.

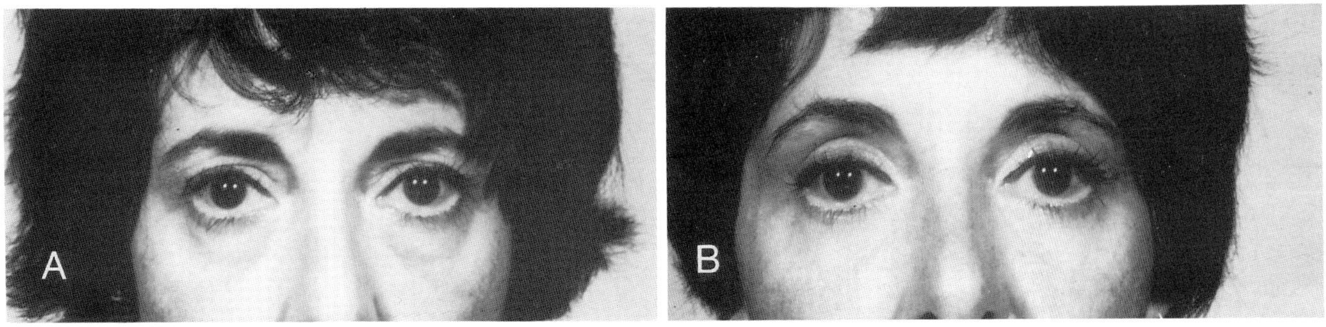

Figure 56.6. *A,* Preoperatively, the patient had marked dermatochalasis with extension temporally. *B,* Post-operatively, following a high lid crease reformation technique and extension of incision slightly beyond the orbital rim, elimination of the rhitides and restoration of a youthful appearance was achieved.

aponeurosis, the needle is passed through a few fibers of the aponeurosis 2 mm superior to this lower skin edge. This is necessary so as to create natural tension on the pretarsal skin, which keeps it flat against the tarsus and gives the lashes an upward direction. The needle is then passed through the properly aligned upper skin edge, which also includes a few fibers of orbicularis (Fig. 56.5). This exact procedure is repeated across the incision. Temporally, near the brow, where levator aponeurosis is absent, no deep bite is necessary. The running lock stitch affords the same ideal cooptation of edges as interrupted sutures but takes less time in placing and in removing them. The locking approach reduces the curling in of skin edges and loosening of each bite as compared with a simple running type closure. The suture is left in for 5 days to permit adequate adhesion between the levator fibers and the orbicularis fibers. Postoperatively, the patient uses continuous wet ice-saline compresses (tapering off in 3 to 4 days) and Erythromycin ointment along the incision two to three times daily. Suture tracks or abscess are rare with this approach. The above technique permits an excellent crease reconstruction while permitting the lid crease to be inconspicuous on downgaze (Fig. 56.6). Lid crease technique using through-and-through sutures may create an adequate crease, however, the crease is not as even and natural and quite often has unsightly dimples. This technique may be difficult to be used in the Orientals who require low lid crease for reconstruction.

When unilateral lid crease repair is needed, such as in trauma cases, where skin grafts have been used or when a more prominent crease is desired, it can be achieved by the following technique: Prior to the skin closure, a separate suture of either 7.0 Prolene or 8.0 virgin silk is placed in a running lock fashion attaching only the lower skin edge orbicularis fibers and securing them to the levator aponeurosis as above (Fig. 56.7). The skin edges are then closed separately with 6.0 Ethibond in running lock fashion without picking up any orbicularis or aponeurotic fibers. When there is absence of levator function, then a bite of the underlying tarsal tissue is engaged to fix the orbicularis skin edge, i.e., "anchor blepharoplasty." This can sometimes simulate a crease and still keep the skin tissue flat against the tarsus.

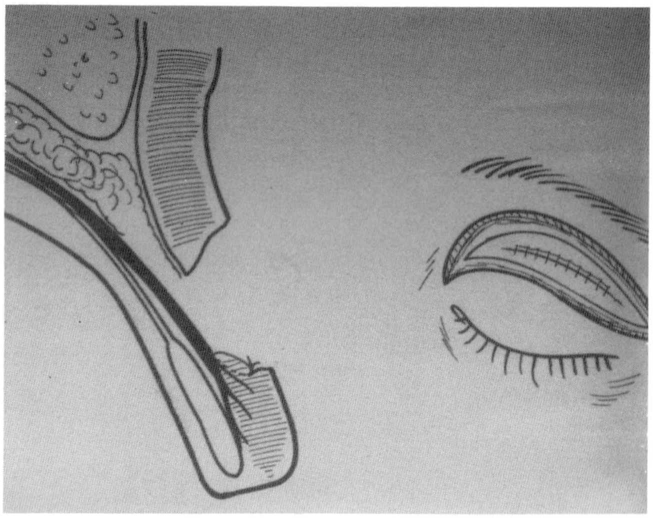

Figure 56.7. Cross section of the lid. Shown is the placement of a running lock suture to fix the lower edge of orbicularis to the levator aponeurosis using a separate suture.

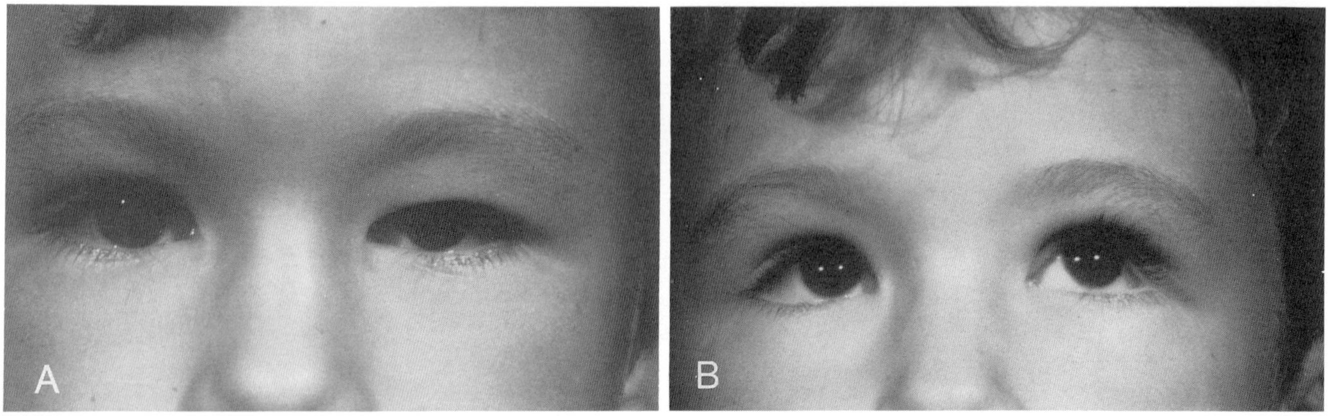

Figure 56.8. This patient demonstrates a typical Occidental eyelid and fold and on the right and a classic Oriental "single lid" on the left. There was no ptosis for which he was referred. A symmetrical Caucasian eyelid crease and fold was achieved with the described technique. *A*, Preoperative. *B*, Postoperative.

EYELID CREASE IN THE ORIENTAL

The most important aspect of this surgery is to appreciate the anatomic variations in each individual patient. Preoperatively, try to show the patient by either lifting the brow or using a fine probe placed under the lid fold. Place it in such a way as to simulate the new lid position. One also needs to predetermine the extent of the incisions, especially nasally, so as not to bridge the canthal sulcus or alter any fold present. Where the present lid crease is or was adequate (by examining all photographs), one simply marks this off, then the excess skin is pinched and outlined proportionately, making sure not to extend it nasal to the punctum. The skin and adjacent orbicularis are excised exposing the low-lying orbital septum. It is incised and whatever fat bulges forth is excised as described above, but not aggressively, as this might lead to a superior sulcus formation that could alter the Oriental characteristic. Close the skin incision similarly to the technique described under "Eyelid Crease in Blepharoplasty"; i.e., by incorporating the levator fibers with "good bites" (Fig. 56.8).

When a higher lid crease is desired (Fig. 56.9), the level is carefully marked off proportionately. If the patient is young and has little excess skin, then mark off only 1 mm of an ellipse of skin above the primary lid crease position. After excising skin, underlying orbicularis and orbital fat, the surgeon must disinsert any prominent attachments of the levator aponeurosis inferior to the incision (new crease

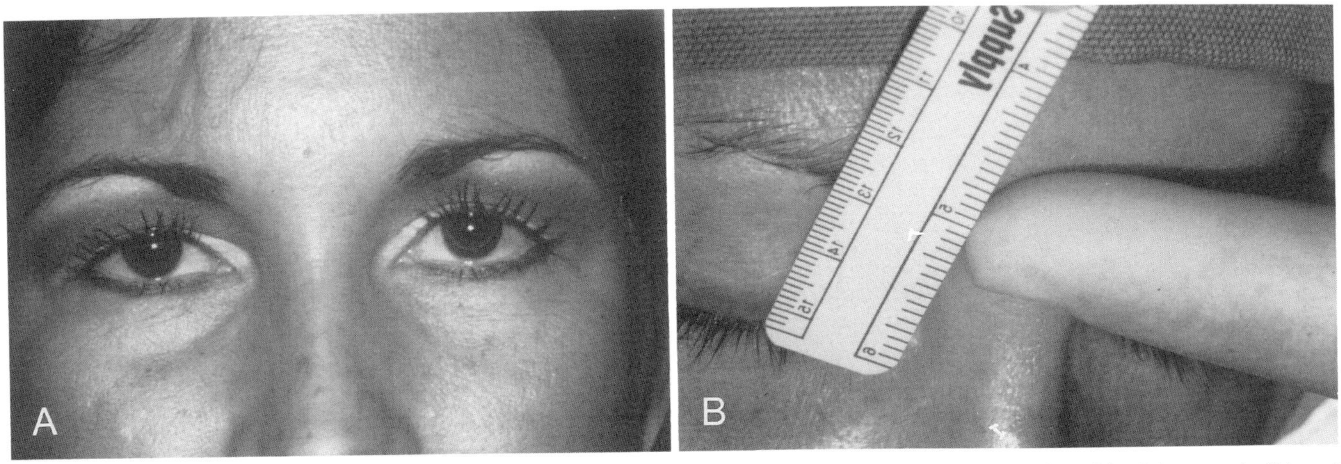

Figure 56.9. This young patient had a blepharoplasty 5 years ago but remained unhappy with the results. Various second opinions and recommendations for repeat blepharoplasty were turned down. On examination, there was an obvious iatrogenic low lid crease with the eyelid fold almost touching the lashes. She tried to mask this with makeup techniques seen in *A*. *B* shows at surgery the old incision site, barely 4 mm above the lash line. On downgaze, no excess lid skin was present.

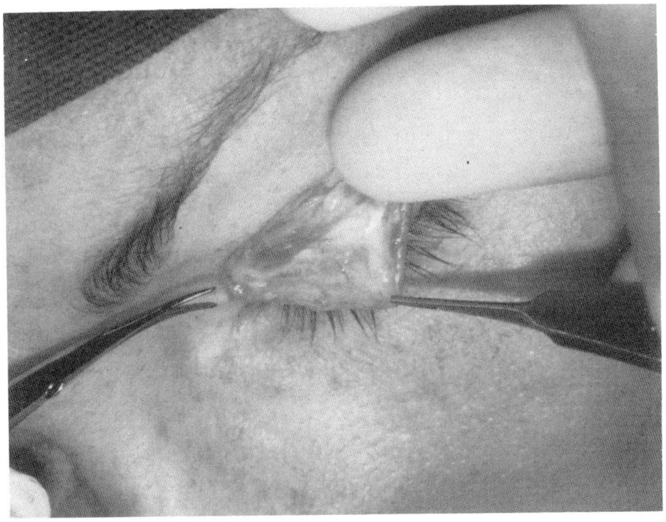

Figure 56.10. Elimination of a low-positioned palpebral crease is accomplished by dissecting a skin muscle flap as low down as the lashes across the full lid.

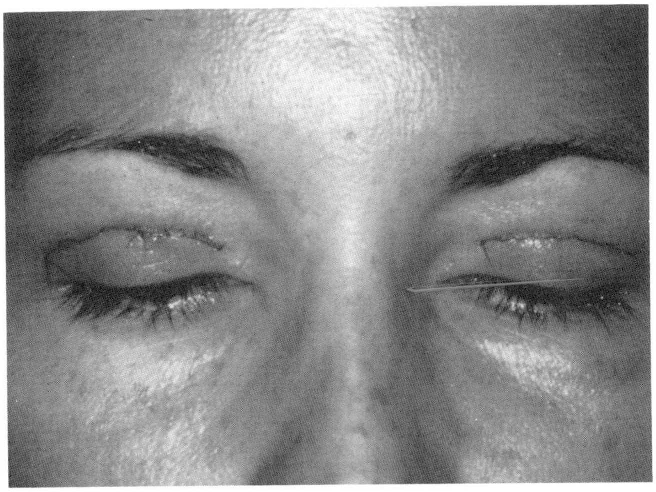

Figure 56.11. Postoperative appearance of the running lock suture in place on both upper lids. Note the height of the newly created lid crease.

line) by dissecting a skin muscle flap as low down as the lashes, so as to undo and prevent any low-lying crease or dimpling of the skin postoperatively (Fig. 56.10). The skin can be closed in one stage as in the blepharoplasty technique described earlier, or in order to create a more definite crease, one should fix the lower skin edge orbicularis to the underlying levator aponeurosis separately, using either Prolene or virgin silk suture. Be certain that the bite is not picking up tarsus as this could create dimpling. The skin edges are then closed separately with 6–0 Ethibond, using a running lock stitch (Fig. 56.11). Surgeons can test the adequacy of the crease height, smoothness of skin anterior to the tarsus, and appropriateness of the lid fold by asking the patient to look up at different intervals while they close the incision, thus allowing the surgeon to naturally alter bites as necessary (Fig. 56.12). As you can see, raising or forming a lid crease is easy, but lowering or undoing a high lid crease, where trauma or previous blepharoplasty has eliminated most or all of the preaponeurotic orbital fat, is an elusive goal. One needs a true fat graft to keep the septum/orbicularis from adhering to the underlying aponeurosis at points higher than designated crease position. In restoring a lid crease after ptosis surgery, one simply closes the incision and picks up the advanced levator fibers as described. Again, this approach is more physiologic than the through-and-through chromic sutures described in the old literature.

In marked blepharoptosis where a sling procedure is indicated, the goal should be to place the horizontal passage of the fascia at such a level that a natural and appropriate skin *fold* will ensue; specifically, the lid incision should be made 6–8 mm from the lash margin

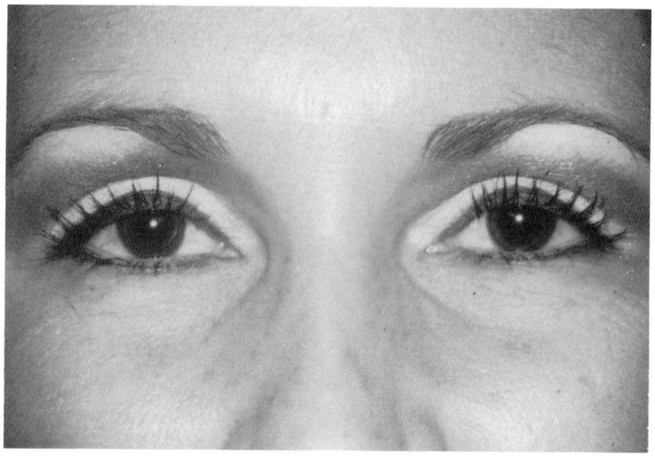

Figure 56.12. The patient now 2 months postoperatively, showing the restoration of the typical Occidental lid with a good amount of skin shown beneath the lid fold. This patient thanked me for "giving my eyes back."

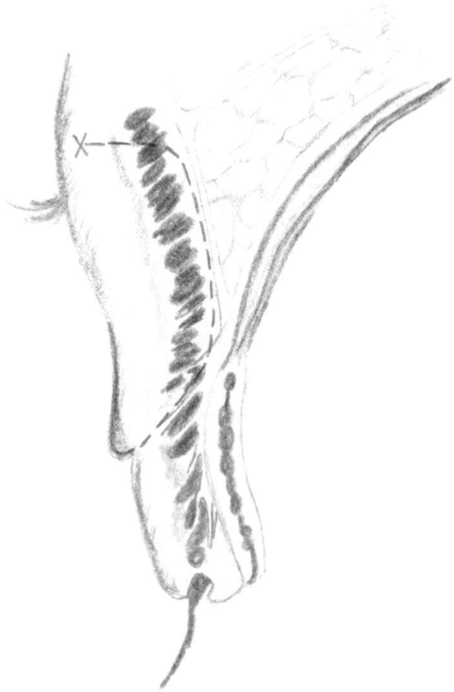

Figure 56.13. Schematic shows how the brow suspension suture should be placed to create a natural appearing lid fold in an eye without any levator action.

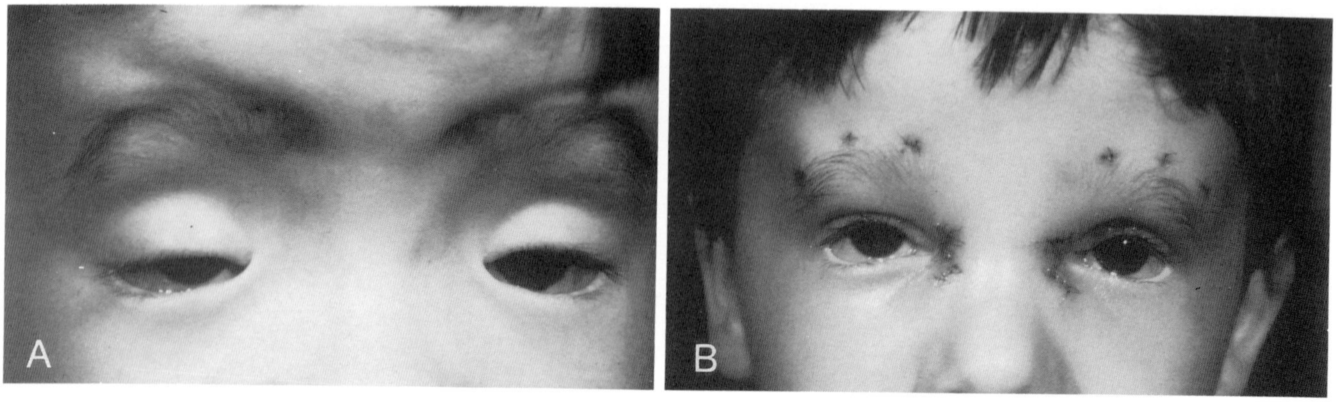

Figure 56.14. *A*, Preoperative photograph of a blepharophimosis patient with marked ptosis and lack of palpebral crease and fold. *B*, Postoperatively, appropriate placement of the skin incisions resulted in a very natural looking eyelid following a sling procedure.

centrally, 4–6 nasally, and 5–7 temporally or proportionate to the opposite lid if unilateral. As the fascial sling is pulled upward by the brow, or just "slung" there, it retains flatness of the skin inferiorly while allowing for a small eyelid fold to form, which results in a very pleasing and natural look in primary gaze (Figs. 56.13 and 56.14) and gives even the lashes an upward direction. The above result will not be achieved if the surgeon places the skin incision 2–3 mm or closer to the lash line as recommended in the classic writings. This will lead towards multiple folds and distortion or irregularly directed lashes.

LOWER EYELID CREASE

Remember that the lower lid is an analogous structure to the upper lid (1). Restoring lower lid crease in a typical blepharoplasty patient is not necessary, besides it would be difficult especially since many surgeons use a subciliary approach. However, in younger individuals such as professional models, it might be necessary to create one. Where excess skin is present, one would still use a subciliary incision, remove fat and so forth, but before closing the skin edges, the orbicularis, usually 4–5 mm below the lashes, is attached to the underlying capsulopalpebral fascia with either 8.0 virgin or 7.0 Prolene sutures. The skin excision is then modified to permit a very small excess of skin to remain; this results in a slight roundness, especially when patient laughs or gazes down. In children or patients with a good crease already present, one should consider making the incision on the crease so as not to disrupt the

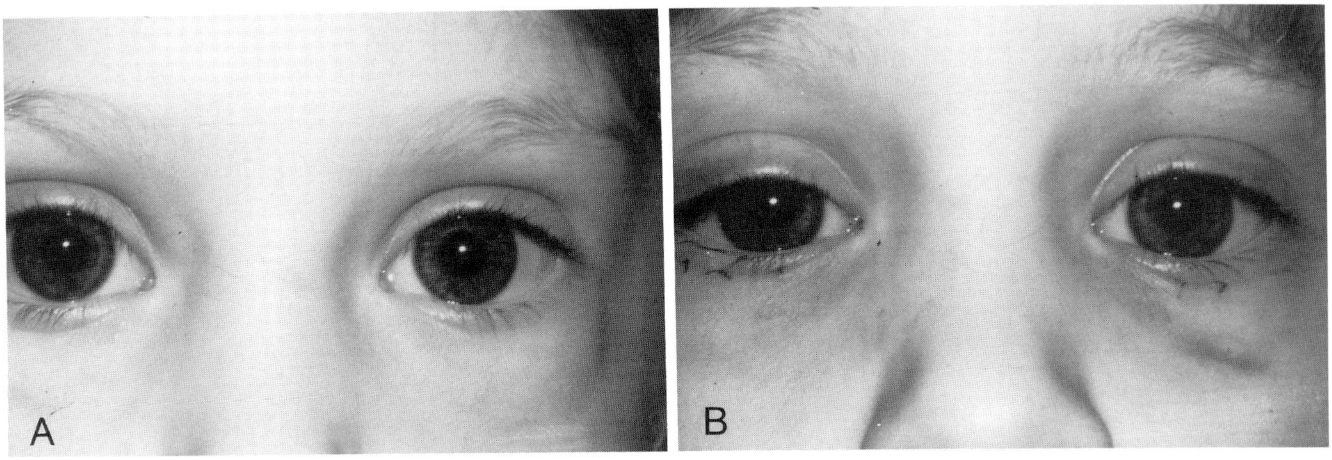

Figure 56.15. This 7-year-old had recurrent lid edema with early onset blepharochalasis of the lower lids as seen in *A*. *B*, Retention of lower lid crease was accomplished by making skin incision onto the original crease and dissecting a skin muscle flap inferior to the retractor attachments.

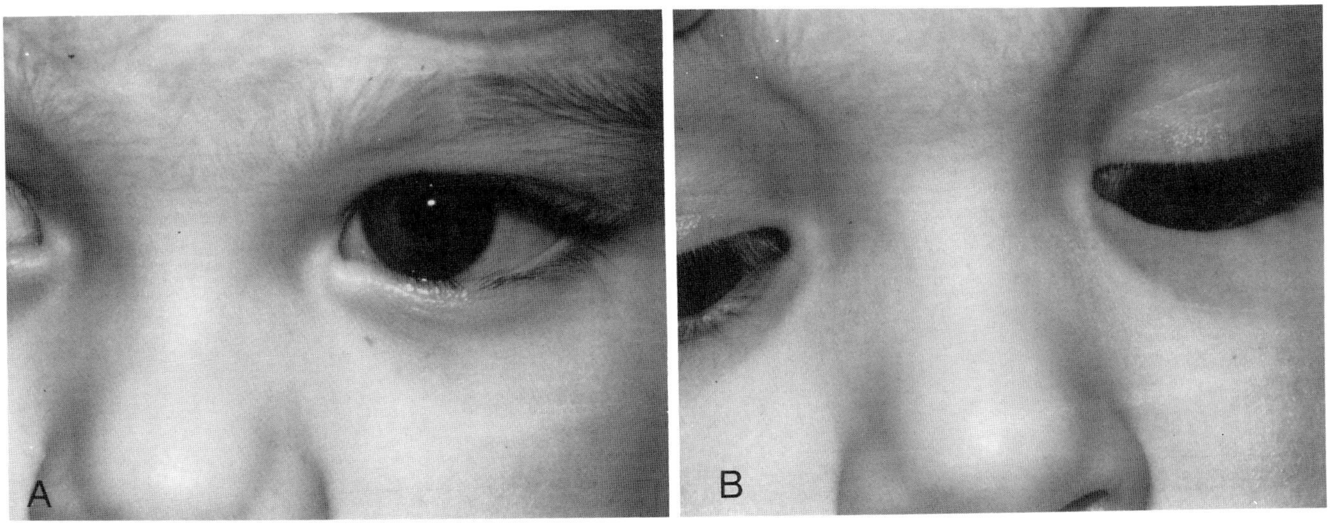

Figure 56.16. *A*, This young patient demonstrates a unique presentation of a normal lower lid crease on the right and absence of such on the left lower lid. *B*, It resulted in trichiasis especially upon reading or downgaze, somewhat like a pseudoepiblepharon.

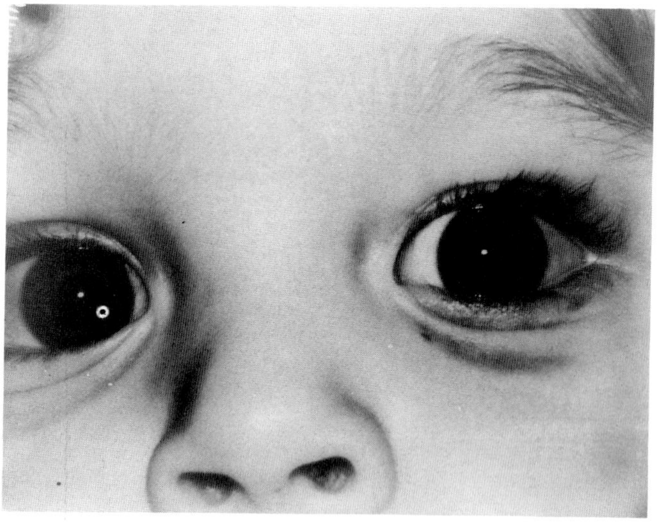

Figure 56.17. The same patient's postoperative appearance after reattachment of the pretarsal orbicularis to the left lower lid retractors, which corrected the trichiasis and the pseudoepiblepharon, and reformed a symmetrical crease. No skin was excised in this repair.

lower lid retractor. Here the skin edges alone are apposed for closure (Fig. 56.15). When the eyelid crease is absent or weak, it can lead to pseudoepiblepharon or trichiasis (Fig. 56.16). Correction involves merely reattaching the capsulopalpebral fascia to the orbicularis skin as done in the upper lid (Fig. 56.17).

REFERENCES

1. Hawes MJ, Dortzbach RK: The microscopic anatomy of the eyelid retractors. *Arch Ophthalmol* 100: 1313–1318, 1982.
2. Doxanas MT, Anderson RL: Oriental eyelids: an anatomic study. *Arch Ophthalmol* 102: 1232–1235, 1984.
3. Boo-Chai K: Plastic construction of the superior palpebral fold. *Plast Reconstr Surg* 31: 556, 1964.
4. Hisatami C, Fujino T: Anatomical considerations concerning blepharoplasty in the Oriental patient. *Adv Ophthal Plast Reconstr Surg* 2: 151–163, 1983.
5. Shein JH: A change in technique of supratarsal fixation in upper blepharoplasty. *Plast Reconstr Surg* 59: 831–834, 1977.
6. Shein JH: Supratarsal fixation in upper blepharoplasty. *Plast Reconstr Surg* 54: 424–431, 1974.
7. Putterman AM: Reconstruction of the upper eyelid crease and fold. *Arch Ophthalmol* 94: 1941–1954, 1976.
8. Shein JH: Tarsal fixation in lower blepharoplasty. *Plast Reconstr Surg* 62: 24–31, 1978.

CHAPTER 57

Oriental Eyelids: Anatomic Difference and Surgical Consideration

DON LIU, M.D., Ph.D.

The difference between the Oriental eye (of the Mongolian race) and the Occidental eye has stirred a great deal of interest recently. Although there are some excellent anthropological and morphological studies on the subject (1–6), most of the clinical studies were done within the past few decades. Generally, the Occidental eye is exemplified by the Greek eye. It is horizontally set, with a deep superior sulcus. It has wide palpebral fissures and long lashes tilted upward. On the other hand, a somewhat obliquely set, almond-shaped eye with acute corners has been taken as representative of the Oriental eye. When compared with the Occidental eye, the Oriental eye has a narrower palpebral opening with fullness in the upper eyelid. Frequently, there is also an epicanthal fold. The slanted Oriental eye is said to give a mysterious, charming, and exotic look; the big round Occidental eye gives a cheerful and energetic impression (Fig. 57.1).

Ever since the Second World War, there has been a tremendous global spread of Western influence. Consequently, some of the Western beauty standards have become well accepted in the traditional minds of the East. Notably, the Western-type of upper eyelid has come to be the ideal in some strata of the societies.

The creation of an upper eyelid crease has been for a long time the most popular cosmetic surgical procedure in many Asian countries. It is looked upon by the Orientals as a method to enhance the beauty of the eyelids but not as an attempt to "Westernize" their facial features. Various techniques of constructing an upper eyelid crease have long been used by ophthalmologists and nonophthalmologists in the Far East. Even nonsurgical means such as glue or tape have been tried. It is only in recent years that these types of operations are documented in the English language. Already there has been some confusion in the terminology for this operation. It has been variously called cosmetic blepharoplasty, duplication of eyelid operation, double eyelid operation, construction of an upper eyelid fold, revision of the Oriental eyelid, and Westernization of the Oriental eye. "Double eyelid" is used extensively in the lay public in most parts of Asia. "Westernization of Oriental eyelid" may sound patronizing, therefore, objectionable to some people. We believe "plastic construction of an upper eyelid crease" is probably the most accurate term and will use it throughout this chapter.

The facial features of Orientals differ from Occidentals in many respects. Depending on the objectives and motivation of the patient and surgeon, several surgical procedures may be necessary. We very rarely find any Oriental wanting his or her facial features entirely Westernized; besides it is technically impossible. Most likely, they will want to have an upper eyelid crease and/or a deeper superior sulcus. Frequently, the patient is not even aware of the presence of an epicanthal fold.

A small child may be brought in by parents who are under the impression that the child has a convergent strabismus. Sometimes this turns out to be a pseudoesotropia due to epicanthal folds and a relatively flat nose. The parents usually refuse surgery to correct the folds unless they are truly prominent.

Epiblepharon is seen more commonly in the Oriental

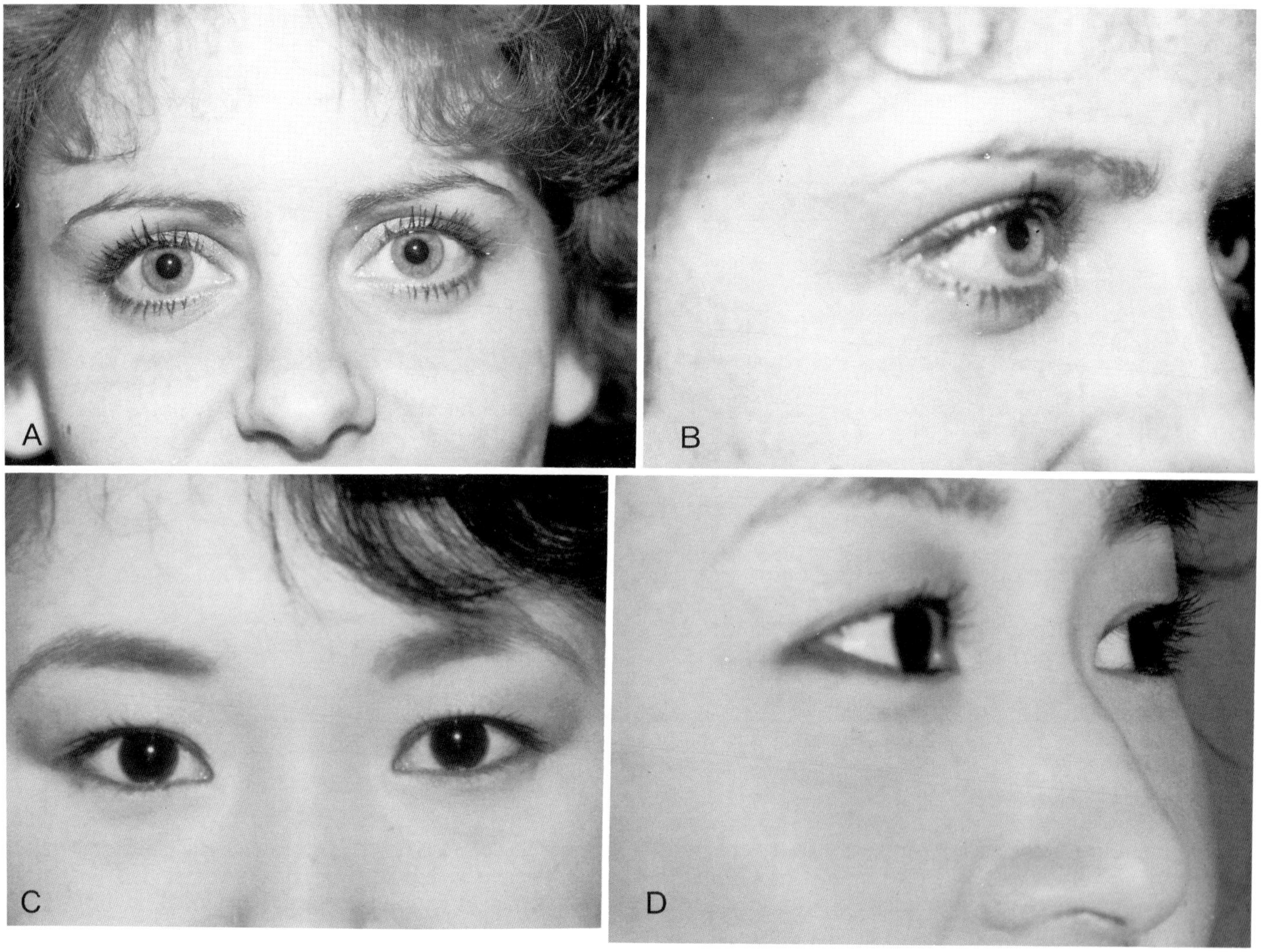

Figure 57.1. *A,* Occidental eyelids, frontal view. *B,* Occidental eyelids, side view. Note distinct crease, deep superior sulcus. *C,* Oriental eyelids, frontal view. *D,* Oriental eyelids, side view. Note absence of crease and fullness in upper eyelid.

than in the Occidental children. Usually, very little evidence of corneal damage is seen despite tearing and occasional conjunctival injection. Epiblepharon should be distinguished from congenital entropion, which worsens with the passage of time.

Discussion in this chapter shall be limited to the anatomic difference between the Oriental and Occidental upper eyelids and the surgical techniques of constructing an upper eyelid crease, deepening the superior sulcus, eliminating prominent epicanthal folds, and correcting epiblepharon in an Oriental patient.

ANATOMY

The Mongolian race consists of many different ethnic groups, with each group having its characteristic features and regional variations. Nevertheless, the typical Oriental eyelid is considered to have some or all of the following features: (*a*) absence of an upper eyelid crease with fullness in the upper eyelid, (*b*) a narrower palpebral fissure, and (*c*) the presence of epicanthal folds.

UPPER EYELID CREASE

Although there are many papers published on this subject, they are mostly based on clinical experiences (7–19). This is because of the Confucian philosophy and reverence for ancestors, making surgical procedures and cadaver dissection virtually nonexistent in the Orient for thousands of years. Only recently, definitive anatomical works by excellent cadaver dissections are provided by both Hisatomi and Fujino in Japan, and Doxanas and Anderson in the United States (20–22).

A cross section through the upper eyelid from superficial to deep reveals the following layers:

Skin

The eyelid skin is probably the thinnest in the body. It measures 0.6 mm or less than 1 mm (23–27). Liu and

Hsu (28) have studied the thickness of the eyelid skin clinically and histologically and found that the Oriental eyelid skin is slightly thicker than the Occidental's. The thickness of the Oriental upper eyelid skin ranges from 0.30 to 0.80 mm (depending on the age of the patient), with an average of 0.65 mm. The difference is mainly due to the presence of a thicker subcutaneous areolar layer and occasional small amounts of subcutaneous fat found in the Oriental's skin layer.

Muscle

Liu and Hsu also found that in almost 85% of the Orientals, a submuscular fat pad exists. This is in accordance with the experiences of other authors (7, 15, 16, 22, 29).

Fascia Layer

The fascia layer consists of the orbital septum, orbital fat and the levator aponeurosis. It is the difference in this anatomic layer that results in the clinically different appearance between the Occidentals and the Orientals. Mainly, the eyelid crease and fold are a result of the relationship between the orbital septum and the levator aponeurosis. A detailed description of the Occidental eyelid can be found in any standard textbook. To summarize, the levator muscle becomes aponeurotic approximately 10–12 mm above the superior tarsal border. The levator aponeurosis fuses with the orbital septum a few millimeters above the superior tarsal border, and this fused complex continues inferiorly. At the inferior extent of the fused complex, the aponeurotic fibers extend anteroinferiorly and pass interdigitally in the fibrous septa of the orbicularis muscle and then insert into the subcutaneous tissues. The formation of the eyelid crease is the result of the subcutaneous insertion of the most superior fibers.

The lower eyelid is a structure analogous to the upper eyelid, with the capsulopalpebral fascia as the retractor. In the lower eyelid, an autonomous retractor analogous to the levator muscle of the upper eyelid does not exist. Since very little difference in the lower eyelid exists clinically between Occidentals and Orientals, there will be no further discussion of the lower lid.

In Orientals, the levator aponeurosis fuses with the orbital septum below the superior tarsal border. This results in two major clinical differences. First, with the preaponeurotic fat extending closer to the eyelid margin, an appearance of fullness of the eyelid results. Second, the more inferior extension of the orbital septum prevents a well-defined subcutaneous insertion of the anterior portion of the levator aponeurosis fibers. This results in a less well developed or a somewhat lower eyelid crease in Orientals (Fig. 57.2).

Tarsus

This dense connective tissue plate contributes to the form and support of the eyelid.

Conjunctiva

Conjunctiva is the posterior layer of the eyelids. This mucosal membrane is firmly adherent to the tarsus and loosely adherent to Müller's muscle.

In the Orient, an upper eyelid without a crease is generally called a "single eyelid" and an eyelid with a crease, a "double eyelid." Written in the Chinese idiogram, this term defies translation. The double eyelid is further classified into three categories.

Outer Double Eyelid. The "outer double eyelid" is a distinct upper eyelid crease lying anywhere from 7 to 10 mm above the lash margin. It resembles very much a typical Occidental eyelid crease. This type of double eyelid is called the "parallel type" by Mutou (30).

Inner Double Eyelid. The "inner double eyelid" is a relatively low-lying eyelid crease. It may be located anywhere from 3 to 5 mm above the lash margin. It usually disappears when the patient looks up and the overlying skin fold touches the eyelashes. This type of double eyelid is called the "unfolded fan" by Mutou (30). The eyelid crease in this case, follows the curvature of the epicanthal fold, or as pointed out by Johnson (31, 32), is an exaggeration of the epicanthus tarsalis. Because of the hooding of the low-lying skin fold, the inner double eyelid sometimes can be mistaken for ptosis; conversely, a ptotic eyelid can give a patient the appearance of having an inner double eyelid.

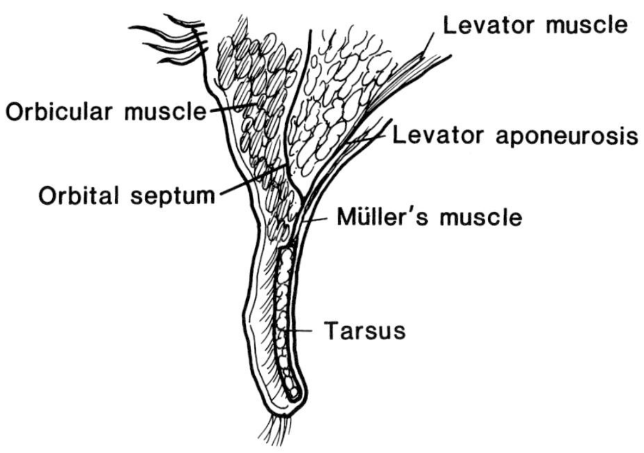

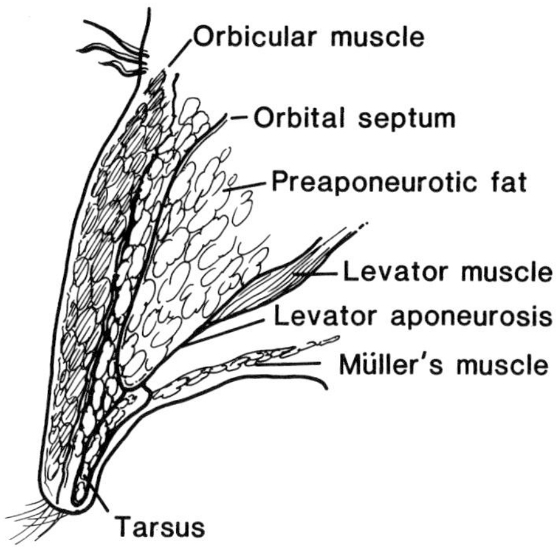

Figure 57.2. On the *left* is a typical Occidental eyelid. Note the fusion of levator aponeurosis and orbital septum is above the superior border of the tarsal plate. On the *right* is a typical Oriental eyelid. Note the fusion takes place below the superior tarsal border. There is also a small submuscular fat pad.

Unilateral Double Eyelid. Present only in one eye, the majority of this type of double eyelid has a low-lying crease. Frequently, this type of double eyelid is present intermittently depending on the presence or absence of edema. There have been various estimates of the prevalence of double eyelid in the Orientals, ranging from 30 to 90% (7, 11, 13, 17, 30, 33). In a recent collaborative study including more than 3000 Chinese people residing in Taiwan and the United States, Liu and Hsu (34) found 67.2% of the population studied have the outer double eyelid, 4.9% have the inner double eyelid, 4.7% have the unilateral double eyelid, and 23.2% have no eyelid crease. Of those patients without the eyelid crease, about 60% of them prefer the inner double eyelid or the low-lying eyelid crease to the outer double eyelid or the high-lying eyelid crease. This preference is also noted by Mutou and Mutou (30) (Fig. 57.3).

PALPEBRAL FISSURE

The palpebral fissure measures about 28–30 mm × 12–14 mm in Caucasians (23, 25, 34, 35). Liu and Hsu concluded that the palpebral fissure in the studied Oriental population is 27.2 ± 1.2 mm × 8.5 ± 0.9 mm. These numbers agree with the previously reported numbers (9, 10, 36). Liu and Hsu also concluded that the eyelid crease in the Orientals in the populations studied ranged from 3.0 to 9.5 mm, with an average of 6.5 ± 0.7 mm.

EPICANTHAL FOLD

The term "epicanthal fold" was first coined by Von-Ammon in 1831 (37) and was first described by Schon in 1828 (38). This is a semilunar fold of skin extending from the upper eyelid across the medial canthal area to the margin of the lower eyelid medially. It is present in fetal life from the third month to the sixth month in all races. In whites, blacks, and some Eskimos, it usually disappears before birth. However, in the Mongolian race it remains as a characteristic feature. It is generally accepted that the epicanthal fold is present in 70–90% of the population in the Mongolian race and in only 2–5% of Caucasians (41). However, Liu and Hsu found it is present only in about 40.7% of the population studied (34).

Epicanthus is almost invariably bilateral but occasionally may be asymmetrical, and rarely it may be unilateral. In the Mongolian race, the combination of epicanthal folds and a relatively flat nose frequently results in an esotropic appearance. In Caucasians, epicanthus may be an isolated anomaly or may be associated with ptosis or blepharophimosis syndrome. There are four types of epicanthus described (41).

Epicanthus Supraciliaris

The epicanthal fold arises from the region of the eyebrow and runs towards the tear sac or the nostril.

Epicanthus Palpebralis

In epicanthus palpebralis, the epicanthal fold arises from the upper eyelid, above the tarsal region, and extends to the lower margin of the orbit.

Epicanthus Tarsalis

In epicanthus tarsalis, the fold arises from the tarsal fold and loses itself in the skin close to the medial canthus.

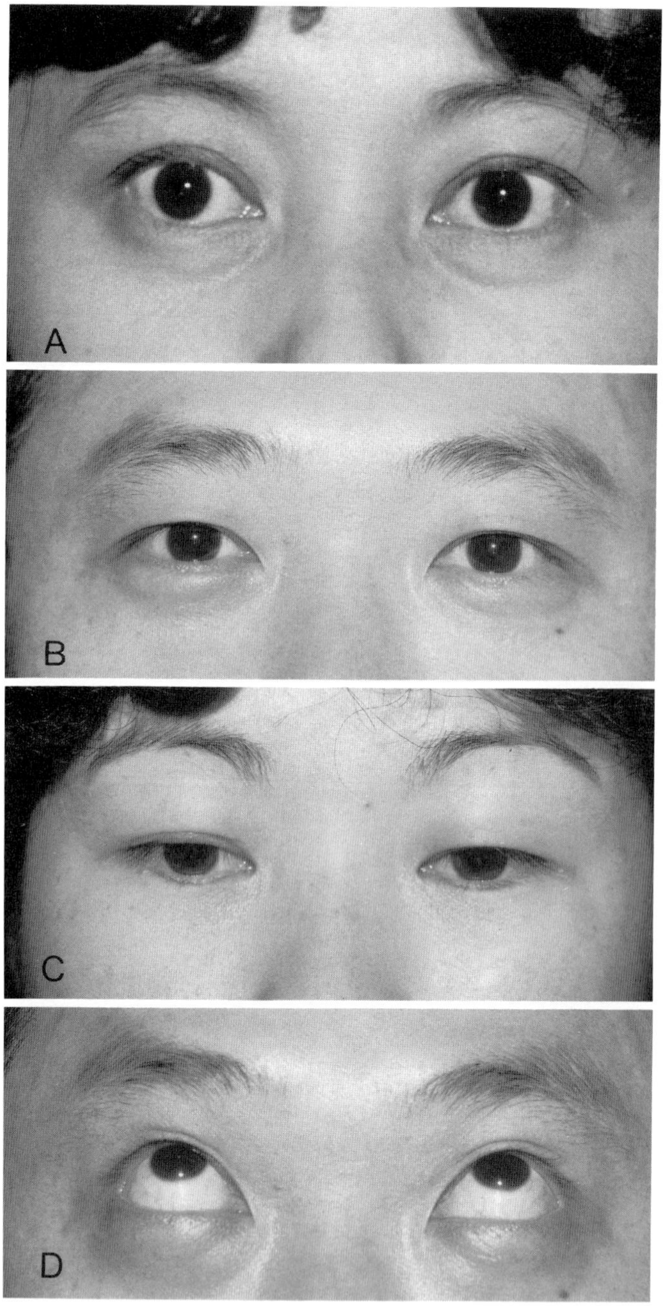

Figure 54.3. *A,* Outer double eyelid. Lid crease is 8–10 mm above lash margin. This resembles the Western eyelid very much. *B,* Inner double eyelid. Note its low position, curvature and its relationship with the epicanthal fold. *C,* Unilateral double eyelid. Note the low-lying crease on right that follows the curvature of the epicanthal fold. *D,* Same patients as in panel *B.* Curiously, there exists a partial lid crease that is only present on upgaze.

This type is most commonly seen in the Orientals. In fact, the double eyelid that many Oriental patients prefer is related to this type of epicanthal fold; namely, the eyelid crease is looked upon as the extension of the epicanthal fold and is located 3–5 mm above the lash margin.

Epicanthus Inversus

In epicanthus inversus, a small fold arises in the lower eyelid and extends upward to partially cover the medial

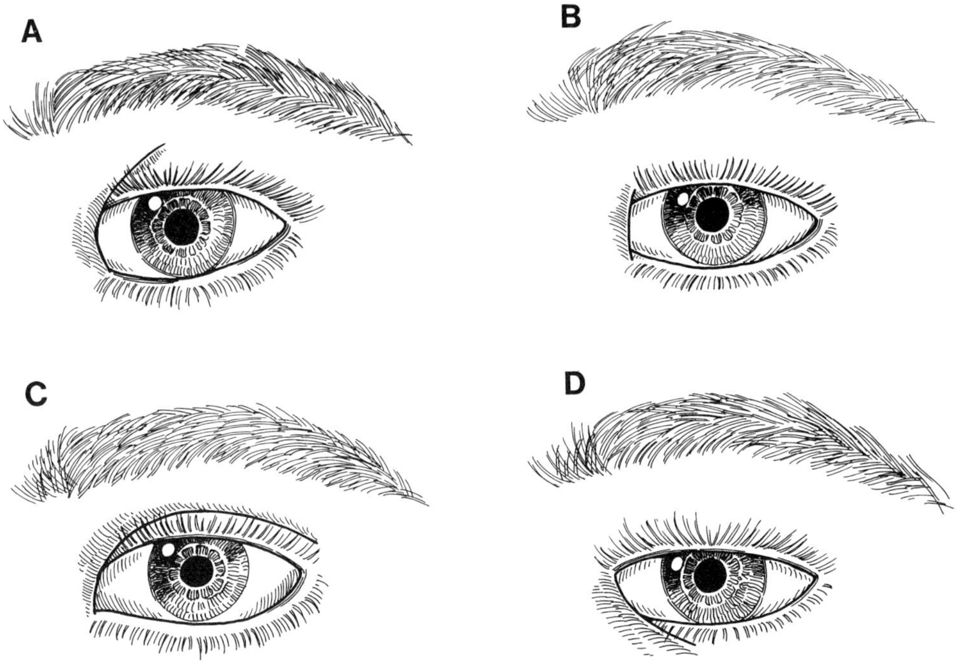

Figure 57.4. Four types of epicanthus. *A,* Epicanthus superciliaris. *B,* Epicanthus palpebralis. *C,* Epicanthus tarsalis. *D,* Epicanthus inversus.

canthus. It is frequently associated with blepharophimosis syndrome. There may be hypoplasia of the caruncle and semilunar fold, ptosis, ectropion and telecanthus (Fig. 57.4) (23, 31, 32).

EPIBLEPHARON

Epiblepharon is an extra-tented-up fold of eyelid skin that extends horizontally from the medial canthus to the lid laterally. There may be a band of orbicularis muscle underlying the skin fold. It is frequently associated with epicanthal folds. It is typically present bilaterally, more frequently in the lower eyelid than in the upper eyelid.

Usually, epiblepharon does not cause any problem. However, when the accessory eyelid skin fold becomes too exaggerated, the lashes may be pushed against the cornea. This is easily seen in Orientals with eyelashes pointed straight forward. In Occidentals with long curly lashes, it may be detected only when the patient is in upgaze or downgaze (39). However, the Oriental's cornea seems to be much more resistant to the irritation of the lashes. There usually is very little evidence of corneal damage despite the lashes rubbing against the cornea. If there is punctate staining of the cornea, symptoms are usually minimal and the patient rarely complains.

In all races, epiblepharon is considered a developmental anomaly. The cause of it is in dispute. Some believe a maldevelopment in the fascial planes or an anomalous insertion or insufficiency of the inferior rectus muscle is responsible for this condition. Others believe that a kink in the tarsal plate, the closeness of the lid margin to the subcutaneous insertion of the levator fibers, or a combination of hypertrophied muscle with an extra skin fold is responsible for this condition (23, 31, 32, 40, 41).

Epiblepharon should be distinguished from entropion. Epiblepharon usually disappears by the age of 2, whereas entropion worsens with age. Entropion of the lower eyelid is due to a different mechanism or etiology. It also involves the inturning of the entire lower eyelid margin.

PREOPERATIVE EVALUATION

As is true for any cosmetic surgery, careful patient selection is the first step toward successful surgery. First of all, the surgeon should elicit the patient's expectation and motivation for the surgery. A candid discussion is held between the doctor and patient, and what can be realistically expected is carefully delineated.

The surgeon should obtain a pertinent medical history and perform an eye examination even when there is no psychiatric contraindication to surgery. Cosmetic eyelid surgery (except when simple suture technique is used) is considered only if thyroid, cardiac, and renal disorders have already been ruled out and if the patient is not a keloid former. An eye examination should include recorded visual acuity, funduscopic examination, slitlamp examination, and lacrimal function evaluation. The upper eyelid height and its contour and the direction of the lashes should be noted. If brow ptosis, eyelid ptosis, or an epicanthal fold is present, it should be taken into consideration in the surgical planning. If the patient desires a deeper superior sulcus, removal of orbital fat and/or subcutaneous tissues should be kept in mind. All surgical candidates (except when simple suture technique is used) who are on aspirin or Coumadin are instructed to discontinue taking these drugs for at least 2 weeks prior to the scheduled surgery.

For the patient who desires having an upper eyelid crease, the position or the height of the eyelid crease is often the most important concern. What can be achieved realistically may be demonstrated to the patient by gently pressing on the upper eyelid skin at the proposed height with the aid of a small paper clip. Sometimes photographs or sketches may be helpful.

If an adult patient does not complain about the presence of the epicanthal folds, surgery is not suggested. If the patient brings up the subject, the removal of them may be demonstrated to the patient by pulling the nasal skin medially. Small children are usually brought in by parents who are under the impression that they have esotropia. Similar digital manipulation of the nasal skin will eliminate the child's esotropic appearance. This will convince the parents that removal of the epicanthal fold is the corrective surgery needed. The patient or parents should be advised of a possible temporary hypertrophic scar in that area.

If an adult has epiblepharon, the patient usually relates a history of corneal irritation, foreign body sensation, conjunctival injection, or constant tearing. In addition to the ocular examination just described, the surgeon should ask the patient to look up and down and to close the eyelids tightly. This will help determine whether epiblepharon, trichiasis, or entropion may be the cause of the problem. Such a maneuver is especially important in a small child brought in by parents with history of epiphora or chronic conjunctivitis not resolved by antibiotic drops (39).

Epiblepharon is to be distinguished from congenital entropion. True entropion usually worsens with time, while epiblepharon usually disappears by the age of 1 or 2 years in most Occidentals, while it occasionally persists into adulthood in Orientals.

ANESTHESIA

General anesthesia is usually necessary to perform any of these surgical procedures on small children. If there is no contraindication, the surgeon can use a small amount of local anesthetic with epinephrine 1:100,000 in the proposed surgical field for better hemostasis. For adults or older children who can cooperate, local anesthesia supplemented by intravenous sedation is preferred. Sedatives and analgesics are given intramuscularly approximately 2 hours preoperatively. Additional intravenous sedation with diazepam is given in the operating room. After all measurements and all the necessary skin markings have been made and the patient is sufficiently sedated, local infiltration with 2% Xylocaine with epinephrine 1:100,000 is given with a No. 27 needle immediately beneath the skin. This facilitates dissection of the tissue planes and improves hemostasis.

CONSTRUCTION OF AN UPPER EYELID CREASE

If the construction of an upper eyelid crease alone is desired, the proposed new eyelid creases are to be marked first. (If other associated conditions are to be corrected, such as epicanthal fold, telecanthus, epiblepharon, see discussion in the appropriate sections.)

As stated before, the patient's preference for the location of the new upper eyelid crease may vary anywhere from 3 to 10 mm above the lash line. If a relatively low-lying crease (as an extension of the epicanthal fold) is desired, the location of such a crease is determined as follows: By digitally pulling the nasal skin inframedially to accentuate the epicanthal fold, the surgeon can follow the epicanthal fold laterally, and hence determine the location of the new eyelid crease.

If an epicanthal fold is not present or the patient desires a relatively high-lying upper eyelid crease, this can be outlined by direct measurement. Finally, if the patient has a unilateral existing eyelid crease, the proposed crease in the fellow eye should match the existing crease as closely as possible.

SURGICAL TECHNIQUES

SUTURE TECHNIQUES

These suture techniques are all based on the principle that some adhesion or scarring between the skin and the deeper tissues is created by the suture (30, 42). These techniques do not involve any skin incision, are simple to perform, and can be repeated when necessary. For the patients who do not want more extensive surgery or when radical surgery is not indicated, suture technique is a very effective method of creating an upper eyelid crease.

Pang's technique uses three doubly armed silk sutures (42). These sutures are placed in a mattress fashion through the full thickness of the eyelid tissue in a similar manner as that used for the correction of entropion. The eyelid crease thus created tends to be somewhat temporary, and the exposed suture on the conjunctival side may cause some corneal irritation. In Mutou's technique, doubly armed 6-0 buried silk suture is used (30).

My own technique is as follows: The proposed eyelid crease is first outlined with the marking pen. A small amount of local anesthetics is given just beneath the skin along the entire length of the proposed crease. The eyelid is then everted. A small amount of anesthetic is administered subconjunctivally along the entire superior tarsal border. A 5-0 chromic suture is first anchored in the skin at the medial end of the eyelid crease. The needle is then passed through the full thickness of the eyelid tissue and exits on the conjunctival side. From the conjunctival side, the needle is picked up and reentered the eyelid tissue through the same conjunctival exit wound. Moving temporally, this needle is placed just under the skin and comes out 3–4 mm away from the first exit wound. The needle is picked up again and reentered through the next exit wound. The process is repeated until the needle comes out of the temporal end of the skin marking. The suture is pulled tight and anchored in the skin temporally. The suture is left in place until it falls out. [Sutures with straight needle may be used, but it is more difficult to control the depth of penetration and the curvature of the crease (Fig. 57.5).]

This technique has several advantages over the other suture techniques: (*a*) There is no corneal irritation since there is no exposed suture on the conjunctival side. (*b*) The entire length of the eyelid crease is sutured, therefore, one can better control the curvature and the length of the crease. (*c*) There are eight to 10 sutures placed in the eyelid tissue, which provide stronger adhesions. The eyelid crease remains distinct for many years, and to date, we have not had to repeat the operation for anyone.

Postoperative Care

Suture techniques are so simple to perform that most of our patients have them performed in the office. The patient goes home with instructions to apply Maxitrol ointment and cold compresses. The first postoperative visit is on the seventh day. The vision is recorded and the cornea is carefully examined under the slitlamp. The creases and the sutures are inspected.

Complications

A temporary eyelid crease that needs reoperation is probably the most frequent complication with the suture technique (8, 16, 30, 42). Although not reported in the literature, we have heard of complications such as eyelid infection, suture or foreign body granuloma formation, and unsightly scars. A suture technique that also entails a skin incision designed by Mutou and Mutou (30) has cyst formation as the most common complication. In addition, loss of the eyelid crease, asymmetry, neurosis syndrome, and eyelid infection are also reported.

INCISIONAL TECHNIQUES

Although many techniques have been described, in principle they all resemble that of a blepharoplasty procedure (6–18, 33, 43–47). Depending on the individual patient, the proposed eyelid crease may be high or low in its position and various amounts of skin, muscle, subcutaneous or orbital fat may be removed. A new contour is thus sculptured.

If only a small amount of "redundant" skin is present and no large amount of soft tissue resection is planned, the pinch technique is recommended. Otherwise, the drape technique is recommended. (If there are associated conditions to be corrected surgically such as epiblepharon or epicanthal fold, see discussion under the appropriate heading.)

Pinch Technique

The proposed eyelid crease is first marked with a marking pen. Repeated measurements are carried out to ensure exactness and symmetry in the two eyelids. The marked eyelid crease is used as the inferior border of the area to be excised. The superior border is determined by the pinch technique. With one blade at the eyelid crease, the skin is grasped with a smooth forceps. The amount of skin that can be grasped when the lashes first evert is the amount that can be excised safely. Medially, the markings should be no closer than 3 mm from the eyelid margin. The angle at the junction of the inferior and superior incision should

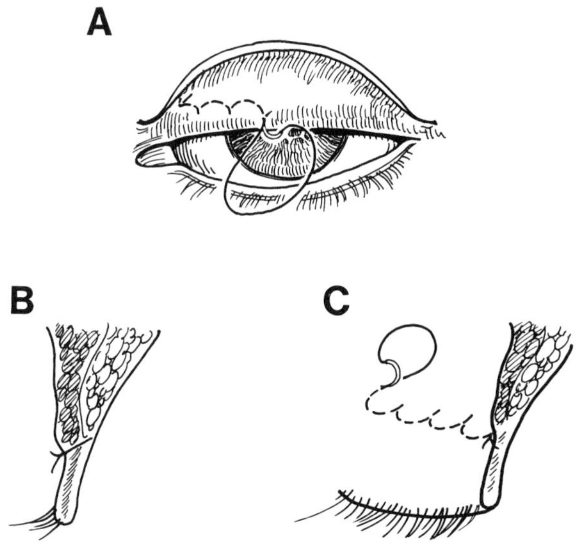

Figure 57.5. Suture technique to create upper eyelid crease (see text for details). *A*, Chromic suture (5-0) is used. Eyelid is anesthetized and everted. Suture is anchored on skin side first and then run continuously within the eyelid tissue by reinserting the needle through the previous exit wound. *B*, Side views. *C*, Side views.

be no more than 30° to avoid dog ear and extending the incision. Laterally, the lower incision should curve slightly superiorly at the lateral canthus. It should be at least 5 mm above the horizontal midline and form an angle of 30° or less when it joins with the superior incision. Both upper eyelids should be marked at the same time to ensure symmetry. After injection of local anesthetics, the patient's face is gently prepared and draped.

The incisions are carried out and the skin undermined and excised. A small strip of the underlying orbicularis muscle is also removed. If submuscular fat pad is encountered, it is removed also. Unless brow fixation is intended, no extensive dissection superiorly should be performed (48). If a small amount of orbital fat is also to be removed, an incision is made into the orbital septum and the orbital fat is gently prolapsed. This is grasped with a small mosquito clamp. The fat is excised and the pedicle cauterized lightly. The fat pedicle is allowed to retract into the orbit. The surgeon inspects the area to be certain that there is no further bleeding. If there is no medical contraindication, the operated area is irrigated with a few drops of Neosporin solution and Triamcinolone suspension.

The creation of the upper eyelid crease is achieved in the following manner: The levator aponeurosis is first identified. A 6-0 silk suture is placed along the midpupillary line through the lower skin edge, taking a bite through the muscular layer. Next, a small horizontal bite into the aponeurosis at the superior border of the tarsal plate is taken. The same needle is brought out through the muscle and then the skin layer in the upper skin edge. Two additional sutures are placed in a similar manner on either side of the first suture about 5 mm away. The sutures are tied tight and cut long. These are the "crease sutures" to be left in place for 10–14 days. The remaining skin wound can be approximated with 6-0 silk or nylon suture in a running or interrupted fashion. Usually sutures of a different material or color are used to aid later in the identification of the crease sutures.

Maxitrol ointment is placed over the incision and in the eyes. The eyes are left unpatched. Immediate cold compresses are applied in the recovery room to both eyes.

Drape Technique

When a deep superior sulcus is desired and a large amount of soft tissue removal is planned, the drape technique is recommended. The proposed new upper eyelid crease is first marked. The incision is begun after anesthetics have been administered. The skin is widely undermined up to the superior orbital rim. If brow fixation is planned, this can be accomplished by using a 4-0 Mersilene suture to anchor the subcutaneous tissue of the eyebrow to the periosteum at the desired level. A strip of the underlying orbicularis muscle superior to the eyelid crease incision is then carefully removed. In Orientals there is often a submuscular fat pad. This fat pad may very well be an extension of the brow fat pad (48, 49). Resection of this fat pad alone is not enough to give an Oriental person a deep superior sulcus; some orbital fat needs to be removed as well. The orbital septum is then incised, and the orbital fat pad gently prolapsed. The fat is grasped with a small clamp and excised, and its pedicle is cauterized lightly. Before the surgeon proceeds with the skin closure, the fat pedicle is allowed to retract into the orbit and the area is inspected to be certain of no further bleeding. In general, the central fat pad is found along with a smaller medial fat pad. The lateral fat pad is the smallest of all, which sometimes cannot be found in an Oriental person (7, 15, 16, 45). When excising tissue laterally, the surgeon should take care to avoid damage to the lacrimal gland.

It is usual practice to put aside the excised skin and fat pad from one eyelid to compare with that excised from the fellow eyelid. After irrigating the surgical field with Neosporin and Kenalog solution, the skin flap is gently draped over the lower skin edge. Because of the removal of large amounts of subcutaneous tissue, a new contour is carved out. In order to cover this new contour without tension in the skin and prevent overcorrection, one should perform very little or no skin resection. When closing the wound, the surgeon should not suture the orbital septum and orbicular muscle. The creation of the eyelid crease and closure proceed as previously described. At the conclusion of the operation, a small amount of Maxitrol ointment is applied in both eyes and over the incision. Immediate cold compresses are started in the recovery room. No eye patches are used.

Postoperative Care

Most of our incisional techniques are done on a one-day surgery basis. When the patient is ready to be discharged home by the anesthesiologist, we check the patient's vision and inspect the wound in the recovery room. The patient is instructed to apply cold compresses over the wound for the next 48 hours continuously. Patients and relatives are instructed to look out for possible signs of an orbital hemorrhage. If such signs or symptoms are present, they are to alert the physician immediately, and the physician acts accordingly (50).

The first postoperative visit is usually on the fifth day. Visual acuity is recorded, the cornea examined with slit-lamp, and the wound is inspected. Symmetry, eyelid closure, and the direction of the lashes are assessed. The nonabsorbable skin sutures are all removed at this time. The eyelid crease sutures are left in place for an additional 7–10 days.

Complications

For the more radical, incisional techniques, the best management of complications is their prevention by careful planning, conservative management, atraumatic surgical techniques, and meticulous closure. As in cosmetic blepharoplastic procedures, complications may include blindness, ectropion, ptosis, extraocular muscle palsy, epiphora, unacceptable scars, asymmetry, overcorrection or undercorrection, dry eyes, and loss of lashes (50).

Edema or ecchymosis is a commonly seen postoperative sequela, especially when resection of large amounts of soft tissue is performed. This can be minimized by atraumatic surgical technique, good hemostasis throughout the procedure, and meticulous wound closure. Making certain that the patient is off aspirin and Coumadin also prevents excessive bleeding intraoperatively and prolonged ecchymosis postoperatively. Subconjunctival hemorrhage is occasionally seen with extensive removal of the orbital fat. Wound gaping may be due to excessive swelling, undue tension in the wound, or faulty suture technique. It can be amended by applying a sterile strip for healing with secondary intention.

Asymmetry may be prevented by careful planning. Exposure keratitis or ectropion may be prevented by conservative skin and soft tissue resection. Abnormal folds may be a result of overambitious undermining of the skin and/or removal of the subcutaneous tissue. This may be also caused by overzealous application of cautery and faulty suture technique.

Shallow eyelid crease or temporary crease has been reported. Understandably, a hematoma or edema immediately postoperatively may disinsert some or all of the sutures that are used to create the adhesion between the skin and the deeper tissues. Additionally, the sutures may not be tied tight enough or not left in long enough to form a good adhesion. Sayoc also has another explanation for this (8, 9). He feels that the lower skin flap may be anchored to the orbital septum, especially when the lid incision is made higher than 10 mm from the lid margin. With the passage of time, the supraorbital fat pushes the septum forward and downward and eventually removes all the adhesions that haved been formed between the skin and the deeper tissue, hence a shallow crease. This should not happen if the surgeon knows eyelid anatomy.

EPICANTHAL FOLD

SURGICAL TECHNIQUES

In 1932, Blair stated that the crux of the problem lies in the rearrangement of the tissue and not in the resection of the defect itself (51). Based on his principle, many techniques have been developed for the correction of epicanthal folds (31, 32, 51–59). For correction of nontraumatic ethnic epicanthal fold, I have most often used the Y-V operation (31, 32, 51). This is simple, of sound design, and very effective. However, it occasionally results in a cosmetically undesirable horizontal scar that extends over the nasal skin.

The new medial canthal commissure is first determined and marked on the skin. This usually is 5–7 mm medial to the old commissure. Starting from this point, the surgeon draws a horizontal line measuring about 5 mm medially to the bridge of the nose. Starting again from this new commissure, one draws two arms approximately 10 mm long running parallel to the lid margin, which results in a "Y" lying horizontally on the canthus. Following the incisions, the skin is widely undermined to allow movement of the canthal angle toward the nose. The medial canthal tendon is exposed. A doubly armed 4-0 nonabsorbable (Mersilene, Supramid) suture is used to tuck the tendon. One needle is placed through the bony insertion of the tendon, and the other, near the old canthal angle.

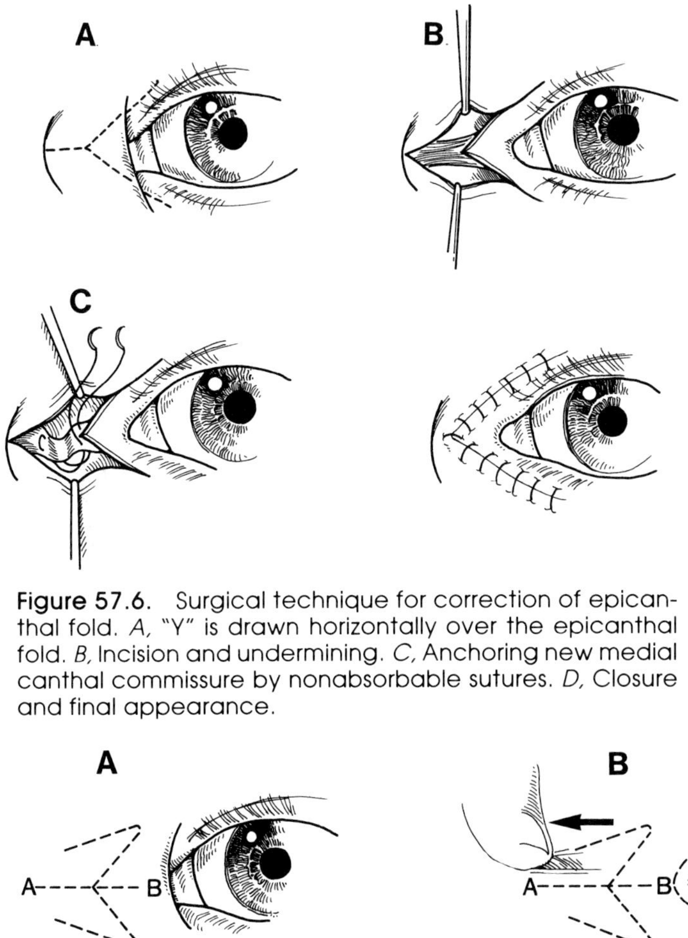

Figure 57.6. Surgical technique for correction of epicanthal fold. *A,* "Y" is drawn horizontally over the epicanthal fold. *B,* Incision and undermining. *C,* Anchoring new medial canthal commissure by nonabsorbable sutures. *D,* Closure and final appearance.

If excessive subcutaneous tissue is present, this should be removed to allow room for the fixation of the new medial canthus. Additional buried subcutaneous 6-0 Dexon sutures will help reduce tension on the tissue. The skin is approximated with 6-0 silk or nylon sutures (6-0 chromic sutures in small children) (Fig. 57.6).

The Mustardé four-flap technique for correction of the epicanthal fold gives excellent results (55). It is especially effective when the epicanthal fold is prominent or is associated with blepharophimosis syndrome. The resultant scar is in a vertical line; it passes through the inner canthus and does not lie in the nasal skin.

The location of the proposed new medial canthal commissure is based on the rule that the intercanthal distance is one-half the interpupillary distance (Fig. 57.7). This site is marked (point A) without any pull upon the nasal skin. A second point (point B) is placed at the old canthus, and the two points are now joined. This line is measured, giving the basis for the other lines, which are all drawn 2 mm shorter. Beginning at the midpoint of this line with an angle of 60° toward the eye, the surgeon draws two straight lines 2 mm shorter than line AB. At the end of each of these two lines, an additional line is drawn at a 45° angle back toward the nose. Next, from the second point (point B), two lines are drawn parallel to the upper and lower eyelid margins at 2 mm from the margins. These lines are drawn with the old canthal angle being pulled medially by keeping tension on the nasal skin.

Following the incisions, all flaps are carefully and thoroughly undermined. Usually, some subcutaneous tissue needs to be removed in order to make room for the fixation of the new medial commissure. Mersilene or Supramid suture (size 4-0) is used to anchor the medial commissure at the desired point (point A). The four flaps are now transposed and sutured in place. In adults, 6-0 nylon or silk is preferred; for small children, 6-0 chromic is used. Some trimming of the flaps may be necessary to achieve a good fit without bunching up.

At the conclusion of the surgery, a small amount of Maxitrol ointment is given in both eyes, as well as over the incision. A small piece of Telfa is first placed over the wound. A dental roll and some narrow elastoplast bandage complete the wound dressing. Moderate pressure is exerted against the new medial canthal angle. Care is taken so that nothing is rubbing against the globe, and the patient is

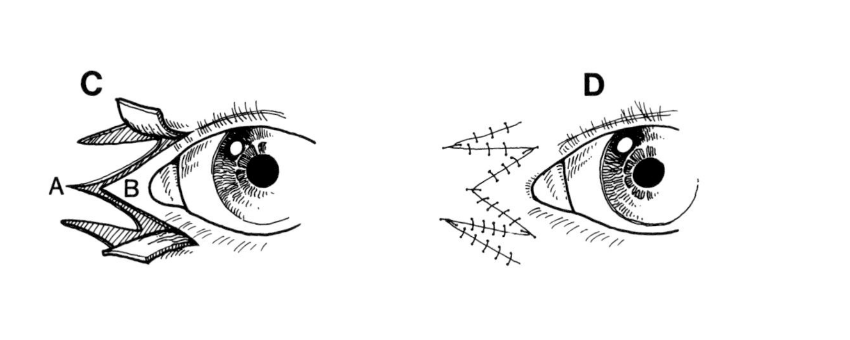

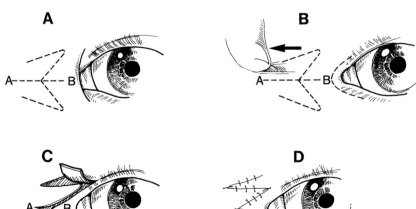

Figure 57.7. Mustardé four-flap technique (see text for details). *A,* Point A and B are determined and the lines drawn. *B,* Pulling of the skin medially and drawing of the remaining lines near the eyelid margin. *C,* Incisions and undermining. *D,* Closure and final appearance.

able to use both eyes immediately postoperatively. This dressing is to be kept in place undisturbed for 5 days.

POSTOPERATIVE CARE

For the majority of our patients, the surgery is performed on an outpatient basis requiring no hospital stay. The occasional inpatient is usually discharged the next morning.

The first visit is generally on the fifth to the seventh postoperative day. Visual acuity is recorded, and the dressing is removed. The symmetry and the viability of the skin flaps are carefully assessed. Slitlamp examination of the cornea to check for possible staining is also performed. All nonabsorbable skin sutures are removed on the same day.

COMPLICATIONS

Careful planning, atraumatic surgical technique, and meticulous closure help prevent complications. No serious complications have been reported in the literature, nor have I seen any so far. The most commonly seen complication is a hypertrophied scar in the medial canthus. This usually reaches its peak in the first 4–6 postoperative weeks (31, 32, 45, 59). Application of warm compresses or topical steroid preparation or cocoa butter with gentle massage in this area help to generally fade away scarring without any sequelae. I have never seen any keloid formation. Minor asymmetry may be due to poor design or loosening up of the anchoring sutures. Small wound gaping can be amended by applying a sterile strip. No infection or necrosis of the flap has ever been seen.

EPIBLEPHARON

SURGICAL TECHNIQUES

When epiblepharon is the single condition to be corrected surgically, simple excision of the skin in the form of a crescent or ellipse usually will be sufficient (Fig. 57.8). Frequently, a strip of orbicularis muscle is removed at the same time to prevent overriding of the muscle or bunching up of the wound. To avoid ectropion, one should take care not to remove excessive skin. This is accomplished by carefully applying the pinch technique. This is done by using a forcep to grasp the skin, placing one blade of the forcep at the proposed incision site. The location of the other blade at the point when the lashes just begin to evert is the limit of the skin that can be excised safely. This location is also marked, resulting in a crescent-shaped or elliptical-shaped area of skin to be excised. Conservatism in skin and muscle resection prevents complications.

Still simpler but just as effective is the suture technique for the correction of lower eyelid epiblepharon described by Quickert and associates (60). In their technique, several doubly armed 4-0 chromic sutures are placed at the inferior tarsal border from the conjunctiva out through the skin. The sutures are tied tightly in a horizontal plane and left in place to create adhesion. However, I have found that in more severe cases of epiblepharon, it is necessary to place the suture in the same manner as for the correction of entropion; that is, the exit site on the skin is closer to the lid margin than the entrance site on the conjunctival side.

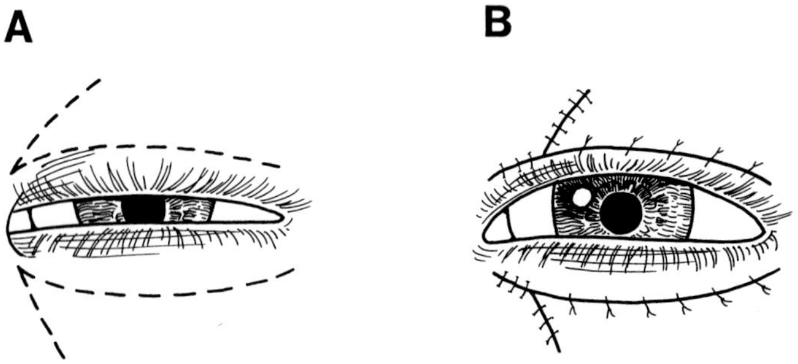

Figure 57.9. *A,* Markings on both upper and lower eyelids for Johnson's V-Y technique. *B,* Closure and final appearance.

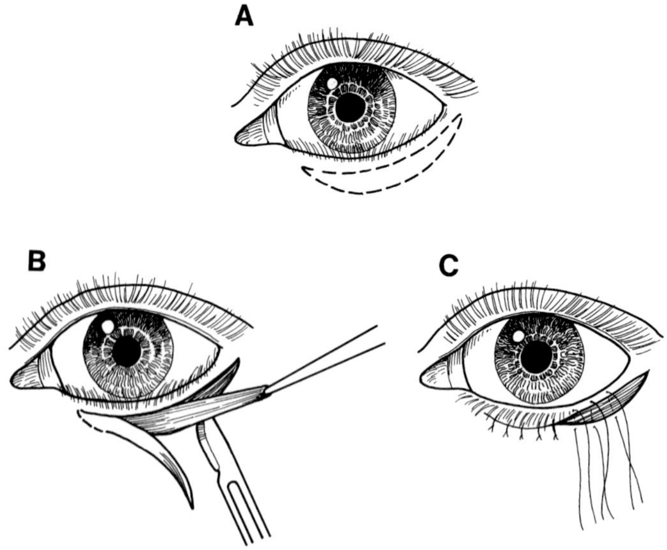

Figure 57.8. *A,* Excess amount determined by pinch technique and marked. *B,* Excision of skin and muscle. *C,* Closure.

When epiblepharon is associated with an epicanthal fold and/or absence of an upper eyelid crease, the correction of each of these conditions may be approached separately (see the appropriate sections in this chapter). However, by using the V-Y technique described by Johnson, the correction of all these three conditions may be achieved simultaneously (31, 32) (Fig. 57.9). The technique is as follows: When the creation of an eyelid crease in the upper eyelid is desired, the proposed eyelid crease is first marked. The medial end of this marking is at the apex of the medial epicanthal fold. From this apex, the shorter arm of a "V" is drawn. Depending on the extent of the epicanthal fold, it measures 10–15 mm running in a curvilinear fashion superomedially to the eyelid crease. A similar design is used in the lower eyelid. However, rather than creating a lower eyelid crease, ones uses a subciliary incision, with the shorter arm of the "V" inferomedial to it. This subciliary incision can best hide the lower eyelid scar. The pinch technique is used to estimate the amount of excess skin to be removed.

The incisions are made and the skin undermined and resected. If the surgeon prefers, rather than using the pinch technique, he or she can estimate and resect the excess skin by using the drape technique. In the upper eyelid, the skin is undermined superiorly. Draping this flap over the inferior cut edge without tension, the surgeon can estimate the amount of skin that can be safely excised. In the lower eyelid, the inferior flap is draped over the superior cut edge. Frequently, a strip of orbicularis is also excised. The skin closure is begun at the temporal end of the incision with each suture placed through the tarsus. The correction of the epicanthal fold is achieved by the relaxation of the skin at the medial canthus. To maximize the effect, the surgeon advances each suture through the upper skin edge slightly and progressively toward the nose. Hence, the "V" at the medial canthus is converted to a "Y."

In adults, nonabsorbable sutures such as 6-0 silk or nylon are used to close the skin wound. In small children, absorbable sutures such as 6-0 chromic are used. At the conclusion of the procedure, a small amount of Maxitrol ointment is applied in the eye and over the incision. Cold compresses to both eyes are applied immediately while the patient is in the recovery room.

POSTOPERATIVE CARE

Generally, all patients are discharged on the same day of the surgery. Cold compresses are applied for the initial 48 hours continuously. The first postoperative visit is on the fifth to seventh day. Vision is checked and recorded. The cornea is examined with a slit lamp, and the wound is inspected. The lid margin and the direction of the lashes are carefully inspected. The patient, if able to cooperate, is asked to look up and down to better assess the surgical result. All nonabsorbable skin sutures are removed at this time.

COMPLICATIONS

To date, I have not seen any complications, nor are there any serious complications reported in the literature. The possible complications may include overcorrection, undercorrection, residual epicanthal fold, and minor asymmetry. Other minor complications such as ecchymosis, wound dehiscence, or corneal irritation are possible. These can be prevented and treated accordingly.

REFERENCES

1. Adachi B: Mikroshopische untersuchunger uber die augenlider der affen und des Menschen im Kyoto-Igakkai (1906). *Mitt Med Fak Toyko* 7: 47, 1908.
2. Fortuyn: *Q Rev Biol* 7: 298, 1931.
3. Skeller: *Anthropological and Ophthalmological Studies of Angmagssalik Eskimos.* Copenhagen, 1954.
4. Aichel O: Ergebnisse einer forschungreise nach Chile-Bolivien. *Beit Anthropol Sudamer Anthropol Inst Univ Kiel* 123: 31, 123, 1933.
5. Yoshii A: A morphological and genetic study of the upper eyelids. *Jpn J Anthropol* 3: 108, 1958.
6. von Siebold: *Nippon (Leyden)* 2: 3, 1832.
7. Fernandez LR: Double eyelid operation in the Oriental in Hawaii. *Plast Reconstr Surg* 25: 257–264, 1960.
8. Sayoc BT: Anatomic consideration in the plastic construction of a palpebral fold in the full upper eyelid. *Am J Ophthalmol* 63: 155–158, 1967.
9. Sayoc BT: Surgery of the Oriental eyelid. *Clin Plast Surg* 1: 157–171, 1974.
10. Sayoc BT: Surgical correction of the Oriental eyelid. *Plast Reconstr Surg* 2: 947–956, 1977.
11. Furukawa M: A blepharoplasty technique for refinement of Oriental eyelid with lateral fold. *Aesthet Plast Surg* 3: 123–127, 1979.
12. Millard DR: Oriental peregrinations. *Plast Reconstr Surg* 16: 319–336, 1955.
13. Uchida J: A surgical procedure for blepharoptosis vera and for pseudoblepharoptosis Orientals. *Br J Plast Surg* 15: 271–276, 1962.
14. Rubenzik R: Surgical revision of the Oriental lid. *Ann Ophthal* 11: 1189–1192, 1977.
15. Hin LC: Oriental blepharoplasty—a critical review of technique and potential hazards. *Ann Plast Surg* 7: 362–372, 1981.
16. Boo-Chai K: Plastic construction of the superior palpebral fold. *Plast Reconstr Surg* 31: 74–78, 1963.
17. Hiraga Y: The double eyelid operation and augmentation rhinoplasty in the Oriental patient. *Clin Plast Surg* 7: 553–567, 1980.
18. Ohmori S: Transformation of Oriental eye into the Western eye. In Goldwyn RM (ed): *Unfavorable Result in Plastic Surgery.* Boston, Little, Brown, & Co, 1972.
19. de Castro O, Colares JH, Mortari S: Blepharoplasty to form the orbitopalpebral sulcus and nasal bone graft in Oriental subjects (Occidentalization). *Aesthet Plast Surg* 4: 287–294, 1980.
20. Hisatomi C: Thoughts on ophthalmic plastic surgery. *Jpn J Clin Ophthalmol* 30: 481–489, 1976.
21. Hisatomi C, Fujino T: Anatomical considerations concerning blepharoplasty in the Oriental patient. *Adv Ophthal Plast Reconst Surg* 2: 151–165, 1983.
22. Doxanas MT, Anderson RL: Oriental eyelids—an anatomic study. *Arch Ophthal* 102: 1232–1235, 1984.
23. Duke-Elder S: *System of Ophthalmology.* St. Louis, CV Mosby, 1961, vol 2, p 499, 841, 849, 857.
24. Iliff CE, Iliff WJ, Iliff NT: *Oculoplastic Surgery.* Philadelphia, WB Saunders, 1979, p 20.
25. Wolff E: *Anatomy of the Eye and Orbit,* ed 7. Philadelphia, WB Saunders, 1961, p 183–185.
26. Beard C: *Ptosis,* ed 3. St. Louis, CV Mosby, 1981, p 12.
27. Whitnall SE: The structure of the eyelids. *Anat Hum Orbit* 2: 124, 1932.
28. Liu D, Hsu DM: A study of eyelid dimensions. Presented at the First Taiwan Regional Congress of Ophthalmology, November, 1984.
29. Boo-Chai K: Surgery for Oriental eyelids: some refinements in technique. *Aesthet Plast Surg* 1: 57–60, 1976.
30. Mutou Y, Mutou H: Intradermal double eyelid operation and its follow-up results. *Br J Plast Surg* 25: 258–291, 1972.
31. Johnson CC: Epicanthus and epiblepharon. *Arch Ophthalmol* 96: 1030–1033, 1978.
32. Johnson CC: Epicanthus. *Am J Ophthalmol* 66: 939–946, 1968.
33. Weingarten CZ: Blepharoplasty in the Oriental eye. *Tr Am Acad Ophthalmol Otolaryngol* 82: 442–446, 1976.
34. Liu D, Hsu WM: Oriental eyelids. *Ophthal Plast Reconstr Surg* 2(2): 59–64, 1986.
35. Kestenbaum A: *Applied Anatomy of the Eye,* New York and London, Grune and Stratton, 1963, p 250.
36. Kikkawa Y: Measurements of corneal diameter and size of palpebral aperture. *J Jpn Contact Lens Soc* 21: 76–79.
37. von Ammon FA: Epicanthus und das epiblepharon. *Behr Hildebr J Kinder* 34: 313–393, 1860.
38. Schon: Hb path anat d auges. Hamburg, 60: 1828.
39. Lemke BN, Stasior OG: Epiblepharon—an important and often missed diagnosis. *Clin Pediatr* 20: 661–662, 1981.
40. Wen: *Chin Med J* 43: 1216, 1934.
41. Karlin DB: Congenital entropion, epiblepharon, and antimongoloid obliquity of the palpebral fissure. *Am J Ophthalmol* 50: 487, 1960.
42. Pang HG: Surgical formation of upper lid fold. *Arch Ophthalmol* 63: 783–784, 1961.
43. McCurdy JA: Westernization of the Oriental eyelid. *Otolaryngol Head Neck Surg* 90: 142–145, 1982.
44. Harahap M: Blepharoplasty for Orientals. *J Dermatol Surg Oncol* 7: 334–339, 1981.
45. Boo-Chai K: The Mongolian fold (plica mongolia). *Singapore Med J* 3: 132–136, 1962.
46. Wiratmadja RM: Notes on aesthetic surgery in the Indonesian. *Clin Plast Surg* 1: 173–178, 1974.
47. Horibe K, Horibe EK, Nery GBL, Suzuki T, Castro H: Construcción del surco órbito palpebral superior en ojos Orientales. *Cirug Plast Ibero-Latinoam* 5: 387–393, 1979.
48. Lemke BN, Stasior OG: The anatomy of eyebrow ptosis. *Arch Ophthalmol* 100: 981–986, 1982.

49. Zide BM: Anatomy of the eyelid. *Clin Plast Surg* 8: 623–634, 1981.
50. Liu D, Stasior OG: Cosmetic blepharoplasty. *Persp Ophthalmol* 5: 203–209, 1981.
51. Blair VP, Brown JB, Hamm WG: Surgery of the inner canthus and related structures. *Am J Ophthalmol* 15: 498, 1932.
52. Hughes WL: Surgical treatment of congenital phimosis: the Y-V operation. *Arch Ophthalmol* 54: 586, 1955.
53. Taylor WOG, Cameron JH: Epicanthus and the intercanthal distance. *Trans Ophthal Soc (UK)* 83: 371, 1963.
54. Spaeth EB: Further consideration of the surgical correction of blepharophimosis and epicanthus. *Am J Ophthalmol* 41: 61, 1956.
55. Mustarde JC: The treatment of ptosis and epicanthal folds. *Br J Plast Surg* 12: 252, 1960.
56. del Camp AF: Surgical treatment of the epicanthal fold. *Plast Reconstruct Surg* 73: 566–571, 1984.
57. Field LM: Repair of a cicatricial epicanthal fold by a double z plasty (Spaeth). *J Dermatol Surg Oncol* 8: 215–216, 1982.
58. McCord CD: The correction of telecanthus and epicanthal folds. *Ophthal Surg* 11: 446–454, 1980.
59. Boo-Chai K: Some aspects of plastic (cosmetic) surgery in Orientals. *Br J Plast Surg* 22: 60–69, 1969.
60. Quickert MH, Wilkes DI, Dryden RM: Nonincisional correction of epiblepharon and congenital entropion. *Arch Ophthalmol* 101: 778–781, 1983.

CHAPTER 58

Lateral Canthal Considerations in Cosmetic Surgery

PHILIP L. CUSTER, M.D.
RICHARD R. TENZEL, M.D.

Cosmetic eyelid surgery is generally designed to provide the patient with an appearance of relative youth. The procedures employed by cosmetic surgeons usually incorporate the excision of prolapsed orbital fat and excessive eyelid skin. The creation of symmetrical and naturally contoured palpebral fissures is an additional consideration in these cases. The integrity, position, and shape of the lateral canthus and its associated structures contribute to the formation of the eyelid fissure. Abnormalities of the lateral canthus may compromise the cosmetic and functional results in eyelid surgery.

The lateral canthal angle is formed by the relatively acute juncture of the upper and lower eyelids near the lateral orbital rim. The eyelid margins are normally well approximated, with no overlap in the anteroposterior dimension. Firm lateral attachments of the eyelids are provided by the lateral canthal tendons, which extend from the pretarsal orbicularis muscles to the periosteum of the lateral orbital tubercle. The medial and lateral canthal tendons are indirectly connected to the tarsus. The complex formed by these structures creates a "tendon tarsal" sling that suspends the lower eyelid from the orbital rim.

POSITION OF THE CANTHAL ANGLE

The lateral canthus is normally at the same level or up to 2 mm higher than the medial canthus (1). Antimongoloid or mongoloid slants of the lid fissure occur if the lateral canthus is located unusually high or low. Vertical malposition of the canthus can either be congenital or acquired in nature. Displaced lateral orbital rim fractures may draw the canthal tendons inferiorly. Extreme hypotropia of the lateral canthus can occasionally contribute to the etiology of blepharoptosis, secondary to a tethering effect on the eyelid. The vertical position of the lateral canthus can be surgically adjusted using the Z-plasty technique (2).

TECHNIQUE OF LATERAL CANTHAL Z-PLASTY

The present and desired positions of the lateral canthal angle are marked on the skin. These two points are utilized in drawing the Z-plasty transposition flaps. Larger distances will require longer flaps. One flap will include the canthal angle and lateral portion of both eyelids. The second flap is based laterally and includes the desired new canthal position.

Infiltrative local anesthesia is administered and incisions are made through the skin and muscle layers with a razorblade knife. Blunt and sharp dissection is employed to elevate the myocutaneous flaps. Wet-field cautery is utilized for hemostasis. The lateral canthal tendon is usually easily isolated by palpating a band of tissue between the lids and the lateral orbital rim. The tendon is transected close to the periosteum. The eyelids should now be freely mobile. If this is not the case, the lateral attachments of the lower eyelid retractors may also have to be divided.

A permanent suture (5-0 nylon) is passed in a whipstitch fashion through the periosteum of the inner edge of

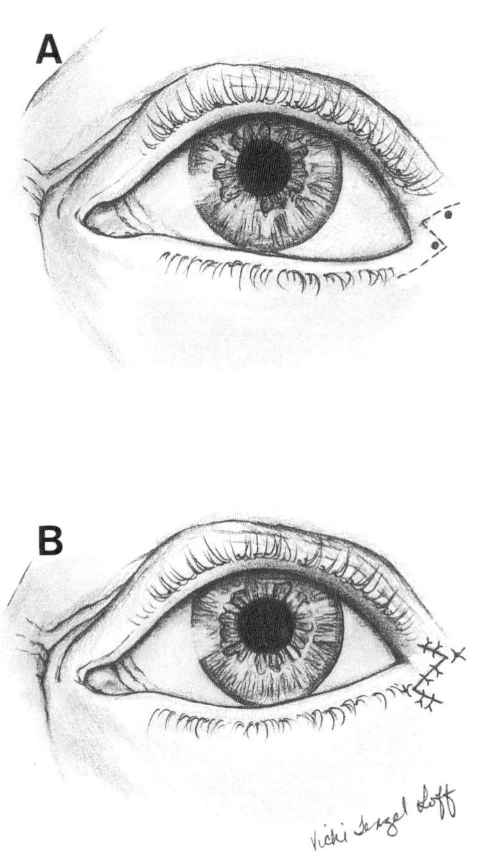

Figure 58.1. Z-Plasty for vertically changing position of lateral canthus. *A*, Z-plasty marked out on skin. The lower dot will interchange places with the upper dot on flap transposition. The two dots are placed first and the Z-plasty is drawn around the dots. *B*, elevation of lateral canthus after transposition of flaps.

the lateral orbital rim at the new canthal position. This suture is employed to reattach the canthal tendons at this location. Additional sutures may be required to reattach the lower eyelid retractors. The transposition flaps are closed in layers. Absorbable sutures (6-0 Vicryl) unite the muscle layer. The skin incisions are closed with interrupted sutures (7-0 silk). The ends of the flaps generally require subcuticular closure to prevent necrosis of the flap tips. The skin sutures are removed in approximately 5 days (Fig. 58.1).

LOWER EYELID LAXITY

The lateral canthal region is intimately involved in blepharoplasty surgery. It is in this area that the skin of the eyelids becomes thicker with increased subcutaneous tissue. The lateral portion of the blepharoplasty incision can frequently be hidden in one of the laugh lines, which run temporally past the lateral canthus. In the upper eyelid, it is imperative that at least 5 mm separate the lower edge of the blepharoplasty incision and the canthal angle. Placing the incision in this location will avoid interruption of lymphatic drainage of the eyelid and development of prolonged postoperative edema.

The examination of every lower eyelid blepharoplasty patient should include the preoperative evaluation for eyelid laxity. This condition frequently results from the detachment or dehiscence of the lateral canthal tendon. Failure to recognize and correct lower eyelid laxity will place the patient at high risk for developing a postblepharoplasty ectropion. Mild eyelid laxity is corrected by shortening the eyelid. The lateral canthus is the preferred site of lower eyelid resection, since this will permit the reattachment of the canthal tendon. Surgery isolated to the lateral portion of the eyelid will sacrifice less of the tarsus and maximize the support provided by this structure. Lid notching and trichiasis may occur with intramarginal eyelid resections and are avoided if the scar is confined to the lateral canthal region.

TECHNIQUE OF LOWER EYELID TIGHTENING AT THE LATERAL CANTHUS

Eyelid tightening during lower eyelid blepharoplasty is performed following the creation of the skin muscle flap and excision of excessive orbital fat. A small (1–2 mm) horizontal lateral canthotomy is created. It is usually possible to isolate the detached end of the lateral canthal tendon in the inferior portion of the canthotomy. The correct localization of this structure can be confirmed by grasping the tendon with a forceps and placing medial traction. If the canthal tendon has been isolated, a firm band of tissue can be palpated between the forceps and the orbital rim. A vertical incision dividing the eyelid margin is made at the point where the intact tendon is located. The degree of eyelid laxity is now determined by using two forceps to overlap the cut end of the tendon and the free eyelid margin. Moderate lateral traction is placed on the eyelid and the point of overlap is marked. A second vertical eyelid marginal incision is made at this location and the segment of eyelid is resected in a pentagonal block fashion. Wet-field cautery is used to achieve hemostasis.

The eyelid is reattached to the lateral canthal tendon with three interrupted sutures (6-0 Vicryl). These sutures pass through the upper, middle, and lower tarsus and corresponding points of the tendon. Failure to suture the lid to intact lateral canthal tendon may lead to an early recurrence of the eyelid laxity, lateral canthal deformity, or poor apposition between the eyelid and the globe. Localization of the canthal tendon is facilitated by recognizing that the tendon is usually located just temporal to the cut edge of the conjunctiva. The lower eyelid retractors and the pretarsal orbicularis muscle are reattached laterally with interrupted sutures. Careful placement of these sutures is required to prevent abnormal rotation of the eyelid margin and a resultant entropion or ectropion. Excess skin and orbicularis muscle can be excised. To prevent unsightly scarring, closure of these tissues in the lateral

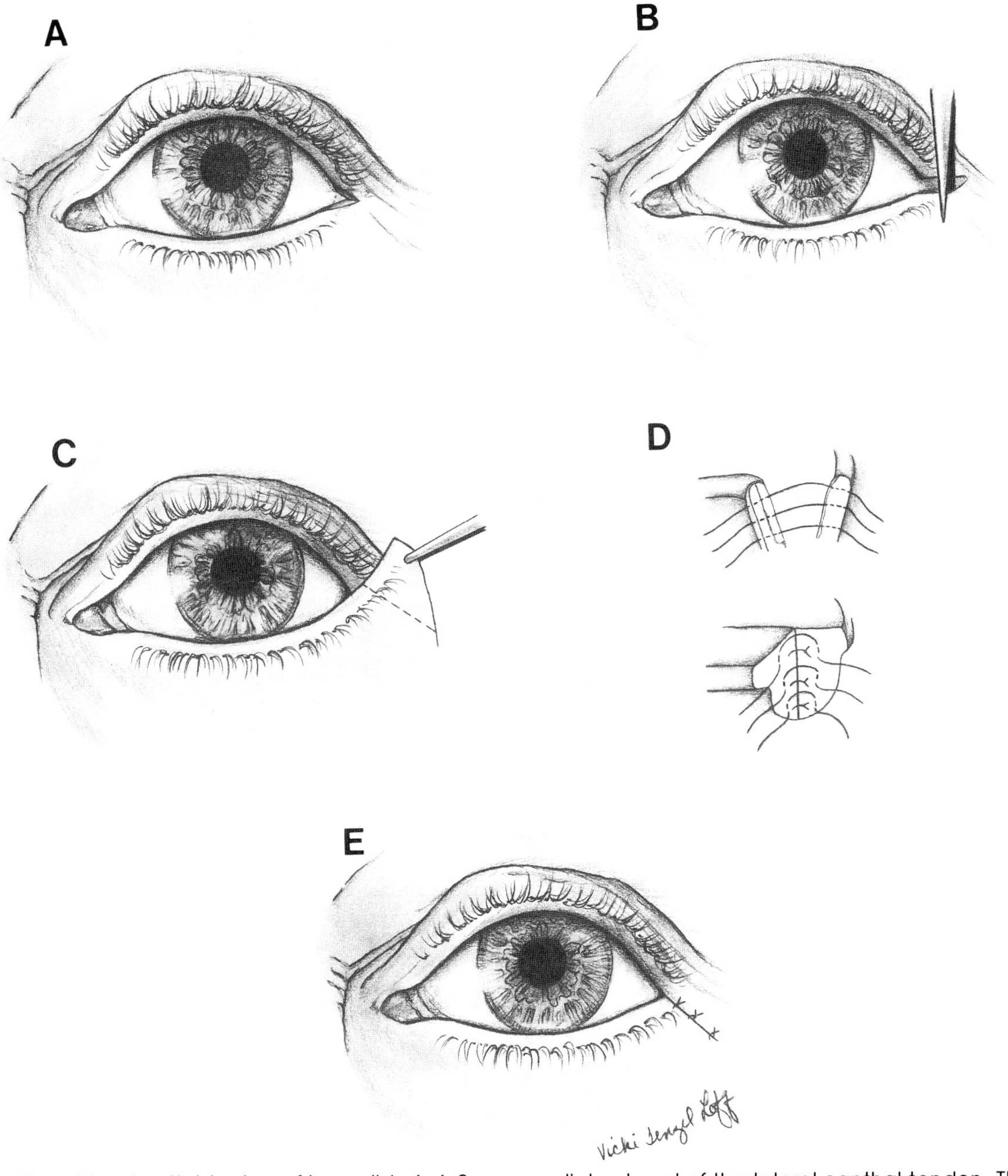

Figure 58.2. Tarsal tendon tightening of lower lid. *A*, A 2-mm canthotomy has been made at the lateral canthus. *B*, Cantholysis of inferior arm of the lower lid. *C*, Overlapping lid and dotted lines indicate the extent of horizontal lid shortening. *D*, Suturing. Three interrupted 7-0 Vicryl sutures are placed partial thickness in the tarsus and into the medial cut end of the lateral canthal tendon. The tendon is just anterior to the conjunctiva. The muscle layer is closed with interrupted 7-0 Vicryl sutures with knots buried deep in the wound. *E*, the skin is closed with interrupted wipe off sutures of 7-0 silk.

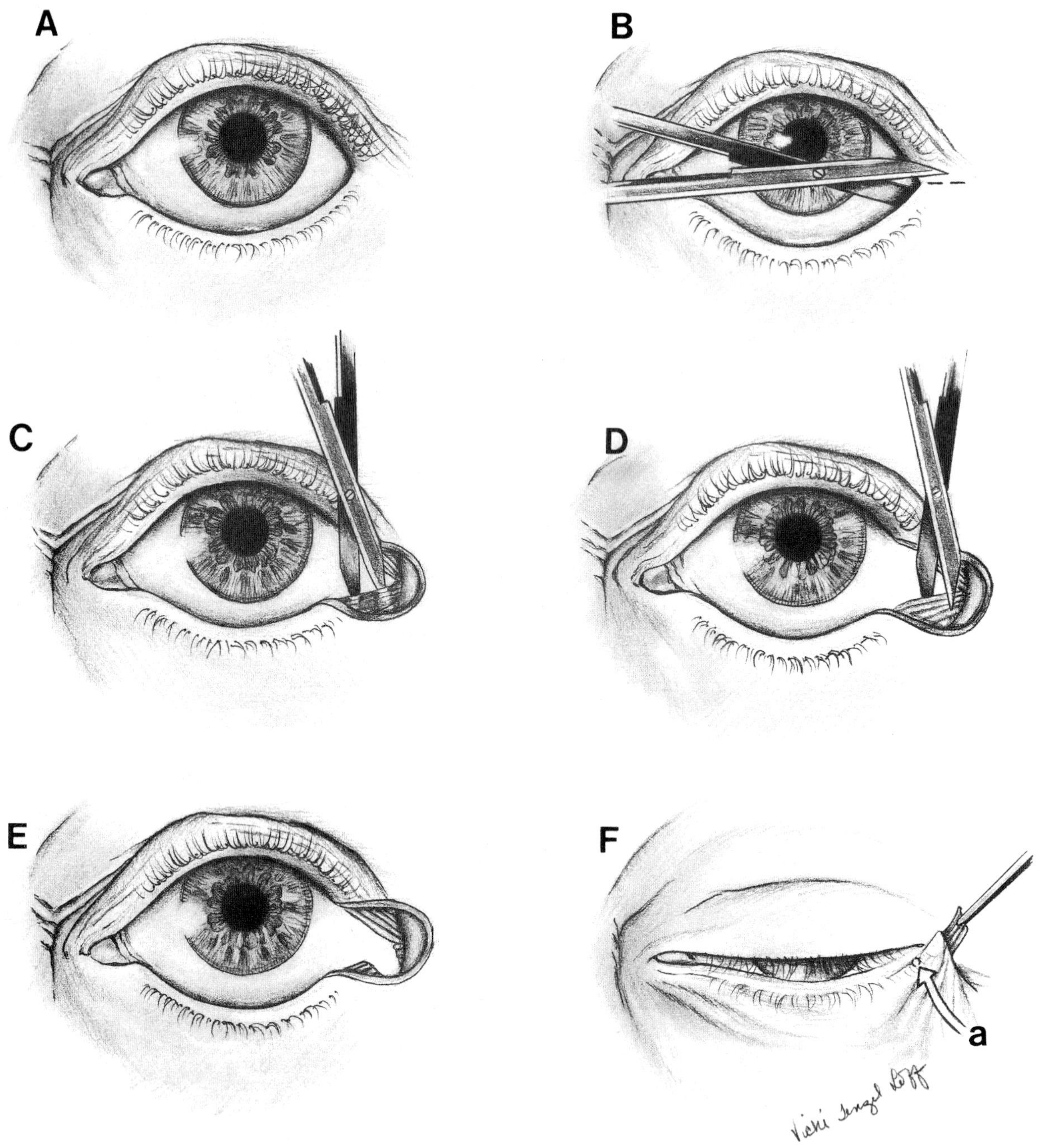

Figure 58.3. Lateral canthal sling. *A*, Lagophthalmos of lower lid and rounding of lateral canthus is shown. *B*, Canthotomy is made temporal. *C*, Skin and conjunctiva is freed off lower canthal tendon. *D* and *E*, Lower canthal tendon is cut at the orbital rim. *F*, Lower lid is pulled over upper lid to determine amount of elasticity involved. The lower lid is marked at point of crossing upper lid, when desired amount of tightness has been obtained (*a*). *G*, Conjunctiva is freed from canthotomy up to mark (*a*) made on lid. *H*, Skin is freed up to lash margin from canthotomy to same point (*a*) on lid. *I*, Lid margin and then lashes are excised to previously marked point (*a*). *J*, Skin is undermined from periosteum superior and temporal to upper canthal tendon. *K*, Upper canthal tendon is buttonholed in lid margin as close to original canthal angle as possible. A suture of nylon or prolene is placed at the end of the tarsal tendon strap for easier manipulation. *L*, Canthal tendon and tarsus is brought through upper canthal tendon buttonhole. *M*, Double-armed 5-0 dermalon on a d01 needle is placed as a whip stitch in the periosteum and brought through lower lid tarsus (preferrably) or canthal tendon. *N*, Suture is tied. Previously placed suture in lower canthal tendon is also inserted into periosteum and tied, giving reinforcement of closure. *O*, The lateral canthal angle is reconstructed with a full-thickness lid vertical mattress suture tied over a cotton pledget to facilitate removal. Skin is closed with interrupted vertical mattress sutures or deep, then running, skin sutures.

canthal region is accomplished either with a vertical mattress-style suture or separate closure of the skin and muscle layers. Skin sutures are removed in about 5 days. This method of eyelid shortening is also easily incorporated into the surgical correction of either entropion or mild ectropion (Fig. 58.2).

Postoperative eyelid fissure deformities in patients with blepharoplasty are usually related to positional abnormal-

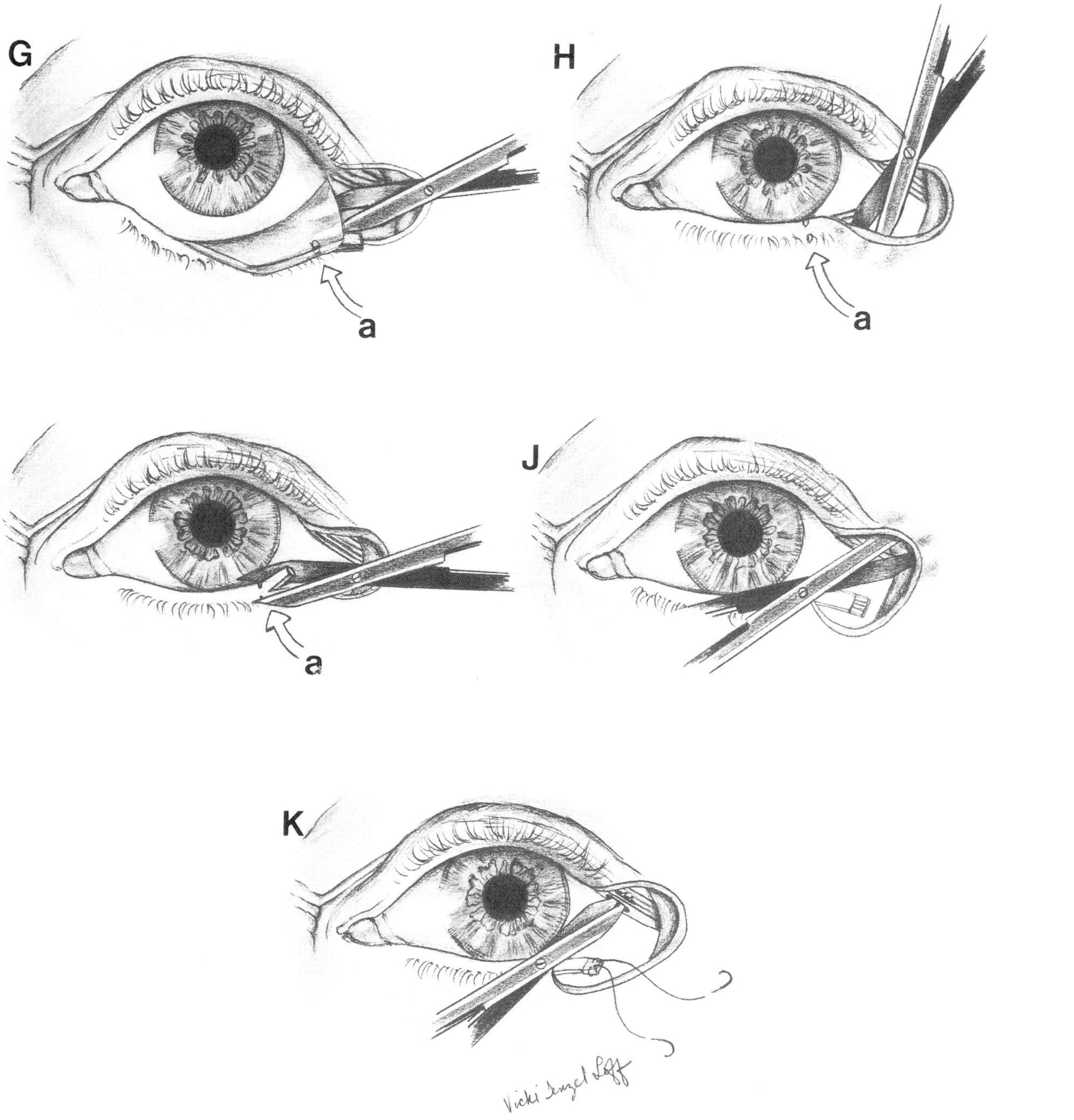

Figure 58.3. *G–K.*

ities of the lower eyelid. Failure to correct lower eyelid laxity may result in sagging of the eyelid margin or actual ectropion. Unrepaired lateral canthal tendon dehiscence frequently leads to a rounded deformity of the canthal angle. Excessive skin excision will tether the eyelid inferiorly and cause varying degrees of inferior scleral show, lagophthalmos, or ectropion.

Mild eyelid laxity or lateral canthal deformities are repaired with the above described method of eyelid shortening and tendon reattachment. Skin shortage coexisting with lid laxity can effectively be treated with a lateral canthal sling procedure (3, 4).

TECHNIQUE OF LATERAL CANTHAL SLING PROCEDURE

After infiltrative anesthesia is administered, a lateral canthotomy is performed, which divides the lateral canthal tendon horizontally down to the orbital rim (Fig. 58.3). The inferior arm of the tendon is transected close to the periosteum, freeing the eyelid from its deep lateral attachments. The lid is drawn temporally, and the point where the eyelid margin crosses the edge of the canthotomy of the upper eyelid is marked. A tendon tarsal strip is fashioned from this segment of excess eyelid by excising the lid margin and eyelashes to this point. A skin muscle flap

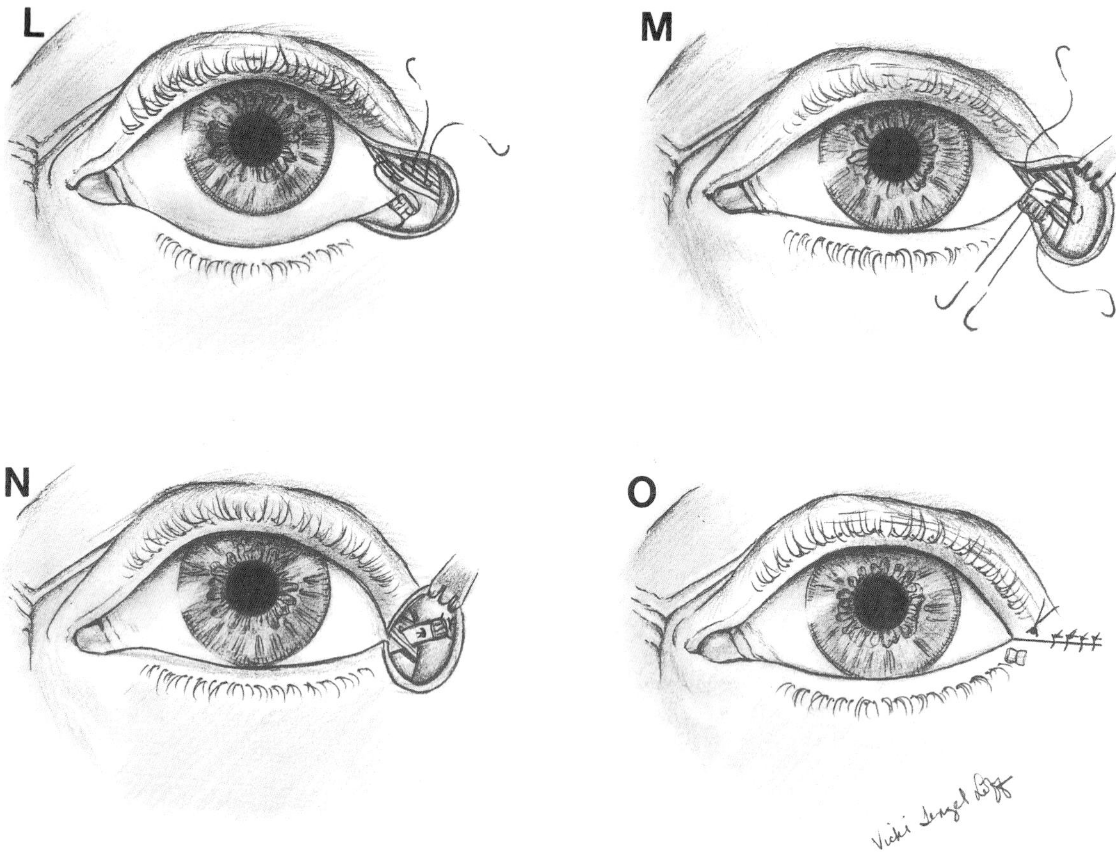

Figure 58.3. *L–O.*

is elevated off of the surface of the tarsus. A similar conjunctival flap is created. Frequently it is necessary to excise conjunctiva that is adherent to the tarsus. A 3-mm-wide strip of tendon and tarsus is finally created by dividing the lower eyelid retractors along the length of the excessive segment of eyelid.

Blunt dissection is employed to isolate the periosteum covering the lateral orbital rim in the region of the lateral canthus. A "buttonhole" is made in the intact superior arm of the lateral canthal tendon near the cut edge of the canthotomy. The tendon tarsal strip is passed through this buttonhole and sutured to the edge of the orbital rim. The correct location of this fixation is determined by manually holding the tendon at various positions on the orbital rim and observing the two eyes for symmetry. The tendon is sutured to the rim with permanent sutures (5-0 nylon) that have been passed through the periosteum in a whip-stitch fashion. Any excess skin and orbicularis can be excised, and the wound is either closed in layers or with vertical mattress-style sutures. A sharp lateral canthal angle is insured by placing a vertical mattress suture (6-0 Prolene) at the edge of the canthal angle. This suture first takes a full-thickness bite of both eyelids, then exits at the posterior edge of the lid margins. The suture is then reversed, passed through the midpoint of both lid margins, and tied over a cotton pledget. This suture must be left in place for 10–12 days, while the skin sutures can be removed in approximately 5 days.

Anderson (5) has described a tarsal strip procedure that is very similar to the lateral canthal sling. However, in the tarsal strip technique only a tongue of tarsus is created. This is sutured to the inner edge of the lateral orbital rim without being passed through a buttonhole in the superior arm of the canthal tendon.

Schorr (6) has modified the tarsal strip procedure to treat the scleral show of postblepharoplasty patients who have had excessive skin excision. Following the canthotomy and creation of a tarsal strip, any subcutaneous cicatricial bands in the lower eyelid are divided. Sutures are used to attach the tarsal strip and the deep subcutaneous tissue of the cheek to the lateral orbital rim and zygomatic arch. This effectively advances and suspends the eyelid and cheek tissues, which relieves the inferior traction on the eyelid margin.

The "Madame Butterfly" procedure is a modification of the above method, which Schorr (6) has employed to relieve postblepharoplasty lagophthalmos secondary to excessive skin excision in the upper eyelid. The tarsal strip is attached higher than usual on the rim, which creates an antimongoloid slant of the palpebral fissure. The lower eyelid is thus elevated, and more complete eyelid closure is permitted.

Cases with more extreme skin shortage of the lower eyelid cannot be corrected with eyelid tightening and suspension alone. In these patients an infraciliary incision is created and a skin flap is dissected inferiorly until all scar bands have been released. The eyelid tightening procedure is now performed. Failure to tighten the eyelid in these cases will result in a high recurrence rate of the ectropion or lagophthalmos. The amount of skin shortage will be apparent at this stage of the procedure. If the deficit is small (less than 3 mm), it is frequently possible to recess the skin edge and leave the area of shortage bare. The defect will gradually epithelialize, generally with good cosmetic results. Larger defects will require a full-thickness skin graft, which can be obtained either from the upper eyelids or the retroauricular area.

Every cosmetic or ophthalmic surgeon should be familiar with the method of using a lateral canthotomy in the treatment of a retrobulbar hematoma. This condition may result from injections, surgery, or trauma. The globe will be noted to be proptotic and the lids may be ecchymotic. Ocular motility is reduced and vision can be compromised by the mass effect of the hematoma either on the optic nerve or the orbital vessels. Successful management of this disorder depends upon its rapid recognition and treatment. A horizontal lateral canthotomy is performed, and both the upper and lower arms of the canthal tendon are completely dividied from the orbital rim. This procedure simultaneously releases the anterior restriction of the orbital contents and provides a route of drainage for the hematoma.

SUMMARY

Normally contoured eyelid fissures will enhance the appearance of patients who have had cosmetic eyelid surgery. The shape and integrity of the lateral canthal structures frequently affect the configuration of the lid fissure. Abnormalities of the lateral canthus may lead to eyelid deformity. An understanding of the various etiologies of postblepharoplasty eyelid fissure defects will enable the cosmetic surgeon to avoid or manage these complications.

REFERENCES

1. Fox SA: The palpebral fissure. *Am J Ophthalmol* 62: 73–78, 1966.
2. Callahan MA, Callahan A: *Ophthalmic Plastic and Orbital Surgery*. Birmingham, AL, Aesculapins, 1979, pp 18–19.
3. Tenzel RR: Treatment of lagophthalmos of the lower lid. *Arch Ophthalmol* 81; 366–368, 1969.
4. Tenzel RR, Buffam FV, Miller GR: The use of the "lateral canthal sling" in ectropion repair. *Can J Ophthalmol* 12: 199–202, 1977.
5. Anderson RL, Gordy DD: The tarsal strip procedure. *Arch Ophthalmol* 97: 2192–2196, 1979.
6. Shorr N: "Madame Butterfly" procedure. Presented at the Fourteenth Annual Scientific Symposium of the American Society of Ophthalmic Plastic and Reconstructive Surgery, Chicago, Nov 4, 1983.

CHAPTER 59

Management of Prolapsed Lacrimal Glands

RICHARD L. PETRELLI, M.D.

Herniation of the lacrimal gland, while not a common condition, can occur spontaneously or in conjunction with certain pathological processes. The purpose of this chapter is to review the etiology of herniated lacrimal glands, to distinguish the condition from other benign and malignant processes, and to review the surgical correction of this condition.

ANATOMY

The lacrimal gland is a bilobed structure consisting of the orbital lobe (main gland) and the palpebral lobe (accessory gland). The orbital lobe, which is kidney shaped, occupies the lacrimal fossa just posterior to the superotemporal orbital rim (Fig. 59.1). It measures about 20 × 15 mm and is separated from the smaller palpebral lobe by the lateral horn of the levator aponeurosis (Fig. 59.2).

Two to six excretory ducts pass from the orbital lobe into the palpebral lobe and empty into the conjunctival sac at about 5 mm above the lateral tarsal border of the upper lid (1) (Fig. 59.3). Interruption of all ducts as they enter the palpebral lobe or, alternatively, removal of the palpebral lobe could result in the interruption of all reflex secretion to the globe (2, 3; A Hornblass, C. Guberina, unpublished data). Some aberrant ducts, however, may bypass the palpebral lobe and enter the conjunctiva directly.

The orbital lobe is suspended by four sets of ligaments (4). Posteriorly, two bands of fascia attach to the subperiosteal tissue. Superolaterally, additional bands of connective tissue adhere to subperiosteum. Anteriorly, fascial bands extend from the gland to the adjacent upper free border of the lateral horn. Medially, a broad ligament anchors the gland to the superior transverse ligament of Whitnall.

The superior transverse ligament is an important anatomical landmark because of its relation to other orbital structures. It is a check ligament that forms a condensation of the levator muscle just above the equator of the globe. It marks the point where the levator muscle, emerging anteriorly from the orbital apex, begins its inferior descent as an aponeurotic sheath to insert on the tarsus. The superior transverse ligament suspends the aponeurosis in a vertical position as the aponeurosis descends to its tarsal attachments and medial and lateral horn extensions.

In addition to its attachments to the orbital lobe of the lacrimal gland, the superior transverse ligament sends extensions medially to the fascia of the superior oblique muscle's pulley and to the tendon of the superior oblique (5).

ETIOLOGY

Either or both lobes of the lacrimal gland may herniate (6). Herniation is usually the result of aging processes or trauma to the orbit. With aging, the lacrimal suspensory ligaments relax and the lacrimal gland prolapses. When the orbital lobe prolapses, a bulge can be seen in the lateral aspect of the right upper lid. Palpation with the thumb

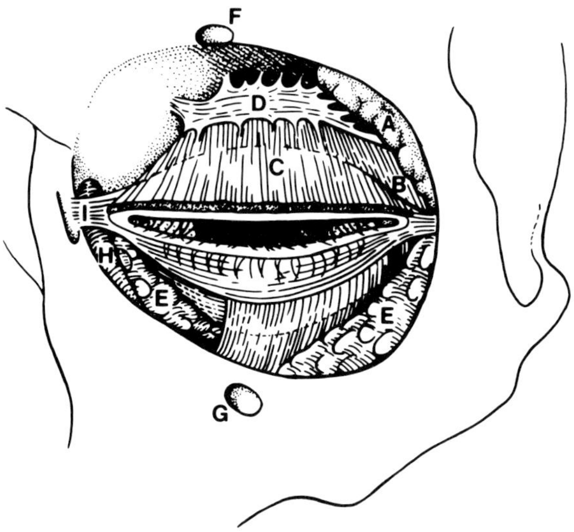

Figure 59.1. View of the orbit devoid of its orbital septum. In this schematic view of the left orbit, the skin and muscle layers of the eyelid have been removed. The entire orbital septum has also been removed, which exposes the contents of the orbit. The orbital lobe of the lacrimal gland (*A*) is seen to rest on the lateral horn (*B*) of the levator aponeurosis (*C*). The superior transverse ligament of Whitnall (*D*) sends extensions to the orbital lobe and the aponeurosis. Fat pads (*E*) fill the space between the globe and the orbital floor. Other structures: *F*, Superior orbital foramen. *G*, Inferior orbital foramen. *H*, Lacrimal sac. *I*, Medial canthal tendon.

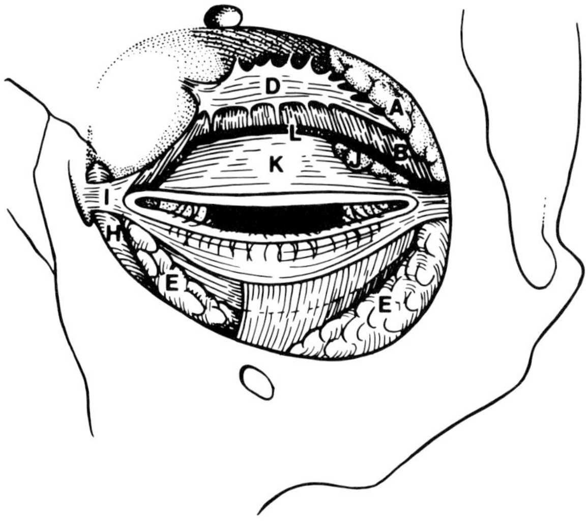

Figure 59.2. Relationship of the orbital and palpebral lobes. Much of the levator has been removed (except for the lateral horn), which exposes the underlying Muller's muscle. The palpebral lobe (*J*) is exposed following removal of the anterior levator, under which lies Müller's muscle (*K*). The cut edge of the remaining levator (*L*) can be followed to the lateral horn of the levator aponeurosis (*B*), which is sandwiched between the orbital lobe (*A*) and the palpebral lobe (*J*).

and forefinger reveals a freely movable mass which can be reposited into the lacrimal fossa. When the palpebral lobe prolapses, a pink mass beneath the conjunctiva can be identified in the lateral fornix (Fig. 59.4).

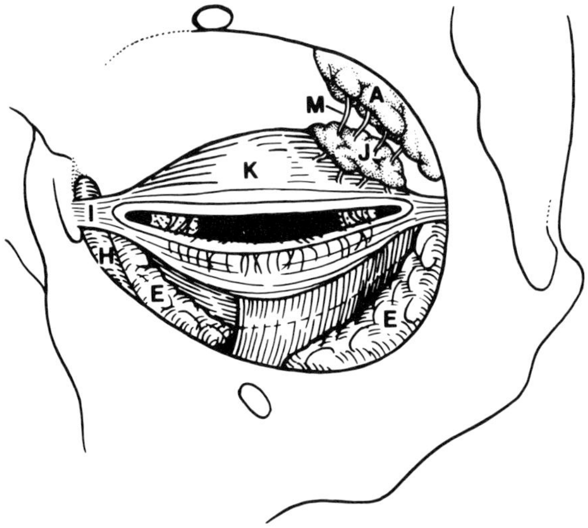

Figure 59.3. The lacrimal lobe excretory ducts. The levator has been removed entirely. The orbital lobe (*A*) is seen with four excretory ducts (*M*), which pass directly to the palpebral lobe (*J*) before entering the conjunctiva in the upper fornix.

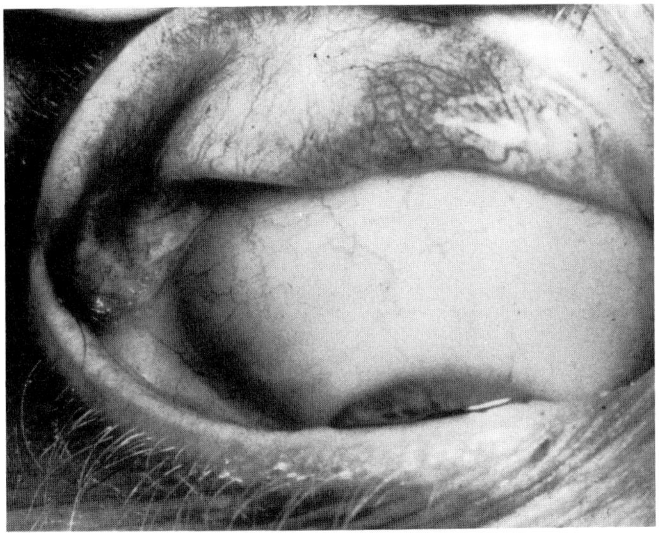

Figure 59.4. Palpebral lobe prolapse. The palpebral lobe is seen to prolapse in the lateral canthus of the right eye of an elderly patient. The upper lid has been everted.

Herniation of the orbital lobe of the lacrimal gland can be associated with blepharochalasis, an uncommon disease of puberty. Patients with blepharochalasis experience recurrent bouts of angioneurotic lid edema (7, 8). More common in blacks, the condition results in stretching of the skin and dehiscence of the orbital septum. The attacks of edema can occur at the time of menstruation. The skin of the lids eventually take on a baggy, attenuated appearance overhanging the lid margin. The orbital lobe of the lacrimal gland can prolapse through the weakened orbital septum and come to rest at the outer lid margin (Fig. 59.5).

Prolapse of orbital fat may also occur and will contribute to the baggy appearance of the upper lid (9). An associated ptosis may be present. Lower lid involvement, while rare,

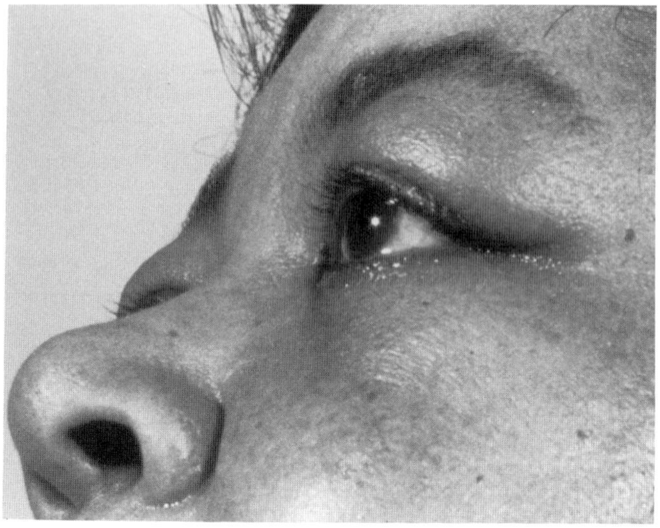

Figure 59.5. Orbital lobe prolapse. This 48-year-old female has bilateral orbital lobe prolapse. Note the bulging prominence in the lateral aspect of the left upper lid.

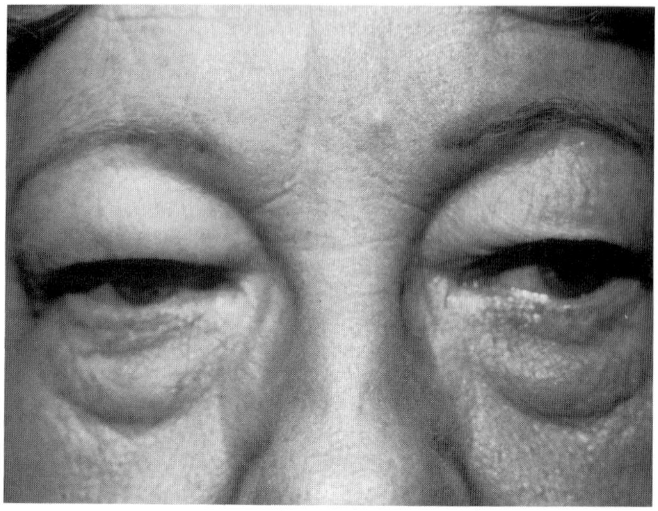

Figure 59.6. Prolapsed orbital fat in an elderly woman.

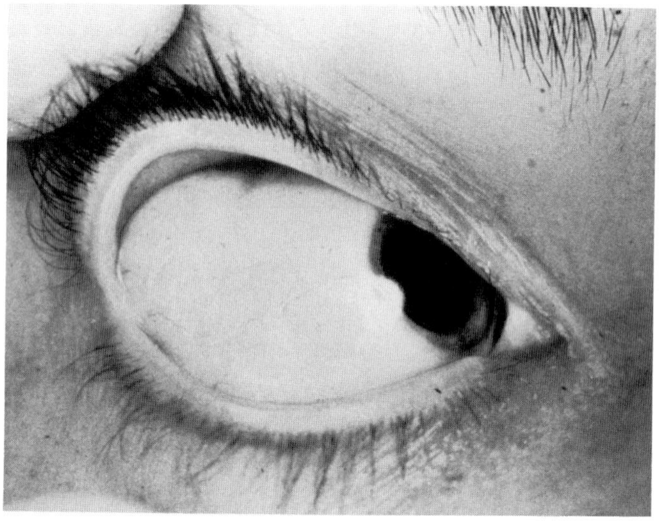

Figure 59.7. Congenital dermolipoma, right eye. A yellow-white smooth soft mass is seen in the superolateral quadrant overlying the globe.

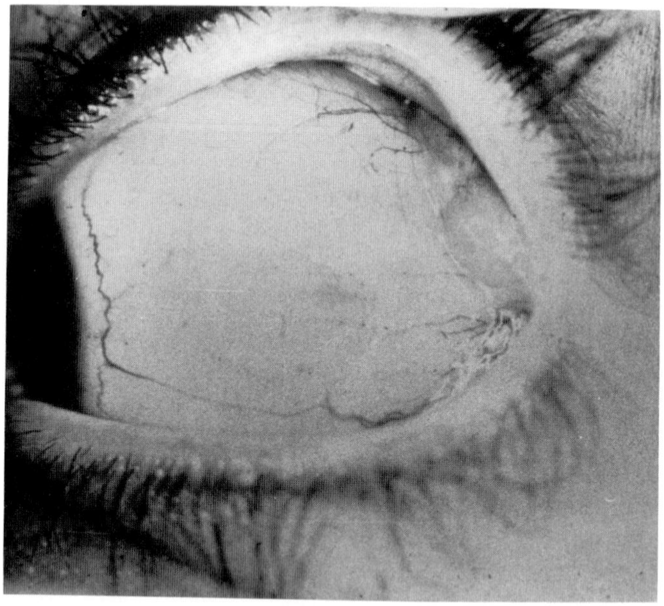

Figure 59.8. Lacrimal gland cyst, left eye. Adjacent to the lateral canthus, the palpebral lobe is loculated and has a cystic appearance.

can occur. Blepharochalasis should not be confused with dermatochalasis, the more common wrinkling of the lid skin due to the skin atrophy and the changes of aging.

Herniation of the lacrimal gland should be distinguished from other benign and malignant conditions. Orbital fat prolapse through the orbital septum may resemble lacrimal gland prolapse. However, fat prolapse usually appears as a diffuse bulge throughout the entire upper lid (Fig. 59.6). Unlike a palpable orbital lobe of the lacrimal gland, prolapsed orbital fat has no defined or discrete borders. Orbital fat that prolapses into the upper fornix may occur in patients with thyroid ophthalmopathy. It has a yellow fatty appearance through the clear conjunctiva. In contrast, prolapsed lacrimal gland appears as a small, pink lobulated mass beneath the conjunctiva in the superotemporal fornix or lateral canthal area.

Congenital epibulbar dermolipomas occurring in the superotemporal quadrant can simulate lacrimal gland masses. Dermolipomas have a fatty appearance and are freely movable masses (Fig. 59.7). They may enter a growth phase should the patient increase body adipose tissue. Dermolipomas are soft to palpation and have a smooth yellow appearance.

Lacrimal gland cyst may present as an enlarged nontender fluctuant mass in the lateral upper lid. The size of the mass may fluctuate as the cystic spaces tend to fill and empty from month to month. Eversion of the lid reveals the palpebral lobe of the lacrimal gland covered with multiple fluid-filled cysts (Fig. 59.8).

Dacryoadenitis and lacrimal gland pseudotumor may also present as a palpable enlarged mass in the upper lid

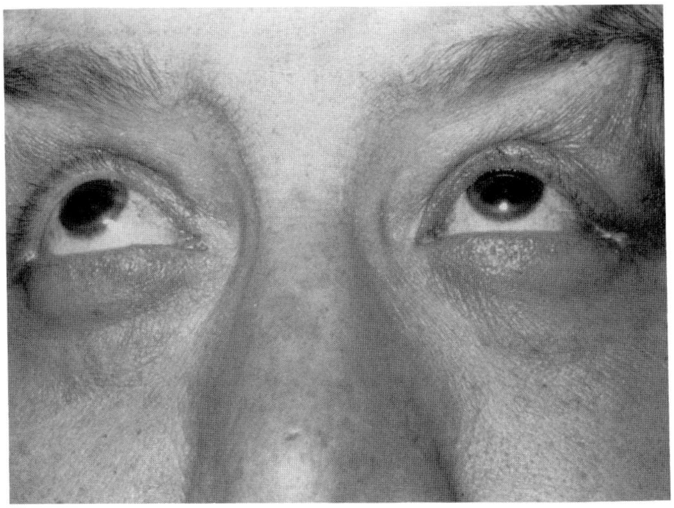

Figure 59.9. Acute dacryoadenitis, left eye. Note the diffuse swelling in the lateral aspect of the left upper lid.

(Fig. 59.9). The condition presents as an acute painful mass beneath erythematous skin and is usually unilateral. In contrast, prolapsed lacrimal gland is neither tender nor erythematous.

Sarcoid is another disease that may include painless swelling of the lacrimal gland. Important features in the diagnosis include the history and clinical picture, anergy to tuberculoprotein, characteristic skin lesions, chest x-ray, and lymph node or lacrimal gland biopsy (10).

Among malignant lesions that should be included in the differential diagnosis are lymphoma, malignant lacrimal gland tumors, and benign mixed lacrimal tumors. Lymphoma causes nontender enlargement of the gland. The lacrimal gland appears as a salmon-pink firm mass beneath the conjunctiva. Proptosis may be present if the lacrimal gland enlargement is deep within the lacrimal fossa.

Epithelial lacrimal gland tumors present as unilateral enlargement of the gland with a history of gradual onset greater than 12 months (benign mixed tumor) or less than 12 months (adenoid cystic and malignant mixed carcinoma). In contrast to lacrimal gland herniation, proptosis is common in epithelial lacrimal gland tumors. The diagnosis is made by the history and clinical features, CT scan, and biopsy (11, 12). When benign mixed tumor is suspected by the history, biopsy should be avoided in favor of en bloc excision to avoid rupture of the tumor capsule.

SURGICAL CORRECTION

The surgical correction of lacrimal gland herniation involves resuspending the gland into its normal anatomic position, the lacrimal fossa (13). A skin incision is made through the supratarsal lid fold approximately 20 mm in length. The upper lip of the incision is undermined deep to the orbicularis muscle (Fig. 59.10). The dissection is carried upward to the origin of the orbital septum where it is attached to the superior orbital rim.

The orbital septum is incised 3 mm below its attachment to the orbital rim (Fig. 59.11). This 3 mm apron extends over the lateral two-thirds of the superior orbital rim and is necessary for the subsequent closure of the orbital septum.

With gentle digital pressure over the globe, the lacrimal gland with preaponeurotic fat will prolapse out of the lips of the incision. The fat is yellow and soft in contrast to the gland, which is pink-grey and firm (Fig. 59.12). Excess fat should be excised and cauterized.

Biopsy of the gland is performed to rule out any pathological process. The area of biopsy should be closed with absorbable suture. Careful attention to hemostasis is mandatory because of the highly vascular nature of the lacrimal gland.

The gland is then resuspended by passing a double

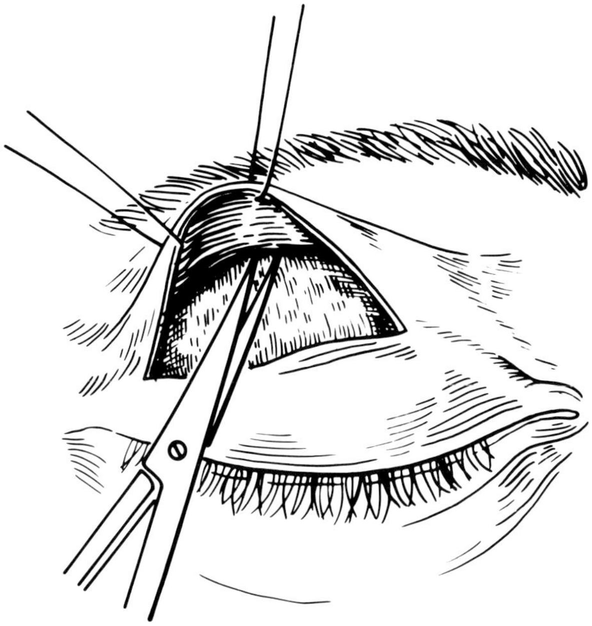

Figure 59.10. Skin incision in the lid fold.

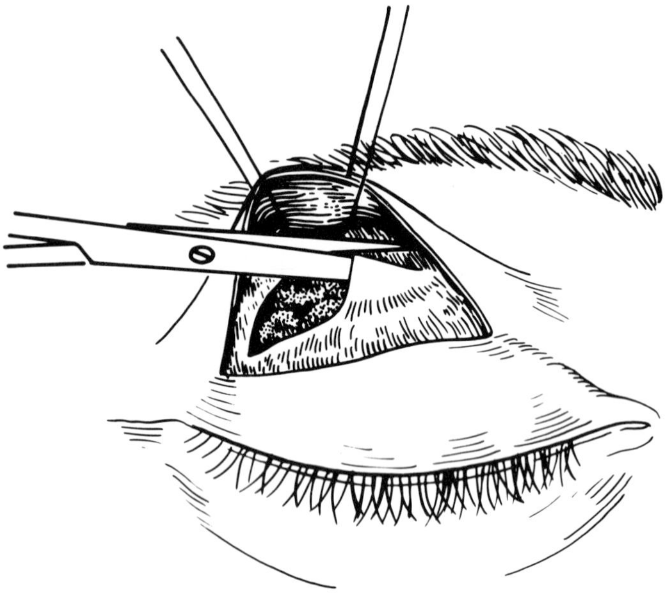

Figure 59.11. Incising the orbital septum.

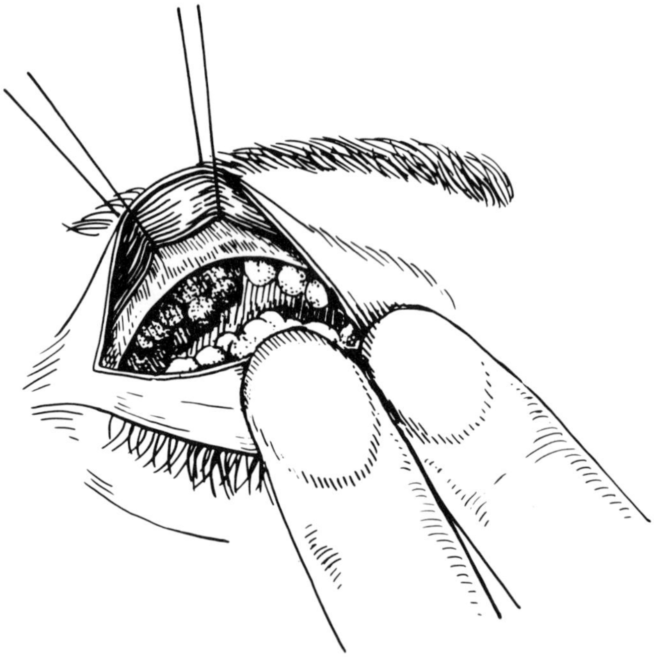

Figure 59.12. Prolapsing the orbital lobe.

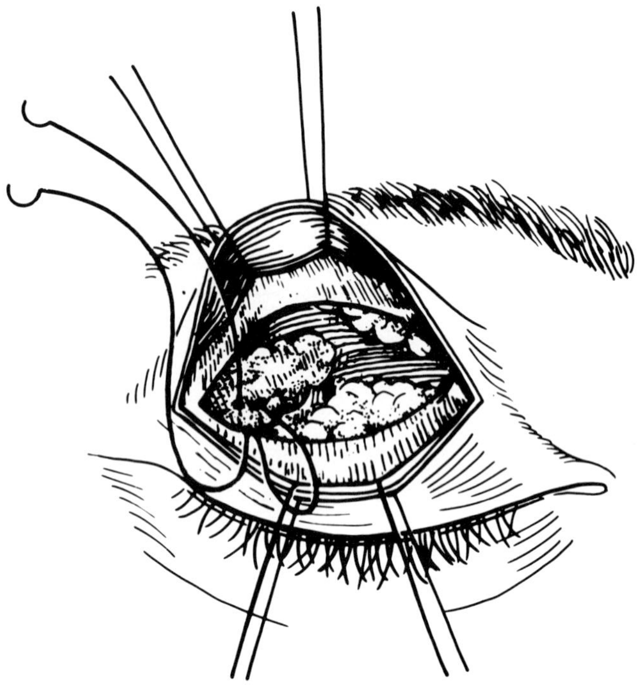

Figure 59.13. Whip stitch through the orbital lobe.

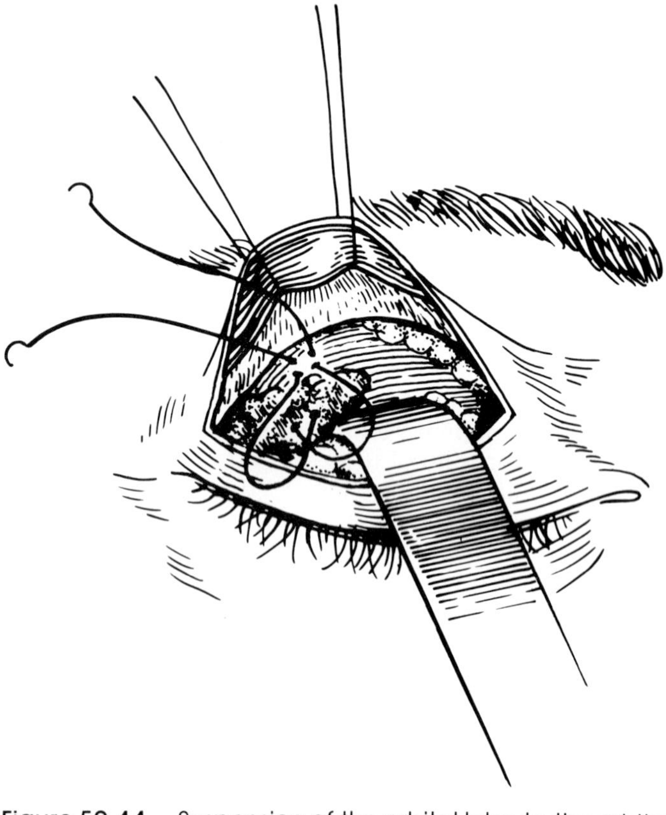

Figure 59.14. Suspension of the orbital lobe to the orbital roof and periosteum.

armed 4-0 chromic gut suture through the inferior surface in mattress fashion to the superior surface of the gland (Fig. 59.13). The suture is tied onto itself to prevent slippage. Each needle is then passed through the periosteum of the orbital roof from a posteroanterior direction close to the orbital rim (Fig. 59.14). The two sutures are then tied onto one another bringing the lacrimal gland in close apposition to the lacrimal fossa (Fig. 59.15).

Small rake retractors are helpful in exposing the lacrimal fossa. Direct visualization of the fossa is enhanced with a nasal speculum. The nasal speculum spreads the tissues apart and enables the proper placement of the sutures in the periosteum.

The orbital septum is closed with interrupted 5-0 chromic gut suture (Fig. 59.16). The lips of the skin incision are apposed, and any excess skin is trimmed appropriately. The skin is closed with interrupted 6-0 black silk (Figs. 59.17 and 59.18).

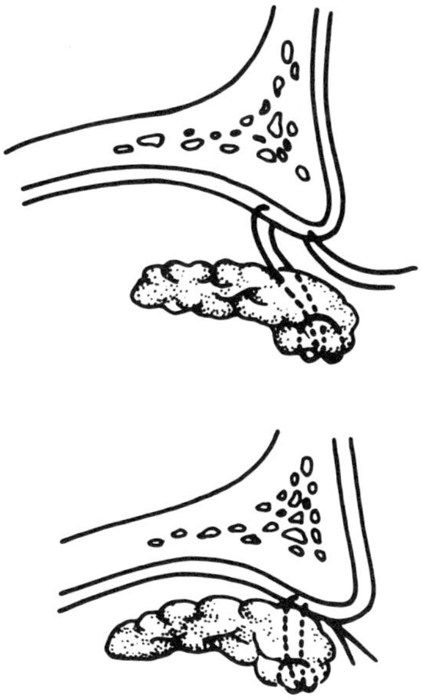

Figure 59.15. Lateral view of the lacrimal gland suspension.

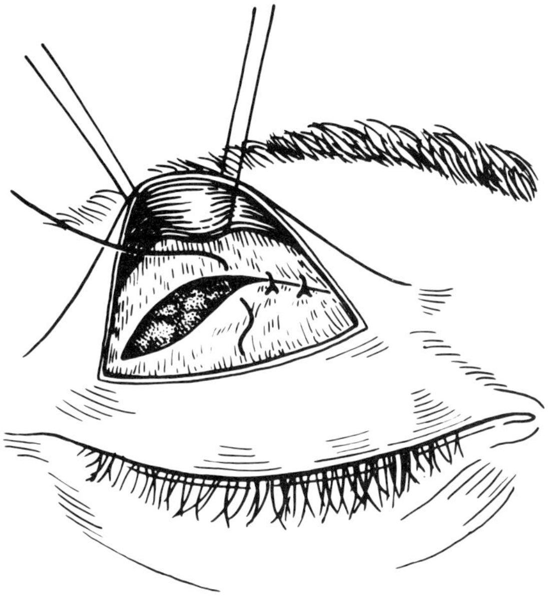

Figure 59.16. Closure of the orbital septum.

In patients who have an associated ptosis, the resuspension may be performed in conjunction with a levator resection or reattachment. Such patients would require a skin incision that runs the entire length of the supratarsal lid fold. Alternatively, the resuspension can be performed with a tarsoconjunctival mullerectomy in patients with minimal ptosis (14). Patients who require an upper lid blepharoplasty occasionally have an associated lacrimal gland herniation. The approach should be through the standard blepharoplasty lid fold incision (15).

In summary, lacrimal gland herniation is a benign, often bilateral, condition that is repaired surgically. Resuspension of the gland requires an understanding of the anatomical landmarks as well as careful attention to hemostasis and suture placement.

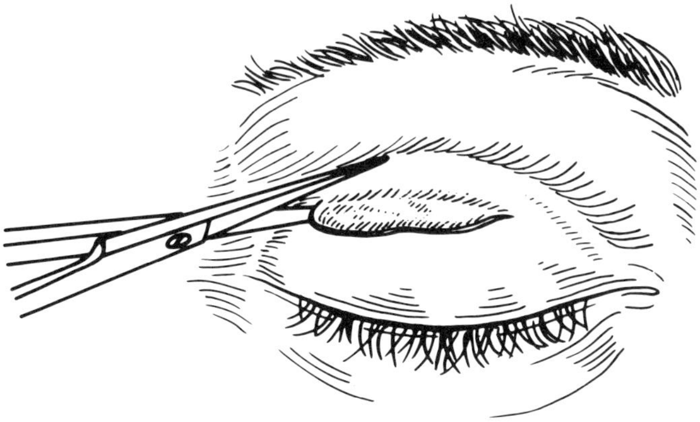

Figure 59.17. Excision of redundant skin.

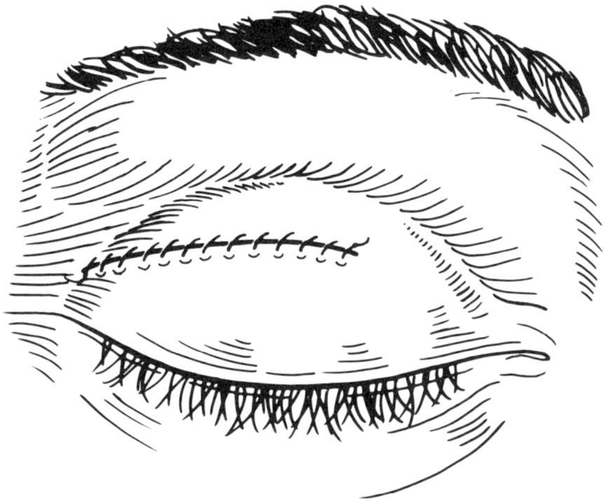

Figure 59.18. Closure of skin.

REFERENCES

1. Jones L, Wobig J: *Surgery of the Eyelids and Lacrimal System*, Birmingham, AL, Aesculapius, 1976, p. 61.
2. Scherz W, Dohlman C: Is the lacrimal gland dispensable? *Arch Ophthalmol* 93: 281–283, 1975.
3. Taiara C, Smith B: Palpebral dacryoadenectomy, *Am J Ophthalmol* 3: 461–465, 1973.
4. Whitnall SE: *Anatomy of the Human Orbit and Accessory Organ of Vision*, London, Humphrey Milford, 1932, 149.
5. Beard C: *Ptosis*. St. Louis, CV Mosby, 1976, p 22.
6. Smith B, Petrelli R: Herniation of the lacrimal glands, *Tr Am Acad Ophth Otol* 84: 988–990, 1977.
7. Fuchs HE: Blepharochalasis. In *Textbook of Ophthalmology*, (ed 7). (Translated by A. Duane.) Philadelphia, Lippincott, 1923, p 407.
8. Rosen FS, Charache P, Pensky J, Donaldson V: Hereditary angioneurotic edema; two genetic variants, *Science* 148: 957, 1965.
9. Stieglitz LN, Crawford JS: Blepharochalasis. *Am J Ophthalmol* 77: 100–102, 1974.
10. James DG, Anderson R, Langley D, Ainslie: Ocular sarcoidosis. *Br J Ophthalmol* 48: 461–470, 1964.
11. Krohel GB, Stewart WB, Chavis RM: *Orbital Disease. A Practical Approach*, New York, Grune and Stratton, 1981, p. 132.
12. Jacobiec FA, Yeo JH, et al: Combined clinical and computed tomographic diagnosis of primary lacrimal fossa lesions. *Am J Ophthalmol* 94: 785–807, 1982.
13. Smith B, Petrelli R: Surgical repair of prolapsed lacrimal glands. *Arch Ophthalmol* 96: 113–114, 1978.
14. Fasanella RM, Servat J: Levator resection for minimal ptosis. *Arch Ophthalmol* 65: 493–496, 1961.
15. Courtiss EH: Selection of alternatives in esthetic blepharoplasty. In Rees TD (ed): *Modern Trends in Blepharoplasty*. Philadelphia, WB Saunders, 1981, vol 8.

CHAPTER 60

Chemabrasion of the Periorbital Area

NICOLAS TABBAL, M.D., F.A.C.S.

Chemabrasion, or chemical peeling, is an effective procedure in treating certain skin disorders. It gained acceptance among surgeons in the early 1960s (1–5) following several reports in the plastic surgical and dermatologic literature. Prior to that period, it suffered from a shady notoriety because of its widespread misuse by lay operators.

Chemabrasion has two separate benefits. It is a very effective method for eliminating fine rhytides of the skin. In addition, it reduces the level of skin pigmentation in the area treated. While this last feature is not always desirable, it can be put to good use in improving localized areas of abnormal pigmentation.

INDICATIONS

Chemical peeling of the eyelids and the periorbital area is indicated for the eradication of fine rhytides of the eyelid skin (Fig. 60.1). When used as a sole procedure, it tightens the skin and significantly improves its texture. When performed in conjunction with a blepharoplasty, it complements the result when preexisting skin lines are not appreciably improved by surgery. In addition, chemical peeling is indicated for the elimination of abnormal hyperpigmentation of the lower lids, a condition that usually resists surgery (Fig. 60.2).

PATIENT SELECTION

Used as a sole procedure, chemical peeling of the eyelids is ideal in patients with fair complexion with sun damaged skin and no periorbital bagginess or eyelid skin excess. In such circumstances, the texture of the eyelid skin is greatly improved and regains a smooth and tight texture (Fig. 60.3). The same effect is achieved when peeling is used to complement the result of a blepharoplasty. Patients with olive skin, however, make poor candidates for chemical peeling, since they tend to show an obvious line of demarcation at the periphery of the area treated. When hyperpigmentation is localized to the lower lids, however, chemical peeling can be very effective in eliminating this abnormal pigmentation. Paradoxically, a beneficial outcome here results from one of the undesirable side effects of the procedure, namely, loss of pigmentation.

CHEMICAL AGENTS

Phenol is the primary ingredient in chemical-peel solutions. It causes an immediate keratolysis of the skin through disruption of the sulfur bridges of the keratoprotein. It is used in a solution containing distilled water, croton oil, and liquid soap. Pure phenol solutions are not as effective since excessive keratocoagulation of the skin

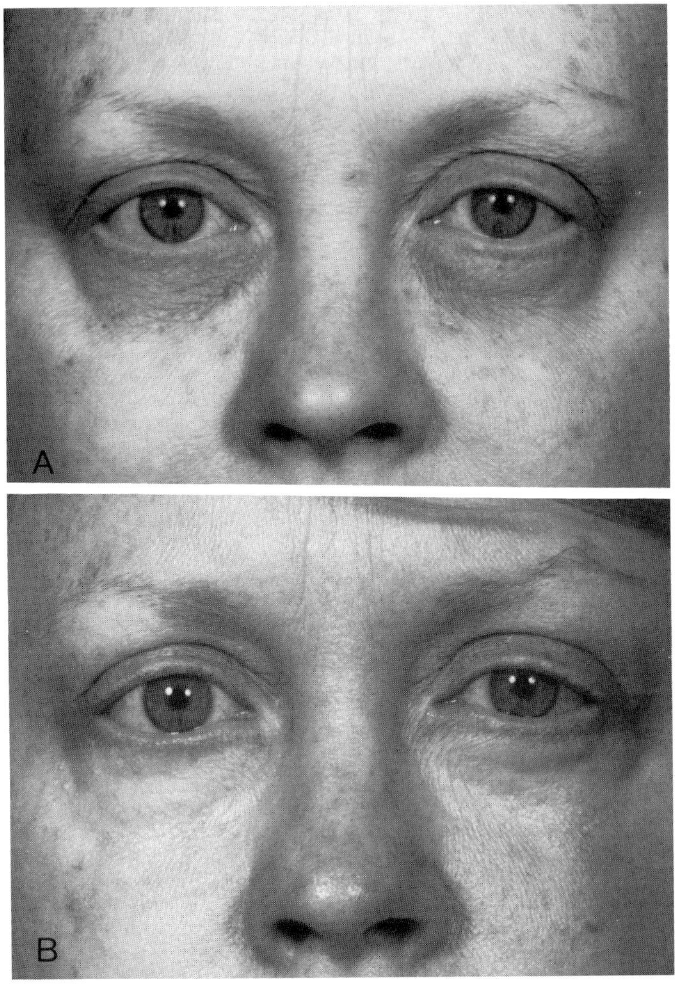

Figure 60.1. *A,* Fine rhytides of eyelid skin do not respond well to blepharoplasty, particularly in patients with sun-damaged skin. *B,* In this patient, chemabrasion of the lower lids was very effective in eliminating these fine skin lines.

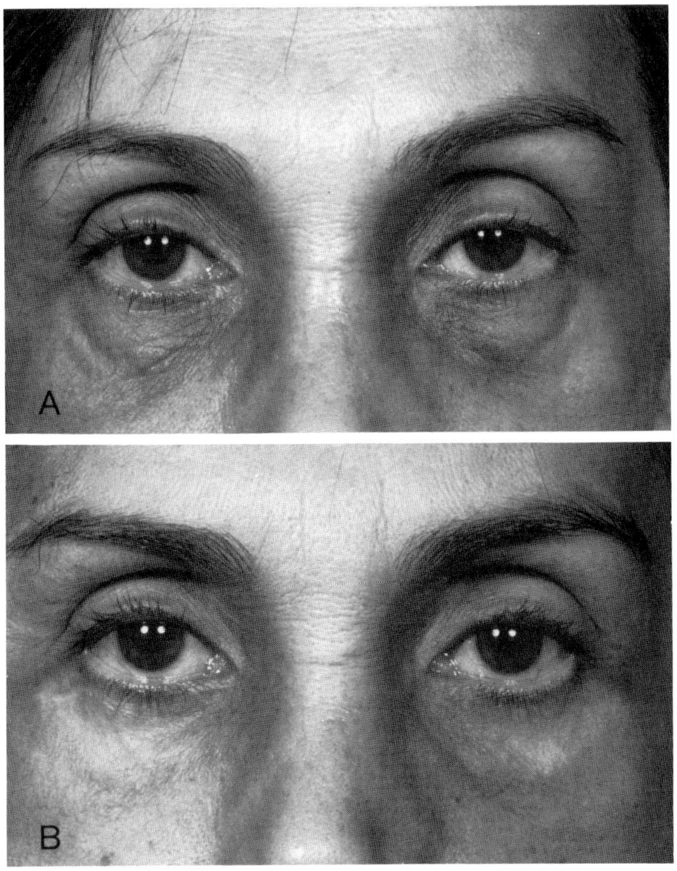

Figure 60.2. *A,* Dark pigmentation of the lower lids is often hereditary. It is more common in patients of Mediterranean origin. Chemabrasion is the only available technique for treating this abnormal pigmentation. This patient had previously undergone a blepharoplasty, but was still distressed by the dark circles under her eyes, which were not easily covered by makeup. *B,* Chemabrasion of the lower lids reduced this hyperpigmentation significantly.

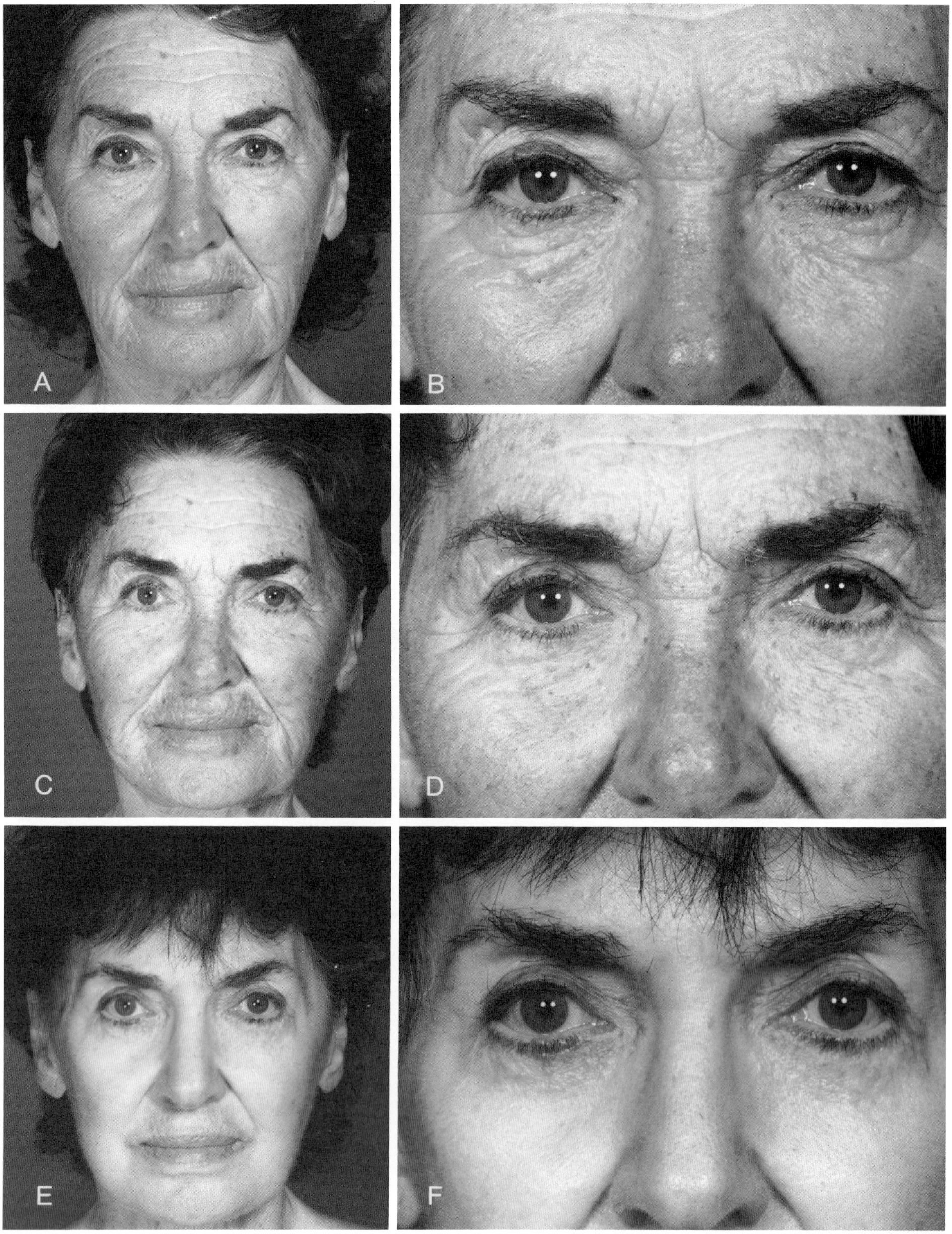

Figure 60.3. *A* and *B*, Deep lines of facial skin secondary to prolonged sun exposure respond poorly to surgery. *C*, *D*, Following a facial plasty and a blepharoplasty, this woman still exhibited significant rhytidosis of the face. *E*, *F*, A full-face chemabrasion practically eliminated all the skin lines and the areas of blotchy pigmentation.

actually forms a barrier against deeper penetration of the substance into the dermis. In addition, the croton oil acts as an irritant, while liquid soap retards phenol penetration and absorption by increasing surface tension. This mechanism enhances the macerative action of phenol by delaying its keratolytic action and preventing its deeper penetration in the tissues. In addition, covering the area with waterproof tape immediately following the application of the solution prevents phenol evaporation and promotes maceration of the skin, allowing a deeper peel. Taping following periorbital peeling, however, is not indicated since it may cause full-thickness burn of the extremely thin eyelid skin.

MICROSCOPIC CHANGES

Following chemabrasion, the microscopic anatomy of the skin shows typically persistent changes. Dermal collagen exhibits reorientation with an increase in fibroblastic density. In addition, melanin-producing cells in the basal layers of the dermis show a marked decrease in number. Finally, an increase in elastic tissue content is usually evident. These changes have been shown to be permanent and do not seem to adversely affect the treated skin (1, 6, 7).

SYSTEMIC ABSORPTION OF PHENOL

During chemical peeling, systemic absorption of phenol takes place. Phenol blood levels depend upon the surface area treated, and the speed of the application. The modest amount of phenol absorbed during chemical peeling of the facial area is readily excreted by the kidneys, either as a free substance or after it is conjugated (8, 9). Only in patients with chronic renal failure does the phenol blood level reach toxic levels following a limited application. On the other hand, cardiac irregularities have been reported during chemical peeling (10). They are caused by cardiac irritability, secondary to phenol absorption. Thus, chemical peeling of large surface areas should not be done precipitously and the patient should be monitored throughout the procedure. Such cardiac rhythm changes, however, are unlikely when only small areas are treated, such as the periorbital region.

PROCEDURE

Chemical peeling of the eyelids should never be performed at the time of a blepharoplasty because of the potential of skin slough, ectropion, or severe prolonged eyelid edema (9, 11). It can be safely performed, however, as early as 8 weeks following surgery.

The patient should be sedated preferably with an intramuscular dose of Demerol or an intravenous dose of Valium. Heavy sedation is not essential, however, when the procedure is restricted to the lower lids since many patients find it quite painless. The peel solution should be freshly mixed according to the following formula:

Phenol 88%, U.S.P. 3 ml;
Croton oil, 3 drops;
Septisol soap, 8 drops;
Distilled water, 2 ml.

Following removal of any oily skin deposit with ether, the peel solution is applied with a cotton-tipped applicator that has been partially dried out to avoid dripping. It is particularly important to avoid holding the bottle containing the mixture in close proximity to the patient since accidental spillage can lead to disastrous consequences. As soon as the substance is applied, the skin acquires a white discoloration. Gentle stretching of the skin while painting the solution allows an even penetration of the substance in all the skin crevices. The peel solution should be applied lightly at the periphery of the treated area in order to avoid a sharp demarcation. The ciliary margin should be carefully avoided in order to avoid conjunctival or corneal burn. An intact strip of skin measuring about 2 mm in width at the ciliary border should thus be left intact. When the full face is being treated, the phenol solution should be applied slowly on one area at a time so that abnormal blood levels of phenol are avoided. In addition, chemical peeling of the upper and lower lids should not be performed simultaneously since the subsequent swelling would temporarily interfere with the patient's vision. Taping is not recommended in the periorbital area, particularly in the lower lids since it may cause an undesirably deep peel of the thin eyelid skin and secondary ectropion.

POSTOPERATIVE CARE

During the application of the peel solution, and for several hours subsequently, patients will complain of a burning sensation in the area treated. This discomfort gradually subsides over the first 48 hours. If used, waterproof adhesive tape is then removed and the area is covered with a thin film of thymol iodide powder in order to promote formation of a thin scab. The powder is applied as long as there is a serous discharge from the treated area. Once a definite scab has formed, usually at about the third or fourth day following the procedure, a bland cream (Crisco) is applied several times a day in order to promote its separation. The "new skin" will appear pinkish. It is mildly edematous and tends to be dry. Moisturizing cream should thus be applied regularly. The discoloration of the areas treated subsides over several weeks. A coverall makeup, however, can be successfully used as soon as the skin is totally healed. Exposure to the sun should be carefully avoided as long as the treated area is showing some discoloration since ultraviolet rays promote blotching and irregular pigmentation. Application of sun-blocking creams is essential during this period.

COMPLICATIONS

Hypopigmentation of the treated skin is the most common complication following chemabrasion. It is more common in patients with dark complexion. An abrupt line of demarcation can be avoided by carefully feathering out the peeling at the periphery of the treated area (6, 11). In addition, limiting the treatment to complete aesthetic units makes such a complication more tolerable since the line of demarcation tends to be less visible.

Redness of the treated skin resolves usually within 2–3 months. When persistent, however, it can be a source of aggravation to the patient. Topical steroid creams are helpful in enhancing its resolution (11). In addition, patients should be warned preoperatively that temporary ectropion of the lower lids may occur following the chemical peeling. In most instances, it resolves spontaneously. Rare persistant ectropion necessitating skin grafting, however, has been reported.

SUMMARY

Chemabrasion, or chemical peeling, of the periorbital area is effective in eliminating fine rhytides of eyelid skin along with any abnormal pigmentation. It is not a substitute for surgery if there is excessive periorbital bagginess or skin excess, but it can complement surgery in specific circumstances.

REFERENCES

1. Brown AM, Kaplan LM, Brown ME: Phenol-induced histological skin changes: Hazards, technique and uses. *Br J Plast Surg* 13: 158, 1960.
2. Baker TJ: Ablation of rhytides by chemical means. *J FL Med Assoc* 47: 451–454, 1961.
3. Baker TJ: Chemical face peeling and rhytidectomy, a combined approach for facial rejuvenation. *Plast Reconstr Surg* 29: 199, 1962.
4. Ayres S, III: Superficial chemosurgery in treating aging skin. *Arch Dermatol* 85: 385, 1962.
5. Ayres S, III: Superficial chemosurgery, its current staus and relationship to dermabrasion. *Arch Dermatol* 89: 395, 1964.
6. Baker TJ, Gordon HL, Mosienko P, Seckinger DL: Long-term histological study of skin after chemical face peeling. *Plast Reconstr Surg* 53: 522, 1974.
7. Spira M, Dahl G, Freeman R, Gerow FJ, Hardy SB: Chemosurgery—A histological study. *Plast Reconstr Surg* 45: 247, 1970.
8. Litton C: Followup study of chemosurgery. *South Med J* 50: 1007, 1966.
9. Litton C, Fournier P, Capinpin A: A survey of chemical peeling of the face. *Plast Reconstr Surg* 51: 645, 1973.
10. Truppman ES, Ellenby JD: Major electrocardiographic changes during face peeling. *Plast Reconstr Surg* 63: 44, 1979.
11. Spira M, Gerow FJ, Hardy SB: Complications of chemical face peeling. *Plast Reconstr Surg* 54: 397, 1974.

CHAPTER 61

Management of Complications of Upper Eyelid Blepharoplasty

DAVID F. KAMIN, M.D.
KEVIN I. PERMAN, M.D.

Upper eyelid blepharoplasty is a surgical procedure that has gained increased popularity in recent years. Complications are relatively rare, but with the increased level of awareness displayed by today's blepharoplasty patients, the surgeon faces a demanding group of patients who will not tolerate the slightest postoperative complication. In this chapter we will discuss the evaluation, management, and prevention of potential complications starting from the preoperative planning stage, including the intraoperative phase, and through the early and late postoperative periods.

PREOPERATIVE MANAGEMENT

The management of potential complications begins at the initial meeting, where the preoperative evaluation is made (1, 2). It is at this time that the potential for complication is discussed. The discussion may touch upon everything from postoperative blindness (3–9) to the smallest wrinkle, but most importantly the patient must come away with a realistic expectation of what benefits will be realized from the surgery. This is why the most important tool at the initial meeting is the hand mirror (Fig. 61.1). With the patient looking straight into the mirror (as others normally see him or her), the surgeon describes what the surgery will offer the patient and reviews with the patient what are indeed realistic expectations. A review of the skin quality and a cautionary note about how surgery can correct upper lid hooding but not crow's feet is always beneficial. A review of lid crease height and even depth is crucial (Figs. 61.2–61.4) (10). This is especially important in reassuring male patients that blepharoplasty will not give them an effeminate appearance with a deep superior sulcus and high lid crease. It is also important to the Asian patient considering blepharoplasty who may not want to look totally Occidental with an elevated lid crease (11–13). Having established a good rapport with the patient during the preoperative evaluation, the surgeon takes a thorough medical history with careful attention to the possibility of thyroid disease; cardiovascular problems, including history of myocardial infarction, hypertension, and coagulopathies (14). The surgeon always asks about any medicines [e.g., aspirin (15] the patient may be currently taking, which may have to be stopped or modified prior to surgery. The possibility of drug allergy is always confronted. A thorough ocular exam including vision motility, lid function (16), and brow height (17) is performed. Tear function testing is also recommended.

Thus, before stepping into the operating room the surgeon has significantly decreased the possibility of blepharoplasty complications. Anesthesia is always a potential risk variable in any surgery, however, a full discussion of sedatives and narcotics is beyond the scope of this chapter. We perform the majority of upper lid blepharoplasty surgery with local anesthesia and intravenous sedation. An anesthesiologist or nurse anesthetist is always in attendance to monitor the patient and advanced life support equipment is always available, whether the surgery is performed in an office or hospital operating room.

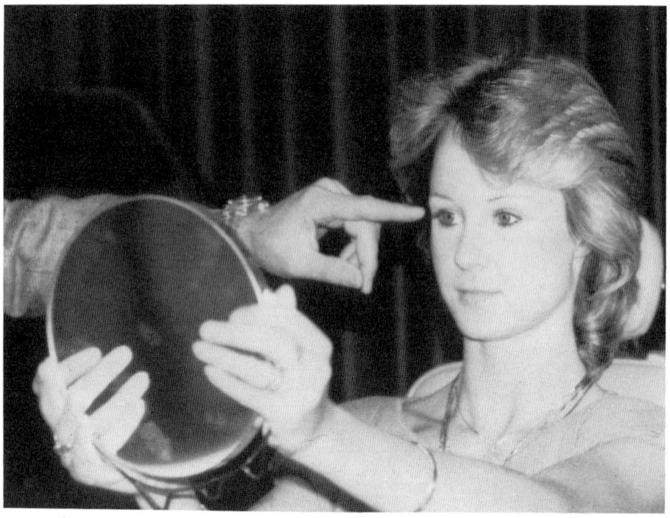

Figure 61.1. The use of a hand mirror aids in pointing out realistic expectations of surgery to the patient.

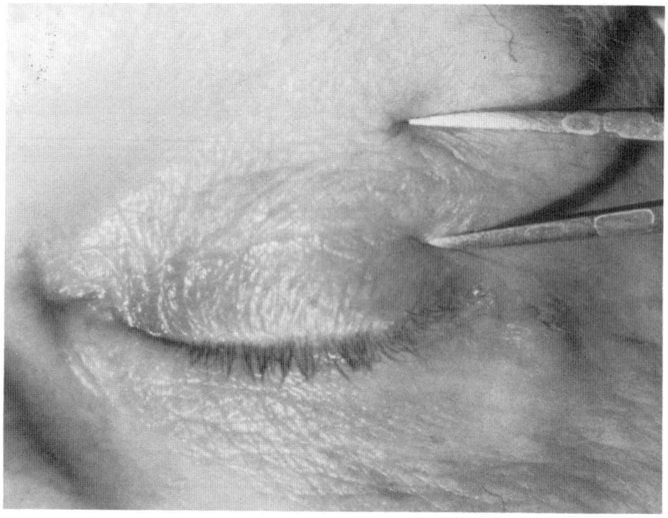

Figure 61.2. Calipers aid in establishing lid crease location, amount of skin to be resected, and act as a safeguard for symmetry between the two lids.

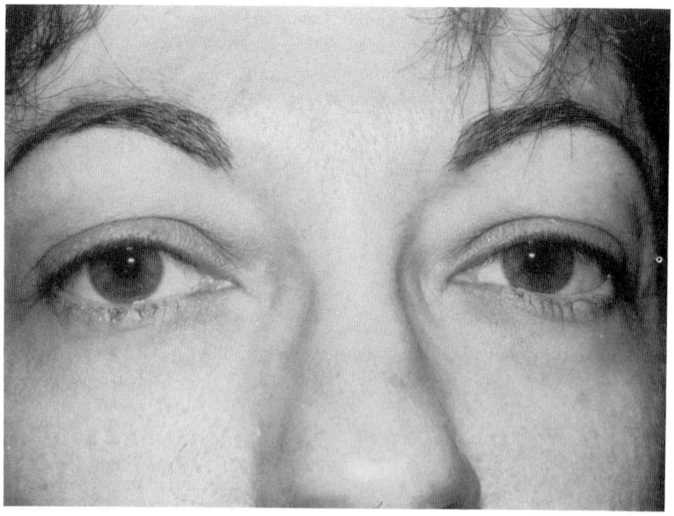

Figure 61.3. Preoperative appearance of blepharoplasty patient.

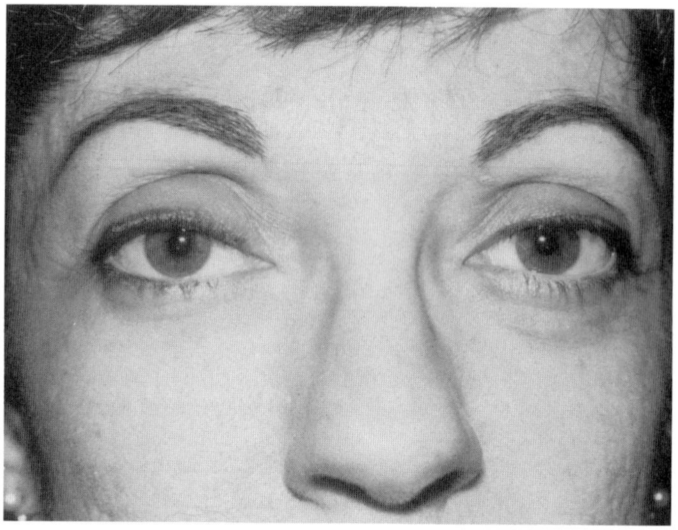

Figure 61.4. Postoperative appearance of same patient as in Fig. 61.3. Notice raised lid crease and deepened sulcus.

SURGICAL MANAGEMENT

TEMPORARY BLINDNESS

The most feared but well-documented complication of blepharoplasty is blindness (1–9). The blindness seen as a result of blepharoplasty surgery is often reversible and rarely permanent but in any event must be addressed immediately. The etiology is a retrobulbar hematoma with bleeding vessels from the cut orbicularis oculi muscle and the vessels coarsing through the orbital fat. This leads to raised intraorbital and intraocular pressure, which compromise the circulation to the optic nerve (7). This has been borne out by electrophysiologic testing (3).

The possibility of a retrobulbar hematoma is a strong case for never allowing postblepharoplasty patients to be with occlusive pressure dressings for prolonged periods (as opposed to brief periods of ice compresses during the immediate postoperative period). If there is any suggestion of severe decrease in vision (not just blurriness), especially with concomitant orbital pain, increased tension to retropulsion with proptosis, lid ecchymosis, and hemorrhage, the incisions should be immediately opened (in the recovery room if necessary) and a lateral canthotomy and cantholysis performed (Figs. 61.5–61.7). At the same time medical treatment should include intravenous injections of mannitol, acetazolamide, and steroids. If more drastic measures prove to be necessary, an orbital decompression should follow, either by the Kronlein approach or preferably the transantral (Ogura) approach, to remove the orbital floor and posterior ethmoids to relieve the hematoma at the orbital apex.

SECONDARY LAGOPHTHALMOS

Having dealt with the worst of the blepharoplasty complications, we will now focus on some of the more com-

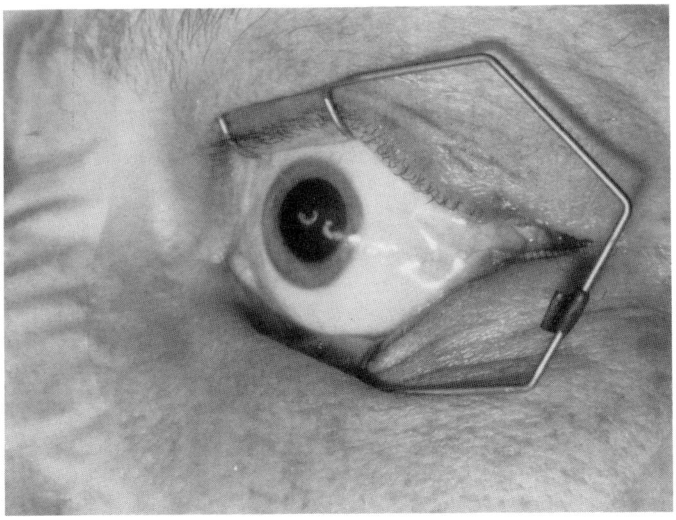

Figure 61.5. Lateral canthotomy.

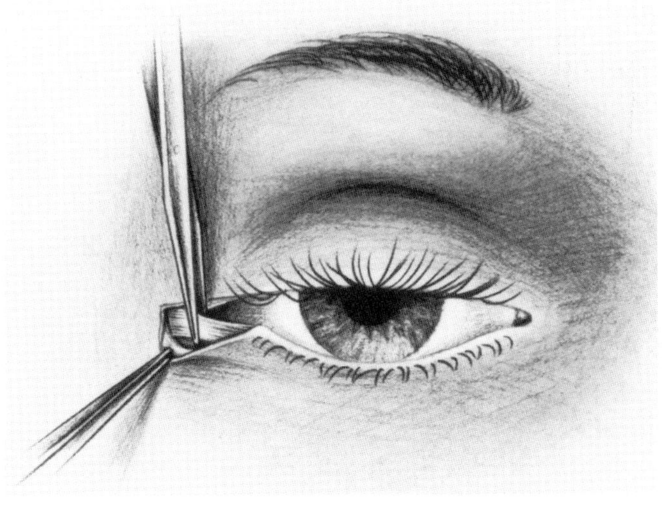

Figure 61.7. Lysis of inferior limb of lateral canthal tendon.

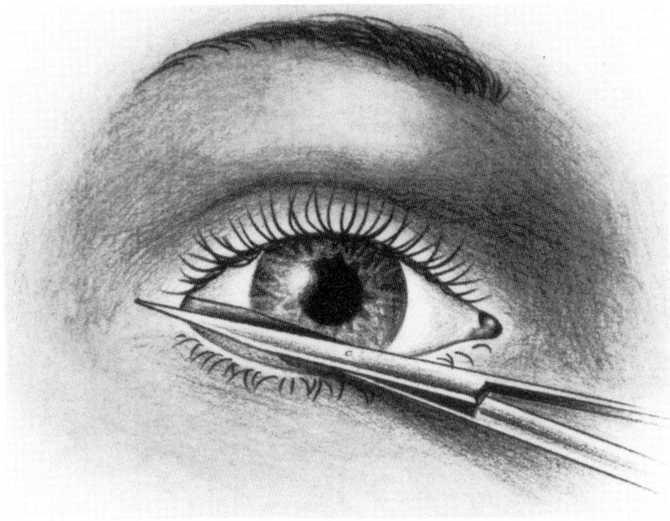

Figure 61.6. Lateral cantholysis.

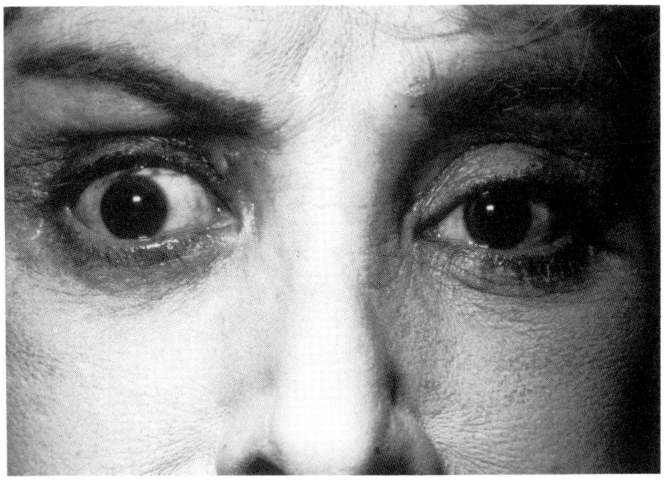

Figure 61.8. Right upper lid retraction following blepharoplasty surgery.

mon complications. These remaining complications are indeed subtle but very real. Excessive skin excision with resultant lagophthalmos and chronic corneal irritation is a serious complication (18–20). These problems are usually handled with tincture of time but it is important for the surgeon to realize that during the preoperative evaluation, these patients had a low lid crease to begin with and that the surgeon was a bit overzealous in the removal of skin (Fig. 61.8). Some patients who have good basic tear function will tolerate the poor closure, yet others will eventually present with keratitis and corneal ulceration. These patients need a skin graft to the upper lid via full-thickness skin graft (Fig. 61.9). The best color match is offered from the retoauricular area, but the supraclavicular may be used. Split-thickness skin grafts may be used but shrinkage is an added variable to be considered here (21).

The other major cause of lagophthalmos and poor lid closure is that the orbital septum has been pulled inferiorly and incorporated into scar (Fig. 61.10). This must be treated by division and release of the orbital septum with recreation of the lid crease (22, 23). With the lid on stretch for easier identification of the septum, the surgical dissection is carried through the orbicularis muscle down to the septum itself. The septum is opened and released from the scar (crease). The lid crease is reformed by skin closure with incorporation of a small bite of levator aponeurosis. The authors do not normally incorporate aponeurosis in the closure of male blepharoplasty patients.

POSTOPERATIVE PTOSIS

Postoperative ptosis is often encountered as a result of direct injury to the levator aponeurosis during surgery (24). Sharp dissection leading to laceration, blunt trauma during manipulation, or postoperative edema can result in temporary or permanent ptosis.

The direct injury is most often encountered during the skin muscle incision. This may be avoided by a ballooning of the tissues with local injection prior to incision (an especially useful technique to the novice blepharoplasty surgeon). The levator aponeurosis might also be injured as the septum is opened and the preaponeurotic fat pad

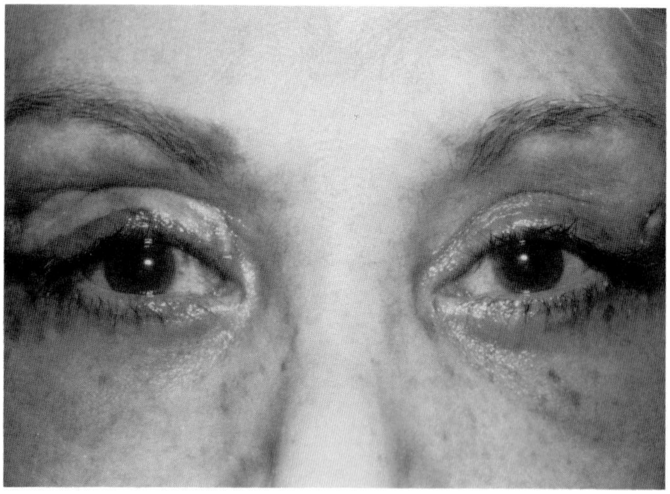

Figure 61.9. Full-thickness skin graft to right upper lid.

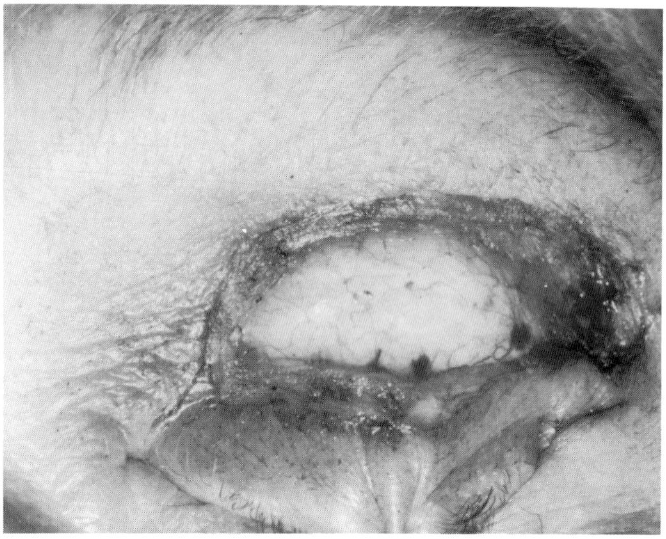

Figure 61.10. Intraoperative view of orbital septum.

identified. We recommend that the less experienced blepharoplasty surgeon open the septum at a higher level, which might preclude levator injury. We advocate that the assistant put a downward traction (gently) on the lid to put the aponeurosis in an orientation away from the dissection.

The ptosis may also be caused iatrogenically during wound closure, where sutures are placed too high into the aponeurosis, which will cause tethering. Of course, in our discussion of ptosis as a postoperative complication, we have taken for granted a thorough preoperative evaluation ruling out preexisting ptosis with or without a levator dehiscence. The best treatment of postblepharoplasty ptosis is also "tincture of time." The patient is observed to see if there is any improvement in lid excursion. If not, the ptosis is best handled surgically either by direct repair of the aponeurosis defect (Fig. 61.11), levator resection for 2–4 mm and full-thickness repair or tarsomyomectomy for 2 mm or less (10).

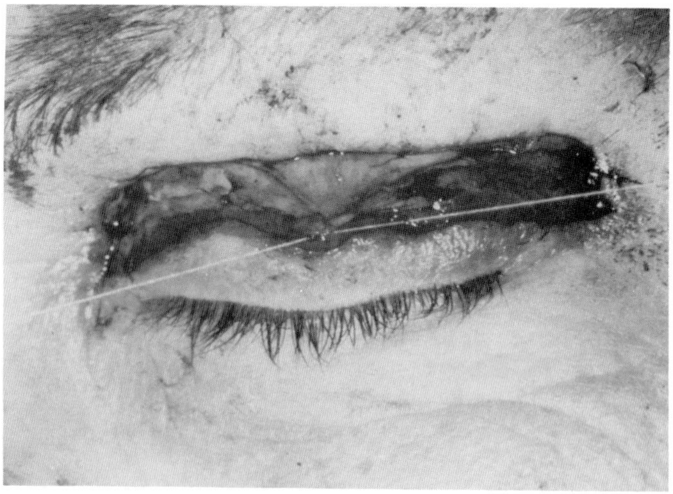

Figure 61.11. Direct repair of aponeurosis defect.

LID ASYMMETRY

Asymmetry of lid contour and fullness, also referred to as "sulcus deformities," are also common postoperative complications. These are encountered as a result of too much fat being excised from one of the upper lids. There is a resulting depressed area that is very difficult to treat. Rotation flaps of orbicularis muscle have been advocated by some, while others have attempted a wide variety of alloplastic and autogenous materials to rectify the volume loss (25–28). If tolerated by the patient, a mild sulcus deformity can be matched by removal of fat from the other side. The best advice on handling this complication is graded fat removal that is measured on the table and constant intraoperative viewing of the preoperative polaroid photographs to remind the surgeon of which fat pockets specifically need removal.

Lid crease abnormalities may be the most commonly encountered complication of upper eyelid blepharoplasty surgery, and to the patient they are probably the most distressing. If the lid crease is too low postoperatively, it is usually a sign of failure to incorporate the levator aponeurosis into the wound closure and will manifest itself as a low crease with a redundancy of skin (usually not real) (16, 28). This is rectified with one of the lid crease procedures usually referred to as "supratarsal fixation techniques" (10, 22, 23). The original description by Sheen has since been modified by others, but the essential goal of any lid crease procedure is to fix the skin edges to either the superior border of the tarsus or levator aponeurosis at a level coincident with the new crease. Parenthetically, we would like to add that our experience in dealing with a lid crease that is too high has been dismal. Our experience with fat grafts and alloplastics cannot be recommended to the reader.

WEBBING

The surgeon often faces webbing or pseudoepicanthal folds medially when the incision has been placed too far medially or too much skin excised medially. This problem can be dealt with by using a Y-to-V plasty.

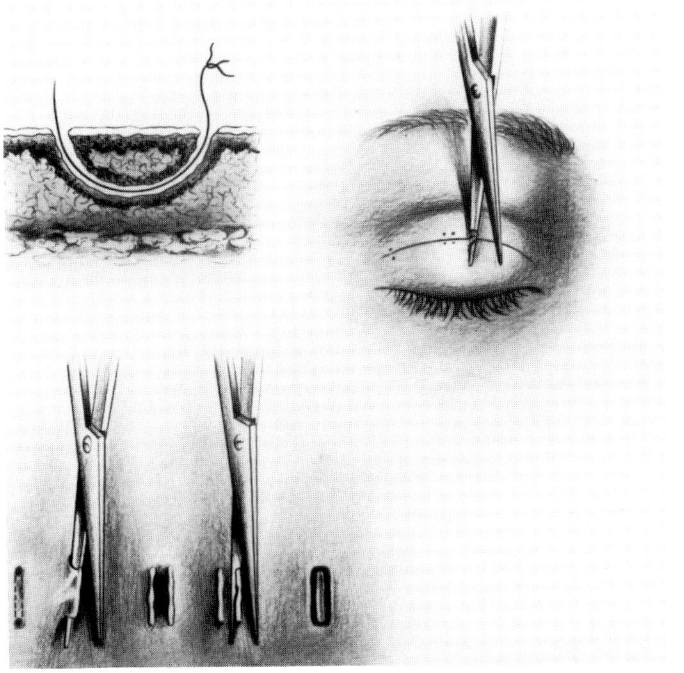

Figure 61.12. Unroofing cysts with sharp scissors. (From Converse JM: Clinical note: treatment of epithelialized suture tracts of the eyelid by marsupialization. *Plast Reconstr Surg* 38: 576, 1966.)

SUBCUTANEOUS HEMATOMAS

Less frequently encountered complications of upper eyelid blepharoplasty include small subcutaneous hematomas, which are best treated with warm compresses. Suture tunnels are a function of epithelialization around the sutures when sutures are left beyond 5 days. Unroofing the tunnel with a scissors or blade and exposing the subcutaneous keratin is the treatment of choice (29). Cysts are similarly treated by unroofing the cyst with a sharp scissors (Fig. 61.12).

WOUND DEHISCENCE

Wound dehiscence is rare, but when it does occur it may be handled either surgically with resuturing of the wound or by observation; the criteria as to how the dehiscence is handled is its location. A wound dehiscence in the central or even medial part of the lid will often close spontaneously. This is due to the natural action of the orbicularis oculi muscle to close the wound. Lateral wound defects near or beyond the lateral canthal angle are under relatively greater tension and need to be closed surgically.

SECONDARY INFECTION AND HYPERTROPHIC SCARRING

Infection secondary to blepharoplasty is very rare, mainly because of the excellent blood supply to the eyelids. Warm compresses and antibiotics are usually sufficient to handle any infection, which is always superficial.

Hypertrophic scars are rarely encountered in the eyelid region, even in scar-forming patients. This is also probably due to the excellent vasculature of the eyelids. When hypertrophic scarring is present, a subcutaneous injection of triamcinolone may be helpful in avoiding a big scar (18).

REFERENCES

1. Putterman A: Evaluation of the cosmetic oculoplastic surgery patient. In: *Cosmetic Oculoplastic Surgery*. New York, Grune & Stratton, 1982, p 12–26.
2. Mustarde JC: Problems and pitfalls in blepharoplasty. *Aesthet Plast Surg* 1: 349–354, 1978.
3. Anderson RL, Edwards JJ: Bilateral visual loss after blepharoplasty. *Ann Plast Surg* 5: 288–292, 1980.
4. DeMere M, Wood T, Austin W: Eye complications with blepharoplasty or other eyelid surgery. *Plast Reconstr Surg* 53: 634, 1974.
5. Hartley J, Lester J, Schatten W: Acute retrobulbar hemorrhage during elective blepharoplasty. *Plast Reconstr Surg* 52: 8, 1973.
6. Heinje J, Huston J: Blindness after blepharoplasty: mechanism of early reversal. *Plast Reconstr Surg* 61: 34, 1978.
7. Hepler R, Sugimora G, Straatsma B: On the occurence of blindness in association with blepharoplasty. *Plast Reconstr Surg* 57: 233, 1976.
8. Putterman A: Temporary blindness after cosmetic blepharoplasty. *Am J Ophthalmol* 80: 1081, 1975.
9. Waller R: Is blindness a realistic complication in blepharoplasty procedures? *Ophthalmology* 85: 730–735, 1978.
10. Putterman A, Urist MJ: Reconstruction of the upper eyelid crease and fold. *Arch Ophthalmol* 94: 1941–1952, 1976.
11. Boo-Chai K: Plastic construction of the superior palpebral fold. *Plast Reconstr Surg* 31: 74, 1963.
12. Fernandez LR: Double eyelid operation in the oriental in Hawaii. *Plast Reconstr Surg* 25: 257, 1960.
13. Pang RG: Surgical formation of upper lid fold. *Arch Ophthalmol* 65: 783–784, 1961.
14. Callahan MA: Prevention of blindness after blepharoplasty. *Ophthalmology* 90: 1047–1051, 1983.
15. Paris GL, Waltuch G: Salicyclate-induced bleeding problem in ophthalmic plastic surgery. *Ophthal Surg* 13: 627–629, 1982.
16. Hornblass A: Ptosis and pseudoptosis and blepharoplasty. In *Clinics in Plastic Surgery, Symposium on Modern Trends in Blepharoplasty*. Philadelphia, WB Saunders, 1981, p 811–830.
17. Tenzel R: Brow lift and upper lid blepharoplasty. In *Symposium on Diseases and Surgery of the Lid, Lacrimal Apparatus, and Orbit*. St. Louis, CV Mosby, 1982, p 216.
18. Rees TD: *Aesthetic Plastic Surgery*. Philadelphia, WB Saunders, 1980, p 534.
19. Jelks G, McCord C: Dry eye syndrome and other tear film abnormalities. *Clin Plast Surg* 8: 803–809, 1981.
20. Rees TD: Dry eye complications after blepharoplasty. *Plast Reconstr Surg* 56: 375, 1975.
21. McCord CD: Complications of upper lid blepharoplasty. In Putterman A (ed): *Cosmetic Oculoplastic Surgery*. New York, Grune & Stratton, 1982, p 250–274.
22. Flowers RS: Anchor blepharoplasty. In *Transactions of the Sixth International Conjunctival Plastic Surgery*. Paris, Masson, 1976, p 471.
23. Sheen JH: Supratarsal fixation in upper blepharoplasty. *Plast Reconstr Surg* 54: 424, 1974.
24. Baylis HI, Sutcliffe RT, Fett D: Levator injury during blepharoplasty. *Arch Ophthalmology* 102: 570, 1984.
25. Smith B, Lisman R: Use of sclera and liquid collagen in the camouflage of superior sulcus deformities. *Ophthalmology* 9: 230–235, 1983.
26. Vistnes LM, Paris GL: Uses of RTV silicone in orbital reconstruction. *Am J Ophthalmol* 83: 577–581, 1977.
27. Soll DB: The anophthalmic socket. *Ophthalmology* 89: 407–423, 1982.
28. Tenzel R: Surgical treatment of complications in cosmetic blepharoplasty. *Clin Plast Surg* 5: 517–523, 1978.
29. Converse JM: Clinical note: treatment of epithelialized suture tracts of the eyelid by marsupialization. *Plast Reconstr Surg* 38: 576, 1966.

CHAPTER 62

Management of Complications of Lower Eyelid Blepharoplasty

NORMAN SHORR, M.D., F.A.C.S.
STUART R. SEIFF, M.D.

NORMAL POSITION AND FUNCTION OF THE LOWER EYELID

The normal, unoperated lower eyelid margin lies tangent to the inferior limbus and may be digitally elevated to the superior limbus in the primary position. The normal Occidental lateral canthus is 2 mm superior to the medial canthus. The lower eyelid is made up of three separate lamellae (Fig. 62.1). Each lamella must be evaluated for possible laxity or contraction in both the horizontal and vertical planes.

The anterior lamella is composed of skin and orbicularis. Its vertical length may be thought of as the distance from the lower eyelid margin to the nasal labial fold and corner of the mouth. It is for this reason that many surgeons have the patient open the mouth before trimming excess anterior lamellar tissue in lower eyelid blepharoplasty.

The middle lamella is composed of the orbital septum,

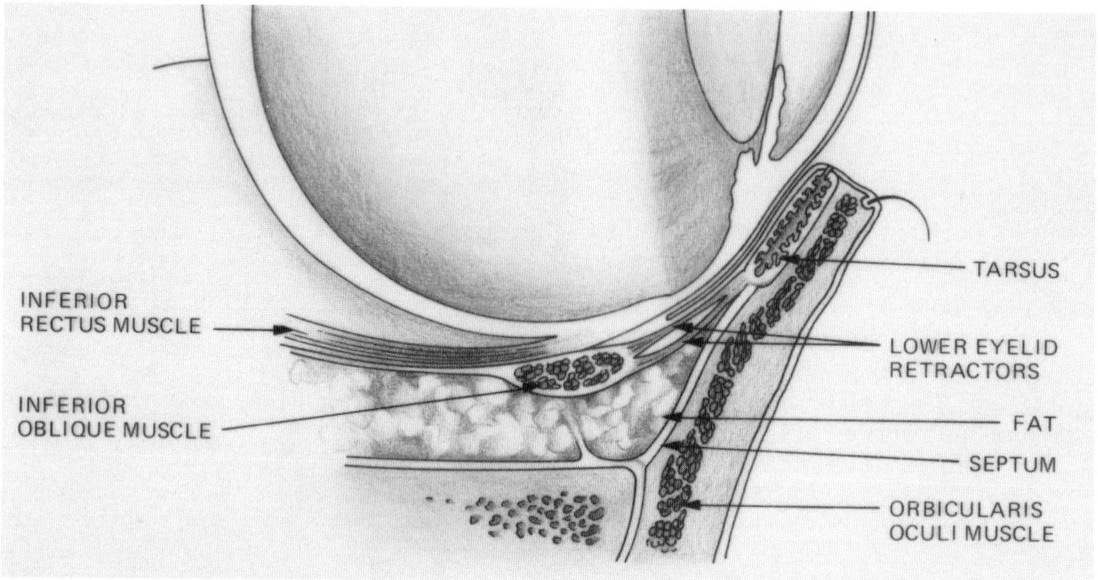

Figure 62.1. Normal lower eyelid anatomy.

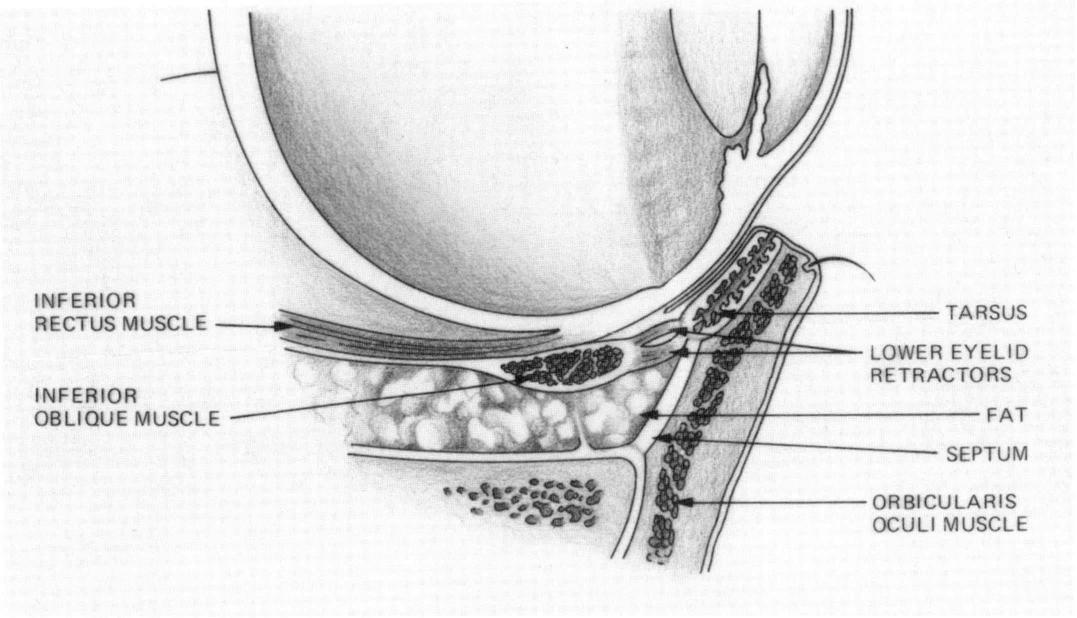

Figure 62.2. Lower eyelid retraction with anterior and middle lamellar vertical shortening.

which extends from the inferior border of the tarsus to the orbital rim. The middle lamella may be shortened if it is inadvertently included in a skin muscle flap or sutured after fat removal, if a cicatrix develops, or if the technique of infratarsal fixation is employed (1). It has been postulated that middle lamellar cicatrix may occur due to excessive cautery, accumulation of blood at this level, or patching of the lower eyelid in an inferior position (Fig. 62.2).

The posterior lamella consists of conjunctiva and the lower eyelid retractors. Unlike either anterior or middle lamellar problems, posterior lamellar abnormalities are rarely seen following blepharoplasty.

A normal, unoperated upper eyelid usually protects the cornea regardless of any lower eyelid malposition. However, when the upper eyelids have undergone blepharoplasty, the lower eyelids are necessary to provide corneal protection and comfort. In the presence of vertically shortened upper eyelids and a lower eyelid malposition, lagophthalmos and exposure keratopathy may result.

GOALS OF SURGERY

In lower eyelid blepharoplasty, the maintenance of a normal position of the lower eyelid is far more important than the creation of a tight, smooth lower eyelid. In the upper eyelid, a lid fold allows enough skin for eyelid movement. The lower eyelid, however, because it does not have a lid fold, must have enough redundant skin to allow for superior motion of the eyelid in upgaze. The priorities of lower eyelid blepharoplasty are (*a*) to remove the reductant fat bags; (*b*) not to distort the anatomy and leave an unattractive, uncomfortable eye; and (*c*) to remove some of the redundant skin and muscle.

Identifying horizontal eyelid laxity decreases the incidence of lower eyelid blepharoplasty complications. This is determined with the "distraction test" and the "snap test."

The lower eyelid distraction test is performed by grasping the lower eyelid and pulling it anteriorly away from the globe. The distance between the globe and the central eyelid margin is measured or estimated. If this distance is greater than 8 to 10 mm, lower eyelid laxity exists and the lateral canthal tendon is attenuated. This patient will be at increased risk for developing any of the lower eyelid malpositions (Fig. 62.3).

The snap test, also called the "snap-back test", is performed in the following manner. The patient is instructed to look straight ahead and not to blink. The lower eyelid is pulled inferiorly by the examiner's finger and released. If the eyelid does not spontaneously return to its normal apposition to the globe before the patient's next blink, the test is positive (Fig. 62.4). The lower eyelid therefore has inadequate tone, and the patient is at increased risk for developing lower eyelid retraction (scleral show), ectropion, or round lateral canthus (2).

Horizontal eyelid margin shortening procedures should be included with the lower eyelid blepharoplasty when either of these tests are positive.

COMPLICATIONS

The most common complication of lower eyelid blepharoplasty is lower eyelid retraction (scleral show) with or without a rounded lateral canthal angle (2). Frank ectropion is more infrequent (3–6). Infection and loss of vision are extremely rare and will not be discussed further here.

Anterior lamellar shortage problems result in inferior

and anterior rotation of the tarsal plate; the former contributes to lower eyelid retraction, and the latter contributes to ectropion. Shortening of the middle lamella is manifest by inferior displacement of the tarsus and, concomitantly, inferior displacement of the lower eyelid margin. Thus, a pure anterior lamellar vertical shortening would result in ectropion. A pure middle lamellar shortening would result in eyelid retraction without ectropion.

A "forced elevation" test of the lower eyelid is mandatory in any preoperative evaluation of a patient with lower eyelid malposition. This procedure may be done digitally in the office or may be performed with forceps at the time of surgery. Stress lines will help determine which of the lower eyelid lamellae is vertically shortened, tethered, or both. Although both isolated anterior and middle lamellar problems can exist, many cases appear to include shortening of both lamellae (Fig. 62.5).

The functional symptoms that result from the combination of lower eyelid retraction and vertical shortening of the upper eyelid center upon lagophthalmos and resultant exposure keratopathy. Even under the best circumstances (good precorneal tear film and no corneal irregularities), comfort may be maintained only with constant daytime artificial tears and ointment and taping the eyelids at night.

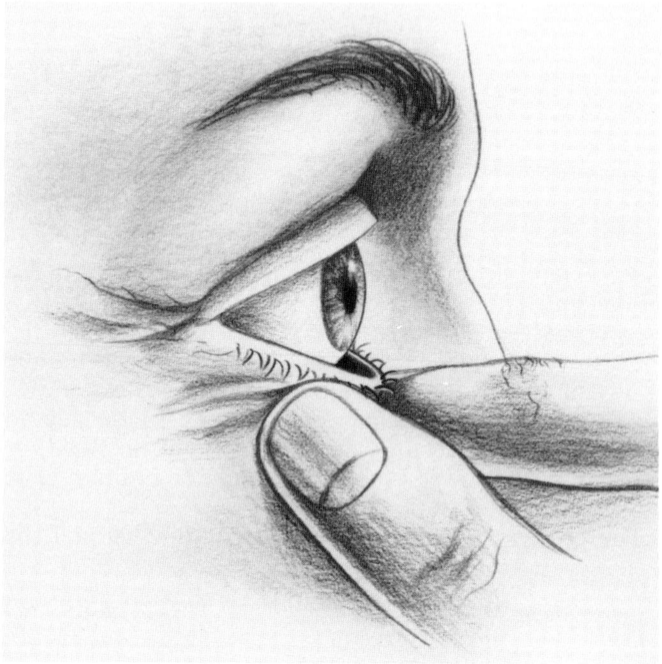

Figure 62.3. The lower eyelid "distraction test," which is used to identify horizontal eyelid laxity.

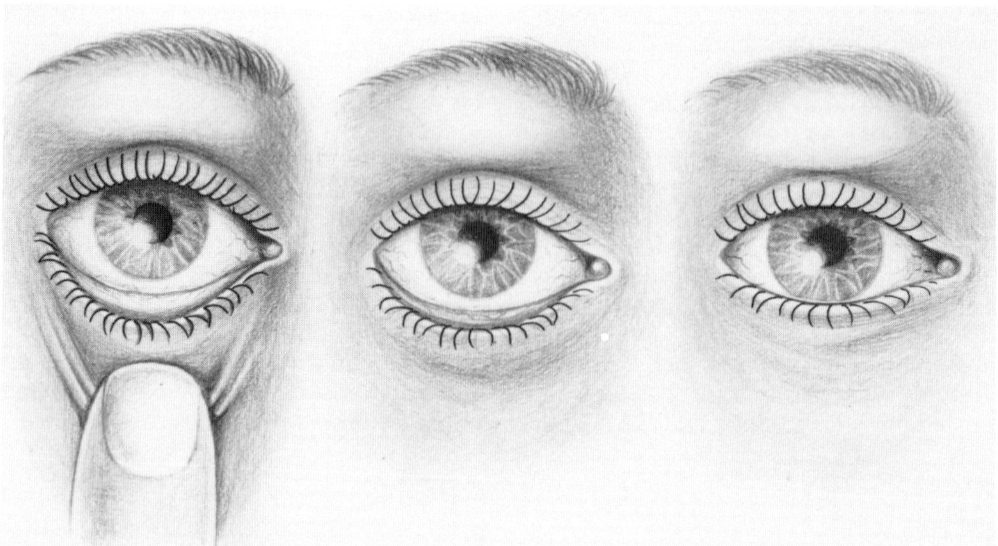

Figure 62.4. The "snap test" is also used to detect horizontal eyelid laxity.

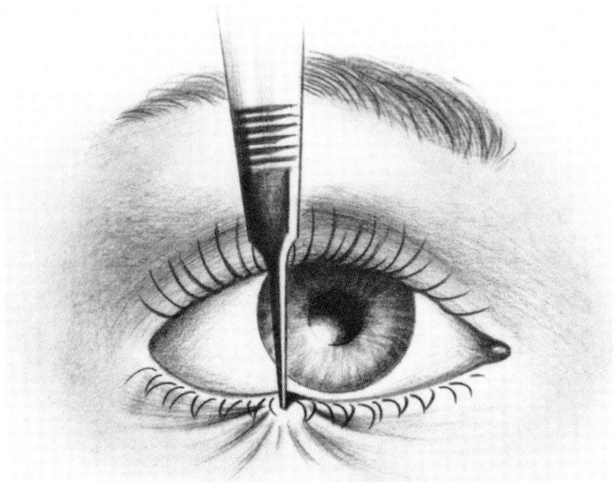

Figure 62.5. "Forced elevation" test is used to determine location and degree of restriction.

SURGICAL CORRECTION OF COMPLICATIONS

There are several techniques for dealing with round lateral canthus, lower eyelid retraction and ectropion which may result from lower eyelid blepharoplasty (Fig. 62.6) (7, 8). The traditional method includes the use of a skin graft with or without a horizontal shortening and lateral canthal resuspension. An alternative method is the "Madame Butterfly" procedure (9), which can be performed with or without an ear cartilage graft (10). In this procedure, the need for a skin graft, which may be cosmetically unacceptable, is eliminated. Occasionally a skin graft may also be needed for the upper eyelid to eliminate severe lagophthalmos. These methods are outlined in the following sections.

LOWER EYELID SKIN GRAFTING

The traditional method of treating lower eyelid retraction, round lateral canthus, and ectropion utilizes a full-thickness skin graft. A carefully performed lower eyelid skin graft procedure will often result in an excellent functional and cosmetic outcome. Although surgeons can present an optimistic attitude, they must stress possible postoperative problems with thickness, color, and corrugation. Approximately 75% of patients who require lower eyelid skin graft also have severe lower eyelid laxity and will benefit from lower eyelid horizontal shortening and lateral canthal resuspension. This decision is made only after the cicatrix is lysed and the graft bed created.

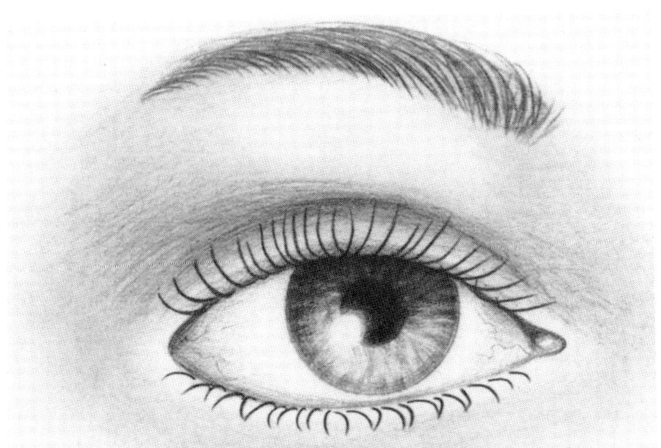

Figure 62.6. Preoperative appearance of lower eyelid retraction and rounded lateral canthal angle.

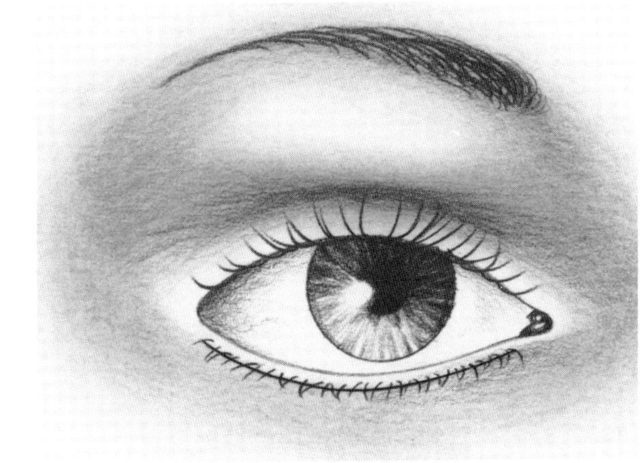

Figure 62.7. Infralash incision.

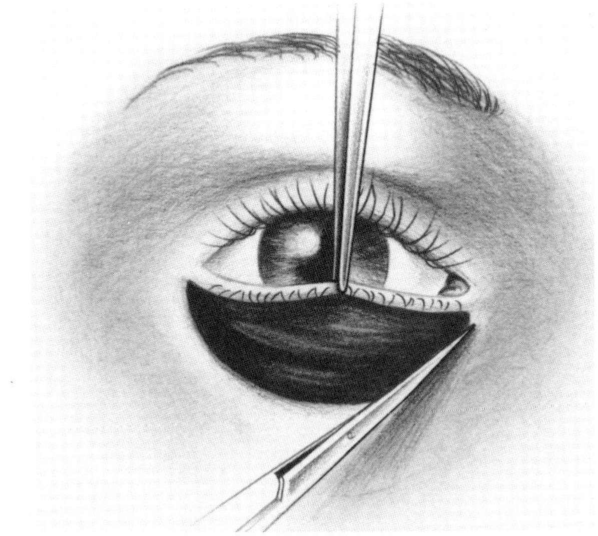

Figure 62.8. Creation of bed with lysis of cicatrix.

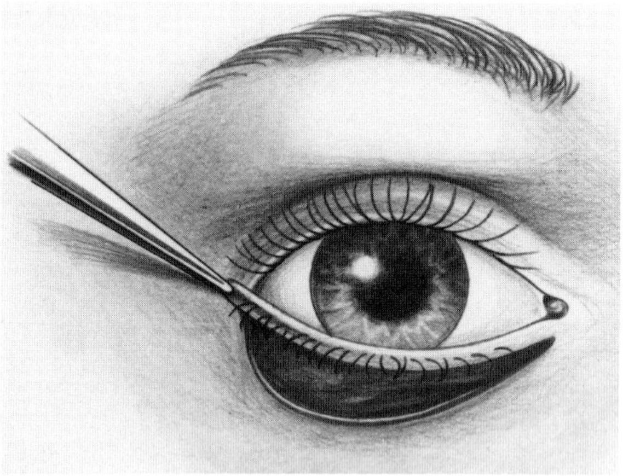

Figure 62.9. Determination of horizontal eyelid laxity.

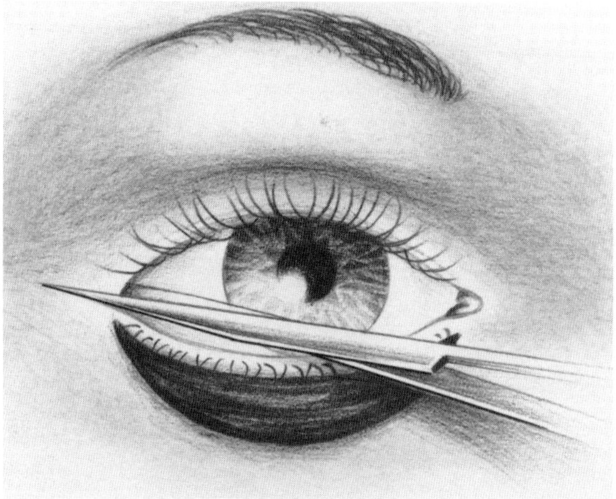

Figure 62.10. Lateral canthotomy.

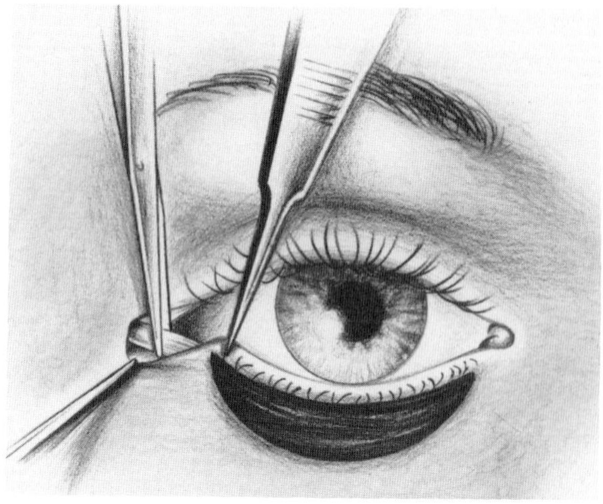

Figure 62.11. Lysis of inferior limb of lateral canthal tendon.

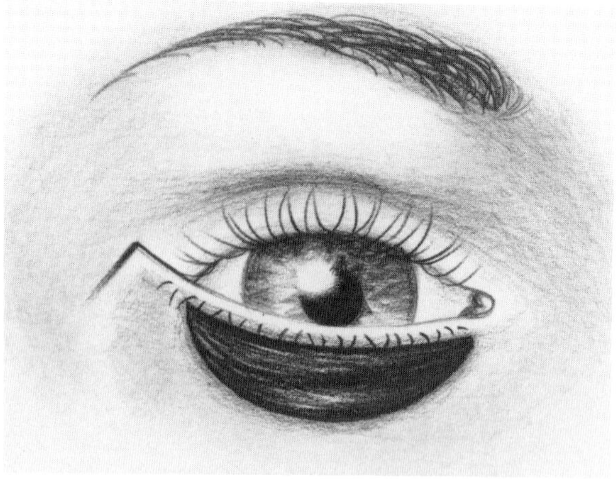

Figure 62.12. Determination of new lateral canthal position.

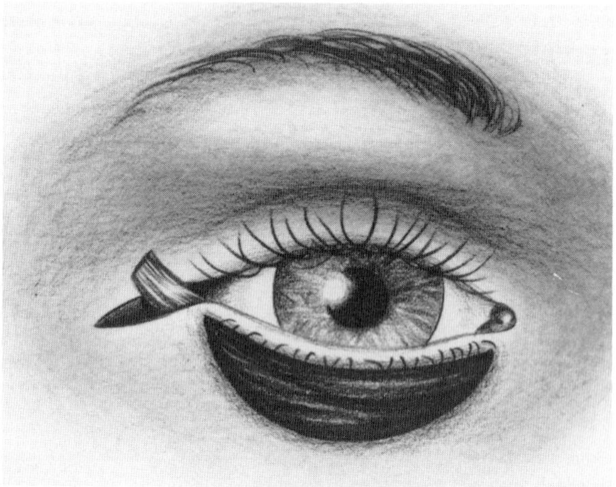

Figure 62.13. Creation of lateral tarsal tongue.

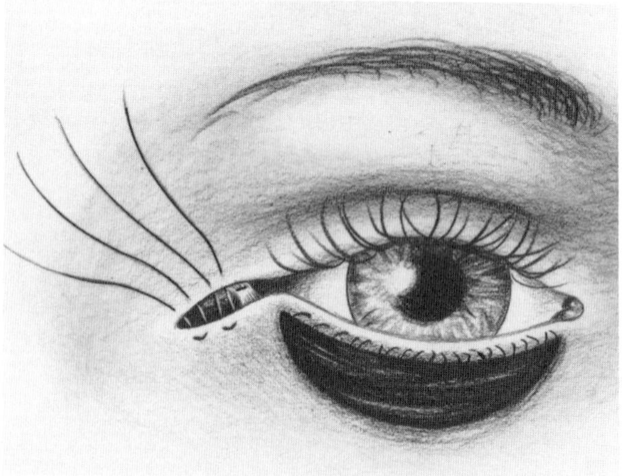

Figure 62.14. Suturing of tarsal tongue to periosteum and closure of lateral canthus.

An infralash incision is made from the punctum medially to a point just below the lateral canthus (Fig. 62.7). With superior traction on the lower eyelid margin, the cicatrix of both the anterior and middle lamellae is dissected until the lower eyelid margin can be elevated to the middle pupil in primary position (Fig. 62.8). At this point, the lower eyelid is evaluated for laxity (Fig. 62.9). If there is no horizontal laxity, a skin graft may be placed as described below. If horizontal eyelid laxity is present, a lateral canthotomy is made and the inferior limb of the lateral canthal tendon is lysed (Figs. 62.10 and 62.11). The lower eyelid is draped over the lateral canthus to determine the amount of horizontal laxity (Fig. 62.12). A tarsal tongue is created by excision of the surrounding tissue (Fig. 62.13). The tongue is trimmed to the appropriate length and sutured to the periosteum at the lateral orbital rim. This creates a sharp lateral canthal angle. A 5-0 Dexon suture on a ½-circle needle is used (Fig. 62.14). The canthus is closed with a 6-0 mild cuticular chromic or 6-0 nylon suture. Stay sutures are passed from the eyebrow, through the upper and lower eyelid margin, back through the eyebrow, and tied. These sutures place the lower eyelid on a moderate stretch. Do not pull the lower eyelid margin above the pupil or a corrugation of the lower eyelid may result.

The exact size of the graft bed should be measured and a full-thickness skin graft should be obtained. The upper eyelid, posterior auricular region, supraclavicular region, and inner upper arm are the donor sites in order of preference for color and texture match. The graft is placed in the bed and trimmed to the exact size necessary. Do not use a larger graft in anticipation of shrinkage. A graft that is too large will invariably corrugate and thicken. A smooth flat graft of good texture and color that is just a little small is far better than a corrugated graft. Do not cut holes in the graft. The graft should be sutured in place with 6-0 black silk or any suture of choice (Fig. 62.15). Do not tie the suture over a bolster or a crater may be created in the middle of the graft. Place a piece of Telfa over the graft and then use a firm dressing of two eye patches, benzoin and paper tape. Leave the dressing undisturbed for 5–7 days.

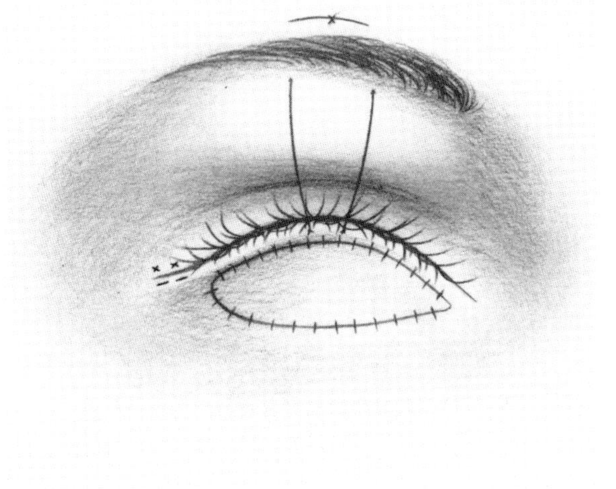

Figure 62.15. Placement of lower eyelid skin graft.

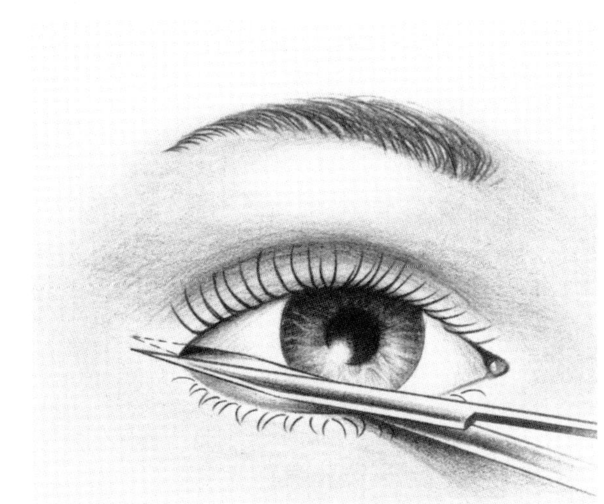

Figure 62.16. Lateral canthotomy.

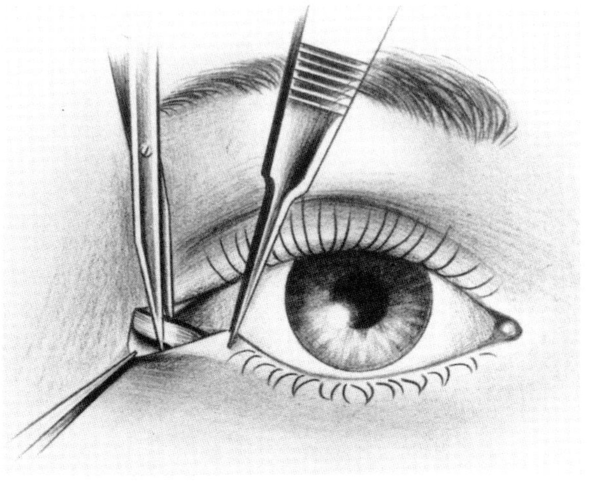

Figure 62.17. Lysis of inferior limb lateral canthal tendon.

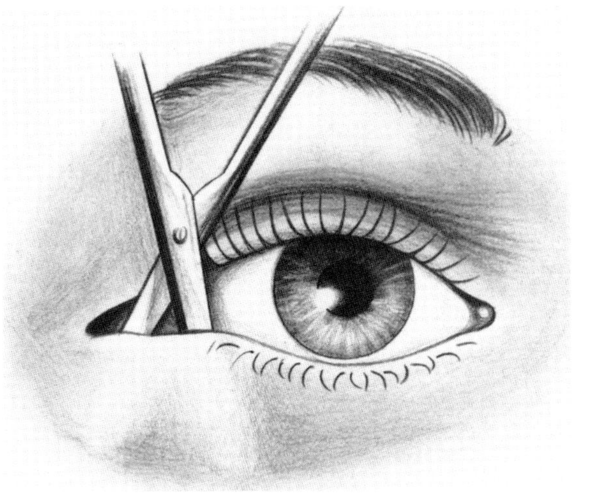

Figure 62.18. Lateral and inferomedial undermining of cheek tissues.

"MADAME BUTTERFLY" PROCEDURE

This procedure is an alternative to using a skin graft in the patient with lower eyelid retraction and a vertically shortened upper eyelid. The goal is to afford a functional improvement in eyelid closure and elevation of the lower eyelid and lateral canthus without the use of a skin graft. The typical patient presents with lower eyelid retraction, a rounded lateral canthal angle, horizontal laxity of the lower eyelid, and vertical shortening of the upper eyelid, which all work together to create the obvious cosmetic and functional defects. This procedure eliminates the middle lamella cicatrix that tethers the tarsus to the inferior orbital rim. The lower eyelid is elevated such that it protects the inferior aspect of the cornea from exposure keratopathy, and the previously inferiorly displaced and rounded lateral canthal angle is elevated and reconstructed in a position 4 mm higher than the medial canthus. This creation of an exaggerated Mongolian slant gives the procedure its name.

The Madame Butterfly procedure may be performed either under local infiltrative anesthesia or general anesthesia. On the operating table, a forced elevation test of the lower eyelid is performed. This maneuver should be repeated at intervals throughout the procedure. The first surgical step is a lateral canthotomy and severing of the inferior limb of the lateral canthal tendon (Figs. 62.16 and 62.17). Through this incision, a pair of Stevens scissors is used to undermine the cheek tissue at the level of periosteum and temporalis fascia, laterally and inferomedially to the lateral canthal angle (Fig. 62.18). The lateral extent of this undermining is directly proportional to the amount of lower eyelid elevation required. Once the cheek tissues have been undermined, the cheek over and lateral to the malar eminence may be elevated. This relieves all tension on the anterior lamella. If the lower eyelid is still fixed on forced traction elevation, the resistance must be at the middle lamella.

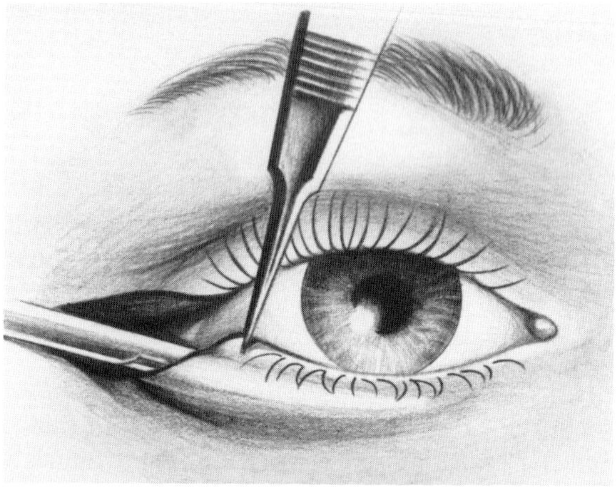

Figure 62.19. *In glove* lysis of middle lamellar cicatrix.

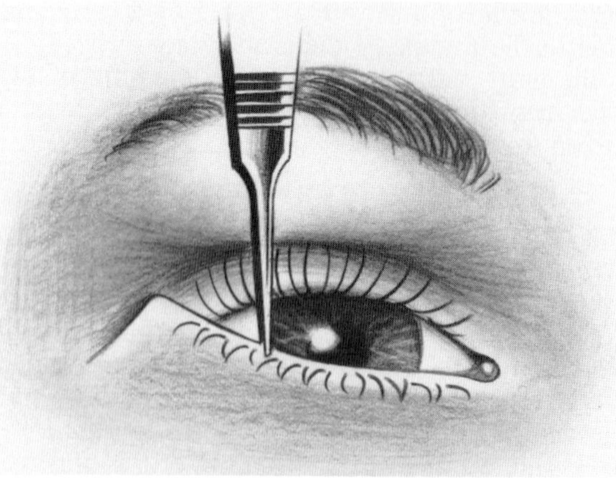

Figure 62.20. Improved mobility of lower eyelid. (Illustrated with eyelid forced elevation test).

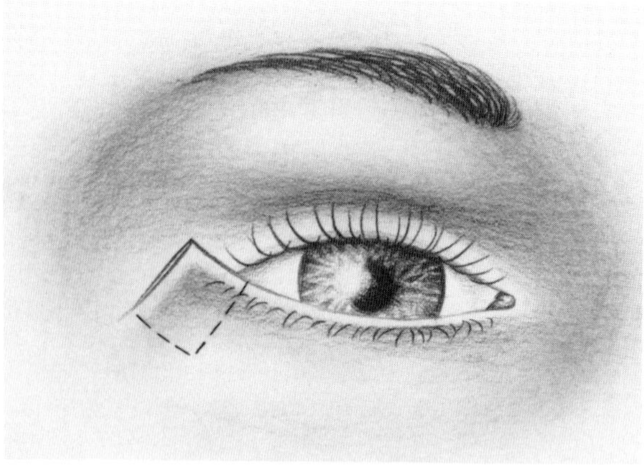

Figure 62.21. Determination of new lateral canthal angle position.

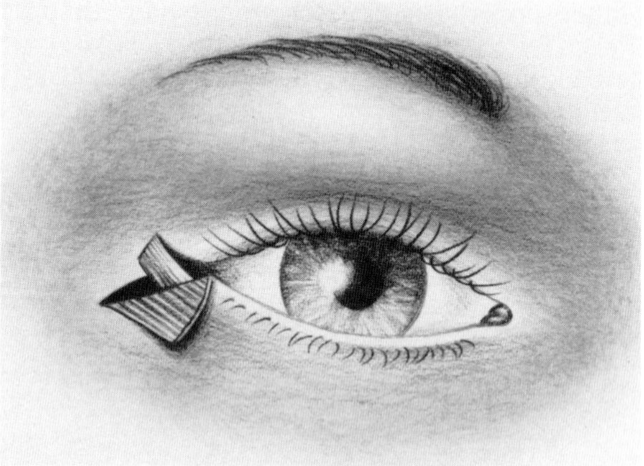

Figure 62.22. Creation of lateral tarsal tongue.

Attention is then turned toward lysis of the middle lamella (orbital septum) cicatrix. The Stevens scissors are inserted through the original canthotomy incision. A combination of blunt and sharp dissection through the deepest layers of the orbicularis and orbital septum is performed in an "in glove" fashion, such that the skin and the majority of the orbicularis remains anterior to the anterior scissor blade and the conjunctiva remains posterior to the posterior scissor blade (Fig. 62.19). The lower eyelid retractors are intimately attached to the conjunctiva and damage to them is unlikely. However, no harm will come from division of the lower eyelid retractors. The endpoint of this dissection is determined by the eyelid forced elevation technique in which the lower eyelid margin is grasped by a pair of forceps and elevated. Successful dissection and lysis of the middle lamella cicatrix is indicated by the ability to elevate the lower eyelid margin to at least the middle pupil, if not the superior limbus (Fig. 62.20).

At this point, the operation leaves the traditional bounds of eyelid surgery, and the original canthotomy incision is extended 1–4 cm laterally to the lateral canthal angle at the level of the periosteum. The extent of this incision beyond the lateral canthal angle is determined by the amount of necessary cheek and lower eyelid elevation. With sufficient cheek elevation, the anterior lamella be-

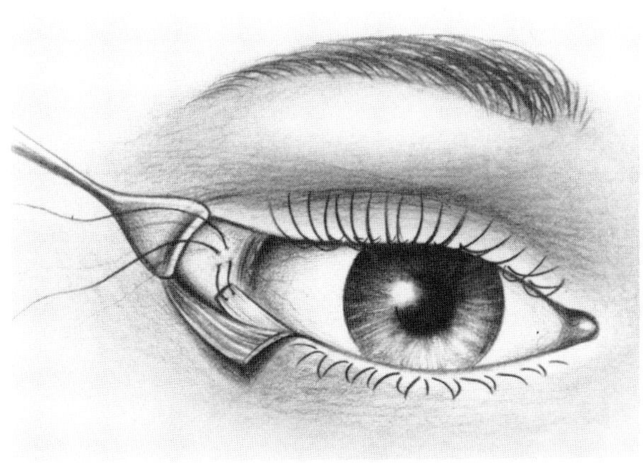

Figure 62.23. Periosteal suspension of lateral tarsus.

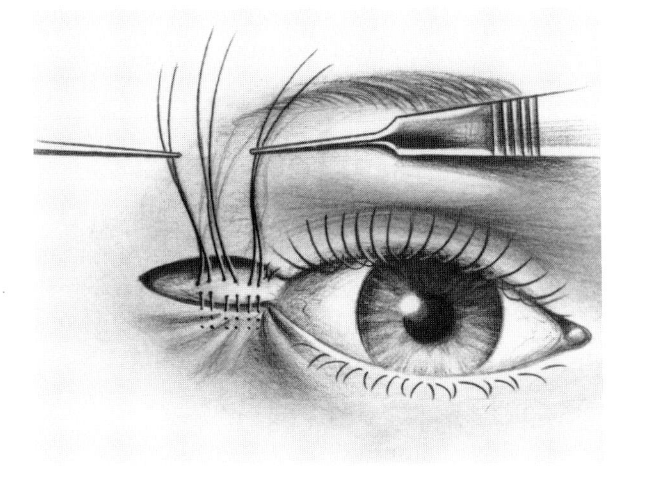

Figure 62.24. Periosteal suspension of deep cheek tissue.

comes adequate. The middle lamella is lysed and the posterior lamella is stretched.

The next step is the lower eyelid horizontal shortening and reconstruction of the lateral canthal angle. A tongue of tarsus is fashioned from the most lateral aspect of the lower eyelid, and the periosteum is identified on the lateral orbital rim. The exact location of the resuspension site is determined by the degree of lower eyelid elevation being sought (Fig. 62.21). Generally, the lateral canthal angle is elevated 2 mm higher than its normal anatomic position, resulting in a lateral canthal angle 4 mm higher than the medial canthal angle. The tongue of tarsus is placed in position and horizontally shortened to provide appropriate lower eyelid tension (Fig. 62.22). The resuspension procedure involves suturing the tongue of tarsus to the periosteum with a 5-0 Dexon or Vicryl horizontal mattress suture (Fig. 62.23).

Attention is once again turned to the cheek flap. Using double-armed, 5-0 Dexon or Vicryl horizontal mattress sutures, the surgeon firmly affixes the deep tissues of the cheek to the underlying periosteum at a level that provides sufficient elevation of the lower eyelid (Fig. 62.24). Finally, the skin is closed with great care to reform the lateral canthal angle. In contrast to the preoperative condition, the cheek and eyelid now resist inferior traction (Figs. 62.25 and 62.26).

The net result of this procedure should be to impart a slightly greater than normal Mongoloid slant to the eyelids (Fig. 62.27). With time, the tissues involved in the elevation of the cheek tend to relax and return the lateral canthal region to a more normal Occidental appearance. However, an elevated lower eyelid, sharp lateral canthal angle, and coverage of the lower cornea are maintained (Fig. 62.28).

"MADAME BUTTERFLY" PROCEDURE WITH EAR CARTILAGE GRAFT

The Madame Butterfly operation is performed with the surgeon's full understanding that two natural phenomena are always working against the procedure during the healing phase. First, gravity will tend to pull the cheek and eyelid inferiorly. The cheek and eyelid have been sutured to bone at the orbital rim and lateral to the orbital rim. If the deep tissues return to the preoperative position, they will drag the anterior lamella and eyelid margin inferiorly

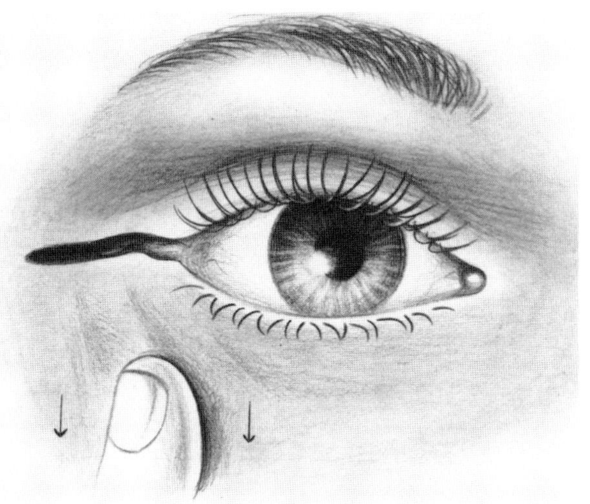

Figure 62.25. Suspended cheek and eyelid resist inferior traction.

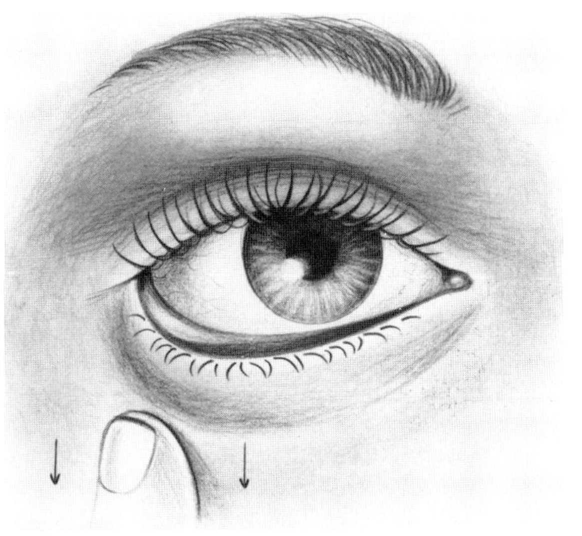

Figure 62.26. Preoperatively, cheek and eyelid yield to inferior traction.

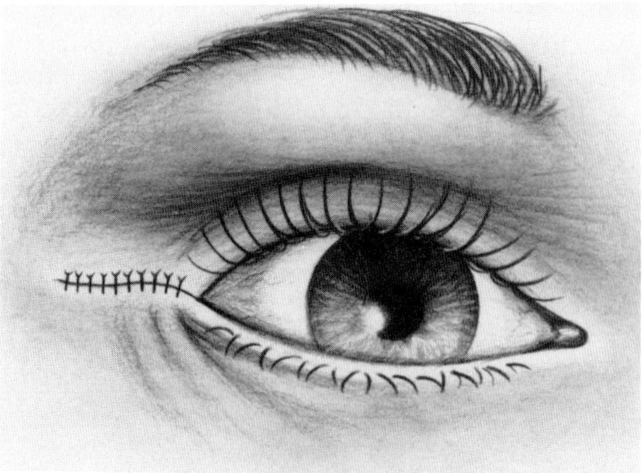

Figure 62.27. Immediate postoperative appearance. (Note overcorrection of lateral canthal angle elevation.)

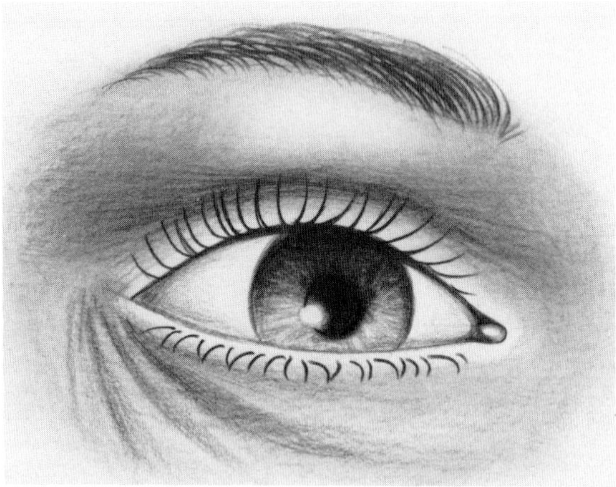

Figure 62.28. Final result. (Note lower eyelid protects inferior cornea).

with them. Second, the middle lamellar cicatrix, which has been lysed by the in-glove method and then pulled apart and left to heal by secondary intention, may contract and reapproximately itself. This may pull the lower eyelid margin inferiorly once again.

In the great majority of patients undergoing the Madame Butterfly procedure, these two phenomena have not resulted in surgical failure. However, they always come into play to some degree. Initial planned surgical overcorrection is used to help compensate for this.

In cases in which there appears to be adequate or marginally adequate anterior lamella (skin), but the middle lamella is extensively involved with cicatrix, good judgement may suggest the placement of a middle lamellar spacer. An ear cartilage graft placed through a conjunctival approach is a method of placing such a spacer. It does not shrink and is cut to the exact size and shape. This graft is not visible and therefore not aesthetically offensive. It must be stressed that this procedure depends upon stretching an existing anterior lamella (skin) or combining the stretching with a cheek lift (Madame Butterfly procedure).

The procedure is performed just as the previously described Madame Butterfly procedure. The in-glove lysis of the middle lamellar cicatrix is replaced by the transconjunctival approach to the middle lamella (Fig. 62.29). The conjunctiva and lower eyelid retractors are divided and the lower eyelid margin is placed on a superior stretch. Continued dissection of the middle lamella is carried out as far inferiorly and as close to the skin as necessary to offer free elevation of the lower eyelid margin. At this point, the vertical and horizontal dimensions of the graft bed are measured. A graft of the exact size is taken from the ear. In preparing an ear cartilage graft, the ear is injected beneath the skin of the pinna anteriorly and posteriorly with 2% Xylocaine, 1:100,000 epinephrine and Wydase (Fig. 62.30). The ear is reflected anteriorly so that the margin and posterior surface are visible. A marking pencil inscribes an incision line on the posterior superior skin. A No. 15 blade incises the skin and Stevens scissors are used to reflect the skin posteriorly (Fig. 62.31). The exact size and shape of needed cartilage is marked with a

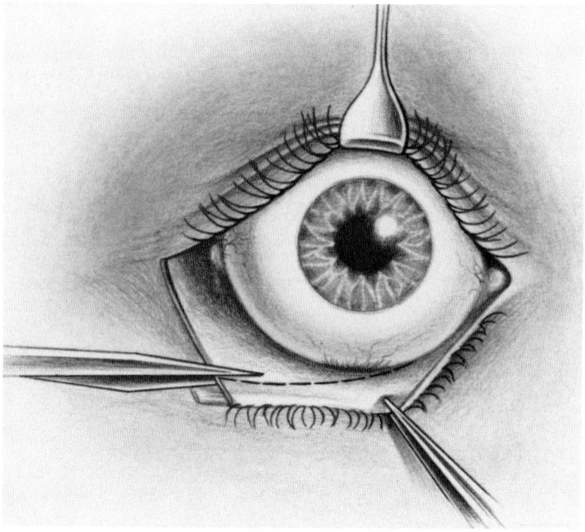

Figure 62.29. Transconjunctival approach to midlamella.

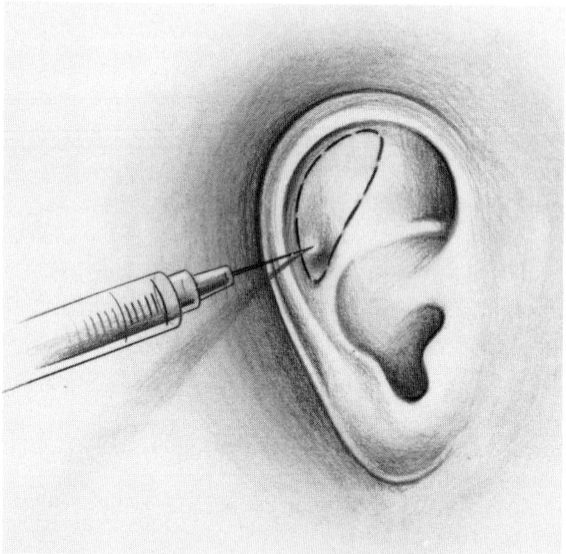

Figure 62.30. Outline of ear cartilage graft and infiltration of local anesthetic anteriorly and posteriorly.

marking pencil; then using a scalpel blade, the surgeon incises the cartilage with great care not to perforate the anterior skin (Fig. 62.32). The anterior skin may be ballooned at this point to avoid perforation. The full-thickness ear cartilage is removed (Figs. 62.33 and 62.34). The ear skin is closed with a running 4-0 cuticular chromic, or other, suture after hemostasis has been obtained. Hemorrhage may result in a "cauliflower ear." The ear will heal and no noticeable defect will remain. The ear cartilage may be split with a dermatome, or full-thickness ear cartilage may be used.

Plain gut absorbable suture, or a running "pull-out" 6-0 Prolene suture, may be used to secure the graft (Fig. 62.35). The remainder of the operation is identical to the previously described Madame Butterfly procedure.

UPPER EYELID SKIN GRAFT

Vertical shortening of the anterior lamella of the upper eyelid may result in lagophthalmos after upper eyelid blepharoplasty has been performed. This may be well tolerated when the lower eyelid is normal. However, in the presence of lower eyelid malposition, lagophthalmos often becomes symptomatic with exposure keratopathy. When treating these patients, a surgeon should first consider lateral canthal or lower eyelid surgery because of the possible unacceptable aesthetic results from upper eyelid skin grafts. In cases that require vertical lengthening of the upper eyelid anterior lamella, a skin graft should be performed with the least amount of skin, which will allow the upper eyelid to cover the lower limbus.

Before surgery, the surgeon should carefully evaluate eyebrow position. In most cases, the eyebrows have been too low before the blepharoplasty (11); that is, in retrospect, the patient may have been better off with eyebrow and forehead elevation and a very modest upper eyelid blepharoplasty. If the eyebrows are low, it will be easier and require a smaller graft to simply leave the eyebrows alone. If eyebrow elevation is performed with a skin graft, better general structure will be achieved, but a larger upper eyelid graft will be required.

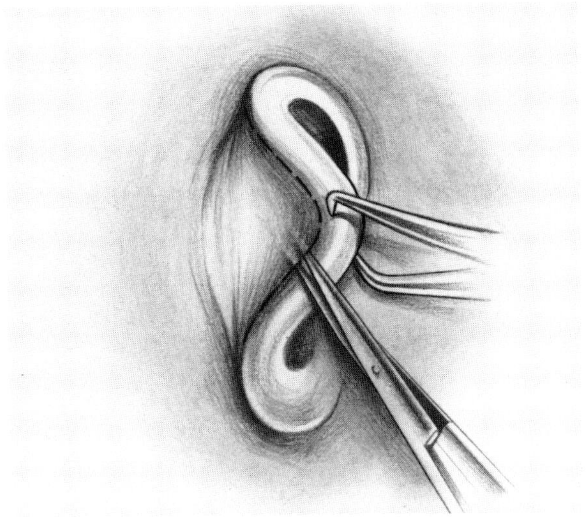

Figure 62.31. Skin incision and dissection of posterior skin from cartilage.

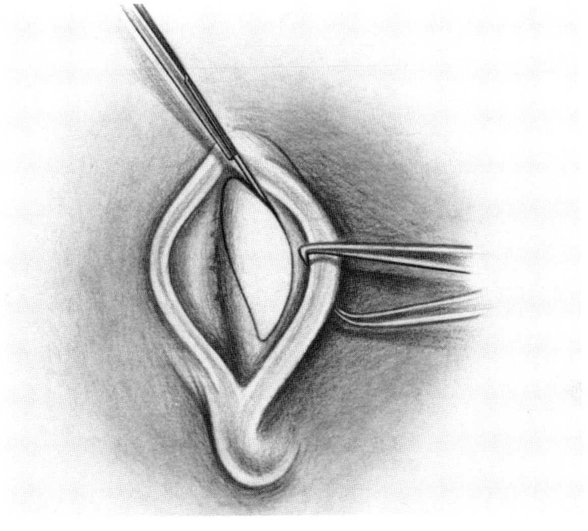

Figure 62.32. Incision of ear cartilage graft is done with care not to perforate the anterior skin.

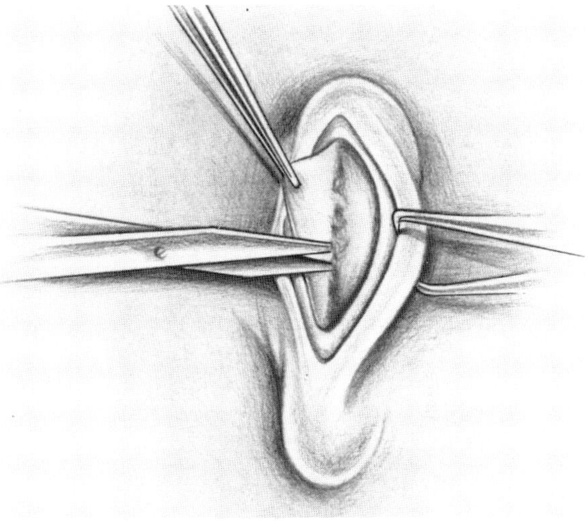

Figure 62.33. Dissection of ear cartilage from the anterior skin surface.

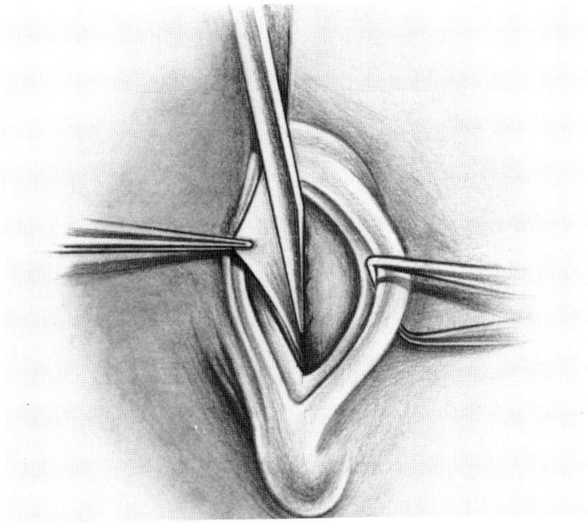

Figure 62.34. Excision of ear cartilage from donor.

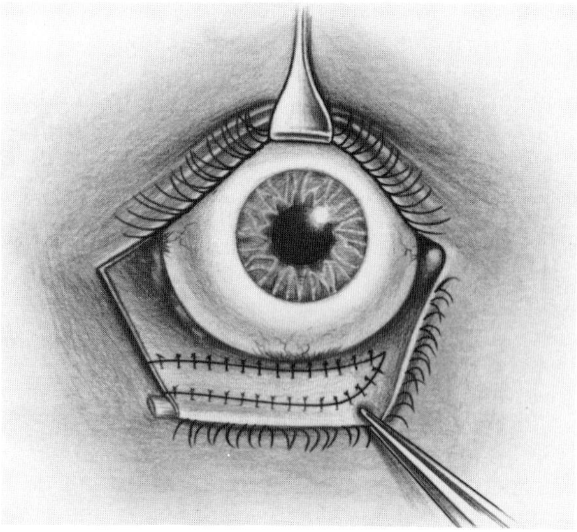

Figure 62.35. Placement of ear cartilage graft.

The surgical technique is as follows: Make an incision just superior to the lash line along the upper eyelid. Undermine the skin and lyse the cicatrix superiorly; proceed carefully so as not to cut the levator aponeurosis (Fig. 62.36). If necessary, carry the dissection superiorly to the lid crease. Constantly pull the lid margin inferiorly until it will cover the inferior limbus. At this point, obtain hemostasis primarily with pressure. If the lid crease is involved in the dissection, place three double-armed 6-0 black silk horizontal mattress sutures from the conjunctival surface through full-thickness eyelid and out the lid crease. Now, use three "reverse Frost" sutures from the cheek, through lower and upper eyelid margins, and back to the cheek. This will hold the upper eyelid on a stretch, with the upper eyelid margin at the lower limbus. Now, obtain a full-thickness skin graft of the exact dimensions of the bed. If necessary, place the eyelid crease sutures through the graft and tie them on themselves. Suture the skin graft in place with 6-0 black silk sutures (Fig. 62.37). Place a piece of Telfa on the graft. Tying a bolster over the skin graft is usually counterproductive. Place two eye patches firmly with benzoin and paper tape and do not disturb the patches for 7 days.

Time will usually improve all problems associated with skin grafts. If there is unsatisfactory thickening, whitening, or corrugation of the graft after 3 months, one must consider removing and replacing the graft. Of course, the replacement graft may not be as good as the graft you have replaced. At approximately 6 weeks, areas of hypertrophic graft thickening may be injected with 0.1 ml of Kenalog (10 mg/cc). These injections may be repeated once or twice at monthly intervals to soften and flatten the hypertrophic areas of the graft.

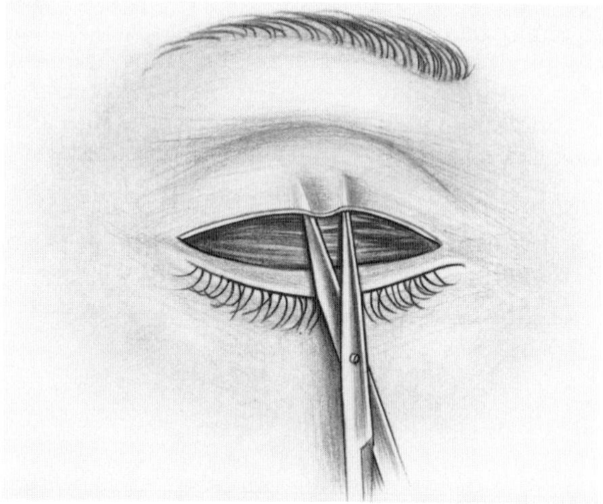

Figure 62.36. Preparation of upper eyelid skin graft recipient site.

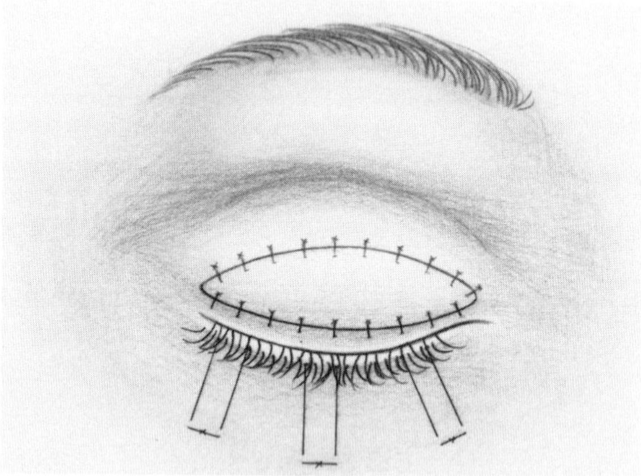

Figure 62.37. Placement of upper eyelid skin graft.

CONCLUSION

The three most frequently encountered complications of lower eyelid blepharoplasty are lower eyelid retraction, round lateral canthus, and ectropion. Skin grafts to the upper and lower eyelids, horizontal shortening, lateral canthal resuspension, and Madame Butterfly procedures may all help alleviate these problems. However, none of these are as satisfactory as prevention of these complications. Proper preoperative evaluation of brow position, horizontal eyelid laxity, lateral canthal tendon position, precorneal tear film, and skin excess may greatly decrease the incidence of dissatisfaction with the lower eyelid blepharoplasty procedure.

ACKNOWLEDGMENT

The authors thank David Hinkle for creating the illustrations used in this chapter.

REFERENCES

1. Sheen JH: Tarsal fixation in lower blepharoplasty. *Plast Reconstr Surg* 62: 24–30, 1978.
2. Hamako C, Baylis HI: Lower eyelid retraction after blepharoplasty. *Am J Ophthalmol* 89: 517–521, 1980.
3. Edgerton MT: Causes and prevention of lower lid ectropion following blepharoplasty. *Plast Reconstr Surg* 49: 367–373, 1972.

4. Smith B: Postsurgical complications of cosmetic blepharoplasty. *Trans Am Acad Ophthalmol* 73: 1162–1164, 1969.
5. Tenzel RR: Complications of blepharoplasty. *Clin Plast Surg* 8: 797–802, 1981
6. Neuhaus RW, Baylis HI: Complication of lower eyelid blepharoplasty. In Putterman AM (ed): *Cosmetic Oculoplastic Surgery.* New York, Grune & Stratton, 1982.
7. Tenzel RR: Treatment of lagophthalmos of the lower eyelid. *Arch Ophthalmol* 81: 366–368, 1969.
8. Wilkins RB, Hunter GJ: Blepharoplasty: cosmetic and functional. In McCord CD (ed): *Oculoplastic Surgery.* New York, Raven Press, 1981.
9. Shorr N, Fallor MK: Repair of the post blepharoplasty round eye and lower eyelid retraction: combined cheek and lateral canthal resuspension. In Ward PH, Berman WE (eds): *Plastic and Reconstructive Surgery of the Head and Neck.* St. Louis, Mosby, 1984.
10. Baylis HI, Rosen N, Neuhaus RW: Obtaining auricular cartilage for reconstructive surgery. *Am J Ophthalmol* 93: 709–712, 1982.
11. Webster RC, *et al*: Blepharoplasty: when to combine it with brow, temple, or coronal lift. *J Otolaryngol* 8: 339–343, 1979.

CHAPTER 63

Ptosis and Pseudoptosis in the Blepharoplasty Patient

ALBERT HORNBLASS, M.D.
NEIL D. GROSS, M.D.

Ptosis or pseudoptosis may be coexistent in a patient who is undergoing blepharoplasty. In order to treat these patients properly, surgeons must ascertain first the presence of a ptosis or a pseudoptosis. In this chapter, the etiologies of ptosis will be briefly reviewed. The discussion will primarily focus upon involutional ptosis, as this is the most common type of ptosis encountered in patients undergoing blepharoplasty. Two surgical approaches aimed at correcting this problem will be detailed. The causes of pseudoptosis with selected treatment plans will also be outlined. Finally, ptosis as a complication of blepharoplasty will be described.

HISTORY AND CLINICAL FEATURES

Ptosis is commonly divided into the categories of congenital ptosis, acquired ptosis, and pseudoptosis (1) (Table 63.1). Congenital ptosis is recognized at or soon after birth. Its clinical features and treatments are well described.

Most blepharoplasty candidates who have ptotic lids suffer from involutional ptosis (2). Involutional ptosis is thought to be due to a dehiscence or disinsertion of the levator aponeurosis (3–5) and/or myoatrophy of the levator muscles.

Patients who are suspected of having an involutional ptosis should be queried specifically about previous lid trauma, prior intraocular surgery, or previous bouts of lid swelling. All of these conditions may contribute to a dehiscence or disinsertion of the levator muscle.

The size of the palpebral apertures must be measured with respect to the pupil and limbus (6). Levator function should always be measured. During this portion of the examination, it is critical that the contribution of the frontalis muscle be neutralized. This is accomplished by applying one or two fingers against the frontalis just above the eyebrow during the measurement. The position of the lid creases should be carefully noted. Patients with a higher lid crease on the affected side may owe this asymmetry to a dehiscence or disinsertion of the levator aponeurosis. Wilkins (2) observes the lines of tension developed as the patient forcefully looks up, while downward traction is applied to the eyelashes. He claims that the pull of the eyelid retractor will appear superior to its normal position at the upper border of the tarsus in patients with involutional ptosis.

It is axiomatic that prior to the surgery all blepharoplasty/ptosis patients undergo a thorough ophthalmological examination with Schirmer's testing, evaluation of the Bell's phenomenon, and measurement of horizontal lid laxity (7). Preoperative visual field testing, orthoptic evaluation and Tensilon injections (8, 9) should also be considered, as indicated.

SURGICAL APPROACHES TO PTOSIS AND BLEPHAROPLASTY

Adults with poor levator function, such as those with congenital ptosis or neurogenic ptosis, present difficult problems. It is recommended that they first undergo ptosis repair (10, 11). After an acceptable lid position has been achieved, a standard blepharoplasty may be performed at the same operation.

Patients with involutional ptosis generally possess excellent levator function. These patients are candidates for simultaneous ptosis repair and blepharoplasty.

MINIMAL INVOLUTIONAL PTOSIS AND BLEPHAROPLASTY

Patients with 2–4 mm of ptosis with good levator function will benefit from a combined Fasanella-Servat/blepharoplasty procedure. The Fasanella-Servat procedure will lift the upper lid 2–3 mm. The blepharoplasty skin excision will add 1 mm of lid elevation. This is usually quite sufficient to improve the patient's visual field, as well as improve his or her cosmetic appearance. A drop of 2.5% Neo-Synephrine in the ptotic eye may help raise the lid by stimulating the contraction of Mueller's muscle. This technique helps to preview the singular contribution of the Fasanella-Servat procedure or conjunctivo-Muellerectomy, prior to surgery.

This combined procedure is performed under local anesthesia. A frontal nerve block is established under the roof of the orbit. The amount of skin to be excised is outlined first, and the superior palpebral fold is measured from the lid margin. Symmetry of both upper lids is crucial. The amount of skin to be excised is then picked up with a tooth forceps until slight eversion of the margin of the lid is induced. A 25-gauge needle is used to inject 2% lidocaine with epinephrine subcutaneously. The skin is then excised (Fig. 63.1). A methylmethacrylate contact lens is placed on the eye for protection, and a 5-0 nylon suture is passed from the skin through the superior palpebral fold above the tarsus on the conjunctival surface on the temporal third of the lid. A Desmarres retractor is then used to evert the upper lid. Two curved hemostats are placed 3 mm from the superior tarsal border of the everted lid. The tissues enclosed by the clamps are conjunctiva, Mueller's muscle, tarsus, and the levator aponeurosis. The suture is run under the curved clamps and brought nasally from the conjunctival surface of the skin of the superior palpebral fold (Fig. 63.2). The clamps are removed one at a time, and a Westcott spring-handle

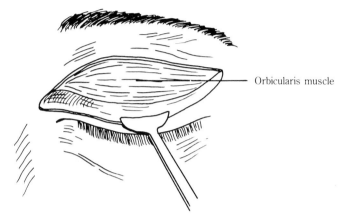

Figure 63.1. The excess upper lid skin has been outlined and excised, revealing the underlying orbicularis muscle.

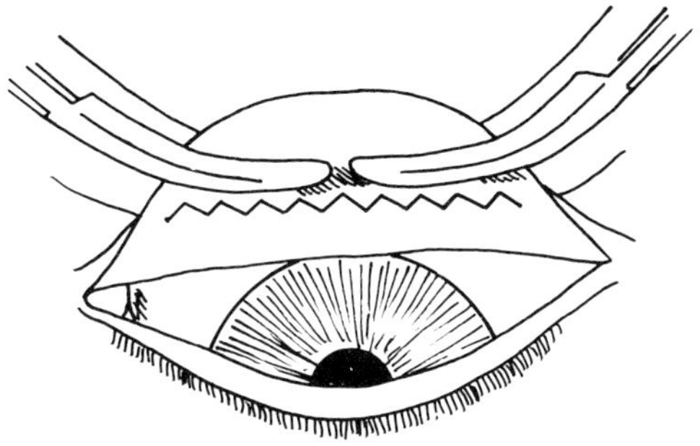

Figure 63.2. The everted tarsus with attached Mueller's muscle and levator aponeurosis is captured by the two identical curved hemostats. A running 5-0 nylon suture is passed, in running fashion, at 45° angles beneath the clamps.

Table 63.1.
Beard's Classification of Ptosis

Congenital Ptosis
- With normal superior rectus function
- With superior rectus weakness
- With blepharophimosis syndrome
- Synkinetic ptosis (Marcus Gunn "jaw-winking" ptosis)
- Misdirected third nerve ptosis

Acquired Ptosis

Neurogenic Ptosis
- Traumatic ophthalmoplegia
- Disease caused by lesions of the third cranial nerve
- Ophthalmoplegic migraine
- Horner's syndrome
- Multiple sclerosis ptosis

Myogenic Ptosis
- Senile ptosis
- Late acquired hereditary ptosis
- Progressive external ophthalmoplegia
- Hyperthyroidism
- Steroid ptosis

Traumatic Ptosis

Mechanical Ptosis
- Lid tumor
- Blepharochalasis
- Cicatricial ptosis

Pseudoptosis
- Due to anophthalmia, microphthalmia, and phthisis bulbi
- Due to hypotropia
- Due to dermatochalasis

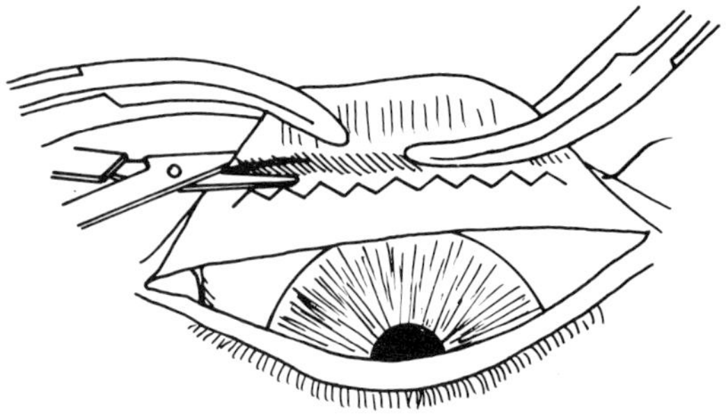

Figure 63.3. The medial hemostat is repositioned and the tarsus is cut along the crushed edge.

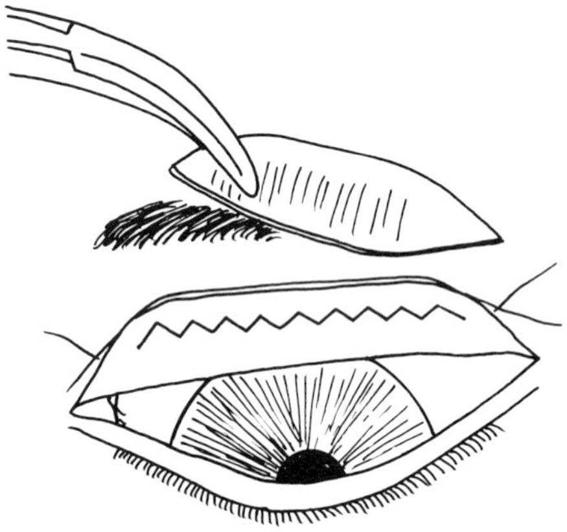

Figure 63.4. Amputation of tarsus with attached Mueller's muscle and levator aponeurosis is captured without disruption of the preplaced 5-0 running nylon suture.

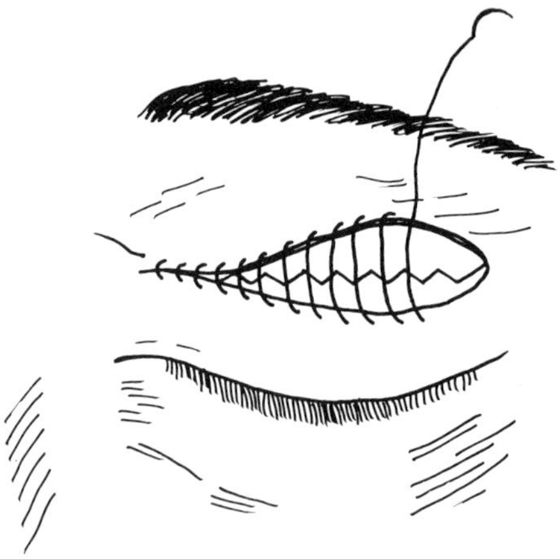

Figure 63.5. Upon completion of the Fasanella-Servat procedure, the superficial skin wound is closed with 5-0 nylon suture.

scissors is used to excise the crushed tissue (Figs. 63.3–63.5). The suture is then tied on the skin and removed 2 weeks later. The skin incision is closed with 5-0 nylon in subcuticular fashion and bolstered with interrupted 6-0 black silk suture. These sutures can be removed in 2–4 days (Figs. 63.6 and 63.7).

Dortzbach has an alternate procedure for mild acquired ptosis (12). He resects the superior tarsal muscle in patients who have satisfactory elevation of the eyelid on preoperative testing with the phenylephrine eye drop test. Advan-

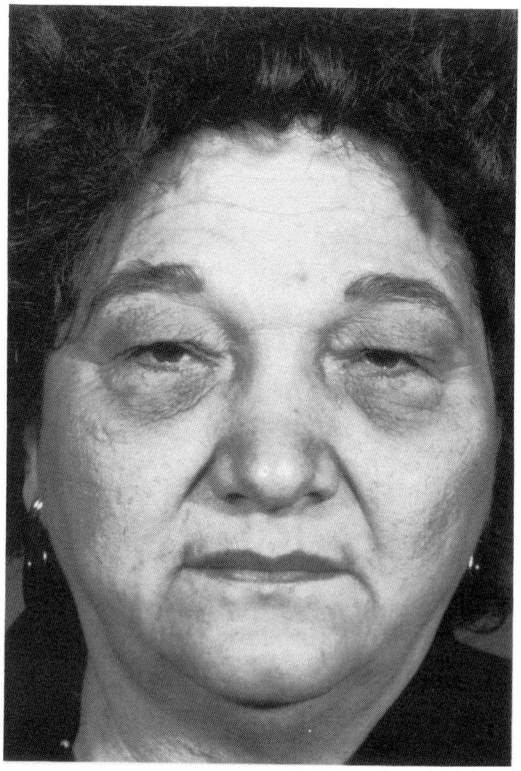

Figure 63.6. A 67-year-old female with ptosis of the right upper lid and dermatochalasis of both upper lids.

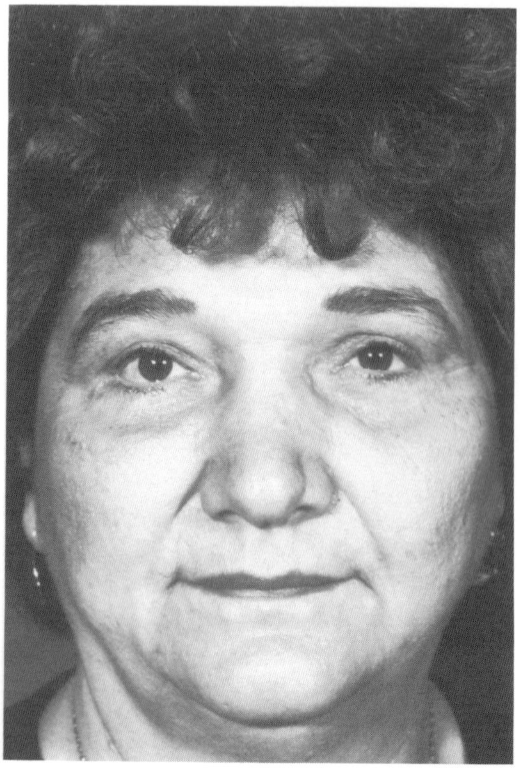

Figure 63.7. Correction of the ptosis and dermatochalasis via the combined Fasanella-Servat/blepharoplasty procedure. Postoperatively, the untouched left upper lid is slightly lower presumably secondary to Hering's Law.

tages of this procedure are that, while the superior tarsal muscle is resected, the conjunctiva and basic lacrimal secretors are preserved and tarsal stability is maintained.

The A-frame operation is another alternative procedure in the blepharoplasty patient with ptosis (13). It can be performed easily and rapidly with a minimum of dissection: corneal irritation is not a complication, tarsus is not disturbed, and it can be easily mastered. This operation consists of a block resection of levator aponeurosis, Mueller's muscle, and conjunctiva. The term *A-frame* was adopted to describe the use of temporary traction sutures to pull up the layers to be resected, a configuration that suggests an A-frame building.

MODERATE TO SEVERE INVOLUTIONAL PTOSIS AND BLEPHAROPLASTY

If the ptosis is greater than 3–4 mm in patients with good levator function, surgery of the levator aponeurosis is combined with a blepharoplasty. To combine levator surgery with a blepharoplasty, the surgeon makes the initial incision in routine fashion. The preseptal orbicularis muscle is undermined, and the orbital septum is incised. The levator aponeurosis, with its glistening surface, is identified. If disinsertion is apparent, it should be repaired with interrupted double-armed 6-0 black silk sutures (14). Two to three sutures are placed through the anterior tarsal surface at its superior margin. Each arm of the suture is then placed through the disinserted end of the levator.

If a dehiscence of the levator is encountered, a levator tuck is employed (Fig. 63.8). Again, two or three 6-0 black silk sutures are placed through the anterior surface of the tarsus at the superior border. An adequate portion of the levator aponeurosis is included with each bite of the suture, so the lid will rest at the superior limbal border with a good contour (Fig. 63.9). These sutures can be placed on slip knots and readjusted. Some surgeons sit the patient up to verify the level of the lid in this position. Typically, the lid will drop 1–1.5 mm postoperatively. The sutures are tied when the lid is deemed to be in the appropriate position (Fig. 63.10). Further skin is excised to facilitate an even closure, if necessary. If a large tuck is required, an unsightly bulge in the lid near the margin can

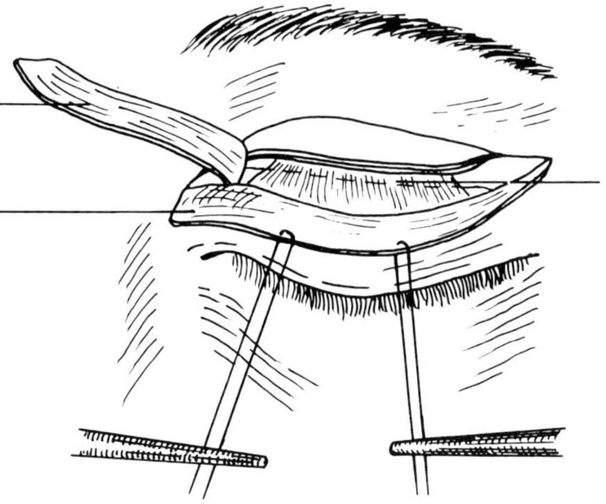

Figure 63.8. The excess upper lid skin has been outlined and excised. A strip of orbicularis muscle, still attached medially, is removed, which reveals the orbital septum/aponeurosis of the levator muscle.

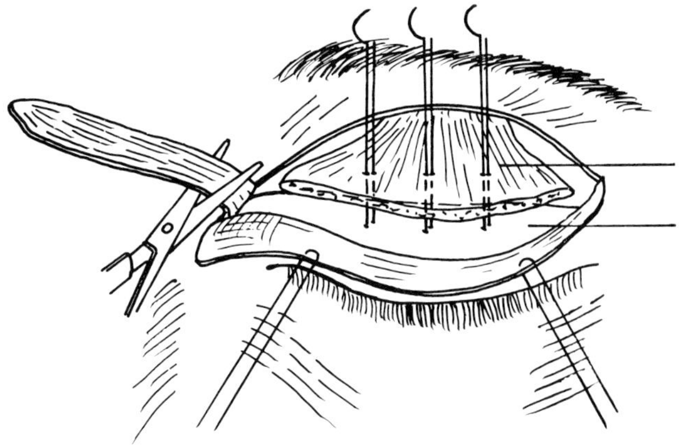

Figure 63.9. The levator aponeurosis has been detached from the tarsus and resected. Three double-armed 5-0 silk sutures are placed through the tarsus and anchored to levator muscle.

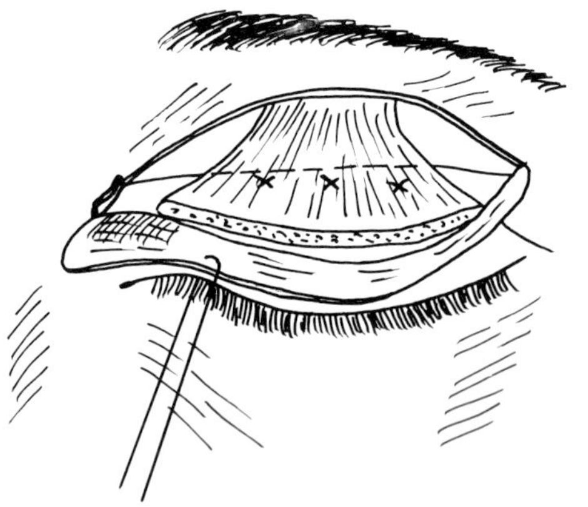

Figure 63.10. The levator aponeurosis is tightly secured to the superior tarsus. Closure of the superficial skin wound should then ensue.

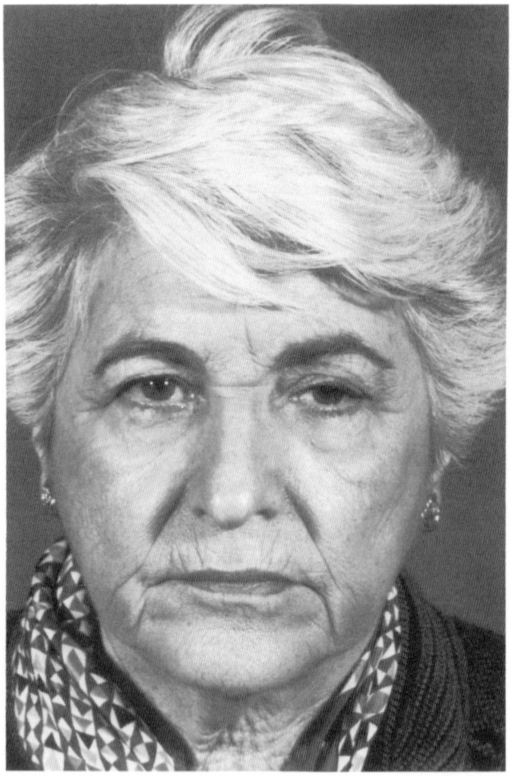

Figure 63.11. A 52-year-old female with ptosis of the left upper lid secondary to dehiscence of the levator aponeurosis. Bilateral upper lid dermatochalasis is also present.

occur. In those instances, a levator resection is preferred. The skin incision is closed with 5-0 subcuticular nylon (Figs. 63.11 and 63.12).

During skin closure, the appearance of the eyelid crease must be evaluated. In some individuals, superficial closure will provide adequate definition to the lid crease. However, conventional blepharoplasty without upper lid crease fixation sutures may lead to early redundancy of the skin that hangs low on the lid. One technique of lid crease fixation involves the imbrication of the orbicularis to the levator muscle to create a higher supratrasal fold (15). Putterman has also shown several other techniques for reconstruction of the upper lid fold (16).

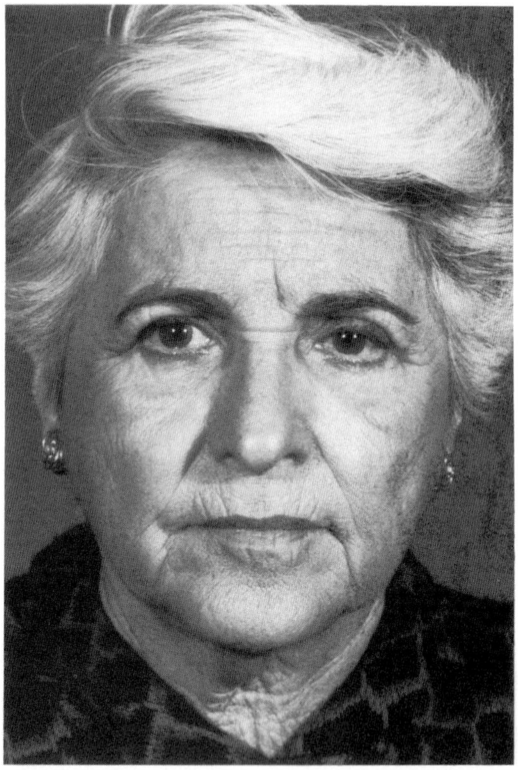

Figure 63.12. Repair of the left levator dehiscence with concomitant bilateral excess of redundant skin rectifies the left upper lid ptosis and bilateral upper lid dermatochalasis.

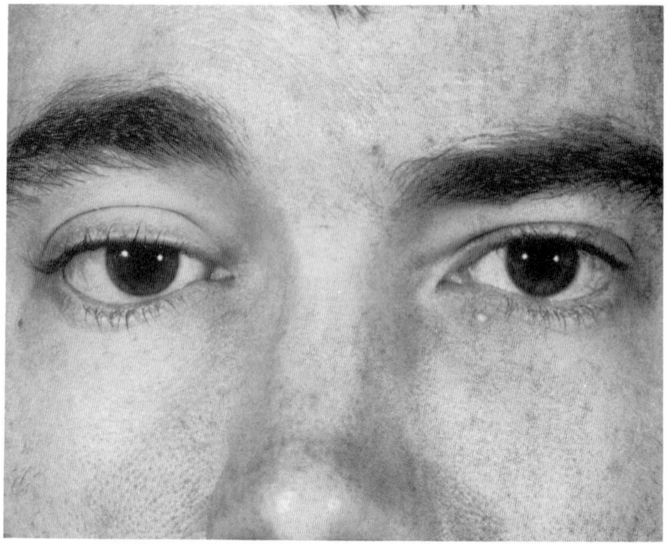

Figure 63.13. A 23-year-old male with anophthalmos, OD, secondary to trauma 6 years prior to presentation. Several progressively larger prostheses failed to correct the ptosis. Moderate flattening of the superior sulcus secondary to volume loss is visible.

PSEUDOPTOSIS AND BLEPHAROPLASTY

Pseudoptosis is associated with microphthalmos, enophthalmos, phthisis, and anophthalmia. The loss of volume within the socket permits the levator complex to migrate anteriorly (17); this forward movement decreases interpalpebral width and gives the appearance of ptosis (Fig. 63.13).

A patient with pseudoptosis in the presence of a poorly fitting prosthesis may undergo blepharoplasty after an attempt is made by the ocularist to correct the pseudoptosis with prosthetic aids. The ocularist may use an extended shelf on the prosthesis to keep the lid open (18).

It must be remembered that true ptosis can coexist with pseudoptosis. In patients with true ptosis in an anophthalmic socket, a McCord tarsectomy (19) will provide a good correction without shortening the cul-de-sac. The combination of ptosis and pseudoptosis is also recognized in association with hypotropia (20). A two-stage surgical correction is generally favored for these patients. Initially, a Kanpp procedure with or without inferior rectus recession is undertaken in affected eyes, depending upon the etiology of the hypotropia (21). After the pseudoptosis secondary to the hypotropia is resolved, the ptosis is treated by levator surgery, tarso-Muellerectomy, or a frontalis sling.

Finally, brow ptosis should also be suspected as a component of pseudoptosis or true ptosis (22). Evaluation and treatment of this condition are described elsewhere in this volume.

PTOSIS AS A COMPLICATION OF BLEPHAROPLASTY

Permanent ptosis can occur from injury to the levator muscle or aponeurosis caused by thrusting the blades of the scissors into the orbit in an attempt to divide the septum and the orbital fat pockets prior to removal (23, 24). In a very high (12–14 mm) supratarsal fixation, the pull from the lateral skin attachments to the underlying levator aponeurosis can cause mild ptosis. This usually resolves by itself in 6–8 weeks. If the skin sutures to the aponeurosis are removed, the ptosis clears promptly. Secondary repair of ptosis cannot be performed until 6 months after the initial surgery. Frequently, there is complete resolution without surgical intervention.

An unusual type of ptosis or flattening of the lid can occur after excision of fat from the upper nasal pocket. This usually heals spontaneously without problems. However, a permanent lid flattening and a deep sulcus of the nasal upper lid may result. Treatment requires release of adhesions to the superior oblique muscle with use of the orbicularis muscle as a flap to fill in the sulcus and elevate the nasal portion of the lid.

REFERENCES

1. Beard C: *Ptosis*. St. Louis, CV Mosby Co, 1976.
2. Wilkins RB, Patipa M: The recognition of acquired ptosis in patients considered for upper eyelid blepharoplasty. *Plast Reconstr Surg* 70: 431–434, 1982.
3. Dortzbach RK, Sutula FC: Involutional blepharoptosis: A histopathological study. *Arch Ophthalmol* 98(11): 2045–2049. 1980.
4. Dryden RM, Leibsohn J: The levator aponeurosis in blepharoplasty. *Ophthalmology* 85: 718–725, 1978.
5. Pearl RM: Acquired ptosis: a reexamination of etiology and treatment. *Plast Reconstr Surg* 76: 56–64, 1985.
6. Fox, S: *Surgery of Ptosis*. Baltimore, Williams & Wilkins, 1980.
7. Hornblass A: Blepharoplasty and its complications. Presented at the Annual Meeting of the American Academy of Ophthalmology Instruction Section, 1978.
8. Miller M: Myasthenia gravis: Systemic and ocular considerations. *Ophthalmology* 86: 2165–2174, 1979.
9. Anderson RL, Dixon RS: Neuromyopathological ptosis: A new surgical approach. *Arch Ophthalmol* 97: 1129, 1979.
10. Fasanella RM, Servat J: Levator resection for minimal ptosis; Another simplified operation. *Arch Ophthalmol* 65: 493, 1971.
11. Putterman AM, Urist MJ: Müller muscle-conjunctiva resection. *Arch Ophthalmol* 93: 619, 1975.
12. Dortzbach RK: Superior tarsal muscle resection to correct blepharoptosis. *Ophthalmology* 86: 1883, 1979.
13. Small RB: The A-frame operation for acquired blepharoptosis. *Arch Ophthalmol* 98: 516, 1980.
14. Jones LT, Quickert MH, Wobig JL: The cure of ptosis by aponeurotic repair. *Arch Ophthalmol* 93: 629, 1975.
15. Sheen JH: A change in the technique of supratarsal fixation in upper blepharoplasty. *Plast Reconstr Surg* 59: 831, 1977.
16. Putterman AM, Urist MJ: Reconstruction of the upper eyelid crease and fold. *Arch Ophthalmol* 94: 1941, 1976.
17. Vistnes LM: Mechanism of upper eyelid ptosis in the anophthalmic orbit. *Plast Reconstr Surg* 58: 539, 1976.
18. Allen L: Reduction of upper eyelid ptosis with the prosthesis. In Guibor P, Guibor M: *Technique of Anophthalmic Cosmesis*. Miami, Symposia Specialists, 1976.
19. McCord CD, Jr: An external minimal ptosis procedure-external tarsoaponeurectomy. *Trans Am Acad Ophthalmol* 79: 683, 1975.
20. Pap AV: Congenital unilateral pseudoptosis of the upper eyelid. *Plast Reconstr Surg* 70: 483–484, 1982.
21. Flicker LA, Collin JR, Lee JP: Management of ipsilateral ptosis with hypotropia. *Br J Ophthalmol* 70: 732–736, 1986.
22. Dingman RD, Peled I, Izenberg D: Forehead and brow lifts and their relationship to blepharoplasty. *Ann. Plast. Surg* 2: 32, 1979.
23. Baylis HI, Sutcliffe T, Fett DR: Levator injury during blepharoplasty. *Arch Ophthalmol* 102: 570–571, 1984.
24. Tenzel R: Upper lid complications of cosmetic blepharoplasty. In Aston A, Hornblass A, Meltzer, M, Rees M: *Third International Symposium of Plastic and Reconstructive Surgery of the Eye and Adnexa*. Baltimore, Williams & Wilkins, 1982.

CHAPTER 64

Orbicularis Oculi in Blepharoplasty: A Balancing Act with the Levator Palpebrae[a]

DAVID W. FURNAS, M.D.
DONALD I. ALTMAN, M.D.

ANATOMY

MUSCLE

In 1876, Duchenne described the anatomy of the orbicularis oculi muscle and emphasized its role in facial expression and function (1). He divided the muscle into orbital (*orbiculaires palpébraux supérieur et inférieur*) and palpebral (*palpébraux supérieur et inférieur*) portions (Figs. 64.1 and 64.2). He further endowed each segment with emotional qualities. He called the superior orbital segment the muscle of *réflexion*; the upper and lower palpebral segments, the muscles of *mépris* (scorn); and the inferior orbital segment, the muscle of *bienveillance* (kindness). Among neighboring muscles, the nasalis muscle was endowed with qualities of *lasciveté* or *lubricité*.

The orbital part of the orbicularis oculi muscle inserts on orbital bone medial to the superior orbital notch and the infraorbital foramen. Elsewhere along the orbital rim are firm attachments, so that a submuscular plane is not easy to develop. The orbital portion of the orbicularis oculi muscle forms a continuous oval sphincter without interruption, except at the medial canthal tendon (Fig. 64.3).

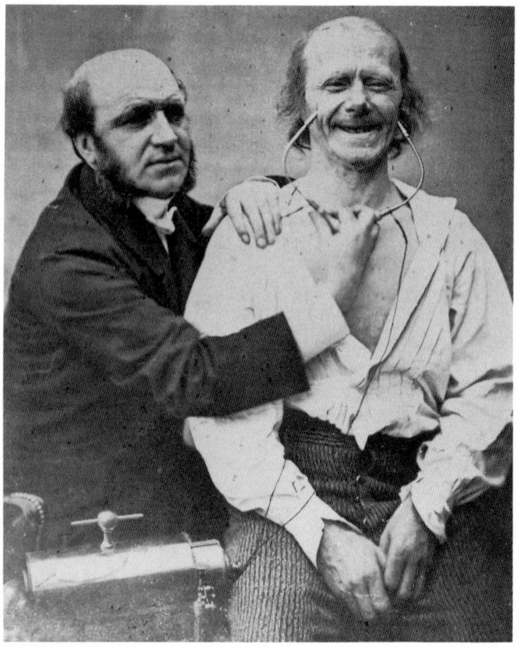

Figure 64.1. Duchenne stimulating muscles of facial expression with his *appareil voltafaradique à double courant.*

[a] The illustrations in this chapter and the text, which appears here in a different form, were published earlier under the title "The Orbicularis Oculi Muscle—Management in Blepharoplasty" (*Clin Plast Surg* 8: 687–715, 1981) by the W. B. Saunders Co.

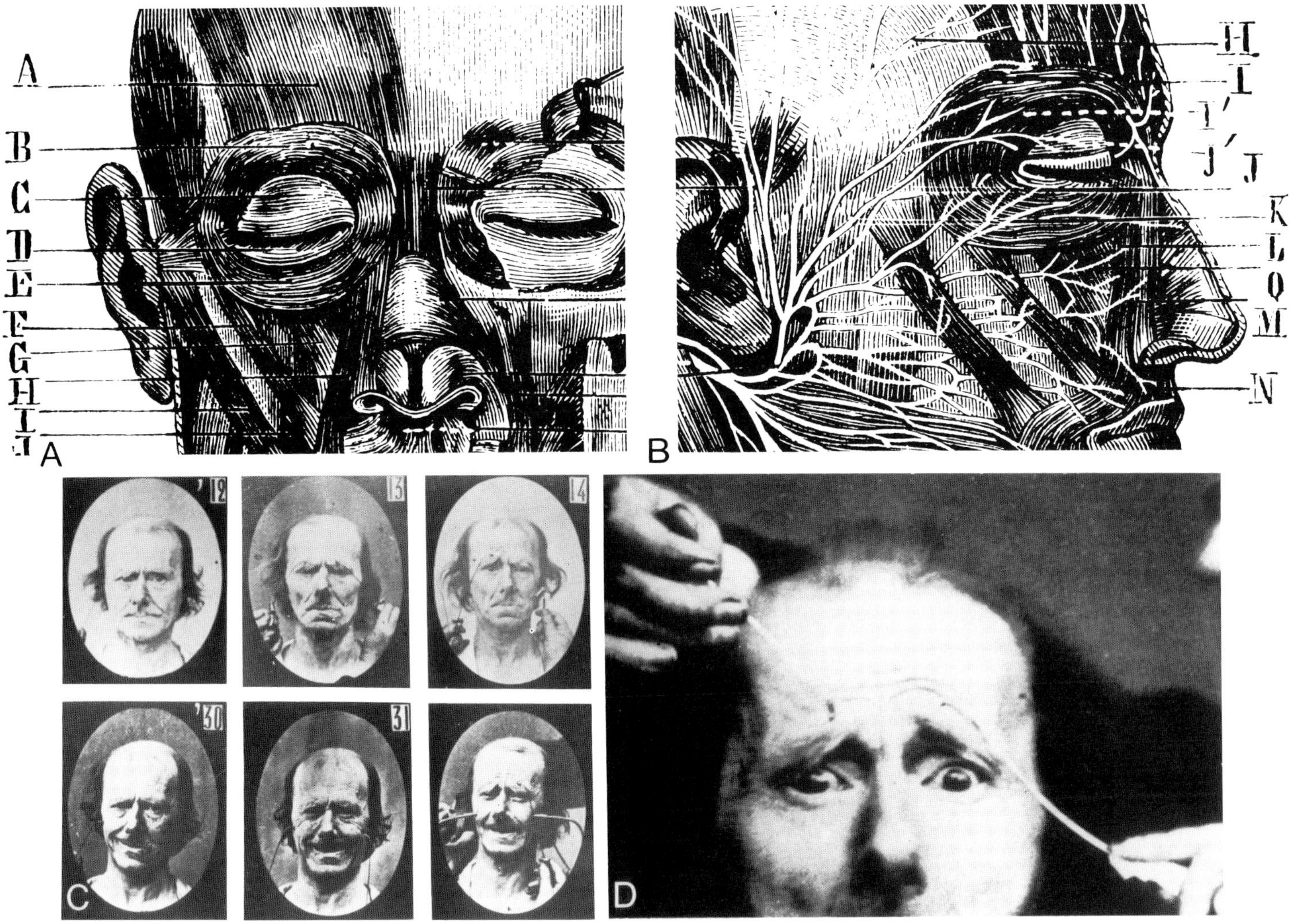

Figure 64.2. Duchenne's studies on orbicularis oculi and facial muscles. *A*, Duchenne divided the orbicularis oculi into orbital segments (**B** and **E**) and palpebral segments (**C** and **D**). *B*, He made detailed studies on the branches of the facial nerve supplying the orbital area (**I–K**). *C*, He studied the anatomy and function of the facial nerve and tried to analyze expression of the human face in terms of anatomic and physiologic components. *Top three frames* show stimulation of the superior orbital part of the orbicularis oculi, with moderate stimulus, then stronger stimulus, then maximal stimulus. *Lower three frames* show stimulation of the inferior palpebral portion of the orbicularis along with the zygomaticus major: *First frame*, strong stimulus on the right and none on the left. *Second frame*, stronger stimulation bilaterally. *Third frame*, maximal stimulation with the additional stimulation of the frontalis. *D*, Simultaneous application of three electrodes gives maximal stimulation to the frontalis, corrugator, and upper orbicularis oculi (and additionally the platysma and depressors of the jaw), producing the appearance of fright and pain. The patient shows what is sometimes called the "the setting sun" sign (4), in which sclera shows above and iris is hidden below. This sign can occur as an operative complication if there is excessive tightness of lower lid repair coupled with retraction of the upper lid.

The palpebral portions are much thinner and are particularly thin where they are joined by fibers of the levator aponeurosis. The palpebral portions are divided into preseptal and pretarsal fibers. The preseptal fibers make a pseudoraphe laterally; medially the upper preseptal muscle inserts on bone on either side of the lacrimal sac. The lower preseptal fibers insert on the lacrimal diaphragm. The pretarsal fibers are tethered to the lateral orbital tubercle by the lateral canthal tendon, which is thinner and much more mobile than the medial canthal tendon (Figs. 64.3*B* and 64.4). As they attach to the medial canthal ligaments the pretarsal fibers form several insertions that pass on either side of the lacrimal sac and attach to both sides of the canaliculus.

On the basis of electromyographic findings, Gordon (2) described three functional groups of fibers in the orbicularis oculi: (*a*) *blink fibers* located principally in pretarsal muscles; (*b*) *mixed blink and volitional fibers* located principally in preseptal muscle; and (*c*) *volitional fibers* located in the preseptal and orbital areas. The number of fibers per neuromuscular unit for these bundles is estimated to be 25 (as for facial muscles) (3) as compared with five to ten for extraocular muscles and 30 to 300 for skeletal muscles (4). The action of closing the eyelids is so

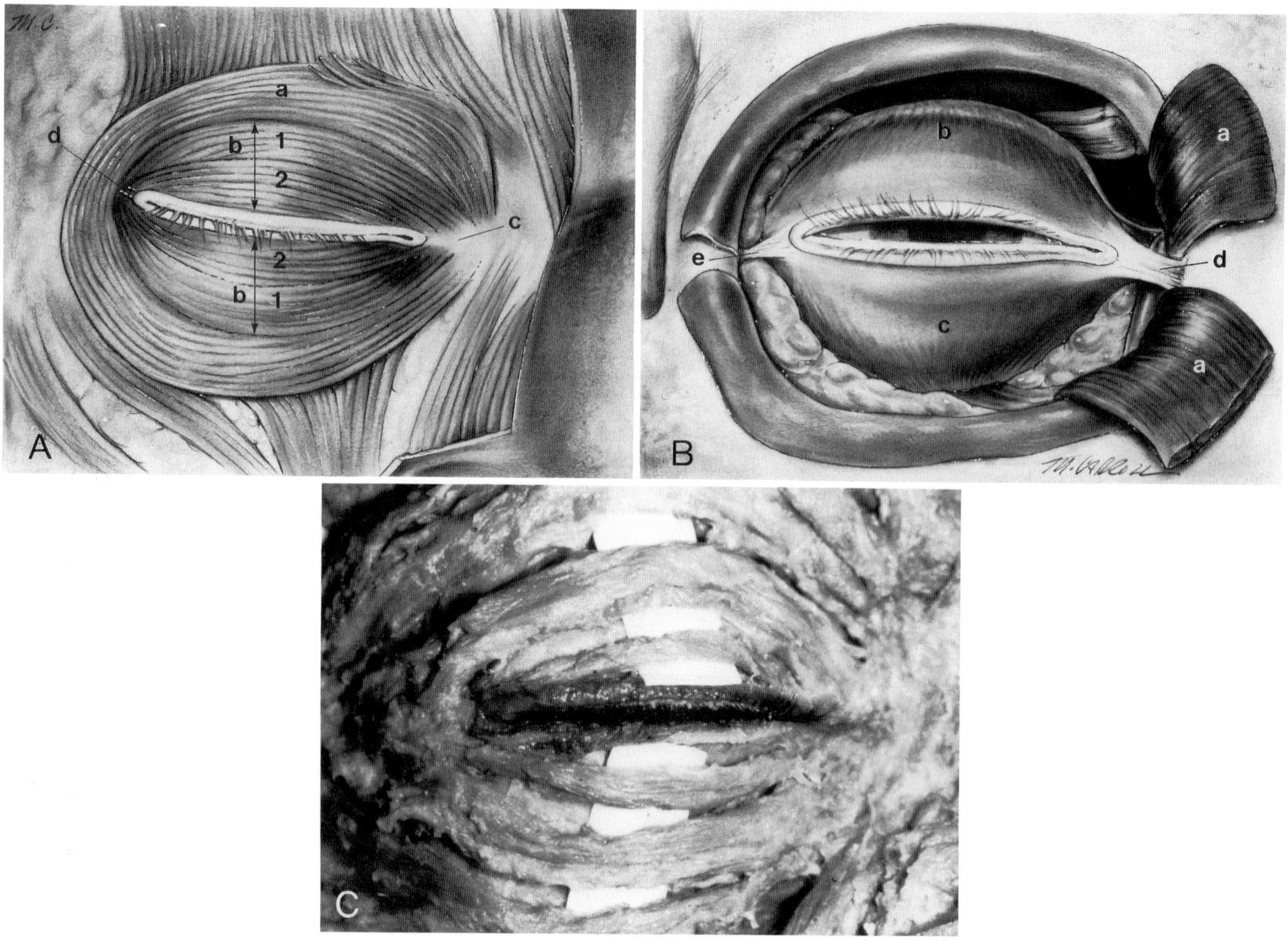

Figure 64.3. *A*, Anatomy of the orbicularis oculi muscle. Most peripheral are the orbital fibers (*a*). Covering the lid structures are palpebral fibers (*b*), which are divided into preseptal (*1*) and pretarsal (*2*). A strong medial canthal tendon secures the insertion (*c*). The lateral origin is relatively free, and the muscle fibers form a continuous ring laterally in a pseudoraphe (*d*). *B*, Aponeurosis of the levator palpebrae (*b*) and the capsulopalpebral head of the inferior rectus (*c*). The orbicularis fibers (*a*) have been reflected forward from their attachments around the lacrimal sac and medial canthal tendon (*e*), which attaches at the lacrimal crests. The lateral canthal tendon (*d*) attaches at the orbital tubercle. The levator functions as a totally independent muscle, whereas the capsulopalpebral head of the inferior rectus functions only in a downward gaze. Both are lid retractors. *C*, Dissection of the right orbicularis oculi muscle. The fibers have been split according to the scheme cited by Whitnall (see A). The peripheral bundle is the orbital portion; the remaining muscle is the palpebral segment, which is subdivided into the pretarsal and preseptal portions.

finely graded that the movement of the upper lid can vary from a fleeting miniature blink that does not even encroach on the pupil (5) to an active sustained contraction of all segments of the orbicularis oculi in which the eyelashes are buried by preseptal skin (4).

SUPPORTING STRUCTURES

The posterior surface of the orbicularis is invested with a delicate fascia, the extensions of which pass between the orbicularis fibers, securing the muscle intimately to the overlying skin. Deep to these fibers is the thin orbital septum, which attaches circumferentially to the orbital rim as an extension of the periosteum. Webs and weak points of the septum have been systematized as the *orifices adipeux*, where orbital fat tends to bulge forward (6). The orbital septum fuses with the levator aponeurosis. The level of fusion depends on the amount of fat in the preaponeurotic space (or vice versa).

Behind the septum is a fine capsule that encloses the lobes and lobules of the fatty reticulum of the orbit (7). The fat that is peripheral to the recti muscles is divided into four lobes placed between the recti muscles (8). The space within the muscular cone is also filled with fat.

BLOOD SUPPLY

The orbicularis oculi muscle is served by a rich blood supply. The classic patterns shown on dissections by Jones (7), Wolff (8), and Whitnall (6), have been amplified by

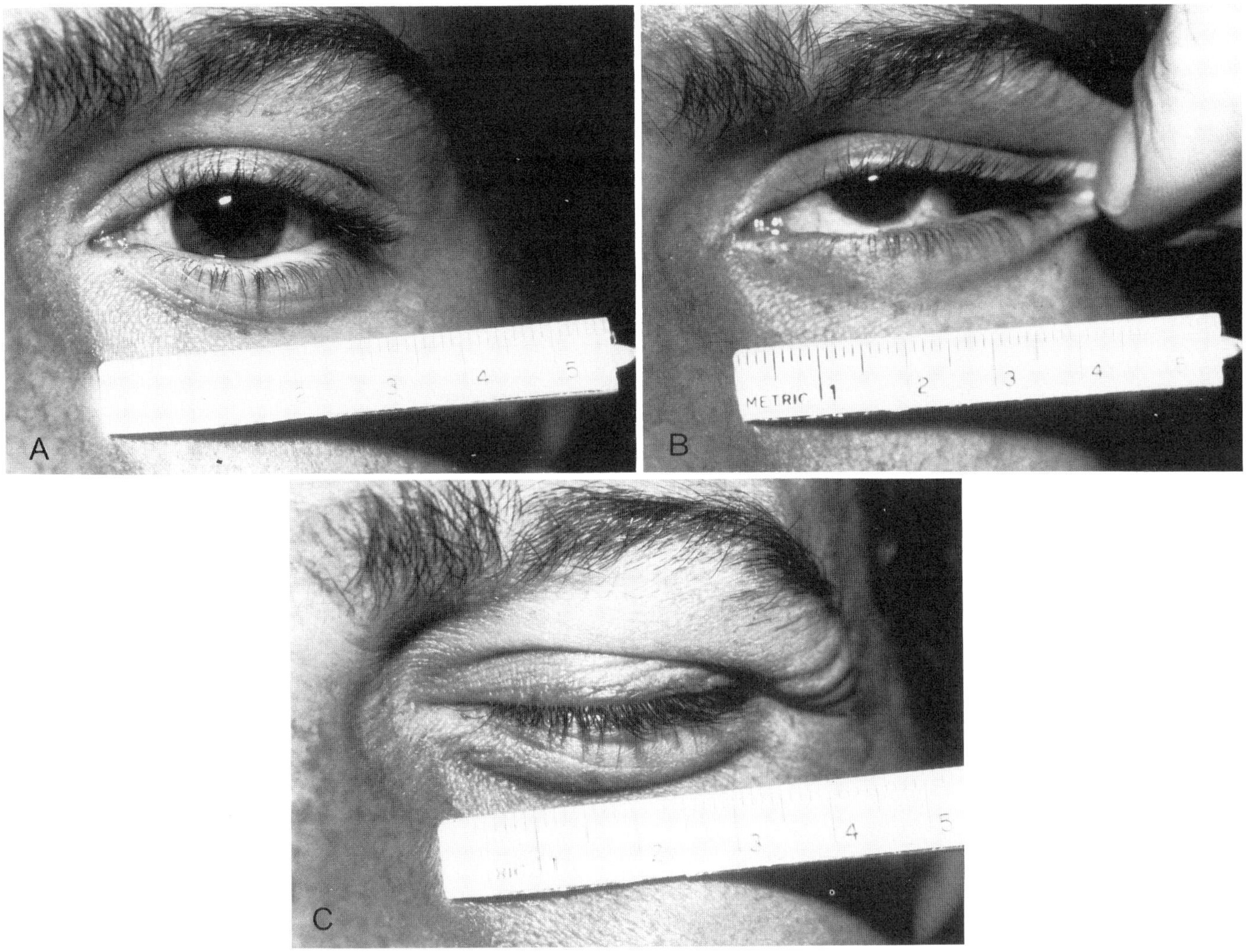

Figure 64.4. Displacement of canthi in an 18-year-old man. *A*, Eyelid in repose. The palpebral fissure is 30 mm wide. *B*, Lateral traction on lids. The palpebral aperture is 40 mm wide. The medial canthus is moved from 2 mm laterally, and the lateral canthus has been displaced about 12 mm. (The lateral canthus is much more mobile.) *C*, Maximal contraction of orbicularis oculi muscle. The palpebral fissure is 27 mm wide. The lateral canthus is displaced 3 mm; medially, the canthus is essentially undisplaced. Orbital and upper preseptal fibers of upper lid overlap the lower preseptal and pretarsal fibers.

dynamic models constructed by Lasjaunias (9) (Fig. 64.5) from the patterns of selective angiograms of the facial, the superficial temporal, and the internal maxillary arteries. Extensive overlap and interchangeability of flow are the rule, conforming to the *angiotome* model described by Taylor (10). That the orbicularis oculi can be separated from both the underlying orbital septum and the overlying skin without compromise was shown by Klatsky in his muscle flap technique for blepharoplasty (11).

FACIAL NERVE

The variability of the pattern of the buccal and zygomatic branches of the facial nerve is well known (12). These branches freely interconnect as they course through the areolar layers of the cheek toward the undersurface of the orbicularis (Fig. 64.6). Ninety percent of these branches exchange rami with one another. Thus orbicularis paresis caused by local injury to these nerves is usually followed by recovery in 3–6 months; this contrasts to the infrequent recovery seen after injury to the nerve of the frontalis muscle, where the branches exchange rami less than 15% of the time (13).

EMBRYOLOGY, VARIATIONS, AND ANOMALIES

The orbicularis oculi originates as mesoderm of the second branchial arch; it migrates forward, bending around the orbit like a horseshoe, and inserts above and below the medial canthus (7). This muscle is subject to numerous variations: accessory bundles from neighboring muscles are common; union of one orbicularis with the other by a *transversus glabella* muscle is known; interconnection with an upward bound platysma occurs. The

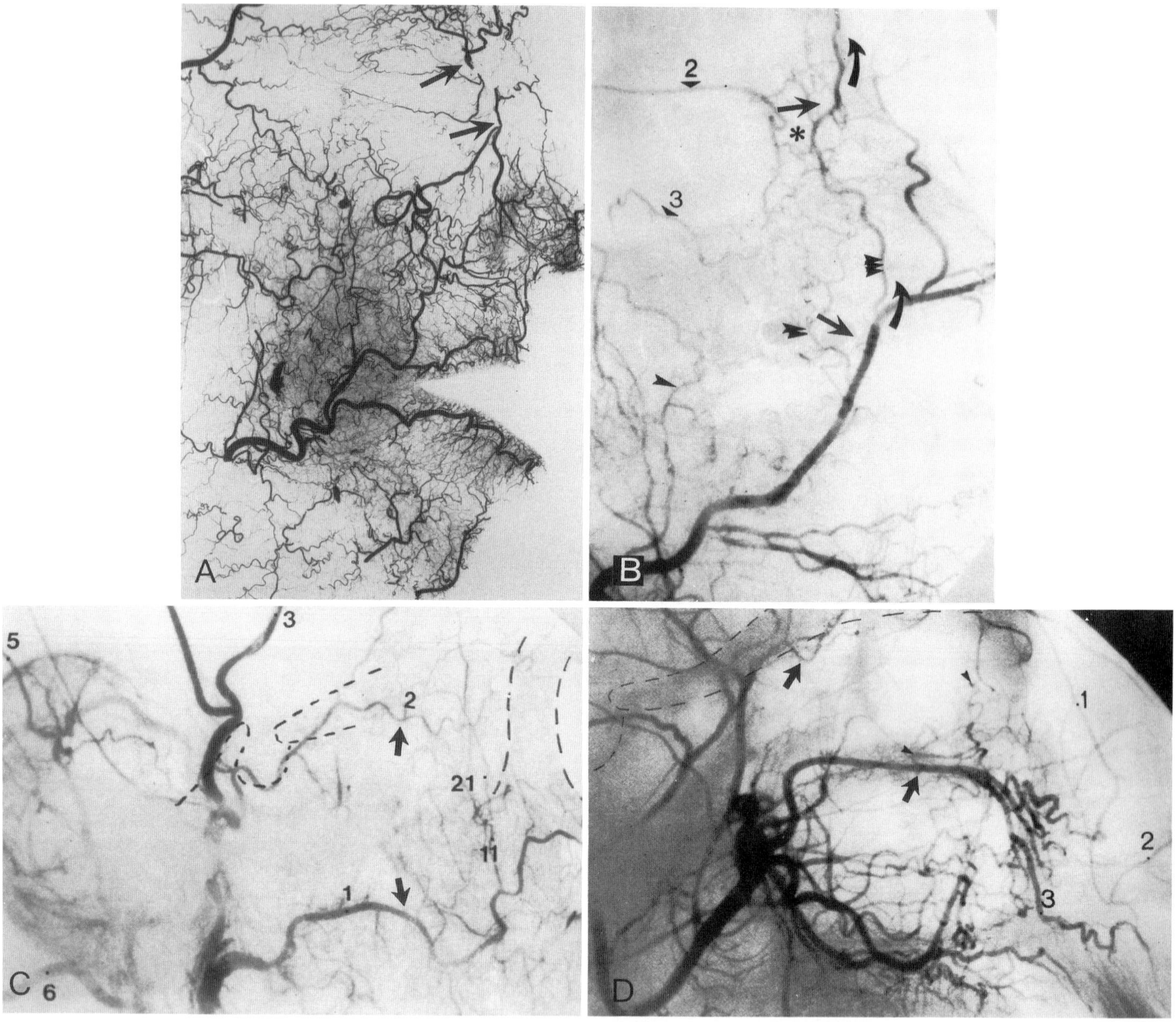

Figure 64.5. Arterial supply to orbicularis oculi. *A*, The orbicularis oculi is richly supplied with arterial circulation from three major sources with abundant collaterals. In this radiogram of a cadaver specimen injected with radiopaque plastic, note the network to orbital area (*arrows*). *B*, Facial artery: selective angiogram in which feeding vessels to orbicularis can be seen (*large arrow*). *C*, Superficial temporal artery: selective angiogram in which vessels supplying the orbicularis can be seen (*arrows*). *D*, Internal maxillary artery: in this selective angiogram, note the vessels to the orbital area (*arrow*). (From Lasjaunias PL, Berenstein A: *Craniofacial and Upper Cervical Arteries*. Baltimore, Williams & Wilkins Co., 1981.)

palpebral portion of the orbicularis may be completely separate from the orbital portion; and partial or complete absence of either of these portions has been described (6). Jones (7) described a patient in whom the embryonic palpebral muscles had stopped short at the middle of each eyelid, failing to attach medially. The patient could barely close his lids and he had constant epiphora because of a nonfunctioning lacrimal pump.

FUNCTION

Duchenne (1) studied the function of the orbicularis and analyzed some of his findings in terms of facial expression (Figs. 64.1 and 64.2). With mild electrical stimulation an expression of "reflection" was noted, with modest stimulation "attention" was seen. Stronger stimulation showed "vehemence," and very strong stimulation

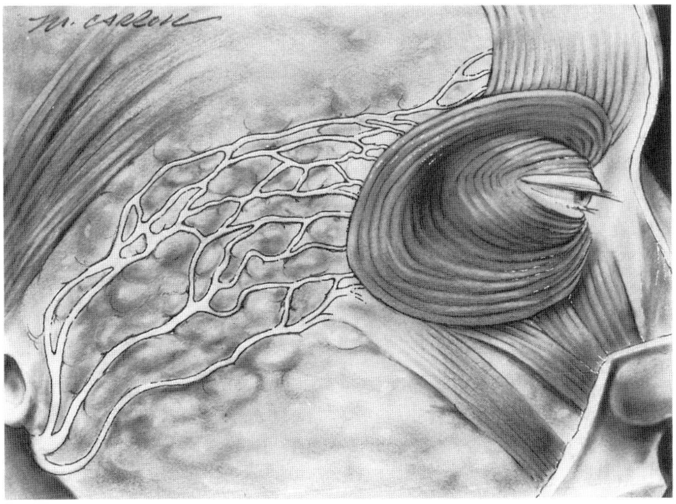

Figure 64.6. Nerve supply to the orbicularis oculi. Several rami of the temporal facial branch of the facial nerve break up into a number of filaments to enter the inferior surface of the orbicularis oculi. Because of numerous interconnections, permanent paresis from nerve injury is uncommon.

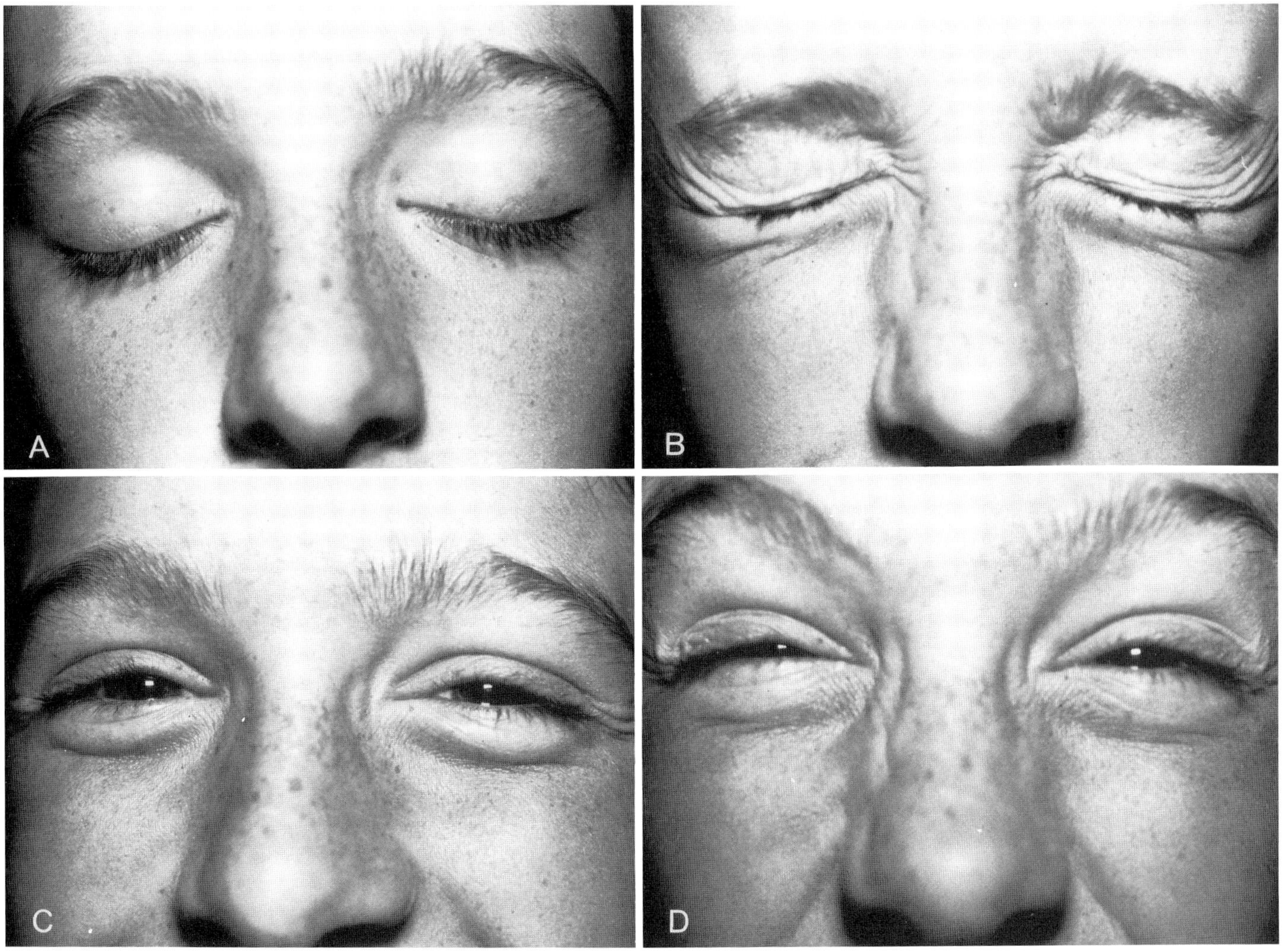

Figure 64.7. Actions of the orbicularis oculi in a 14-year-old boy. *A*, Gentle closure of lids as in sleep, with reciprocal tonus of the orbicularis oculi and the levator palpebrae. *B*, Maximal contraction of the orbicularis. *C*, Contraction of the palpebral fibers of the orbicularis of the lower lid in a smile. *D*, Contraction of the orbital and palpebral fibers of the lower lid, and partial contraction of the orbital and palpebral fibers of the upper lid, with reciprocal contraction of the levator and frontalis fibers as in a reaction to glare or smoke.

showed "displeasure and gloom." The lower orbicularis yielded an "insincere smile" on limited stimulation, a "marked smile" with stronger stimulation, and the appearance of "agreeable surprise" with maximal stimulation. Using several electrodes for simultaneous stimulation of several facial muscles, Duchenne achieved some artificial expressions worthy of the stage.

The orbicularis oculi contracts in three modes of volition (Fig. 64.7): voluntary, automatic [blinking to moisten cornea, also called "periodic blinking" (4)], and reflex (blinking of the eyes in response to a bright light or a threat of danger). Movements of the upper lid during blinking are almost completely vertical. Horizontal motion is seen in the lower lid, however, and during active contraction, the medial motion exceeds the vertical motion (4). When the orbicularis acts as a whole as a protective sphincter (6), voluntary and involuntary movements may be concurrent. Also, a monocle can be held in place by the voluntary contraction of the orbital part of the orbicularis, while the pars palpebralis retains the independent automatic function of moistening the cornea.

During sleep, there is a persistent tonic contraction of the orbicularis that keeps the eyelids closed (7). If the motor nerves are blocked by local anesthesia, the upper lid will open due to the tone of the levator. Neither lid can move completely independently of the other since they are connected at their common canthi (6). The orbicularis oculi works in concert with the other muscles of expression and with the levator palpebrae. When the orbicularis oculi, frontalis, and corrugator supercilii contract together, they are collectively called the "accessory muscle of accommodation." Persons with normal vision commonly contract these accessory muscles when they are doing close work, whereas those who are myopic may contract them when looking into the distance (6).

The orbital portion of the orbicularis oculi is an antagonist of the frontalis muscle; the palpebral portion of the orbicularis is an antagonist of the levator muscle. The pretarsal fibers of the orbicularis are active in tensing the margin of the eyelids, shortening the palpebral fissure, and helping with lid closure. The preseptal fibers are the fibers chiefly responsible for reflex eyelid closure. The preseptal and pretarsal muscle both contribute to the lacrimal pump mechanism for "milking" tears from the conjunctival sac into the lacrimal drainage system.

Electromyography of the upper eyelid shows that on gradual forced closure of the eyelids, the pretarsal fibers come into play first with the greatest frequency and amplitude, and then in a graduated manner they are followed by the lower preseptal fibers, the upper preseptal fibers, and finally the orbital fibers.

FESTOONS AND OTHER SURGICAL PROBLEMS

The orbicularis oculi muscle, the orbital septum, and the other supporting structures of the eyelids are interdependent in their function. With attenuation, degeneration, and involution several structures often relax simultaneously and the weakest link in the chain is not always evident. Festoons of the orbicularis muscle in their infrequent pure form involve only skin and muscle (Figs. 64.8 and 64.9). Owing to the efforts of gravity, age, and idiosyncrasy, the orbicularis sags like a hammock, carrying skin with it (14). The pathologic anatomy of these pure muscle festoons can be verified in the operating room by elevating a skin flap to expose the anterior face of the orbicularis oculi (Fig. 64.9*C*). More commonly the lax orbicularis is only a contributing cause of bags of the eyelids and simply adds muscle bulk to the bulge of protruding fat. The orbicularis also plays a role in the upper temporal visual field block caused by lateral ptosis of the brow and upper lid (also called *deckfalte*, *pli de recouvrement*, *lateral epicanthis*, or *ptosis adiposa* (6) (Fig. 64.10).

An undesired badge of seniority is the *bourrelet sénile* (6). This protrusion of fat from the medial portion of the upper orbit, just below the superior oblique muscle, is due to weakness of the orbicularis and a gap in the orbital septum. Bell's palsy presents an "experiment in nature" in which the interdependency of the supporting structures of the eyelid is demonstrated. If the orbicularis is paralyzed for many months in an older person, the supporting tissues may sag because of the absence of this important muscular reinforcement, which causes a bulge of the orbital fat. The stretching of the orbital septum and fascia may persist even after return of muscle function (Fig. 64.11).

In the case of a cheek bag due to the combined effect of a drooping orbicularis and stretched skin and connective tissue, surgical correction can be directed chiefly at tightening up the skin, combined with limited orbicularis excision (Fig. 64.12) or, on the contrary, the major effort can be directed at the muscle itself with limited excision of skin. Hinderer (15) called attention to the usefulness of raising and tightening the lateral canthal tendon in blepharoplasty, which indirectly effected change on the orbicularis. An anatomic variation of the orbicularis muscle that is associated with youth rather than age is bulging of a bulky pretarsal orbicularis. This can sometimes diminish the quality of the result of a blepharoplasty, and trimming may be helpful (16).

CLINICAL TESTS

SQUINCH TEST

When examining the patient with baggy eyelids, the surgeon observes carefully the patterns of orbicularis contraction. In the squinch test, the muscle is tightly contracted, or "squinched," and the floppy festoons, or bags, are effaced (Fig. 64.13). The festoons then reappear as the muscle relaxes. If the orbital fat has been suspended as a passenger in an orbicularis bag, the position of the fat will change as the muscle contracts: it moves toward the ciliary

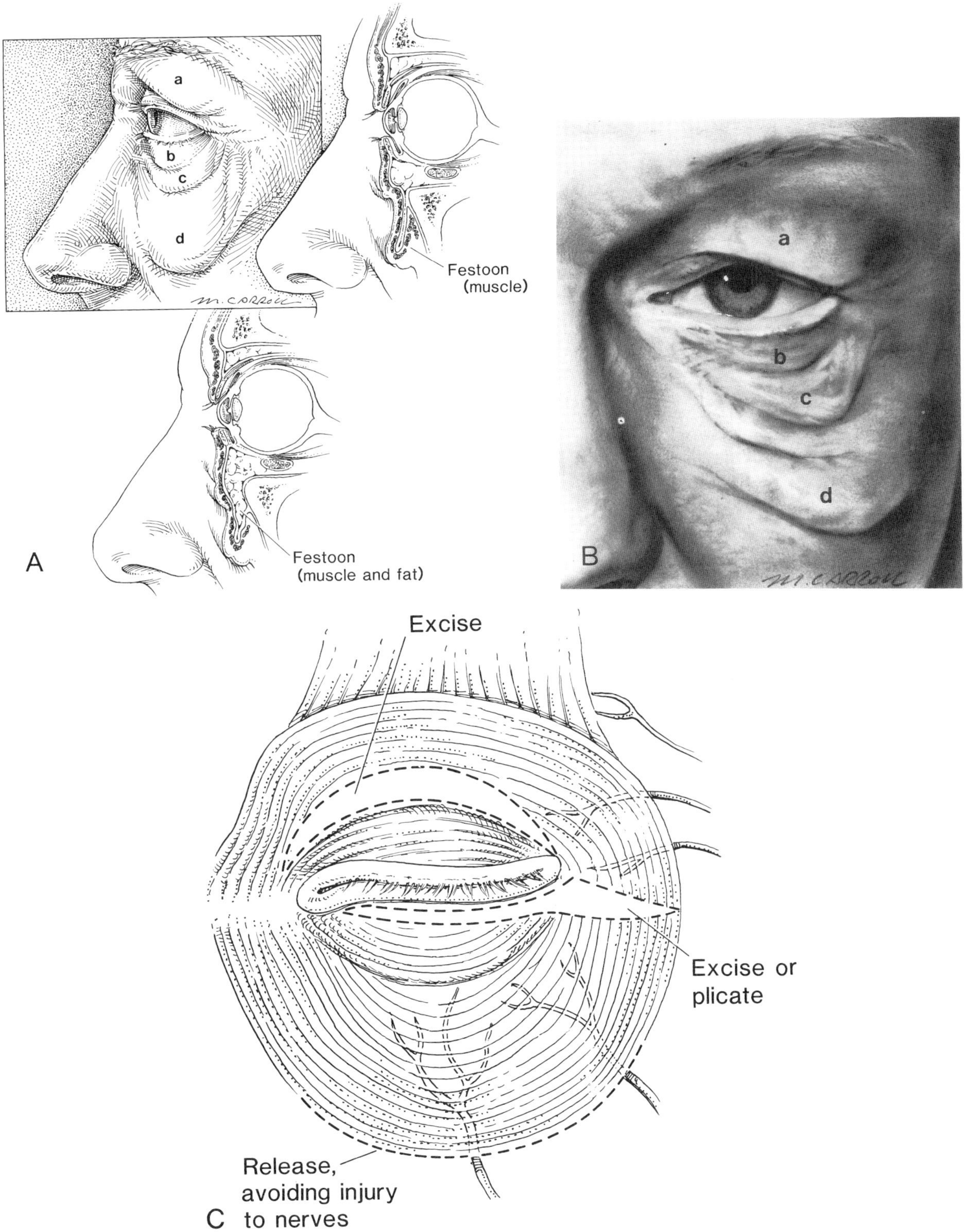

Figure 64.8. *A*, Orbicularis muscle festoons (*upper left*): *a*, upper lid; *b*, pretarsal; *c*, preseptal; *d*, orbital and jugal. Lax orbicularis muscle sags, which creates a hammock of skin and muscle if it is a pure muscle festoon (*upper right*), or contains within it protruding orbital fat (*middle*). *B*, Common sites of muscle festoons of the orbicularis: *a*, upper lid; *b*, pretarsal; *c*, preseptal; *d*, jugal. *C*, The muscle excisions are planned to minimize excision of active *protractor* muscle. Orbital portion can be excised freely. Sufficient muscle is excised to efface the festoons.

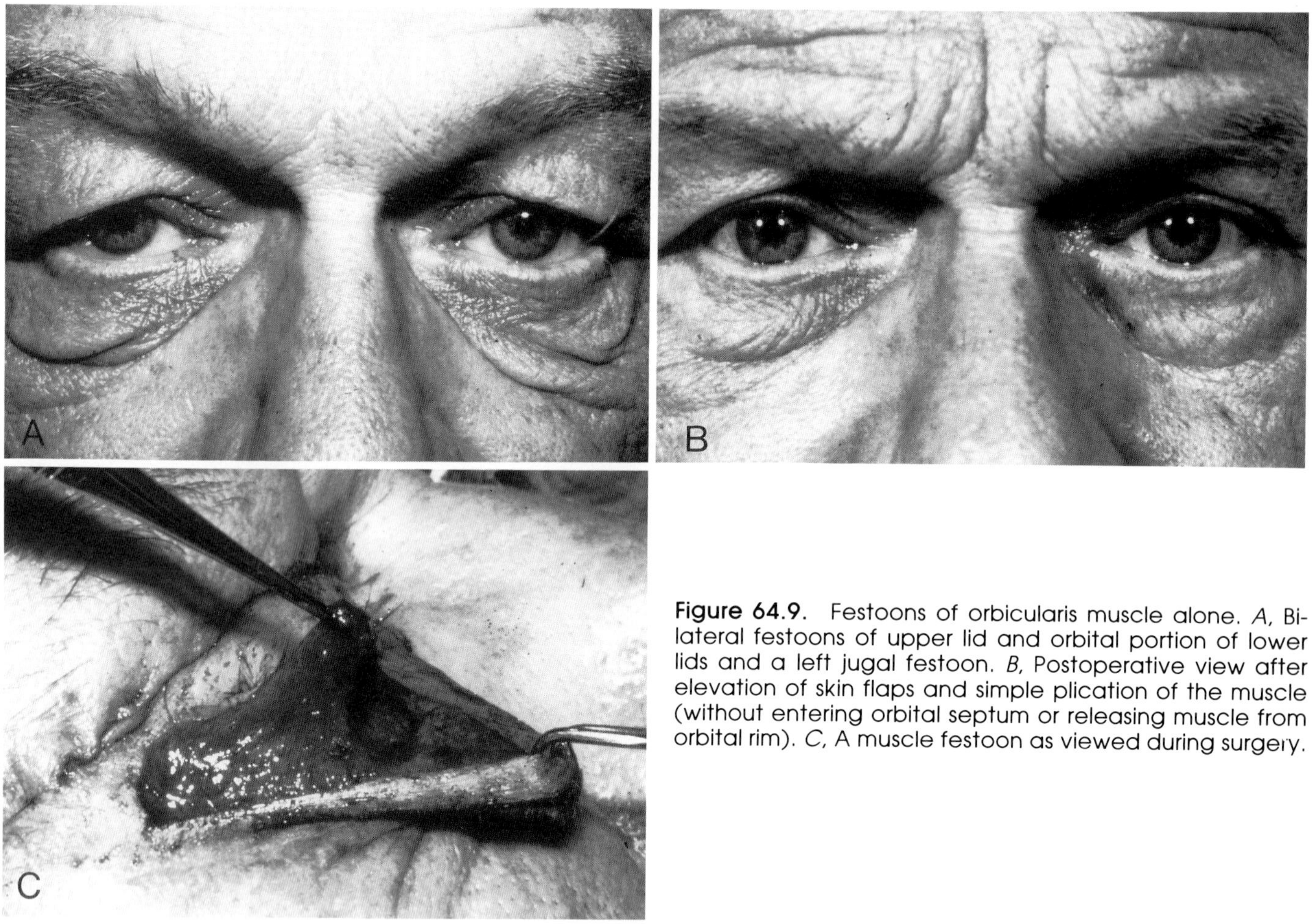

Figure 64.9. Festoons of orbicularis muscle alone. *A*, Bilateral festoons of upper lid and orbital portion of lower lids and a left jugal festoon. *B*, Postoperative view after elevation of skin flaps and simple plication of the muscle (without entering orbital septum or releasing muscle from orbital rim). *C*, A muscle festoon as viewed during surgery.

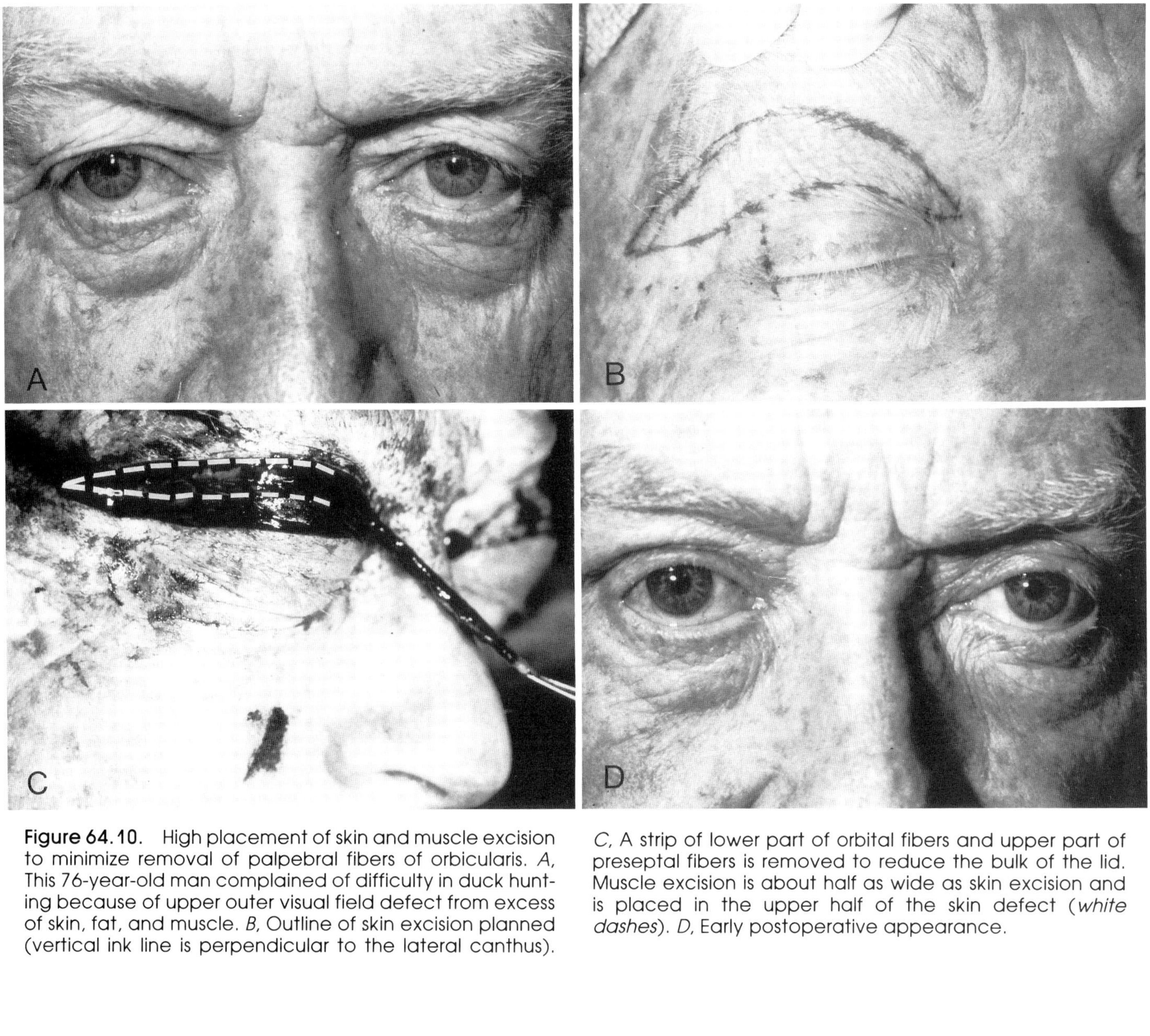

Figure 64.10. High placement of skin and muscle excision to minimize removal of palpebral fibers of orbicularis. *A*, This 76-year-old man complained of difficulty in duck hunting because of upper outer visual field defect from excess of skin, fat, and muscle. *B*, Outline of skin excision planned (vertical ink line is perpendicular to the lateral canthus). *C*, A strip of lower part of orbital fibers and upper part of preseptal fibers is removed to reduce the bulk of the lid. Muscle excision is about half as wide as skin excision and is placed in the upper half of the skin defect (*white dashes*). *D*, Early postoperative appearance.

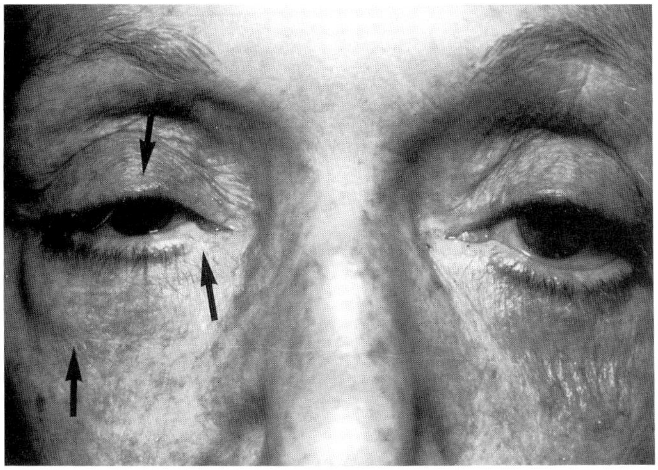

Figure 64.11. Bulging orbital fat, epiphora, and ptosis associated with Bell's palsy (history of previous blepharoplasty). This 76-year-old woman underwent an upper and lower blepharoplasty 20 years ago. Eighteen months ago, she had Bell's palsy, with 80% recovery. Three permanent problems resulted from the transient paralysis and the residual paresis: prominent bulges of the intraorbital fat in the lower lid from lack of support of the orbital septum (*lower left arrow*); epiphora from loss of capillarity from failure of the lower punctum (*lower right arrow*) to meet the globe and partial loss of the pumping action of the pars lacrimalis of the orbicularis (44); and ptosis of the right upper lid (*upper arrow*), the onset of which was probably aggravated by the patient's habit of wiping tears from her eye in a downward direction.

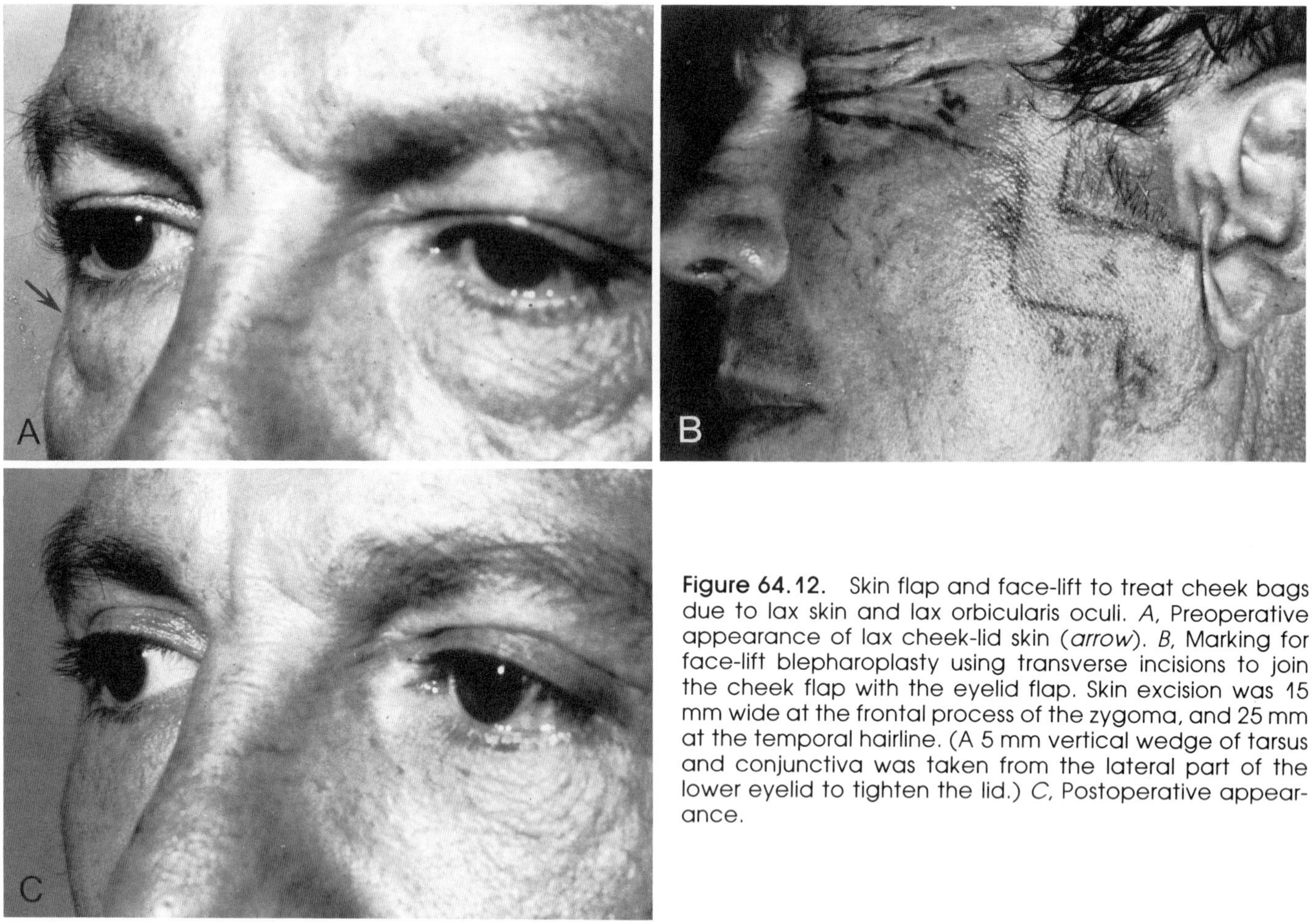

Figure 64.12. Skin flap and face-lift to treat cheek bags due to lax skin and lax orbicularis oculi. *A*, Preoperative appearance of lax cheek-lid skin (*arrow*). *B*, Marking for face-lift blepharoplasty using transverse incisions to join the cheek flap with the eyelid flap. Skin excision was 15 mm wide at the frontal process of the zygoma, and 25 mm at the temporal hairline. (A 5 mm vertical wedge of tarsus and conjunctiva was taken from the lateral part of the lower eyelid to tighten the lid.) *C*, Postoperative appearance.

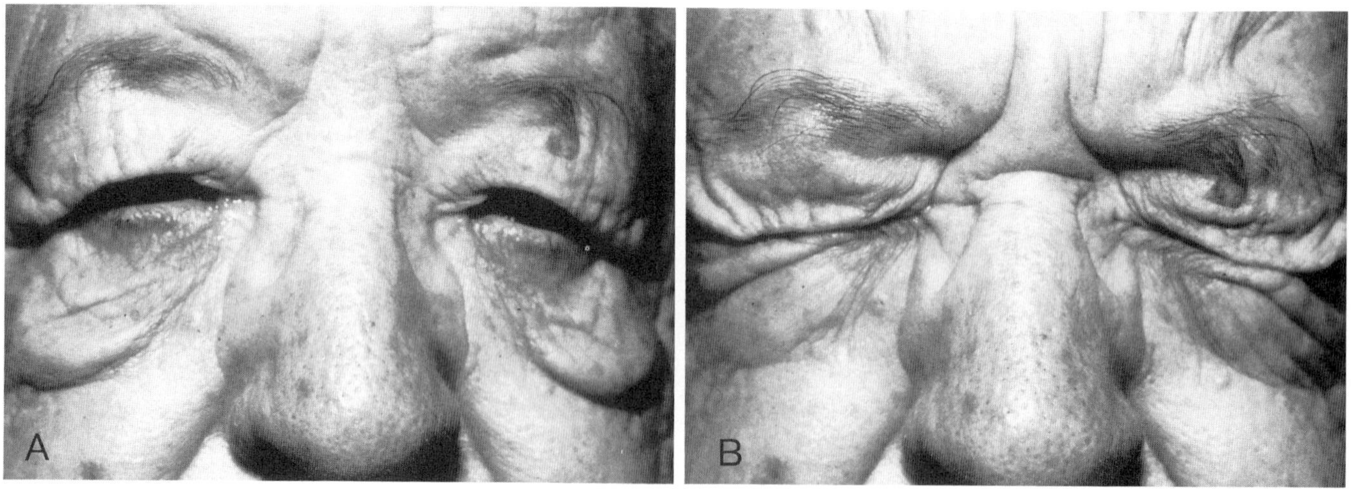

Figure 64.13. The squinch test, which is used to demonstrate muscle festoons. *A*, In repose. *B*, When the lids are squinched, the festoons are effaced.

margin and is effaced by muscle tension. When the orbicularis relaxes, the bag of fat resumes its previous position.

This pattern of contraction has been called "screwing up the eye" by Wolff, "occlusion effort" by Whitnall, and "squeezing" by Jones—terms that seem poorly descriptive; the term "squint" is confusing because in ophthalmology it refers to strabismus. The word "squinch," exhumed from the Oxford English Dictionary, means "to forcefully, but partially, screw shut the eyes," and appears useful in describing this forceful movement if the meaning is slightly amplified to include either open or shut eyes.

PINCH TEST

To determine the extent of the attachments between the skin and the underlying orbicularis muscle, the examiner gently picks up the skin and the attached muscle using the

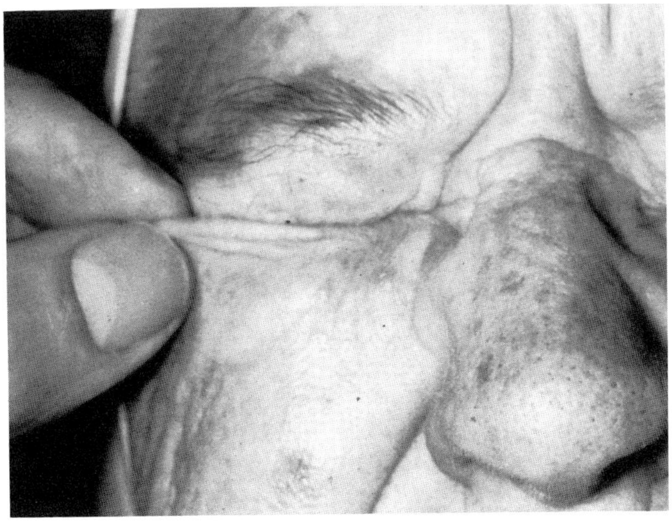

Figure 64.14. The pinch test. The movement, tension, and the adherence of the skin to the underlying orbicularis are tested in repose. Then the patient forcefully contracts the orbicularis against the resistance of the examiner's pinch.

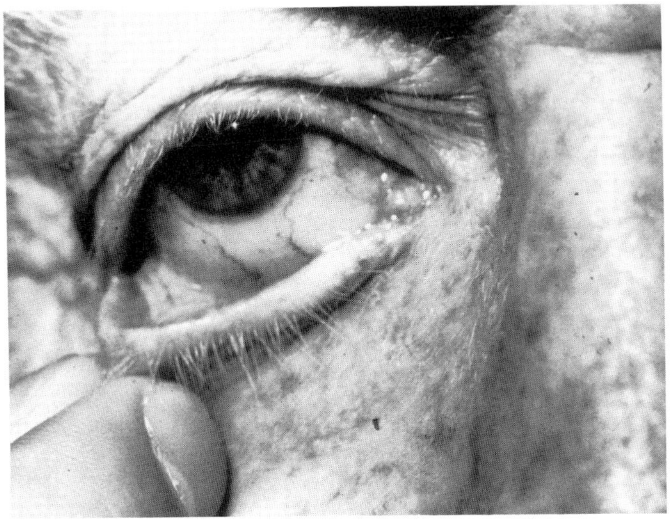

Figure 64.15. Lid distention test for lid laxity (Stasior). By pinching the skin of the lower lid and distending it away from the globe, one can determine the laxity of the supporting structures. Stasior suggests that if the lid can be pulled 8 mm away from the globe in a candidate for blepharoplasty, a tarsal wedge resection should be considered as an adjunctive procedure.

thumb and index finger and stretches the skin at selected sites while the patient performs expressive movements (Fig. 64.14). The examiner evaluates the resistance of the skin and muscle, the firmness of attachments, and the muscle bulk. This aids in distinguishing which of the features are due to muscle changes and which are due to skin.

LID DISTENTION TEST (STASIOR)

The lid distention test is of paramount importance in detecting excess laxity of the supporting structures of the lower lid prior to a blepharoplasty. The test is performed by pinching the skin and soft tissues of the lower lid and pulling the lid margin directly away from the globe (Fig. 64.15). Stasior advised that a gap of greater than 8 mm strongly suggests the need to incorporate a tarsal wedge excision with the blepharoplasty (17).

LEVATOR STRENGTH TEST

Since the levator and orbicularis are intimately related, evaluation of the strength of the levator is an important step. With the patient looking down, the lashes of both eyelids are grasped simultaneously by the examiner (Fig. 64.16). The patient is told to look strongly upward, and the tension of the levator is evaluated. As a further check, the examiner then tests each lid separately with the dominant hand. Examination of photos of the eyes in primary position, upward gaze, and downward gaze are also important.

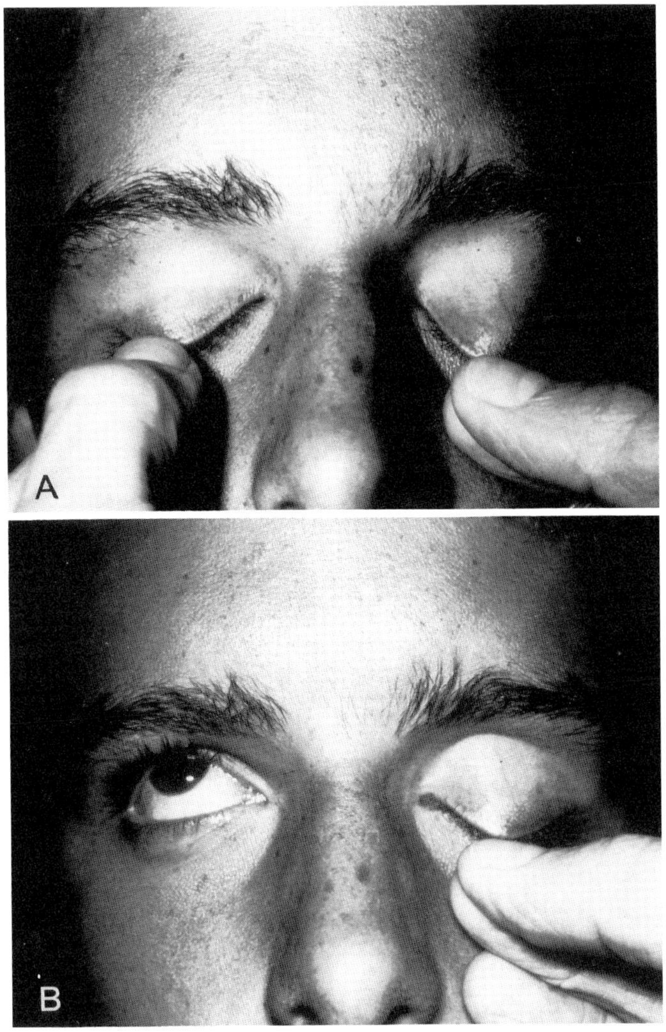

Figure 64.16. Levator traction test for levator strength. *A*, Examiner places gentle forward traction on lashes of upper eyelids while patient tries to look up. The relative strength of levators is estimated. Right and left lids are tested simultaneously. *B*, For further comparison, right and left lids are then tested sequentially with the examiner's dominant hand.

PROTRACTOR-RETRACTOR RELATIONSHIP

When planning alterations on the orbicularis oculi muscle, surgeons must consider the "protractor-retractor" relationships of the eyelids (Fig. 64.17). Jones referred to the orbicularis muscle fibers as the *protractors* of the upper and lower eyelids (7). The antagonists of these protractors are the *retractors*, which are the levator palpebrae in the upper eyelid and the capsulopalpebral head of the inferior rectus muscle in the lower lid. Of these muscles, the orbicularis is by far the stronger. [It is difficult to open the eye of an uncooperative baby but easy to hold an eyelid shut with gentle finger pressure (18).] The greater tone of the orbicularis is responsible for the fact that the level of the eyelid is lowered during sleep.

Cogan believes that the relationship between the orbicularis and levator is analogous to that between any other reciprocal pairs of extraocular muscles (19), and Van Allen and Blodi have confirmed the similarity based on electromyographic studies (20). This relationship can be demonstrated with a unilateral lidocaine block of the nerves to the orbicularis oculi (Fig. 64.18). Once the orbicularis is paralyzed, retraction of the unopposed levator palpebrae is seen. Mustardé has exploited this phenomenon in his most recent ptosis procedure, in which he excises some orbicularis muscle to diminish the load on the levator (21).

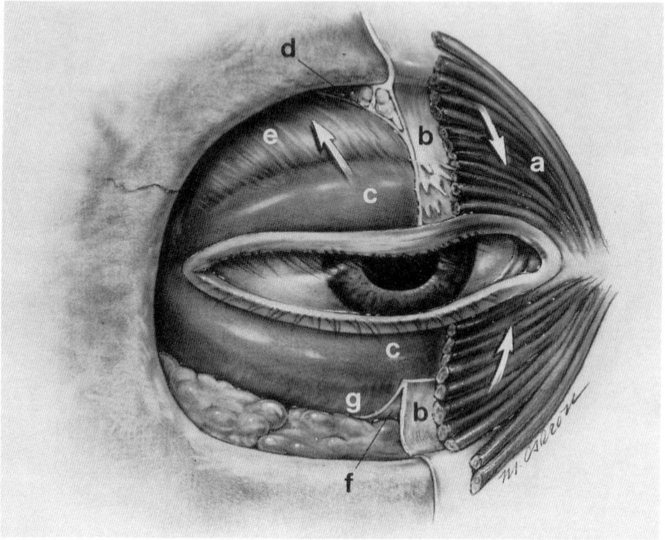

Figure 64.17. Anatomy of the protractors and retractors. Antagonistic retractor action of the aponeurosis of the levator palpebrae (*d*) and the superior tarsal muscle (*e*), and the protractor action of the orbicularis oculi muscles of the upper lid (*a*) are portrayed. The orbicularis is by far the stronger muscle, but a delicate balance is achieved. The orbicularis of the lower lid (*a*) is counteracted by a combination of gravity and the action of the aponeurosis of the capsulopalpebral head of the inferior rectus (*f*) and the inferior tarsal muscle (*g*) inserting into tarsus (*c*). The fusion of posterior fascia of the orbicularis, the orbital septum, and the protractor aponeurosis is seen at (*b*) above and below: in the lower lid, the area of fusion is cut away at its junction for clarity.

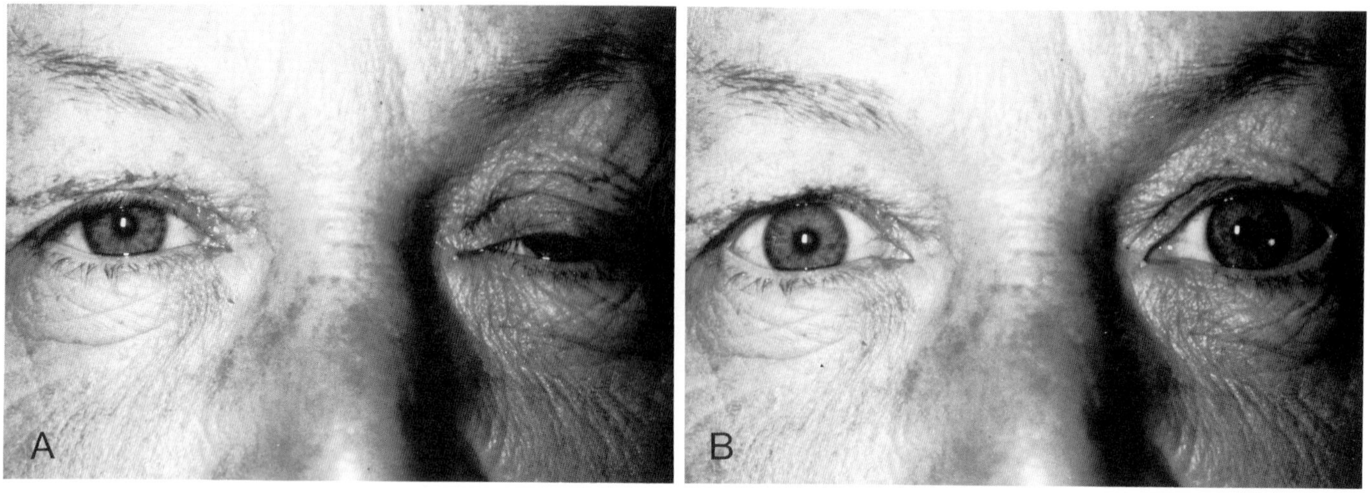

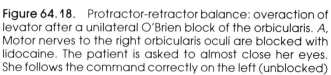

Figure 64.18. Protractor-retractor balance: overaction of levator after a unilateral O'Brien block of the orbicularis. *A*, Motor nerves to the right orbicularis oculi are blocked with lidocaine. The patient is asked to almost close her eyes. She follows the command correctly on the left (unblocked) side, but on the right the eyelid stays open because the tonus of the levator palpebrae is unopposed by any protraction of the orbicularis oculi. *B*, The patient is asked to focus her gaze on the camera lens. Overreaction of the right levator is again seen for the same reason.

RETRACTION OF UPPER EYELID

Not only form but also function of the orbicularis must be carefully considered in eyelid operations, particularly when one considers that the most common site of sagging is in the preseptal fibers, which are the fibers most active in automatic lid closure. A mild change in the protractor-retractor balance can give an aesthetic improvement in some patients. If the ciliary margin of the upper eyelid is low at the outset, a procedure that leaves it at a slightly higher level is acceptable, indeed desirable (Fig. 64.19). However, in the patient with a tendency toward levator retraction, even 0.5 mm of increased elevation of the upper lid may show a scleral rim above the limbus in neutral gaze and thus be unattractive (4). In such a case, another method of correcting the sagging orbicularis muscle of the upper lid, such as a forehead-lift or excision of local skin, should be selected (Fig. 64.20).

An increase in lid load from redundant fat and soft tissue can cause ptosis (22); conversely, a diminished lid load from excision of excess tissues can cause upper lid elevation. If orbicularis fibers are included in this excision, the balance can tip in favor of the lid retractors, resulting in an unexpected lid retraction syndrome (Fig. 64.21).

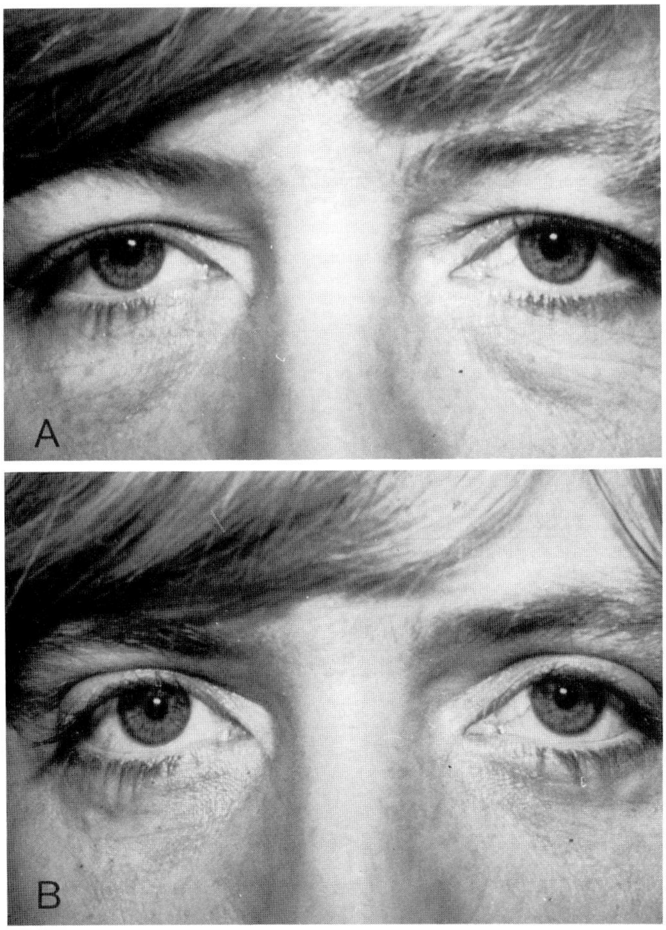

Figure 64.19. Change in level of upper lid margin following resection of preseptal fibers. *A*, Preoperative level. *B*, Postoperatively, the lid margin rests at a very slightly higher level. In this case the change is desirable.

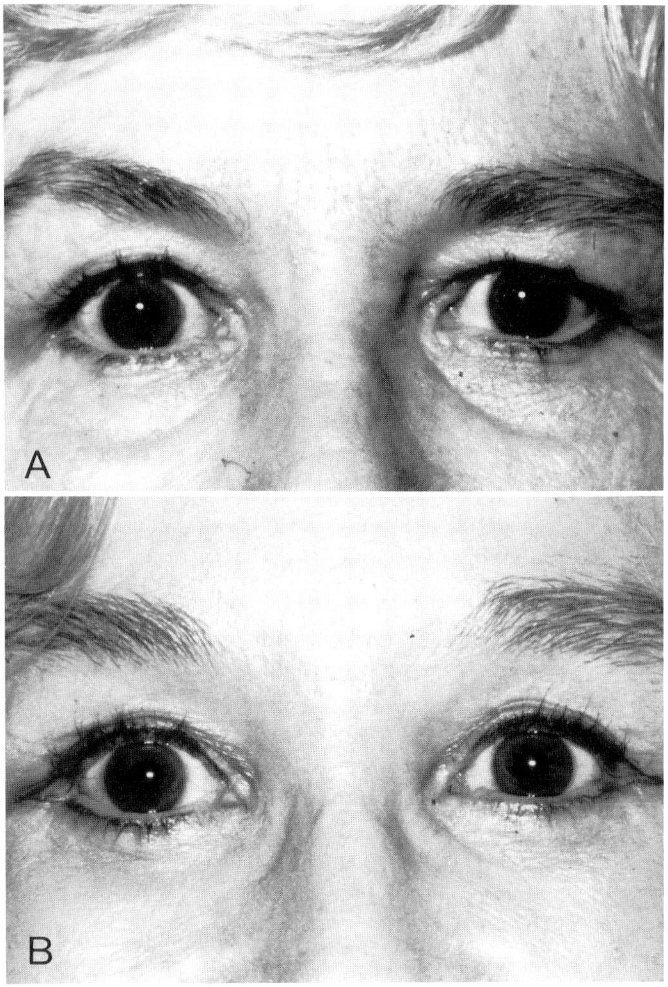

Figure 64.20. Preoperative levator retraction. To correct the upper eyelids, surgeon used a forehead-lift instead of excision of orbicularis. *A*, Preoperative mild levator retraction on the right. Further elevation of the ciliary margin would be undesirable; therefore, a forehead-lift was carried out in conjunction with excision of eyelid fat. *B*, Postoperative appearance.

A tendency to postoperative lid retraction can be treated by encouraging the patient to retrain "eyelid habits" during the early postoperative period. He or she can place a sign on the bathroom mirror as a reminder to keep the eyelids relaxed at all times. I have found this effective on several occasions. Patients who have a tendency toward lid retraction are often those who preoperatively have animated facial movements and active shifts of the upper lid margin when they carry on conversation.

Flowers has suggested a carefully calculated levator myotomy as a means of correcting persistent lid retraction (23). Numerous techniques of levator tenotomy have been described for treatment of lid retraction associated with hyperthyroidism. Eye drops of guanethidine, or other β-adrenergic drugs, have been useful for the lid retraction of hyperthyroidism.

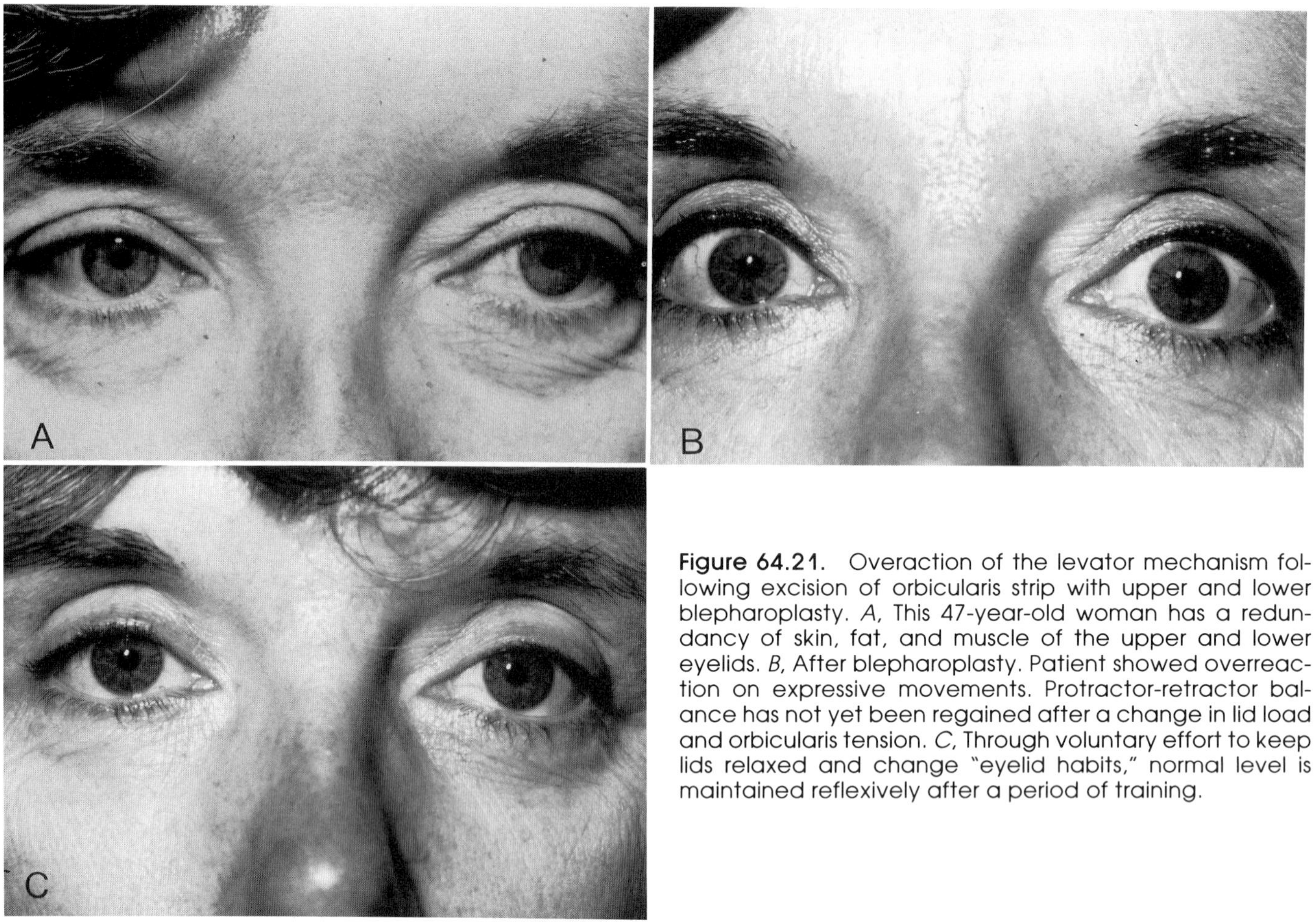

Figure 64.21. Overaction of the levator mechanism following excision of orbicularis strip with upper and lower blepharoplasty. *A,* This 47-year-old woman has a redundancy of skin, fat, and muscle of the upper and lower eyelids. *B,* After blepharoplasty. Patient showed overreaction on expressive movements. Protractor-retractor balance has not yet been regained after a change in lid load and orbicularis tension. *C,* Through voluntary effort to keep lids relaxed and change "eyelid habits," normal level is maintained reflexively after a period of training.

PTOSIS OF UPPER EYELID

Of all the muscles in the orbital area, by far the greatest number of anomalies are found in the levator palpebrae (7). At least 20% of the population has anomalies of the levator, which usually occur without signs or symptoms. The most common symptomatic anomaly is dehiscence of the levator aponeurosis; as long as the superior tarsal muscle (of Müller) is normal, ptosis may not be evident. However, if the aponeurotic defect is coupled with a weak superior tarsal muscle then the ptosis becomes evident.

In aging patients one sees attenuation, dehiscence, and sometimes detachment of the levator aponeurosis due to involutional changes of the tissues (24). The details of the pathologic anatomy and therapeutic strategies of this type of ptosis have been the subject of several recent studies (25–29). The tarsal muscle also loses strength with age, which further predisposes the individual to ptosis (Fig. 64.22).

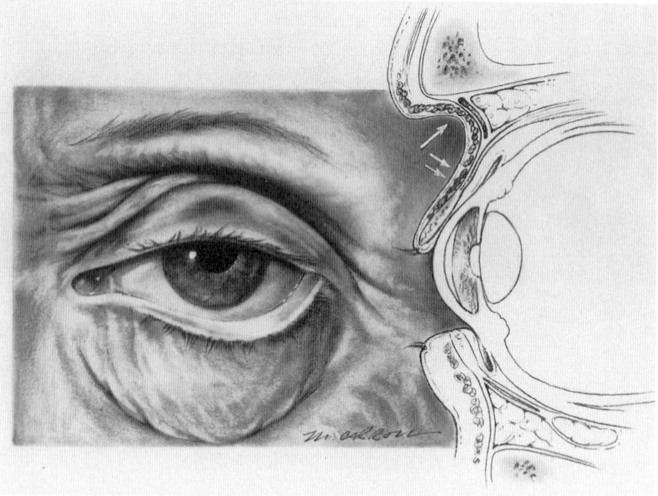

Figure 64.22. Absorption of preaponeurotic fat and attentuation of structures of the lid in an older patient. The thinness of the lid structures and the relative compression of the connective tissues of the lid (*arrows*) put the levator mechanism at risk during surgical procedures.

Intraoperative ptosis is a startling complication that I have encountered (Fig. 64.23). A marked unilateral ptosis was noted during a routine blepharoplasty and face-lift at the time the patient sat up for her dressings. Immediate exploration showed that the insertion of an attenuated aponeurosis had been detached. A repair was carried out

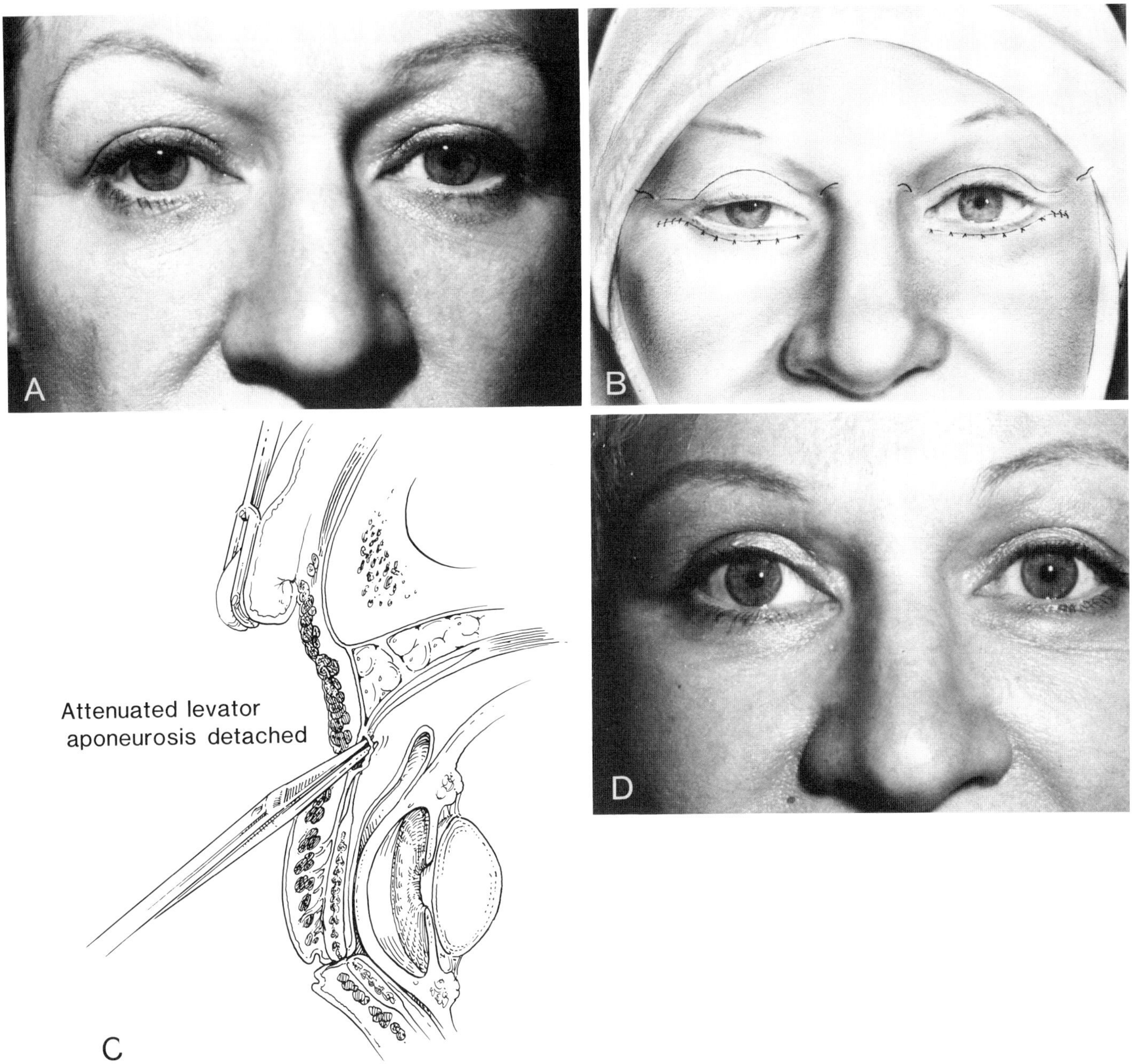

Figure 64.23. Intraoperative ptosis, a complication of blepharoplasty. *A*, This 52-year-old woman has an excess of skin, muscle, and fat of the upper eyelid; there is no sign of ptosis. *B*, Artist's impression of eyelids immediately after a blepharoplasty and face-lift (ptosis on right). *C*, In the course of spreading the tissue planes of the lid, attenuated levator aponeurosis was detached from its insertion. Immediate exploration was carried out. The aponeurosis was identified. Trial sutures were placed three times to obtain symmetry of the lids with the patient in a sitting position, and finally the wound was closed. *D*, Four months postoperatively, the right eyelid has higher tarsal fold due to repair.

as described by Jones (7). Ellenbogen (30) and Wilkins (31) have emphasized the preoperative diagnosis and the systematic treatment of patients who have problems amenable to combined blepharoplasty and ptosis repair.

I have seen several patients with late onset of involutional ptosis years after a bilateral upper blepharoplasty was performed. In one patient, the ptosis was bilateral (Fig. 64.24) and had developed slowly. Examination of previous preoperative and postoperative photographs showed no suggestion of ptosis. A bilateral Lester Jones repair was performed with successful results; the dissection was only slightly hampered by residual scar tissue. Another patient (Fig. 64.25) presented 8 years after blepharoplasty with disinsertion of both levators. In addition, Müller's muscle was disinserted from the left tarsus. A trial with levator reattachment caused excessive lid retraction. Therefore, aponeuroses were left untouched and Müller's muscle alone was reinserted, which gave asymmetry.

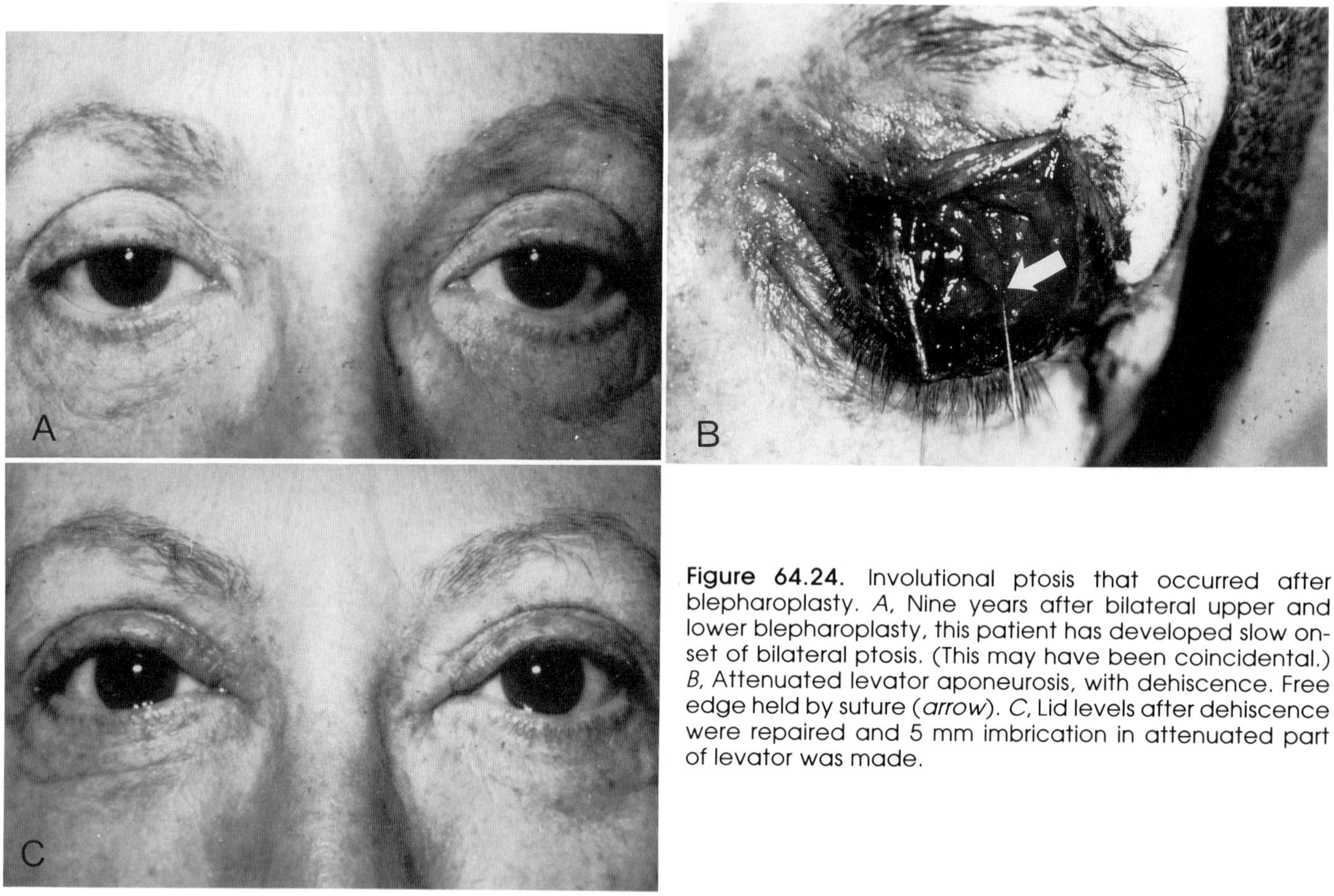

Figure 64.24. Involutional ptosis that occurred after blepharoplasty. *A*, Nine years after bilateral upper and lower blepharoplasty, this patient has developed slow onset of bilateral ptosis. (This may have been coincidental.) *B*, Attenuated levator aponeurosis, with dehiscence. Free edge held by suture (*arrow*). *C*, Lid levels after dehiscence were repaired and 5 mm imbrication in attenuated part of levator was made.

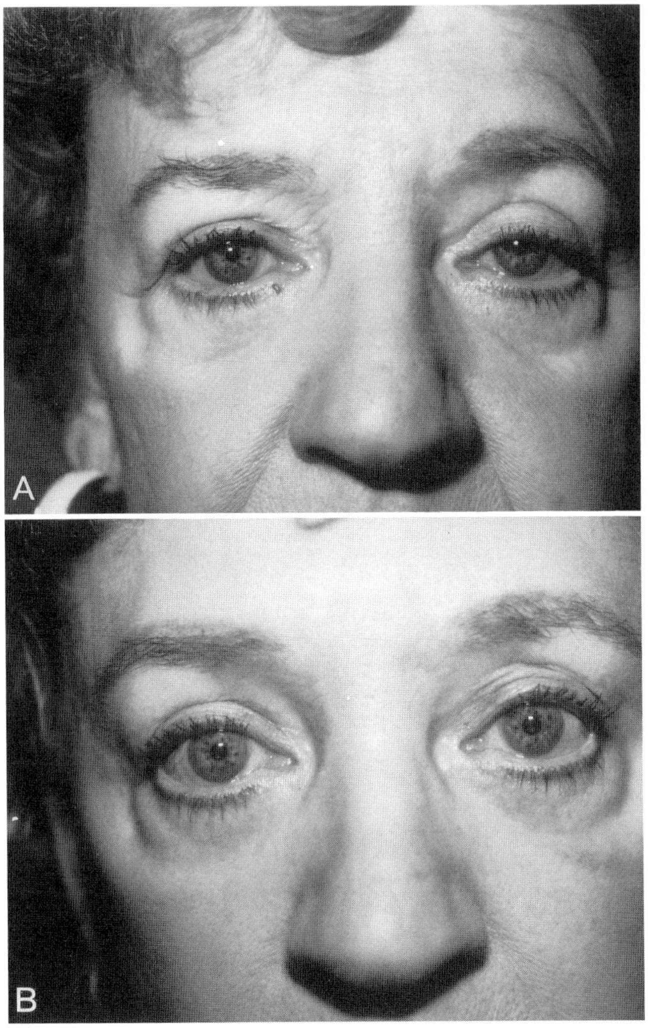

Figure 64.25. Bilateral levator disinsertion with unilateral disinsertion of Müller's muscle 8 years after blepharoplasty. This 73-year-old woman developed asymmetrical ptosis 8 years after a routine blepharoplasty. At operation, bilateral disinsertion of the levator aponeurosis was identified. The insertion of Müller's muscle was detached from the tarsus on the right but not on the left. A trial reinsertion of the levators caused what appeared to be hyperretraction at surgery. Therefore, only the detached Müller's muscle was repaired. The levator aponeuroses were left untreated. *A*, Disinserted Müller's muscle on left, disinsertion of both levator aponeuroses. *B*, Müller's muscle only reinserted (simultaneous secondary face-lift and forehead lift).

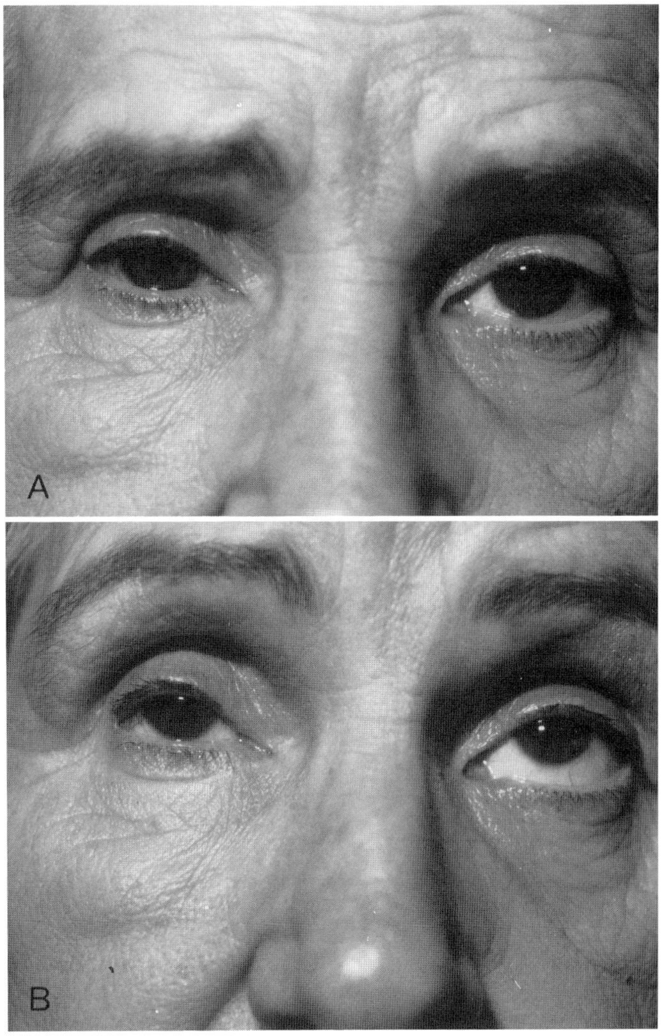

Figure 64.26. Ptosis and narrow palpebral aperture (pseudoenophthalmos) after Bell's palsy, blepharospasm, and ocular surgery. Woman, age 64, with onset of blepharospasm of right orbicularis associated with recovery period of Bell's palsy at age 19. Epiphora was present for many years and then ceased. Ptosis of the upper lid was noted for years and increased after cataract extraction and scleral buckle at age 55. Palpebral aperture is short and narrow. Hertel exophthalmometer values are 13 mm on right and 14 mm on left. Right ptosis is symptomatic. Right lower eyelid is higher than left. Upward gaze of right eye is diminished. Our analysis was that constant spasms of the orbicularis oculi stretched the canthal tendons, thereby shortening and narrowing the palpebral aperture and contributing to the ptosis and elevated lower lid. Stretching of the upper lid from rubbing during period of epiphora, ocular surgery, and senile changes may have contributed. The scleral buckle interferes with upward gaze. *A*, Primary gaze. *B*, Upward gaze.

Another patient (Fig. 64.11) had acute onset of a right Bell's palsy 20 years after a bilateral upper and lower blepharoplasty. Because of paresis of the orbicularis, she was bothered by epiphora. After 18 months, 80% of facial nerve function was recovered in a spotty distribution (some branches were even hyperactive). During the recovery period, right unilateral ptosis plus bulging of the intraorbital fat of her right lower lid developed. We suspect that the ptosis was due to stretching of a weak aponeurosis by repeated wiping of tears, and that the bulge of fat was from a stretching of the orbital septum that had been unsupported by the orbicularis. Another patient with recovered Bell's palsy but persistent blepharospasm developed shortening and narrowing of the palpebral aperture (Fig. 64.26).

Other causes of postoperative ptosis are adherence of the overlying eyelid skin to the superior oblique muscle, where excess fat has been excised from the medial pocket, and also excessive postoperative swelling in the presence of involutional changes in the eyelid (32).

OTHER SYNERGISTIC MUSCLES

The frontalis is an accessory elevator of the upper eyelid. The levator palpebrae acts in unison with the frontalis in expressing astonishment. We have seen transient lid retraction from synkinesis (*secondary deviation*) (33) of these movements in a postblepharoplasty patient with superimposed Bell's palsy (Fig. 64.27). All three muscles act together in looking upward at the extreme (6).

The inferior rectus muscle, through its capsulopalpebral head, retracts the lower eyelid about two-thirds of the distance that the globe rotates downward. In primary position, the margin of the lower eyelid is about level with the lower limbus of the cornea. As the eye rotates downward about 10 mm, the lower eyelid follows roughly half this distance. In a position of direct gaze, this muscle, unlike the levator, does not have any effect on the lower eyelid.

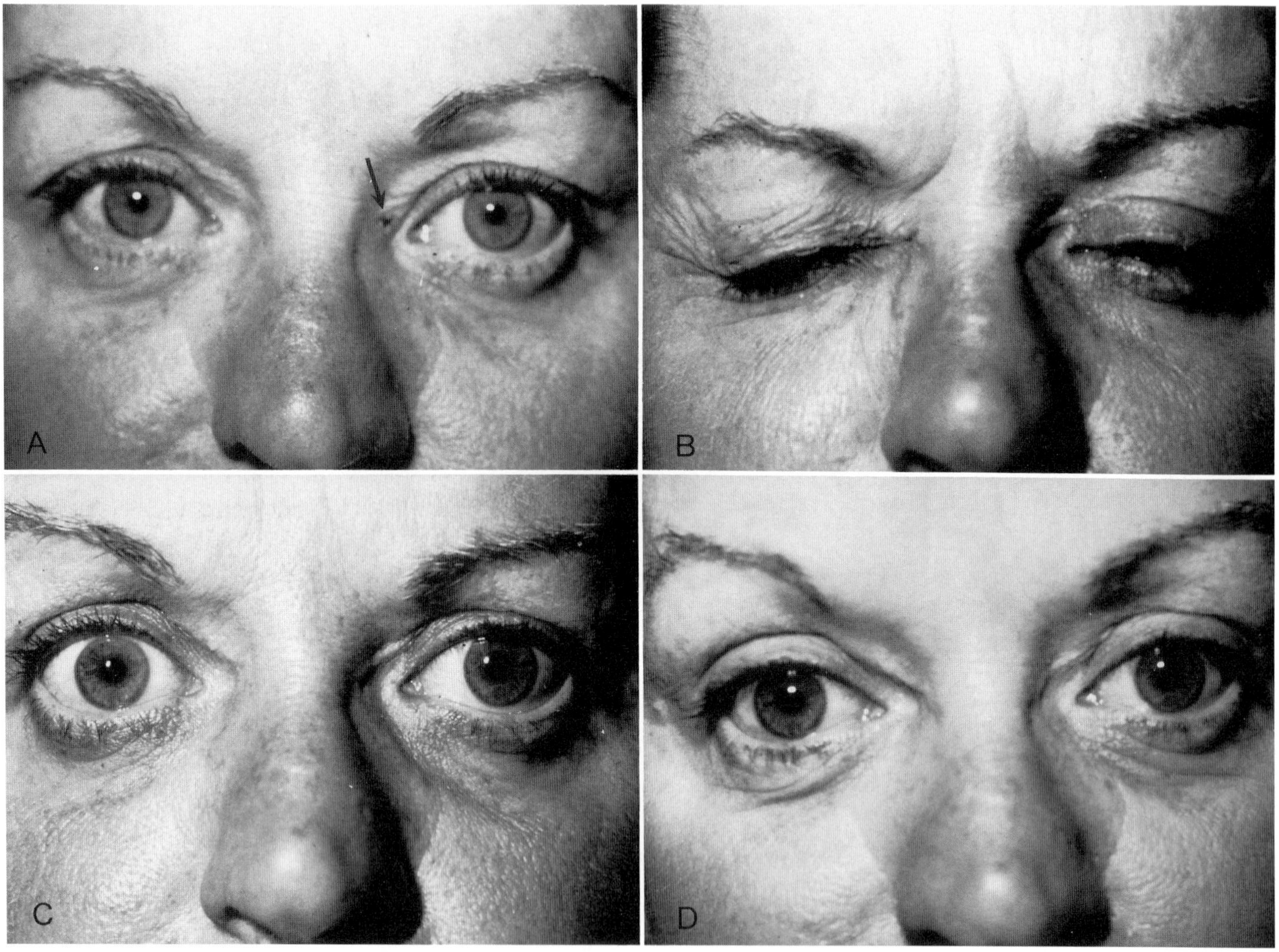

Figure 64.27. Lid retraction from synkinetic movements of the right frontalis and levator due to left Bell's palsy (previous blepharoplasty; secondary deviation of nonparetic lid) (15). *A*, This 51-year-old woman has a basal cell carcinoma of left nasoorbital area (*arrow*). Bilateral upper blepharoplasties were done to obtain a skin graft and simultaneously to correct the excess skin, muscle, and fat. *B*, One year after blepharoplasty and skin graft, the patient had acute onset of Bell's palsy on the left side. One week after onset, the patient uses maximal effort to close both eyelids; the left lid lags. *C*, Patient showed overreaction (secondary deviation) of right levator and right frontalis in direct gaze. The right eye is the dominant eye. Patient has always had animated expression ("I can talk with my face"). Skin was quite adequate and there was no tethering effect between the levator and the skin or orbicularis. The lid retraction appeared to be from a synkinesis of the right levator and the frontalis in response to the patient's efforts to make her usual expressive movements on the left. *D*, Eyelid findings completely cleared 1 year later, after 90% return of nerve function.

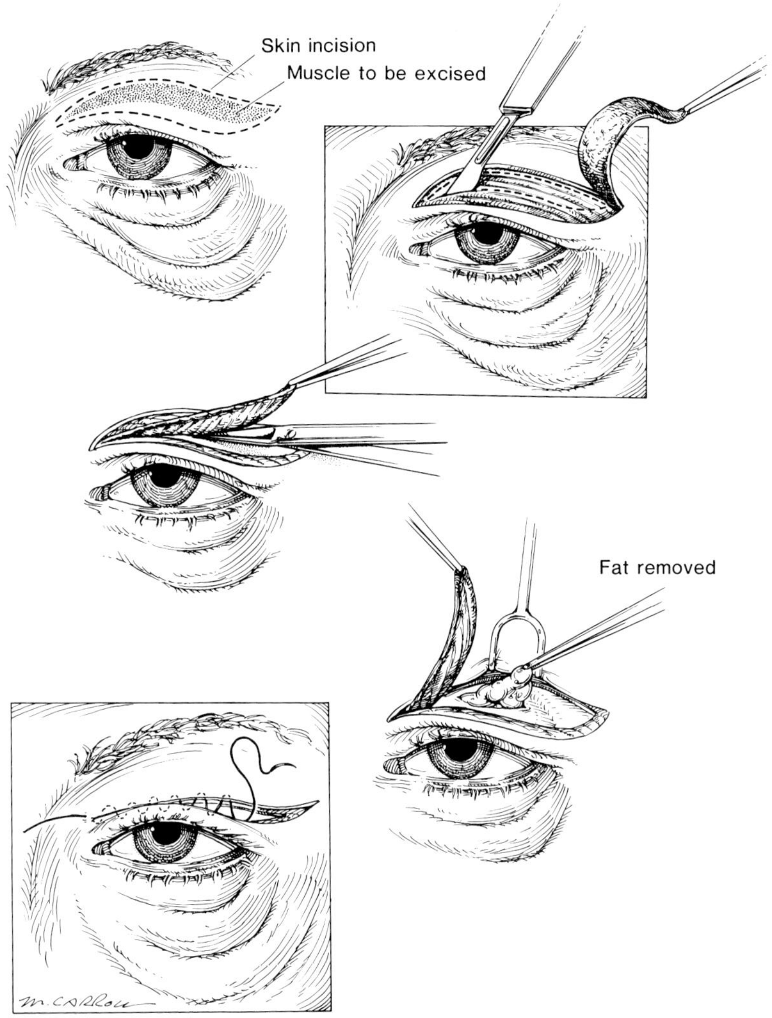

Figure 64.28. Surgical treatment of festoon of upper lid. Festoon blocks the upper outer visual field. The orbicularis muscle is excised conservatively and relatively high but in sufficient quantity to diminish the obstruction to vision.

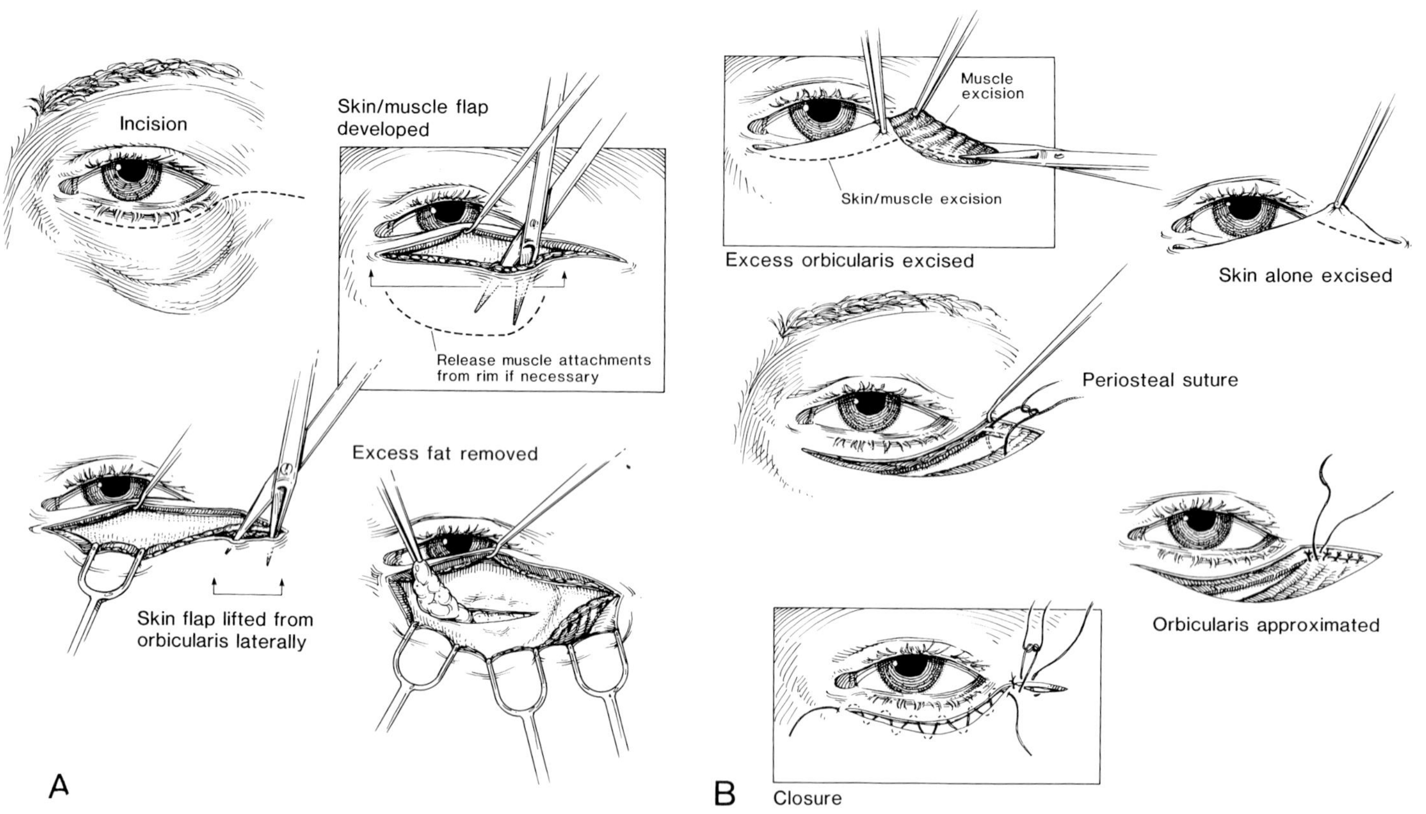

Figure 64.29. Muscle excision technique for festoon of lower lid. *A*, A *split flap* dissection is used (skin-muscle flap medially, skin flap alone laterally). With severe festoons, release of the muscle from the inferior orbital rim is sometimes helpful. Great care is exercised to avoid injury to the entering rami of the facial nerve. *B*, Sufficient muscle is excised to take up the slack of the festoon. The tension of the muscle is taken up on the lateral closure line.

Figure 64.30. Muscle plication technique for festoon of the lower lid (an alternate technique). A skin flap is elevated. The orbicularis muscle is freed along the ciliary margin, then the excess is simply plicated. A key suture is placed through periosteum, then muscle-to-muscle sutures are placed. Excess skin is excised.

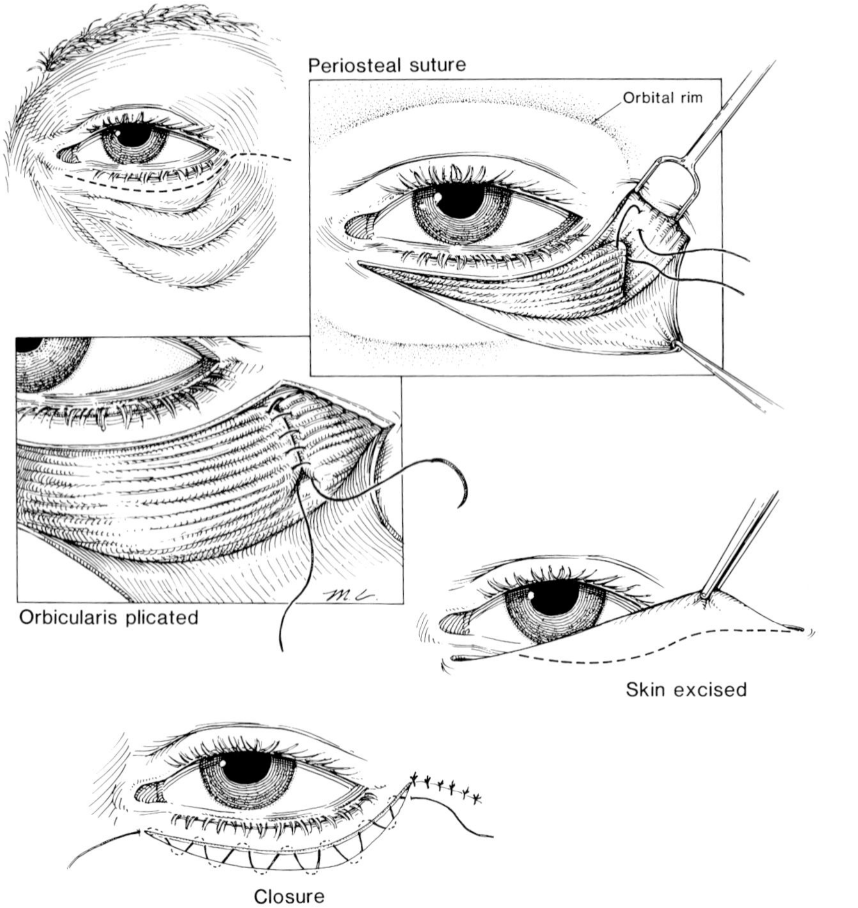

OPERATIVE TECHNIQUES

Operative manipulation of the orbicularis as part of esthetic and reconstructive surgery of the orbit has stimulated increasing interest. McIndoe and Beare developed the skin muscle flap with excision of orbicularis of the lower lid (34). Flowers sometimes thins the pretarsal muscles when needed in blepharoplasties (35). Flowers (23) and Sheen (36) described techniques for fixation or anchorage of the orbicularis to the levator; but Baker could determine no final postoperative difference between "anchor" or "fixation" techniques when compared with a blepharoplasty with simple removal of a strip of orbicularis and fat (37). Loeb described reduction of bulky orbicularis muscles of the lower lid (16). Klatsky described use of a muscle flap technique for orbicularis (11). Skoog laid out, split, and resected the lateral parts of the orbicularis to reduce "crow's feet" (38). Aston has elaborated on Skoog's technique (39). Leber and Cramer used a transfer of a bundle of orbicularis to treat entropion (40). Spira (41) and Owsley (42) have added refinements to management of the orbicularis. Adamson devised a technique for treatment of orbicularis festoons, in which the unwanted orbicularis muscle was moved laterally and then used as an overlapping sling to support the lower lid (43).

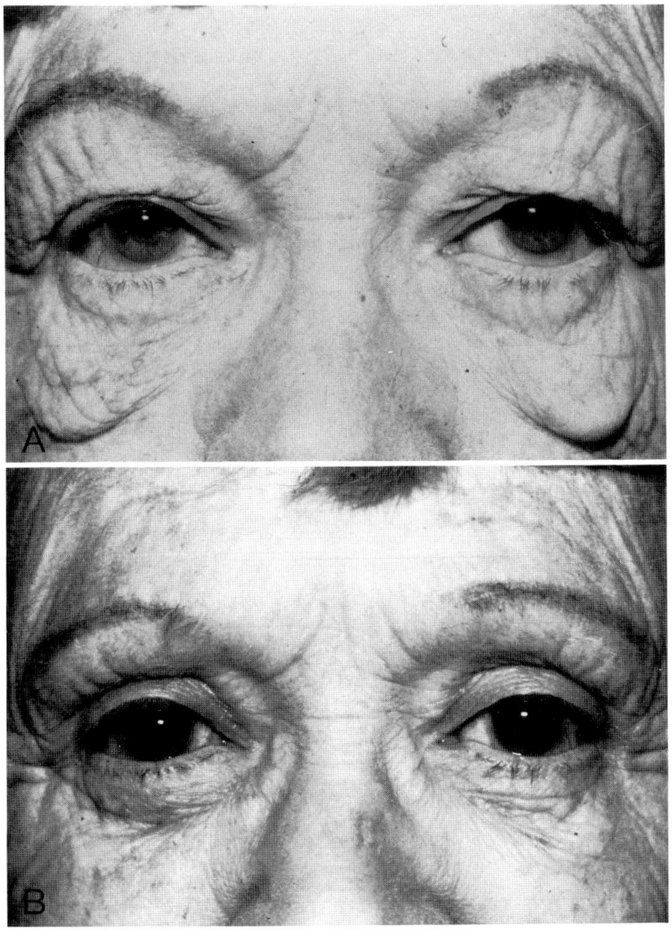

Figure 64.31. Jugal festoons. *A*, Preoperative appearance. *B*, Appearance after skin, muscle, and fat of the upper and lower eyelids were trimmed using orbicularis excision.

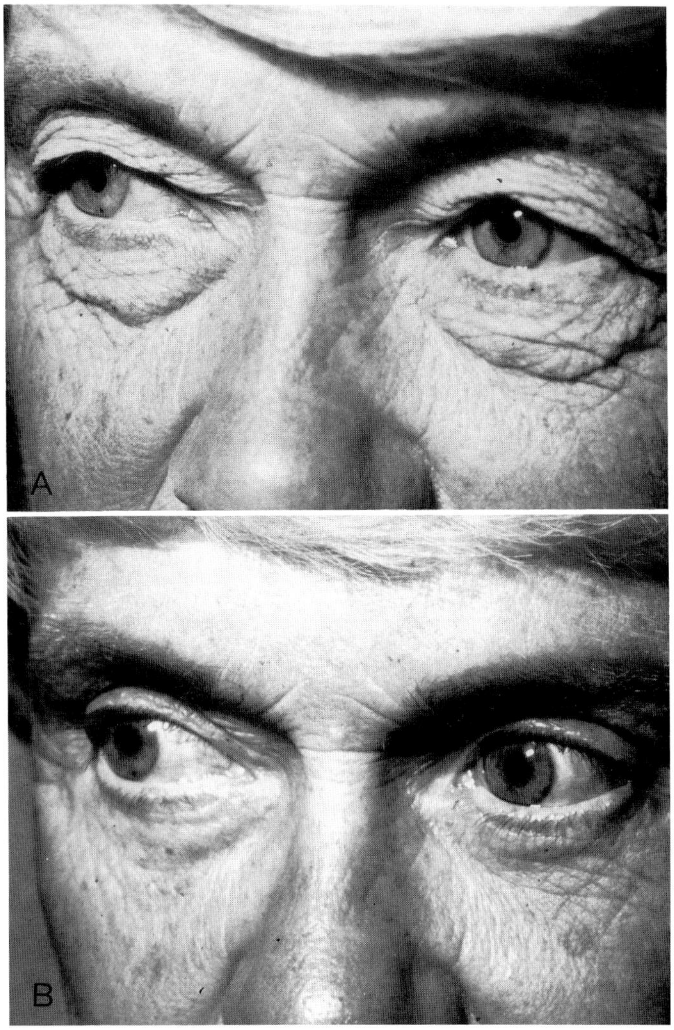

Figure 64.32. Mild orbital festoons of orbicularis with important component from orbital fat, upper and lower lids. *A*, Preoperative appearance, *B*, Appearance after resection of muscle, fat, and skin.

Two other techniques of treating muscle festoons are illustrated (Figs. 64.28–64.30). I believe it is important to do as much advance planning of the excisions as possible. The patient is examined upright just before making the marks. I mark out the proposed skin excisions and then scratch them in as soon as the local anesthesia has been injected. Any deviation from this original plan must be done with great deliberation. Pilot cuts and temporary sutures are helpful guides. One must bear in mind that the local anesthesia paralyzes the orbicularis during surgery and that the combination of the muscle flaccidity and the supine position diminishes the quality of any decisions made during surgery. Using these dicta and the techniques

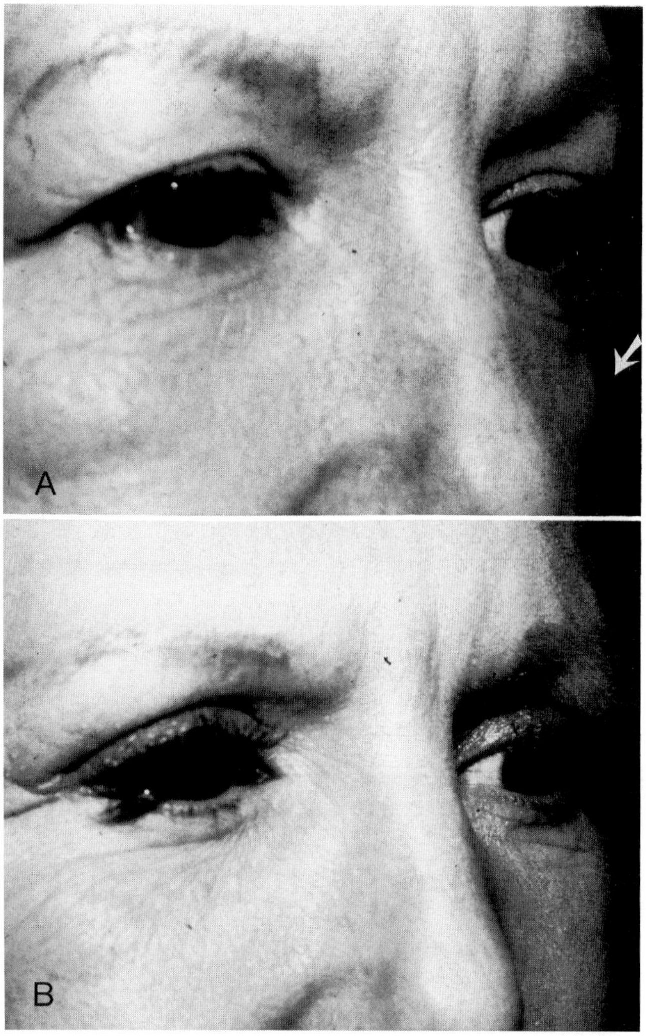

Figure 64.33. Mild jugal festoons. *A,* Preoperative appearance. *B,* Appearance after release of orbicularis and upward advancement of muscle-skin flap (upper blepharoplasty at the same time).

described herein, we believe that our surgical control over orbicularis festoons and their permutations have been improved (Figs. 64.31–64.33).

REFERENCES

1. Duchenne GB: *Mécanisme de la Physionomie Humaine.* Paris, Libraire J.B. Baillieŕe et Fils, 1876.
2. Gordon G: Observations Upon the Movements of the Eyelids. *Br J Ophthalmol* 35: 339–351, 1951.
3. Feinstein B, Lindegard B, Nyman E, *et al*: Morphologic studies of motor units in normal human muscles. *Acta Anat* 23: 127–142, 1954.
4. Walsh FB, Hoyt WF: *Clinical Neuro-Ophthalmology,* ed 3. Baltimore, Williams & Wilkins, 1969.
5. Kennard DW, Glaser GH: An analysis of eyelid movement. *J Nerv Ment Dis* 139: 31-48, 1964.
6. Whitnall SE: The anatomy of the human orbit and accessory organs of vision, ed 2. London, Oxford University Press, 1932.
7. Jones LT, Wobig JL: *Surgery of the Eyelids and Lacrimal System.* Birmingham, AL, Aesculapius, 1976.
8. Last RJ: *Wolff's Anatomy of the Eye and Orbit,* ed 6. Philadelphia, WB Saunders, 1968.
9. Lasjaunias PL, Berenstein A: *Craniofacial and Upper Cervical Arteries.* Baltimore, Williams & Wilkins, 1981.
10. Taylor GI, Corlett RJ, Boyd JB: The versatile deep inferior epigastric (inferior rectus abdominis) flap. *Br J Plast Surg* 37: 330, 1984.
11. Klatsky SA, Manson PN: Separate skin and muscle flaps in lower-lid blepharoplasty. *Plast Reconstr Surg* 67: 151, 1981.
12. Le-Quang C: Le plexus génien du nerf facial: anatomie et conséquences cliniques. *Ann Chir Plast* 21: 5, 1976.
13. Baker DC, Conley J: Avoiding facial nerve injuries in rhytidectomy. *Plast Reconstr Surg* 64: 781, 1979.
14. Furnas DW: Festoons of orbicularis muscle as a cause of baggy eyelids. *Plast Reconstr Surg* 61: 540, 1978.
15. Hinderer UT: Blepharocanthoplasty with eyebrow lift. *Plast Reconstr Surg* 56: 402, 1975.
16. Loeb R: Necessity for partial resection of the orbicularis oculi muscle in blepharoplasties in some young patients. *Plast Reconstr Surg* 60: 176, 1977.
17. Stasior O: Cicatricial ectropion. In Aston SJ, Hornblass A, Meltzer MA, Rees TD (eds): *Third International Symposium of Plastic and Reconstructive Surgery of the Eye and Adnexa.* Baltimore, Williams & Wilkins, 1982, p 126.
18. Iliff CE, Iliff WJ, Iliff NT: *Oculoplastic Surgery.* Philadelphia, WB Saunders, 1979, p 20.
19. Cogan DG: *Neurology of the Ocular Muscles,* ed 2. Springfield, IL, CC Thomas, 1970.
20. Van Allen MW, Blodi FC: Electromyographic study of reciprocal innervation in blinking. *Neurology* 12: 371–377, 1962.
21. Mustarde JC: The role of Müller's muscle in ptosis surgery. In Ely JF (ed): *Transactions of the Seventh International Congress of Plastic and Reconstructive Surgery, São Paulo, Sociedade Brasileira de Cirurgia Plástica, 1980,* p 355–357.
22. Rees TD, Tabbal N: Lower blepharoplasty. *Clin Plast Surg* 8: 643, 1981.
23. Flowers RS, Boo Chai K, Furukawa M, et al: Aesthetic surgery of the eyelids. In Marchac D (ed): *Transactions of the Sixth International Congress of Plastic and Reconstructive Surgery.* Paris, Masson, 1976, p 470–475.
24. Beard C: *Ptosis,* ed 3. St. Louis, CV Mosby, 1981.
25. Lemke BN, Stasior OG: The anatomy of eyebrow ptosis. *Arch Ophthalmol* 100: 981, 1982.
26. Morax S: Le Vieillissement des paupières. *Ann Chir Plast Esthet* 29: 115, 1984.
27. Nabil M, O'Keefe M, Romano JH, Casey TA: The septum orbitale in ptosis surgery. *Br J Plast Surg* 36: 507, 1983.
28. Pearl RM: Acquired ptosis—a reexamination of etiology and treatment (abstract). American Association of Plastic Surgery. 63rd Annual Mtg., Chicago, 1984, p 63–64.
29. Siegel R: Surgical anatomy of the upper eyelid fascia. *Ann Plast Surg* 13: 263, 1984.
30. Ellenbogen R, Swara N: Correction of asymmetrical upper eyelids by measured levator adhesion technique. *Plast Reconstr Surg* 69: 433, 1982.
31. Wilkins RB, Patipa M: The recognition of acquired ptosis in patients considered for upper-eyelid blepharoplasty. *Plast Reconstr Surg* 70: 431, 1982.
32. Tenzel R: Complications of blepharoplasty. In Aston SJ, Hornblass A, Meltzer MA, Rees TED (eds): *Third International Symposium of Plastic and Reconstructive Surgery of the Eye and Adnexa.* Baltimore, Williams & Wilkins, 1982, p 323.
33. Gay AJ, Salmon ML, Windsor CE: Hering's law, the levators, and their relationship in disease states. *Arch Ophthalmol* 77: 157–160, 1967.
34. Beare R: Surgical treatment of senile changes in the eyelids: the McIndoe Beare technique. In Smith B, Converse JM (eds): *Proceedings of the Second International Symposium on Plastic and Reconstructive Surgery of the Eye and Adnexa.* St. Louis, CV Mosby, 1967, chap. 44.
35. Flowers RS: Anchor blepharoplasty. Presented at the Third International Symposium, Plastic and Reconstructive Surgery of the Eye and Adnexa, New York, 1980.
36. Sheen JH: A change in the technique of supratarsal fixation in upper blepharoplasty. *Plast Reconstr Surg* 59: 831, 1977.
37. Baker TJ: Upper blepharoplasty. *Clin Plast Surg* 8: 635, 1981.
38. Skoog T: *Plastic Surgery.* Philadelphia, WB Saunders, 1974, p 317.

39. Aston SJ: Orbicularis oculi muscle flaps: a technique to reduce crow's feet and lateral canthal skin folds. *Plast Reconstr Surg* 65: 206, 1980.
40. Leber DC, Cramer LM: Correction of entropion in the elderly. *Plast Reconstr Surg* 60: 704, 1977.
41. Spira M: Lower blepharoplasty—a clinical study. *Plast Reconstr Surg* 59: 35, 1977.
42. Owsley JQ, Jr: Functional upper eyelid anatomy as applied to aesthetic blepharoplasty. *Aesth Plast Surg* 5: 115, 1981.
43. Adamson JE, McCraw JB, Carraway JH: Use of a muscle flap in lower blepharoplasty. *Plast Reconstr Surg* 63: 359, 1979.
44. Duke-Elder S: *Textbook of Ophthalmology,* London, Kimpton, 1952, vol 5, p 5165–5166.

CHAPTER 65

Management of Eyebrow Ptosis

NORMAN SHORR, M.D., F.A.C.S.
STUART R. SEIFF, M.D.

GRAVITATIONAL SYNDROME

With time and gravity, all individuals will develop structural sagging and loose, redundant facial tissue to some degree. The structural sagging, or *gravitational syndrome,* represents a spectrum. At the early end of the spectrum, the only problem may be just enough lower eyelid horizontal laxity to surprise the unwary blepharoplasty surgeon with a postoperative ectropion. At the other end of the extreme, there may be the patient with such dramatic eyebrow ptosis that the eyebrow hairs obstruct vision and must be routinely trimmed.

In the gravitational syndrome, the multicontoured areas of the medial and lateral canthi have both horizontal and vertical redundancy. These redundancies are always associated with eyebrow and lateral canthal ptosis. Correction of redundancy in the multicontoured areas represents the greatest challenge to the aesthetic surgeon. It is well recognized that upper eyelid surgery on patients with marked eyebrow ptosis will pull the eyebrow down and suture the eyebrow to the eyelashes (Fig. 65.1). The reestablishment of the structural integrity of the eyebrow is fundamental to achieving an aesthetically acceptable surgical result.

By digitally elevating the medial and lateral eyebrow during the consultation, the surgeon can show the patient a beautiful multicontoured medial and lateral canthus. Surgically, the same results can be obtained with eyebrow resuspension. An eyebrow-lift that returns the eyebrow to a normal position resolves all or most of the redundancy in the multicontoured areas. The remaining redundancy is treated as in patients who have a foundation of normal structural anatomy.

NORMAL POSITION AND COSMETIC ASPECTS OF THE EYEBROW

The eyebrow is an often neglected part of facial anatomy. It, however, is critical in establishing the patient's mood, as determined by facial expression. Upward-slanting eyebrows denote surprise or sadness, downward-slanting eyebrows denote anger, flat eyebrows hanging over the eyes denote fatigue, and eyebrows with a proper arch denote happiness (Fig. 65.2) (1).

It is critical that the eyebrows have a graceful arch. Both medial and lateral aspects of the brow should rest 1 cm above the supraorbital rim, with the high point of the arch being directly above the lateral aspect of the limbus. The medial aspect of the brow should end at a point directly above the alae of the nose, and the lateral aspect of the brow should end on a line drawn between the alae of the nose, lateral canthus, and brow (Fig. 65.3).

The male brow is heavier than the female brow in hair content, occupies a more inferior position, and is less arched laterally. The female brow thins as it arches laterally.

Cosmetic and functional blepharoplasty must first restore the anatomic position of the eyebrows and lateral canthus. In gravitational syndromes, upper eyelid and lateral canthal skin surgery alone pull down the lateral brow. In men, this is totally unacceptable. In women, the brow can be plucked and painted on in a higher position, but the thicker eyebrow skin is pulled down to the eyelid. This is a poor compromise and results in a more rapid, progressive eyebrow ptosis.

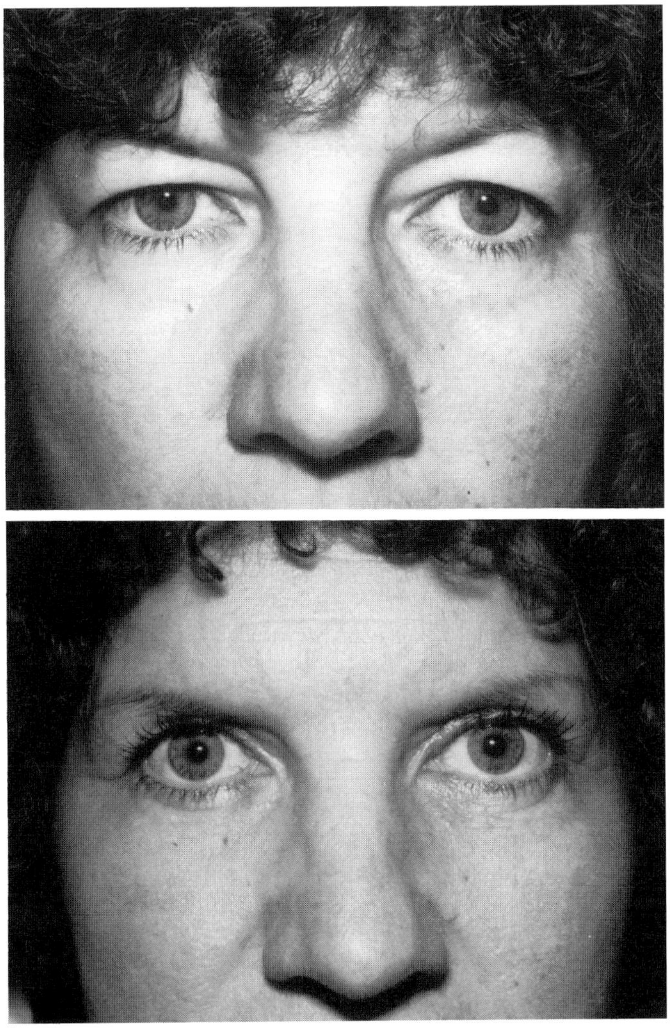

Figure 65.1. *A*, Patient with eyebrow ptosis preoperatively. *B*, Patient with eyebrow "sutured" to eyelashes after upper eyelid blepharoplasty without appropriate attention to eyebrow ptosis.

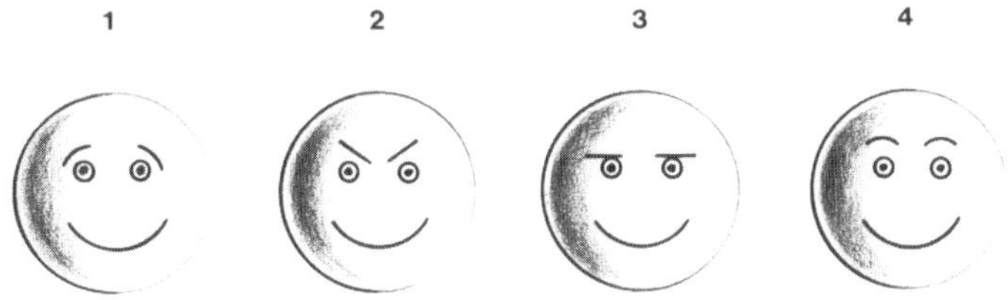

Figure 65.2. Importance of the eyebrow in facial expression.

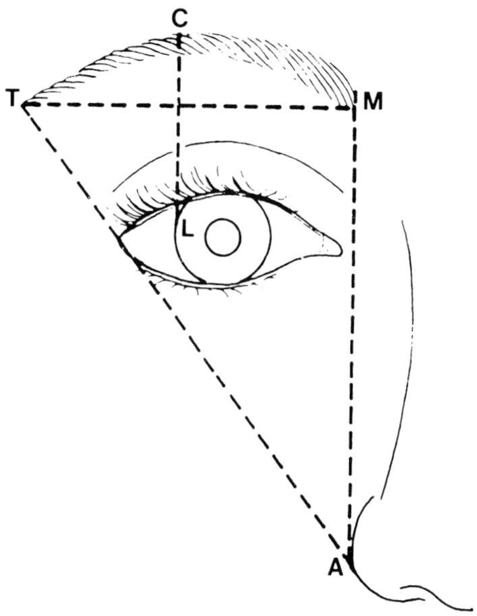

Figure 65.3. Eyebrow arch model.

As patients and surgeons become more sophisticated, an increasing percentage of blepharoplasty is performed in conjunction with the eyebrow lift. Often, after eyebrow elevation, an upper eyelid blepharoplasty is not necessary or becomes a straightforward cosmetic procedure, as in the youthful patient with modest skin excess but normal structural position.

ANATOMY OF THE FOREHEAD AND EYEBROW

The four major muscles of the forehead and eyebrow are the occipitofrontalis, orbicularis oculi, corrugator supercilii, and procerus.

The occipitofrontalis consists of four bellies, two occipital and two frontal, connected by the epicranial aponeurosis, or galea aponeurotica. Each occipital belly arises from the highest nuchal line on the occipital bone. It passes forward and inserts on the galea. The frontal portions arise with the skin and superficial fascia of the eyebrow and pass superiorly to again insert on the galea about midway between the coronal suture and the brow. The action of the occipitofrontalis allows the scalp to move anteriorly and posteriorly. Specifically, the frontal bellies are used to elevate the brows. The occipital bellies are supplied by the posterior auricular branch of the facial nerve, whereas the frontal bellies are supplied by the temporal branch (Fig. 65.4).

There are three parts to the orbicularis oculi: the orbital, preseptal, and pretarsal orbicularis (Fig. 65.5). The orbital portion overlies the orbital rim and arises from the anterior limb of the medial canthal tendon and the periosteum around it. The fibers sweep superiorly and inferiorly around the eye and meet over the zygoma laterally. The preseptal portion has superficial heads from the medial canthal tendon and deep heads from the posterior lacrimal crest. Again, the fibers sweep laterally and form the lateral palpebral raphe. The pretarsal fibers arise from the medial canthal tendon and the tensor tarsi (Horner's muscle). The fibers pass laterally to unite at the lateral canthal tendon (2).

The orbicularis closes the eyelid. In so doing, it pulls the skin of the forehead, temple, and cheek. The superior portions are supplied by the temporal branch of the seventh nerve, while inferiorly, it is innervated by the zygomatic branch.

The corrugator supercilii has its origin from the perios-

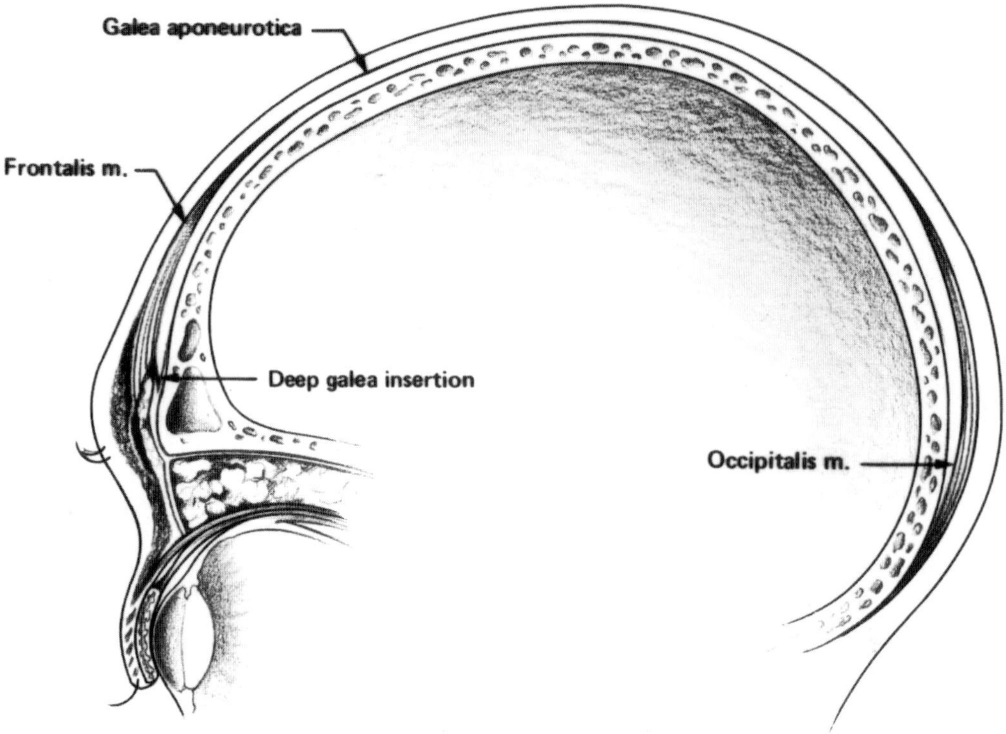

Figure 65.4. The occipitofrontalis-aponeurotic complex.

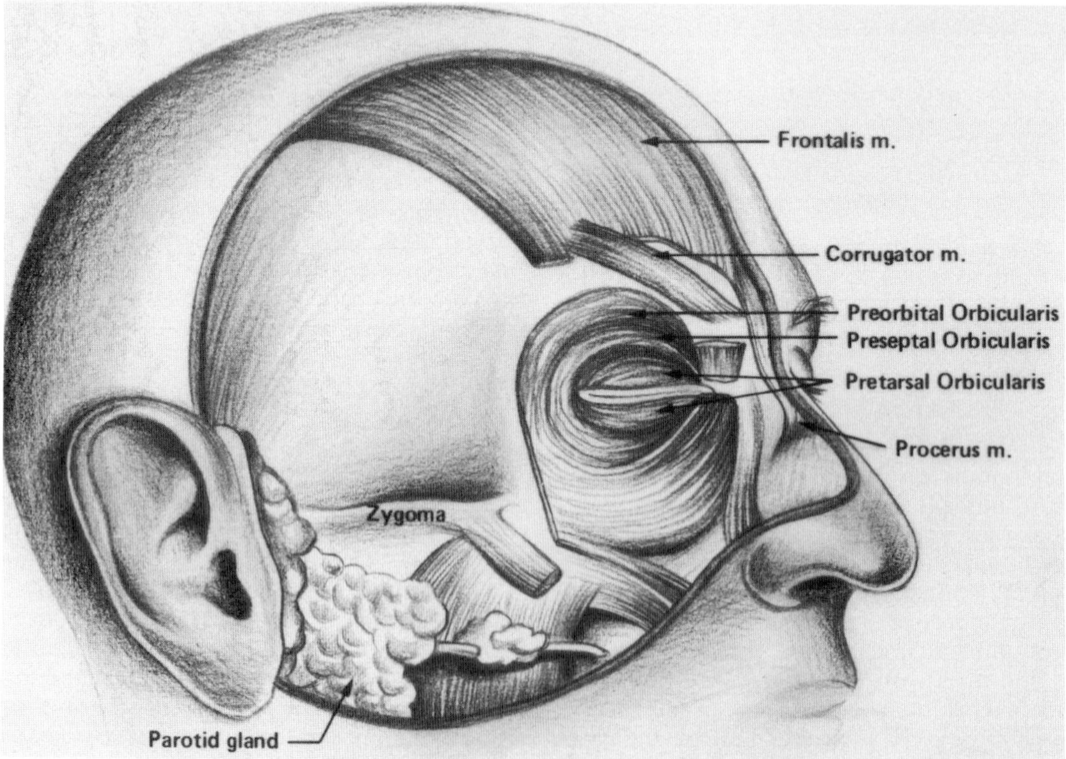

Figure 65.5. The muscles of the eyebrow and forehead.

teum of the nasal process of the frontal bone. The corrugator fibers blend with the deeper portions of the frontalis and orbital orbicularis. The fibers insert into the skin of the medial eyebrow. The action of this muscle produces vertical wrinkles of the forehead. It is supplied by the temporal branch of the facial nerve (Fig. 65.5).

The procerus is continuous with the inferior medial margin of the frontalis. Its origin is from the lower part of

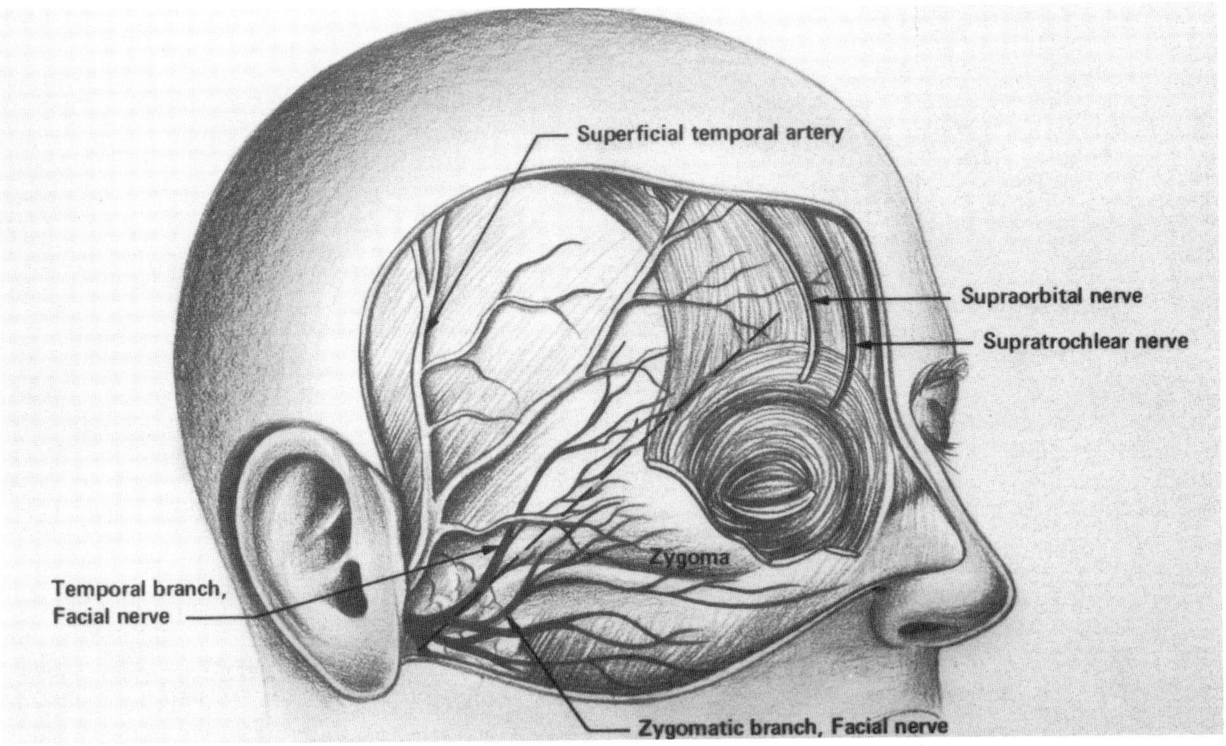

Figure 65.6. The motor and sensory innervation of the forehead and eyebrow. The temporal branch lies along a line from the earlobe to a point along the zygoma below the anterior temporal hairline and continues through a point 1.5 cm lateral to the eyebrow.

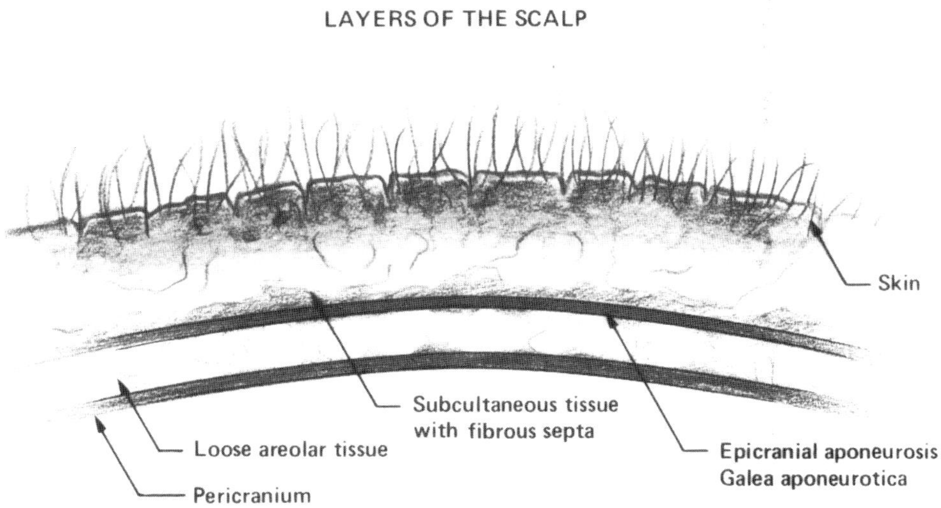

Figure 65.7. The layers of the scalp.

the nasal bone. The muscle is innervated by the buccal branch of the facial nerve, and its action pulls down the medial end of the eyebrow and wrinkles the skin of the nose (Fig. 65.5).

As discussed, the motor function of these muscles is derived from the facial nerve. The facial nerve emerges from the stylomastoid foramen and enters the anteromedial surface of the parotid gland. It passes forward within the gland, superficial to the retromandibular vein and external carotid artery, and divides into five terminal branches (Fig. 65.6).

The *temporal branch* emerges from the upper border of the gland and supplies the anterior and superior auricular muscles, the frontal belly of the occipitofrontalis, the orbicularis oculi, and the corrugator supercilii (3, 4). The *zygomatic branch* emerges from the anterior border of the gland and supplies the inferior orbicularis (3, 4). The *buccal branch* leaves the anterior border of the gland below the parotid duct and runs near the lower border of the zygoma. It supplies the buccinator, procerus, and muscles of the upper lip and nostril (3–5). The *mandibular* and *cervical branches* emerge from the anterior border of the gland and lower border of the gland respectively (3, 4).

The temporal branch travels superiorly in the musculoaponeurotic layer. Temporal to the nerve in this layer are the superficial temporal vessels. The temporal branch lies along a line from the earlobe, to a point along the zygoma below the anterior temporal hairline. The line continues through a point 1.5 cm lateral to the eyebrow (Fig. 65.6) (5–8).

Sensory innervation to the brow is derived from the supraorbital and supratrochlear branches of the ophthalmic nerve. These cross the orbital rim anterior to the periosteum and move into more superficial layers as they course superiorly (Fig. 65.6).

The scalp consists of five layers (Fig. 65.7). The first layer is the skin, which tends to be quite thick. The second layer is the superficial fascia or subcutaneous tissue, which is a fibrofatty layer, adherent to the skin and to the underlying muscle and its aponeurosis. The third layer consists of the tendinous epicranial aponeurosis (galea aponeurotica) and its associated occipitofrontalis muscle. The galea splits to form a sheath around the muscles. The fourth layer consists of loose areolar tissue that occupies the subaponeurotic space. This loosely connects the epicranial aponeurosis to the periosteum of the skull (the pericranium). The areolar tissue contains a few small arteries, but it also contains some important emissary veins. The fifth layer is the periosteum of the skull, or the pericranium. These layers may be recalled by the mnemonic *SCALP*: *S* for skin, *C* for connective tissue, *A* for aponeurosis, *L* for loose areolar tissue, and *P* for pericranium.

It is best to regard the first three layers as a single layer, since when surgically turned down, they remain firmly connected to each other. A wound that does not involve the galea aponeurotica does not gape. The blood vessels that lie in this tissue do not contract when wounded, and therefore hemorrhage from scalp wounds is often considerable. The subaponeurotic areolar tissue is surgically important. It is loose and lax. It is along this plane that surgical dissection may be readily performed. The vessels are in the more superficial layer, and since they anastomose freely, sloughing of such a flap is unusual.

In the region of the eyebrow, the muscle plane is firmly fixed to the skin of the forehead. The frontalis muscle inserts into the eyebrow, where it interdigitates with the orbicularis oculi and corrugator supercilii muscles. Laterally, the muscle is firmly attached at the lateral raphe. Medially, the corrugator supercilii originates from the frontal bone at the superomedial orbital rim. This muscle then inserts in the medial cutaneous portion of the eyebrow. The corrugator produces vertical glabellar creases (Fig. 65.8) (9, 10).

A fat layer lies posterior to the muscle at the brow. The muscle forms the anterior boundary of the eyebrow fat pad. The posterior boundary of the eyebrow fat pad continues into the eyelid as the superior orbital septum. The fat pad continues into the eyelid as the areolar posterior orbicularis fascia.

The muscle plane of the eyebrow is secured to the frontal bone periosteum by a firm attachment on the underside of the fat pad. The fat above these bony attachment sites permits vertical sliding of the overlying skin and muscle. These attachments primarily extend over the medial one-half to two-thirds of the orbit along the supraorbital rim. Weaker connections exist laterally.

ANATOMY AND PATHOLOGY OF EYEBROW PTOSIS

The relative lack of deep attachments of the brow laterally results in earlier and greater ptosis of this portion of the eyebrow. Medial eyebrow ptosis may be explained in the older age group by relative atrophy of the eyebrow fat pad, which allows the overlying skin and muscle layer to move inferiorly by gravity (9, 10). When eyebrow ptosis occurs; the frontalis muscle helps to elevate the brow. This causes deep forehead furrows. However, due to the lack of frontalis fibers laterally, lateral eyebrow ptosis persists in spite of frontalis contraction.

When the eyebrow becomes ptotic, the orbicularis and thin upper eyelid skin also droop. This gives a clinical appearance similar to that of dermatochalasis. Therefore, as previously stated, eyebrow position must be evaluated prior to performing a blepharoplasty.

PREOPERATIVE EVALUATION AND PATIENT PREPARATION

A general eye examination, best corrected vision, tear film evaluation, and a bleeding and allergy history is taken. Preoperative photographs from the front, side, and oblique views are taken. Polaroid close-ups, which can be discussed immediately with the patient, are taken to avoid the difficulties of explaining surgical goals while looking in the mirror. The structural position of the eyebrows (arch and ptosis), eyelids (ptosis and redundant skin), lateral and medial canthi (ptosis and redundancy), and the entire face are examined and discussed with the patient. Specific attention is also paid to areas of herniating orbital fat and redundant or hypertrophic orbicularis muscle.

All abnormalities and asymmetries are fully discussed when the patient. It is stressed that the eyelids must be in keeping with the context of the entire face and a "tight surgical appearance should be avoided." For women, the upper eyelid crease is discussed; the need for creating a smooth upper eyelid below the crease to provide a platform on which to apply makeup is stressed. Finally, skin types are reviewed. The patient with thick, oily skin, colloid milia, and fine wrinkles can expect far less improvement than the patient with smooth, modestly pigmented skin. Similarly, the very fair-complexioned patient is advised that postoperative incision scars may appear slightly more erythematous and raised than in other patients. The patient is then examined in the supine position. This latter point is of particular importance since the patient will eventually be operated on in this position.

Once the surgical procedure and expectations have been reviewed, the patient is told about the anticipated postoperative course, which includes avoiding sunbathing while "black and blue," and not wearing contact lenses for up to several weeks. The patient is also advised to avoid all aspirin-containing compounds for 2 weeks prior to surgery. A specifically written consent form is used. The risks, complications, and reasonable expectations are reviewed.

DIRECT EYEBROW ELEVATION

Pierce (11), Bames (12), and Castanares (13) have described variations on the direct eyebrow elevation. This procedure affords the most lift per millimeter of excised tissue. It is a straightforward procedure and is the best approach for segmental brow elevation. It is useful in men when coronal or temporal lift are ill advised due to a tendency toward male-pattern baldness. The procedure is not likely to inadvertently damage motor function of the brow; however, numbness of the forehead may rarely result, because of interruption of sensory fibers from the supraorbital and supratrochlear nerves by the dissection. A faint scar usually persists along the top of the brow.

The patient should be examined in a sitting position and the extent of brow ptosis determined. The patient should also be observed in the supine position, as this is the way the patient will appear on the operating table.

In the sitting position, the proposed incision site is marked out. The lower border should lie just within the most superior row of eyebrow hairs. The brow is then elevated to the desired level digitally. The marking pen is placed over, not touching, the new superior brow border. The brow is released, and the point under the pen tip

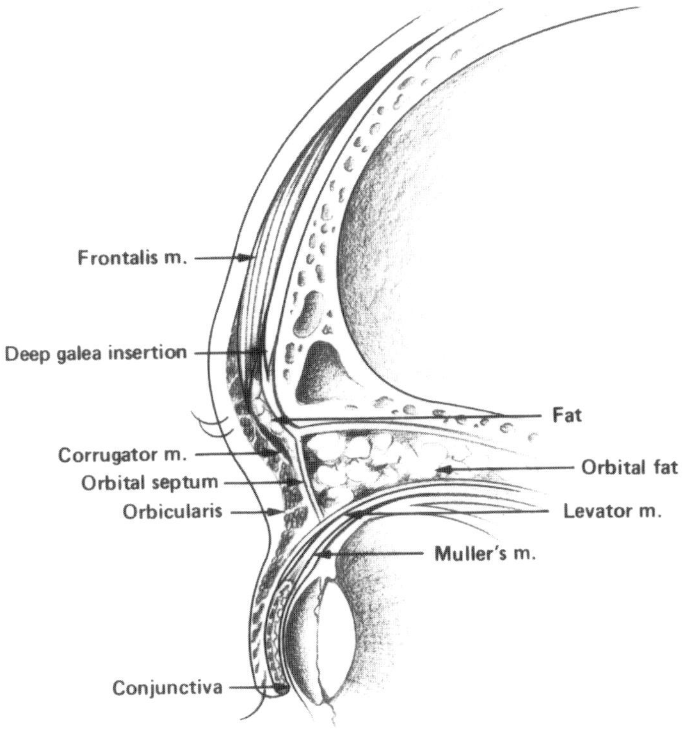

Figure 65.8. Cross section anatomy of the eyebrow.

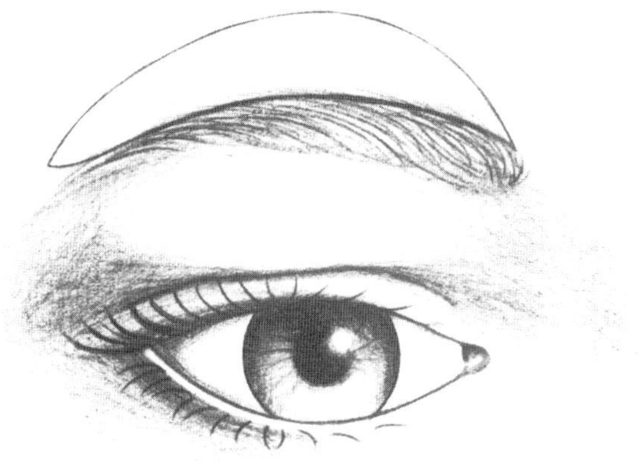

Figure 65.9. Skin marking

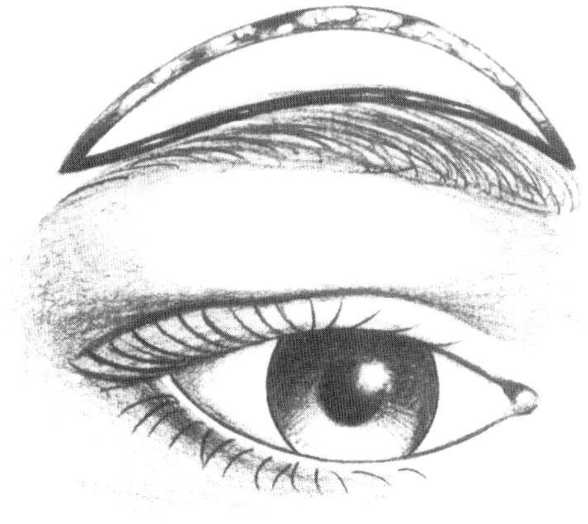

Figure 65.10. Incision of skin muscle tissue.

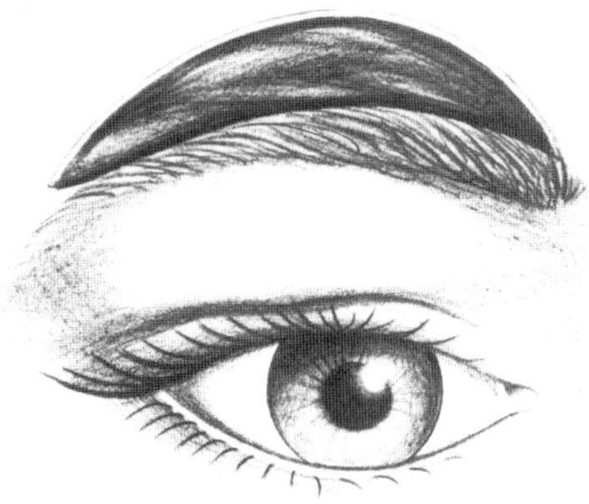

Figure 65.11. Excision of skin muscle tissue.

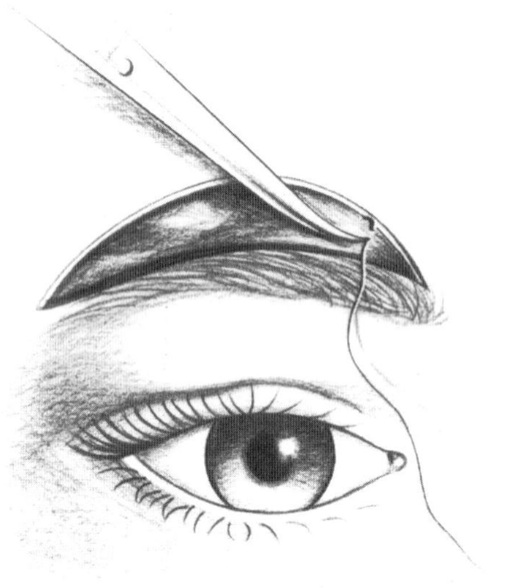

Figure 65.12. Subcutaneous closure (first layer).

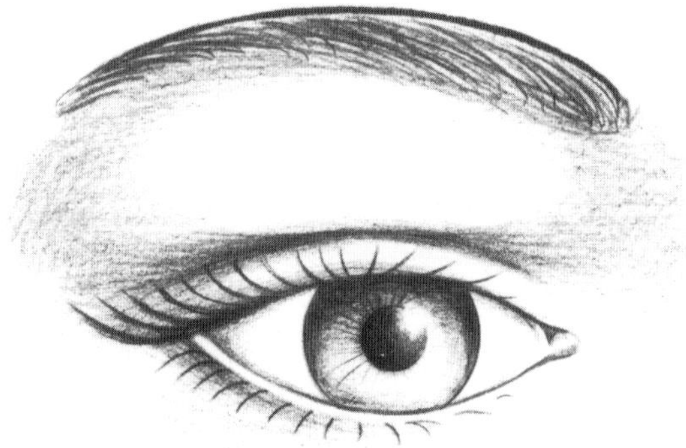

Figure 65.13. Apposed tissue edges following subcutaneous closure.

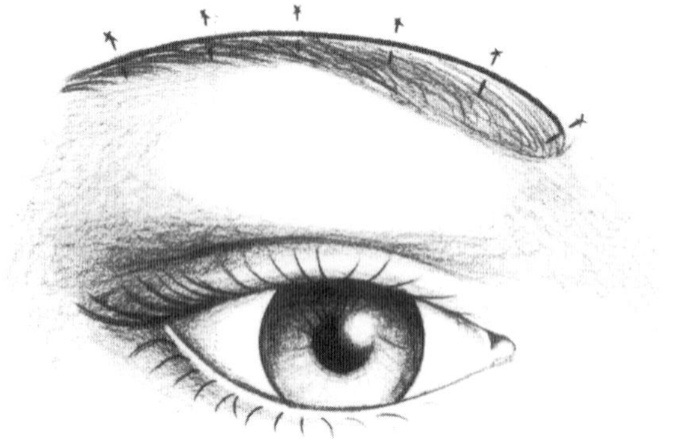

Figure 65.14. Vertical mattress suture closure (second layer).

represents a point on the superior incision line. This procedure is repeated segmentally until the entire incision line is constructed. The final incision is illustrated in Fig. 65.9.

The surgical area is then injected at all levels down to the periosteum with a solution of 2% lidocaine with 1:100,000 epinephrine with Wydase. Additionally, supraorbital nerve blocks are often used. Fifteen minutes are allowed to pass until hemostasis occurs. The incision is made with a No. 15 blade. Along the inferior margin of the incision, an attempt is made to bevel the blade in the direction of the hair follicles so as not to cut off brow hairs (Fig. 65.10) (14). An attempt is made to keep the incision shallow over the supraorbital nerve, with the dissection plane at a level deep to the frontalis muscle. Scissors remove the ellipse of tissue (Fig. 65.11). Meticulous punctate hemostasis is maintained. The wound is then closed with a deep layer of interrupted 5-0 Vicryl suture (Figs. 65.12 and 65.13). Multiple interrupted vertical mattress sutures of 5-0 Prolene or nylon are used to approximate the incision (Fig. 65.14). A running 5-0 Prolene suture is used to evert and close the skin edges (Fig. 65.15). The proposed incision for lateral brow ptosis is shown in Fig. 65.16. The wound should be dressed with antibiotic ointment and ice packs, which are applied for 4 days. After the fourth day, hot compresses may be beneficial in resolving edema and ecchymosis. The sutures may be removed between the fifth and seventh day as evidence of loosening appears.

The primary disadvantage of the direct eyebrow lift is the presence of the fine scar above the brow. If fixation to periosteum is not performed (as described for a paralytic brow), immobility of the brow has not been a problem. Anesthesia of the forehead and scalp may pose a potential difficulty, although we have not seen this to be a permanent problem.

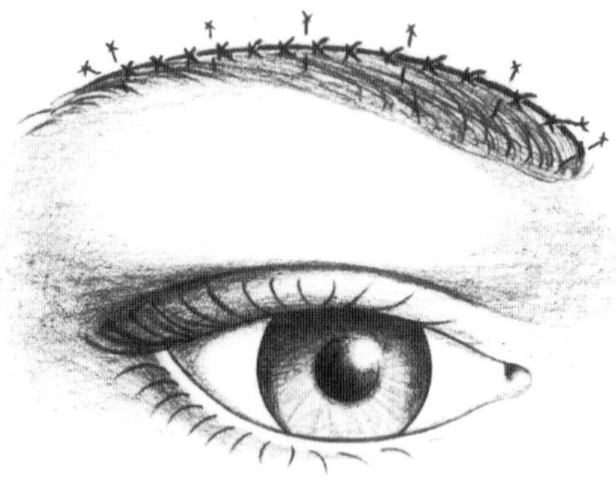

Figure 65.15. Continuous suture closure (third layer) with running "baseball" stitch.

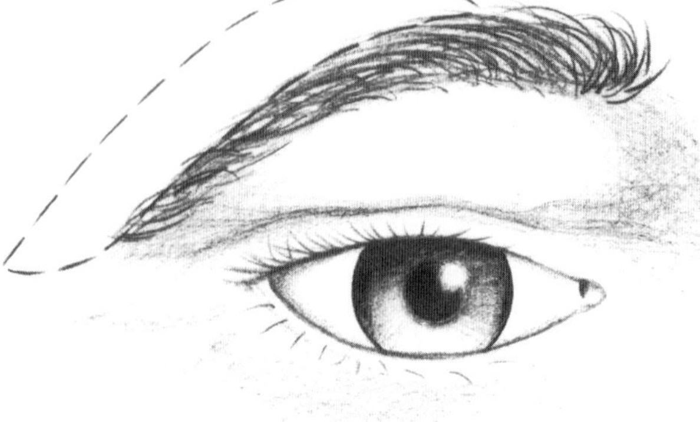

Figure 65.16. Design of incision for lateral brow ptosis.

MIDFOREHEAD BROW LIFT

Variations of the midforehead brow lift have been described by Brennan (15), Rafaty (16), and Ellenbogen (17). This particular approach may be preferred in cases of isolated brow ptosis, glabellar ptosis, and midforehead

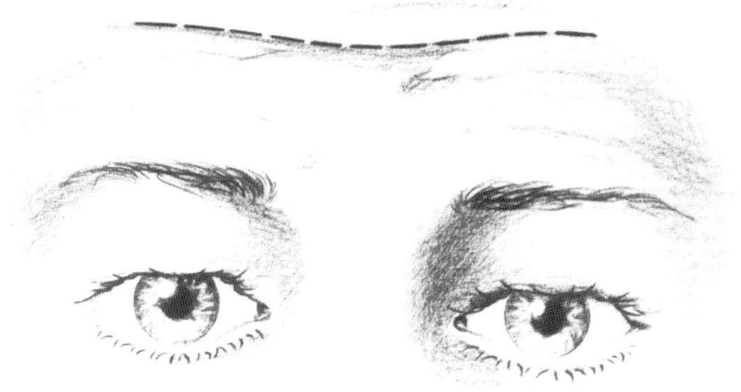

Figure 65.17. Incision for midforehead eyebrow life.

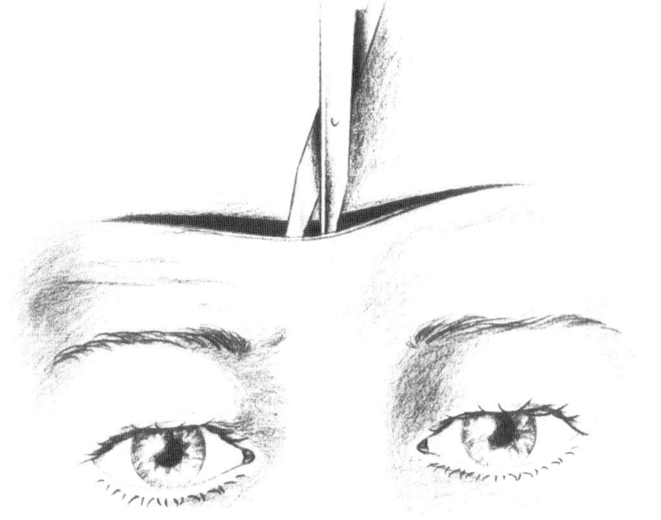

Figure 65.18. Inferior dissection.

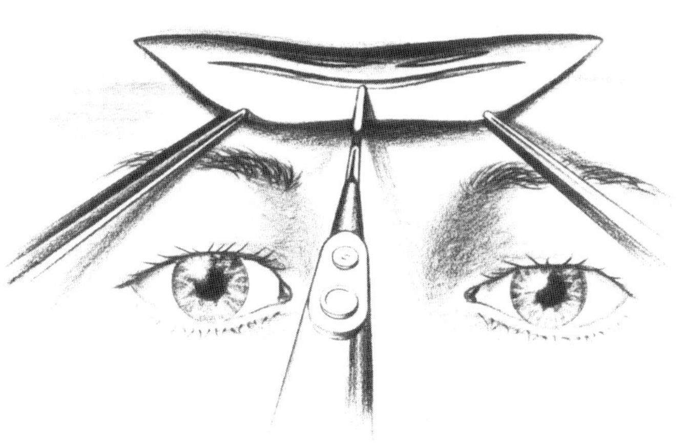

Figure 65.19. Cautery dissection of procerus-corrugator complex.

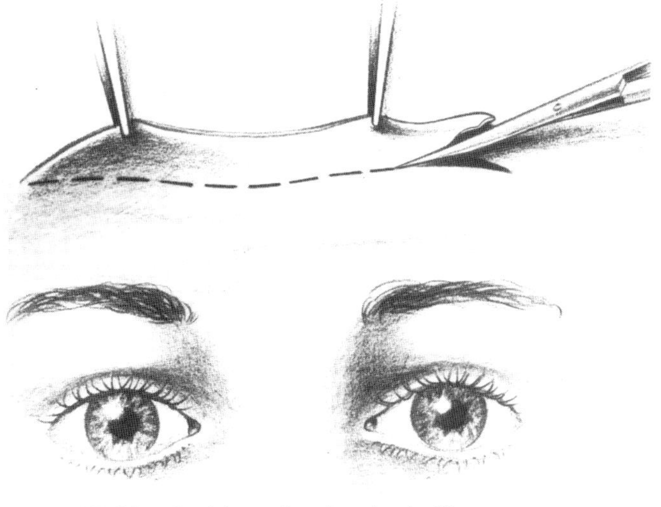

Figure 65.20. Excision of redundant ellipse.

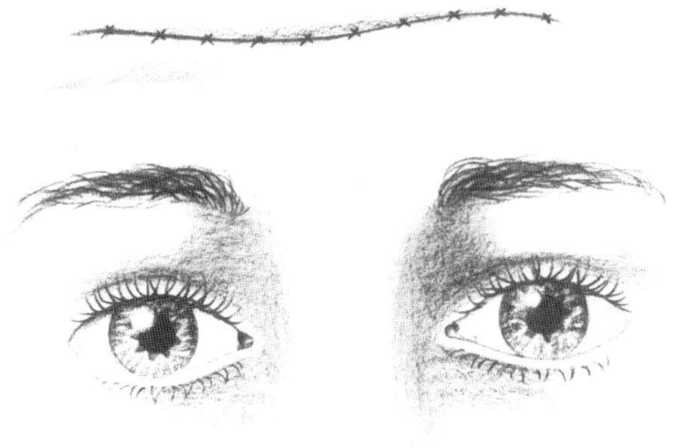

Figure 65.21. Skin closure.

frown lines. The procedure may be especially ideal in cases of high or sparse frontal hairlines, as the hairline appears to be lowered by the procedure. However, patients with unfurrowed brows may be poor candidates for this due to a prominent hyperemic scar that may persist for many months.

The incision is marked in a central forehead crease (Fig. 65.17). Two-percent lidocaine with 1:100,000 epinephrine with Wydase is injected in the manner of bilateral supraorbital nerve blocks and along the incision line. The anesthetic is allowed to cause vasoconstriction over approximately a 15-minute period. The incision line is then made full thickness. Undermining is carried slightly superiorly and inferiorly to the superior orbital rims (Fig. 65.18). Specific dissection of the corrugator and procerus muscles may be undertaken as indicated to eliminate glabellar furrows. Posterior lamella horizontal relaxing incisions may be performed with cautery (Fig. 65.19). The flap is then elevated to the desired height. A full-thickness redundant forehead ellipse is excised (Fig. 65.20). The wound is closed in two layers. The deep layer is closed with 5-0 Vicryl suture. The superficial layer is closed with a combination of vertical mattress sutures of 5-0 Prolene and a running 5-0 Prolene or 5-0 cuticular chromic to evert the skin edges (Fig. 65.21). Antibiotic ointment is applied, and the sutures are removed in 5–7 days as they loosen.

TEMPORAL LIFT

The temporal lift procedure for brow elevation has been described by Gleason (18). It is especially useful in patients with early brow ptosis and lateral canthal ptosis. Disadvantages include minimal elevation of the medial brow and slight elevation of the temporal hairline, which may be undesirable in some patients.

The surgical technique is as follows: The hair is parted along a vertical line above each ear. Then 0.5% lidocaine with 1:200,000 epinephrine with Wydase is injected along the part line and in supraorbital nerve blocks. After 15 min, a vertical incision approximately 12 cm long is made above each ear with a scalpel to the level of temporalis fascia (Fig. 65.22).

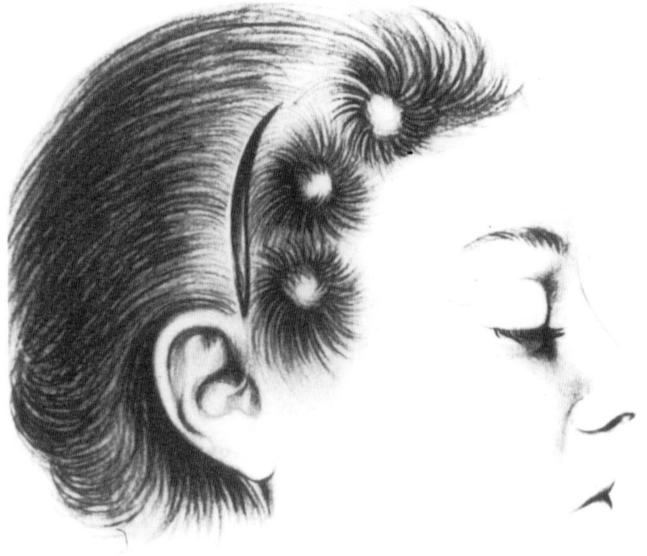

Figure 65.22. Temporal brow life incision.

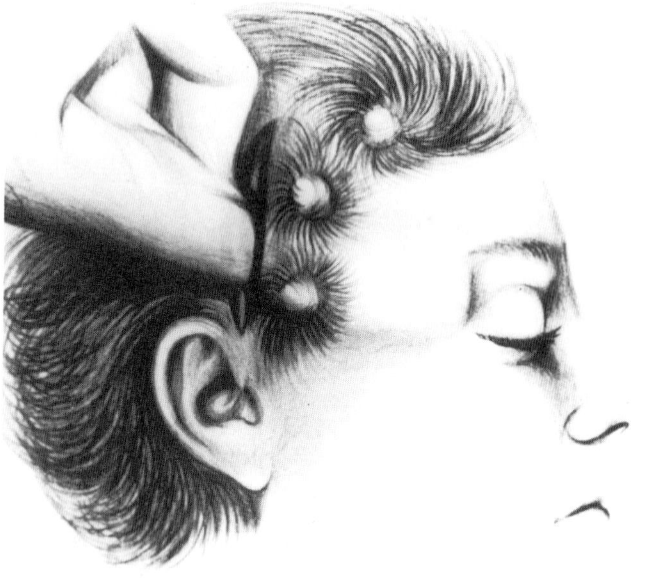

Figure 65.23. Blunt dissection of temporal brow flap.

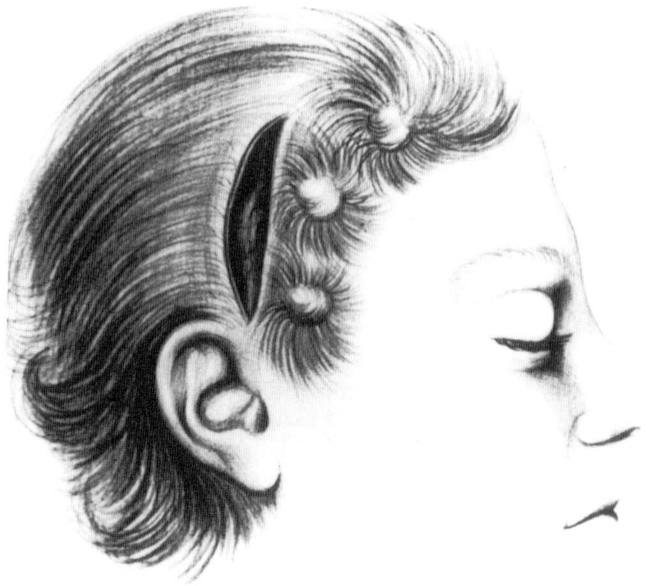

Figure 65.24. Excision of redundant scalp tissue.

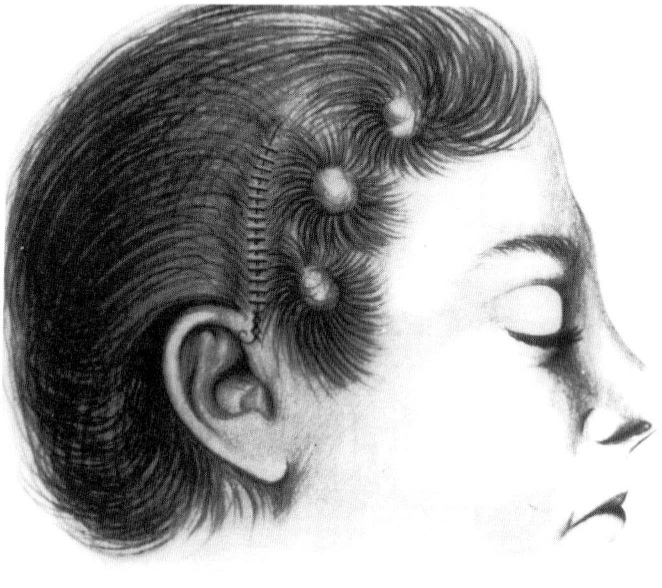

Figure 65.25. Staple closure.

Blunt dissection, using either a finger or a large scissor, is carried along the plane of the temporalis fascia toward the eyebrow. At the scalp hairline, the level of dissection is changed to that of a very thin skin flap. The dissection at this level is superficial to the temporal branch of the facial nerve. With more blunt than sharp dissection, the temporal flap is undermined to just below the level of the brow and lateral canthus (Fig. 65.23). Nerves have more tensile strength than does connective tissue and therefore can tolerate gentle, blunt dissection better than sharp dissection (19). A gauze-wrapped finger may be used to dissect under the thin skin flap by pressing down on the deeper tissue and peeling the layers gently apart. The gentle dissection tends to push the stronger nerve fibers aside while separating the weaker connective tissue in which they lie. Hemostasis is cautiously obtained or damage to the nerve may occur with cautery. After the skin flap is freed, it is advanced and rotated slightly. The redundant tissue is excised (Fig. 65.24). A single-layer closure, using skin staples, is made (Fig. 65.25). Occasionally, the inferior aspect of the skin incision, just superior to the ear, may be sutured in order to better evert the wound edges. A light headwrap is applied and no drain is used. The staples are removed in 10–14 days.

CORONAL EYEBROW AND FOREHEAD LIFT

The coronal eyebrow and forehead life is the most aesthetically pleasing of the brow lifts. Kaye (19) beautifully outlined the history of this technique. Lexer (20), Hunt (21), Joseph (22), and Passot (23) described procedures to elevate the forehead and eyebrow many years ago. More recently, Pangman and Wallace (24) and Gonzalez-Ulloa (25) have described similar procedures. The incision is entirely within the hair-bearing scalp, which covers the scar. The procedure, however, is used primarily in women, since men have, or may develop, male-pattern baldness. The hairline may also be elevated somewhat by the procedure.

The hair is parted and braided along the proposed coronal incision line with the use of K-Y jelly as needed. The incision line extends from the most superior point where the ear touches the scalp to the most superior point where the other ear touches the scalp (Fig. 65.26). In the midline, the incision is 5 or 6 cm posterior to the hairline.

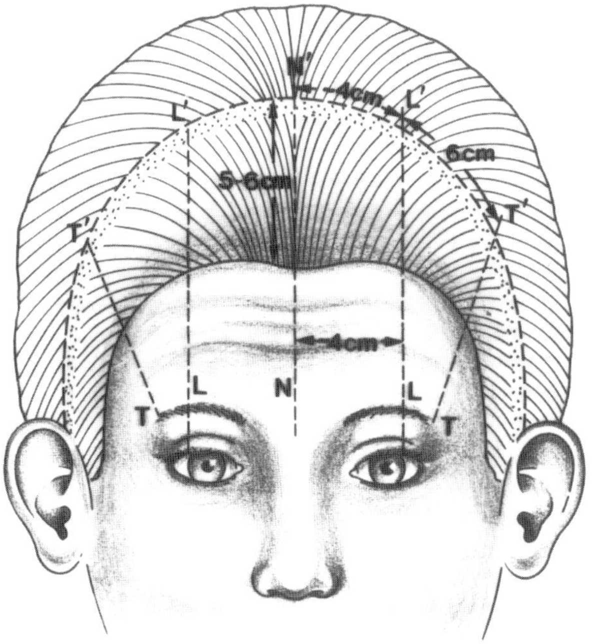

Figure 65.27. Presurgical markings.

A line is drawn (Fig. 65.27) from the midline of the nose (*N*) up to the central point of the incision (*N'*). A line is drawn from the lateral limbus on each side (*L*) to a point along the incision line 4 cm from *N'* (*L'*). A line is then drawn bilaterally from the temporal portion of the brow (*T*) to a point 6 cm along the incision from *L'* (*T'*). These lines form the lines of traction for elevating the brow. The hair is then clipped just anterior to the incision line.

The local anesthetic consists of 40 ml of 0.5% lidocaine with 1:200,000 epinephrine with Wydase; 10 ml are injected along the right incision line, 10 cm along the left incision line, and 10 ml along a line from each ear to the nasal midline including supraorbital nerve blocks. This effectively forms a vascular tourniquet. Excellent hemostasis is obtained.

The incision is made to the level of periosteum with a No. 15 blade. Dissection between the periosteum and the galea is performed with the surgeon's fingers or scissors. The scalp and forehead flap are elevated down to the superior orbital rims (Fig. 65.28). At the orbital rim, care

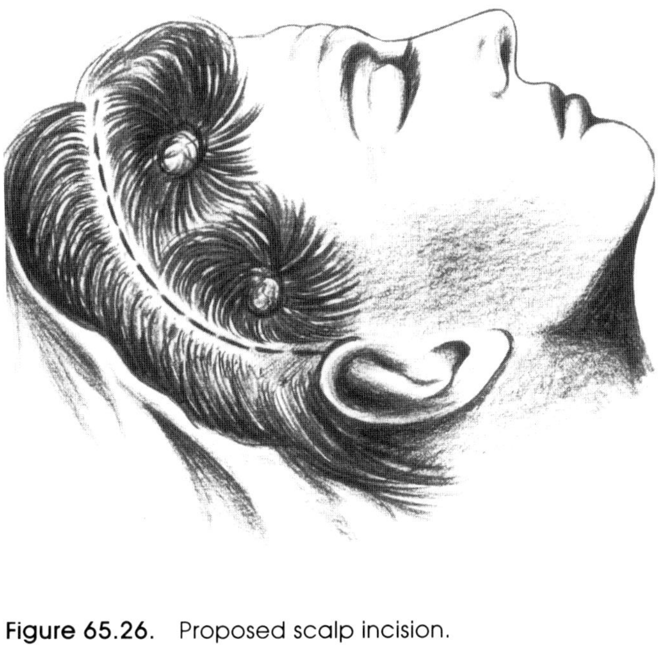

Figure 65.26. Proposed scalp incision.

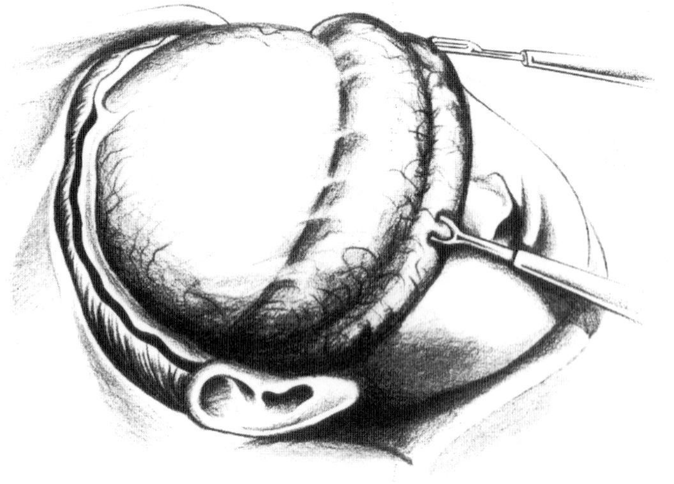

Figure 65.28. Dissection of the forehead flap.

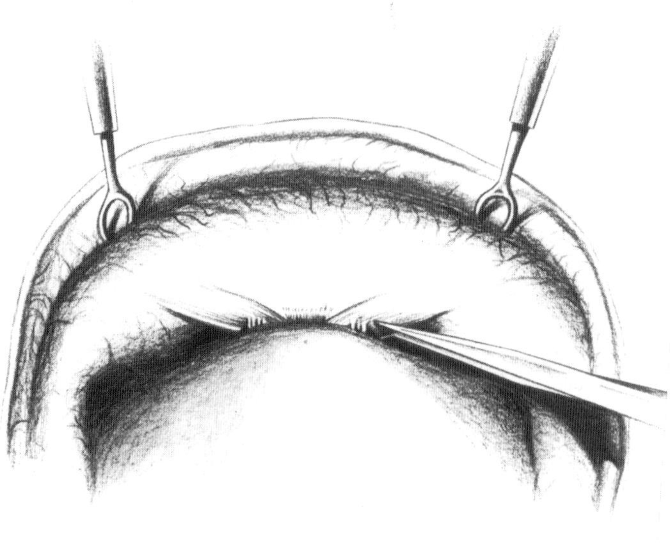

Figure 65.29. Dissection of procerus-corrugator muscle complex with sparing of the neurovascular bundle.

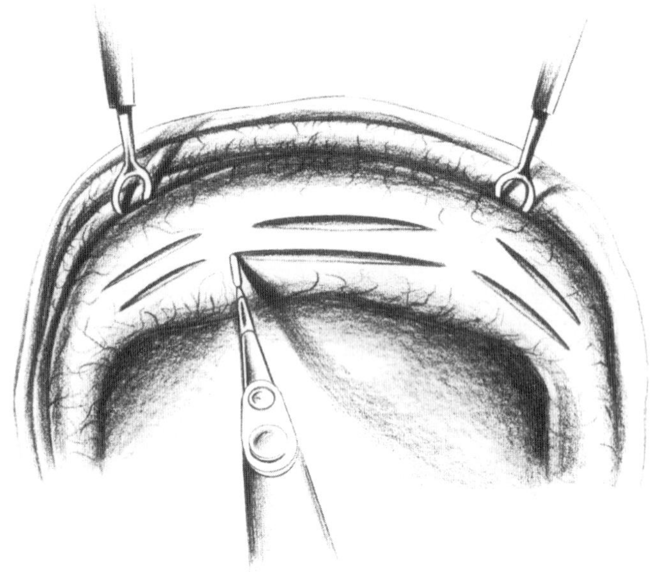

Figure 65.30. Horizontal relaxing incisions in posterior muscle lamella.

is taken to preserve the supraorbital neurovascular bundles.

Special attention must be paid to the dissection bilaterally over the area of the temporalis fossa. The dissection is carried over the temporalis fascia. The dissection plane is thus posterior to all branches of the seventh cranial nerve, which is the motor nerve for the forehead and eyebrow. If the temporal branch of the seventh nerve is cut or injured, temporary or permanent paralysis of the eyebrow and forehead may result. Superior traction on the scalp will lift the brows but will not remove creases and furrows between the brows and in the forehead. Therefore, the procerus-corrugator muscle complex (between the brows) must be cut or dissected out (Fig. 65.29). Additionally, one or more horizontal relaxing incisions must be made in the posterior muscle lamella of the forehead flap. This allows the posterior lamella to relax such that the anterior skin layer can be smoothed out to obliterate forehead furrows. This is done with cutting cautery, but care should be taken to keep the cuts at least 3 cm superior to the lateral orbital rim. This places the incisions in the surgically safe zone for the seventh nerve (Fig. 65.30). (19).

Using a D'Assumpcao clamp, the surgeon advances the posterior scalp and overlaps the forehead flap over the posterior scalp wound margin in the midline. A cut is made anteriorly in the flap to indicate the desired extent of excision. This procedure is repeated along each of the previously marked-out lines (Fig. 65.31). The redundant flaps are then excised with Metzenbaum scissors. A gradually tapering incision in the last segment is performed laterally toward the ears. Staples are used to close and evert the skin margin in a single-layer closure (Fig. 65.32). No drains are used postoperatively. If indicated, attention can be turned now to blepharoplasty, as described by Ellenbogen (1). The hair is then rinsed with 1% hydrogen

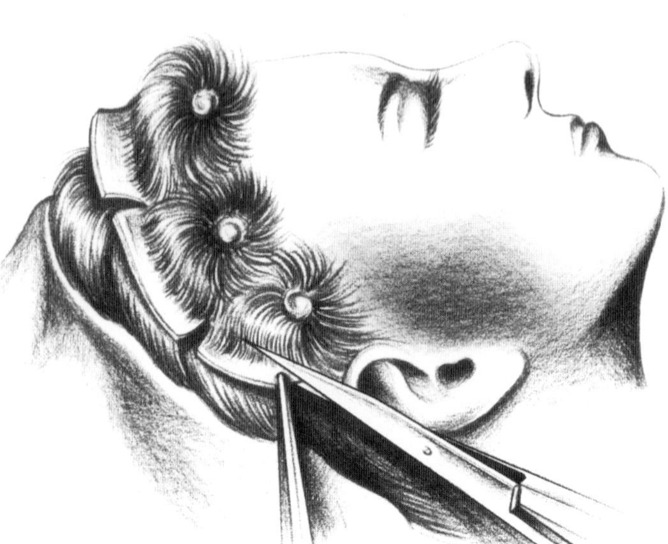

Figure 65.31. Segmental scalp excision.

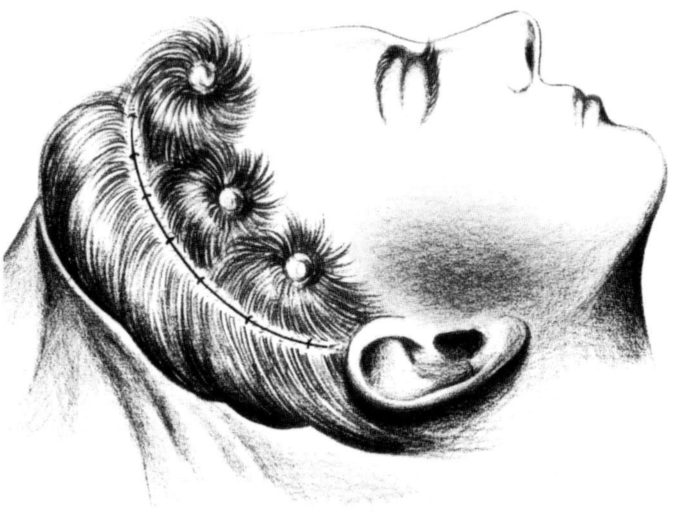

Figure 65.32. Staple closure of skin margins.

peroxide to remove accumulated blood. It is then gently dried. A head dressing is placed at the end of the procedure. The staples are removed between 7 and 10 days.

The authors perform this procedure only in women or in men with no family history of male-pattern baldness. Additionally, the anterior hairline is raised, which may be considered an advantage or disadvantage, depending on the individual patient. Alopecia may occur along the incision line; however, we feel that through meticulous staple closure, this can be minimized. Several patients have reported numbness of the forehead and anterior scalp; however, this usually resolves over several weeks. Additionally, an occasional patient may have a temporary immobility of the brows. In our experience, this has not been permanent, yet there are reports of occasional permanent damage to the seventh nerve with this procedure. Finally, there are rare reports of necrosis of the coronal flap. We have not seen this complication.

CORRECTION OF PARALYTIC BROW

Eyebrow ptosis may also be present in seventh nerve palsies. When the paralysis is longstanding, surgical intervention to elevate the brows is indicated. Beard (26) advocates elevation of the brow incorporated with lateral and medial canthoplasty to better position the eyelids as well. An incision is made just above the hairline of the eyebrow as in the direct brow lift. A crescent of skin may be excised, as described for the direct brow lift, but others (26) suggest that omission of the skin excision forces the skin into some semblance of normal brow wrinkles. Supramid suture (4-0) or equivalent is used in the placement of interrupted permanent buried sutures between the brow in the elevated position and the periosteum of the frontal bone. The muscle layer of the incision is closed with interrupted sutures of 4-0 plain catgut or equivalent. The skin is then closed with subcuticular suture of 4-0 monofilament nylon.

The essential step in this procedure is the placement of sutures between the eyebrow and periosteum to overcome the effects of gravity after the brow ptosis repair. An alternative method involves the placement of three permanent sutures through three stab-wound incisions above the brow. The brow is elevated to the desired position and then the sutures anchor it to periosteum. The knots are buried, and the skin is closed with interrupted sutures.

ACKNOWLEDGMENT

The authors thank David Hinkle for creating the illustrations used in this chapter.

REFERENCES

1. Ellenbogen R: Transcoronal eyebrow lift with concomitant upper blepharoplasty. *Plast Reconstruc Surg* 71: 490–495, 1983.
2. Beard C, Quickert M: *Anatomy of the Orbit*, ed 2. Birmingham, AL, Aesculpaius, 1977, p 4–11, 18–21.
3. Snell RS: *Clinical Anatomy for Medical Students.* Boston, Little, Brown & Co., 1973, p 613–809.
4. Warwick R, Williams PL: *Gray's Anatomy*, ed 35, Philadelphia, WB Saunders, 1973, p 496–497.
5. Furnas DW: Landmarks for the trunk and the temporofacial division of the facial nerve. *Br J Surg* 52: 694–696, 1965.
6. Correia P, Zani R: Surgical anatomy of the facial nerve, as related to the ancillary operations and rhytidoplasty. *Plast Reconstruc Surg* 52: 549–552, 1973.
7. Loeb R: Technique for preservation of the temporal branches of the facial nerve during face lift operations. *Br J Plast Surg* 23: 390–394, 1970.
8. Pitinguy I, Ramos AS: The frontal branch of the facial nerve: the importance of its variations in face lifting. *Plast Reconstruct Surg* 38: 352–356, 1966.
9. Lemke BN, Stasior OG: The anatomy of eyebrow ptosis. *Arch Ophthalmol* 100: 981–986, 1982.
10. Doxanas MT, Anderson RL: *Clinical Orbital Anatomy.* Baltimore, Williams & Wilkins, 1984, p 57–62.
11. Pierce G: Useful procedures in plastic surgery. *Plast Reconstr Surg* 2: 361, 1947.
12. Bames HO: Frown disfigurement and ptosis of eyebrows. *Plast Reconstr Surg* 19: 337–340, 1957.
13. Castanares S: Forehead wrinkles, glabellar frown and ptosis of the eyebrows. *Plast Reconstr Surg* 34: 406–413, 1964.
14. Tardy ME, Tom LWC, Aesthetic correction of the ptosis brow. In Putterman A (ed): *Cosmetic Oculoplastic Surgery.* New York, Grune & Stratton, 1982, p 147–176.
15. Brennan HG, Rafaty FM: Mid forehead incisions in treatment of the aging face. *Arch Otolaryngol* 108: 732–734, 1982.

16. Rafaty FM, Goode RL, Abramson NR: The brow lift operation in a man. *Arch Otolaryngol* 104: 69–71, 1978.
17. Ellenbogen R: Medial brow lift. *Ann Plast Surg* 5: 151–152, 1980.
18. Gleason MC: Brow lifting through a temporal scalp approach. *Plast Reconstr Surg* 52: 141–144, 1973.
19. Kaye BL: Forehead and brow. In Rees TD (ed): *Aesthetic Plastic Surgery,* Vol. II, Philadelphia, WB Saunders, 1980, p 731–748.
20. Lexer E: Zur Gesichtsplastik. *Arch Klin Chir* 92: 749, 1910.
21. Hunt HL: *Plastic Surgery of the Head, Face, and Neck.* Philadelphia, Lea & Febiger, 1926.
22. Joseph J: *Nasenplastik und Sonstige Gesichtsplastik: nebst Einen Anhang uber Mammaplastik.* Leipzig, 1931, Curt Kabitzsch, p 507–509.
23. Passot R: Quelques generalites sur l'operation correctif des rides du visage. *Rev Chir Plast* 3: 23, 1933.
24. Pangman JW, Wallace RM: Cosmetic surgery of the face and neck. *Plast Reconstruc Surg* 27: 544, 1961.
25. Gonzalez-Ullao M: Facial wrinkles, integral elimination. *Plast Reconst Surg* 29: 658, 1962.
26. Beard C: Canthoplasty and brow elevation for facial palsy. *Arch Ophthalmol* 71: 386–388, 1964.

SECTION IX

RECONSTRUCTION OF THE EYELIDS

CHAPTER 66

Reconstruction of the Upper Eyelid: Major Defects

DONALD J. BERGIN, M.D., F.A.C.S.
CLINTON D. McCORD, MD., F.A.C.S.

Hammurabi's code written in the 18th century BC provides ample evidence that eyelid surgery has been practiced for centuries. Ten silver shekels was the reward for successful surgery, and cutting off of the hand ended the career of the unsuccessful surgeon. Until 1869, distant flap techniques of Gaspara Tagliacozzi were the rule in eyelid reconstruction. In 1829, Fricke described the temporal flap for eyelid reconstruction. Eyelid flap techniques were expanded by Burow (1838), Blasius (1842), and Diffenbach (1845). In 1869, Riverdin reported his revolutionary work on transplantation of free pinch grafts, and subsequently full-thickness and split-thickness skin grafting became accepted practice. Teale (1860) first described mucous membrane grafting of conjunctival flaps for the correction of symblepharon. This concept was expanded in 1872 by Houze de L'Aulnoit, who published his work on autogenous buccal mucous membrane grafts. In 1881 and 1885, Landolt designed procedures to share tarsus and conjunctiva on a pedicle flap between the lids. Ear cartilage was used as a free graft to replace the tarsus by Budinger in 1902. These early innovations have been adapted, modified, refined, and incorporated into the modern practice of eyelid surgery we know today.

Full-thickness defects of the upper eyelid encountered by surgeons are usually caused by trauma or created by removal of eyelid tumors. Other causes of upper lid defects are congenital colobomas, loss of tissue following irradiation, postinflammation as in herpes zoster, and chemical or thermal burns.

The art of reconstructing an upper eyelid defect requires meticulous and atraumatic management of injured tissues so that proper eyelid function is restored in an aesthetically pleasing manner. Loss of even the entire lower eyelid may be associated with relatively uncompromised normal eye function. However, even small upper eyelid defects can lead to corneal exposure and threaten vision. Occasionally, patients with a strong Bell's phenomenon and good tear film may tolerate an upper eyelid defect temporarily. For an upper eyelid to function properly it must be of sufficient size to cover the cornea in sleep, but must possess sufficient mobility to elevate above the pupil. It therefore, must, have muscular power to elevate it and be thin and supple enough to allow elevation and conformation to the contour of the globe. It must be lined by mucous membrane, especially the lid margin, to prevent keratitis and maintain comfort, while being of sufficient rigidity to retain its shape.

Irradiation, alkali or thermal damage, or other pathologic changes within tissues may compromise the healing process. Autogenous free grafts of skin or other tissues may not take as well in these tissues, and it may be necessary to use flaps that bring in their own blood supply in order to prevent shrinkage or necrosis of tissue. Stretchability is another factor to be considered in upper eyelid reconstruction. In older individuals the lids are usually much more lax and the defect can be reduced by simple stretching. In others, the lids may not possess this elasticity. This is especially true in younger individuals or eyelids damaged by irradiation, burns, or fibrosis as in scleroderma or after repeated surgeries. In general, the best rule of thumb to use is that the defect can be reduced by 15% more in an older patient with lax tissue than in a younger patient. For grouping purposes, defects can be classified as "small" if they involve 25% of the eyelid, "moderate" if 40% is involved, and "large" if 55% to all of the eyelid is involved.

The availability of tissue for reconstruction is an important consideration of the surgeon planning reconstruction of an upper eyelid defect. Adjacent tissue is an excellent source of tissue that can be advanced directly or with undermining and incision. Direct closure, advancement, and rotational flaps are examples of this. It is not uncommon for this adjacent tissue to be markedly limited or absent, such as in patients who have undergone extensive Moh's surgery. The lower eyelid may be used for repair of the upper eyelid and is the underlying principle of the Cutler-Beard procedure. The availability of free graft tissue, either full-thickness skin, autogenous cartilage, or mucous membrane, is important. The integrity of the recipient bed must be considered. In cases with absence of adjacent tissue or opposing eyelid tissue, remote flaps must be used to restore the upper eyelid.

To evaluate the upper eyelid defect properly, the surgeon must classify it as to size, location, and configuration. Alternative procedures are available for reconstruction of the upper eyelid, determining which procedure to use depends on the factors mentioned above and the expertise and experience of the surgeon. This chapter will include descriptions of eight upper eyelid reconstruction techniques: (*a*) direct closure of full-thickness upper eyelid defects, with lateral cantholysis if needed; (*b*) Tenzel advancement flap; (*c*) sliding tarsal flap with skin graft or musculocutaneous flap; (*d*) Cutler-Beard, or bridge flap, technique; (*e*) transposition forehead flaps, either temporal or medial; (*f*) split-level grafts; (*g*) composite eyelid grafts; (*h*) pedicle graft from lower lid margin.

DIRECT CLOSURE OF UPPER EYELID DEFECTS

Common upper lid defects that the ophthalmic surgeon encounters and that may be closed directly are from tumor excision, trauma, or congenital malformations. Ideally most eyelid tumors can be detected early while still amenable to direct-closure techniques. These tumors should be excised in a pentagonal fashion with sharp instruments, such as the surgical scalpel, which creates sharp wound edges to allow accurate would approximation (Figs. 66.1*A* and 66.2*A*). Using modern swedged-on sutures and sharp spatula needles, the surgeon is able to close lid defects in two layers, which leaves an almost imperceptible scar. Up to 25% full-thickness eyelid defect can be closed directly in younger patients. Increased laxity in older patients allows direct closure in up to 40% of the upper lid or more with the use of lateral cantholysis. Postoperatively, the eyelid may appear tight and ptotic when the upper lid tissue has been stretched, but over a few weeks the lid will relax and assume a normal appearance and position. Direct closure of upper lid defects is valuable since it allows for continuity of the lash line. The most important part of the direct-closure technique is approximation of the tarsal plate. The edges of the tarsus are sutured in as an exact a manner as possible; the use of magnification greatly enhances this closure. Certain traumatic cases will present an irregular or friable tarsal margin; in these cases the tarsal edges should be sharply trimmed so that they

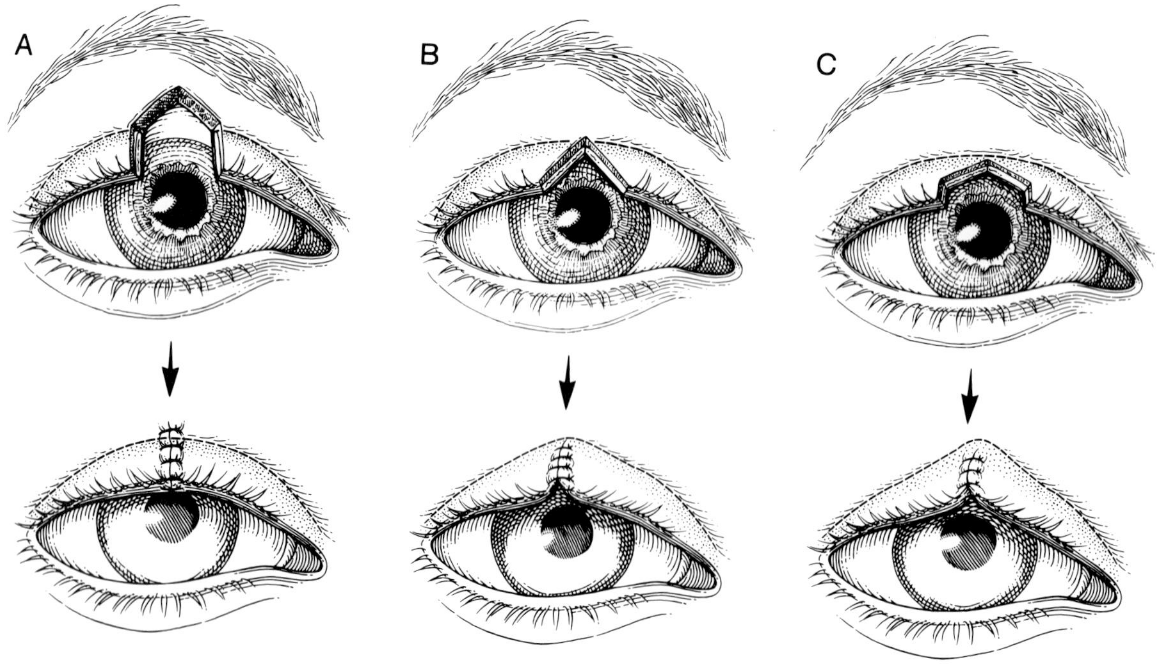

Figure 66.1. *A*, Proper pentagonal incision of the upper lid carries the vertical tarsal incision to the superior border of tarsus. *B,C*, Nonvertical incisions in tarsus result in poor wound approximation with buckling of the tarsus and lid notch formation (superior border of tarsus depicted by *dotted line*).

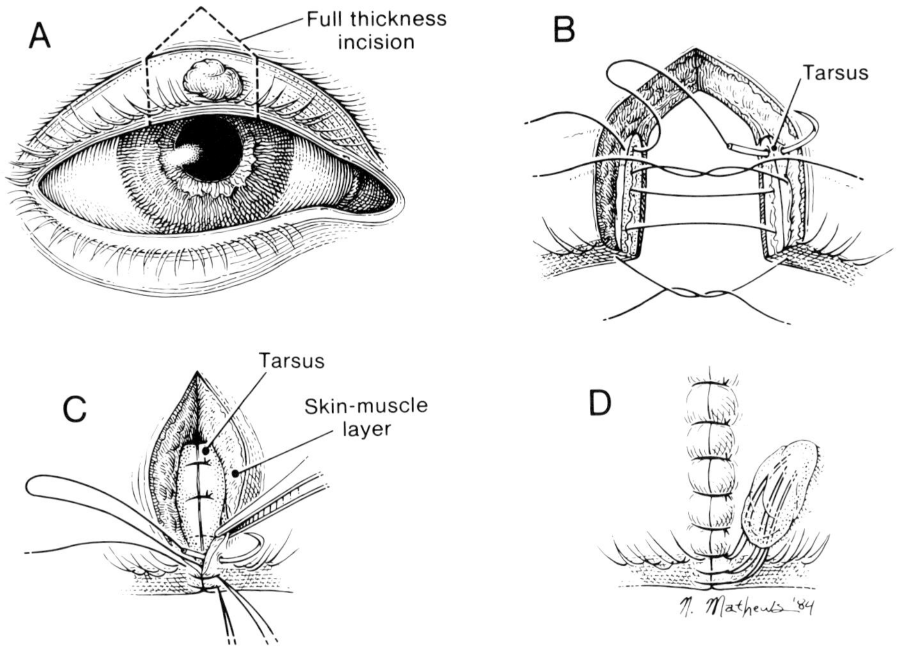

Figure 66.2. *A*, Tumor involving about 25% of the upper eyelid is outlined with adequate margins for pentagon excision. *B*, Central tarsal suture of 6-0 silk is used to reapproximate the lid margin, checking tension on the wound edges. The tarsal plate is closed with three 7-0 silk sutures, and care is taken not to penetrate the conjunctiva. *C*, A posterior and anterior 6-0 silk suture aligns the lid margin. These are left long to keep sutures off the cornea. *D*, The skin muscle layer is closed with interrupted or running 7-0 silk suture.

are vertically parallel and extend the entire vertical height of the tarsus to help exact reapproximation. With tumor removal the wound edges can be made electively. Hesitation on the part of the surgeon to create a full vertical excision of the tarsal segment extending to the superior border will result in notching of the margin or buckling of the upper lid with an abnormal contour. This buckling is caused by the residual bridge of overlapping tarsus left superiorly (Fig. 66.1*B*,*C*). With proper lid reconstruction techniques, trichiasis and lid notching are rare. It is important to remember when freshening the wound edges to get good vertical approximation of tarsus and to save as much lid tissue as possible. Tissue that is blue and apparently necrotic may become viable because of the excellent vascularity of the lids.

TECHNIQUE

Sharp wound edges are created perpendicular to the lid margin, and before closure of the tarsal plate an initial lid margin suture of 6-0 silk is passed through the central tarsus at the lid margin to see if the margin can be brought together with a moderate amount of tension (Fig. 66.2*B*). This suture must pass equally distant from the wound edge on each side. If the eyelid tension is excessive with this suture, a lateral cantholysis must be performed. To perform a lateral cantholysis, the surgeon makes an incision horizontally at the lateral canthus down to the orbital rim. Sharp scissors are then passed between the skin and conjunctiva to sever the superior crus of the lateral canthal tendon. This maneuver is facilitated by grasping the lateral lid margin with forceps, providing medial traction, and feeling the relaxation as the tendon is cut. This relaxation is obtained in a piecemeal manner until the desired amount of laxity is obtained.

The vertical cut edges of the tarsal plate are now closed using three 7-0 silk sutures with a G-7 Ethicon needle placed half-thickness through the tarsus so the sutures will not abrade the cornea (Fig. 66.2*B*). It is helpful to separate the orbicularis muscle fibers from the tarsal plate before the sutures are passed; this insures that only the tarsus is included in this layered closure. Other sutures may be used, but silk causes minimal tissue reaction and has withstood the test of time. A 6-0 silk suture is then placed through the tarsus approximating the posterior lid margin, and another 6-0 silk suture is placed just above the lashes approximating the lash line. All three 6-0 silk marginal sutures are cut long so they can be kept out of the eye with ointment or by placing them under the skin sutures (Fig. 66.2*C*). The conjunctiva requires no sutures and is well apposed due to the meticulous closure of the tarsus. The skin muscle layer is then closed with interrupted or running sutures of 7-0 silk (Fig. 66.2*D*). Sutures can be removed 7 days postoperatively under the usual healing conditions. The three deep 7-0 silk tarsal sutures will maintain tarsal integrity and would apposition. In certain problem cases, especially if there is upward traction on the lid, such as in a laceration extending to the rim, a reverse-Frost suture may be placed from the tarsal lid margin to provide downward traction on the lid for 1–2 weeks.

TENZEL LATERAL SEMICIRCULAR ROTATIONAL FLAP

Upper eyelid defects of 40–60% can be corrected by the Tenzel semicircular flap rotated into the defect. This technique has the advantage of not using tissue of the opposite lid. As the scar heals, it usually falls in natural crease lines and the arched flap helps prevent lateral upper lid retraction. The upper lid defect must be fashioned so that the tarsal edges are perfectly perpendicular, extending the entire vertical length of the tarsus, and the lesion is excised in a pentagon (Fig. 66.3*A*). An inferior arching line is drawn with methylene blue beginning at the lateral canthus. This should extend laterally to the lateral extension of the brow and be confined to the periorbital skin. The horizontal diameter of the flap should be 20–22 mm (Fig. 66.3*A*). The skin and muscle flap is then dissected and widely undermined and a lateral canthotomy performed (Fig. 66.3*B*). The lids are not denervated because the branches of the seventh nerve run lateral to this. The superior crus of the lateral canthal tendon and lateral orbital septum are sharply freed up; the conjunctiva is mobilized; and the flap is brought nasally, which closes the defect. Some orbital fat may prolapse; this is of no consequence; however, care must be taken not to damage the lacrimal gland as this may result in profuse bleeding or damage the lacrimal ductules. The lateral lid tissue containing tarsal remnants is advanced to the medial edge of the defect and closed in the manner described under "Direct Closure." The conjunctiva is mobilized or a mucous membrane graft sutured to the posterior surface of the new lateral upper lid. The mucous membrane is fixated anteriorly with running 6-0 nylon suture and should overlap the lid margin (Fig. 66.3*C*). The lateral canthus is reformed by suturing the flap tissue to the periosteum at the lateral orbital rim with a 4-0 silk vertical mattress suture. This step of lateral canthal fixation is necessary to prevent retraction and elevation of the lateral portion of the lid. If the sides of the lateral incision are not equal, a small dog ear may be excised at the temporal portion of the wound edge. The skin and muscle layer is closed with interrupted 7-0 silk (Fig. 66.3*D*). All the sutures are removed at 5 days postoperatively with the exception of the vertical mattress suture which is removed at 10 days.

This is an excellent technique for closure of small to moderate defects in the upper lids, particularly in patients with loose tissue. It is an identical principle to the Tenzel flap that is used in the lower lid and has withstood the test of time. If the flap is used for defects larger than it can encompass, difficulty in reforming the lateral portions of the lid may occur.

CUTLER-BEARD LOWER LID BRIDGE FLAP

The Cutler-Beard bridge flap technique is used to reconstruct full-thickness eyelid defects that include from 60% to the entire upper lid. This procedure borrows skin, muscle, and conjunctiva from the lower eyelid, which is

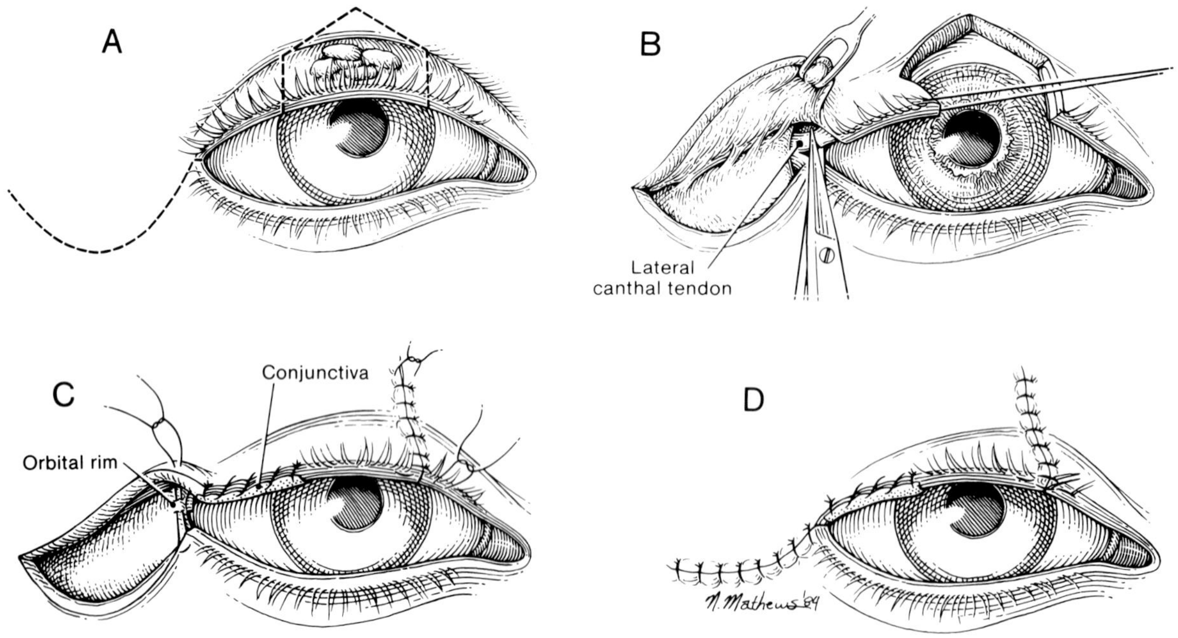

Figure 66.3. *A*, The lesion is outlined in a pentagon. The semicircular flap is marked arching inferiorly, extending about 20–22 mm in horizontal diameter, and not extending beyond the lateral extension of the brow. *B*, The skin and muscle flap is widely dissected. The superior crus of the lateral canthal tendon and septum is sharply dissected, allowing medial rotation of the wound edge. *C*, The pentagonal defect is closed as described in "Direct Closure." The conjunctiva overlaps the lid margin, and a 4-0 silk vertical mattress suture reapproximates the lateral canthal angle. *D*, The upper eyelid is reformed. All the sutures are removed on the fifth postoperative day with the exception of the vertical mattress suture, which is removed on the 10th postoperative day.

advanced into the upper eyelid defect. The incision must be made 5 mm below the lower eyelid margin to preserve the marginal artery, which supplies the lower eyelid and runs along the inferior border of the tarsus approximately 4 mm below the lid margin. If the artery is violated, ischemia and necrosis may develop in the lower eyelid. Because this flap, which is to be advanced into the upper eyelid, contains no tarsus (average vertical height of the lower eyelid tarsus 3.8 mm), tissue such as autogenous ear cartilage must be sandwiched between the advanced skin muscle and conjunctiva. This provides a "skeleton" to the eyelid that maintains stability and prevents upper lid tissue shrinkage. Autogenous cartilage is preferred for this because there is much less shrinkage than with allograft sclera.

TECHNIQUE

Ideally the upper lid defect is rectangular and should be so shaped when removing a tumor. If this is not the case, as in trauma, congenital coloboma, or Mohs' chemosurgery, the defect can be fashioned into a rectangle to receive the flap. The flap of tissue from the lower lid should be approximately the same width as the upper lid defect. However, the medial and lateral margins of the lid defect can be lightly pulled together to reduce the size of the defect and graft needed to correct it. In older individuals with much lid laxity this can make a big difference in the size of the flap.

Five millimeters below the lower lid margin the skin is marked horizontally for the width of the upper eyelid defect. From each end of the mark a vertical line is drawn downward for 10–15 mm. The skin is incised along the marks with a globe protector or lid guard in place. At the lateral ends of the horizontal incision a perforation is made through full-thickness lid and the lid is transected with scissors, taking care to keep them horizontal. Full-thickness incisions are then made through the vertical ends of the flap to the lowest aspect of the inferior fornix on the conjunctival side of the flap (Fig. 66.4*A*).

In younger patients with very elastic tissue, the flap will shrink and not appear to fill the upper eyelid defect. But if the markings have been made of the proper horizontal dimension the tissue will stretch to fill the defect. The flap is then divided into a conjunctivo-capsulo-palpebral layer and skin-orbicularis muscle layer with the Westcott scissors. This step is facilitated by the previous injection of 1% lidocaine with epinephrine 1:100,000 separating the two layers. Both layers are advanced beneath the bridge flap and the conjunctiva is fixated to the conjunctiva of the upper lid defect with a running 6-0 plain gut suture (Fig. 66.4*B*). Relaxing incisions may be needed in the capsulopalpebral fascia to advance the lower eyelid conjunctiva. Autogenous cartilage, which can be harvested by a number of methods, is then fashioned to fit the defect. Ear cartilage from the scaphoid fossa is the best choice because of the ease in obtaining it with minimum morbid-

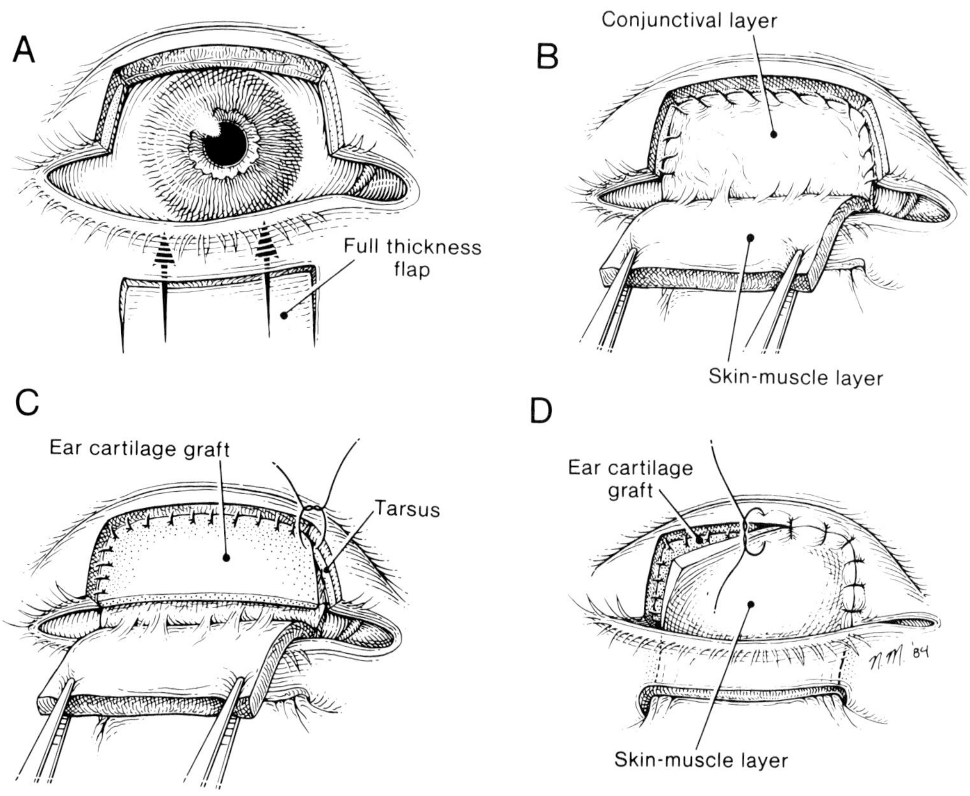

Figure 66.4. *A*, A skin-muscle-conjunctiva flap is prepared 5 mm below the inferior lid margin and extending 10 mm vertically. *B*, The skin and muscle layer has been separated from the conjunctival layer, which is sewn to the conjunctiva of the upper lid defect with a running 6-0 plain suture. *C*, Ear cartilage, conforming to the upper lid defect, is fixated medially and laterally to the edges of tarsus and superiorly to the edge of levator. *D*, The skin and muscle layer is closed to the skin of the upper lid with interrupted 7-0 silk sutures.

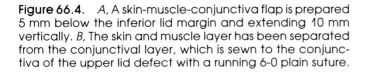

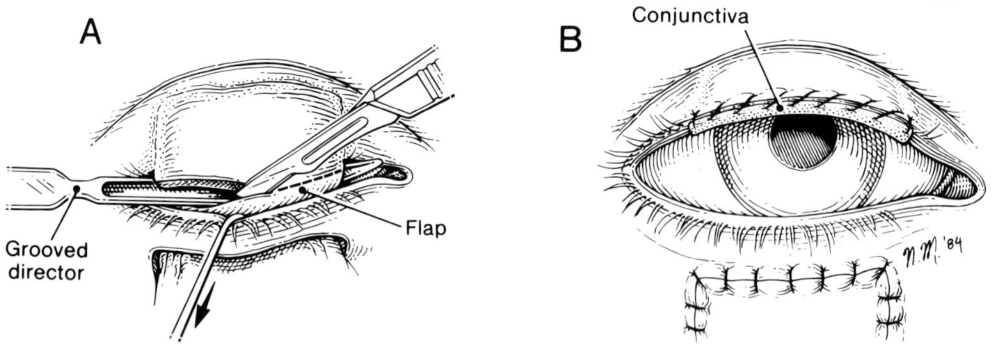

Figure 66.5. *A*, After 2 months the lids are separated 2 mm below the intended upper lid margin. This is accomplished by placing a metal groove director behind the flap and making the incision with a scalpel as the assistant retracts the bridge flap with a hook. *B*, The conjunctiva is overlapped over the superior lid margin, and the lower lid is reapproximated.

ity and because its thinness has greater resemblance to normal upper eyelid tarsus. The cartilage is then sutured medially and laterally with 7-0 silk to tarsal remnants or to the canthal tendons if the tarsus has been completely removed (Fig. 66.4*C*). Superiorly, it is fixed to the edge of levator or, if the levator has been excised, to the orbicularis muscle. The skin muscle flap from the lower lid is then sutured to the skin edges of the defect with interrupted 7-0 silk (Fig. 66.4*D*). Additional undermining of the skin flap over the malar eminence may be necessary to allow the flap to advance. Burrows triangles may be excised at the inferior edges of the advanced flap.

Separation of the flap is carried out 8 weeks later; earlier in very healthy tissue, and later in compromised tissue. Methylene blue is used to mark the flap 2 mm below the desired position of the upper lid margin. As the assistant provides downward traction on the bridge with a skin or muscle hook a groove director is inserted under the flap so a scalpel can be used to make an incision through the bridge flap (Fig. 66.5*A*). One or 2 mm of skin and muscle is then trimmed from the new upper lid margin, leaving conjunctiva that can be rotated anteriorly over the lid margin and fixed to skin with a running 6-0 nylon suture. This provides a smooth surface for the lid margin and provides for mucous membrane to be in contact with the cornea rather than keratinized epithelium or fine skin hairs. The retractors and conjunctiva of the flap are fixated to the inferior border of tarsus of the lower eyelid with 6-0 plain suture, and the skin is united with 6-0 silk (Fig. 66.5*B*).

SLIDING TARSAL FLAP

In this technique a residual layer of tarsus and conjunctiva is slid horizontally into a defect and covered with a skin graft or advanced skin muscle flap. This may be used in lid reconstruction for isolated medial or lateral upper lid defects (Fig. 66.6*A*). The coloboma of the upper lid is usually larger than can be closed with a Tenzel advancement flap, but smaller than would require a two-stage Cutler-Beard procedure.

TECHNIQUE

A 4-0 silk suture is placed vertically through the tarsus and used to rotate the eyelid remnant over a Desmarres retractor. Approximately 4 mm above the remaining lid margin, a scalpel is used to make a horizontal incision through conjunctiva and tarsus parallel to the lid margin. This horizontal incision is the same width as the defect after it has been reduced by mild stretching. A vertical incision is made at the tarsal end of the horizontal incision through tarsus and conjunctiva to the superior border of the tarsus. The tarsoconjunctival flap is sharply freed up, and dissection may need to be carried superior to this through conjunctiva and Müller's muscle to slide the tarsoconjunctival flap into place without tension. The edge of the flap is then fixated to the inside of periosteum near the lateral orbital tubercle (Fig. 66.6*B*). In the case of medial upper lid defects the edge is attached to the periosteum near the posterior lacrimal crest at a site corresponding to the horizontal plane through the visual axis (Fig. 66.7). A nonabsorbable double-armed suture on a small half-circle needle is best used for this. This suture is mandatory to ensure proper lid position and contour. If the lid is fixated anteriorly, the lid will be separated from the globe, which will cause corneal and conjunctival irritation. The superior edge of the tarsus of the flap is fixated with 7-0 silk to the cut edge of levator, which should be below the cut skin edge superiorly. A small notch is removed from the inferomedial tarsoconjunctival flap so that it will fit together with the lid margin of the remaining upper eyelid. The edges are then united at the lid margin with a 4-0 silk suture. All the sutures are placed through three-fourths thickness of the tarsus so that the conjunctiva is not violated with subsequent suture irritation to the cornea (Fig. 66.6*C*). A retroauricular graft or advancement skin or musculocutaneous flap then is sutured to the skin edges, which fills the anterior lamellar deficit (Fig. 66.6*D*). Attention must be given to the lid margin to assure a smooth conjunctival surface and prevent epidermis from rubbing the cornea. The upper lid is splinted to the lower lid with a 4-0 silk double-armed suture in a reverse-Frost

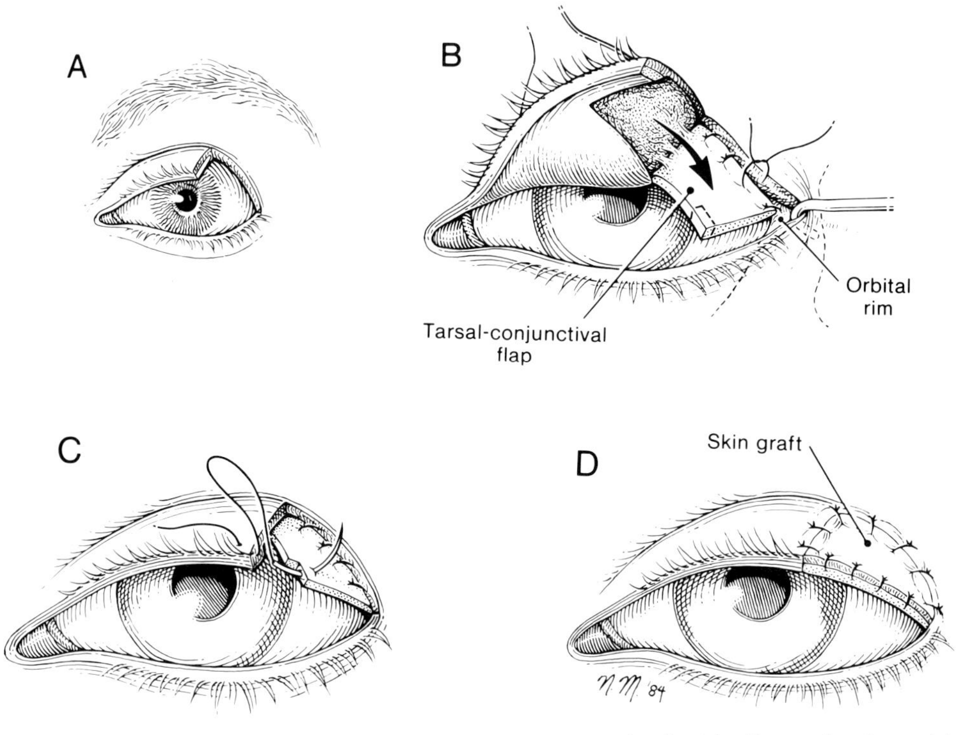

Figure 66.6. *A*, Full-thickness lateral upper eyelid defect involving about 45% of the lid. *B*, A flap of tarsus and conjunctiva is developed 4 mm above the lid margin and rotated into the defect. The edge is fixated to the periosteum inside the lateral orbital rim in the horizontal plane of the visual axis with a 4-0 nonabsorbable suture. The superior border is fixated to the cut edge of levator aponeurosis with 7-0 silk. *C*, A notch has been removed from the inferomedial edge of the flap and the margin sutured medially with a 4-0 silk suture. *D*, A full-thickness skin graft is sutured in place to form the anterior lamella.

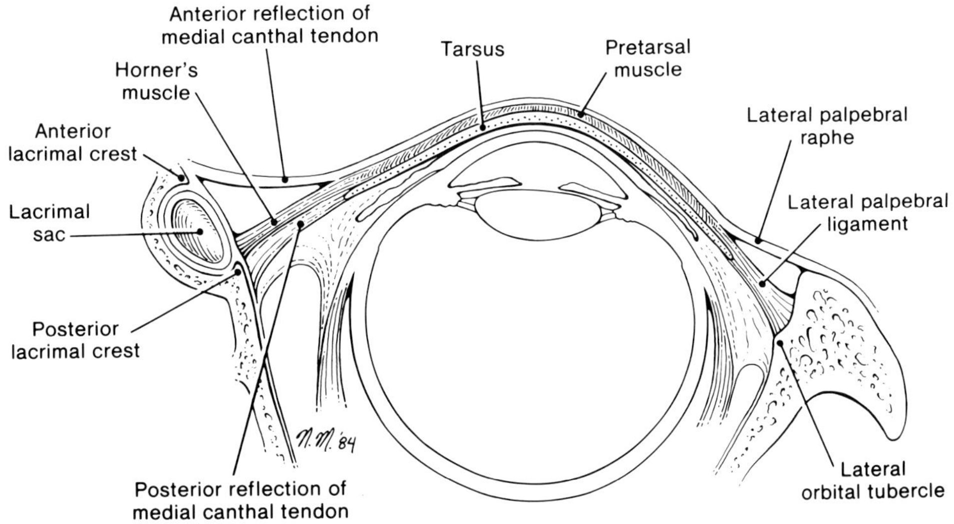

Figure 66.7. The pull of the lid is posterior to the orbital rim. The lateral canthal tendon inserts at the lateral orbital tubercle, and the medial canthal tendon inserts in the anterior and posterior lacrimal crests.

suture that is tied over a cotton bolster on the skin of the lower eyelid. This suture is left for a week. The graft is dressed by covering it with telfa. Dental base plate wax softened in warm water is molded to the graft surface and covered with a pressure dressing. This is left for 7 days if possible. The loss of lashes is more conspicuous nasally than temporally. A lash graft as a second stage may correct this.

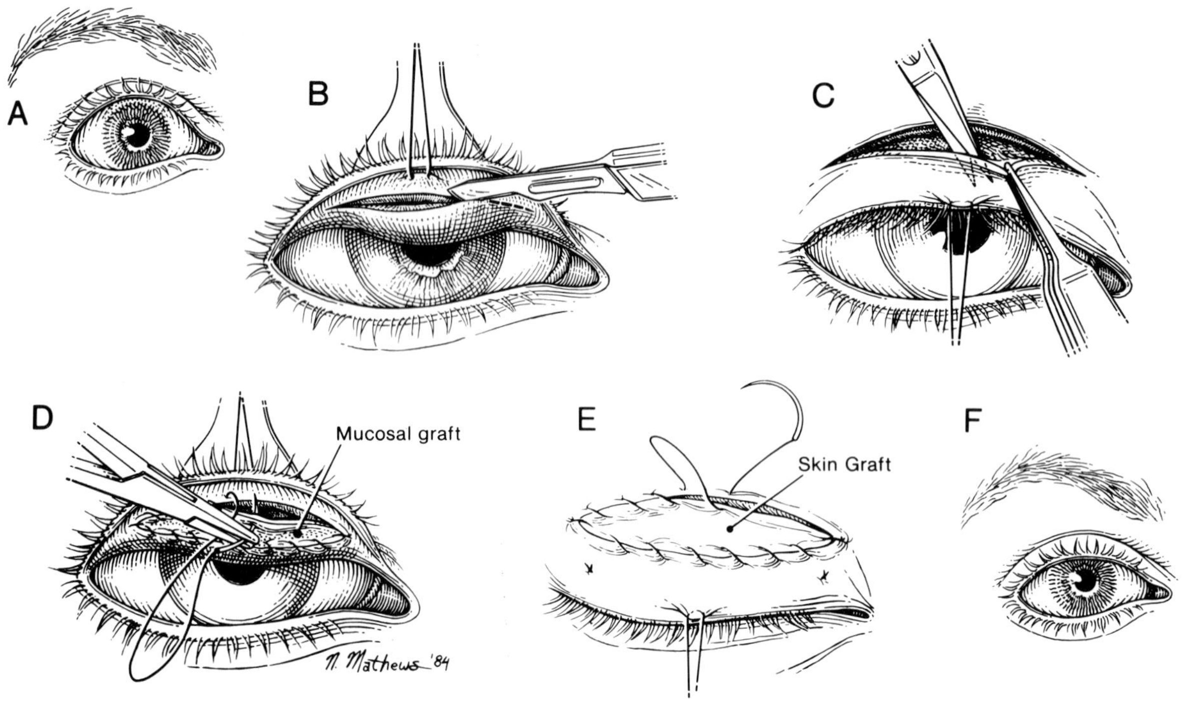

Figure 66.8. *A*, Full-thickness upper eyelid defect with a normal lid margin and retraction of the upper eyelid. *B*, Horizontal incision through conjunctiva and tarsus is made 5 mm above the eyelid margin for the entire width of the eyelid. *C*, The upper eyelid skin is incised horizontally immediately above the superior border of tarsus as the assistant places downward traction on the lid margin. *D*, A chondromucosal or buccal mucosal graft is sutured in place with a running 6-0 plain suture with the knots tied externally. *E*, The upper eyelid has been lengthened full thickness and the lid margin is in normal position.

SPLIT-LEVEL EYELID GRAFTS

Full-thickness eyelid defects that retain a normal upper eyelid margin can be corrected by a technique described by Brown and Beard (Fig. 66.8*A*). These patients have upper eyelid retraction, lagophthalmos, and exposure keratitis. This defect of the upper eyelid may be secondary to removal of excessive amounts of tissue of both lamallae at various times from burns, irradiation, or inflammation such as herpes zoster. A full thickness graft of retroauricular skin or upper lid skin from the opposite eye is used to lengthen the anterior lamella and a full-thickness buccomucous membrane graft or chondromucosal graft lengthens the posterior lamella. Each graft is placed at different levels of the eyelid into its own vascularized bed to ensure viability of the graft.

TECHNIQUE

A 4-0 silk suture is placed through the tarsus at the lid margin, and the lid is rotated over a Desmarres lid retractor. Five millimeters above the lid margin a horizontal incision is made through conjunctiva and tarsus for the entire width of the lid (Figs. 66.8*B* and 66.9*A*). The retractor is removed and inferior traction placed on the 4-0 silk suture as the skin is horizontally incised just above the superior border of tarsus for the entire width of the lid (Figs. 66.8*C* and 66.9*A*). If it is not possible to rotate the lid initially to incise the tarsus, by making the horizontal skin incision first the lid can then be rotated. Undermining between the anterior and posterior lamellae then frees scar tissue and traction bands that caused the lid retraction. The superoanterior and posteroinferior incisions are joined and the lid is lengthened. A 20 × 5 mm buccal mucous membrane graft or chondromucosal graft is fixated with a running 6-0 plain suture, in which the knots are tied externally to prevent corneal irritation (Fig. 66.8*D*). A 30 × 15 mm elliptical retrocurricular skin graft is then sewn into the skin defect with 7-0 silk sutures (Figs. 66.8*E*, 66.9*A*, and 66.9*B*). A 4-0 silk intermarginal suture provides traction on the lid by keeping the grafts stretched. Telfa, dental wax, and a pressure dressing cover the surgical site. The dressing and sutures are removed 7 days postoperatively. The lid may appear ptotic, but this disappears as the lid retracts with shrinkage of the grafts (Fig. 66.8*F*).

MEDIAN FOREHEAD FLAP

In many cases of massive tissue loss of the upper eyelid, when the tissue cannot be borrowed from the apposing lower lid or adjacent areas, or when there is a poorly vascularized recipient bed due to previous irradiation,

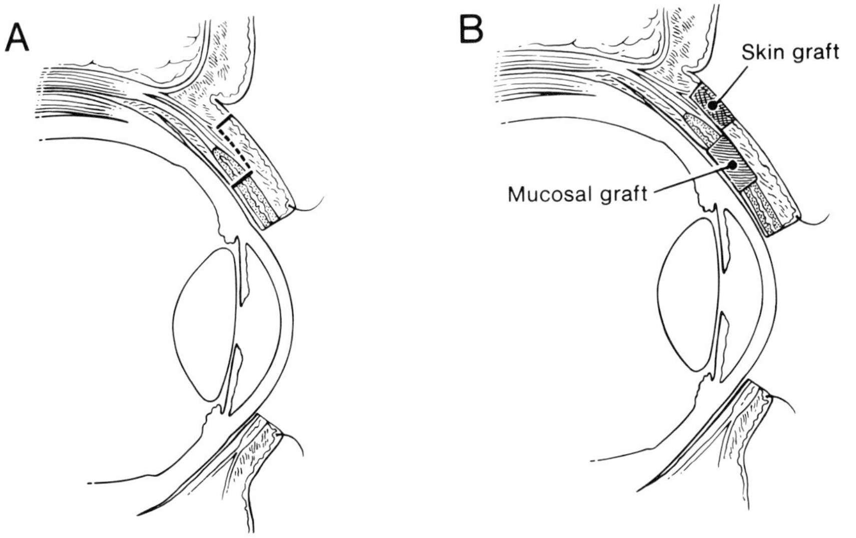

Figure 66.9. *A,* The horizontal tarsoconjunctival incision is made 5 mm above the lid margin, and the skin incision is made just above the superior edge of tarsus. *B,* The posterior buccal mucous membrane graft lengthens the posterior lamella; the skin graft lengthens the anterior lamella. Full-thickness lid has been lengthened, and each graft is in its own vascularized bed.

surgery, or tissue damage, flaps must be brought in from more remote areas. The supraorbital and supratrochlear arteries provide an excellent blood supply to the area of the median forehead, allowing long flaps to be developed without danger of necrosis. Flaps up to 3.5 cm in width and extending to the hairline can safely be made.

TECHNIQUE

Full-thickness buccal mucosa is sutured to the conjunctival edges of the defect with 6-0 plain suture (Fig. 66.10*A*). A piece of suture or plastic drape may be rotated from the root of the nose to the lateral edge of the upper lid defect to determine the proper size of the flap. This should allow for folding at the base of the flap, and the graft should be made 3 mm wider to compensate for shrinkage. The flap is marked off in the midforehead area with methylene blue and incised through the skin and subcutaneous tissue to the frontalis muscle. As much deep tissue as possible is retained at the base. The base should not bc below the intercanthal line, and the side of the incision nearest the defect is extended a little lower than the opposite side to facilitate rotation of the flap. The flap is then rotated into place and attached to the edge of levator aponeurosis or remnants of the levator muscle with 6-0 silk sutures to lend mobility to the lid (Fig. 66.10*B*). Laterally, the tip of the flap is fixated to the remnants of the lateral canthal tendon or periosteum of the lateral orbital tubercle with a 4-0 nonabsorbable suture. Interrupted 6-0 silk sutures unite the skin edges. The graft of mucous membrane is brought around the inferior edge of the flap and fixated with a running 6-0 nylon suture. This ensures that extra mucous membrane overlaps the lid margin, which compensates for shrinkage and allows mucous membrane and not keratinized epithelium to contact the cornea. The area surrounding the flap is widely undermined to allow closure, and a triangle of skin and subcutaneous tissue may be excised at the apex to allow for better closure of the donor site. The donor area is reapproximated in two layers using 4-0 absorbable sutures to close the subcutaneous tissue and 4-0 silk for the skin (Fig. 66.10*B*). After 3–4 weeks the base of the flap should be compressed and the graft inspected for blanching (compression test). If no blanching occurs then sufficient vascularization of the donor tissue by the surrounding recipient tissue has taken place. The flap is divided at the medial edge of the lid and closed with interrupted 6-0 nylon suture. The granulation and fibrous tissue at the base of the flap are excised and only a small portion of the pedicle is returned to close the forehead with interrupted 6-0 nylon sutures (Fig. 66.10*C*).

The upper eyelid will appear tight, and over many weeks the levator muscle will begin to provide vertical motility. The resultant eyelid skin will be abnormally thick and may be cautiously thinned at a later time.

TEMPORAL FOREHEAD FLAP

When there are no other alternatives for reconstructing the upper lid, a temporal transposition graft (Fricke flap) can be used. This is a thick flap and requires lining with advanced conjunctiva or buccal mucous membrane, but no replacement for tarsus is required. This graft has the disadvantage of providing poor eyelid function due to its thickness and stiffness. Besides, the eyebrow is usually noticeably raised, and the procedure requires two stages.

TECHNIQUE

The graft is based on the superficial temporal artery that travels along the lateral orbital rim above the brow. The

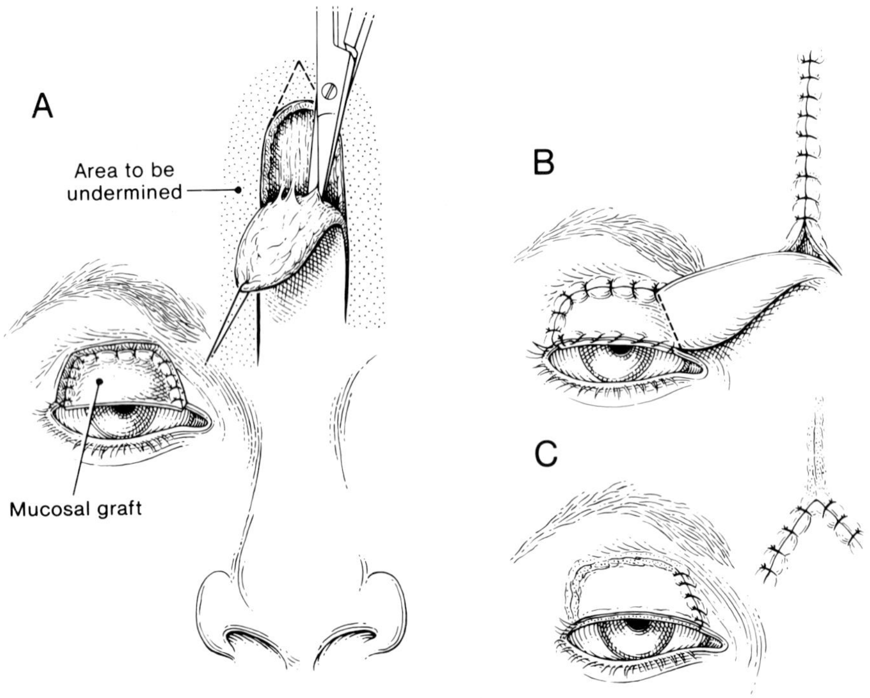

Figure 66.10. The large upper lid defect has been lined with buccal mucous membrane sutured to the edges of conjunctiva with 6-0 plain suture. The pedicle flap has been raised and wide subcutaneous dissection carried out to enable closure of the donor area. A triangle of skin may be removed at the apex of the donor site to facilitate closure. *B*, The graft is fixated to the levator aponeurosis on its superior undersurface with 6-0 silk mattress sutures. The tip is fixated to the lateral canthal tendon or periosteum of the lateral orbital tubercle with a 4-0 nonabsorbable suture. The edges of the flap are united to the skin with interrupted 6-0 silk sutures. The mucous membrane is folded over the lid margin with a running 6-0 nylon suture. The donor site is closed with a 4-0 absorbable suture for the subcutaneous tissue and 4-0 silk for the skin. *C*, The pedicle is incised at the medial margin of the original defect, and the lid granulation tissue is excised at the base of the pedicle excised. Only a small portion of the pedicle is returned to the base; closure is effected with interrupted 6-0 nylon sutures.

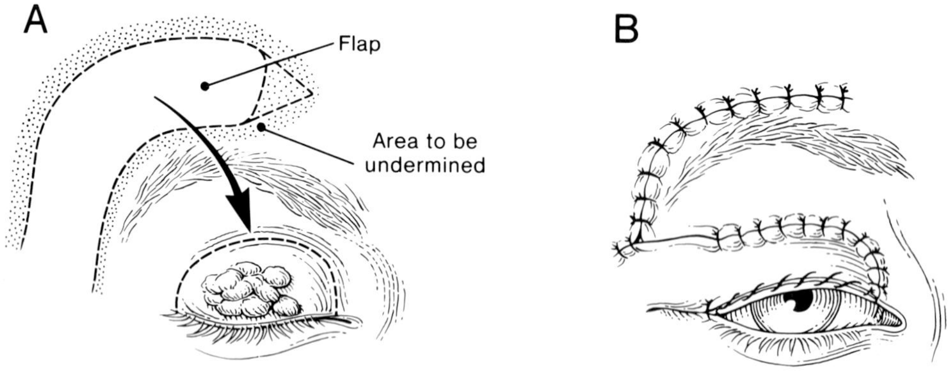

Figure 66.11. *A*, A temporal flap of skin based on the superficial temporalis artery is marked with methylene blue. This must be of sufficient length to cover the horizontal and vertical dimensions of the lid defect. Undermining of the edges and removal of a triangle of skin at the end of the flap simplify the closure. *B*, The temporal forehead flap is in position. It is fixated medially to a remnant of the medial canthal tendon or periosteum of the posterior lacrimal crest with a 4-0 nonabsorbable suture. Mucous membrane lines the graft and lid margin and is fixated with a 6-0 nylon suture with the knots tied on the skin.

artery should be outlined on the skin by palpation or with the use of a Doppler, so that it will be included in the graft (Fig. 66.11*A*). The skin is then marked with methylene blue, and care is taken to include the artery in the base and ensure that the flap is long and wide enough to cover the upper eyelid defect. The skin of the flap is incised, and the flap is developed. Some subcutaneous fat is usually included, but this can be dissected free from the dermis. Care should be taken to avoid cutting the superficial temporal artery. Undermining is usually necessary to allow the flap to turn onto the lid. Buccal mucous membrane graft is fixated to the edges of conjunctiva with interrupted 6-0 plain suture (Fig. 66.10*A*). Obviously, the mucous membrane side should face the globe. The flap is rotated into position. Some buckling will be present at the base of the flap. The flap is fixated medially with a 4-0 nonabsorbable suture to the remnants of the medial canthal tendon or the periosteum near the posterior lacrimal crest (Fig. 66.7). If possible, the levator should be anchored to the superior edge or underside of the flap. The skin of the graft is sutured medially and superiorly to the skin edges of the recipient site with interrupted 6-0 silk sutures. Removing a triangle of skin at the apex of the donor site and wide undermining allow for closure of the donor site. Vertical mattress sutures of 4-0 silk relieve the tension after placing 4-0 deep absorbable sutures (Fig. 66.11*B*). The temporal portion of the brow may be difficult to close, and this can be left open for 3–4 weeks before the base of the flap is separated. After 3 weeks the flap can be divided if the compression test shows no blanching of the flap. If it does, then separation should be delayed for a few more days. Only a small portion of the flap is returned to the temporal brow. The granulation tissue at the base of the flap is excised, and the pedicle of skin not used to rebuild the lid is discarded. The skin is closed with interrupted 4-0 silk sutures.

COMPOSITE GRAFT TO THE EYELID

The best replacement for eyelid tissue is autogenous eyelid tissue. The most important and conspicuous part of the upper lid is the margin, which touches the cornea and contains the lash line. Composite grafting allows for replacement of these two important parts of the lid with normal eyelid tissue. In the past, full-thickness composite grafts have failed because vascularization did not take place soon enough to prevent necrosis and shrinkage of the graft. New techniques that provide more success with composite eyelid grafting have been advanced. The maximum amount of donor lid that can be taken from a normal eyelid is 8 mm. In an older patient with eyelid laxity, a fairly large upper eyelid defect can be closed by utilizing a composite graft.

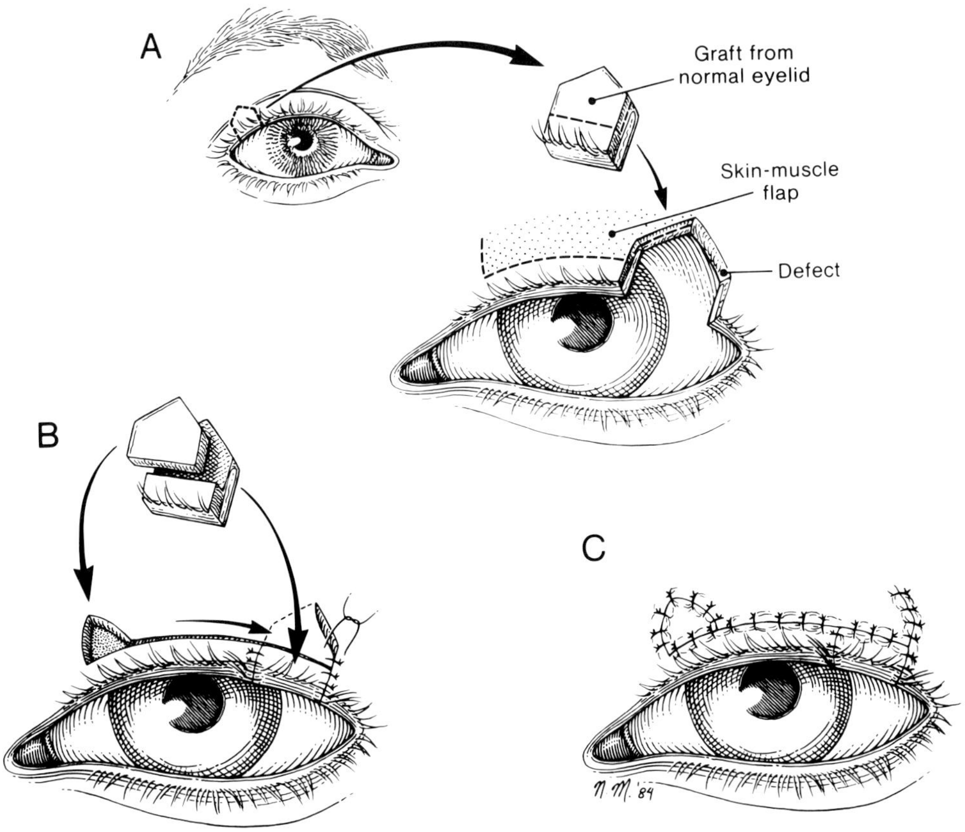

Figure 66.12. *A*, A full-thickness pentagon of tissue is excised from the opposite uninvolved upper eyelid. The vertical lines of the pentagon are 10 mm and extend to the superior edge of tarsus, which provides for accurate lid closure. The defect is modified to accept the graft by mild stretching of the edges and a lateral canthotomy if necessary. A skin muscle advancement flap is outlined. *B,C*, The skin and muscle are excised from the donor eyelid graft 2 mm above the lashes and fixated with interrupted 7-0 silk sutures. The skin and muscle advancement flap is moved over the composite graft, and the skin is closed primarily. If there is a shortage of skin at the distal edge of the advancement flap, the skin from the composite graft can be used as a free skin graft.

TECHNIQUE

A pentagonal section of normal eyelid is removed from the opposite upper eyelid, and it is kept in mind that the parallel vertical lines of the pentagon extend the entire 10 mm vertical height of the tarsus (Fig. 66.12*A*). The defect is closed primarily using the technique described under direct closure of eyelid defects. The anterior skin and muscle of the graft is removed, and the inferior 2 mm above the lashes are spared. This will leave the lash follicles undisturbed (Fig. 66.12*A*,*B*).

This modified composite graft is then sewn into the tarsal defect with interrupted 7-0 silk sutures (Fig. 66.12*B*). If there is some tension on the suture line, a canthotomy must be performed in the recipient eyelid to minimize this tension. A skin muscle flap is then elevated from the recipient lid and slid across or advanced downward to cover the tarsus of the donor portion of the eyelid and is sutured into place (Fig. 66.12*B*,*C*). If there is some shortage of skin in the recipient upper eyelid, some of the skin that has been removed from the composite graft can be placed in the recipient upper lid (Fig. 66.12*B*). It is obvious that the skin muscle flap over the donor composite graft is of primary importance for the graft to be viable. It is possible to use composite grafts from the lower lid to the upper lid, but the lashes are shorter and the tarsal plate will usually not be of adequate vertical dimension.

PEDICLE FLAP FROM LOWER TO UPPER EYELID

The technique of switching a portion of the lower lid margin to the upper lid defect is a useful method for reconstructing broad shallow or margin defects of the upper lid that also replaces lashes and gives an excellent cosmetic result. This technique was described by Mustardé for the reconstruction of total upper lid defects; however, its use seems to be particularly suited for reconstructing margin defects. Patients who have had primarily margin loss from trauma, burns, etc., and who are bothered by the loss of lashes can be rehabilitated with the use of this method. In this technique it is emphasized that the lower lid pedicle should be very broad based (approximately 7–8 mm). The maximum length of lower lid that can be spared without reconstructing the lower lid in most cases is about 6 mm, but this is sufficient to restore lashes and a healthy lid margin in defects that do not involve the majority of the upper lid.

TECHNIQUE

The upper lid edges are shaped in a rectangular manner to receive the pedicle from the lower lid. An outline of the flap is made on the lower lid. The major portion of the flap should come from the central portion of the lower lid since this area contains the longest lashes and it is much easier to close defects in the lower lid that do not include the canthus (Fig. 66.13*A*). In defects not in the center of the upper lid, the lower flap is generally based on the same side as the larger upper lid remnant. The flap is then designed a few millimeters smaller than the upper lid defect, with a pedicle of about 8 mm in width. The lower flap is dissected on its pedicle. The free end of the flap is rotated 180° and set in place without putting undue tension on the pedicle. The edge of the tarsus or deep layers are matched up (Fig. 66.13*B*). Since there is usually resid-

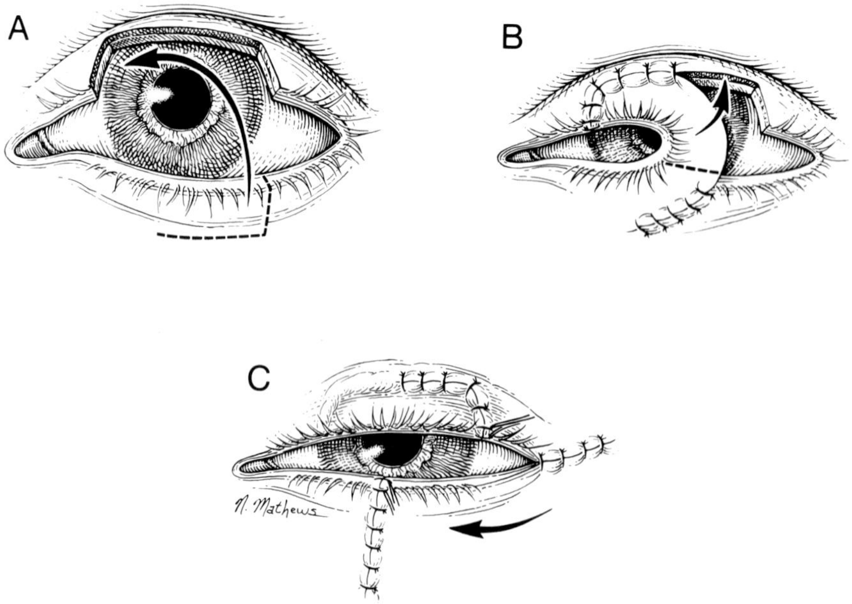

Figure 66.13. *A*, An upper lid defect is present with tarsus still remaining superiorly. A full-thickness pedicle flap of the lower eyelid with an 8 mm base is marked off. *B*, The pedicle flap has been sutured in place superomedially. After 2 weeks the pedicle will be incised and rotated into place. *C*, The pedicle flap has been sutured in place superolaterally after transection of the pedicle. This illustrates that it may be necessary to do a lateral canthotomy and inferior cantholysis and to rotate lateral tissue inward to correct the lower lid defect without undue tension.

ual superior tarsus, the levator is usually not attached to the pedicle. The temporal cut edge of the cut lower lid is then advanced inward and attached to the edge of the flap. It is usually not necessary to perform a canthotomy.

The flap is left in position for at least 2 weeks. In cases of irradiation, fibrosis, etc. it would be preferable to leave it in position longer than this before separation. The base of the flap is divided at the lower eyelid margin. The remaining portion of the lower lid flap is sutured into the defect in the upper lid. There is a tendency to remove tissue from the flap, but this should not be done as there will be some shrinkage and any redundancy can be trimmed at a later date. The lower lid defect can be closed directly with or without lateral canthotomy; inferior cantholysis and some revision of the margin must be carried out to ensure layered approximation (Fig. 66.13*C*). Care must be taken to reconstruct the margin adequately to avoid trichiasis.

This is an extremely reliable and excellent way to reconstruct upper lid margin defects, particularly when one desires to have lashes present. Also, this method is particularly suitable for patients who are not candidates for composite grafts. The disadvantage of the technique is that it is a two-stage procedure and care must be taken in closure of the lower lid, following pedicle removal, to ensure integrity of the lower lid margin. The donation of tissue from the lower lid with this particular technique is not intended to create need for lower lid reconstruction as was described in the original technique by Mustardé. Care must be taken not to transpose excessive tissue from the lower lid to the upper lid; otherwise, secondary reconstructive procedures in the lower lid will be necessary. Should this occur, one could therefore simply perform an advancement flap in the lower lid with cartilage or mucosal graft.

SUGGESTED READINGS

Anderson RL, Edwards JJ: Reconstruction by myocutaneous eyelid flaps. *Arch Ophthalmol* 97: 2358–2362, 1979.

Baylis HI. Rosen N, Nehaus RW: Obtaining auricular cartilage for reconstructive surgery. *Am J Ophthalmol* 93: 709–712, 1981.

Blasius: Neue methode der blepharoplastik. *Med Zeitg* 11: 43–44, 1842.

Budinger K: Eine methode des ersatzes von liddefekten. *Wien Klin Wochenschr* 15: 648–650, 1902.

Brown BZ, Beard C: Split-level full-thickness eyelid graft. *Am J Ophthalmol* 87: 388–392, 1979.

Burow A: Zur blepharoplastik. *Monatsschr Med Augenh Chir* 1: 57, 1838.

Callahan M, Callahan A: *Ophthalmic Plastic and Orbital Surgery.* Birmingham, Aesculapius Publishing Co, 1979, pp 183–209.

Cutler N, Beard C: A method for partial and total upper lid reconstruction. *Am J Ophthalmol* 39: 1–7, 1955.

Dieffenbach JF: *Die Operative Chirurgie.* Leipzig, F A Brockhaus, 1845.

Flanagan JC, Frueh BR, Baylis HI: Tumors of the eyelids. In Silver B (ed): *Ophthalmic Plastic Surgery.* Rochester, NY, American Academy of Ophthalmology and Otolaryngology, 1977, pp 190–206.

Fox S: *Ophthalmic Plastic Surgery,* ed 5. New York, Grune and Stratton, 1976, p 232–255.

Fricke JC: Die bildung never a ugen lider (blepharoplastik) nach zerstorungen und dadurch hervorgebrachten auswartwwendungen derselben. Hamburg, Perthes und Besser, 1829.

Houze de L'Aulnoit: Sur les greffes muqueses. *Gaz Hebd Med Chir* 41, 1872.

Landolt M: Un nouveau cas de blepharoplastie suivant notre procede. *Arch Ophthalmol* 1: 111, 1881.

Landolt M: De quelques operations pratiquees sur les paupieres. *Arch Ophthalmol* 5: 481–498, 1885.

Leone CR: Tarsal conjunctival advancement flaps for upper eyelid reconstruction. *Arch Ophthalmol* 101: 945–948, 1983.

Leone CR: Nasal septal cartilage for eyelid reconstruction. *Ophthal Surg* 4: 68–71, 1973.

Lindberg JV, et al: Preserved irridiated homologous cartilage for orbital reconstruction. *Ophthal Surg* 11: 457–462, 1980.

Lipshutz H: Experiences with upper lateral nasal cartilage in reconstruction of the lower lid. *Am J Ophthalmol* 73: 592–594, 1972.

McCord CD: Surgery of the eyelids. In Duane T (ed): *Clinical Ophthalmology.* Philadelphia, Harper & Row, 1983, vol 5, chap 5.

McCord CD, Wesley RE: Reconstruction of the upper eyelid and medial canthus. In McCord CD (ed): *Oculoplastic Surgery.* New York, Raven Press, 1981, p 175–188.

Montandon D: History of plastic surgery of the orbital region. In Aston S, Hornblass A, Meltzer M, Rees T (eds): *Third International Symposium of Plastic and Reconstructive Surgery of the Eye and Adnexa.* Baltimore, Williams & Wilkins, 1982, pp 2–10.

Mustardé JC: *Repair and Reconstruction in the Orbital Region,* ed 3. Edinburgh, Churchill Livingston, 1980, p 92–151.

Putterman AM: Viable composite grafting in eyelid reconstruction. *Am J Ophthalmol* 85: 237–241, 1978.

Reverdin JL: Greffe epidermique. Experience faite dans le service de M. Le Dr. Guyon a l Hospital Necker. *Bull Imp Soc Chir Paris* 10: 511–515, 1869.

Smith B, Obear MF: Bridge flap technique for reconstruction of large upper lid defects. *Plast Reconstr Surg* 38: 45–48, 1966.

Smith B, Lisman S: Auricular cartilage grafts split thickness. *Ophthal Surg* 13: 1018–1021, 1982.

Smith B: A technique for extirpation and replacement of the lateral canthus. *Trans Am Acad Ophthalmol Otolaryngol* 738–742, 1953.

Smith B: Eyelid reconstruction. In Soll D: *Management of Complications in Ophthalmic Plastic Surgery.* Birmingham, AL, Aesculapius, 1976, p 221–243.

Teale TP: On relief of symblepharon by transplantation of the conjunctiva. *Ophthalmol Hosp Rev* 3: 253, 1860.

Tenzel RR, Stewart WB: Eyelid reconstruction by semicircular flap technique. *Trans Am Soc Ophthalmol Otolaryngol* 85: 1165–1169, 1978.

Wesley RE, McCord CD: Height of the lower tarsus of the lower eyelid. *Am J Ophthalmol* 90: 102–105, 1980.

Wesley RE, McCord CD: Transplantation of eyebank sclera in the Cutler-Beard method of upper eyelid reconstruction. *Ophthalmol* 87: 1028, 1980.

CHAPTER 67

Reconstruction of the Upper Eyelid: Moderate Defects

Kenneth V. Cahill, M.D.
John A. Burns, M.D.

Several surgical techniques for the correction of upper lid disorders are presented in this chapter. Although many of them are quite minor procedures, they are all techniques that will have frequent application for restoring normal lid appearance and function. All these techniques can be performed under local anesthesia in adults. Obviously a general anesthetic may be necessary for children. A skin preparation and draping of the surgical field is necessary for those procedures in which an incision is made.

HYFRECATION

Many small (less than 1 cm diameter) benign cutaneous lesions of the eyelids can be easily eliminated by hyfrecation. Epithelial papillomas, epithelial inclusion cysts, verrucous growths, molluscum contagiosum lesions, and seborrheic keratoses can be effectively treated. Infiltration with a local anesthetic is necessary for all but the smallest lesions. Pedunculated lesions are trimmed flush with the skin prior to hyfrecation. An electrocautery unit is adjusted to produce a moderate electrical arc. The lesion is then reduced to a dark eschar that is level with surrounding tissue. The eschar should be curetted off so the base of the lesion can be observed. If the base of the area treated still appears abnormal, the cycle of hyfrecation and curettage should be repeated. An antibiotic ointment is applied to this eschar for several days. Reepithelialization from remaining deep epithelial appendages and from the adjacent surface usually produces a satisfactory cosmetic result, especially in elderly patients where the skin is lax and hypertrophic scars are unlikely to occur. Skin depigmentation and erythema may be present initially, but these generally improve in several months. Damage to or loss of eyelash and brow cilia can result. This is unlikely unless the hyfrecation is very close to a hair follicle. No specimen for pathological evaluation is obtained when this technique is used, which could be considered a disadvantage.

MARGINAL SHAVE EXCISION

Elevated benign lesions of the eyelid margins that do not have deep extension and that do not involve the eyelash cilia can be shaved off flush to the level of the desired lid margin contour. This is most easily and accurately performed if an extremely sharp blade is used, such as a razor fragment or other microsurgical blade (Fig. 67.1). Adequate anesthesia must be attained so that the lid can be firmly fixated for the most accurate excision. The cut lid-margin surface is then lightly treated with electrocautery to help destroy any remaining abnormal

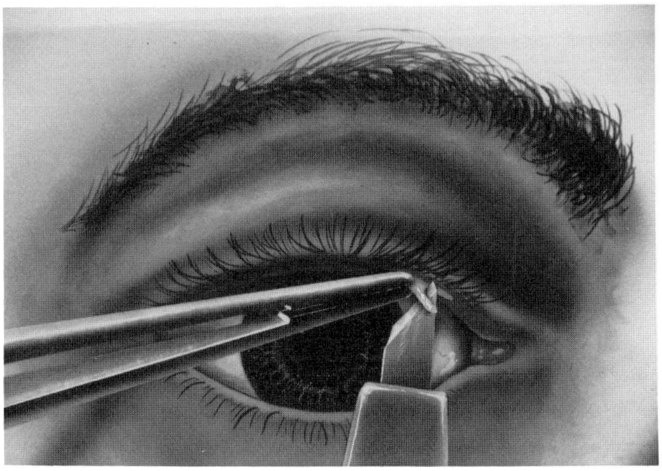

Figure 67.1. A marginal shave excision can be used to eliminate many benign lid-margin lesions.

tissue and to provide hemostasis. An antibiotic ointment should be applied to the excision site for several days. This reduces the potential for corneal abrasion by the eschar at the lid margin. Nevi, epithelial papillomas, epithelial inclusion cysts, verrucous lesions, and molluscum contagiosum lesions may be treated successfully in this way. If the lesion extends anteriorly to involve the follicles of eyelash cilia, its complete removal may result in loss of the cilia, trichiasis, and skin depigmentation. In such situations, the risk of eyelash cilia damage must be weighed against the alternative of performing a full-thickness pentagonal wedge eyelid resection to eliminate the lesion. Generally the benign lesions excised with a marginal shave excision do not recur; however, nevi frequently have some deep extension and residual pigmentation may remain. The lid margin contour following a marginal shave excision should be normal. Notches do not occur unless tissue is excised beyond the level of the desired lid margin or excessive electrocautery is applied.

BIOPSIES

Biopsies should be performed on eyelid lesions that show clinical characteristics of malignancy. If a lesion is very small, it may be completely removed as an excisionsal biopsy. However, this is not practical when the lesion is too large to excise easily with sufficient margins to ensure its total removal. Performing a biopsy has the advantage of confirming the histological diagnosis so that appropriate technique for excision, reconstruction, and further treatment can be planned by the surgeon, patient, pathologist, and other specialists.

The biopsy should be taken so that it samples the full thickness of a representative area of the lesion. If the lesion has a necrotic component, the biopsy should include both vital and necrotic tissue so that tumor cells are not missed. Usually the apparent junction between normal and abnormal tissue is the ideal site. If a lesion is widespread, or if the margins are indistinct, multiple biopsies may be indicated. The source of each biopsy specimen must be carefully recorded. Forceps and cautery should not be used on the biopsy specimen. This avoids tissue damage that could impair the pathological evaluation.

After a skin preparation and local infiltrative anesthesia, the actual tissue incision can be performed using a sharp, pointed surgical scalpel or biopsy punch. A Keyes skin punch[a] works well for this purpose. The skin should be stretched taut and the round cutting surface of the punch is placed at a margin of the lesion. Its handle is turned in alternating clockwise and counterclockwise rotations between the fingertips. Once it has penetrated full thickness epidermis and dermis, a decreased resistance is felt. The punch is withdrawn. The cylindrical-shaped biopsy specimen is then freed from underlying orbicularis muscle with a scalpel blade. A 2–3 mm block of tissue is generally sufficient for diagnosis. It is best to communicate with the pathologist to ensure that the tissue is placed in the proper solution and container and is processed promptly. Small tissue samples such as this do not need to be marked with sutures. It is helpful to document where the biopsy was taken with a sketch or a photograph. The biopsy site may require cautery for hemostasis. A pressure dressing is also helpful for controlling mild bleeding. Suture closure is not necessary. Several days of antibiotic ointment usage are advisable.

[a] American V. Mueller, 600 W. Touhy Avenue, Chicago, IL 60648

CUTANEOUS LESION EXCISION

Eyelid lesions should be surgically excised if they are malignant, too large for hyfrecation, or if hyfrecation alone would produce an undesirable scar. In malignant tumors a free margin of at least 3 mm should be taken to avoid recurrence. Intraoperative frozen-section pathological evaluation is recommended to ensure total removal of the malignancy.

When possible, it is desirable to excise eyelid skin lesions as a spindle shape with the long axis oriented along skin wrinkle lines. The edges of the ellipse should pass perpendicularly through full-thickness epidermis and dermis. If the lesion is malignant it should also include some of the orbicularis oculi muscle. Adjacent skin should be undermined and mobilized to facilitate closing the defect. Primary closure of the ellipse is sufficient unless unacceptable displacement of the margin of the involved eyelid occurs. If the lid margins are separated by less than 3 mm when the patient is asked to gently close the eyes at the conclusion of suturing, then significant lagophthalmos is unlikely to result. If additional skin tissue is needed, advancement and transposition flaps may be used, but generally a full-thickness free skin graft provides the best functional and cosmetic results. The graft may be taken from the opposite upper lid in middle-aged or older adults using a blepharoplasty technique. In younger patients, retroauricular skin provides an excellent match for the eyelids.

TRANSMARGINAL PENTAGONAL WEDGE RESECTION

Lesions involving the lid margin or the full thickness of the eyelid can be excised by performing a pentagonal wedge resection. This is commonly used to excise malignancies occurring on or near the lid margin. It can also be used to revise scars resulting from trauma, eliminate congenital colobomas, and remove benign lesions involving the eyelash cilia. In young patients approximately one-fourth of the upper lid width can be excised and closed primarily. In adults, up to one-third can often be removed with primary closure, without producing cosmetic or functional defects.

The incisions through the lid margins should be made perpendicular to the tangent of the lid margin and should be carried up to the superior edge of the tarsal plate. Heavy tissue scissors can be used to cut the entire lid thickness. Superior to the tarsus, tissue scissors can be used to incise the final two sides of the pentagon. These two incisions do not need to pass more than 2–3 mm above the superior edge of the tarsal plate. They may meet in an oblique angle without risk of producing a permanent skin pucker. The cut tarsal surfaces should be reunited with three 5-0 absorbable sutures (Fig. 67.2*A*). These should pass through approximately 75% of the thickness of the tarsal plate, avoiding the posterior 25% of the tarsus and the conjunctiva. Full-thickness sutures can produce corneal abrasions and other serious corneal complications. Each suture should be pulled up temporarily after it is placed to ensure that it produces proper alignment of the lid margin. Additional confirmation that the sutures have been correctly placed can be obtained by observing if each suture is perfectly parallel with its neighbor. It is best to preplace all three tarsal sutures before tying them permanently. This allows each of the sutures to be placed accurately.

Once the tarsal sutures are tied, 6-0 black silk suture is used to secure the lid margin. Sutures should be placed to align the gray line, posterior lid margin, and anterior lid margin. Again, it is best to draw each suture up temporarily to test the lid margin alignment. After all three sutures are placed, they should be tied permanently. They should be tied tight enough to provide a slight bulge of the lid margin. This prevents lid margin notching. The slight overcorrection of the lid margin closure will resolve spontaneously. The ends of the lid margin sutures should be left long. The pentagonal wedge resection has now been reduced to a vertical linear closure. The skin can be closed with interrupted 6-0 black silk sutures. The long ends of the lid margin sutures can be gathered and secured under additional throws of the skin suture closest to the lid margin (Fig. 67.2*B*). This prevents corneal irritation from the ends of the lid margin sutures. The use of an antibiotic ointment is recommended. The skin sutures can be removed in 5 or 6 days; the one that secures the ends of the lid margin sutures is left. The lid margin sutures should remain in place for 10–14 days.

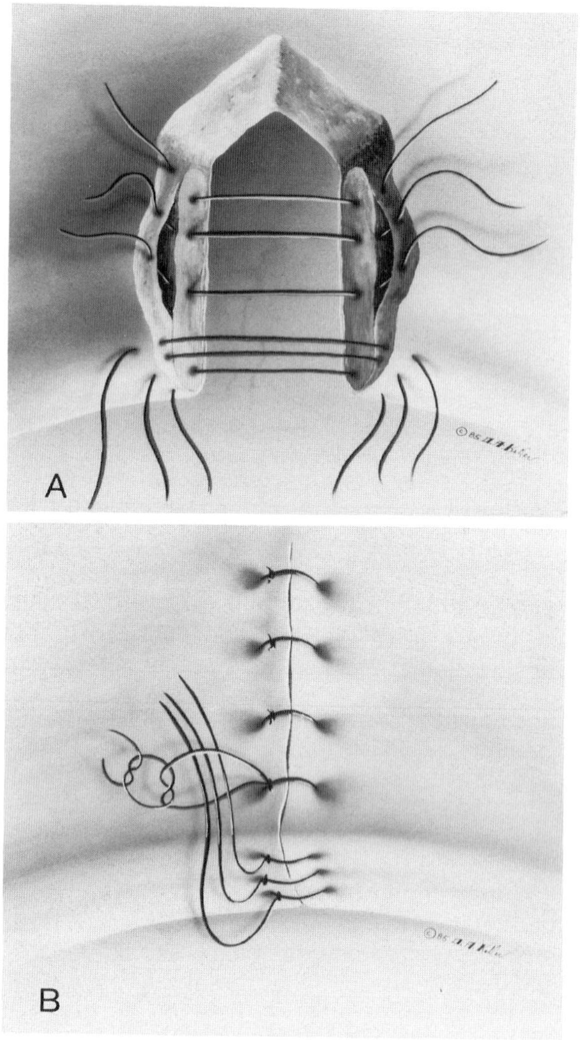

Figure 67.2. Transmarginal pentagonal wedge resection. *A*, The defect is first closed with partial-thickness absorbable tarsal sutures and silk lid-margin sutures. *B*, The ends of the lid-margin sutures should be secured in the knot of a skin suture to avoid corneal irritation.

LATERAL CANTHOLYSIS

If a pentagonal wedge excision cannot be closed without excessive tension, cantholysis of the lateral canthal tendon should be considered. A horizontal lateral canthotomy alone will only allow about 2–3 mm of additional lid advancement. However, by cutting the upper crus of the lateral canthal tendon, a total of 5–7 mm of lid advancement can be achieved. Cutting the upper crus is most easily performed by introducing tissue scissors into the superior aspect of the laterally canthotomy incision between skin and conjunctiva (Fig. 67.3*A*). The lateral segment of the upper lid is then placed on stretch. The tissue scissors are "strummed" back and forth to locate the stretched upper crus, as is done when one identifies the optic nerve with scissor tips when doing an enucleation.

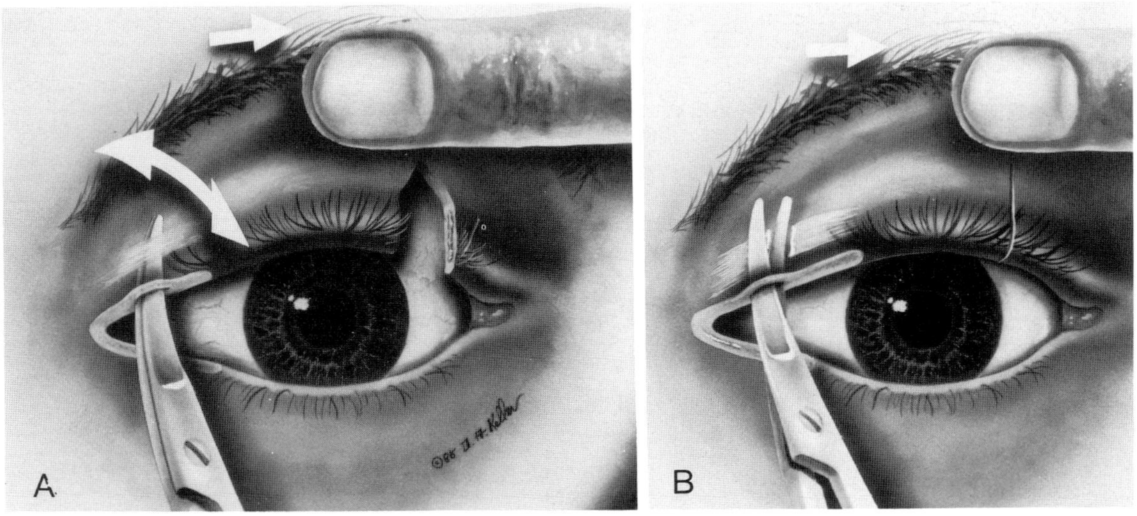

Figure 67.3. Lateral cantholysis. *A*, Following a lateral canthotomy, the upper crus of the lateral canthal tendon can be palpated with closed scissors tips when the lid is stretched. *B*, The upper crus can then be cut with scissors, providing laxity for medial mobilization.

The upper crus is then cut with the scissors. The increased mobilization of the upper lid should be apparent (Fig. 67.3*B*). No closure of the lateral cantholysis is necessary. If it is still not possible to close the cut edges of the pentagon wedge resection site, then more involved reconstruction as described in other chapters will be necessary.

CHALAZIA

An enlarged meibomian gland with an obstructed orifice, retained secretory products, and inflammation is called a *chalazion*. In an acute stage, there may be an element of bacterial infection and even the appearance of an eyelid cellulitis.

The initial management should include hot compresses for 15–20 minutes several times daily to encourage drainage of retained material through the gland's orifice. If the orifice is open, gentle eyelid massage with cotton-tip applicators or smooth glass rods may be attempted to express the retained material. If there is an appearance of eyelid cellulitis, a course of oral antibiotic, such as erythromycin or tetracycline, should be considered. Topical antibiotics or antibiotic-corticosteroid combinations are indicated when an underlying blepharitis is present. But this is probably more beneficial for preventing future chalazia than for treating the one that is present. Small volumes (0.1–0.2 ml) of a parenteral steroid (triamcinolone 10 mg/ml) may be injected directly into a chalazion cyst using a 25- or 27-gauge needle. This appears to facilitate the resolution of the lesion in some cases. Many chalazia will resolve without significant residua after 1 or 2 months when the above management is followed. However, there will be a few that leave persistent nodules that induce astigmatism or produce a cosmetic blemish. Excision can then be used to remove the remaining cyst.

Since a chalazion originates in the tarsal plate, nearly all chalazia can be excised from a posterior approach. A regional anesthetic block (lacrimal, frontal, supratrochlear) or local subcutaneous infiltration can be utilized. Occasionally it will be necessary to evert the upper tarsal plate and inject a small volume of anesthetic subconjunctivally superior to the tarsus. Excessive local infiltration should be avoided since this distorts the tissues and may make the excision more difficult. An appropriate size chalazion clamp is used to stabilize and evert the upper lid. A vertical incision is made into the cyst from the conjunctival side using a blade (e.g., Bard Parker No. 15). This incision should not be extended closer than 2 mm to the lid margin or a marginal deformity may result. The contents of the cyst can be removed using a curette. The walls of the cyst should be gently dissected out using 0.5-mm toothed forceps and scissors. The chalazion clamp should be slowly loosened. Any prominent sources of bleeding should be cauterized. When the clamp is removed, the lid should be palpated between two fingers to ensure that the entire cyst has been removed. Distortion from the local anesthetic and from the clamp sometimes makes this difficult to determine. Rarely it will be noted that the skin has been perforated by the dissection of the capsule. Usually this will not require any sutures and fistulization will not occur.

Occasionally the cyst assumes an anterior position and is not readily accessible from a posterior approach. In these cases a similar anesthetic is used, but the chalazion clamp is placed to allow a horizontal incision to be made through the upper lid skin. This incision can be placed directly over the lesion, but should be at least 2 mm superior to the eyelash cilia to avoid eyelash damage. The cyst can then be dissected out. Several interrupted skin sutures may be necessary to ensure optimal skin healing.

TRICHIASIS

Trichiasis is a condition in which eyelash cilia are misdirected. This is a common problem in elderly patients that may result from eyelid infection, inflammation, and trauma. Lashes that abrade the cornea cause discomfort and can lead to more serious complications such as corneal vascularization and corneal ulceration. A few fine cilia are frequently present near the caruncle. These are usually not responsible for discomfort. But even the finest lashes can cause discomfort if they come into contact with the cornea.

Pulling aberrant lashes with a forceps will provide relief for 2–6 weeks until the lashes regrow. Occasionally the lashes will grow back in a more normal conformation after they have been pulled. Usually they grow back in an abnormal position and again cause ocular irritation. Some patients will be able to pull the lashes with forceps and not desire definitive treatment. For patients who need permanent treatment, either electrolysis or cryotherapy can be utilized.

For electrolysis of lashes, we have found the Birtcher Hyfrecator unit set on the low power range to be effective. A special epilation tip is available, which is thin enough to be introduced along the aberrant lash approximately 2 mm into the lash follicle. This should be done with slitlamp visualization or loupe magnification. The rheostat dial of the hyfrecator unit should be adjusted so that small bubbles will emanate from the follicle after approximately 2 or 3 seconds of treatment. Following this, the lash should slide out of the lid margin without resistance. This careful use of electrolysis should permanently eliminate lashes 80% of the time and not induce further cicatrization or trichiasis. Local infiltration with Xylocaine is necessary. The argon laser can be used to ablate lash follicles by directing the beam along the axis of the cilia. However, this takes longer than hyfrecation, is just as uncomfortable for the patient, and alignment of the laser beam with the lash cilia is not always easy to achieve.

When more than a few lashes are aberrant, cryotherapy should be utilized. Local infiltration with 50:50 Xylocaine/Marcaine provides patient comfort for the procedure and for several hours afterward. A topical anesthetic is instilled and a protective plastic scleral shell is placed over the globe. A nitrous-oxide cryotherapy unit fitted with a 1.5-mm retinal tip works well. The freezing tip should be positioned on the conjunctival surface of the lid immediately below the lid margin where abnormal lashes are present (Fig. 67.4). If a thermocouple is available, its needle-point probe should be positioned amongst the lash cilia follicles to be treated. A freeze, thaw, and freeze cycle achieving −25°C on the thermocouple for 45 seconds during each freeze is usually sufficient. If no thermocouple is available, the end point for the freeze cycle can be 60 seconds of freezing after the iceball reaches the anterior lid surface. The temperature of the retinal tip should register −60°C or lower during each 60-second freeze cycle.

The protective scleral shell is removed and an antibiotic ophthalmic ointment is instilled. Analgesics, such as Tylenol No. 3, and a bedtime sedative are usually indicated for the first few days after treatment. The lid margin area forms bullae followed by a scab. The patient continues to use antibiotic ointment several times daily until this scab is shed. One week after treatment the lashes should pull out with no resistance. Resistance to epilation at this time suggests that inadequate cryotherapy was administered. Some skin depigmentation may result from properly performed eyelid cryotherapy. This must be considered before recommending cryotherapy in darkly pigmented patients.

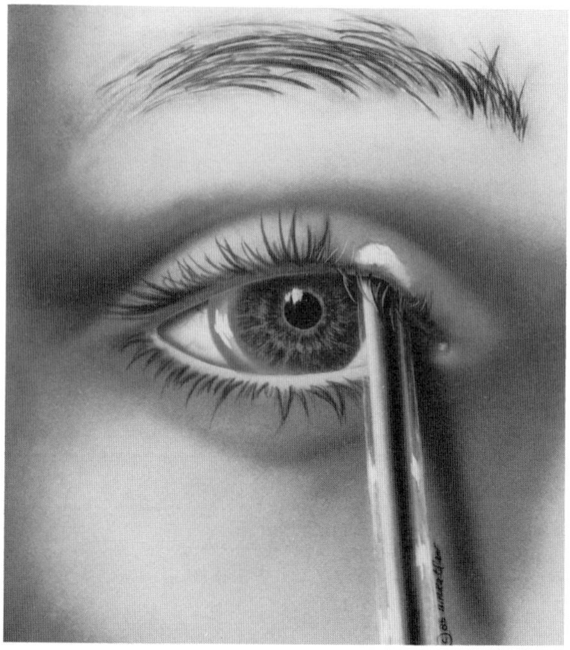

Figure 67.4. Cryoablation of trichiasis. A retinal cryoprobe has been positioned on the tarsal conjunctiva adjacent to the posterior lid margin. Freezing is in progress. A protective plastic scleral shell should be used to protect the globe from the cryoprobe.

When trichiasis is present along with cicatricial entropion, elimination of lashes alone is not sufficient. The lid margin can be split along the gray line forming anterior and posterior lamellae. Cryotherapy of the anterior lamella is performed to destroy the aberrant lash follicles. The anterior lamella is then recessed away from the margin of the posterior lamella. The raw surface resulting from this recession can be covered with a mucous membrane graft. This will eliminate irritation to the globe by keratinized epithelium. However, the mucous membrane often retains a red appearance that will not provide an optimal cosmetic result.

When trichiasis combined with cicatricial entropion is being evaluated, it is important to recognize ocular pemphigoid, because this may be exacerbated by treatment. In such cases it is best to use the least treatment possible to maintain acceptable lid-globe relationships.

DERMABRASION

Skin that has healed with an irregular surface contour and texture may produce an undesirable scar. This is most likely to occur in children and young adults. The thick skin covering the forehead, brow, and cheek, rather than thin eyelid skin, is generally involved. Irregular traumatic lacerations are frequent causes of residual elevated scars.

A raised scar is unlikely to undergo additional spontaneous regression after it has been present for 1 year. At this point, dermabrasion may be considered. Handheld files and sandpaper are ineffective. Instead, a Hall drill with a fine diamond-grit 5–10 mm diameter spherical bit is used. Local infiltrative anesthesia is usually sufficient for adults. The addition of 1:200,000 epinephrine improves hemostasis. General anesthesia is necessary for children. The scar should be abraded down to underlying dermis to a depth even with or just below the level of adjacent normal epidermis. The sculpting effect is provided by the rotational speed of the abrasive diamond bit. Downward pressure of the bit into the skin should not be applied since this increases the chance of skin being pulled and wrapping around the drill bit. This is especially important for thin skin near the eyelids. Dermabrasion of the lids themselves is not advisable. For additional safety, the skin being abraded should be stretched out by an assistant. Irrigation with normal saline prevents heat from building up and keeps the operative field free from blood.

Postoperatively an antibiotic ointment is used for several days. If necessary, Telfa gauze covered with a pressure dressing may be left in place for the first 24 hours after surgery to ensure hemostasis. The abraded areas are re-epithelialized by deep epidermal appendages in the dermis and by surrounding epidermis. A period of at least 3–6 months will pass before the maximum cosmetic improvement is achieved.

CHAPTER 68

Reconstruction of the Lower Eyelid: Moderate Defects

BERNICE Z. BROWN, M.D.

REPAIR OF SMALL-SIZE DEFECTS OF THE LOWER EYELID

In the description that follows we are assuming that these reconstructions are of defects of clean, straight sides and full thickness of the lid. If they are not, then adaptations of the procedure will have to be made.

Small defects can usually be closed by layered primary closure, and if carefully done no deformity will be apparent. In fact, after the lid is healed the site of the surgery can be undetectable.

The two cut edges are brought together, each held by a forceps, to test the tension that will be produced by this type of closure. If a deformity is not induced by this test, one can continue with the procedure as follows.

In a young person, a 5–6 mm defect can be treated in this manner. In an older person with more laxity in the lids, a centimeter or more defect is amenable to this type of closure.

The lateral lid segment is sutured to the medial lid segment with three 6-0 black silk sutures (on a 780 needle) on the lid margin. These lid margin sutures should be carefully placed. The first one should be placed in the middle of the margin, and bites of equal width and depth on each side of the defect should be taken. The needle should enter the lid margin 1.5 mm from the cut edge, exiting from the vertical cut edge of the tarsus about 2 mm from the top of the lid. The needle should then enter the tarsus on the other side of the defect at 2 mm from the top edge of the lid and exit from the lid margin about 1.5 mm from the cut edge.

Two more sutures should be placed on the lid margin. One is placed at the posterior edge of the lid margin and the other at the anterior edge, next to the cilia. These sutures should be placed, taking bites with the needle similar to that described for the first placed suture. These three sutures should be left untied temporarily, to make access to the vertical edge of the tarsus easier. Interrupted 5-0 chromic catgut, "S" polyglycolic acid (Dexon) or polyglactin 910 (Vicryl) suture can be used for this part of the closure.

In the lower lid, the vertical height of the tarsus allows only one or two of these interrupted sutures to be placed. These are placed to pull the edges of the tarsus together. Then the margin sutures are pulled up and tied, leaving the tails of the black silk sutures 1 cm long. If necessary, additional interrupted sutures can be placed in the conjunctiva below the tarsus, but in most cases it is not necessary. The subcutaneous tissues are closed with the same interrupted suture material as was used to close the tarsus.

If the skin is bunched up below the defect, it is excised as a triangle with the base up. The skin is now closed with running, locking, or interrupted 6-0 black silk or 6-0 nylon. One should be careful if using a running suture, not to pull it up too tight and imbricate the tissues vertically. This can cause lid retraction. Before tying the skin suture closest to the margin, place the long tails of the margin sutures down under it to be held down against the skin. This keeps the margin sutures from flipping into the eye.

It is wise to keep this healing incision on traction vertically for a few days to prevent retraction. This can be done with a 4-0 black silk suture placed as a Frost suture and taped to the forehead.

REPAIR OF MODERATE-SIZE DEFECTS OF THE LOWER EYELID

Defects of the lower lid measuring 10–20 mm can be repaired by several methods. It is important for all surgeons doing eyelid surgery to have a repertoire of procedures for lower lid defects. Lesions of the lower lid are far more prevalent than those seen in other eyelid areas. Most of these lesions are of moderate size.

There are several methods of repair I have found useful. The following gives the best results in the author's hands.

TENZEL-STEWART PROCEDURE (MINI-MUSTARDÊ)

The Tenzel-Stewart procedure is a modification of the Mustardé procedure (1, 2). This modified lateral advancement is most successful when a few millimeters of tarsus remain on each side of the defect. It is useful in many moderate-size lower lid defect repairs, and is illustrated in Figures 68.1–68.10.

A skin and muscle flap is outlined lateral to the canthus (Figs. 68.1, 68.2). The diameter of the curve is about 10–20 mm but should remain within the orbital rim or only a few millimeters beyond it. A horizontal lateral canthotomy is done beneath the flap (Fig. 68.3). The inferior limb of the lateral canthal tendon and its lateral and inferior attachments are separated from the orbital rim (Fig. 68.4).

The skin is undermined temporally and inferiorly sufficiently to allow the remaining lateral segment of the lid to be advanced medially for closure of the defect (Fig. 68.5). Undermining the cutting of the fibrous attachments is continued until the segment of lateral lid can be moved medially without much resistance. A "V" of skin and muscle below the defect is excised (Fig. 68.6).

The lateral lid segment is sutured to the medial lid segment with three 6-0 black silk sutures on the lid margin (Fig. 68.7). The vertical segments of tarsus are closed with interrupted 6-0 chromic catgut, "S" polyglycolic acid (Dexon), or polyglactin 910 (Vicryl) sutures. The subcutaneous tissues are closed with interrupted 5-0 or 6-0 plain or chromic catgut sutures. The skin is closed with 6-0 black silk or nylon. The author prefers running locking 6-0 silk. Locking it makes it easier to remove.

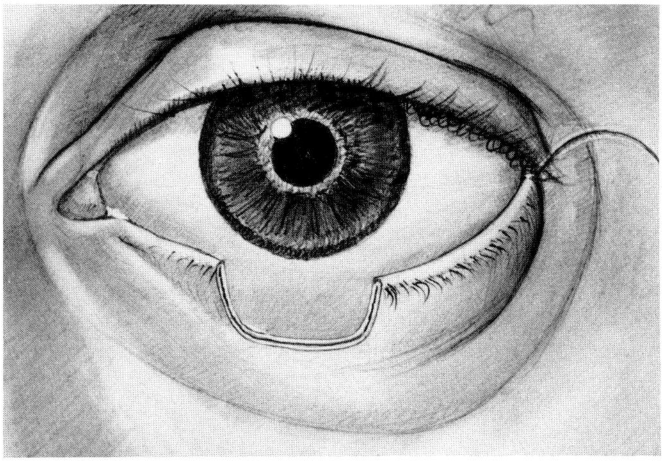

Figure 68.1. A curved skin and muscle flap is outlined lateral to canthus, extending just onto the rim of the orbit.

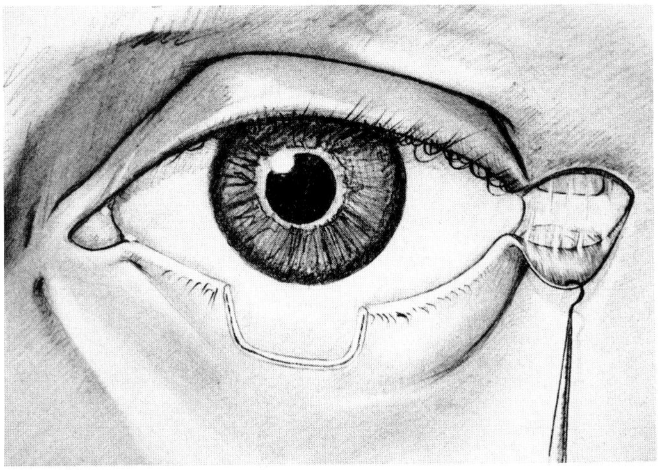

Figure 68.2. Lateral canthal tendon is exposed.

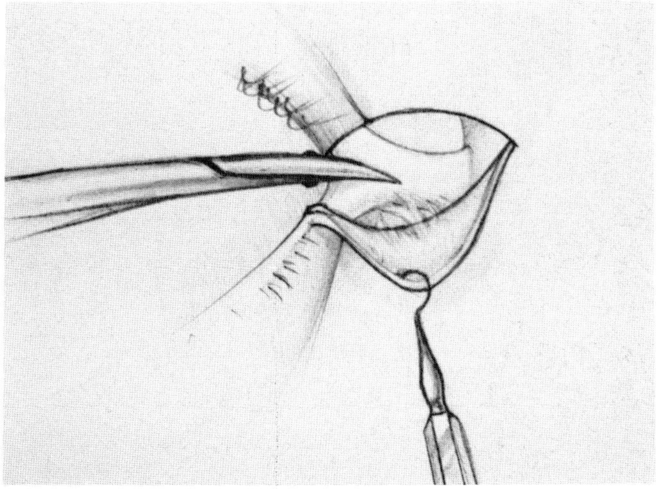

Figure 68.3. Lateral canthal tendon is divided horizontally.

If the vertical height of the lesion spares 2 mm of the inferior part of the tarsus (it seldom does), this segment can be advanced superiorly to reconstruct the margin at the lateral angle. If not, a graft of conjunctiva and tarsus can be obtained from the middle or top of the superior tarsus (Fig. 68.8). No closure of the donor site is necessary.

The lateral canthus should be reformed with care (Fig. 68.9). The tarsal segment and conjunctiva are used to back the skin muscle flap in this region. Medially a Dexon or Vicryl suture is used to join the tarsal graft to what remains of the lower limb of the lateral canthal tendon and tarsus that has been moved medially. A 5-0 Dacron suture is used to fix the tarsal segment graft to the upper limb of the lateral canthal tendon. Size 6-0 plain catgut is used to join the skin to the transposed tarsal segment along the lid margin. An additional 5-0 Dacron should be placed between the upper and lower lid margins at the extreme

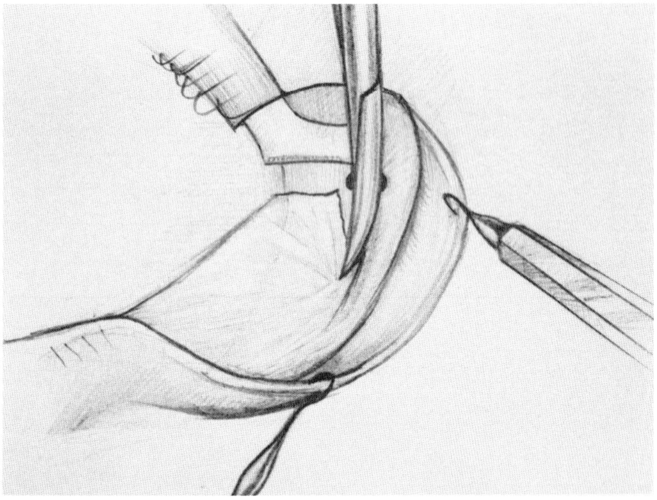

Figure 68.4. Lower limb is detached from the rim of the orbit and the lower lid is freed from all lateral rim attachment.

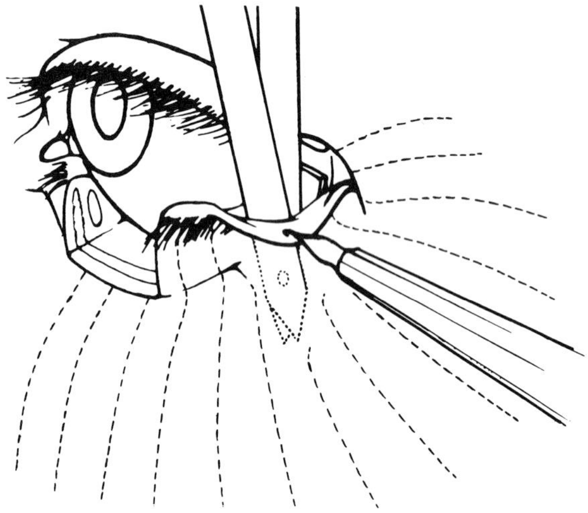

Figure 68.5. Surrounding skin-muscle layer is mobilized to allow the lateral lid segment to be moved medially.

corner to reform the lateral canthus and give it a sharp angulation.

The remainder of the skin closure can be done with a running, locked 6-0 black silk suture (Fig. 68.10). The lid margin should fit the eye snugly but without tension. The skin sutures may be removed in 4 or 5 days. The lid margin and canthal angle sutures should remain in place for 10 days.

There are a number of other useful procedures to repair moderate-size lid defects. Each surgeon, after trying several different methods, will develop a favorite. Other techniques are described next.

REVERSE CUTLER-BEARD PROCEDURE

The reverse Cutler-Beard procedure (3) has the advantage of obscuring the visual axis for a period of 6–8 weeks. There are times when this inconvenience is of secondary importance to a good functional and cosmetic result that could not be obtained by other methods. Extensive shallow central lid involvement in a young individual might present such a situation. This procedure is a full-thickness flap from the opposing lid and spares the lid margin, which remains in place as a bridge.

Technique

A full-thickness, horizontal incision is made in the upper lid, 5 mm above the lash line. Vertical parallel incisions are made upward from its two ends. The flap thus formed includes 4 or 5 mm of the upper tarsus. The horizontal measurement should be less than the width of the lesion. The donor tissue should be only wide enough to fill the defect when the edges are brought toward each other by forceps traction with moderate tension.

The tongue of tissue from the upper lid is passed under the marginal bridge of the upper lid and sutured into the lower lid defect. The tarsal edges are sutured securely with

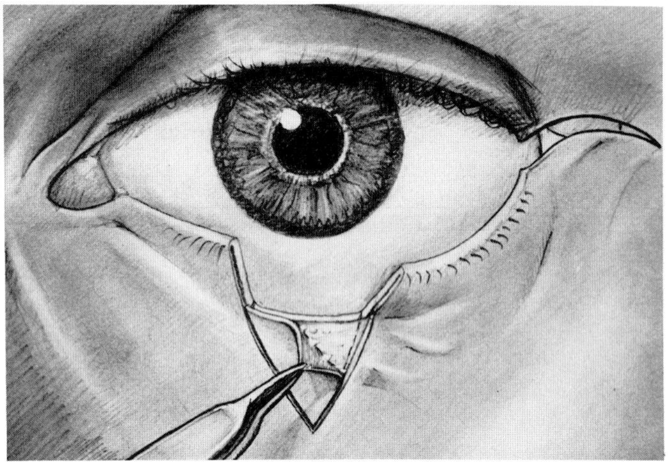

Figure 68.6. Triangle of skin below the area of the excised lesion is removed to avoid bulkiness.

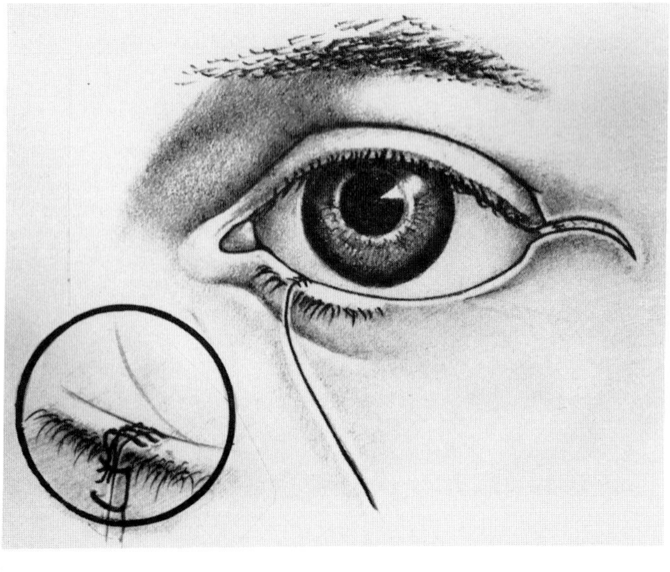

Figure 68.7. Lateral lid segment is sutured to the medial lid segment; careful attention is given to alignment of the margin edges and layered closure.

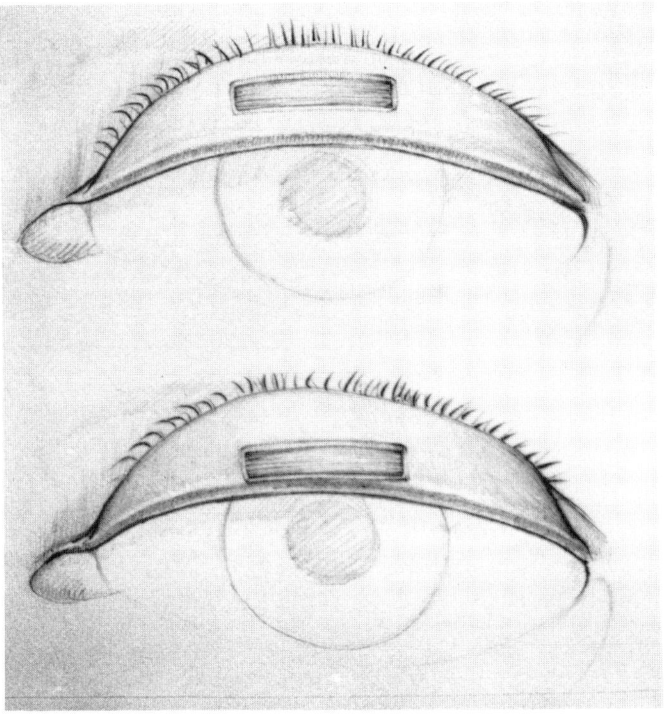

Figure 68.8. Free tarsal graft is removed from ipsilateral or contralateral upper lid; the donor site is not sutured.

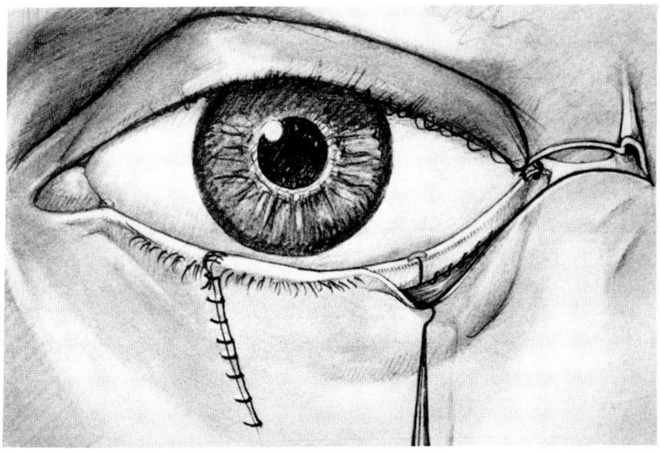

Figure 68.9. This tarsal graft is sutured to the lateral aspect of the tarsus in the lateral lid segment. It is also joined to the upper limb of the lateral canthal tendon and lateral orbital tubercle; this should fit snugly.

6-0 Dexon, Vicryl, or chromic catgut.

Subcutaneous tissue may be joined with interrupted 5-0 or 6-0 chromic catgut. Skin edges close well with running, locking, or interrupted 6-0 black silk sutures. It is not necessary to suture the margins of the upper lid bridge, although some prefer to join the conjunctiva loosely to the skin.

The lid fissure can be opened after 6–8 weeks. The flap is cut rather high as some retraction of the new lid margin will occur. The conjunctival edge should be slightly higher than the skin edge. It will contract more than will the skin.

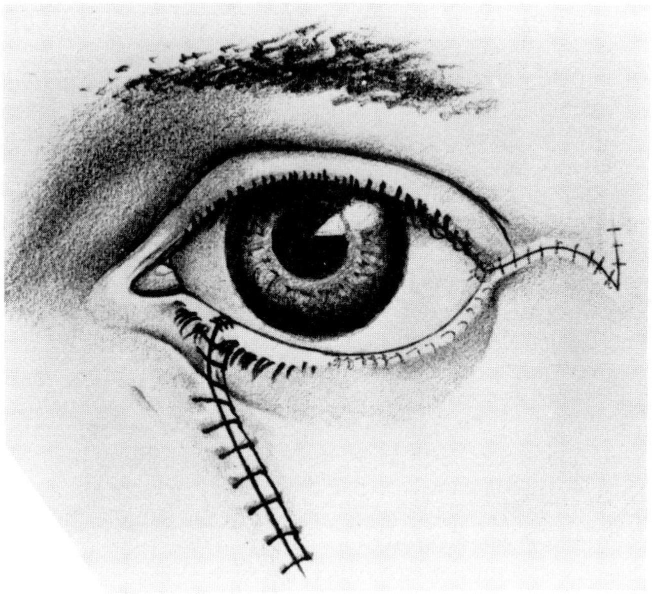

Figure 68.10. Skin muscle flap, which has been moved medially from the simicircular flap, is sutured to the tarsal graft with 6-0 plain gut and the lateral skin edges are closed appropriately with Burrow's triangles, as needed to avoid redundant skin. The tarsal graft helps to support the lateral skin segment.

The new lid margin conjunctiva is sutured to the skin with 6-0 plain catgut, placed in running fashion. The upper border of the bridge is freshened. The remnant of the flap is sutured to it in two layers. The conjunctiva is closed with 6-0 plain catgut and the skin with 6-0 black silk.

HUGHES PROCEDURE (MODIFIED)

The modified Hughes operation (4, 5) consists mainly of a tarsoconjunctival graft that is brought from the upper to the lower lid. It is combined with a sliding, rotating, or transposition flap or a free skin graft to supply the anterior lid layer, depending on the specific needs of the case. This procedure also has the disadvantage of obscuring the vision for 6–8 weeks.

Technique

The upper lid is everted and the tarsoconjunctival flap is fashioned starting 5 or 6 mm from the lid margin. The horizontal measurement of this flap should be wide enough to fill the defect when its edges are brought toward each other with moderate tension.

Müller's muscle is divided from its tarsal attachment. The palpebral conjunctiva is undermined from Müller's muscle to the height of the fornix.

The advancement flap of the tarsus and conjunctiva is sutured into the defect in the lower lid with 6-0 Dexon, Vicryl, or 5-0 chromic catgut sutures at the four corners. Additional sutures can be used to close the sides and inferior edges of the posterior defect.

If the skin is lax enough below the defect, vertical parallel incisions can be made downward from the corners of the lid defect. Undermining the skin and the removal of Burrow's triangles may be sufficient to allow advancement superiorly of the skin to fill the anterior layer of the defect.

Four other options of advancing the skin are available: (*a*) The skin can sometimes be advanced horizontally from one or both sides. (*b*) A free skin graft can be sutured over the tarsoconjunctival flap. The latter, when properly prepared, should provide adequate circulation for the graft to survive. (*c*) A transposition skin flap from the upper lid can be used to furnish an anterior layer. (*d*) A horizontal incision can be made over the orbital rim, and the skin muscle layer above it can be advanced superiorly. The skin defect that develops over the orbital rim can be covered with a full-thickness supraclavicular graft.

After healing, and perhaps a period of massage to reduce fibrosis, the lid fissure can be opened. The delay is usually about 6–8 weeks. The separation is done similarly to that done for the upside-down Cutler-Beard procedure. The incision should bow upward slightly at the center, and the conjunctival edge should be slightly higher than the skin edge. The conjunctiva is sutured to the skin at the lid margin with 6-0 plain catgut sutures. The cut conjunctiva of the upper lid will retract into position and will need no sutures.

HEWES-SULLIVAN-BEARD TARSAL TRANSPOSITION

The Hewes-Sullivan-Beard tarsal transposition (6, 7) was devised to overcome the disadvantage and inconvenience of having to obscure the vision in the operated eye. The operation is done in one stage. It is most useful if the defect is temporal, but a nontemporal defect can be extended to the lateral canthus, making it possible to reconstruct even a total lower lid by this operation (Fig. 68.11).

Technique

A defect extending to the lateral canthus is formed by tumor removal or by freshening traumatic or congenital defect edges.

A transposition flap of tarsoconjunctiva, which is hinged at the lateral tendon, is fashioned. The upper half of the tarsus is used for the flap. It is prepared by making two parallel horizontal incisions: one at midtarsal level, and one at the upper tarsal border. The nasal ends of the incision are joined by a vertical cut. The flap is elevated. The flap should be 2 or 3 mm shorter than the lower lid defect in order that it will hug the globe when sutured in place.

The flap is rotated 180° around its long axis to maintain alignment of the conjunctival surfaces. It is not necessary to close the donor defect in the upper lid. The flap is then sutured into position to replace the posterior layer of the lower lid defect. Plain catgut (6-0) is used, except for the corner sutures where 6-0 Dexon or Vicryl are preferred.

A skin flap, advanced superiorly, can be used to reconstruct the anterior lamella of the lower lid, using 6-0 plain catgut to suture the skin to the lid margin and 6-0 black silk elsewhere. Skin can also be obtained as in the Hughes operation variations.

It is not likely that a free skin graft would take over a long tarsoconjunctival flap, such as this one, but transposition skin flaps have been successfully used (back to back).

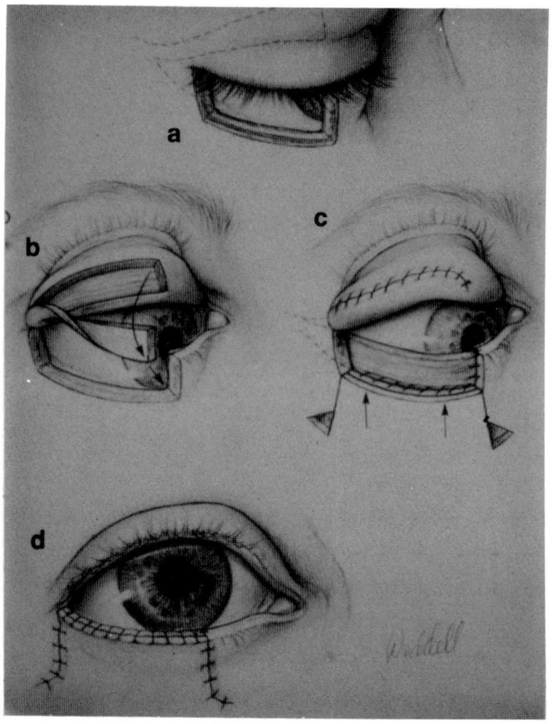

Figure 68.11. *A, B,* Transposition flap of tarsus and conjunctiva is prepared from the ipsilateral upper lid, leaving it hinged at the lateral tendon. It is not necessary to suture the donor defect. The flap should fit snugly when sutured in place. An advancement skin graft can be used to create the anterior lamella. (From Hewes EH, Sullivan JH, Beard C: Lower eyelid reconstruction by tarsal transposition. *Am J Ophthalmol* 81: 512–514, 1976.)

FULL-THICKNESS COMPOSITE GRAFT

The full-thickness composite graft of Gorney and associates (8) is somewhat similar to the Hewes-Sullivan-Beard transposition flap procedure. The skin is carried from the upper to the lower lid as a transposition skin-muscle flap; but it carries at its tip such tarsoconjunctiva as is needed to form the posterior layer of the lid. The flap is therefore full-thickness at its distal portion.

Technique

The size of the graft is outlined with its full-thickness portion slightly smaller than the defect in order that the new lower lid will not be loose or sag.

The nasal part of the flap is full thickness. The lateral part of the flap is skin and muscle only and is hinged laterally. The flap is elevated and transposed to the lower lid. The tarsoconjunctiva is sutured into the posterior layer of the defect with 6-0 Dexon or Vicryl at the corners and 6-0 plain catgut on the inferior border. The upper border of the transposed tarsus is sutured to its overlying skin edge with 6-0 plain catgut.

The skin is closed with 6-0 black silk sutures. The tarsal donor area need not be closed.

FULL-THICKNESS ADVANCEMENT FLAP

Occasionally, only the lid margin is involved by tumor, or a shallow traumatic defect exists. If the inferior border of the tarsus can be safely spared, a full-thickness superior advancement of the remaining lower lid can be used to fill the defect.

Technique

Parallel full-thickness vertical incisions are made inferior to the defect. Next, the two lamellae are undermined separately. The posterior lamella should consist of tarsus and conjunctiva only, the lower lid retractors being separated from the lower edge of the tarsus. The skin muscle layer is undermined to the level of the orbital rim, or below it.

The tarsoconjunctival flap is advanced superiorly and attached to the medial and lateral tarsal remnants with 6-0 Dexon or Vicryl at the corners. The lateral conjunctival closures are done with 6-0 plain or chromic catgut.

The skin and orbicularis muscle flap can now be advanced and sutured in place with 6-0 black silk.

An additional useful procedure is described by Stephenson (9). It reconstructs the lid defect by using an advancement flap of skin and muscle called a "myocutaneous island." The significant difference is the fact that the muscle portion of the advanced flap is left attached to its source so that a vascular supply is still intact and can thus aid healing.

These are all useful procedures and each one can be used successfully. The quality of the repair is enhanced by repeated use of the same or similar procedures and variations thereof, thus improving the skill of the surgeon.

REFERENCES

1. Tenzel RR, Stewart WB: Eyelid reconstruction by the semicircular flap technique. *Ophthalmology* 85: 1164–1169, 1978.
2. Tenzel RR: Reconstruction of the central one half of an eyelid. *Arch Ophthalmol* 93: 125–126, 1975.
3. Hecht SD: An upside-down Cutler-Beard bridge flap. *Arch Ophthalmol* 84: 760–764, 1970.
4. Hughes WL: *Reconstructive Surgery of the Eyelids.* St. Louis, CV Mosby Co, 1943, p 84.
5. Callahan M, Callahan A: *Ophthalmic Plastic and Orbital Surgery.* Birmingham, AL, Aesculapius, 1979, p 188–191
6. Hewes EH, Sullivan JH, Beard C: Lower eyelid reconstruction by tarsal transposition. *Am J Ophthalmol* 81: 512–514, 1976.
7. Leone CR, Gernert JV: Lower eyelid reconstruction with upper eyelid transpositional grafts. *Ophthal Surg* 11: 315–318, 1980.
8. Gorney M, Falas E, Jones H, Manis JR: One-stage reconstruction of substantial lower eyelid margin defects. *Plast Reconstr Surg* 44: 592–596, 1969.
9. Stephenson C: Reconstruction of eyelid using a myocutaneous island flap. *Ophthalmology* 90: 1060–1065, 1983.

CHAPTER 69

Reconstruction of the Lower Eyelid: Major Defects

ROBERT M. DRYDEN, M.D.
ALLAN E. WULC, M.D.

The approach to reconstruction of major lower lid defects is described in this chapter. The full spectrum of procedures will not be examined extensively. Instead, a systemic and effective approach to reconstruction of the lower lid based on simple surgical principles will be described. These principles have been used successfully in a large ophthalmic plastic practice for more than 14 years. Surgical decisions in lower eyelid reconstruction for the majority of cases can be based on the techniques herein described.

Reconstruction of major lower lid defects demands a familiarity with a variety of procedures. While knowledge of many surgical techniques is essential, experience is invaluable. It is highly disconcerting to choose a reconstructive technique, make initial incisions, and mobilize tissues only to find that the flaps are inadequate for effective wound closure. Similarly, it is disadvantageous to perform unnecessary surgery to reconstruct a defect that can be closed with a simpler technique.

Larger lower lid defects are most commonly created after the excision of an eyelid tumor. When excision is based on frozen-tissue technique, complete irradication of tumor is ensured. A significant defect is often created unexpectedly when a tumor involves more of the eyelid than is initially clinically apparent. Eyelid avulsion from trauma, extensive scarring from alkali burn, or inflammatory disease also may cause large lower lid defects. Rarely, congenital coloboma of the lower lid may require reconstruction.

Anatomically, the lower eyelid may be considered as having anterior and posterior lamallae. The anterior lamella consists of skin and orbicularis. The orbicularis muscle is directly involved in the dynamics of lid closure and the pumping of tears. The posterior lamella consists of conjunctiva, tarsus, and the lower eyelid retractors. The posterior lamella provides support and stability for the lower lid and a mucosal surface vital to tear dynamics and corneal integrity.

The eyelid must be reconstructed respecting its bilamellar configuration. Lost mucosa must be replaced by mucosa. Lost skin should be replaced with skin. The loss of tarsus and/or retractors require lid support with an equally firm replacement such as tarsus, nasoseptal cartilage, or donor sclera.

The anterior and posterior limbs of the medial palpebral tendon anchor the lower lid medially with posterior as well as nasal traction. If the nasal lid and medial palpebral tendon must be sacrificed at surgery, the tendinous attachments must be recreated with the use of fine nonabsorbable suture to firmly reattach the tarsus to the stump of the remaining medial palpebral tendon. If the stump contains tumor, the periosteum in the area of the posterior lacrimal crest should be used as a point of fixation, or natural granulation should be allowed to recreate posterior eyelid traction (1).

The lateral palpebral tendon anchors the lid laterally. Cantholysis of the lower limb of the lateral palpebral tendon mobilizes the lower lid. Lateral canthal position is minimally affected by canthotomy and cantholysis. However, after canthotomy and cantholysis, the lateral canthal angle should be re-established with 6-0 silk sutures and the canthus should be re-created when possible using a nonabsorbable suture attached to the periosteum of the lateral orbital rim to create horizontal tension on all lower lid structures.

The excision of medial lower lid defects may involve

the canaliculus. If the canaliculus can be salvaged, canalicular intubation with silicone tubes should be performed prior to closure of the lid defect to create a new punctum. If the canaliculus contains tumor, free margins must be obtained prior to planning the repair. If the entire lower canaliculus is sacrificed, the lower eyelid should be reconstructed without lower canalicular repair in the hope that the upper canaliculus will provide adequate tear drainage. A Jones tube should not be placed at the time of surgery. Tumor may migrate into the nose subsequent to Jones tube placement. Therefore, significant time should elapse to rule out tumor recurrence prior to violating the natural bone barrier of the orbit.

Large defects greater than one-half the eyelid are classified and repaired as "marginal", i.e., involving the eyelid margin, or as "extramarginal" defects.

DEFECTS INVOLVING THE LID MARGIN

DIRECT CLOSURE

In elderly individuals with redundant and loose tissue, it is often possible to close major defects primarily. If the two edges of the defect can be approximated using toothed forceps, even if under tension, the wound may be closed primarily with the pentagonal closure technique described in the preceding chapter. Wound edges should be carefully prepared. The closure should be layered with excellent approximation of all corresponding parts (Figs. 69.1 and 69.2). A major eyelid defect repaired by this simple technique initially may appear overly taut. Often the lid is elevated and the vertical fissure is diminished in size. However, horizontal traction forces in the eyelid appear to cause stretching and, within several months, the fissure widens and a satisfactory cosmetic and functional result is achieved (Fig. 69.3).

DIRECT CLOSURE WITH CANTHOTOMY AND CANTHOLYSIS

If the defect is almost reapproximated by the technique of apposition under tension, release of the lateral attachments of the lower limb of the lateral palpebral tendon may mobilize enough tissue to allow direct closure. A lateral canthotomy alone may be sufficient, but more frequently, cantholysis is also required.

A canthotomy is performed initially to see if mobilization is sufficient prior to proceeding to cantholysis. Local anesthesia with epinephrine is infiltrated subcutaneously from the lateral canthal angle to the lateral orbital rim. Sharp straight scissors are placed horizontally at the lateral canthal angle, with one blade on the skin and one blade on the conjunctiva. A full-thickness horizontal cut, measuring approximately 8 mm, is made (Fig. 69.4). If more mobilization is needed, a cantholysis of the inferior limb of the lateral palpebral tendon is then performed. The tendon is identified with palpation. The sharp scissors are passed beneath the orbicularis, with one blade just inside the conjunctival surface. The tendon is "strummed" with the anterior blade. With the scissors directed inferolaterally, the tendon is cut (Fig. 69.5). An immediate increase in lateral lower lid mobility is observed and should allow closure of the eyelid defect. The lower eyelid is closed with the standard technique of pentagonal closure (Figs. 69.1 and 69.2). Size 6-0 silk sutures are placed in interrupted fashion along the canthotomy site at the lateral canthus, and a running suture approximates conjunctiva to the new lateral lower lid (Fig. 69.6). The lateral canthal angle is reformed with an integrated 6-0 silk suture (Fig. 69.6). The tendon is not repaired. The skin sutures are removed 5–6 days postoperatively, and the lid margin and canthal angle sutures are removed 10–14 days postoperatively.

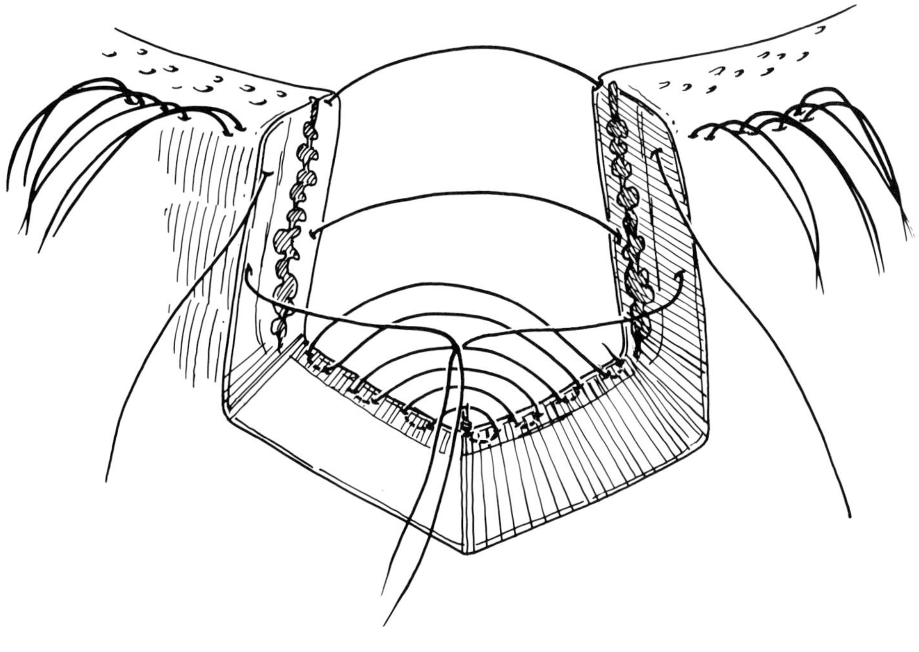

Figure 69.1. Layered closure of pentagonal full-thickness lid defect. Running Vicryl suture is placed through retractors of lower lid. Two additional Vicryl sutures are placed through tarsus. Vicryl is passed through apex of posterior lid margin.

Figure 69.2. Layered pentagonal closure. Size 6-0 silk sutures are passed through greyline, through posterior lash line, and cut extremely short. Skin and orbicularis are approximated with near-far/far-near sutures.

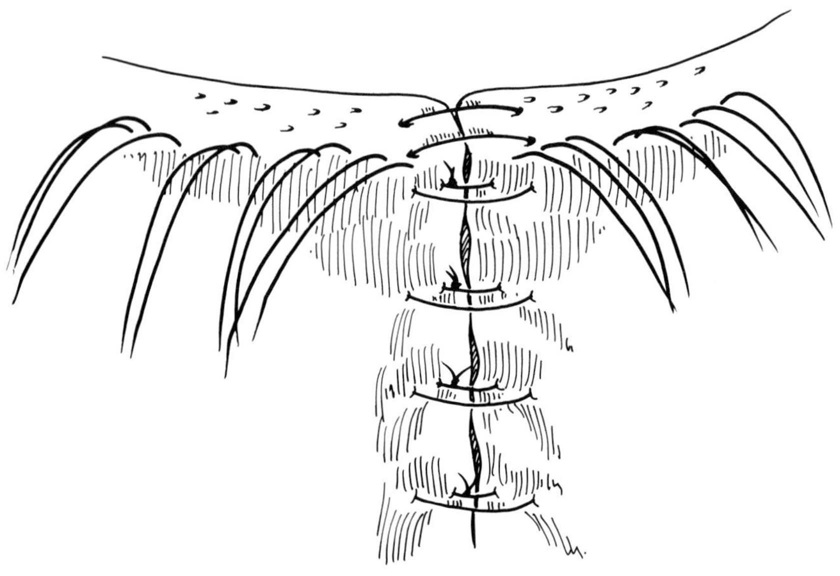

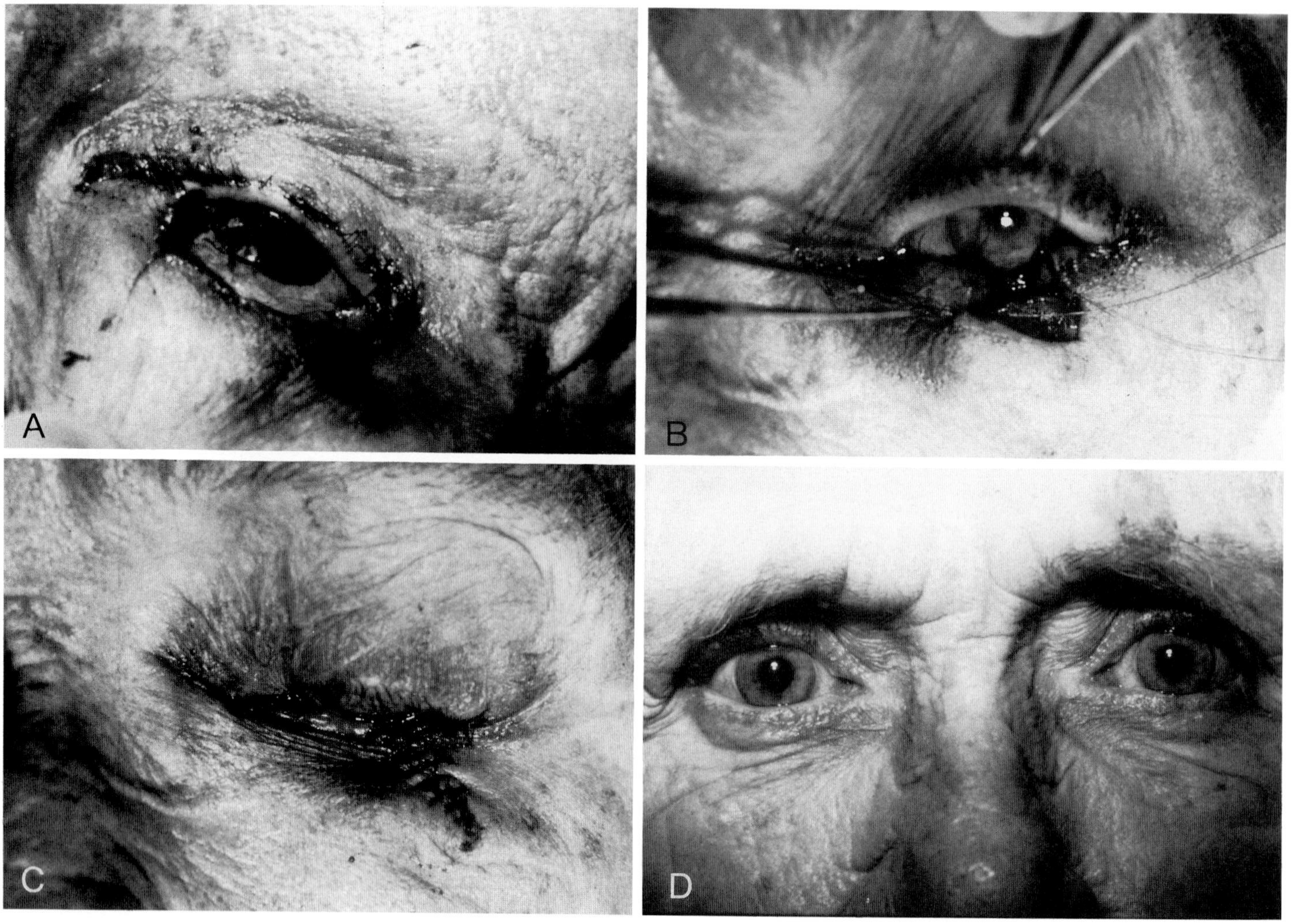

Figure 69.3. Closure of major eyelid defect with primary repair. *A*, Left lower lid defect at surgery measuring 17 mm. *B*, Lower lid defect with Vicryl tarsal sutures in place. *C*, Lid defect following closure, appears overly tight. *D*, Four months following surgery, lid position is satisfactory.

DIRECT CLOSURE WITH SEMICIRCULAR FLAP

Defects of the central or lateral portions of the lid involving as much as 75% of lax lower eyelids can be closed by creating a semicircular advancement flap (3). The technique of direct closure with a semicircular flap allows a greater length of tissue for eyelid replacement than a horizontal incision. A circular flap of approximately 20 mm in diameter, beginning at the lateral canthus and arching superiorly, is outlined (Fig. 69.7). After infiltration with a local anesthetic and epinephrine, an incision is made along the outlined site and a skin or skin-muscle flap is raised. Inferior cantholysis is performed by the technique previously described. The flap is then advanced. Primary closure of the eyelid defect is performed. A lateral canthal tendinous attachment is re-created by passing a double-armed, nonabsorbable suture such as 6-0 Prolene, from dermis to the periosteum of the inner aspect of the lateral orbital rim. The suture is tied and cut short. The conjunctiva is then advanced to the new lid margin attempting not to compromise the fornix. It is sutured to the inner lid margin with a running 6-0 silk suture. A mucosal graft rarely may be needed. The lateral canthal angle is re-created with a 6-0 silk suture in near-far-far-near fashion (Fig. 69.8). The skin is closed with interrupted sutures. The skin sutures are removed 7 days postoperatively, and the lateral canthal and lid margin sutures are removed at 10–14 days.

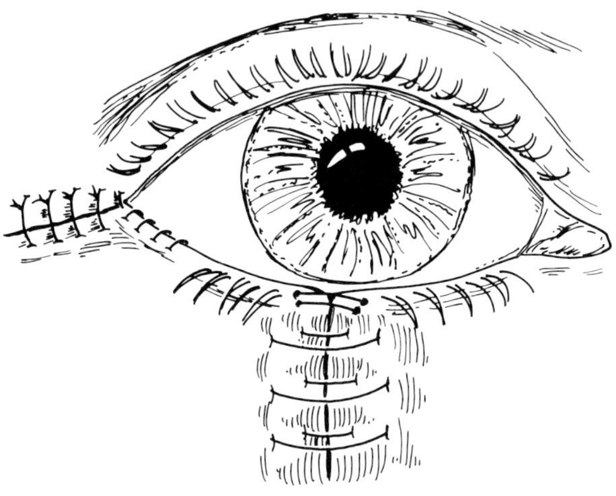

Figure 69.6. Lateral lower lid is mobilized medially, and wound edges are closed with standard primary repair techniques. Lateral canthal angle is re-formed with single 6-0 silk suture cut short and running suture from conjunctiva to anterior lamella of lid.

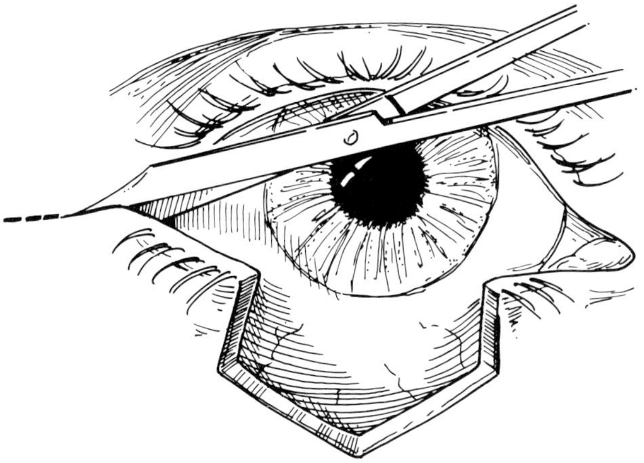

Figure 69.4. Lateral canthotomy. Full-thickness canthotomy is performed with sharp scissors at lateral canthal angle.

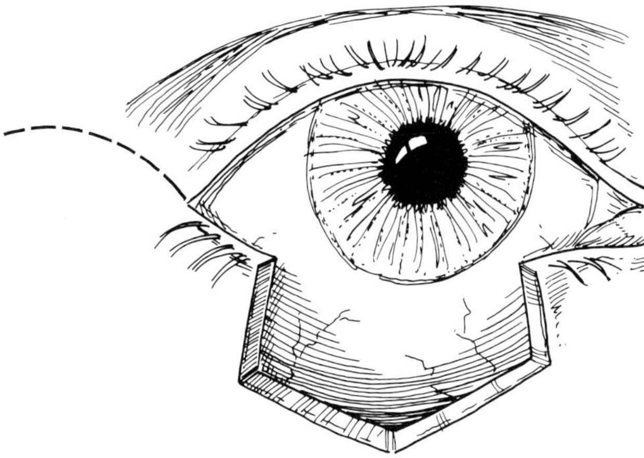

Figure 69.7. Semicircular flap. Semicircular defect approximately 20 mm diameter is outlined, involving lateral canthus to close large lower lid defect.

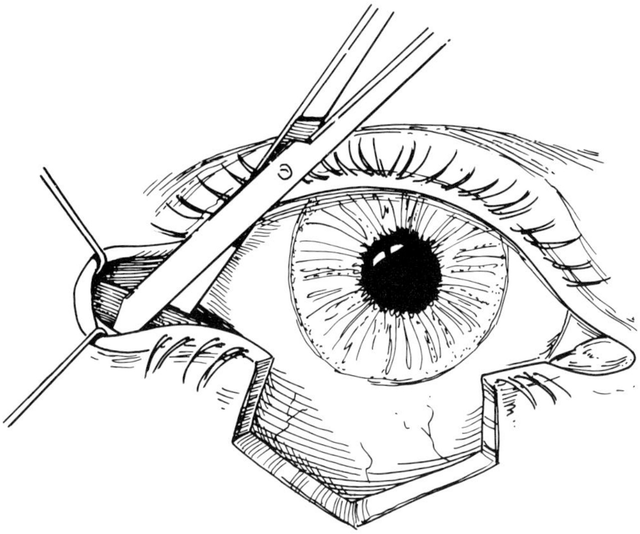

Figure 69.5. Inferior limb cantholysis. Lateral canthal tendon and attachments to orbital septum are cut without incising conjunctiva or skin.

TARSOCONJUNCTIVAL FLAP (MODIFIED HUGHES PROCEDURE)

Direct reapproximation of eyelid defects involving 50% or more of the lower eyelid may be technically impossible in the presence of inadequate horizontal eyelid laxity, especially if greater than 75% of the lid is involved. A lid sharing procedure involving tarsus and conjunctiva from the upper eyelid (4, 5) can be utilized where direct reapproximation is judged to be impossible. However, because this procedure involves occlusion of the eye for a period

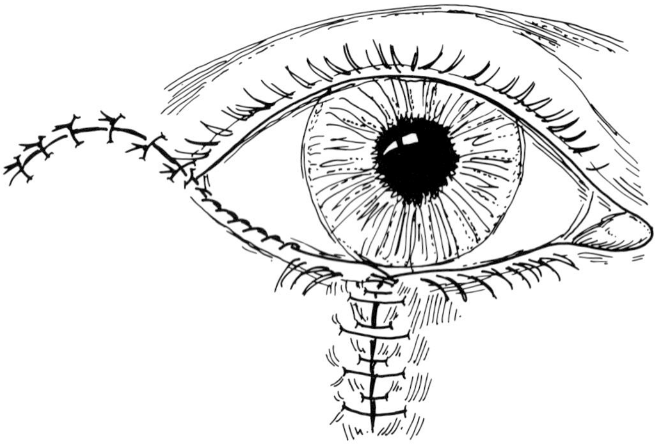

Figure 69.8. Semicircular skin muscle flap advanced into defect for primary closure of lower lid defect. Running conjunctival skin suture at lateral lid. Flap is closed with interrupted sutures. Angle suture is placed to re-form lateral canthal angle.

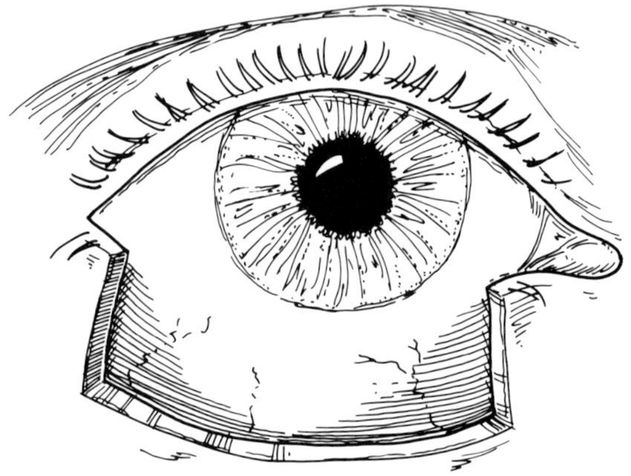

Figure 69.9. Full extent of lower lid defect following excision of lid tumor.

of 8 weeks, it is used only with great reluctance in the repair of large defects in children, where the visual system has not yet matured, as amblyopia may ensue.

In the tarsoconjunctival flap procedure, the horizontal extent of the lower eyelid defect should be measured under tension to determine the horizontal length of tarsus to be advanced (Figs. 69.9 and 69.10). The upper eyelid is everted with a Desmarres retractor and local anesthetic with epinephrine is injected subconjunctivally and deeply into the pretarsal space. An upper eyelid horizontal incision is made parallel to and approximately 3 mm from the upper eyelid margin (Fig. 69.11). Thus, the stability and proper position of the upper eyelid margin is ensured, and the complications of retraction, entropion, trichiasis, and lash loss from dissecting too near the lash follicles are prevented. Two vertical tarsoconjunctival incisions are extended into the fornix as far apart as the measured defect (Fig. 69.11). The tarsoconjunctival flap is dissected with Iris scissors from the levator aponeurosis in the pretarsal space. Upon reaching the upper edge of the tarsus, the surgeon should cut away Muller's superior tarsal muscle from the tarsus and the conjunctiva (Fig. 69.12). Tarsus and conjunctiva are advanced without the superior tarsal muscle to avoid upper eyelid retraction after subsequent separation of the flap. Any buttonholes made in the flap should be repaired with fine absorbable suture as they may enlarge considerably in the postoperative period and compromise the success of the tarsoconjunctival flap. The margins of the original defect are examined. The defect in the lower eyelid should have the cut edges of the tarsus perpendicular to the eyelid margin. The upper eyelid tarsoconjunctival flap is pulled inferiorly into the lower eyelid defect. The upper eyelid tarsus is initially attached medially and laterally to the inferior border of the defect of the tarsus of the lower eyelid using 6-0 Vicryl sutures (Fig. 69.13). An additional tarsal suture may then be placed medially and laterally. The lower

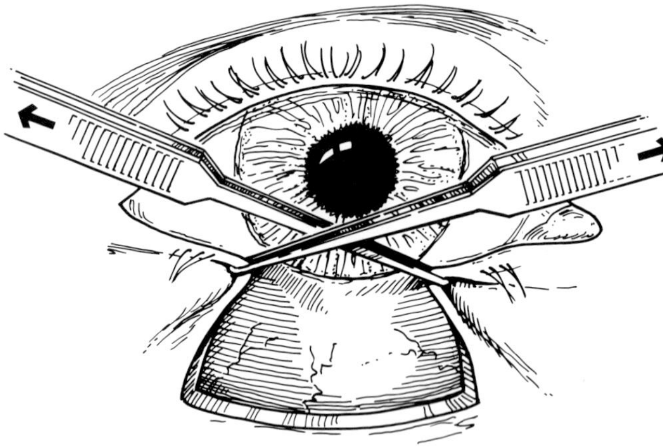

Figure 69.10. Forceps are used to narrow defect under tension to determine horizontal length of tarsus to be advanced.

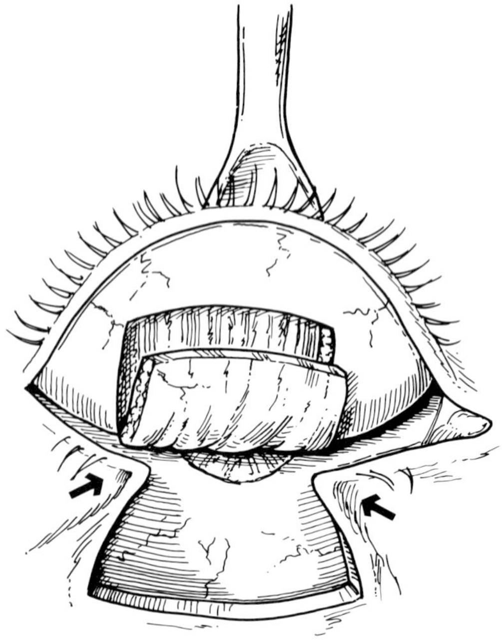

Figure 69.11. Tarsoconjunctival flap. *Arrows* represent horizontal tension on lower lid.

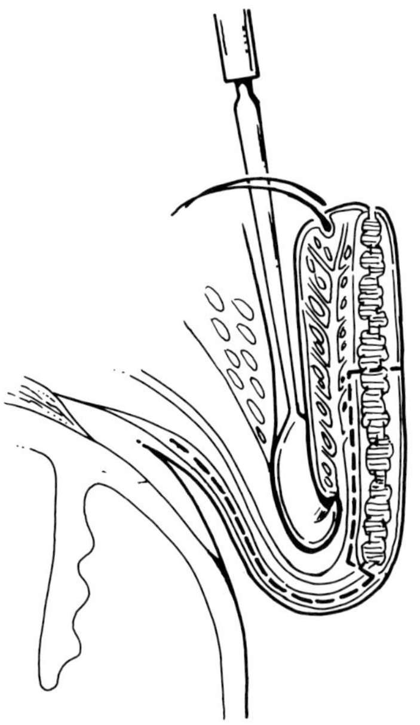

Figure 69.12. Hughes procedure. Cross section of tarsoconjunctival flap is shown. Dissection is made through tarsus in pretarsal space. Removal of aponeurotic fibers from surface of tarsus avoids lid retraction. Dissection is carried beyond superior margin of tarsus. Conjunctiva without Mueller's muscle is advanced with flap.

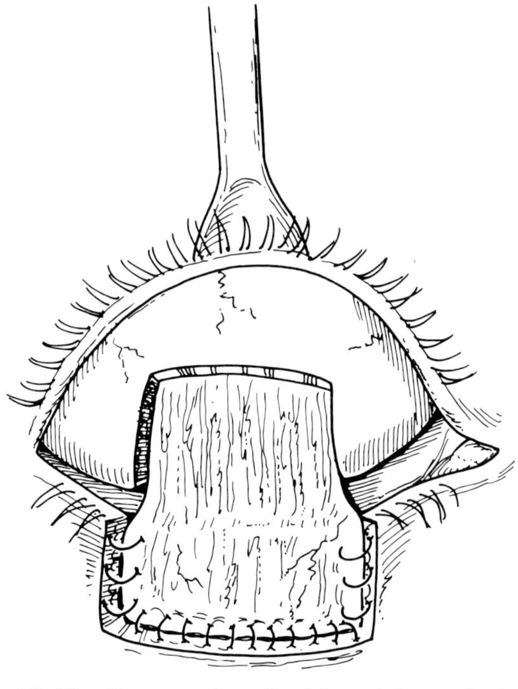

Figure 69.13. Tarsoconjunctival flap. Interrupted partial-thickness 6-0 Vicryl sutures are passed through donor flap and margin of defect, avoiding corneal irritation.

eyelid margin should be sutured to the upper edge of the donor tarsus. The lower eyelid conjunctiva and retractors should be sutured to the lower edge of the upper eyelid tarsoconjunctival flap if possible. The lower eyelid orbicularis may be placed anterior to the upper eyelid donor tarsus to provide support and additional vascular supply. The orbicularis is migrated superiorly while maintaining its nasal and lateral extensions.

If no lateral palpebral tendon remains, the flap may be attached to the periosteum of the inner aspect of the lateral orbital rim using 6-0 Prolene. If no anterior medial palpebral tendon remains, the flap may be attached to the posterior limb of the medial palpebral tendon with 6-0 Prolene, or alternatively to the periosteum in the area of the posterior lacrimal crest with a plicating suture.

A free skin flap or a full-thickness skin graft may provide the anterior lamella of the eyelid defect. A vertical lower eyelid defect up to 3 or 4 mm may be repaired with skin advancement if adjacent skin is available. Alternatively, a postauricular or preauricular skin graft may provide an excellent new skin surface.

A skin flap is undermined inferiorly (Fig. 69.14). Two vertical relaxing incisions may be necessary at the edges of the lower lid advancement flap if the skin cannot be placed over the defect directly and stabilized with horizontal traction. The flap is advanced superiorly (Fig. 69.15) and attached to the site of the new lower eyelid margin. The skin flap is sutured to the lateral and medial skin margins with 6-0 silk under horizontal traction (Fig. 69.16). Vertical traction is to be avoided. Skin sutures are removed 5–6 days postoperatively.

A graft may be necessary if the lower eyelid defect is vertically too large for the amount of available skin below the new defect. The full-thickness skin graft is harvested by standard techniques from preauricular, postauricular, upper eyelid, or supraclavicular skin. The graft is thinned of subcutaneous tissue and placed over the defect. It is sutured to the tarsoconjunctival flap and adjacent skin using 6-0 or 7-0 silk sutures that are tied and left long (Fig. 69.17). The superior edge is attached at the planned site for the newly created lower eyelid margin. A slight excess of skin may be used but is not usually necessary in the eyelid. The silk sutures are tied over a bolster soaked in antibiotic to maintain close graft/flap contact. A shield

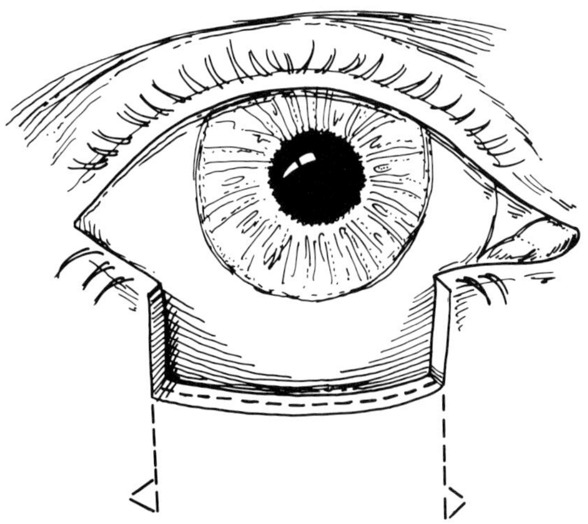

Figure 69.14. Hughes procedures. Skin covering tarsoconjunctival flap is mobilized with inferior incisions parallel to medial and lateral aspects of defect. Burrow's triangles minimize dog ears if needed.

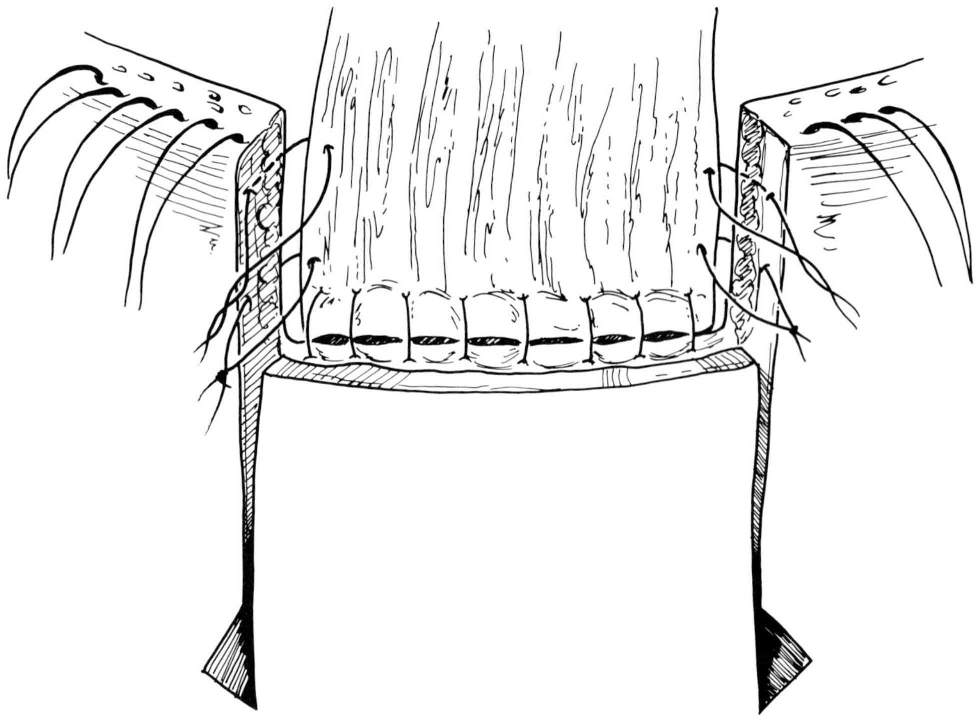

Figure 69.15. Hughes procedure. Tarsoconjunctival flap in place. Skin flap to be advanced inferiorly over tarsoconjunctival flap.

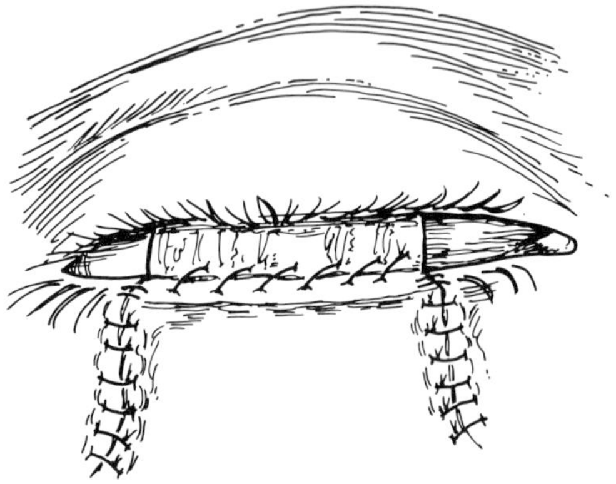

Figure 69.16. Hughes procedure. Tarsoconjunctival graft and skin closed with interrupted sutures. Additional partial-thickness running suture is placed at superior tarsal portion of flap.

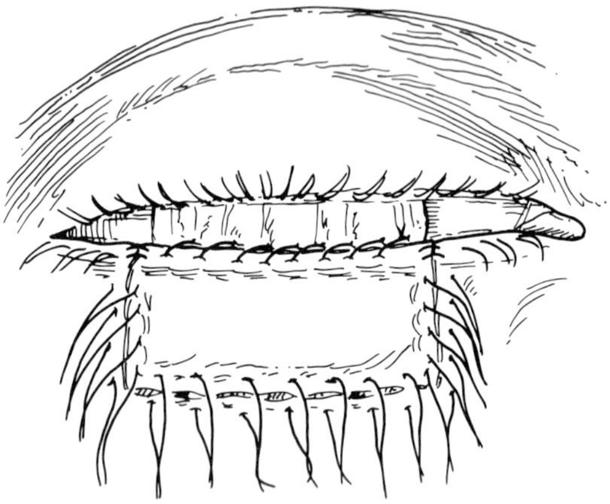

Figure 69.17. Hughes procedure. Skin graft is placed over tarsoconjunctival flap. One suture is left long. Sutures are tied over Dacron bolster to maintain graft-to-flap apposition.

is placed over the wound for protection. The bolster and the sutures are removed approximately 10 days postoperatively. The delicate nature of the graft during healing should be stressed to the patient to avoid graft slough. The bolster should not be touched or moved, particularly the first 4–5 days. The bridge flap and new skin is allowed to develop a new blood supply in the lower eyelid in the postoperative period.

After the new eyelid tissue is pink and soft, in approximately 6–12 weeks, the tarsoconjunctival flap may be divided to reopen the palpebral aperture. Local anesthetic with epinephrine is infiltrated into the flap just above the new eyelid margin. A grooved director is placed beneath the flap to protect the eye. The blade of sharp straight scissors is passed between the grooved director and the conjunctival flap. The flap is incised with the scissors, leaving approximately 0.5 mm of excess lower eyelid tissue (Fig. 69.18). The flap will tend to retract postoperatively and can be trimmed later if needed. The upper eyelid tissue is allowed to retract and may need later trimming. No reundermining of the superior fornix and no reattachment of the lower eyelid mucosa to the anterior eyelid margin is performed. Upper eyelid retraction from Mueller's superior tarsal muscle should not occur if the initial dissections separating Mueller's muscle from conjunctiva were done correctly. Satisfactory attachment of the lower

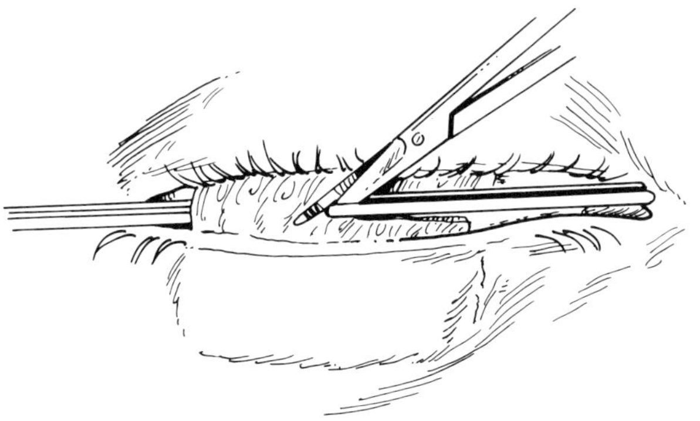

Figure 69.18. Hughes procedure. Division of flap. Grooved director beneath flap. Flap is divided at site of proposed new lower eyelid margin, allowing for slight conjunctival retraction.

eyelid skin to the mucosa is obtained by spontaneous epithelialization. If segmental conjunctivalization of the eyelid margin occurs, it may be corrected at a later date if necessary by cautery, mucosal recession and skin advancement, or skin grafting. Any excess eyelid margin remaining above the desired eyelid margin site may be trimmed as needed. The eyelid recreated by the Hughes technique may look quite normal except for the loss of lashes.

LOCALIZED TARSOCONJUNCTIVAL FLAP

The localized tarsoconjunctival flap can be used to reconstruct a defect involving approximately 50% of the lateral aspect of the lower eyelid (6). In this procedure, a tarsoconjunctival flap is rotated on a lateral base from the upper eyelid to fill the lower eyelid defect. Larger defects can be reconstructed using simultaneous lateral and medial flaps. The major advantage of this technique is the nonocclusion of the visual axis. A double-flap procedure from the nasal and temporal aspects is particularly useful in the reconstruction of the lower eyelids of infants, young children, and one-eyed patients.

The technique is similar to that of the Hughes procedure except for the site of the conjunctival attachment. The upper eyelid is everted over a Desmarres retractor. After subconjunctival and pretarsal infiltration with a local anesthetic containing epinephrine, the lateral or medial conjunctiva and tarsus are incised horizontally from the lateral canthus a sufficient distance to fit the lower eyelid defect under traction. The horizontal incision is made 3 mm above the superior eyelid margin. The ends of the flap are then delimited with a vertical incision to the upper edge of the tarsus. A tarsoconjunctival flap is dissected from the levator aponeurosis at the level of the potential pretarsal space and Mueller's muscle. Mueller's muscle is separated from the conjunctiva so that a sufficient lateral base of conjunctiva is mobilized to fill the soft tissue defect. The flap is sutured into the lower eyelid defect. Laterally, the tarsus should be secured to the lateral orbital rim periosteum or to the lateral palpebral tendon. The tarsoconjunctival flap may be covered with orbicularis and a skin flap or skin graft. If a full-thickness skin graft is used, sutures and bolsters are placed. When the flap is well vascularized, the tarsoconjunctival flap is divided at the lower eyelid margin as is done in the Hughes tarsoconjunctival flap (see preceding section).

PARTIAL DEFECTS

A tumor can involve a single lamella of the lid and not the full thickness of the lid. Reconstruction should involve replacement of the missing tissue only. With defects of the skin, advancement flaps or free grafts can be used. Conjunctival defects alone can be repaired with contralateral conjunctiva or buccal mucous membrane. Loss of the entire posterior lamella of the lid should be reconstructed using a tarsoconjunctival flap from the upper lid. A nasoseptal chondromucosal graft is an alternative if a tarsoconjunctival flap is not available.

The nasoseptal chondromucosal graft is valuable in cases where upper lid graft material is unobtainable. Callahan described a technique for obtaining graft without external nasal dissection (7). However, it is technically simpler to directly view the donor site while obtaining the graft. The mucosal/cartilage interface integrity must be maintained in order to ensure graft survival. It behooves the surgeon to open the ala to gain better control of the dissection. Both nostrils are packed with cocaine pledgets along the nasal septum. After 5–10 minutes has elapsed, the pledgets are removed and local anesthetic containing epinephrine is injected in the nasal ala. The ala is cut along the alar groove (Fig. 69.19). Hemostasis is achieved. The tissue to be harvested, measuring 4–15 mm or the full extent of the defect, is outlined with a marking pen. A rectangular strip is outlined parallel to the nasal floor (Fig. 69.20). Submucosal local anesthetic containing epinephrine is injected on the contralateral side to facilitate separating the mucosa from the cartilage. The ipsilateral mucosa and cartilage are carefully incised with a No. 15 blade. An attempt should be made to avoid perforation of the contralateral perichondrium and mucosa. The blunt end of a Freer elevator is passed posteriorly to the contralateral side after an initial incision is made to separate the cartilage from the underlying mucosa (Fig. 69.21). The incision is then completed along the previously outlined area. The septum does not need to be sutured and will heal if a single layer of mucosa remains contiguous over it. If a large perforation is created, it is necessary to suture it or to mobilize a flap to avoid a septal hole with its attendant complications of whistling, bleeding, and rhinitis. The nose is not packed postoperatively unless active bleeding is observed. The nasoseptal cartilage is thick and must be trimmed to approximately one-half its thickness before use. Alternatively, 80% vertical scoring allows the thickened cartilage to conform to the shape of the globe (Fig. 69.22). The graft of cartilage and mucosa is placed into the surgical defect and sutured to the remaining lid margins. The mucosa should be trimmed so that approximately 1 mm of mucosa, without cartilage, remains at the superior border of the lid margin. The recipient conjunctiva is then sutured to the nasoseptal mucous mem-

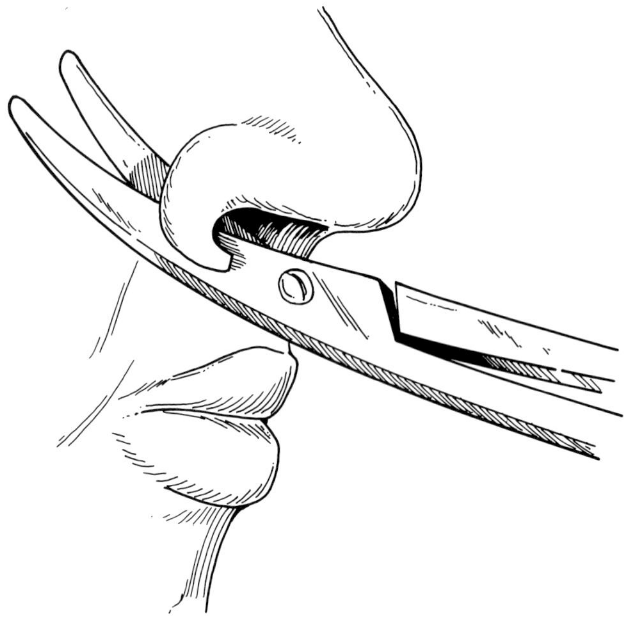

Figure 69.19. Obtaining nasoseptal chondromucosa. Large scissors are used to cut along alar groove.

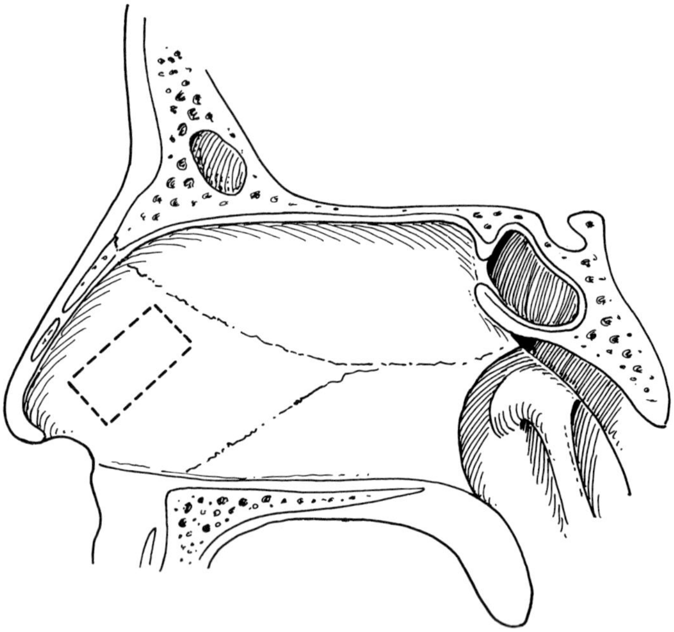

Figure 69.20. Area of proposed graft is marked.

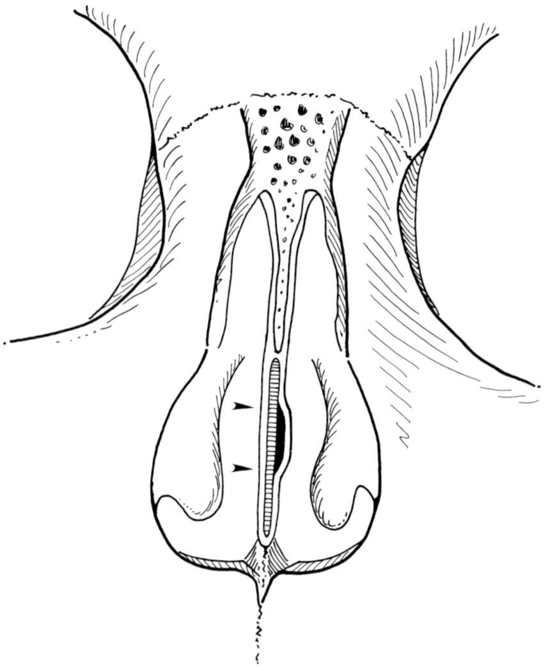

Figure 69.21. Nasal septal chondromucosal graft perforated without lacerating contralateral mucosa. Periosteal elevator immediately behind cartilage bluntly dissects away mucoperichondrium (sling).

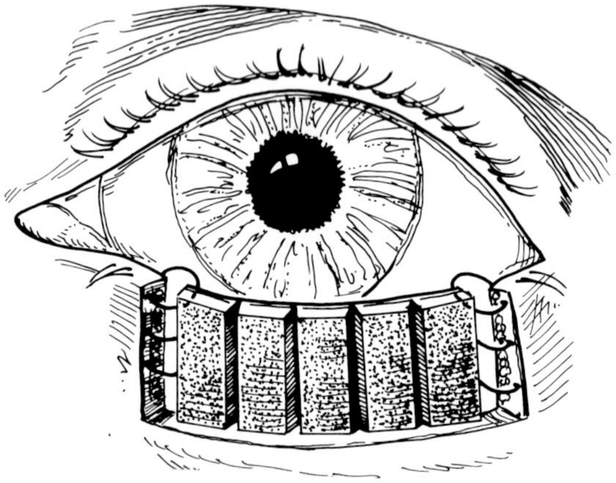

Figure 69.22. Nasal septal chondromucosal graft is scored vertically to allow shape to conform to curve of globe, and then is sutured into place.

brane with interrupted absorbable sutures (Fig. 69.22). The skin and orbicularis from below or laterally are undermined. The skin muscle flap is then advanced into place over the chondromucosal graft and sutured. A free skin graft may not be used over the mucocartilaginous free grafts unless vascularized orbicularis can be mobilized between the skin graft and the mucocartilaginous graft. The nasoseptal graft is available to the surgeon, but fortunately is seldom needed.

OTHER METHODS OF LOWER EYELID CLOSURE

REVERSE CUTLER BEARD

The reverse Cutler Beard described by Hecht (8) uses a full-thickness flap brought from about 4 mm above the upper lid margin. The flap passes beneath the upper lid margin and is placed into the lower lid defect under horizontal tension. It is divided in a second-stage procedure when well vascularized. As this procedure provides no distinct advantages over the Hughes procedure, it is seldom necessary.

"Bucket handle" flaps from the upper eyelid, rotating full-thickness flaps from the lateral upper eyelid or brow, sliding full-thickness flaps from the temporal area, and the medial forehead flap have been used by various authors to reconstruct the lower eyelid (7, 9). We have not needed these procedures to date, but their usage can be considered in the very unusual situation when more satisfactory tissues are not available.

COMPOSITE GRAFTING

Composite grafting, first described by Callahan (11), employs full-thickness, pentagonal sections of the eyelid from the contralateral lid. The free, full-thickness graft is transposed to the area of the eyelid defect. The donor site is then closed. Large defects may require contralateral canthotomy and cantholysis. The recipient graft is then consecutively sutured with grayline sutures, tarsal sutures, and sutures to the retractors of the lower eyelid and the skin. Graft survival is unpredictable. If the graft does survive, lashes are usually lost.

An alternative method involves a composite partial-thickness graft from the contralateral lower eyelid in which eyelid skin is removed (12). The adjacent skin of the recipient site is undermined (Fig. 69.23). The undermined skin is advanced and sutured to the new eyelid margin to provide additional blood supply to the composite graft. While graft necrosis is reported to occur less frequently, lash loss is still a significant complication.

MUSTARDÉ ROTATIONAL CHEEK FLAP

The Mustardé rotational cheek flap (13) is mentioned for the sake of completeness. A large amount of normal lower eyelid tissue in the shape of a triangle that extends above the lateral canthus must be sacrificed in order to rotate in a large temporal cheek flap (Figs. 69.24–69.26. The sacrificed triangle is an isosceles triangle measuring

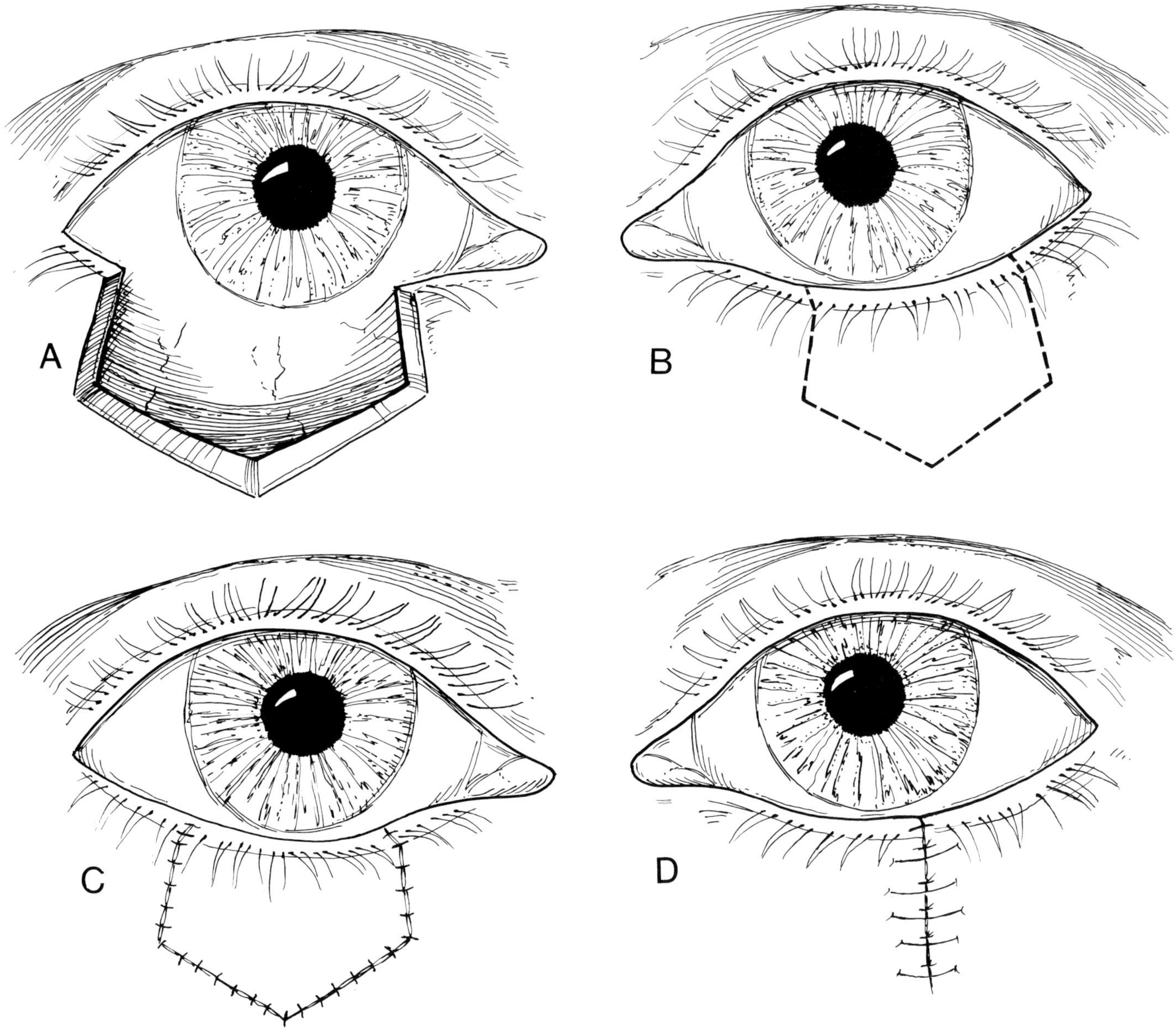

Figure 69.23. Composite graft. *A*, Defect. *B*, Donor source. *C*, Sutured in place. *D*, Donor lid closed.

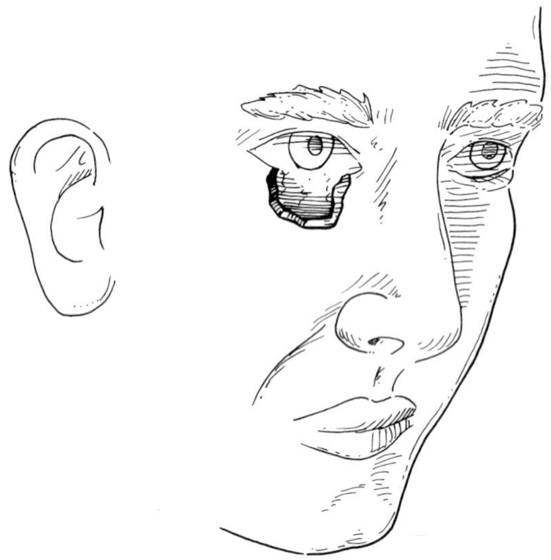

Figure 69.24. Mustardé Flap No. 1. Large eyelid defect to be corrected by Mustardé flap.

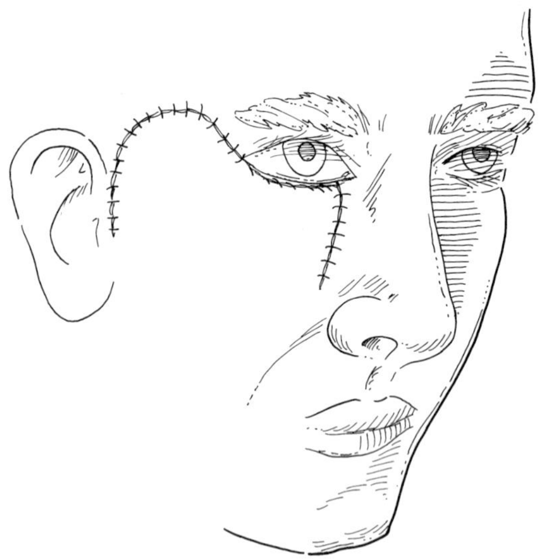

Figure 69.26. Mustardé Flap No. 3. Nasal septal chondromucosal graft sutured in place and cheek rotational flap advanced.

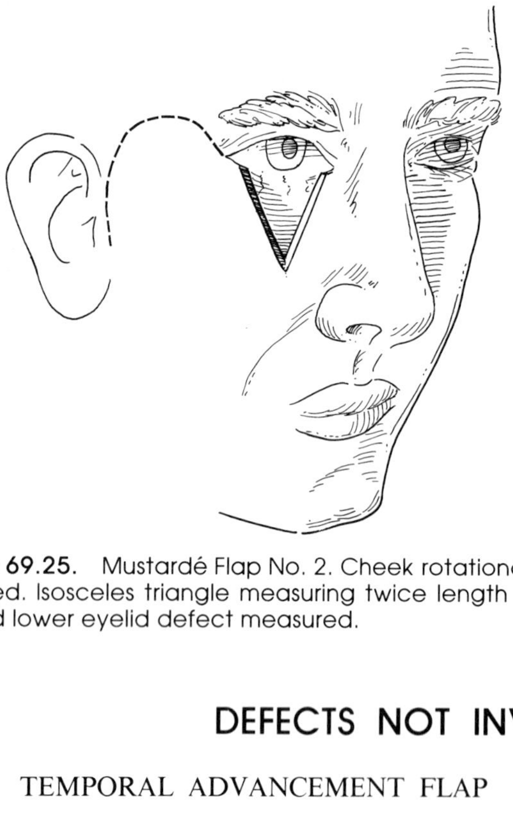

Figure 69.25. Mustardé Flap No. 2. Cheek rotational flap outlined. Isosceles triangle measuring twice length of affected lower eyelid defect measured.

twice the length of the affected lower eyelid defect. The large temporal cheek flap requires extensive undermining Cheek skin is not a good replacement for the lower eyelid as it often contains facial hair which may cause trichiasis and corneal irritation. A graft of nasoseptal cartilage must be obtained to resurface the posterior lamella of the lower lid defect.

The procedure produces a significant facial scar. The lateral aspect of the graft frequently sags, producing lateral canthal dystopia and ectropion. The complication occurs despite attachment of rotated skin to the periosteum high on the orbital rim. The arching of the incision high above the lateral canthus is also helpful in preventing lateral canthal sag.

Other potential complications of the Mustardé cheek rotational flap include seventh nerve palsy and its attendant problems of exposure keratopathy, poor lid closure, ectropion, necrosis of the flap, and unsightly facial and lid scarring. A satisfactory functional and cosmetic reconstruction is difficult to achieve with the cheek rotation flap.

DEFECTS NOT INVOLVING THE LID MARGIN

TEMPORAL ADVANCEMENT FLAP

Large lower eyelid defects that do not involve the eyelid margin usually cannot be closed primarily. In such defects, primary closure may result in ectropion. If skin and muscle alone are deficient, a skin graft is indicated, or a skin muscle flap may be advanced as outlined in Fig. 69.27. If all layers of skin must be sacrificed with no tumor extension posterior to the orbital fat, an advancement flap in combination with a buccal mucosal graft is necessary. In addition, a flap is the procedure of choice in reconstructing individuals who because of previous irradiation have a poor prognosis for graft survival.

After infiltrating with local anesthetic containing epinephrine, an infraciliary incision is made along the residual lower eyelid and extended in arcuate fashion beyond the lateral canthus. A skin muscle flap is raised laterally and extended medially to the area of the defect (Fig. 69.28). If the full thickness of the lid is involved, the posterior side of the muscle is lined with buccal mucosa. The flap is secured with near-far-far-near sutures under tension to the medial edges of the defect (Fig. 69.28). The skin is then closed with interrupted 6-0 nonabsorbable sutures which are removed ten days postoperatively.

DEFECTS INVOLVING THE MEDIAL CANTHUS

A large lower eyelid nonmarginal defect that cannot be repaired with a lateral advancement flap alone can utilize the modification of the Gillies Bishop Mitre V-Y flap (14). The glabellar frown lines caused by the corrugator muscle are outlined on the median forehead. Subcutaneous local anesthetic in conjunction with epinephrine is injected. The incision is made with a No. 15 blade obliquely in the marked brow furrows to the lateral aspect of the medial brow. The incision is made through skin with concurrent undermining to form an upside-down V-shaped defect (Fig. 69.29). After thorough undermining is completed, one edge of the defect may be rotated into the nasal defect. The brow defect is then closed in a "Y" configuration (Fig. 69.30).

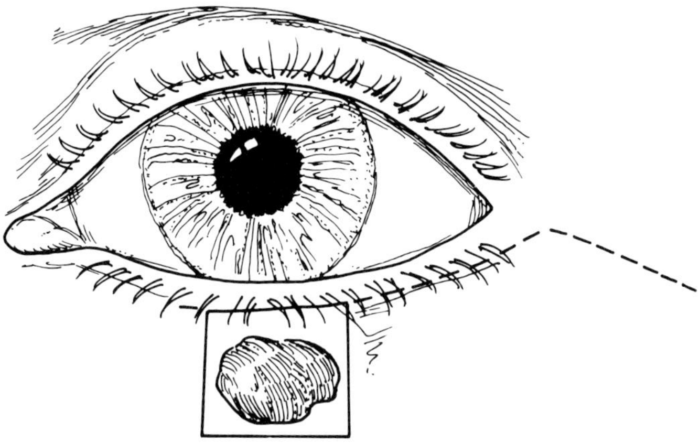

Figure 69.27. Defect of lower eyelid not involving lid margin. *Solid line* indicates size of defect following frozen-section removal of tumor. *Dotted lines* indicate planned flap.

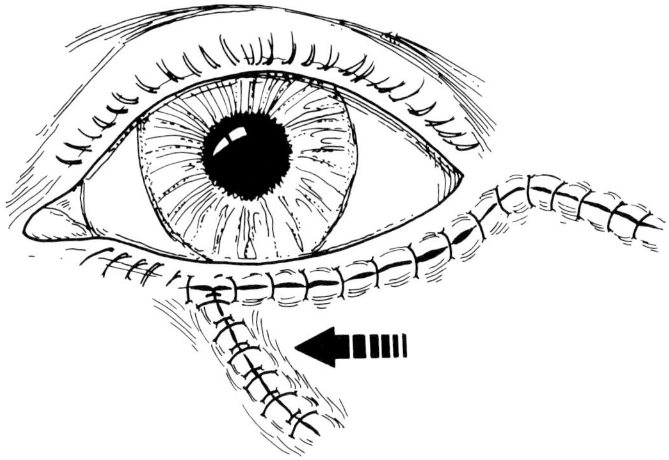

Figure 69.28. Advancement flap for defects not involving lid margin. Skin or skin muscle flap is advanced from lateral to medial to fill excised defect. If mucosa is deficient, conjunctival or buccal mucosa graft resurfaces posterior lamella of lid. Placement of near-far/far-near sutures along margins of wound under tension evert wound and prevent postoperative gape.

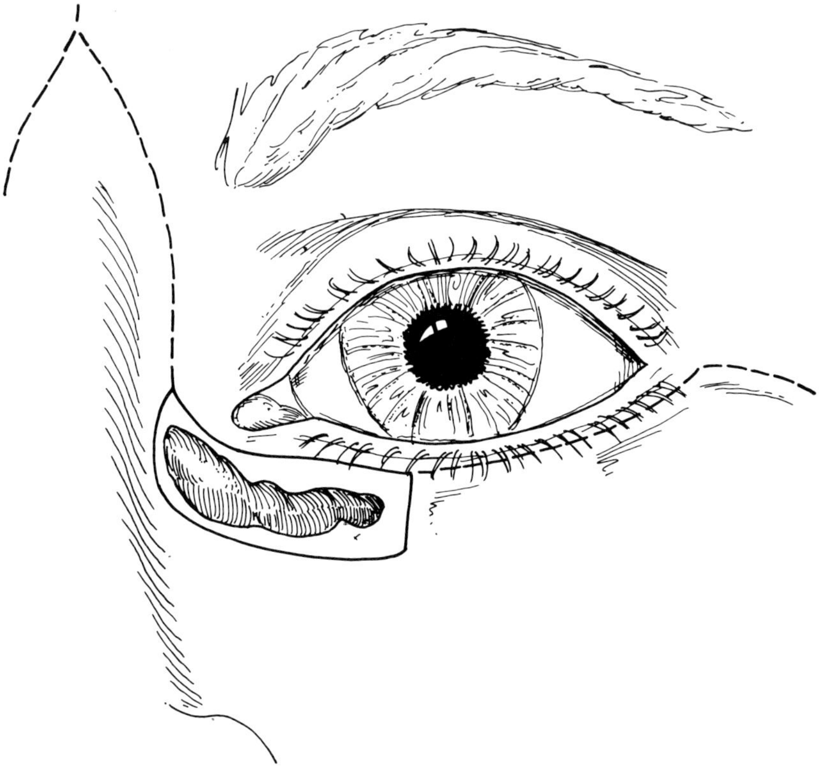

Figure 69.29. Bishop-Mitre flap in conjunction with lower lid advancement flap. *Solid lines* indicate marginal defect involving lower lid medial canthus. *Dotted lines* indicate area of skin flap. Laterally, infracilliary incision beyond lateral canthus. Bishop-Mitre flap is marked along glabellar frown line. *Asterisk* marked at level of brow indicates movement of skin in "VY" pattern to final position in Figure 69.25.

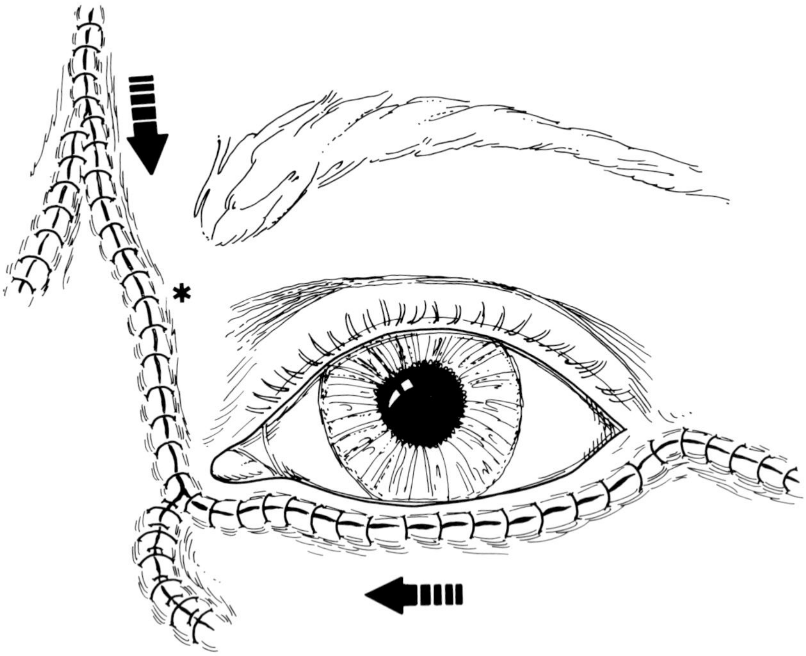

Figure 69.30. Bishop-Mitre flap in conjunction with lower lid advancement flap. Final result. *Arrows* show predominant area and direction of flap advancement. *Asterisk* marks new position of intrabrow skin. Margin of defect closed under tension with near-far/far-near sutures.

SUMMARY

Closure of defects measuring greater than 50% of the eyelid margin demands, above all, a thorough understanding of the principles of various reconstructive techniques. As might be inferred intuitively, simpler surgery is more successful, with fewer complications. An understanding of the anatomy of the eyelids and the dynamics of lid closure provides surgeons with a full armamentarium that will increase their ability to obtain optimal results.

REFERENCES

1. Fox SA, Beard C: Spontaneous lid repair. *Am J Ophthalmol* 58: 947, 1964.
2. Dryden RM, Meronk F: Primary closure of major eyelid defects. In press.
3. Tenzel RR, Stewart WB: Eyelid reconstruction by the semi-circular flap technique. *Ophthalmology* 85: 1164–1169, 1978.
4. Ceis WA, Bartlett RE: Modification of the Mustarde and Hughes methods of reconstruction of the lower lid. *Ann Ophthalmol* 7: 1497–1502, 1975.
5. Hughes WL: *Reconstruction of the Lids.* St. Louis, CV Mosby Co, 1958.
6. Smith B: A technique for extirpation and replacement of the lateral canthus. *Trans Am Acad Ophthalmol Ontolaryngol* 57: 738–742, 1953.
7. Callahan MA, Callahan A: *Ophthalmic Plastic and Orbital Surgery.* Aesculapius, AL, 1979, p 23–25.
8. Hecht SD: An upside down Cutler-Beard bridge flap. *Arch Ophthalmol* 84: 760–764, 1970.
9. Iliff CE, Iliff WJ, Iliff NT: *Oculoplastic Surgery.* Philadelphia, Saunders, 1979, pp 242–265.
10. Callahan MA, Callahan A: *Ophthalmic Plastic and Orbital Surgery,* Aesculapius, AL, 1979, pp 192–193.
11. Callahan A: Free composite lid graft. *Arch Ophthalmol* 45: 539, 1954.
12. Putterman AM: Viable composite grafting in eyelid reconstruction. *Am J Ophthalmol* 85: 237–241, 1978.
13. Mustarde JC: *Repair and Reconstruction in the Orbital Region,* Edinborough, Churchill-Livingstone, 1979.
14. Gillies H, Millard DR: *The Principles and Art of Plastic Surgery.* Boston, Little Brown & Co, vol 1, 1957, p 17.

CHAPTER 70

Mohs Fresh-Tissue Technique for Periorbital Skin Cancer

MICHAEL A. CALLAHAN, M.D., F.A.C.S.
ALSTON CALLAHAN, M.D., F.A.C.S.
GARY D. MONHEIT, M.D.

In 1941, Frederick Mohs described a unique technique (1) for removing cutaneous cancer that has only recently become recognized for its superior cure rate. As performed by Mohs, the lesion first underwent a biopsy or was debulked, then zinc paste was spread over the involved area, which fixed a 1–2 mm thickness layer of tissue (9). In a few days the tissue-paste complex would slough and the specimen could be studied systematically for surgical margins to make a histographic map of the tumor's growth. Successive applications were made in the areas of residual positivity until the tumor was extirpated. Healing occurred by granulation. This process took days to accomplish and precluded immediate reconstruction because the surrounding tissues were inflamed. Unacceptable functional and cosmetic results were obtained often, especially when the lesion was in the periorbital region. A major modification of this method is the fresh-tissue technique, which omits the chemical fixation (2). Successive layers of tissue 1–2 mm thick are excised with a scalpel, immediately studied, and a systematic map constructed. Cures by this method (96–99%) pioneered by Tromovitch (2) equal the results of the Mohs zinc chloride technique. Lesions can be completely removed within hours, so that immediate reconstruction can be performed. The term *Mohs chemosurgery* has evolved into *Mohs chemosurgery: fresh-tissue modification* with this change in technique. Other terms are *microscopically guided histographic surgery* and *microscopically controlled excision*. In this chapter, we use "Mohs technique" to refer to the presently performed fresh-tissue modification. Although several series (3–5) document the effectiveness of conventional frozen-section control of surgical margins, we have found it unreliable, especially with deep medial canthal skin cancers. Our cure rate with conventional frozen sections was approximately 85%, in contrast to our 99.8% cure rate with the Mohs technique.

ADVANTAGES

The greatest advantage of the Mohs technique is its 99% cure rate for basal cell carcinoma (BCC) (6, 7) and 94% (6) for squamous cell carcinoma (SCC). The sheer number of patients in the Mohs series (6) (more than 10,000) combined with the high cure rates have more weight than the results in smaller series of conventional frozen section (3–5). The Mohs technique has also been successfully used for meibomian gland carcinoma, hemangioendothelioma, malignant fibrohistiocytoma, leiomyoma, dermatifibroma protubuans, and adenocystic carcinoma.

Complete resection of skin cancer with histologic proof is a major advantage over radiation (8) or cryotherapy (9, 10). With neither of these modalities can a cure be proved except by the absence of recurrence after years have passed. Radiation is probably as effective as cryotherapy in curing skin cancer, but often leads to undesirable com-

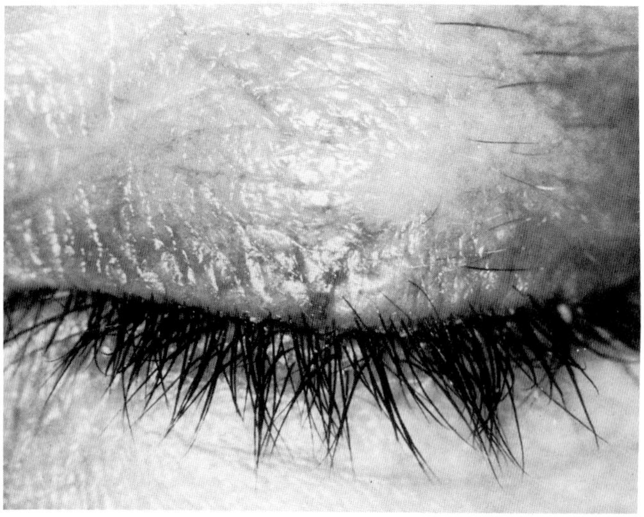

Figure 70.1. Recurrent squamous cell carcinoma in the left upper lid of a 67-year-old female.

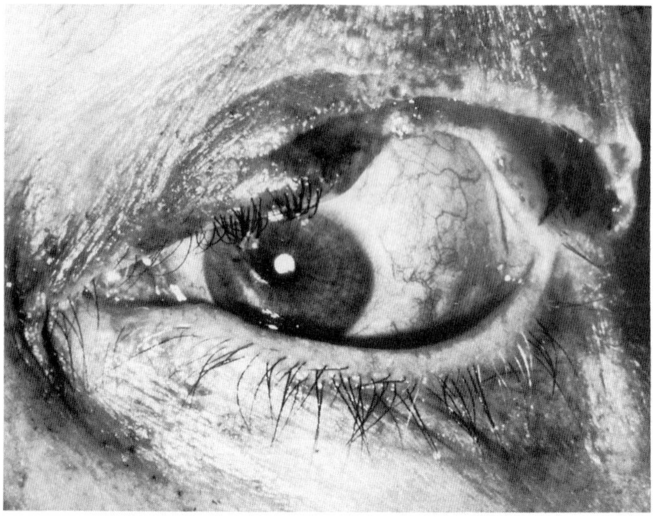

Figure 70.2. After Mohs technique excision, a 15 × 16 mm elliptical tarsal defect was present on the lateral half of the left upper lid. Repair consisted of a vertical sliding flap of tarsus and conjunctiva and a free skin graft. This relatively simple reconstruction was possible because of the retention of a generous amount of tarsus and conjunctiva.

plications, such as canalicular fibrosis, loss of cilia, or teleangiectasis of the skin. Fortunately, with modern radiotherapy techniques, radiation cataract and radiation retinopathy are infrequent complications. Both cryotherapy and radiation have a limited but definite niche in

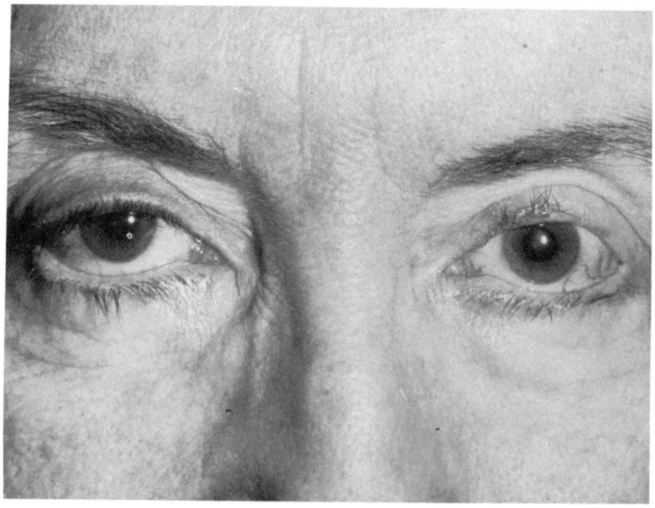

Figure 70.3. Postoperative appearance 3 months after tarsoconjunctival posterior lamellar flap and free skin graft repair.

treatment of skin cancer for debilitated patients too infirm to undergo surgical excision involving local anesthesia.

With the Mohs technique, a greater amount of uninvolved tissue is saved for reconstruction than with the conventional frozen-section control. When we previously used the frozen-section method, we excised a generous margin of normal-appearing tissue beyond the clinical extent of the tumor to try to "get it all." Frequently, this led to the unnecessary sacrifice of precious amounts of eyelid tissue, necessitating more advanced reconstruction techniques. Since we have utilized the Mohs technique exclusively, the functional and cosmetic nature of our results has improved greatly because many defects can be closed primarily or by local flaps or small grafts (Figs. 70.1–70.3).

Since our patients are managed first by a dermatologic surgeon and then by an ophthalmic reconstructive surgeon, there is usually an interval ranging from 2 to 24 hours between completion of excision and repair. During this time, reconstructive alternatives can be considered by the surgeon (and residency staff) and discussed with the patient and family; cancer surgery is psychologically brutal, and we have found that such communication allays fear and anxiety. The patient's expectations can be explored and the timing and necessity of repair explained. For example, if a large, deeply invading tumor in the lateral canthus has been removed, split-thickness skin grafting may be preferable to repair with a more cosmetically pleasing flap so the area can be more carefully observed for recurrence. Definitive repair in such cases may be delayed for 5 years, and this should be discussed with the patient.

OPERATIVE TECHNIQUE

There are seven basic steps to the Mohs technique (Fig. 70.4):

1. Conservative gross excision (or debulking) of the full clinical extent of the neoplasm is performed, followed by hemostasis.

2. (Level 1) The first microscopic section is excised. The knife blade is angled 30° to the skin so that a horizontal sheet of tissue—without discontinuity—is removed from the entire base of the defect.

3. This sheet of tissue is cut and divided into smaller

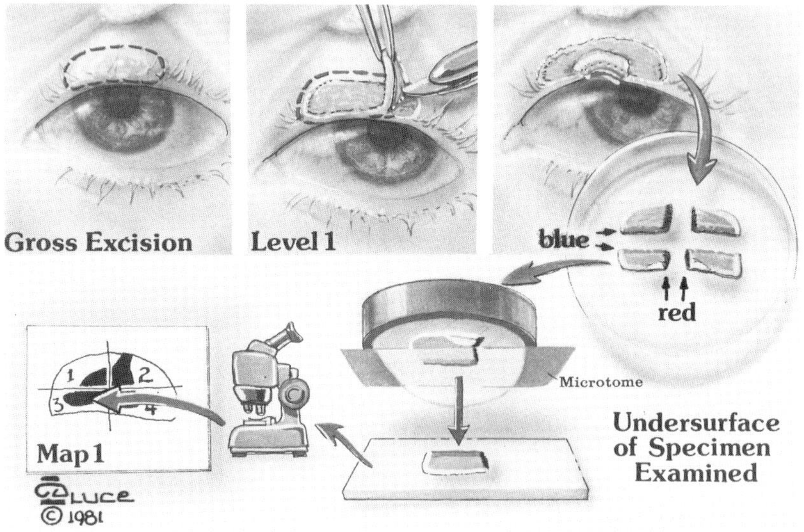

Figure 70.4. Seven steps of the Mohs fresh-tissue technique, from gross excision to mapping (see text).

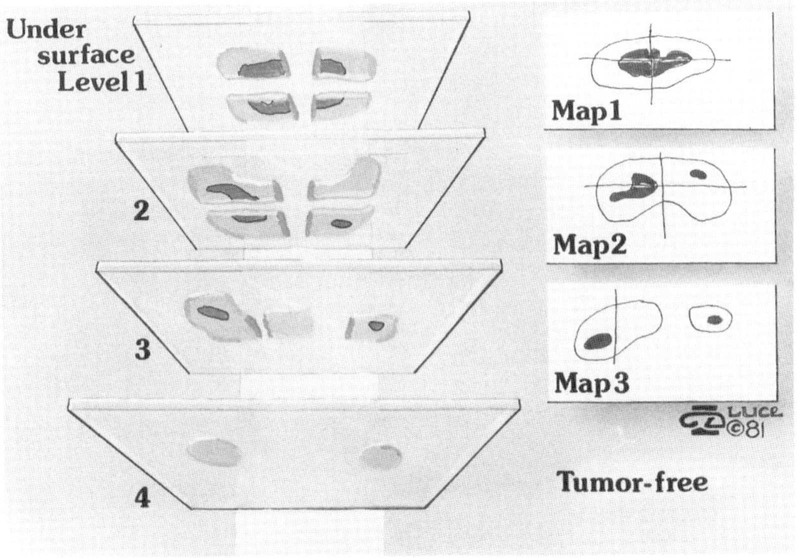

Figure 70.5. Undersurface of levels 1–4 is depicted (*at the left*) on glass slides. The corresponding maps 1–3 (*on the right*) show remaining positivity. Since the undersurface of level 4 is negative, the patient would be declared tumor free. Note that at the deeper level, specimens become progressively smaller as they are taken only from areas of remaining positivity (shown as *dark spots* on the levels and maps); this saves a greater amount of normal tissue for reconstruction.

specimens, which are serially numbered for identification. They are color coded with blue and red supravital dyes (so that the margins can be seen microscopically) and placed in a petri dish.

4. The specimens are transferred to the laboratory, where the technician processes them by turning them upside down in a molded cup and flattening them out with a small weight so that they do not curl up. After freezing, 7- to 10-μm thick sections are cut with a microtome.

5. The microscopic sections are mounted and stained (with hematoxylin and eosin) in an orientation that allows the undersurface of the original sheet of tissue to be examined.

6. The sections are delivered to the Mohs surgeon for microscopic review of the surgical margins.

7. The areas of residual tumor are charted on the map (Map 1).

Steps 1–3 are performed in the operating room by the dermatologic surgeon, and steps 4–7 are performed in the laboratory. This entire process for one layer usually takes 15–20 minutes. When there are any remaining positive areas, steps 2–7 are repeated as needed. The successive layers are directed at the areas only of remaining positivity, according to the defect map (Fig. 70.5).

Another important advantage is that we have been able to pinpoint and remove tumor extensions near the globe, and thus avoid the mutilation of exenteration. We have a prospective ongoing study (see appendix) of 14 such patients with deeply infiltrative tumors referred to us for exenteration, but who instead underwent the Mohs technique. With an average follow-up of 6 years, only one has recurred, which necessitated exenteration.

DISADVANTAGES

Availability of dermatologic surgeons trained in the Mohs fresh-tissue technique appears a major obstacle to widespread acceptance and utilization of this treatment modality. To date, there are approximately 75 dermatologic surgeons who have received this special postgraduate training and there are 15 training centers approved by the American College of Chemosurgery.

In this ever-increasing cost-conscious world, we have found that this procedure has a 10–15% higher cost for the extra laboratory time and histotechnician fees, compared with conventional frozen-section control. These economic factors cannot be ignored, but must be weighed against the Mohs technique's superior cure rate and as well as the other advantages.

The popularity of this procedure has been adversely affected because of the hideous deformities that sometimes results from the healing of wounds by secondary intention. This disadvantage is becoming less important since now 95% of the Mohs technique is by the fresh-tissue modification with immediate reconstruction.

Multiple injections of local anesthesia are administered if more than one layer is excised, and this disadvantage may cause discomfort. However, we have had no cases in which patients were unwilling or unable to complete the excision once the process was started.

Mapping out subcutaneous tumor projections with the Mohs technique has given us better insight into their pathological nature and predilection for subcutaneous extensions. Once the epithelial, subepithelial aggregation, and dermal invasion stages are over, the posterior spread of BCC may be thwarted by the underlying subcutaneous fascial plane. From here it demonstrates a propensity to extend along the longitudinal axis of the orbicularis muscle fibers rather than burrowing perpendicularly through them. Having broken the orbicularis muscle barrier, a posteriorly spreading skin cancer next encounters the tarsal plate and orbital septum. Fascial and aponeurotic planes resist neoplastic spread; thus deflected tumor cells either spill over the lid margin to invade the conjunctiva or slide inferiorly along the orbital septum to the arcus marginalis and periosteum of the orbital rim. Proliferation and extension of neoplastic cells along the metabolically active periosteum appears to be preferential to orbital connective tissue septae and fat, which have a relatively poor blood supply and lower metabolic rate. When given an equal opportunity of extending medially or laterally, most basal cells prefer to go toward the medial canthal area. This so-called embryological fusion plane is a favorite site for deep invasion of BCCs (11), probably because of the orientation of connective tissue planes to the skin surface. The vascularity of the medial canthus provides a rich supply of metabolic fuel for proliferating cancer cells and the adventitial sheaths of the numerous small penetrating vessels in this region provide conduits for tumor spread (Figs. 70.6–70.9).

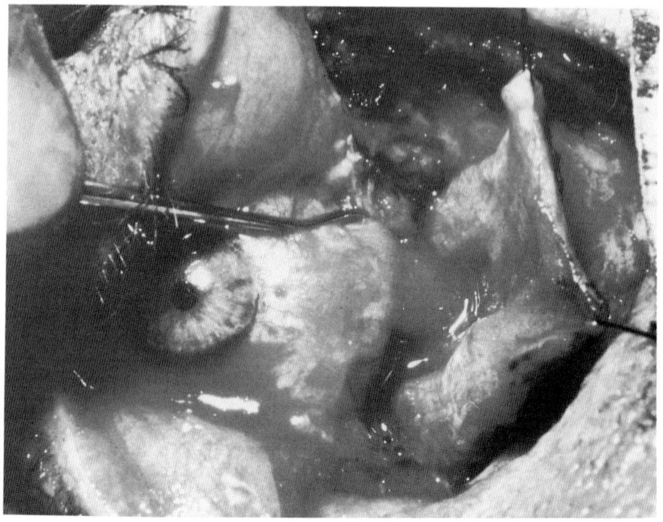

Figure 70.7. Deep orbital microscopic layer following debulking of the tumor and two microscopic levels. Superficial tumor invasion present in medial rectus muscle capsule (held to right by two ligatures). A Jamieson muscle hook is under the insertion of the medial rectus muscle.

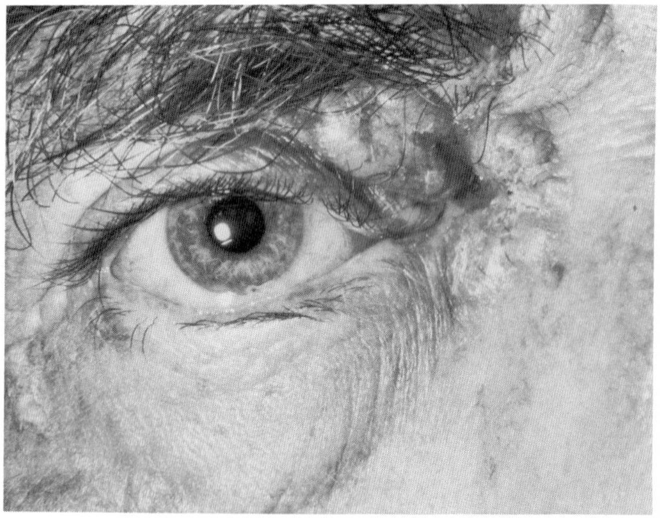

Figure 70.6. Londstanding ulcerative basal cell carcinoma of the right medial canthus, which had been enlarging over the previous 7 years. This 65-year-old patient had not previously sought medical help.

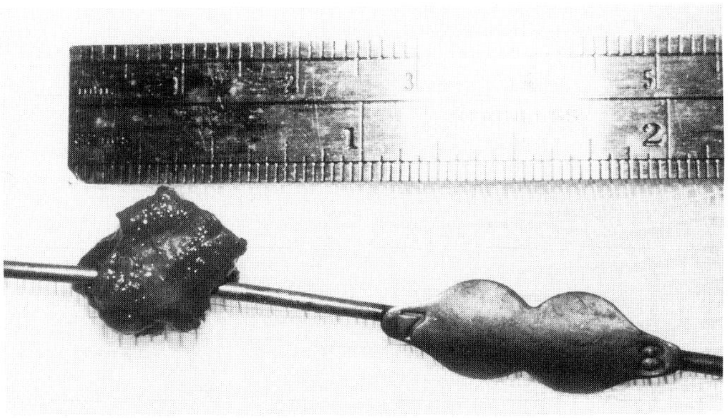

Figure 70.8. The tumor was traced into the proximal portion of the interosseous nasolacrimal duct, shown here with a Bowman probe through the nasolacrimal duct.

A further example of skin cancer's biological drive to seek the path of least resistance is its tendency to spread around or away from the irradiated tissue rather than through it. The superficial scarring of an incompletely irradiated skin cancer acts like a nutritional, mechanical, and metabolic cap, and thus recurrences following this treatment modality tend to be deep and are usually associated with greater morbidity and occasional mortality.

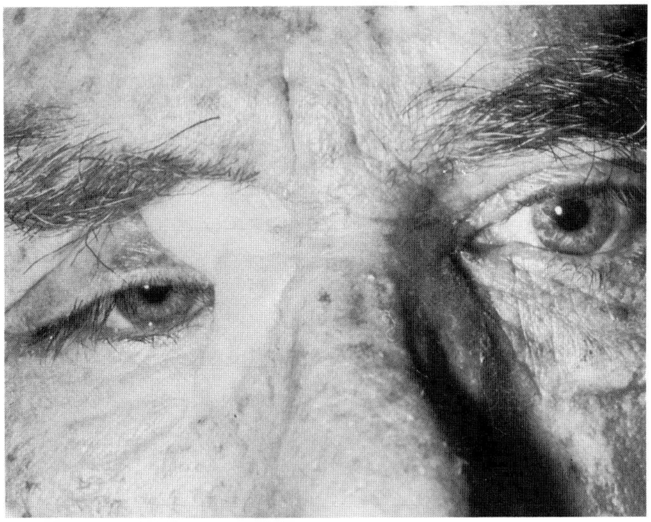

Figure 70.9. Four-year postoperative appearance following midforehead flap repair. Patient has limited versions and diplopia, but prefers vision in the immobile right eye to the cataractous left eye.

External factors may also influence the direction of the tumor growth—even the nose pads of patients who wear spectacles have been known to influence the spread of tumor cells (6).

HISTOPATHOLOGICAL ANALYSIS

The ophthalmologist lacking extensive training in skin pathology should be attuned to the influence of histologic characterization in the treatment of skin cancer. Sclerosing BCC (morpheaform) is more aggressive than nodular BCC, and deserves special consideration (12, 13). Clinically, it has ill-defined borders and may exhibit multicentricity; histologically, it can send out finger-like sinuous extensions up to 7.2 mm in length, which can result in incomplete excision and recurrence (14). Many reports on recurrent BCC document a higher percentage of morpheaform BCC. For example, 35% of BCC recurred in less than 2 years when tumor involved the surgical margin (15). Thomas (16) found an 82% recurrence rate for incompletely excised eyelid, perianal, and nasal BCC. Recurrent BCC has a 96% cure rate (6) when treated by Mohs technique compared with a 50% cure rate when treated by conventional means (17). Basal-squamous cell carcinoma is another aggressive form of BCC that has a similar clinical behavior to SCC and has a high recurrence rate similar to morpheaform BCC (18).

WHEN MOHS TECHNIQUE SURGEON IS UNAVAILABLE

Under the following circumstances, the patient should be referred to a center where the Mohs technique is available:

1. Deep orbital invasion of BCC, especially when there is bony fixation of the tumor or invasion of the lacrimal fossa and lacrimal sac;
2. Longstanding BCCs and SCCs 3 cm or greater in diameter in the medial canthal area.

When a skin cancer is confined to the lid, a modified frozen-section controlled technique can be considered in lieu of the Mohs technique. A hypothetical case would be a 5-mm nodular BCC located in the middle of the lower lid margin. This should be excised 2 mm beyond the area of clinical extension, leaving a 9 by 7 mm rectangular defect. This primary block of tissue is studied microscopically and the tumor's histologic appearance confirmed. Three 1- to 2-mm strips of tissue should then be excised from the base, medial, and lateral walls of the defect. These should be numbered and a map drawn in the operating room corresponding to their location. Preferably, the map should be drawn by the pathologist observing the procedure. The specimens should then be sectioned longitudinally, and remaining nests of positivity should be marked on the map. This method is far superior to vertical sections through the primary block (as is commonly used in conventional frozen-section analysis), which frequently miss the "silent" strand-like extensions of skin cancer.

CONCLUSION

All physicians who undertake the responsibility of managing a patient with periorbital skin cancer should know that the primary goal is complete extirpation of the cancerous process. The reconstructive effort is of secondary importance, but should not be neglected. When compared to the Mohs technique as performed by a surgeon having extensive postgraduate training in this technique, conventional frozen-sections lack control in deep extensions, especially near the orbital septum, around the peribulbar fat, along the orbital rims, and into the lacrimal excretory apparatus. Several studies document that exenteration may be required to remove carcinomas that have invaded the orbit; even this mutilating procedure has not been uniformly effective in preventing mortality. In fact, 2–10% tumor death rates from periorbital skin cancer have been reported (19, 20), so they should not be taken lightly. We believe that the Mohs technique provides state-of-the-art modality for managing periorbital skin cancer.

Prospective Pilot Study of Fourteen Patients Referred for Exenteration Who Instead Underwent Mohs Excision

In our study of 14 patients, there are seven males and seven females. The average age is 65.6 (range 32 to 87) years. The skin lesion's average size (when the patient was seen by us) was greater than 3 cm in 10 patients, approximately 2.5 cm in one patient, 2 cm in two patients, and 2 mm in another patient. The medial canthal area was involved in seven patients (50%), the lower eyelid in four patients (29%), the upper eyelid in two patients (14%), and the lateral canthal area in one patient (7%). The average length of time the lesion was known to be present was 13 years (6 months to 46 years); the median time was 6 years. One patient with an extensive nodular basal cell carcinoma (BCC) was unsure as to the length of time the lesion had been present.

Sclerosing BCC was present in six patients, and nodular BCC was present in five; one patient had a pigmented BCC, and two patients had squamous cell carcinoma (SCC). Eleven of the 14 patients (79%) underwent previous treatment with radiation, excision, or both; thus we first saw these lesions when they were recurrences. Of these 11 recurrent tumors, five were sclerosing BCC, four nodular BCC, and two SCC.

Two of the five patients with recurrent sclerosing BCC underwent previous radiation; the other three had incomplete excisions, although this was not recognized at the time. One of the four patients with nodular BCC had been previously irradiated, and the other three had inadequate excisions. One of the two patients with BCC had been irradiated, and the other had incomplete excision.

Eleven of these 14 patients had clinical tumor fixation to the orbital rim; seven underwent resection of the orbital rim together with the adjacent orbital wall. Removal of the periosteum was effective in removing all microscopic extensions of the tumor in the other four patients. The ethmoid and lacrimal were the most frequently resected bones. One patient underwent resection of one-half of the maxilla in addition to the inferior orbital rim. Other resected bones were the nasal bone and superior orbital rim.

Two patients had tumor extension along nerve sheaths. BCC invaded the infraorbital nerve in one, which was traced from the infraorbital foramen 20–25 mm posterior to the inferior orbital rim. The other patient had SCC with invasion of the supraorbital nerve; it extended 15 mm posterior to the rim along the orbital roof subperiosteally. We were able to resect both tumors with the Mohs technique and have so far avoided exenteration.

Seven of the 14 patients had involvement of the lacrimal excretory system including the common canaliculus, fundus of the lacrimal sac, and proximal nasolacrimal duct. (All of those patients that underwent resection of the ethmoid and lacrimal bones were in this group.)

Three patients had postoperative diplopia with limitation of ocular motility. One of the patients had invasion of the inferior oblique muscle's capsule, and the other two had extensive invasion and scarring of the palpebral and bulbar conjunctiva which caused the restriction.

Only one recurrence, which required exenteration, has occurred in this group during the follow-up period, which averages 6 years (range 5 to 8 years). This patient had a pigmented BCC and enjoyed the use of his 20/20 eye for 5 years after reconstruction. After exenteration he has lived for 2 years without recurrence.

REFERENCES

1. Mohs FE: Chemosurgery: a microscopically controlled method of cancer excision. *Arch Surg* 42: 279–295, 1941.
2. Tromovitch, TA, Stegman SJ: Microscopically controlled excision of skin tumors: chemosurgery (Mohs): fresh-tissue technique. *Arch Dermatol* 110: 231–232, 1974.
3. Older JJ, Quickert MH, Beard C: Surgical removal of basal cell carcinoma of the eyelids utilizing frozen section control. *Trans Am Acad Ophthal Otolaryngol* 79: 658–663, 1975.
4. Cole JG: Histologically controlled excision of eyelid tumors. *Am J Ophthalmol* 70: 240–244, 1979.
5. Doxanas MT, Green WR, Iliff CE: Factors in the successful management of basal cell carcinoma of the eyelids. *Am J Ophthalmol* 91: 726–736, 1981.
6. Mohs FE: Chemosurgery: *Microscopically Controlled Surgery for Skin Cancers.* C C Thomas, Springfield, IL, 1978.
7. Mikhail GR: Chemosurgery in the treatment of skin cancer. *Int J Dermatol* 14: 33–38, 1975.
8. Cobbett JR: Recurrence of rodent ulcers after radiotherapy. *Br J Surg* 52: 347–349, 1965.
9. Zacarian SA: Cryosurgery of skin cancer: improper prospective. *J*

Dermatol Surg Oncol 1: 33–38, 1975.
10. Fraunfelder FT, Zacarian SA, Wingfield DL, et al: Results of cryotherapy for eyelid malignancies. *Am J Ophthalmol* 97: 184–188, 1984.
11. Panje WR, Ceilley RI: Influence of embrology of the midface on spread of epithelial malignancies. *Laryngoscope* 89: 1914–1920, 1979.
12. Cottel WI, Proper S: Mohs surgery, fresh-tissue technique: our technique with a review. *J Dermatol Surg Oncol* 8: 576–586, 1982.
13. Robins P: Chemosurgery: my 15 years of experience. *J Dermatol Surg Oncol* 7: 779–789, 1981.
14. Salasche SJ, Amonette R: Morpheaform basal cell epithelomas: a study of subclinical extension in a series of 51 cases. *J Dermatol Surg Oncol* 7: 387–392, 1981.
15. Gooding C, White TG, Yatsuhashi M: Significance of marginal extension in excised basal cell carcinoma. *N Engl J Med* 273: 923–925, 1965.
16. Thomas P: Treatment of basal cell carcinoma of the head and neck. *Rev Surg* July-August, 1970, pp 293–294.
17. Menn J, Robins P, Kopf AW, et al: The recurrent basal cell epithe-loma. *Arch Dermatol* 103: 628–631, 1971.
18. Swanson NA: Mohs surgery: technique, indications, applications, and the future. *Arch Dermatol* 119: 761–774, 1983.
19. Payne JW, Duke JR, Bunner R, et al: Basal cell carcinoma of the eyelids: a long term follow up study. *Arch Ophthalmol* 81: 553–558, 1969.
20. Birge HL: Cancer of the eyelids. *Arch Ophthalmol* 19: 700–708, 1939.

CHAPTER 71

Medial Canthal Reconstruction

JAY JUSTIN OLDER, M.D.

Most cases of tissue loss in the area of the medial canthus are related to tumor removal. When trauma does occur in this region, the reconstruction usually follows the same principles of repair as after tumor removal. One of the basic principles of skin cancer surgery is to remove the entire malignancy without regard to the difficulty that may be encountered when performing a subsequent reconstruction. This principle is particularly important when a tumor arises in the medial canthal area. Incomplete excision of a basal cell or squamous cell carcinoma in the area of the medial canthus might result in spread to the adjacent sinuses and, possibly, to the brain with mortality as the end result. Complete excision should be done with microscopic evaluation of all the margins, including the deep margin. When there is no evidence of any microscopic tumor invasion in the area of resection, the reconstruction should begin.

Certain structures, when sacrificed, will increase the difficulty of reconstruction. One or both canaliculi may be interrupted or completely excised. The lacrimal sac itself may be partially excised. Excision of the medial canthal tendon or excision of the medial aspect of one or both eyelids can adversely affect the final cosmetic appearance. The method of repair must consider the structures that have been removed or interrupted. The technique will depend upon the amount of excess skin available in the area and the elasticity of the skin, which is usually directly proportional to the age of the patient. The position of the medial canthal angle must be compared with the other side when considering the repair. Avoidance of telecanthus is important. Preservation of the indentation in the area of the medial canthus must be considered. A person with a prominent bridge of the nose will have a larger depression in the area of the medial canthus than a person with a flat bridge.

Large defects with involvement of one or both eyelids might require compromises when considering the type of repair intended. Reconstruction of the lacrimal drainage system will be less important in the older person since tear production decreases with age. In an older person with excess skin, advancement flaps or primary closure might be sufficient to close a large defect. However, the advancement flaps might cause anterior malposition of the medial canthal angle unless there is sufficient laxity to allow the flaps to "drop" into the area in which the medial canthal tendon attaches to the lacrimal crest.

One has to consider the direction of forces associated with scar formation. If the upper and lower horns of the medial canthal tendon are intact, but there is skin loss in the medial aspect of either eyelid, this defect must be covered. If spontaneous granulation is allowed to occur in these areas, the result will probably be ectropion of the affected eyelid.

If either one or both eyelids have full-thickness resection in the medial aspect, the eyelids have to be repositioned to the area of the medial canthal tendon so that a downward or upward malposition of the medial canthal angle will not occur. Certain flaps or grafts in the area of the medial canthus can cause blunting of the medial canthal angle if the eyelids are not placed in proper position with consideration to the forces of scar formation that will occur during the healing process.

RECONSTRUCTION TECHNIQUES

SPONTANEOUS GRANULATION

Spontaneous granulation was described in 1964 by Fox and Beard (1). The technique was first used in cases with significant bleeding after removal of large tumors in the area of the medial canthus. The reasoning at the time was that increased bleeding would cause failure of a graft to

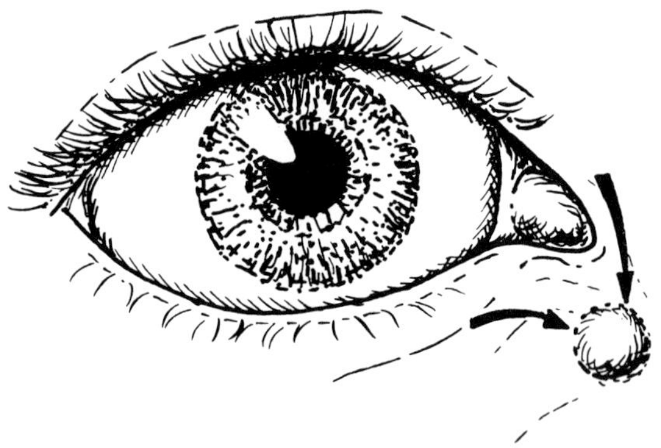

Figure 71.1. *Arrows* indicate the direction of pull by the healing process when spontaneous granulation is allowed to occur. Note that medial ectropion on the lower lid could occur with sufficient cicatrix formation in the direction of the *lower arrow*.

the involved area. Other authors (2, 3) have found this technique useful in repairing defects in the area of the medial canthus. If the defect does not involve any aspect of the upper or lower lid and is situated more toward the side of the nose than toward the lid itself, good results can be obtained by simply placing antibiotic ointments in the defect and placing a nonstick dressing[a] over the involved area. A protective crust will usually form in 5–6 days, and most defects will be well healed in 2–3 weeks.

The laxity in the tissues in the surrounding area has to be considered with this type of repair. The skin along the side of the nose is firmly attached to the underlying structures and will probably not migrate. The skin near the eyelids and near the brow will migrate toward the center of the defect, causing a tendency toward ectropion. The medial canthal angle will have a tendency to migrate in a medial to downward direction. These forces must be understood when allowing spontaneous granulation to occur (Fig. 71.1). If it appears that the final result might give a cosmetic deformity, then auxiliary repair such as advancement flaps or full-thickness skin grafts, might be employed to augment the spontaneous granulation.

If the defect involves one or both eyelids, then appropriate repair of the eyelid defects must be done in conjunction with the spontaneous granulation technique. If there is a defect in a lower lid that is less than 5 mm wide, then the lower lid can be brought medially and attached to the remains of the medial canthal tendon. If the defect is larger, then a lateral canthotomy and a cheek rotation flap or other advancement flap that releases the lateral canthal tendon attachment and allows the lid to advance medially must be employed (Fig. 71.2). The same approach applies to defects in the upper lid. However, larger defects in the upper lid may not be repaired in this way if migration of the lid medially would cause too much tension and not allow the lid to open properly (see "Advancement Flaps"). A medial tarsorrhaphy or simple attachment of the upper and lower lids medially might have to be employed instead.

In some cases there will be no medial canthal tendon or other periosteal tissues for attachment of the medial aspects of the eyelids. In these instances additional advancement flaps may have to be used for attachment of the medial aspects of the lids, or permanent sutures from the medial aspects of the upper lids to some tissue in the area of the anterior or posterior lacrimal crest could be implemented. If spontaneous granulation does not seem appropriate to fill in a large defect, the defect could be partially filled by other techniques, and spontaneous granulation could be allowed to fill in the remaining defect. (Fig. 71.3).

The texture of the skin after spontaneous granulation is usually very similar to the surrounding skin. Spontaneous granulation maintains the depression within the medial canthal angle, as well as the rest of the shape of the medial canthal angle. This is in contrast to glabella flaps, which may give a thickened medial canthal angle, or free skin grafts, which might be elevated by underlying bleeding and result in lack of definition of the depression of the medial canthal angle.

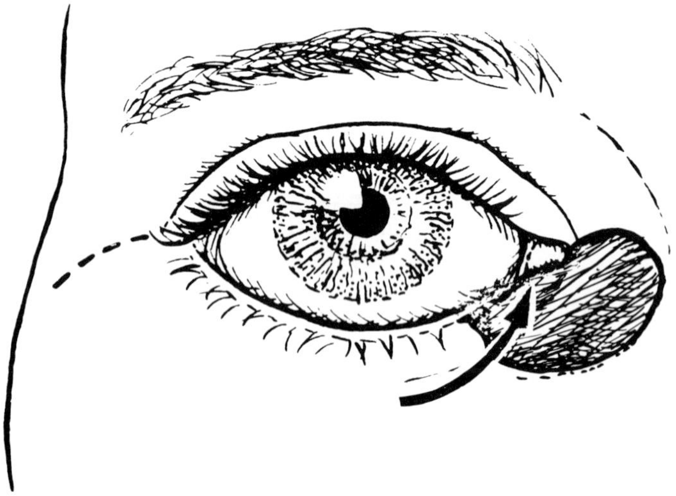

Figure 71.2. When the defect involves full-thickness eyelid as well as the medial canthal area, the eyelid should be advanced medially with release of appropriate attachments as described in the text.

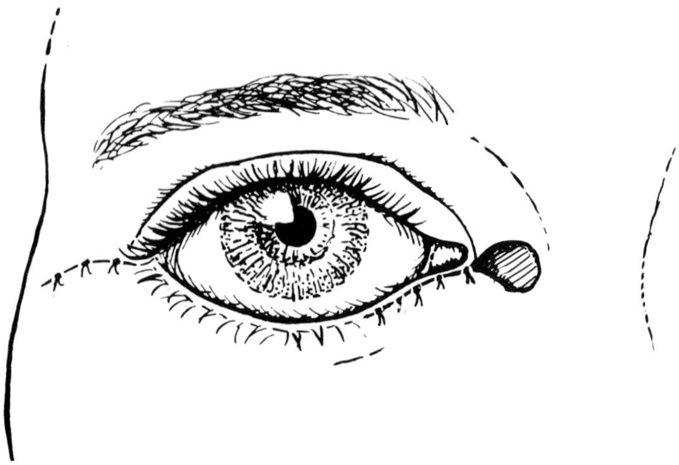

Figure 71.3. This advancement may not completely fill a defect, and spontaneous granulation can be allowed to supplement the lower lid advancement.

[a] Such as Telfa, which will not adhere to the granulating tissue.

Scar formation can cause migration of the medial canthal angle in a medial, upward, or downward direction. It can also cause ectropion of one or both eyelids. Conjunctival granulation tissue might form in the medial canthal angle. This can easily be excised. In some cases, spontaneous granulation will result in an elevated, thickened area of skin in the medial canthus rather than a smooth, contoured depression. Complete healing usually takes several weeks (Figs. 71.4–71.9).

FULL-THICKNESS SKIN GRAFTS

When the medial canthal defect has tissue upon which to place a skin graft, the chance for a good take is quite high. If the base of the defect is bone, then the chance for the skin graft to take is diminished. As with other eyelid defects that are repaired by skin grafts, the best source for skin is another eyelid or the retroauricular area. If the defect is small enough so that skin from another eyelid is

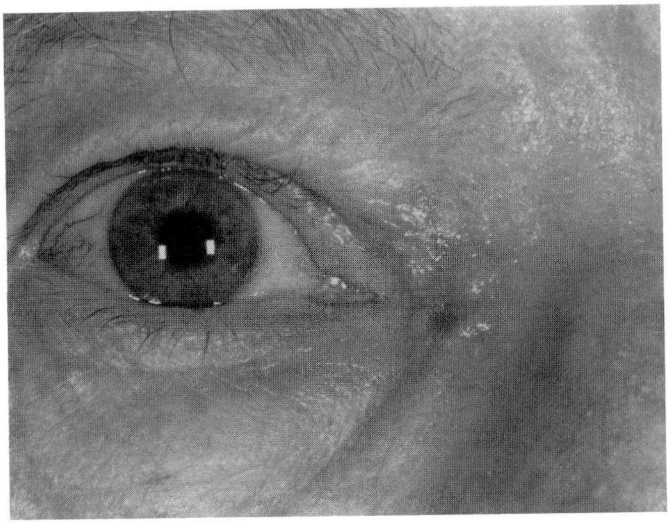

Figure 71.4. A basal cell carcinoma in the right medial canthus of a 68-year-old man.

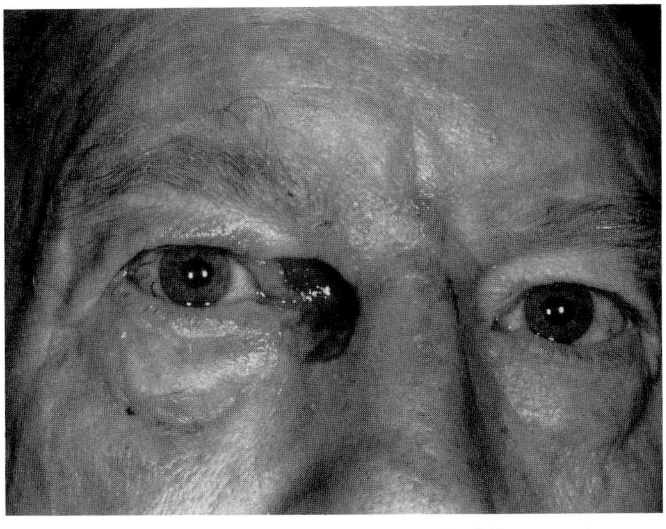

Figure 71.5. Three days after removal of the carcinoma, spontaneous granulation was used to heal the defect.

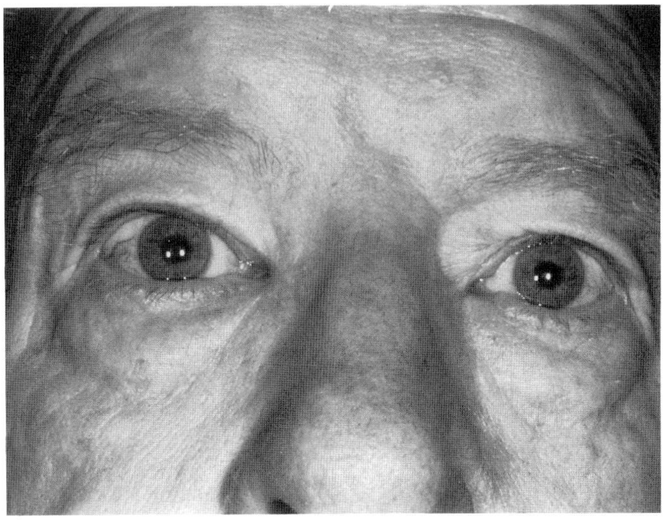

Figure 71.6. Four months after surgery.

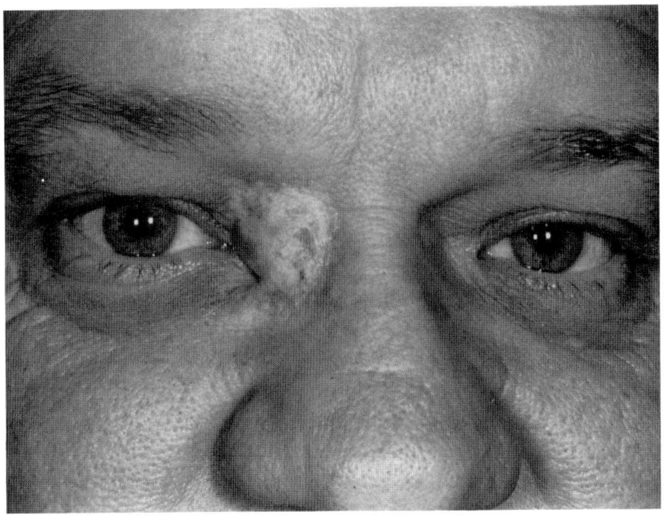

Figure 71.7. A 55-year-old man with a recurrent basal cell carcinoma in the right medial canthus.

readily available, the defect can probably be repaired using advancement flaps or spontaneous granulation. Therefore, the usual need for a skin graft arises with a relatively large defect in the medial canthal area.

After the graft is trimmed of all subcutaneous tissue, it is placed in the recipient bed, which has been prepared so as to minimize the chance for postoperative bleeding under the graft. Absorbable sutures are used to sew the graft into the deep tissues, specifically to the medial canthal tendon and nearby structures (Fig. 71.10). This is done to preserve the depression within the medial canthal angle. The graft is then sewn to the surrounding tissues using small removable sutures, such as 6-0 or 7-0 nylon. A bolster is placed over the graft and tied in place with sutures to keep the graft close to the bed to allow neovascularization to occur. If the skin of the graft has to extend onto the eyelids, care must be taken so that pressure from the bolster is not transmitted to pressure on the globe itself.

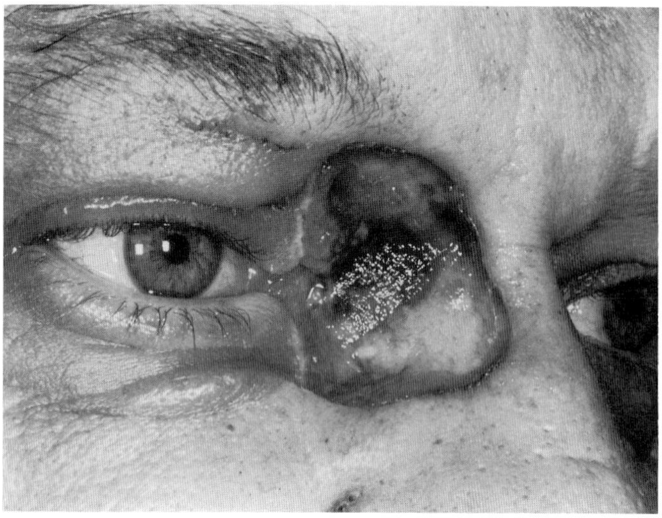

Figure 71.8. Six days after removal of the basal cell carcinoma using spontaneous granulation to fill in the majority of the defect and a small advancement skin flap in the upper lid.

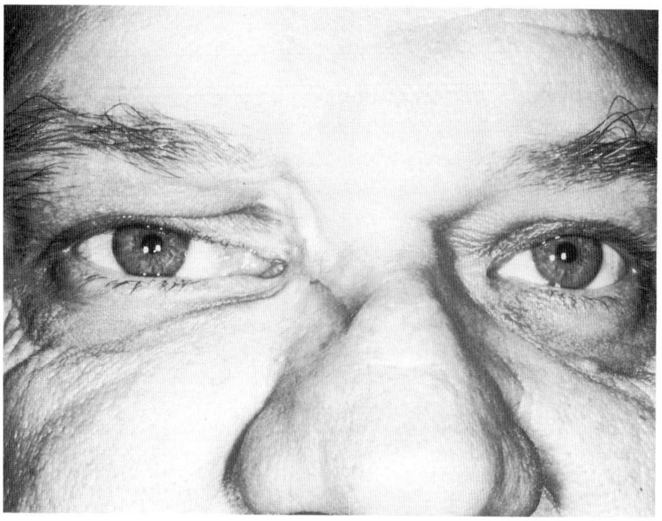

Figure 71.9. Six months after surgery.

ADVANCEMENT FLAPS

Advancement flaps are made from the adjacent tissues. They can be formed by undermining the appropriate area and advancing only skin into the defect or advancing skin and subcutaneous tissue into the defect (Fig. 71.11). If there is not sufficient skin and subcutaneous tissue to stretch properly into the defect, a skin muscle flap can be formed. This allows further advancement of the flap. The muscle and vascular bed are left attached beneath the forward aspect of the skin flap, and the posterior aspect of the advancement flap is freed from the underlying tissues so that the skin can be advanced into the defect. The area from which the flap was taken is closed primarily.

A single skin muscle flap or multiple skin muscle flaps can be used, depending upon the amount of available surrounding tissue and the size of the defect that must be closed. As with free grafts, care must be taken to attach the advanced skin to the underlying medial canthal tendon or surrounding tissues to preserve the depression in the medial canthus. The shape of the skin muscle flaps can very according to the amount of donor tissue available and the shape and size of the defect (Fig. 71.12).

If the medial aspect of the upper and lower lids are involved in a medial canthal tumor, the repair becomes more difficult. The lower lid defect can be repaired with an advancement flap such as a Tenzel type or a mini-Mustardé flap, in which the remaining lower lid is advanced medially by cutting the inferior horn of the lateral canthal tendon and forming the skin muscle flap from the tissue lateral to the lateral canthal angle (Fig. 71.2). If the upper lid is also involved, an advancement flap might be done. However, this is often more difficult and would result in significant ptosis. Therefore, a modification of the tarsoconjunctival flap can be done. The tarsoconjunctival flap can be brought from the superior aspect of the remaining tarsus medially into the upper lid defect and then covered with adjacent skin.

If it does not seem appropriate to do an advancement flap in the lower lid, then the tarsoconjunctival flap can be brought from the upper lid into the lower lid as one would do with a modified Hughes procedure, and the entire defect can then be covered with skin from surrounding areas or a free skin graft. When appropriate healing has occurred, usually in 6 weeks, the tarsoconjunctival flap with appropriate skin covering can then be divided to form the new medial canthal angle.

ROTATION FLAPS

As with the myocutaneous flaps, the rotation flaps depend upon the availability and the relative laxity of the surrounding tissues. The midforehead glabellar flap has been popular for reconstruction of the medial canthal area for many years. This rotation flap is designed in the midforehead region (Figs. 71.13 and 71.14). After the skin and subcutaneous tissue is freed from the forehead, the tissue is rotated into the medial canthal defect. The size of the flap will depend on the size of the defect to be

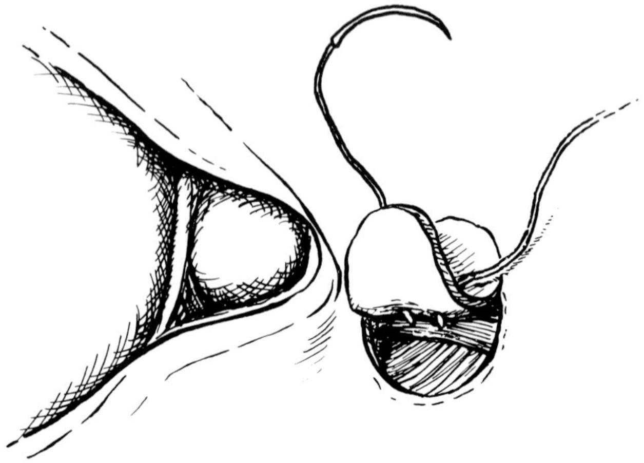

Figure 71.10. The full-thickness skin graft is sewn to the deep tissues using long-lasting absorbable sutures so as to maintain the normal depression within the medial canthal angle.

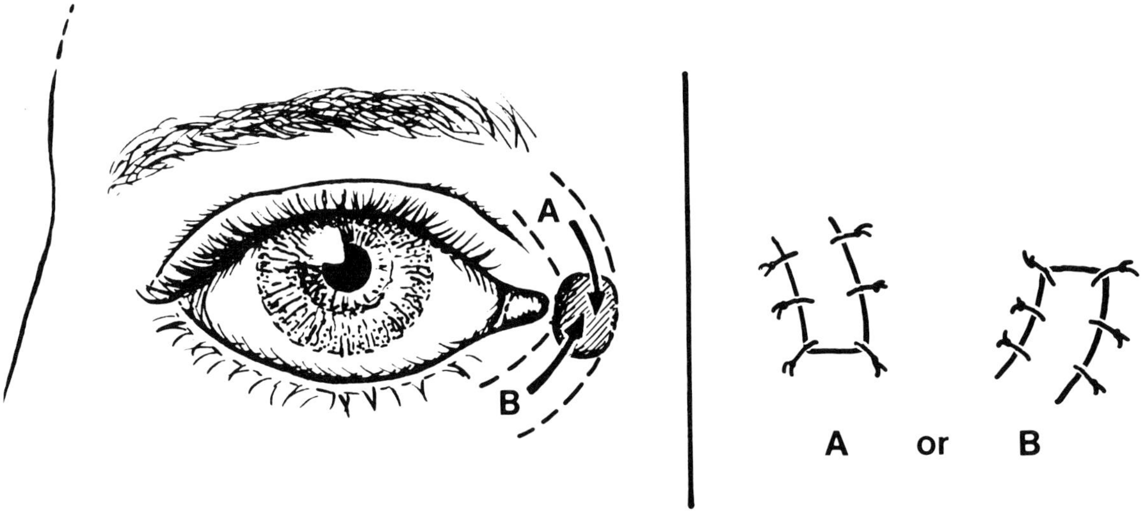

Figure 71.11. Advancement flaps of skin or skin and subcutaneous tissue are shown filling in a medial canthal defect. One flap or multiple flaps can be fashioned to cover the area of surgical incision.

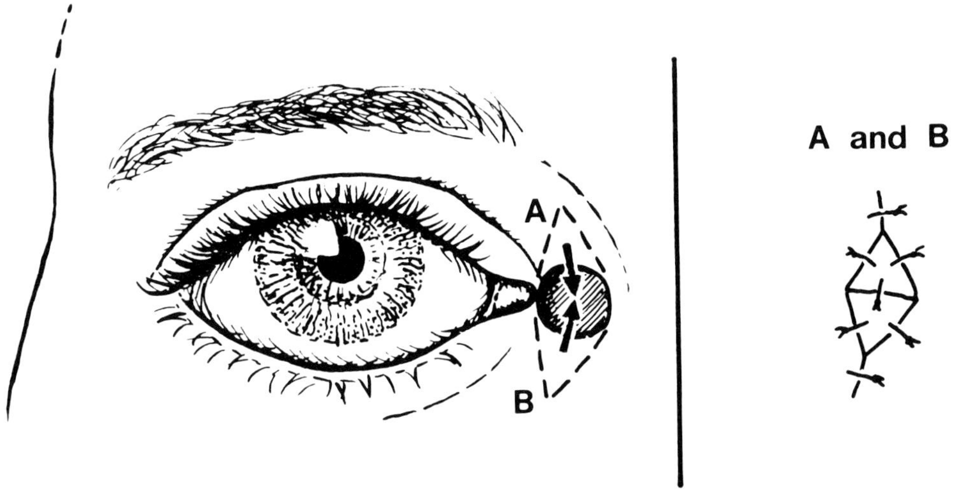

Figure 71.12. Myocutaneous flaps can be fashioned to fill the defect in the medial canthal tumor repair. In this case, the skin is completely freed of surrounding skin. The blood supply is carried with the underlying muscle, which is left attached at the anterior aspect of the myocutaneous flap. As with skin flaps, one or multiple myocutaneous flaps can be used to fill the defect.

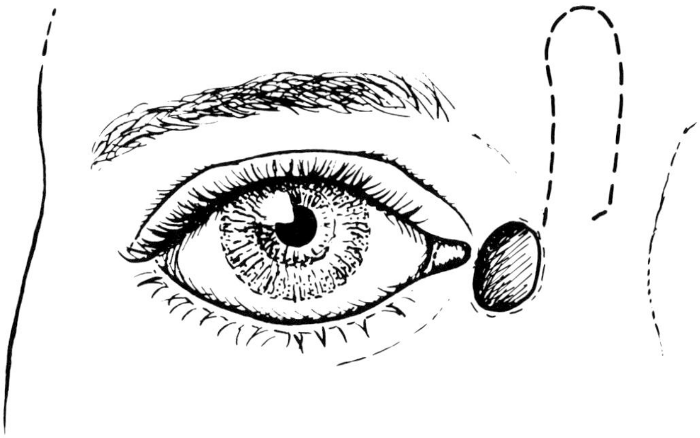

Figure 71.13. A midforehead flap is fashioned and is then rotated into the defect.

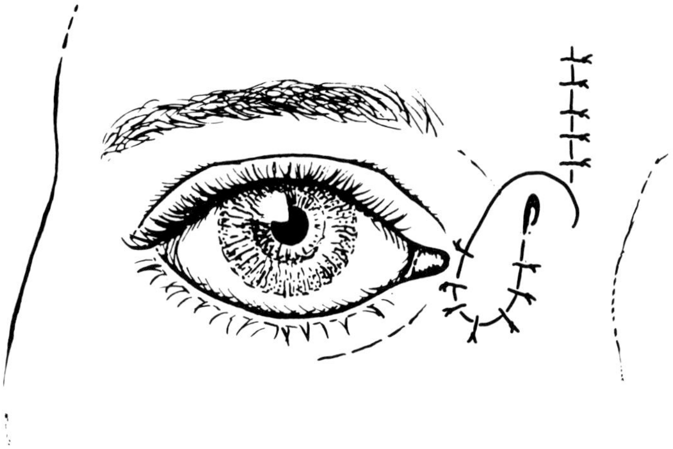

Figure 71.14. The donor site is closed primarily.

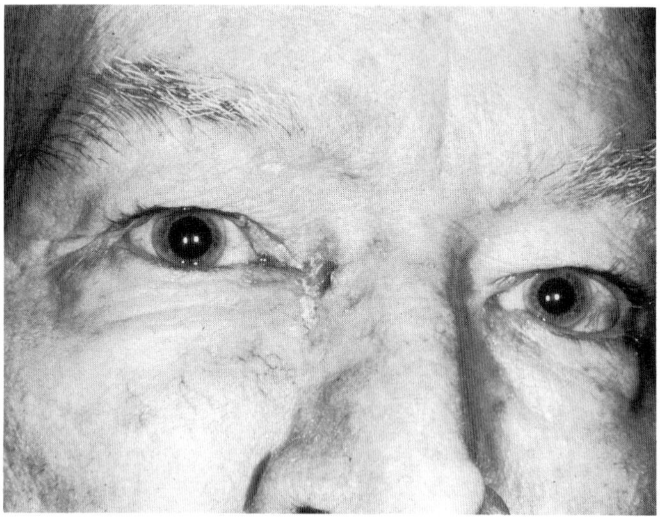

Figure 71.15. A 68-year-old man with a recurrent basal cell carcinoma in the right medial canthus. The lesion was initially treated with surgery and radiation therapy. The lesion extended to the lacrimal sac. The surgical defect, after tumor removal, was approximately 15 × 15 mm and extended to the anterior lacrimal crest and the lacrimal sac fossa.

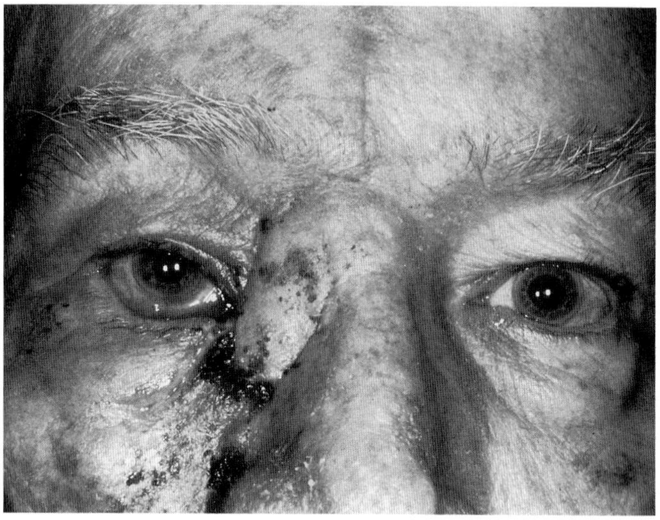

Figure 71.16. Ten days following repair of the defect with a midforehead flap.

covered. The flap is sewn into the defect in the medial canthus, and the area from which the flap has been taken is repaired with primary closure. In some cases, a secondary procedure will be needed to trim the flap in the medial canthal area and in the glabellar region (Figs. 71.15–71.18).

RHOMBOID FLAP

The rhomboid flap is also used in many types of reconstruction where a defect has been created and adjacent skin is available. The rhomboid flap can be taken from the glabellar region or other skin on the nose or forehead. Care must be taken not to rotate this type of flap from an

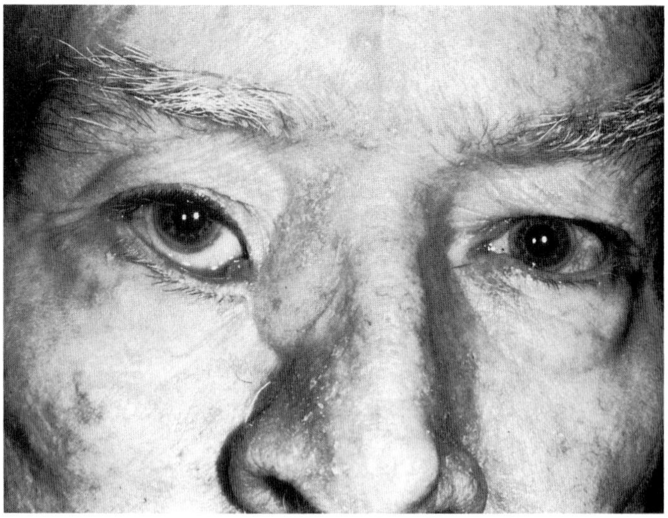

Figure 71.17. Three months following the initial repair. The medial canthus shows an inferiorly directed deformity.

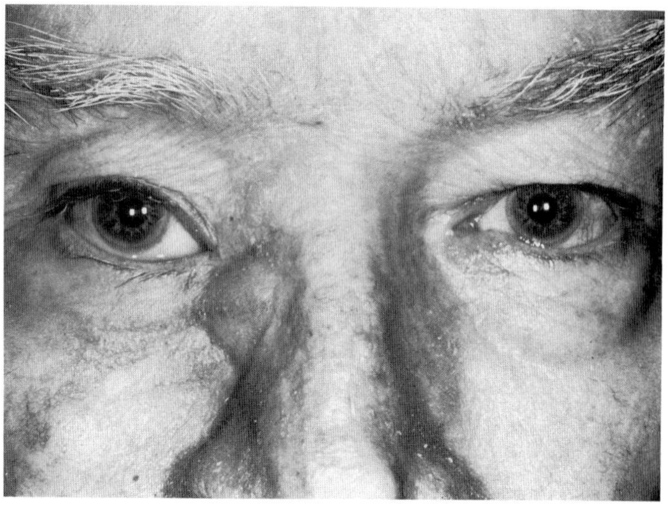

Figure 71.18. Three weeks following medial canthal reconstruction.

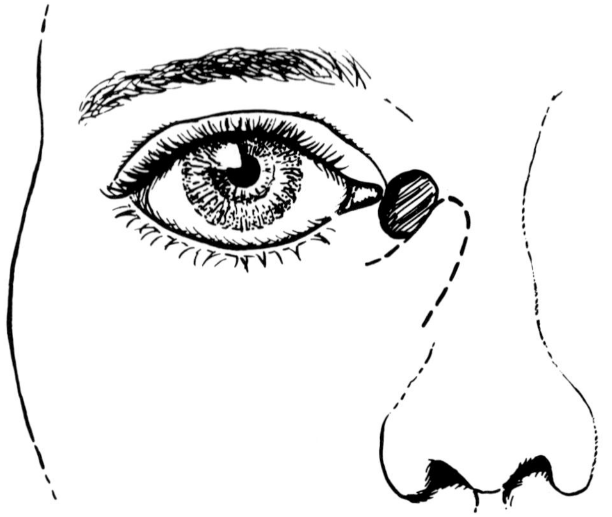

Figure 71.19. A flap from the area inferior to the defect with a base at the eyelid or eyelid cheek junction is rotated into the defect.

eyelid, where closure of the secondary defect will cause a deformity of the eyelid margin.

CHEEK ROTATION FLAP

If the medial canthal defect is in the lower aspect of the medial canthus and/or if the lower lid is involved along with the medial canthus, a rotation flap from the medial aspect of the cheek as it meets the lateral aspect of the nose can be brought superiorly into the defect (Figs. 71.19 and 71.20).

LACRIMAL SYSTEM INVOLVEMENT

Repair of the lacrimal system can be combined with most other types of reconstruction in the medial canthal area. If part of the canaliculus is interrupted, the remains of the canaliculus can be reapproximated over a silicone tube. The silicone tube, with an inside diameter of 0.0125 inches and an outside diameter of 0.025 inches, can be placed in the canaliculus and sutured to the surrounding eyelid tissues and allowed to remain in place for 1–2 weeks. If both of the canaliculi have been excised but the common canaliculus or most of the lacrimal sac remains and if sufficient conjunctiva remains, a tunnel of conjunctiva can be fashioned and wrapped around a silicone tube leading to the remains of the lacrimal system (4) (Figs. 71.21–71.24). This has been referred to as a "conjunctivoductostomy" by Mustardé (5). If these techniques for lacrimal system repair are unsuccessful and if epiphora is a problem after complete healing has occurred, then a conjunctivodacryocystorhinostomy with implantation of a Jones pyrex tube can be done at a later date.

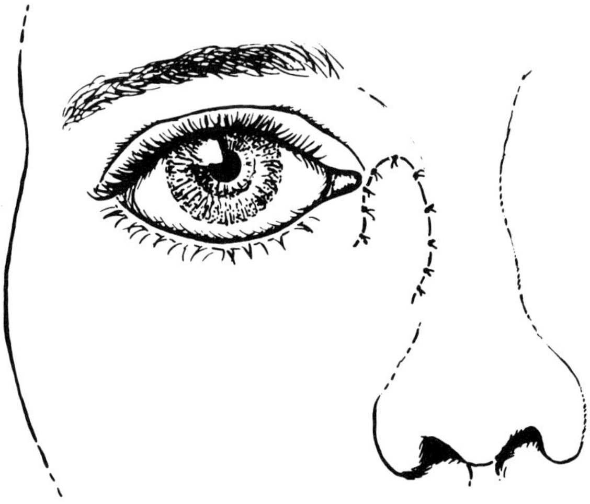

Figure 71.20. The donor site is closed primarily.

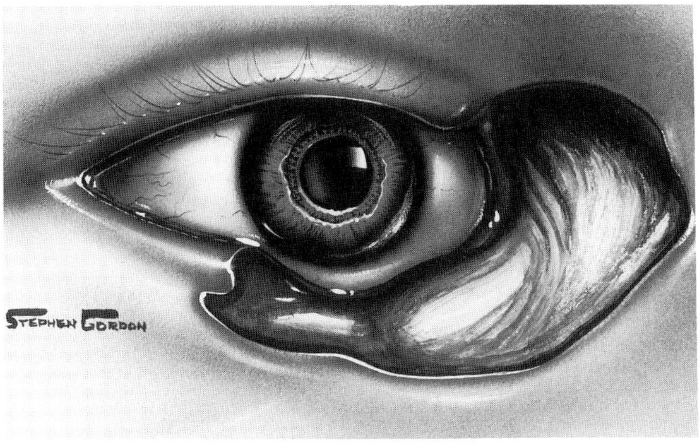

Figure 71.21. Defect left after medial canthal tumor has been resected. (From Older JJ: Treatment of the lacrimal excretory system after resection of medial canthal and eyelid tumors. *Ophthal Surg* 10: 29–34, 1979.)

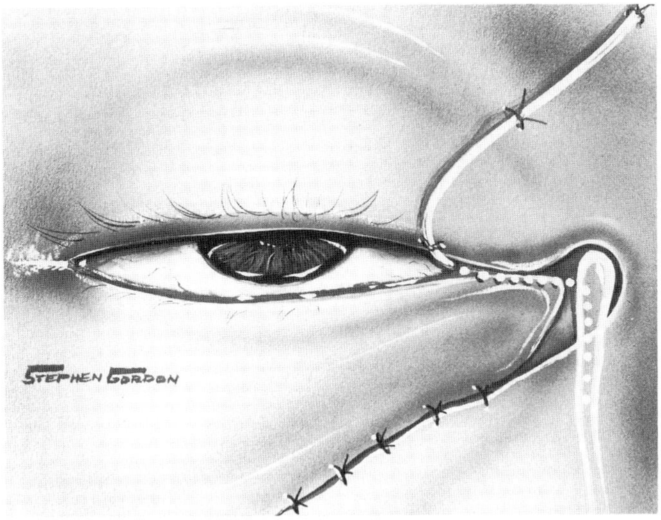

Figure 71.22. Use of silicone tube as a stent to form a reconstructed lacrimal drainage system. (From Older JJ: Treatment of the lacrimal excretory system after resection of medial canthal and eyelid tumors. *Ophthal Surg* 10: 29–34, 1979.)

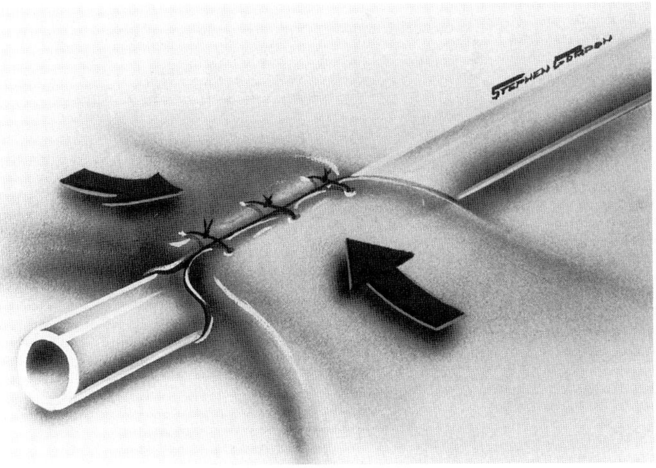

Figure 71.23. Conjunctiva being folded over silicone tube to form passage for drainage of tears. (From Older JJ: Treatment of the lacrimal excretory system after resection of medial canthal and eyelid tumors. *Ophthal Surg* 10: 29–34, 1979.)

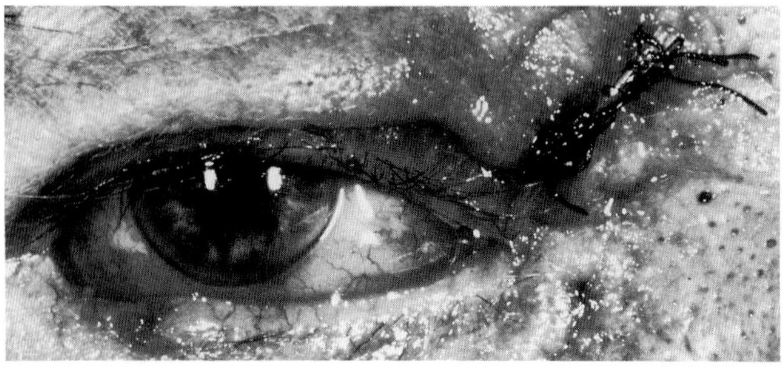

Figure 71.24. Silicone tubing in place sutured to the surrounding tissues. Photograph taken 6 weeks after surgery. (From Older JJ: Treatment of the lacrimal excretory system after resection of medial canthal and eyelid tumors. *Ophthal Surg* 10: 29–34, 1979.)

EDITOR'S COMMENT

Dr. Older describes his techniques in repair of the medial canthal area following tumor removal. It should be emphasized that medial tumors are the most serious tumors that surgeons operating on the periorbital area will encounter, and that this area has the highest morbidity and mortality of any area around the eyelid. It is important to make small perforations in the skin graft to allow for drainage of blood to prevent hematoma formation. Dr. Older emphasizes that bolster should be placed over the graft. I like to use a Telfa bolster, which does not adhere to the skin graft. One could also apply antibiotic solutions to the site of the skin graft.

Dr. Older suggests repairing the lacrimal system at the time of the medial canthal reconstruction. I strongly recommend, as he does, not to put a Jones tube in as a primary procedure. In an elderly patient one could defer any alloplastic implantation, because of the typical age-related drop in tear secretion. In a younger person I try to use some sort of exteriorization of the conjunctiva to allow for drainage. If that fails, Dr. Older has suggested a conjunctivodacryocystorhinostomy.

REFERENCES

1. Fox SA, Beard C: Spontaneous lid repair. *Am J Ophthalmol* 48: 947–952, 1964.
2. Fier RH, Older JJ: Spontaneous repair of the medial canthus after removal of basal cell carcinoma. *Ophthal Surg* 13: 737–740, 1982.
3. Harrington JN: Reconstruction of the medial canthus by spontaneous granulation (laissez-faire): a review. *Ann Ophthalmol* 14: 956–970, 1982.
4. Older JJ: Treatment of the lacrimal excretory system after resection of medial canthal and eyelid tumors. *Ophthal Surg* 10: 29–34, 1979.
5. Mustardé JC: *Repair and Reconstruction in the Orbital Region-A Practical Guide*, ed 2. Edinburgh, Churchill Livingstone, 1980, p 169–182.

CHAPTER 72

Symblepharon

RODNEY W. McCARTHY, M.D.

Of Greek origin, symblepharon (*syn*, together; *blepharon*, eyelid) denotes an adhesion of one or both lids to the eyeball (1). A union of tissue between the lid and globe, sparing the fornix, is termed an *anterior symblepharon*, whereas adhesions involving the fornix describe a *posterior symblepharon*. The symblepharon may be segmental, creating a web configuration, or may be diffuse with complete forniceal obliteration leading to ankyloblepharon (2).

ETIOLOGY

Symblepharon may arise from a disparate group of etiologies including trauma, infection, drugs, inflammation, and autoimmune disease (Table 72.1). Alkali and acid burns (2) and thermal injuries (2) frequently denude wide areas of bulbar and palpebral conjunctiva, forming extensive posterior symblepharon. Combined lid-globe laceration may result in localized anterior symblepharon. Repair of large lid defects following trauma or tumor excision may iatrogenically induce conjunctival adhesions. Symblepharon formation following pterygium excision and β-radiation has been reported at a 6% level in one large series (3). Radiation injury may produce conjunctival shrinkage (2) and cryotherapy for trichiasis has resulted in symblepharon formation or acceleration (4, 5).

In severe deepithelizing membranous conjunctivitides and herpetic zosteriform eruptions, ubiquitous conjunctival adhesions may develop, whereas in late trachoma, usually the upper fornix is preferentially involved as opposed to the lower fornix symblepharon that may follow chronic staphylococcal blepharoconjunctivitis.

Irreversible unilateral conjunctival cicatrization similar to ocular cicatricial pemphigoid may occur from long-term usage of idoxuridine (IDU) (6). Similar chronic toxic or allergic responses have been reported with topical miotics such as echothiophate iodide (phospholine iodide) (7), isoflurophate (DFP), furtrethonium (Furmethide) (8) and pilocarpine (9). Administration of topical epinephrine (10) as well as oral practolol have likewise resulted in conjunctival shrinkage (9).

Noninfectious inflammatory diseases such as sarcoid (11), Sjogren's syndrome (12) and postvaccinal reactions have rarely been reported to form primary symblepharon.

Ocular cicatricial pemphigoid (OCP), the most frequent cause of nontraumatic symblepharon, is the ophthalmic manifestation of a systemic disease, benign mucosal pemphigoid (BMP). The estimated incidence is 1:20,000 ophthalmic cases (2) with an average age of onset at 58 years. Young adults and children are less commonly affected by a severe form of erythema multiforme, the Stevens-Johnson syndrome. This hypersensitivity reaction to many drugs, agents, and infectious organisms (13–15) has also been reported following a typical follicular conjunctivitis secondary to an adenoviral infection with subsequent diffuse mucocutaneous disease (16).

Less commonly, symblepharon formation may occur in epidermolysis bullosa, hydroa vacciniforme and dermatitis herpetiformis; it occurs rarely in pemphigus and toxic epidermal necrolysis.

Table 72.1.
Etiology of Symblepharon

Trauma
Chemical keratoconjunctivitis (alkali, acid)
Thermal keratoconjunctivitis
Laceration of lid and globe
Surgical repair of lid defects
Pterygium excision
Irradiation
Cryosurgery
Infection
Membranous conjunctivitis (diphtheria, β-hemolytic streptococcus, pneumococcus, primary herpes simplex, adenovirus 8,19)
Trachoma, stage IV
Chronic staphylococcal blepharitis (± acne rosacea)
Herpes zoster
Drugs
Idoxuridine (IDU)
Echothiophate Iodide (phospholine iodide)
Isoflurophate (DFP)
Furtrethonium (Furmethide)
Pilocarpine
Epinephrine
Practolol
Inflammation
Sarcoid
Sjogren's syndrome
Postvaccinal
Autoimmune Disease
Ocular cicatricial pemphigoid
Stevens-Johnson syndrome
Epidermolysis bullosa
Dermatitis herpetiformis
Hydroa vacciniforme
Pemphigus
Toxic epidermal necrolysis

HISTOPATHOLOGY

The conjunctiva is composed of a superficial nonkeratinizing stratified squamous epithelium and a submucosal lamina propria. This deep lymphofibrovascular layer is firmly adherent to the entire superior tarsal plate, the upper one-half of the inferior tarsal plate and fuses with anterior Tenon's fascia to the sclera 3 mm posterior to the limbus (17). Early shrinkage of the lamina propria therefore is best observed in the more mobile fornices, notably in the shallower lower fornix.

Regardless of etiology, the common pathological feature of conjunctival shrinkage is hypertrophy of the stromal connective tissue with concomitant acute or chronic inflammation, leading to fibrous scarring and contraction (18). Destruction of only the epithelial layer is easily repaired by mitosis and sliding of the adjacent viable cells without contracture. In severe chemical and thermal burns, however, an ischemic necrosis of the lamina propria occurs with repair by granulation tissue and eventual shrinkage of the fibrovascular scars (2). In membranous conjunctivitis, an exudative fibrinous cellular membrane composed of the entire epithelium may be stripped from the lamina propria with resultant scarring. Drug-induced symblepharon also have shown subepithelial fibrosis (6). The bullae of ocular cicatricial pemphigoid form in a subepithelial location (18) with resultant damage to the epithelial basement membrane. In contrast, acantholysis is present in ocular pemphigus with rare scarring secondary to the interepithelial edema and bullae. Circulating antibodies to corneal and conjunctival epithelium and the deposition of immunoglobulin and complement on the conjunctival basement membrane strongly indicate an immunological process in the chronic progression of ocular cicatricial pemphigoid (19).

The conjunctival epithelium undergoes metaplasia with keratinization, parakeratosis, and the loss of goblet cells (18). Acute inflammation may be present with trauma, infection, and occasionally in OCP, where eosinophils are also noted. Keratinitis sicca and xerosis may ensue because of associated lacrimal duct obliteration exacerbated by trichiasis and entropion. Progressive visual loss may occur secondary to corneal punctate erosions, ulceration, pannus formation, opacification and perforation.

EXAMINATION OF PATIENT

The history of previous trauma, drug use, and severe infection may obviate a search for the cause of symblepharon; however, ocular cicatricial pemphigoid, chronic staphylococcal infection, and stage IV trachoma may present with an insidious onset. Patient complaints include chronic irritation, burning, injection, and mucoid discharge. Large webs may be cosmetically objectionable or may limit ocular ductions with resultant diplopia. The late sequellae may result in vision impairment.

Examination may indicate unilateral [trauma, drugs, herpes zoster and rarely OPC (19)] or bilateral disease. Epithelial defects with staining are seen in acute traumatic etiologies and membranous conjunctivitides but rarely in OPC and other autoimmune diseases. A poor tear film with early break-up time and whitish mucoid discharge is seen on biomicroscopy. The earliest signs of conjunctival shrinkage are finc whitish striae (2) within the lamina propria secondary to perivascular thickening and fibrosis. With further progression, placing external traction upon the lids to extend the fornices will demonstrate contracture bands or webs. (Fig. 72.1). Endstage fibrosis results in xerosis and lagophthalmos with restricted Bell's phenomenon, trichiasis and distichiasis, cicatricial entropion, pseudopterygium, ankyloblepharon, and corneal neovascularization and opacification (Fig. 72.2).

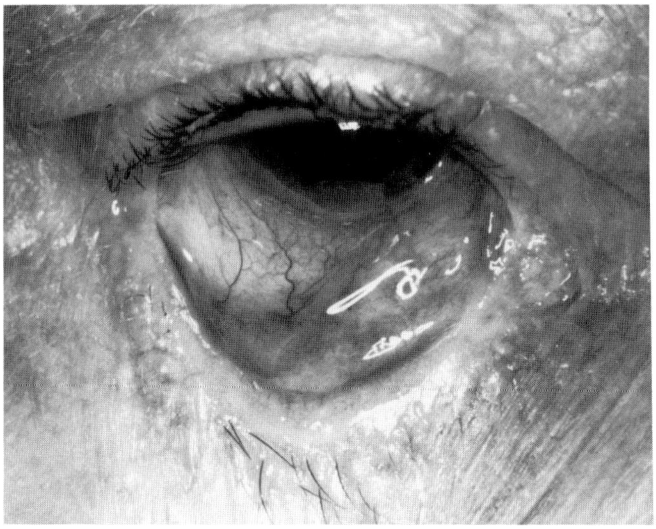

Figure 72.1. Moderate ocular cicatricial pemphigoid with a central posterior symblepharon and extensive symblepharon to the medial plica semilunaris and the lateral canthus.

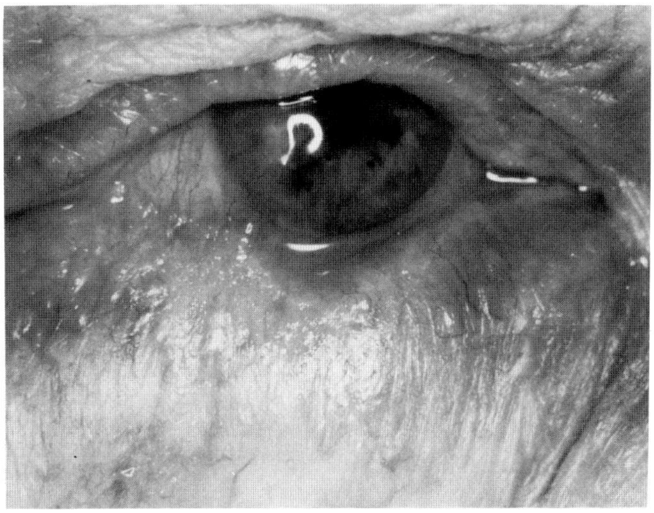

Figure 72.2. Advanced ocular cicatricial pemphigoid with obliteration of inferior fornix, trichiasis (treated by cryotherapy), severe keratitis sicca, and corneal neovascularization.

MEDICAL TREATMENT

Early recognition and appropriate treatment of some causes of symblepharon may prevent their development. The iatrogenically induced disease secondary to IDU or miotics, if recognized, may be ameliorated by their discontinuance prior to significant changes. Attention to avoidance of known sensitizing systemic drugs in selected patients may prevent the often severe ocular sequellae of Stevens-Johnson syndrome.

If trauma leads to conjunctival denuding on either the bulbar or palpebral surface alone, usually no symblepharon will form. However, two opposing raw surfaces will adhere. Therefore interposition of contact lenses (21), "donut conformers" (22) (Fig. 72.3), or both (23), may be required depending on the extent of the injury. The traditional method of lysis of symblepharon with a glass rod, or more recently, a thermometer (24), is usually unsatisfactory unless some form of stent is interposed. In chemical burns, prompt irrigation and debridement followed by antibiotics and corticosteroids (1st week only) may help minimize symblepharon formation.

The progressive nature of ocular cicatricial pemphigoid mandates continuous medical treatment with lubrication drops and ointments and appropriate treatment of superimposed bacterial infections. On occasion, an acute conjunctival inflammatory reaction unrelated to infection or irritation will be noted either as a discrete, hyperemic, ulcerated mound or a diffuse, chemotic, hyperemic reaction. Biopsy or other surgical procedures may initiate this reaction, which appears to respond well to high-dose systemic steroids (80–100 mg) to prevent rapid conjunctival shrinkage (25). Long-term treatment with oral steroids, sometimes in combination with cyclophosphamide, or with azothioprine or Dapsone may delay progression, especially in moderate to severe cases (26, 27). Because of possible toxicity, especially within an older population, this treatment should be carried out in conjunction with an oncologist or hematologist.

SURGICAL TREATMENT

Surgical intervention is mandated in severe conjunctival shrinkage when vision is threatened, when impaired motility results in troublesome diplopia and when scarring is grossly objectionable. If possible, it is best to delay surgery until all contracture of the scarring within the lamina propria has occurred. A rough guideline, in most cases, would include the following waiting periods:

Laceration of lid and globe Pterygium excision Drug-induced contracture Inflammatory etiology	3 months
Thermal burns Cryosurgery	6 months
Irradiation Chemical burns	1 year
OCP and other autoimmune etiologies	During a quiescent period

Although surgical correction of symblepharon may be performed alone, often, because of other associated deformities, a series of planned steps in major reconstruction must be undertaken to achieve the desired result in one or even two surgeries. Depending upon the surgeon's skill and experience, many possible combinations of procedures may be implemented, either alone or within a team (oculoplastic surgeon, optician for contact lens fitting, corneal transplant surgeon, etc.). Table 72.2 outlines some of the more common treatments one would encounter in dealing with conjunctival shrinkage. Our interest is directed toward surgical treatment of the symblepharon themselves. However, prevention of significant symblepharon formation is certainly preferable to its later surgical treatment.

In conjunction with medical therapy, prevention of early symblepharon may be augmented by use of silicone, plastic, or Saran Wrap sheets (23, 28). In place of soft contact lenses and conformers, these materials may be useful in children or uncooperative patients. The material is simply wrapped around the inner and external surfaces of one or both lids and sutured into place from the conjunctival surface with double-armed sutures in the same manner as Snellen sutures. Thin silicone sheets of 0.13 or 0.18 mm thickness are most easily used; they generally cause no corneal irritation and are removed in two weeks.

If the symblepharon is limited to essentially the bulbar or palpebral conjunctiva, relatively simple methods may

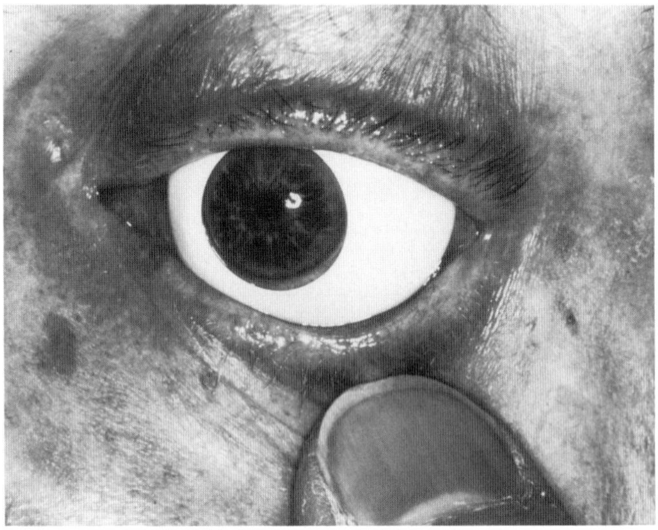

Figure 72.3. A vaulted conformer with a central opening ("donut conformer") prevents bulbar-palpebral adhesions.

Table 72.2
Treatment of symblepharon and its complications

	Symblepharon	Trichiasis	Entropion	Xerosis	Corneal Opacification
Bulbar *or* Palpebral	Z-plasty	Epilation	Tenzel procedure	Topical lubricants	Lamellar keratoplasty
	Sliding flaps	Electrocautery	Lamellar tarsoplasty	Lacri-serts	
	Bare sclera	Cryotherapy	Wies procedure	Punctal occlusion	Penetrating keratoplasty
		Excision with FTMM strip[a]	Wies procedure with full-thickness shortening (Quickert)		Epikeratoprosthesis
					Keratoprosthesis
Bulbar *and* Palpebral	Lysis with silicone sheets				
	Conjunctival transplantation				
	FTMM graft[a]				
	STMM graft[b]				
	Chondromucosal graft				

[a] Full-thickness mucous membrane
[b] Split-thickness mucous membrane

suffice. Although a Z-plasty does not increase the overall mucosal surface area, it may allow for release of strictures that limit ductions or exacerbate lagophthalmos. The central portion of the "Z" is placed along the stricture line and the arms are angled at approximately 60° to lie within the natural confines of the lids and cornea (Fig. 72.4). The subepithelial fibrous bands must be completely excised in all symblepharon surgery with care not to injure the adjacent cornea, extraocular muscles, or adnexal tissues. Forced ductions may aid in determining the adequacy of scar resection. If exposed rectus muscle is encountered, advancement of normal Tenon's tissue over its bared surface may limit subsequent contracture. The arms of the "Z" are well undermined and transposed to achieve an approximate 50% lengthening in the direction of restriction. Absorbable sutures of 6-0 plain or chromic gut must fix the conjunctiva with a deep episcleral bite to stabilize the tissues.

Advancement, rotational, or pedicle flaps (29) of many possible sizes and locations may be used if the segmental symblepharon does not exceed 5–6 mm (30). The adjoining bulbar conjunctiva or upper fornix, if healthy, is usually most suitable in flap formation. The same principles apply as that for a Z-plasty, except that donor site healing may occur by primary closure or by bare sclera technique if there is no deepithelialized opposing surface. In mobilizing the flap, especially in the upper fornix,

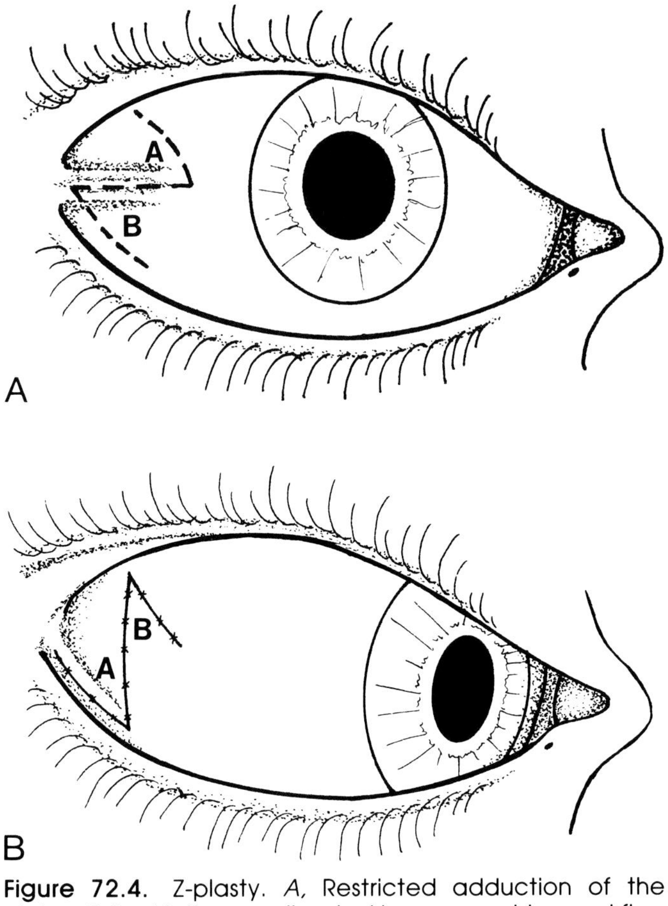

Figure 72.4. Z-plasty. *A,* Restricted adduction of the globe. *B,* Restriction ameliorated by scar excision and flap transposition.

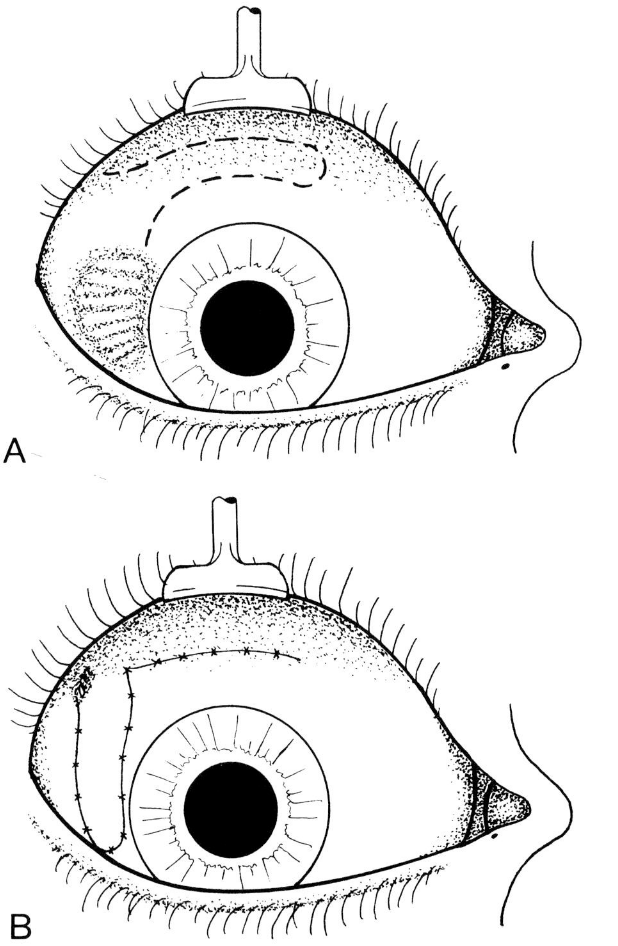

Figure 72.5. Pedicle flaps. *A,* A localized lateral bulbar scar may be excised and the upper fornix mobilized. *B,* The pedicle flap is secured by episcleral fixation with primary closure of the donor site.

injection with Xylocaine 1% with epinephrine will balloon up the conjunctiva away from the superior tarsal muscle and avoid injury. All flaps are handled with 0.12-mm tooth forceps in a gentle manner to avoid traumatizing the wound edges. Interrupted sutures with episcleral fixation usually offer a more secure placement rather than running sutures. A superior fornix donor site requires primary closure to avoid a secondary symblepharon (Fig. 72.5).

A broad but limited posterior symblepharon, especially of the lower fornix (Fig. 72.6), may be relieved by a bare sclera technique. The epithelial layer is ballooned up if possible and dissected free from the underlying scar tissue, which is completely excised. The mucosa is allowed to fill the lower fornix and is then fixed at its bulbar extent with 6-0 chromic sutures. Minimal cautery is applied to the bare sclera for hemostasis. The fornix convexity may be enhanced by a donut conformer or a polyethylene tube fixed to the lid. Postoperatively, topical medication in the form of drops is superior to ointment because of possible poor flap healing secondary to submucosal displacement of ointment.

Where extensive posterior symblepharon or ankyloble-

Figure 72.6. Bare sclera technique. *A,* The conjunctiva overlying the symblepharon is preserved if possible with complete subepithelial scar excision. *B,* The epithelial layer is recessed and fixed allowing the bulbar defect to reepithelialize.

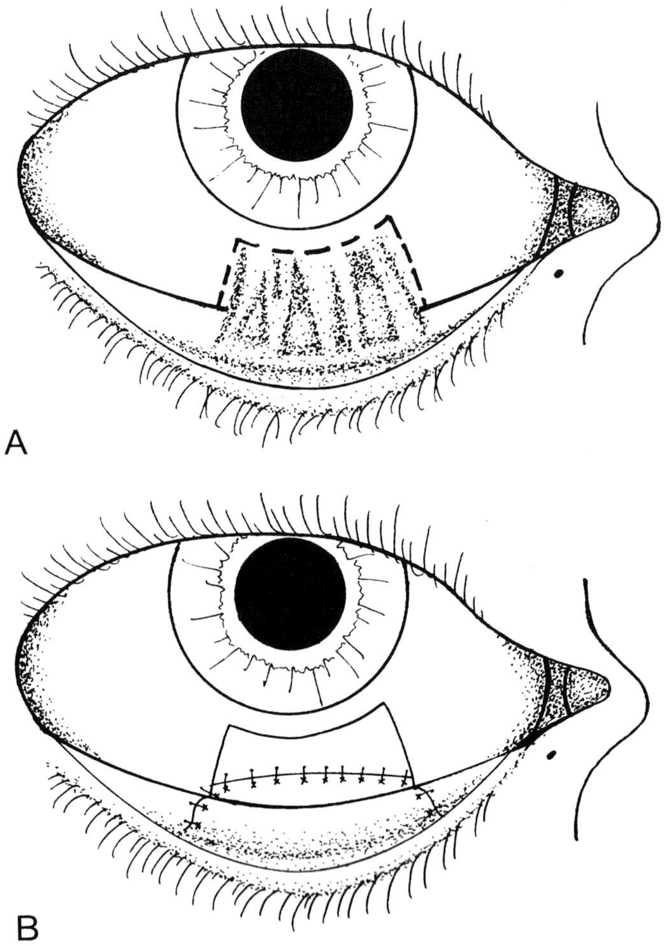

pharon exists, the former methods are inadequate and mucosal replacement is required. Some success has been reported, however, by extensive lysis of symblepharon and placement of a silicone sheet over the internal and external lid as previously discussed (31). However, it is felt that two rows of double-armed mattress sutures are needed to fix the sheets at the level of the fornix and at 4–5 mm from the lid margin. This may offer a partial solution in cases where only local anesthesia is possible and limited surgery may be carried out.

Both split-thickness (0.4 mm) and full-thickness mucous membrane grafts offer an increased mucosal surface to expand contractures and the fornices. When possible, visible bulbar tissue is best replaced by full-thickness conjunctival mucous membrane (conjunctival transplant) or split-thickness labial mucous membrane. Only the *contralateral* upper fornix may be a donor site in unilateral disease when full-thickness conjunctiva is desired. Traction sutures through the lid for eversion and a superior rectus bridle suture for inferior rotation aid in exposure. The mucosa is ballooned up and excised carefully to avoid underlying structures. A suture marker on its epithelial surface will aid in maintaining orientation. Should the free graft become disoriented, observation under high magnification will usually delineate the epithelial and subepithelial surfaces. All grafts are soaked in an antibiotic solution (e.g., Neosporin ophthalmic solution) prior to placement. A suitable systemic antibiotic is routinely administered. Split-thickness labial mucosa is usually harvested with a Castroviejo mucotome and care is taken once again in its orientation. The lip is allowed to heal spontaneously and does so with little discomfort. A last alternative is that of sublingual full-thickness mucous membrane (32), which is finer than buccal or labial mucosa.

Split-thickness grafts, however, undergo a 50% shrinkage, thereby minimizing their use in forniceal and palpebral reconstruction. Full-thickness buccal or labial mucous membranes, which contract approximately 20%, are readily available in most cases. A large buccal donor graft may measure 25–30 mm × 20 mm and allows for complete forniceal reconstruction. The assistant retracts the upper and lower lips with towel clips, and the graft is outlined with a marking pen. A Bowman probe is placed in Stensen's duct orifice to avoid injury. The mucosa is ballooned up with Xylocaine 1% with epinephrine and harvested by incision with a No. 15 Bard-Parker blade and undermining with scissors. Hemostasis is achieved with Bovie cautery on a suction-tip catheter and closure is effected with a running 2-0 chromic suture. Xylocaine jelly and mouthwash are routinely used postoperatively.

In severe contractures (Fig. 72.7), the symblepharon are lysed, all scar tissue excised, and the residual conjunctiva allowed to seek a relaxed position. The oversized (20%)

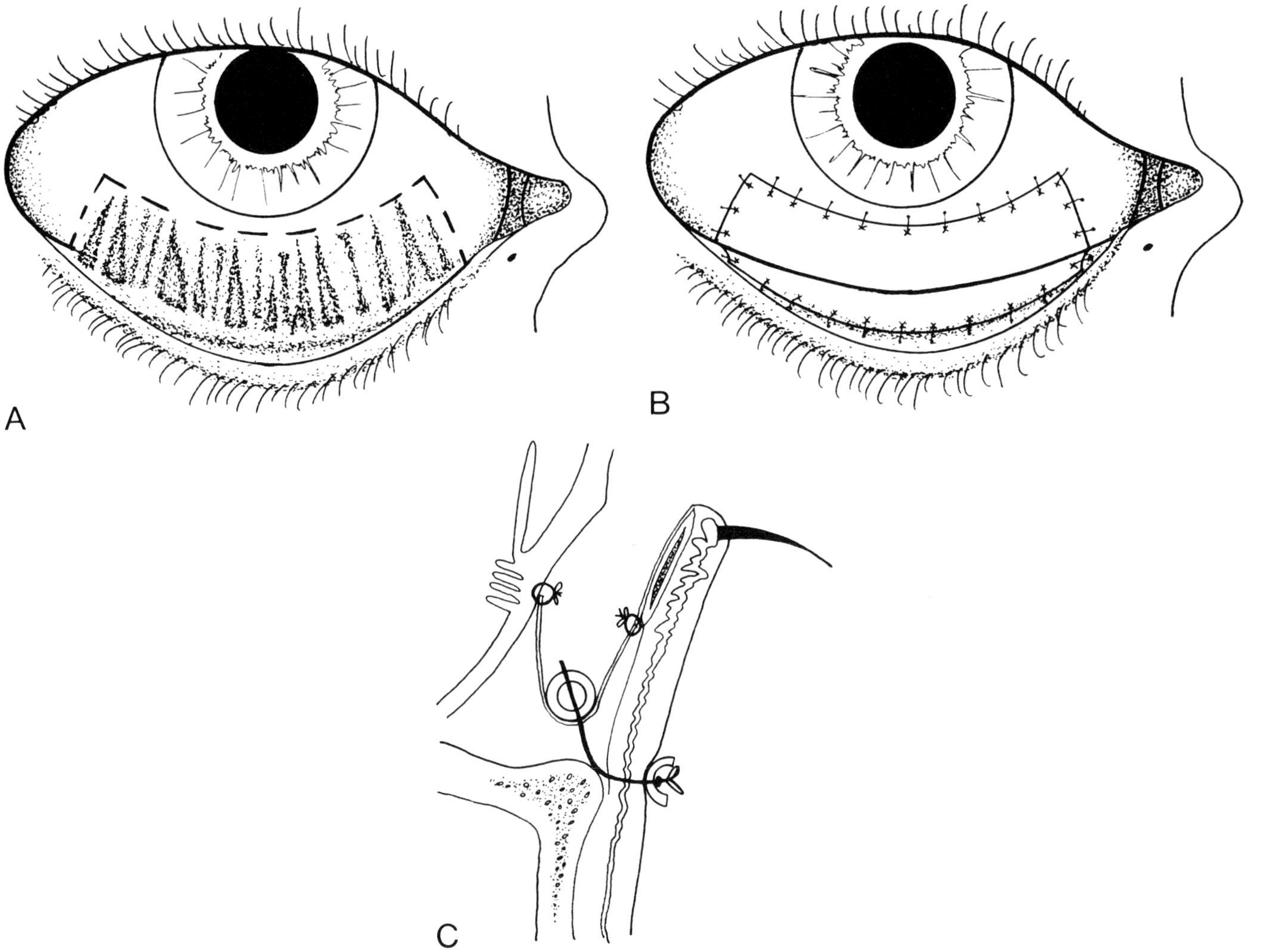

Figure 72.7. Free mucous membrane graft. *A,* The extensive posterior symblepharon is excised preserving conjunctiva where possible. *B,* A free buccal mucous membrane graft is sutured into place with *C,* an inferior stent to secure a deep fornix.

free buccal graft is sutured into place along one side with interrupted 6-0 chromic sutures and molded to the defect. A marking pen aids in delineating that portion that overlaps the normal conjunctiva, and it is excised in increments with advancing interrupted suture placement. Once completed, a stent of synthetic material (e.g., polyethylene tubing) is fixed with double-armed horizontal mattress sutures of nylon and brought out through the inferior rim periosteum and lid and tied over dental rolls or No. 41 silicone bands. The stent is removed in approximately 2–3 weeks, once the graft has become vascularized.

When the tarsal plate has undergone severe shrinkage, especially in the lower lid, a chondromucosal graft from the nasal septum not only offers mucosal expansion but also a new stable posterior lid lamella. The harvesting of the composite graft requires some skill, and its technique is well outlined elsewhere (33). The symblepharon are lysed and scar tissue excised as previously described. The lid is then split along the gray line (Fig. 72.8) to excise the deformed tarsus and overlying conjunctiva. The chondromucosal graft is trimmed to size and thinned to approximately 1–1.5 mm as the cartilaginous portion of the composite graft is usually 2–3 mm thick. An overhanging edge of mucosa 1–2 mm in length is desirable to place at the new lid margin, where it is fixed to the skin edge with 6-0 chromic sutures. The fornix may be reformed with existing conjunctiva, or further mucous membrane grafts may be added. The fornix may be stented with a polyethylene tube and horizontal mattress sutures tied externally over bolsters.

Adjunctive procedures are listed in Table 72.2. It should be noted that in ocular cicatricial pemphigoid, the success of surgical repair is limited by the continuing disease process. Cryotherapy, a very useful tool in the treatment of trichiasis, may initiate an acute inflammatory reaction and rapid shrinkage. Attentive observation and use of systemic steroids may decrease that complication. Entropion of the upper lid, if mild to moderate, may be ameliorated by tarsal wedge excision by the Tenzel technique (34); if entropion is more severe, it may require a lamellar tarsoplasty (35) or a full-thickness lid fracture and rotation (36). In the lower lid, a Wies technique, occasionally with

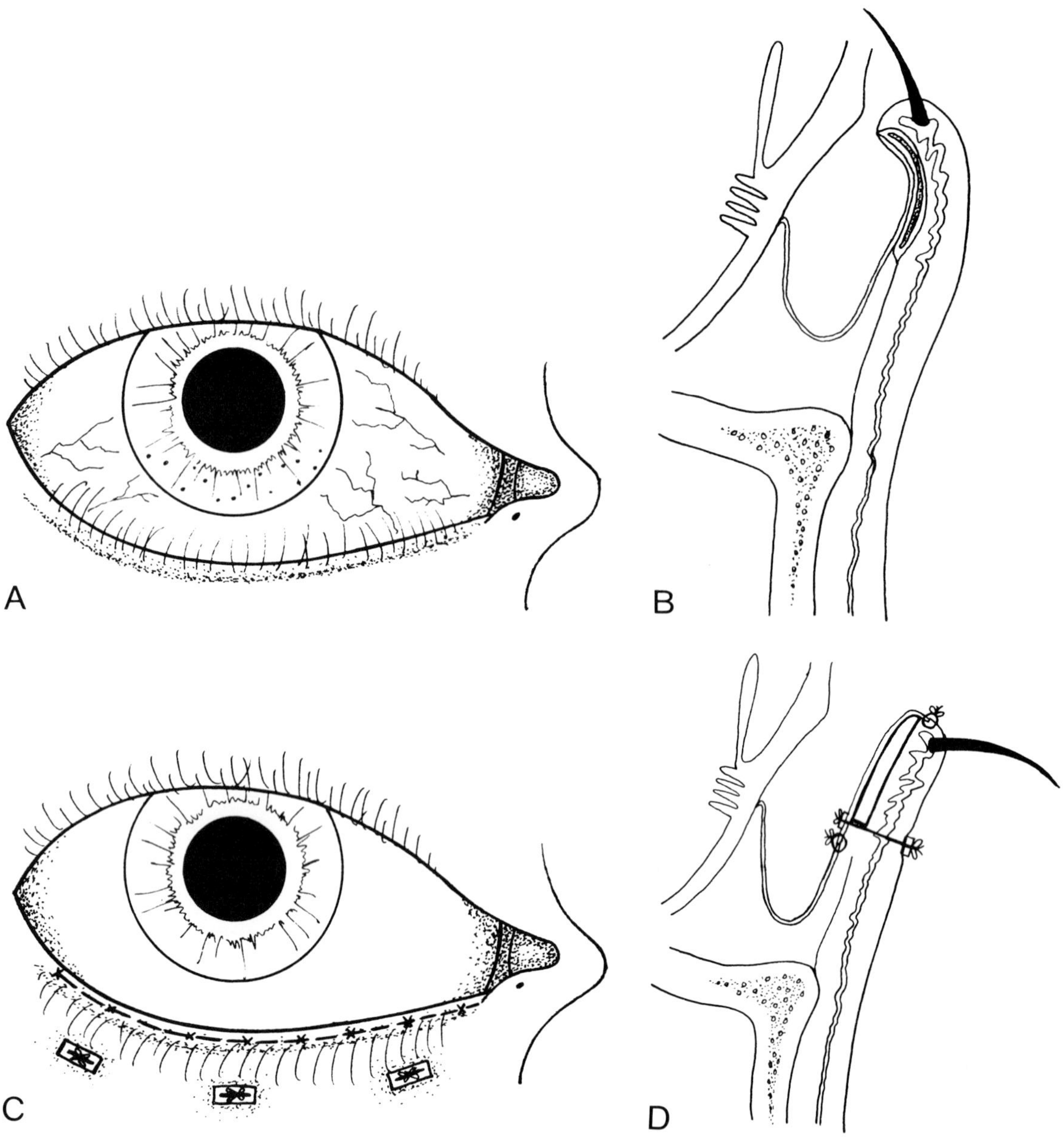

Figure 72.8. Chondromucosal graft. *A* and *B*, Trichiasis secondary to symblepharon with cicatricial entropion. *C* and *D*, A chondromucosal graft replaces both the tarsal plate anteriorly and the conjunctiva posteriorly and is fixed with full thickness mattress sutures.

full-thickness shortening [Quickert technique (33)] may be required. In corneal involvement with a pseudopterygium, a superficial keratectomy may suffice; however, with a large pannus a lamellar keratoplasty may be required (37). A strip peritomy entailing excision of 4 mm of perilimbal conjunctiva circumferentially was advocated by Sir Benjamin Rycroft, but this has not shown to be very effective in preventing corneal neovascularization and, indeed, may exacerbate OCP. Penetrating keratoplasty, epikeratoprostheses (38), and keratoprosthesis (39) may be considered in selected cases.

REFERENCES

1. *Stedman's Medical Dictionary*, ed 2. William & Wilkins, 1966, p 555.
2. Duke-Elder: *System of Ophthalmology*. St. Louis, CV Mosby, 1965, vol 8, pt 1, pp 6, 502–511, 747–776, 965–968.
3. Tarr KH, Constable IJ: Late complications of pterygium treatment. *Br J Ophthalmol* 64: 496–505, 1980.
4. Sullivan JH: The use of cryotherapy for trichiasis. *Trans Am Acad Ophthalmol Otolaryngol* 83: 708–712, 1977.
5. Wood JR, Anderson RL: Complications of cryosurgery. *Amer Ophthalmol* 89: 460–463, 1981.
6. Lass JH, Thoft RA, Dohlman CH: Idoxuridine-induced conjunctival cicatrization. *Amer Ophthalmol* 101: 747–750, 1983.
7. Patten JT, Cavenagh HD, Allansmith MR: Induced ocular pseudopemphigoid. *Am J Ophthalmol* 82: 272–276, 1976.
8. Havener W: *Ocular Pharmacology*, ed 3. St. Louis, CV Mosby, 1977, p 282.
9. Jones DB: Prospects in the management of ten deficiency states. *Trans Am Acad Ophthamol Otolaryngol* 83: 693–700, 1977.
10. Kristensen EB, Norm MS: Benign mucous membrane pemphigoid: 1. Secretion of mucous and tears. *Acad Ophthalmol* 52: 266–81, 1974.

11. Flack A: Symblepharon in sarcoidosis. *Amer J Ophthalmol* 85: 210–14, 1973.
12. Jones BR: The ocular diagnosis of benign mucous membrane pemphigoid. *Proc R Soc Med* 54: 109–110, 1961.
13. Yetiv JZ, Bianchire JR, Owens JA: Etiologic factors of the Stevens-Johnson syndrome. *South Med J* 73: 599, 1980.
14. Tonnesen MG, Soter MA: Erythema multiforme. *J Am Acad Dermatol* 1: 357, 1979.
15. Arstikaitis M: Ocular aftermath of Stevens-Johnson Syndrome. *Arch Ophthalmol* 90: 376, 1973.
16. Kiernan JP, Schamzlin DJ, Leveille AS: Stevens-Johnson syndrome associated with adenovirus conjunctivitis. *Am J Ophthalmol* 92: 543–45, 1981.
17. Wolff E: *Anatomy of the Eye and Orbit*, ed 7. Philadelphia, WB Saunders, 1976, p 205–222.
18. Fine BJ, Yanoff M: *Ocular Pathology, A Text and Atlas*, ed 2. Philadelphia, Harper & Row, 1982, 274–283.
19. Mondino BJ, Brown SI: Ocular cicatricial pemphigoid. *Ophthalmology* 88: 95–100, 1981.
20. Mondino BJ: Cicatricial pemphigoid and erythema multiforme. *Int Ophthamol Acad* 23: 69–79, 1983.
21. Citran J, Dyer JA: The use of therapeutic soft contact lenses in corneal lesions. *Mayo Clin Prac* 50: 443–52, 1975.
22. Guibor P, Smith B: Symblepharon shield. *Trans Am Acad Ophthalmol Otolaryngol* 77: 484–5, 1973.
23. Kaufman HE, Thomas EL: Prevention and treatment of symblepharon. *Am J Ophthalmol* 88: 419–423, 1979.
24. Schwab IR, Stamper RL: Symblepharon lysis with a thermometer (letter). *Am J Ophthalmol* 90: 270–1, 1980.
25. Mondino BJ, Brown SI, Lempert J, Jenkins MS: The acute manifestations of ocular cicatricial pemphigoid: diagnosis and treatment. *Ophthalmology* 86: 543–55, 1979.
26. Mondino BJ, Brown SI: Immunosuppressive therapy in ocular cicatricial pemphigoid. *Am J Ophthalmol* 98: 453–459, 1983.
23. Foster CJ, Wilson LD, Ekins MB: Immunosuppressive therapy for progressive ocular cicatricial pemphigoid. *Ophthalmology* 89: 340, 1982.
28. Choy AU, Asbell RL, Tatorka HE: Symblepharon repair using a silicone sheet implant. *Am J Ophthalmol* 9: 197–204, 1977.
29. Hughes WL: *Ophthalmic Plastic Surgery Academy Manual*, ed 2. 1976, p 70–74.
30. Soll DB: *Management of Complications in Ophthalmic Plastic Surgery.* Birmingham, AL, Aesculapius, 1976, p 70–74.
31. Ralph RA: Reconstruction of conjunctival fornices using silicone rubber sheets. *Ophthalmol Surg* 6: 55–57, 1975.
32. Tessier P, et al: *Plastic Surgery of the Orbit and Eyelids.* New York, Masson, 1981, p 392.
33. Callahan MA, Callahan A: *Ophthalmic Plastic and Orbital Surgery.* Birmingham, AL, Aesculapius, 1979, p 23–25, 88–90.
34. Tenzel RR, Miller GR, Rubenzik R: Cicatricial upper lid ectropion. *Arch Ophthalmol* 93: 999, 1975.
35. McCarthy, RW: Lamellar tarsoplasty--a new technique for correction of horizontal tarsal kink. *Ophthal Surg* 15: 859–860, 1984.
36. Wies FJ: Cicatricial entropion. *Trans Am Acad Ophthalmol Otolaryngol* 59: 503, 1955.
37. Thomas CI, Michel B, Waisman M, Levine M, Bean SF: Treatment of shrinkage disease of the conjunctiva. *Ann Ophthalmol* 6: 1289–94, 1974.
38. Kok-Van Alpen CC: Epikerotoprosthesis: *Ophthalmologica* 171: 46–49, 1975.
39. Rao GM, Blatt HC, Aquavella JV: Results of keratoprosthesis. *Am J Ophthalmol* 88: 190–196, 1979.

CHAPTER 73

Surgery of the Lateral Canthus

EUGENE O. WIGGS, M.D.

Lacerations or tissue defects due to surgery or trauma of the lateral canthus require reconstruction of the lateral canthal tendon. Failure to reconstruct or repair the lateral canthal tendon results in a rounded lateral canthus with medial displacement of the lateral canthus and sometimes ectropion of the lower lid. Where possible, skin closure should be tension free, with clean, debrided and everted edges. Lateral canthal defects also frequently involve defects of the upper and/or lower lid, and this problem is discussed later in this chapter.

RECONSTRUCTION OF THE LATERAL CANTHAL TENDON

If the lateral canthal tendon has been severed or dislocated medially due to injury or surgery, there will invariably be a rounding of the canthus. Y-V operations have been described for rounding of the lateral canthus, but in my hands this maneuver has not been successful except to treat minor skin deformities in this area. The principles are the same in reconstruction of the lateral canthus whether one is dealing with primary repair at the time of injury, late repair, or surgery. The goals are to obtain a sharp lateral canthal angle, a proper length to the palpebral fissure, and correct tension on the appropriate lid or lids. I use one of three methods to repair or reconstruct the lateral canthal tendon. In reconstruction of the lateral canthal tendon, the choice of method is frequently made for the surgeon by a process of elimination in that all but one or two methods may be impossible to use because of tissue loss or damage.

SUTURING LATERAL CANTHAL TENDON TO LATERAL ORBITAL WALL

Through a canthotomy the medial end of the severed lateral canthal tendon is tagged with a 4-0 or 5-0 monofilament nonabsorbable suture. The suture is then passed through the periorbita of the lateral orbital wall several millimeters behind the orbital rim. A rather strong sharply curved needle is needed for this maneuver and I prefer to use a Lane cleft palate needle to make this pass with the suture. The suture is then tightened, tied and cut with slight tension on the tendon so as to firmly approximate the lower lid (Fig. 73.1). If the upper crus of the lateral canthal tendon has been severed, one must be careful not to place excess tension on the tendon as cicatricial ptosis can result.

LATERAL TARSAL STRIP OPERATION

If the lateral canthal tendon has been avulsed, a tongue of tarsus and conjunctiva can be mobilized as recommended by Anderson and Gordy (1). The essence of the procedure is to perform a lateral cantholysis and pull the

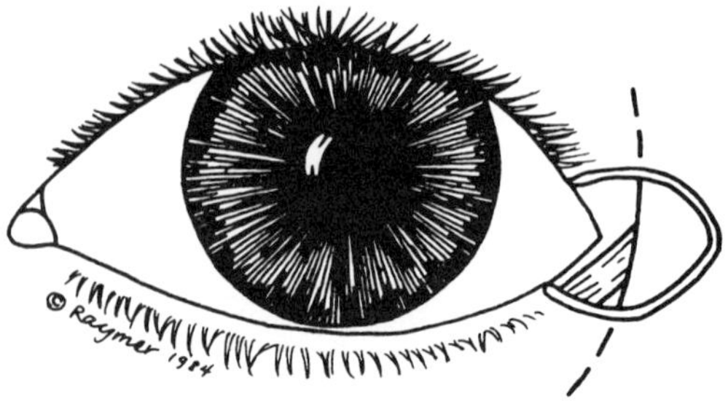

Figure 73.1. Lateral canthal tendon has been sewn to the inner aspect of the lateral orbital wall using a lateral canthotomy approach.

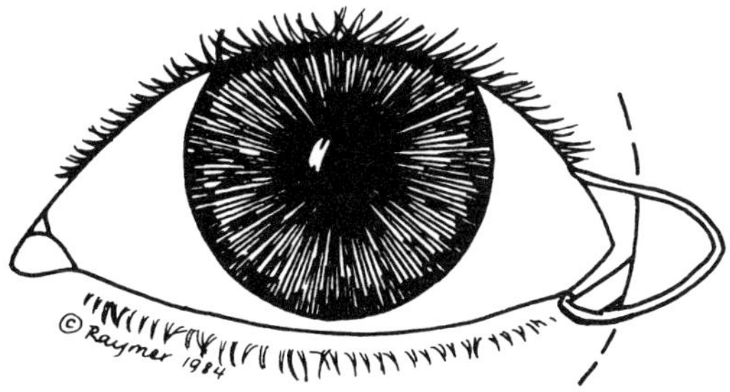

Figure 73.2. A lateral tarsal strip is sewn to the inner orbital wall.

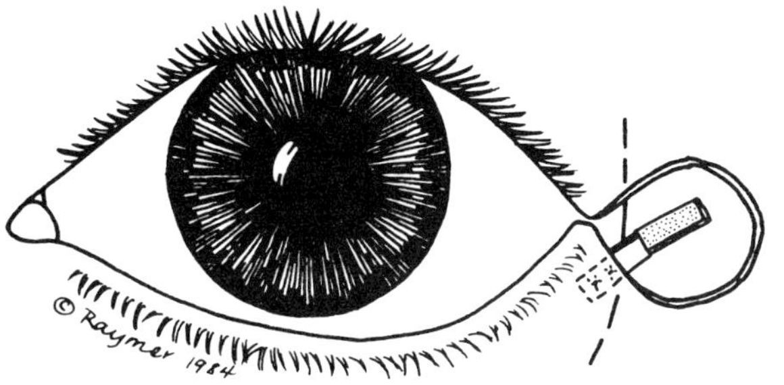

Figure 73.3. Periosteal tongue to suspend and anchor lateral canthus.

eyelid laterally until it is of proper tension against the globe. A mark is made where the eyelid strikes the apposing lid at the lateral canthal angle. Full-thickness lid margin is removed lateral to this mark, and the lid is then split into skin-muscle and tarsoconjunctival lamina. A horizontal cut is made beneath the remaining tarsal strip, and it is then denuded of epithelium posteriorly. The tarsal strip is sutured to the inner orbital wall with nonabsorbable sutures. This method may also be used to horizontally shorten an eyelid for ectropion or to correct a sagging lower lid in anophthalmos (Fig. 73.2).

PERIOSTEAL TONGUE TECHNIQUE

The periosteal tongue operation is particularly useful after tumor resection in which the lateral aspect of the eyelid(s) and lateral canthus have been sacrificed. It is also useful in traumatic avulsions. A strip of periosteum is mobilized from the lateral orbital rim, with the base of the periosteal tongue at the medial aspect of the lateral orbital rim. The periosteal strip is then anchored to the tarsus of one or both lids or to the tarsoconjunctival flap that has been advanced from the upper to the lower eyelid (Fig. 73.3). Details are described under "Repair and Reconstruction of Associated Upper and Lower Lid Defects."

REPAIR AND RECONSTRUCTION OF ASSOCIATED UPPER AND LOWER LID DEFECTS

One of three associated defects may be present with tumor resection or injury of the lateral canthus: (*a*) upper lid defects, (*b*) lower lid defects, (*c*) upper and lower lid defects. Where possible use primary closure in treating these defects rather than using a more complicated procedure.

Associated major upper lid defects can be treated by a Cutler-Beard procedure with a periosteal tongue used for a new lateral canthal tendon.

Associated major lower lid defects, such as canthal tumors that extend onto the lower eyelid or injuries that have produced tissue maceration or avulsion in these areas, can be repaired by applying basic lid and canthal surgery principles. If the lower lid defect cannot be closed by mobilizing the lid laterally, it is best repaired by advancing a tarsoconjunctival flap from the upper lid into this defect as is described for the modified Hughes procedure. It is emphasized that a tarsoconjunctival advancement flap should begin approximately 3 mm from the lid margin so as not to distort the normal lid margin and cause trichiasis. The skin defect in the lower lid can be closed by an advancement flap from below in many elderly patients, but should not usually be done in younger patients because of possible ectropion induction. A skin-muscle transposition flap based laterally can also be used to fill in the anterior laminar defect. It is emphasized that in creating an upper lid transposition flap, one must excise tissue across the whole length of the upper lid as in a blepharoplasty to avoid inducing an upper lid deformity. Unless the defect is extensive in the lower lid, a portion of the skin-muscle transposition flap will have to be sacrificed medially. A full-thickness skin graft may also be used to close the anterior lamina of the lid. The lateral canthal defect can be closed with a rhombic rotation flap (2) or a full-thickness skin graft.

Associated upper and lower lid defects can be repaired using a method by Smith and Cherubini (3). They have described a method in which an upper lid tarsoconjunctival flap is advanced downward and laterally to fill in the posterior lamina of a lower lid defect. Size 5-0 plain gut sutures secure the flap to the lower lid conjunctiva and 5-0 chromic sutures secure the flap to the lower eyelid tarsus medially. A periosteal tongue becomes the new lateral canthal tendon. The anterior lamina is covered with a flap from a contiguous area or full-thickness skin graft (Fig. 73.4).

CANTHOTOMY AND CANTHOLYSIS

LATERAL CANTHOTOMY

A straight scissors is used to cut through the skin and lateral fornix, thus splitting the lateral canthal tendon. Canthotomy has three main uses: (*a*) Canthotomy is useful in lengthening the palpebral fissure in which conjunctiva in the lateral fornix is freed up and sewn to the edges of the canthotomy using horizontal mattress sutures. A symblepharon lens kept in place for 7–10 days will help push

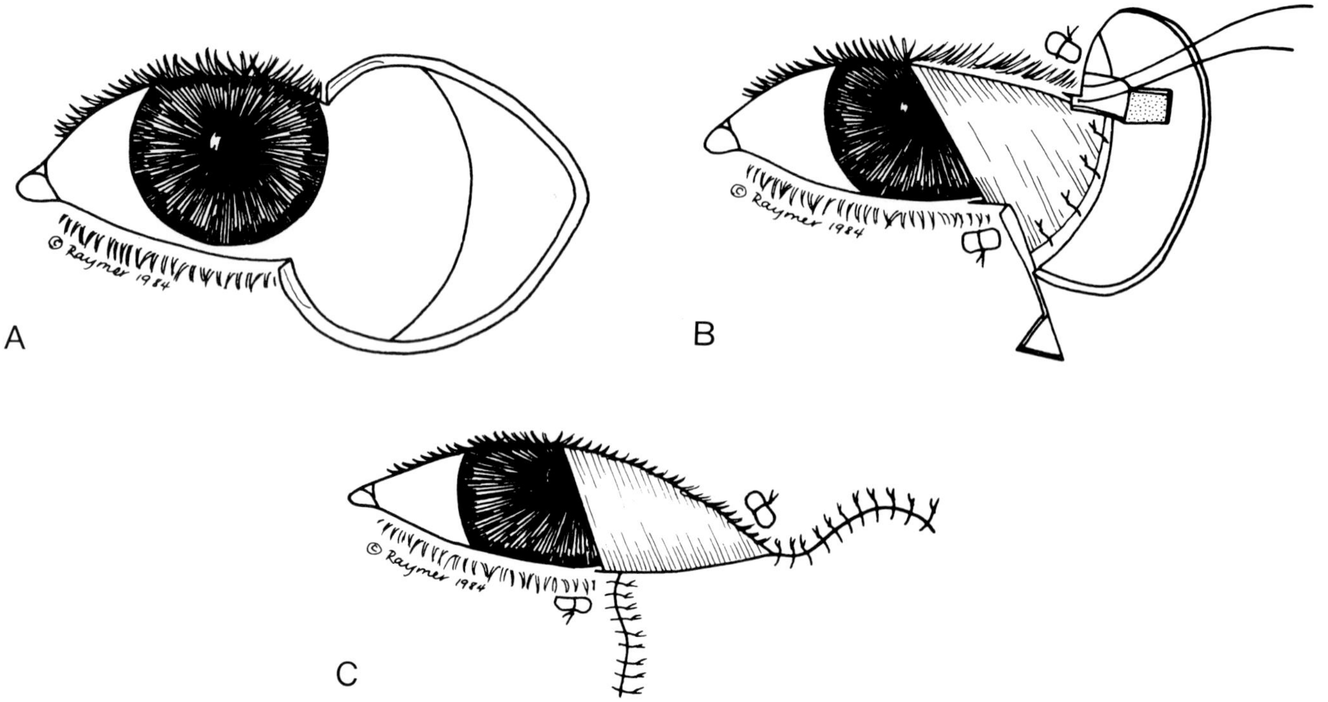

Figure 73.4. *A*, Full-thickness defect of lateral portion of upper and lower lids combined with lateral canthal defect. *B*, Upper lid tarsoconjunctival flap is sewn into defect in lower lid and secured laterally with periosteal strip. *C*, Final skin closure.

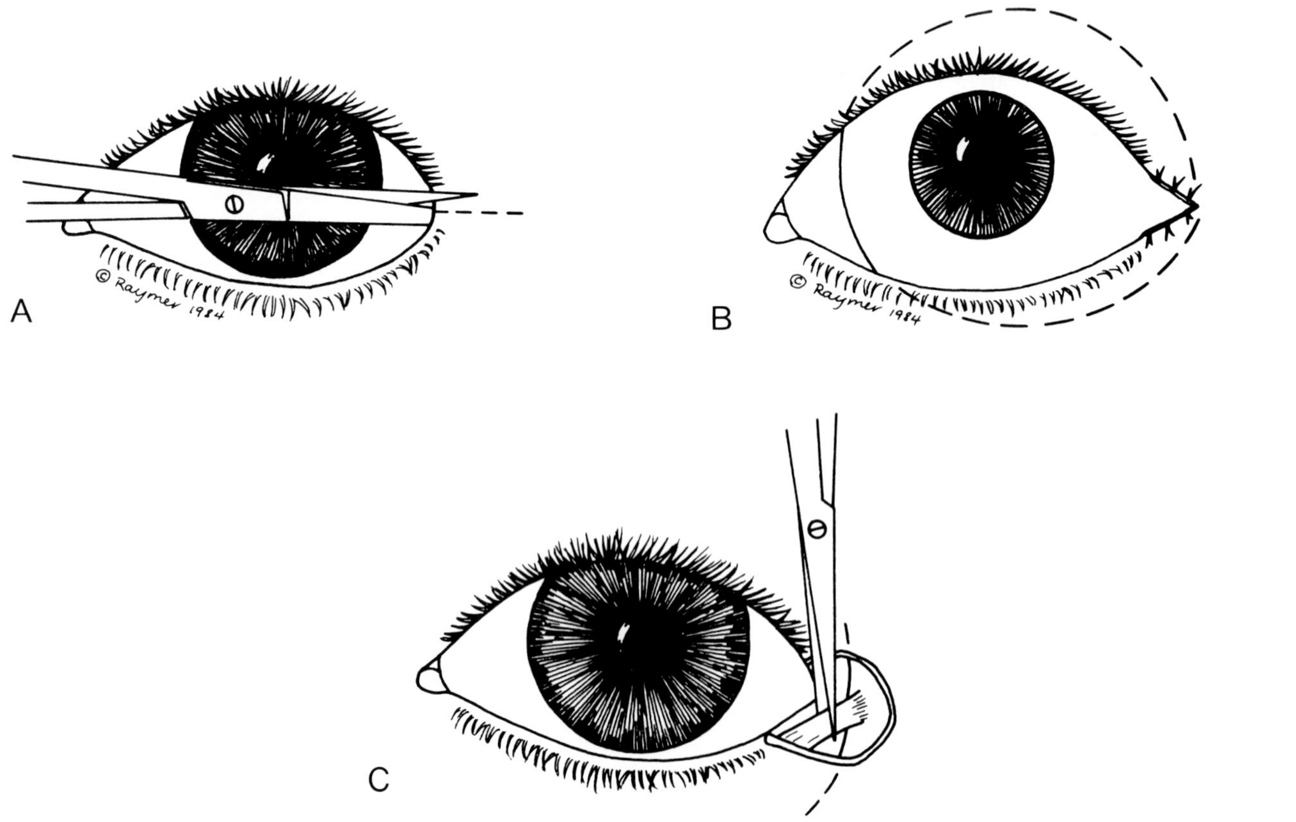

Figure 73.5. *A*, Lateral canthotomy. *B*, Conjunctiva sewn into extended lateral fornix and symblepharon lens placed between the lids and globe. *C*, Severing of inferior crus of lateral canthal tendon.

the conjunctiva into the lengthened fissure (Fig. 73.5 *A*, *B*). This procedure is useful in congenital anophthalmos to help lengthen the fissure horizontally. Congenital horizontal shortening of the fissure occurring in association with the blepharophimosis syndrome can be rectified by a medial canthoplasty or a transnasal fixation. Lateral canthal surgery is not usually necessary in blepharophimosis patients as the surgery on the medial canthus not only lengthens the fissure but reduces the telecanthus as well. (*b*) Canthotomy is useful in exposing the orbital rim and to gain access to the lateral canthal tendon. (*c*) Canthotomy is useful in intraocular surgery in rare instances where there is excessive eyelid pressure on the globe. Skin should be closed after a canthotomy in order to prevent undue postoperative discomfort for the patient. I have not found canthotomy useful in relaxing the eyelid in order to obtain a primary lid closure.

LATERAL CANTHOLYSIS

Lateral cantholysis is a technique for severing the upper or lower crus of the lateral canthal tendon to mobilize the eyelid for primary repair after tumor resection or where there has been lid avulsion due to trauma. A lateral canthotomy is performed. Then by retracting the skin, a whitish band of tissue can sometimes be seen between the skin and conjunctiva at the lateral fornix. Whether or not one visualizes this whitish tissue, the tissue between conjunctiva and skin in the lateral fornix is the lateral canthal tendon. A straight, pointed scissors is used to sever the lateral canthal tendon under direct visualization (Fig. 73.5*C*). After the tendon is severed there is a dramatic relaxation of the eyelid, which in young people mobilizes the lid about 5–6 mm and in the elderly sometimes up to one-half the lid length. The lateral canthal wound should be closed with skin sutures.

ECCENTRIC POSITIONING OF THE LATERAL CANTHUS

Upward or downward displacement of the lateral canthus can occur as a sequela of trauma or as a congenital deformity. A Z-plasty and creation of a new lateral canthal tendon or repositioning of the original tendon are the essentials of a good repair. In the illustrations shown, the lateral canthus has been displaced downward. A mark 10–12 mm long is made 2 mm from and parallel to both upper and lower lid margins laterally. The marks meet at the eccentric lateral canthal angle. A mark is then made on the skin over the lateral orbital rim about 2 mm above the proposed true canthal site. The mark is made slightly higher because the canthus tends to migrate downward postoperatively. This mark is then connected by a line to the medial aspect of the upper lid line. The area is infiltrated with local anesthesia containing epinephrine. Skin is then incised along the "Z" and the flaps are widely undermined. Hemostasis is meticulously maintained. Scar tissue is resected as necessary. Frequently with a traumatically displaced canthus there will be deep adhesions along the orbital rim that involve the septum and periosteum. To fully mobilize the lateral canthal angle one must sever and/or resect all the scar tissue. Flaps are then transposed, and deep closure is made by reconstructing a lateral canthal tendon using one of the methods described previously. Skin is closed with interrupted fine sutures (Fig. 73.6). The tips of the Z-plasty are closed with an epidermal-dermal stitch to prevent tip necrosis. The suture begins by going through the epidermis and then dermis of the recipient angle, through the dermis of the donor angle, and then back out through the dermis and epidermis of the recipient area.

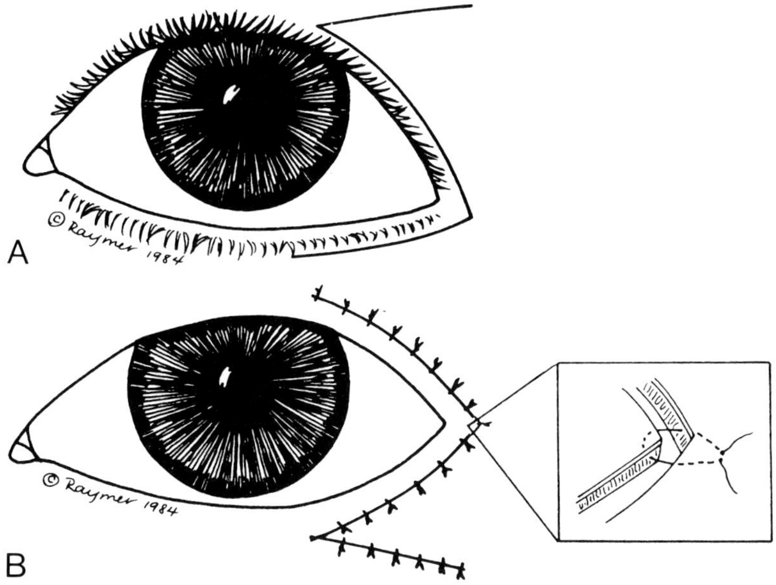

Figure 73.6. *A*, Downward displacement of the lateral canthal angle. *B*, Elevated canthus with skin closure.

LATERAL CANTHAL FLAPS

Larger defects of the lateral canthal angle that cannot be closed primarily or by an advancement flap often can be closed with a rhombic flap (2) or with a rhombus-to-W flap (4).

RHOMBIC ROTATION FLAP

"Rhomboid" is the frequent adjective used to describe this flap, but since most defects are a true rhombus, "rhombic" is a more accurate description than "rhom-

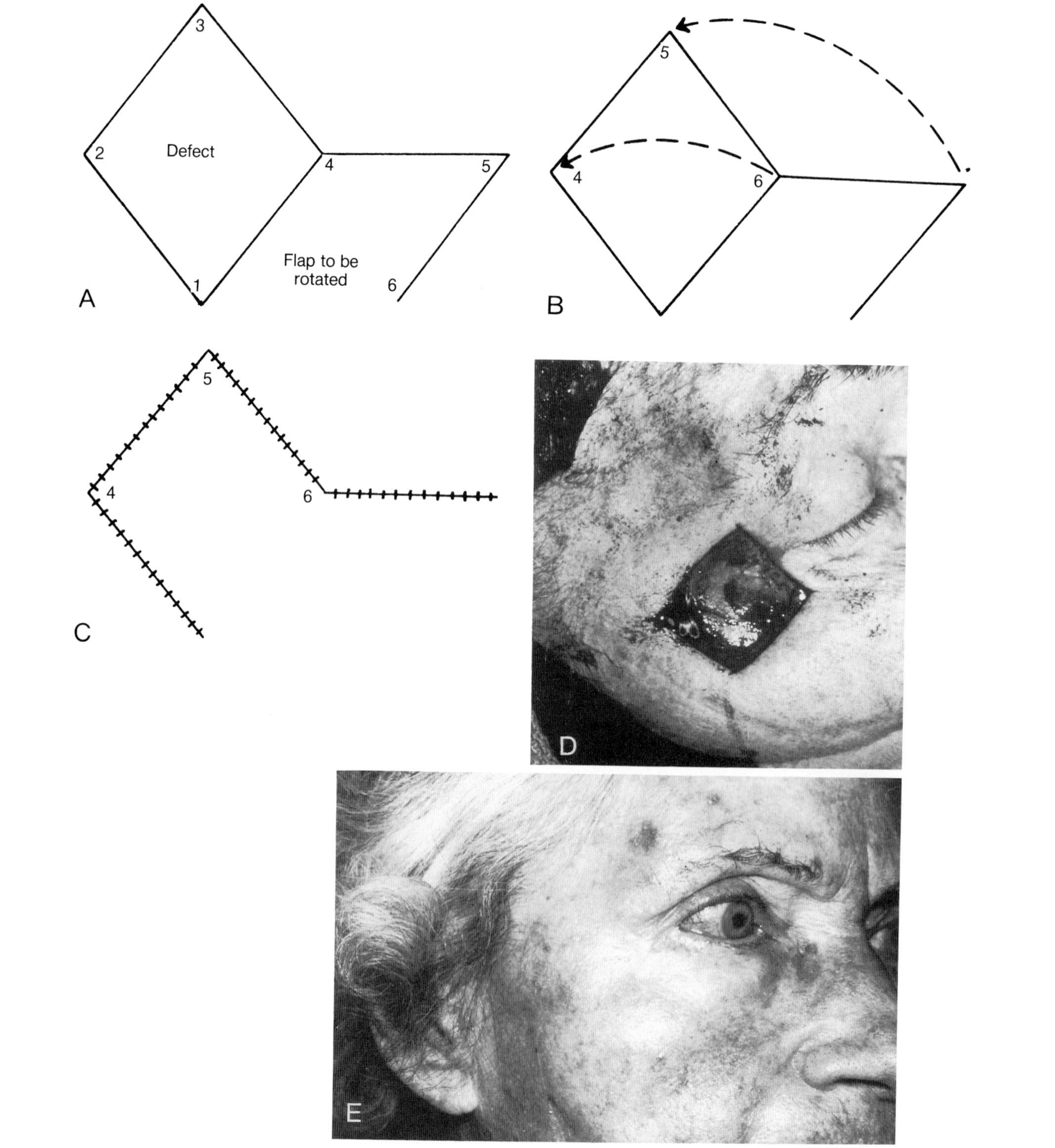

Figure 73.7. *A*, Rhombic defect and flap drawn on skin. *B*, Lines of rotation of rhombic flap. *C*, Final closure. *D*, Lateral canthal defect. *E*, Result of repair with rhombic rotation flap.

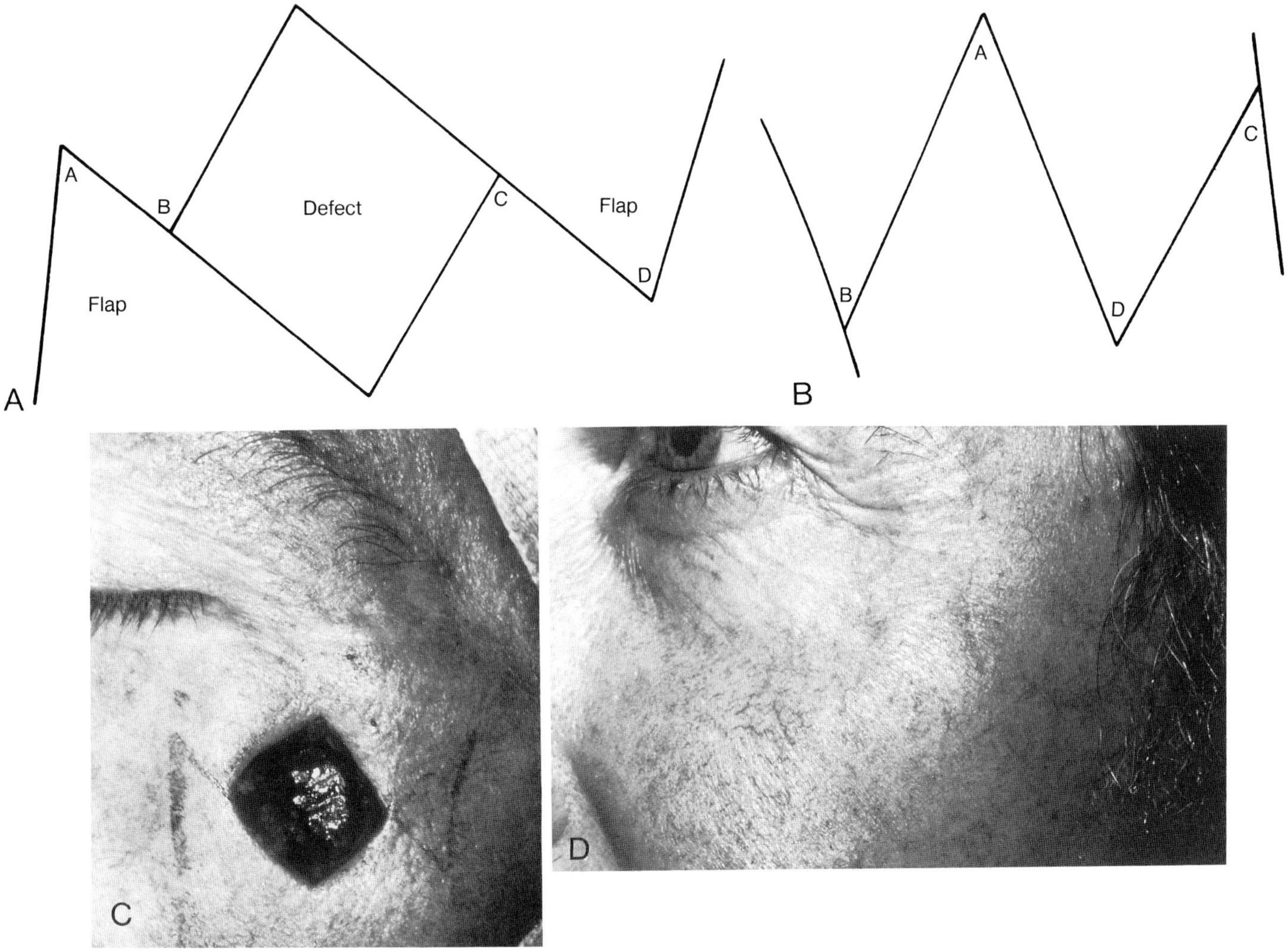

Figure 73.8. *A*, Rhombic defect with flaps drawn for W closure. *B*, Final rhombus-to-W closure. *C*, Defect from basal cell carcinoma over lateral orbital rim below canthus. *D*, Final results 6 months postoperatively. Rhombus-to-W closure.

boid" (5). If possible the lateral canthal defect should be in the shape of a rhombus with adjacent angles of 60° and 120°. Additional minimal tissue excision to convert a defect into this shape is acceptable. With skin stretching and wider undermining of the tissue, essentially square defects can sometimes be filled in with this flap. The flap is developed by drawing a line from the 120° angle into normal tissue (Fig. 73.7*A*). Note that the maximum tension is between *points 4* and *6* in the flap. This maximum tension should, where possible, be located along the line of maximum tissue elasticity. The one exception to this is that in the lower lid the execution of this principle will frequently lead to ectropion of the lower lid. To fulfill this criterion, one obviously must not induce a deformity such as displacement of an eyebrow or hairline, or ectropion. Figure 73.7*B* shows the lines of rotation of the flap into the defect. To make closure easier and reduce tension on the flap, one closes the donor defect first; I frequently use a near/far-far/near suture between *points 4* and *6*. If the skin is fairly elastic a near/far-far/near suture is not necessary. Figure 73.7*C* shows the final closure. Theoretically, one of four possible flaps are available for closing rhombic defects—two per 120° angle. If the defect is more square there are eight possible flaps that can be developed. Nonrhombic defects are generally harder to close than a rhombic defect. From a practical point of view the choice of a flap is limited by the line of maximum elasticity of the skin and the proximity of the eyebrow, hairline, eyelids, etc. An advantage of a flap such as this is that a minimal amount of normal tissue is sacrificed in tumor resection. A large elliptical excision sacrifices an undue amount of normal tissue and frequently produces an unsightly linear scar. Figure 73.7*D*, *E* shows a large lateral canthal defect and the result following a rhombic rotation flap.

RHOMBUS-TO-W CLOSURE

Rhombus-to-W closure allows closure of rhombic defects by using tissue from both sides of the defect (4). It is particularly useful in cases where a rhombic flap would induce a deformity of the eyelid, eyebrow, or hairline. Lateral and medial canthal defects are ideally suited for the rhombus-to-W closure. Figure 73.8*A* shows a tissue defect and flaps drawn on the skin from opposite sides of the defect. The four flaps are undermined, transposed, and sutured into place as shown in Figure 73.8*B*. The scar from this procedure becomes virtually imperceptible after a few months. Figure 73.8*C*, *D* shows the defect from a basal cell carcinoma and the result following the rhombus-to-W closure.

ACKNOWLEDGMENT

The author thanks Susan Raymer for preparing the illustrations for this chapter.

REFERENCES

1. Anderson RL, Gordy DD: The tarsal strip procedure. *Arch Ophthalmol* 97: 2192–2196, 1979.
2. Bullock JD, Koss N, Flagg SB: Rhomboid flap in ophthalmic plastic surgery. *Arch Ophthalmol* 90: 203–205, 1973.
3. Smith B, Cherubini TD: *Oculoplastic Surgery: A Compendium of Principles and Techniques.* St. Louis, C. V. Mosby, 1970.
4. Becker H: The rhomboid-W technique for excision of some skin lesions and closure. *Plast Reconstr Surg* 64: 444–447, 1979.
5. Borges AF: The rhombic flap. *Plast Reconstr Surg* 67: 458–466, 1981.

CHAPTER 74

Tarsorrhaphy

CARL J. HANIG, M.D.
ALBERT HORNBLASS, M.D.

The procedure of tarsorrhaphy, or blepharorrhaphy, is defined as "the suturing together of the eyelid margins" (1). The definition may be extended to include intermarginal sutures, in which the lids are brought into apposition without any actual surgical union. Depending upon the technique used, the indication for the procedure, and the surgeon, this may be a temporary or a permanent union. This chapter will discuss the various reasons for performing a tarsorrhaphy and the various techniques available.

HISTORICAL

Lisfranc is credited with the first recorded tarsorrhaphy in 1836, in which he performed closure of the entire interpalpebral fissure. The temporary paracentral tarsorrhaphy, first described by Bowman in 1892, has been modified by many authors since that time (2).

INDICATIONS

One major function of the eyelids is to preserve the integrity of the corneal surface and to maintain the tear film over it. Compromise of this function may lead to serious ocular complications. Corneal exposure, sometimes leading to ulceration, may result from inadequate lid closure, as in a seventh nerve palsy. This may also cause a paralytic ectropion, with resultant compromise of the corneal tear film and lacrimal pump. These secondary corneal problems, as well as primary corneal disease, may benefit from the protection of a temporary or permanent union of the upper and lower lids.

A tarsorrhaphy or an intermarginal suture may be used as an adjunct to another surgical procedure. In the prevention of keratopathy, this is especially useful after ptosis repair, where increased corneal exposure, sometimes compounded by a poor Bell's phenomenon, may lead to keratopathy or ulceration in the immediate postoperative period. An intermarginal suture may be helpful in enhancing the effect of recession of the upper or lower lid retractors in a patient with lid retraction. It also helps provide a flat recipient bed for skin grafts to the lids (3, 4).

The tarsorrhaphy may be used as the primary procedure in some situations. Mild degrees of upper and lower eyelid retraction, secondary to trauma, prior surgery, and thyroid ophthalmopathy, may be treated with a lateral tarsorrhaphy. The reader is cautioned that in a thyroid patient with progressing exophthalmos, a tarsorrhaphy may place counterpressure on the orbital contents and even compromise the optic nerve. Thus, the patient's proptosis should be stable before this procedure is attempted (5). Finally, in the anophthalmic socket, the lateral tarsorrhaphy may be a simple alternative procedure where prosthetic retention is the problem, secondary to a lax lower lid with adequate conjunctival fornices.

TECHNIQUE

In the evaluation of a patient for a tarsorrhaphy or intermarginal suture, it must first be decided how long the procedure must remain intact. The three variations of the Frost and intermarginal sutures shown are good for at most a few days. These variations are useful adjunct to ptosis repair, lid retractor recession, and other procedures where temporary corneal protection is required (Fig. 74.1).

When a more permanent bonding is required, a variety of procedures are available. It is important to decide how large a segment of the lids need to be joined to produce the desired effect. One must also keep in mind the future possibility of opening the tarsorrhaphy, so that sparing of the cilia (possible in all of the techniques described, excepting the skin flap method) is desirable.

In the first technique shown (Fig. 74.2), the upper and lower lid margins are marked transversely after instillation of topical anesthetic. Pinching the lids together allows one to check that the upper and lower segments are in corresponding positions. Local subcutaneous anesthetic is given, and the marginal epithelium is excised with a razor knife or other blade. Care is taken to spare the ciliary roots. Failure to do this may produce trichiasis later on. Initial use of a chalazion clamp may facilitate the marginal dissection. The denuded area may be split along the grey

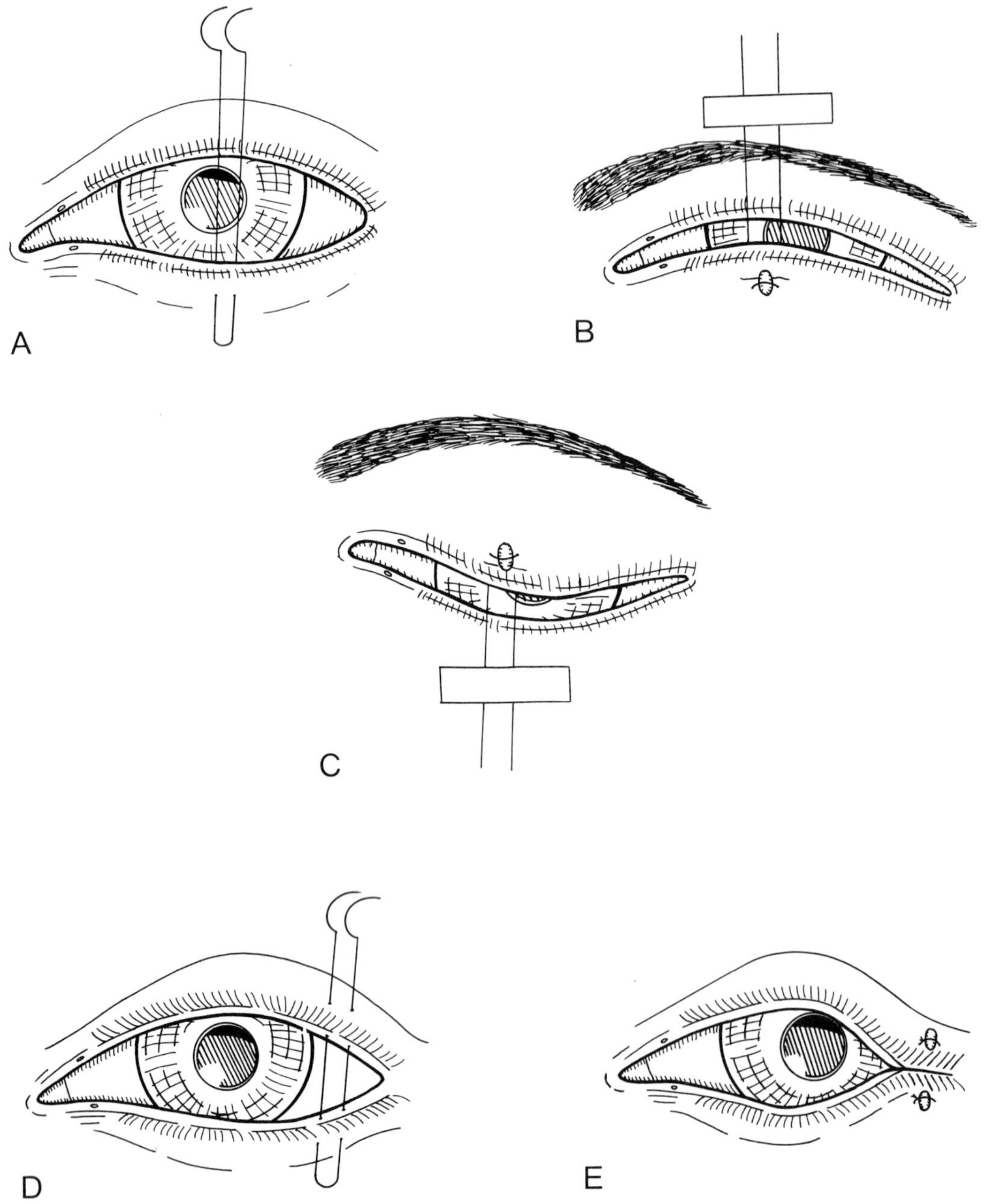

Figure 74.1. *A–C,* Frost sutures. *D, E,* Intermarginal sutures.

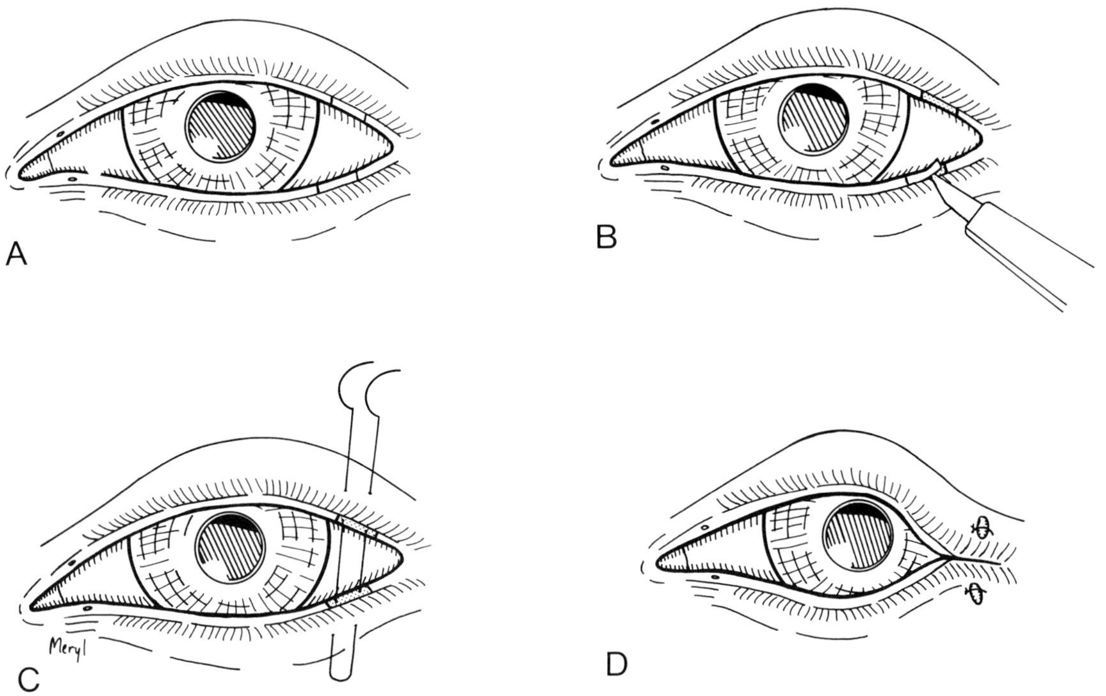

Figure 74.2. Technique of lateral tarsorrhaphy. *A*, Corresponding areas of lid margins are marked. *B*, Excision of marginal epithelium. *C*, Placement of sutures. *D*, Closure over bolsters.

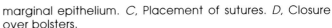

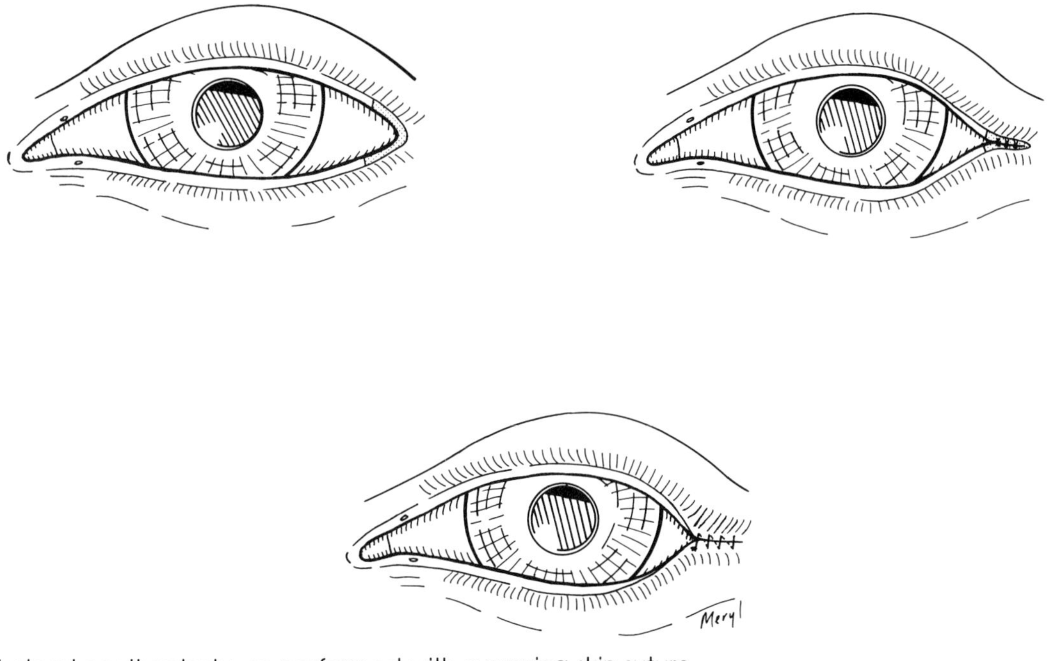

Figure 74.3. Lateral canthoplasty, as performed with a running skin suture.

line to provide a greater surface area of contact. Each needle of a double-armed 4-0 silk suture is then passed successively through lower lid infraciliary skin, lower lid margin (through the midpoint of the denuded area), upper lid margin, and upper lid supraciliary margin; cotton or silicon bolsters are placed at the skin entrance and exit sites to avoid skin erosion. The ends are tied snugly to bring the deepithelialized margins together, and the suture is left in place for about 10–14 days. Alternatively, 5-0 chromic or other absorbable suture may be used, especially in pediatric patients, so that suture removal is not necessary (6). This technique may be used centrally, laterally, and/or medially, and is easily reversed. When used medially, it should be kept lateral to the puncta, so that the tear drainage system remains patent.

In situations where a more permanent bond is desired between the lids laterally, the above method may prove unsatisfactory, both from a functional and a cosmetic point of view. In the following lateral canthoplasty, a more permanent and less easily reversed result is achieved. Denuding of the lateral lid margins is carried to the lateral canthus, and closure is performed in two layers. The conjunctiva and tarsus of the lids are apposed with interrupted 5-0 chromic or other absorbable sutures. The skin margins are then closed with either a running 6-0 nylon or interrupted 6-0 silk sutures. An intermarginal suture placed just nasal to the canthoplasty reduces the tension on the healing area. The sutures are removed in 10–14 days. As some amount of stretching may be expected after suture removal, the initial length of marginal epithelium excised should exceed the desired length of closure by 2–3 mm (Fig. 74.3).

When marked skin tension or lid retraction is present, or when previous tarsorrhaphies have failed, a skin or tarsal flap may be incorporated. In the technique of Elschnig (Fig. 74.4), a triangle of tarsus and conjunctiva is excised from the lower lateral lid. A tarsoconjunctival flap is then formed from the upper lid, with the dissection carried into the superior fornix. A double-armed absorbable suture (e.g., 5-0 Vicryl) is then placed through the

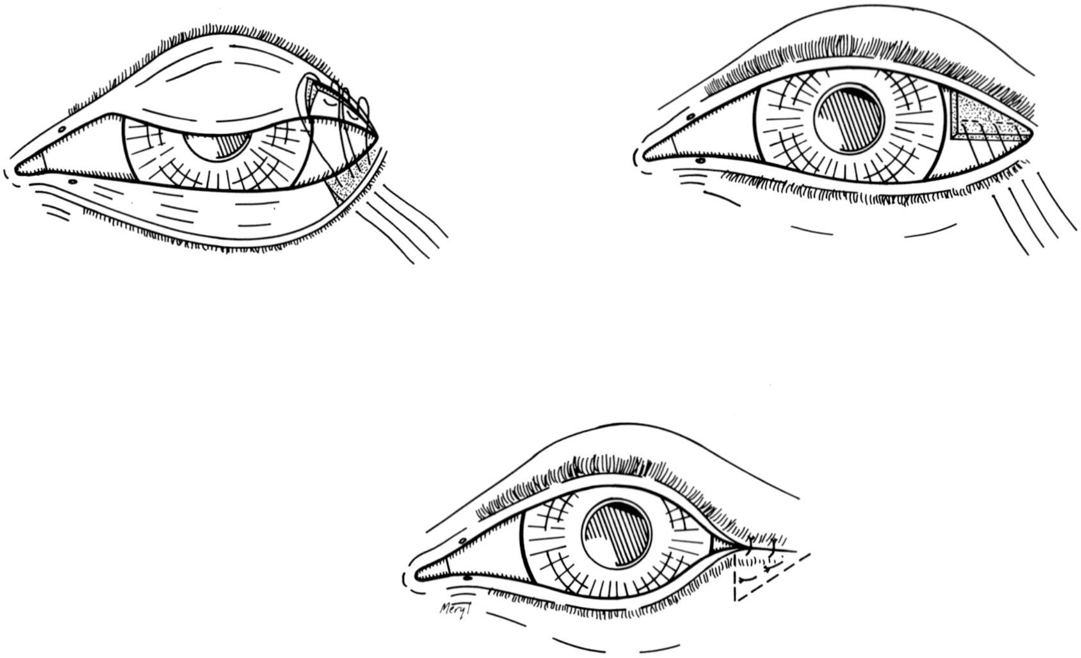

Figure 74.4. Lateral tarsorrhaphy, as performed with a tarsal flap.

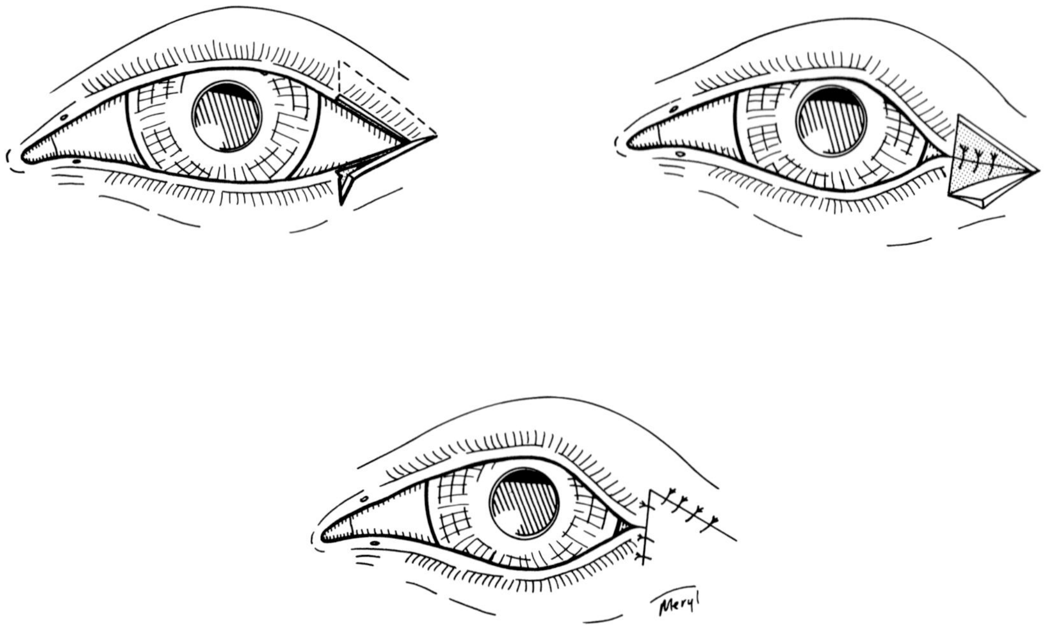

Figure 74.5. Lateral tarsorrhaphy, as performed with a skin-muscle flap. Note the excision of cilia from both lid margins.

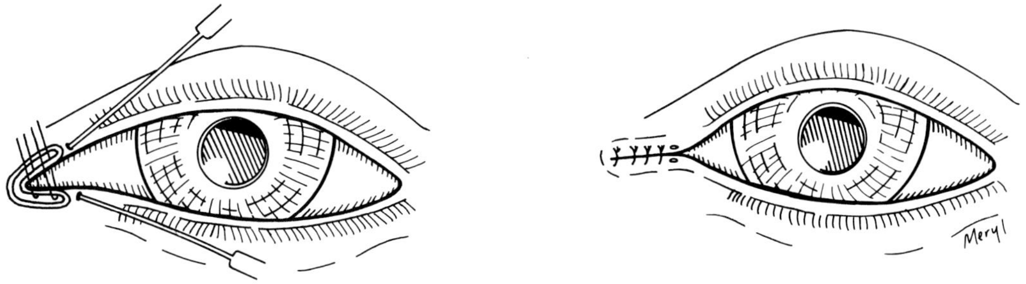

Figure 74.6. Medial tarsorrhaphy.

flap, which is then transposed to the defect in the lower lid. The sutures are now pulled through the lower lid orbicularis and skin, and tied. Skin sutures through the lid margins will reinforce the closure, and excision of cilia is optional. The same method may be used to transpose a flap from the lower to the upper lid, with the same ultimate effect.

The skin flap technique (Fig. 74.5) involves sacrifice of cilia and is less easily reversed. After the lid margins are split, a triangle of skin and orbicularis muscle is excised from either the upper lid (Fuchs technique) or lower lid (Goldstein technique). A flap of skin and muscle from the opposite lid is dissected to fit into the open area. The tarsal margins may be denuded of surface epithelium and joined with 5-0 chromic sutures. The skin muscle flap is closed with interrupted 6-0 silk sutures, which are removed in 7–10 days. This technique may be adapted for use medially as well as laterally, with care taken to preserve the canaliculi (2).

The position of the puncta and canaliculi makes the medial tarsorrhaphy a delicate procedure. In the technique shown (Fig. 74.6), the canaliculi are intubated with Bowman's probes, and the lid margins are split nasal to the puncta. The conjunctival margins are sutured with absorbable sutures; the skin margins are sutured with 6-0 silk sutures. As this technique may prove difficult to reverse, the method outlined in Figure 74.2 may be more practical for a temporary medial tarsorrhaphy (7).

The use of cyanoacrylate is well documented in the treatment of corneal disease. This material has also been used to produce a temporary tarsorrhaphy. The most frequent situation is accidental, often occurring in children. The purposeful application of cyanoacrylate to the lateral cilia produces a tarsorrhaphy that lasts about 3 weeks. The material is relatively well tolerated by the cornea and conjunctiva, producing loss of corneal epithelium, sparing of Bowman's membrane, and localized conjunctival chemosis, injection, and inflammation (8–10).

The reversal of tarsorrhaphies is performed with topical and locally injected anesthetic. Adhesions are lysed with either a blade or scissors, and excess tissue is excised. Hemostasis is usually achieved with pressure alone. Antibiotic ointment is applied to the lid margins, and follow-up care is directed toward ensuring that no adhesions reform.

REFERENCES

1. Stedman's Medical Dictionary, ed 23. Baltimore, Williams & Wilkins, 1976.
2. Fox S: *Ophthalmic Plastic Surgery*. New York, Grune and Stratton, 1976, p 111–120, 215–218.
3. Frost AD: Supporting suture and ptosis operations, *Am J Ophthalmol* 17: 633, 1934.
4. Putterman AM: Suture tarsorrhaphy system to control keratopathy after ptosis surgery. *Ophthal Surg* 11: 577–80.
5. Cooper WC: The surgical management of the lid changes of Graves disease. *Ophthalmology* 86: 2071–80, 1979.
6. Raju VK, Mathalone B: Tarsorrhaphy with catgut. *Ophthal Surg* 11: 625–6, 1980.
7. Stewart WB: *Ophthalmic Plastic and Reconstructive Surgery*, San Francisco, American Academy of Ophthalmology, 1984, pp 149–50.
8. Margo CE, Trobe JT: Tarsorrhaphy from accidental instillation of cyanoacrylate adhesive in the eye. *JAMA* 247, 5: 660–61, 1982.
9. Streit S, Ackerman J, Kanarek I: Cyanoacrylate. *Ann Ophthalmol* 13: 315–16, 1981.
10. Mindlin AM: Acetone used as a solvent in accidental tarsorrhaphy. *Am J Ophthalmol* 83: 136–7, 1977.

CHAPTER 75

Use of Cutaneous Argon Laser in Ophthalmic Plastic Surgery

RICHARD D. LISMAN, M.D.
GLENN W. JELKS, M.D.
PHILIP SILVERSTONE, M.D.

Dermatologists and plastic surgeons have reported the effective uses of cutaneous laser since 1968. Argon laser treatment of port wine stains, mixed cavernous and capillary hemangiomas, small vascular lesions, and cutaneous melanomas have been described.

Selective tissue absorption of argon laser provides the basis for its use on skin lesions. The argon laser emits coherent light with relatively discrete wavelengths of 488 nm and 514 nm. Optical absorption by the superficial 2 mm of epidermis and dermis produces thermal tissue damage. Replacement of necrotic tissue by new tissue ensues. During the past several years, cutaneous argon laser has become a useful treatment modality for the ophthalmic plastic surgeon.

HISTORY OF CLINICAL LASER TREATMENT

Light amplification by stimulated emission of radiation was first described by Maiman in 1960. It is nonionizing, monochromatic, coherent radiation created by photons stimulating the emission of other photons within a gain medium. The property of monochromaticity enables changes of wavelength to provide selective optical absorption and thereby produce relatively specific tissue damage.

The first clinical use of laser on the skin dates back to 1968, when Solomon and colleagues treated port wine stains and studied the histological changes in the thermally burned lesions. They found that a coagulative necrosis of superficial skin layers was followed by fibrosis and reepithelialization of the lesion. Since then, the port wine stain has been the skin lesion with the most extensive treatment and follow-up records.

In the past, the therapeutic goal in cutaneous laser treatment was to produce specific vascular destruction, leaving overlying epidermis and dermis intact. Theoretically, the tunable dye laser, with high-density, short-pulse duration and width, should permit such selective tissue destruction. Conversely, argon and ruby lasers are relatively nonspecific and thermally damage all tissues superficial to the vascular lesion. In a comparison of nonselective skin damage by argon and dye laser sources, Greenwald found that the dye laser results in vascular damage, leaving epidermis and dermal appendages relatively unaltered. Although hemoglobin maximally absorbs at 420 nm, a wavelength of 577 nm was chosen to allow for deeper dermal penetration. In sharp contrast, the argon laser resulted in diffuse epidermal and dermal necrosis. The reason is that hemoglobin absorption is not as complete at the argon wavelength and a wider pulse width allows for extensive heat diffusion throughout the epidermis and dermis. The conclusion of this study was that the dye laser should be more effective in the treatment of highly vascular lesions such as the port wine stain. It is the nonselective nature of the argon laser that fortuitously allows for closure of port wine stains. The diffuse destruction of the dermis, along with its abnormal blood vessels, allows for the establishment of new vessels with a different flow pattern.

The selectivity of destruction of the argon laser is made possible by altering peak powers, pulse width, and wavelength.

PORT WINE STAIN

HISTORY OF TREATMENT

Port wine stains are a subgroup of congenital vascular malformations termed *nevus flammeus*, which most commonly involve the forehead, face, occiput, and nuchal regions. Although they are present in a relatively large percentage of newborns, most lesions disappear within the first year of life. Port wine stains, however, persist into childhood and adulthood.

The term "port wine" derives its name from O'Porto, the chief city in Portugal from which the strong red wine of that country was exported. Medical literature during the 19th century often used the descriptive term "port wine stain" to label these congenital malformations.

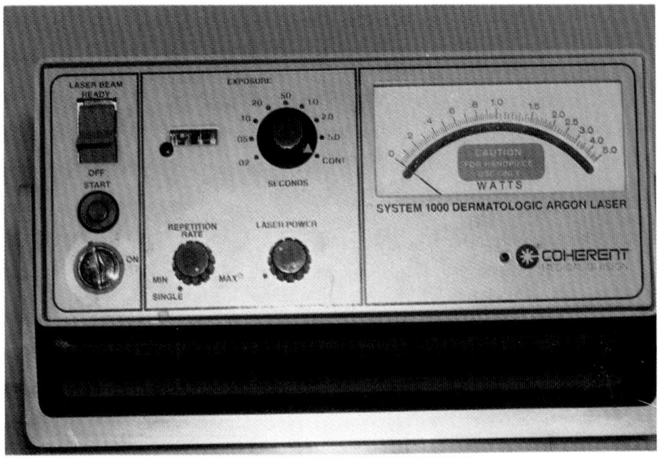

Figure 75.1. Coherent 900 laser control box for cutaneous handpiece is capable of delivering 5 watts of power at rates up to 80–90 burns/min. (Note that the control box for the cutaneous laser differs from the ophthalmic laser in that a rapid repetition control is used. Bursts of laser are provided with only one depression of a foot pedal.)

Prior to the advent of laser therapy, many methods were utilized to treat port wine stains. Partial or total excision with skin grafting or advancement flaps was most widely used. Dermabrasion and grafting, cauterization, irradiation, closure by ligation, injection of sclerosing compounds, liquid nitrogen and carbon dioxide snow, steroids, protamine, and heparin have all been attempted. Laborious cover-up with cosmetics has been used by many patients. Although this may give an acceptable visual appearance, it is time-consuming and far from ideal.

Many aforementioned treatment modalities succeeded by creating subcutaneous scarring. This same principle is the basis for argon laser lightening. Physicians in the 1800s attempted to produce scarring and reduce vascularity by either vaccination within the lesion or by injection of hospital pus. Obviously, these methods had their shortcomings.

The incidence of port wine stains is probably underestimated because of incomplete reporting. Mothers often state that the lesion does not become evident until a few hours after birth. The childhood stain is most often pink in color and darkens to red or purple near puberty. With increasing age, the stain may become nodular with dark purple cavernous regions. It is at this late stage that extreme discomfort and cosmetic deformity cause the patient to seek relief.

TREATMENT GOALS

The benefits of treatment, in addition to lightening of the hemangioma, include breakup of the solid color mass, a change in the texture or elevation of the lesion, and the elimination of hemorrhaging. Complications of treatment are minimal. Scarring occurs in less than 4% of patients.

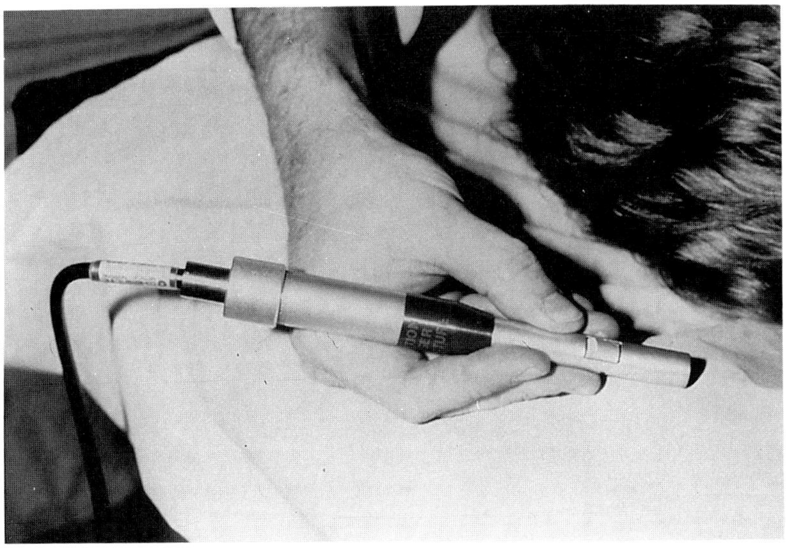

Figure 75.2. Cutaneous laser delivery system. Laser is delivered through a handpiece from the Coherent 900 power source; 1- or 0.5-mm beam size can be used.

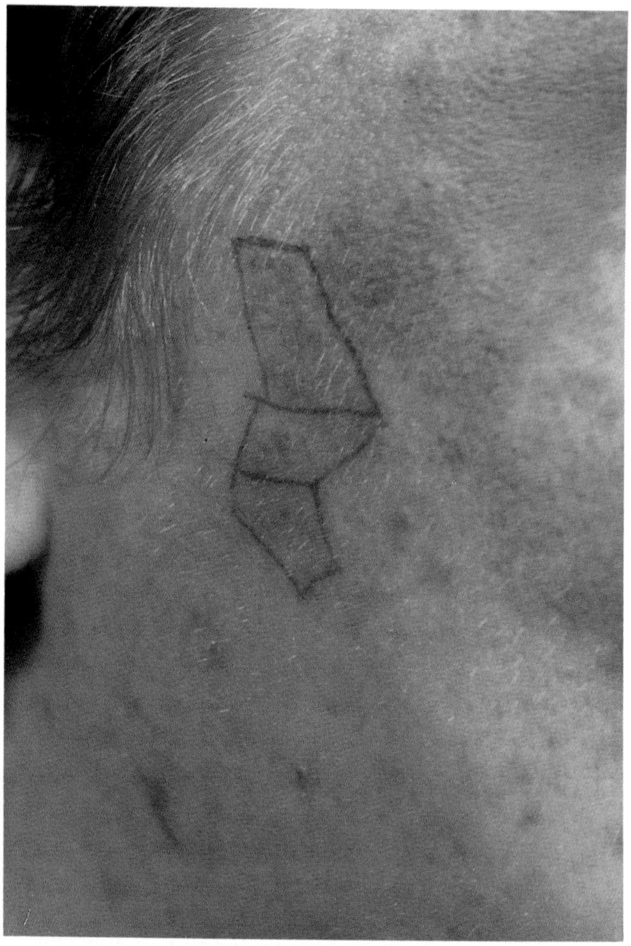

Figure 75.3. Test patch for port wine stain. Multiple areas are mapped over a homogenous area; each grid takes a different laser power and duration to determine the acceptable parameters for treatment.

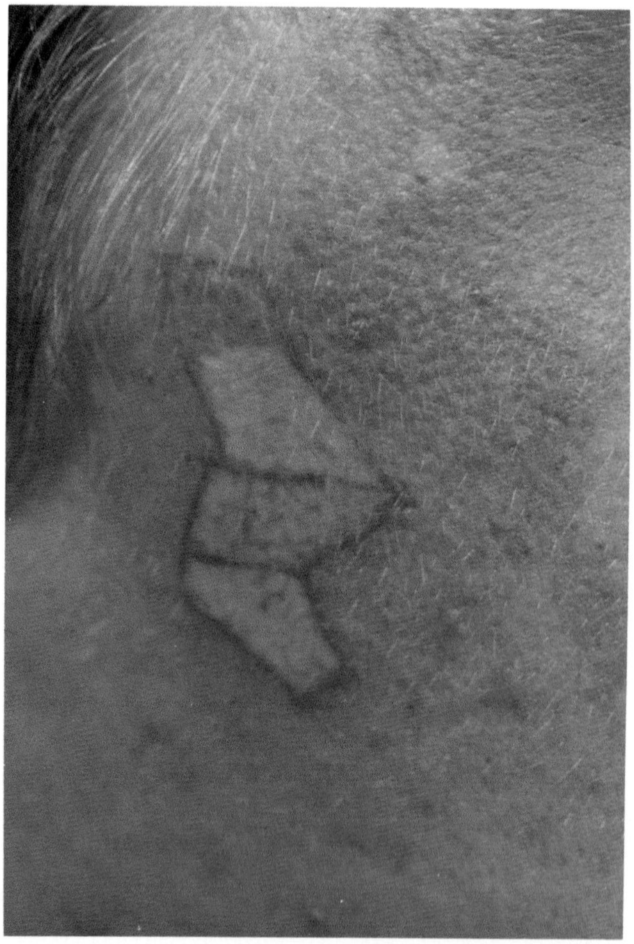

Figure 75.4. Immediate blanching of port wine stain after test patching. *Top grid* received 2.5 watts with 0.5-second burns. *Middle grid* received 1.5 watts with 0.5-second burns. *Lower grid* took 1-watt burns delivered for 0.2 seconds.

The mouth and nasolabial fold appear most sensitive to scarification; therefore these regions are treated lightly. Infection and ocular injury have not occurred in our experience. Discomfort during treatment is variable, and one-half of the patients require local anesthesia in order to complete treatment. If a patient desires outpatient therapy, the overall treatment time may span months. This occurs because eschar formation over the treated area may be extensive, and therefore, 3–5 weeks are allowed between treatment sessions.

Attempts at modifying lesional skin to enhance treatment effect have not been rewarding. Theoretically, reducing the temperature in the vascular lesion should enhance the laser effect by pooling red cells (hemoglobin). Clinically, this pooling is manifested by color changes of lesions noted by patients when exposed to low ambient temperatures. However, Gilchrest has demonstrated that reducing lesional temperature only reduces thermal injury to the nonvascular skin elements and thereby diminishes scarring. Biopsies on patients after treatment with argon laser found no significant difference between dermal vessels in the cooled and noncooled areas.

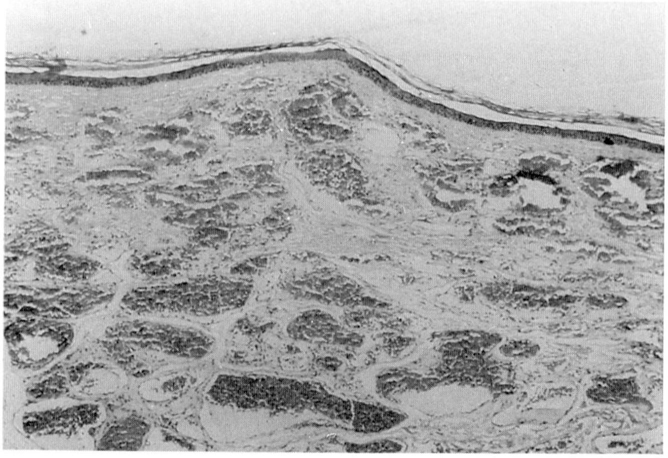

Figure 75.5. Pretreatment biopsy reveals large-caliber vessels, with large quantity of red blood cells per high-powered field. This correlates clinically with a darker lesion in a patient over 17 years of age. Hematoxylin and eosin; original magnification ×60.

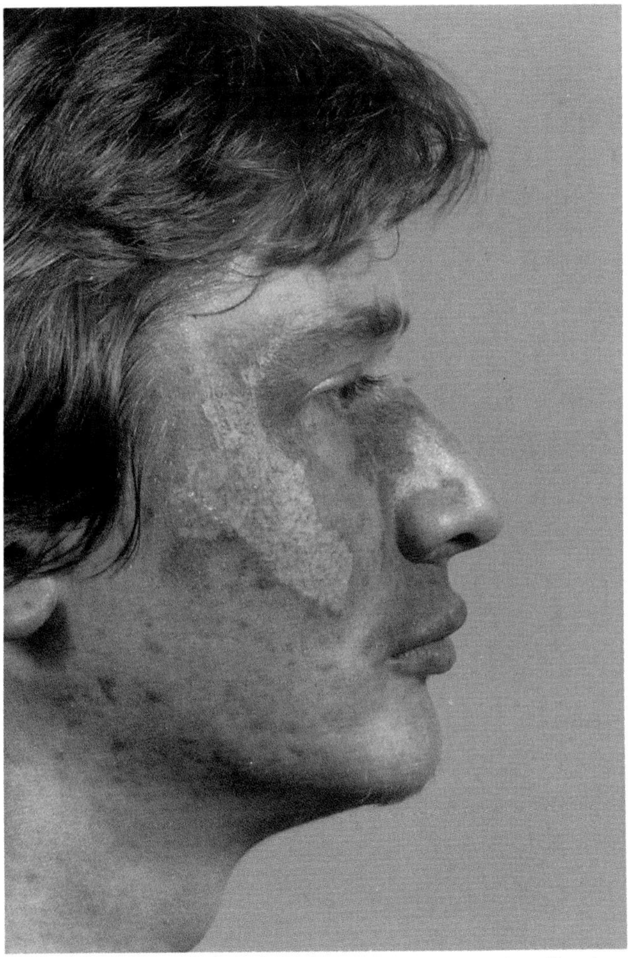

Figure 75.6. Lightening of stain shown 6 weeks after treatment.

GENERAL TECHNIQUE OF TREATMENT

The argon source is used in conjunction with a cutaneous handpiece that (Figs. 75.1 and 75.2) substitutes for a conventional slitlamp delivery system. The barrier filters within the slitlamp are replaced by protective goggles. If the eyelids are treated, the patient must wear opaque contact lens barriers.

The specific parameters used are decided after test patching (Figs. 75.3 and 75.4). Either a 0.5 mm or 1 mm spot size is used. Pulse duration varies between 0.5 seconds and continuous duration, with intensity ranging between 1 and 5 watts.

The degree of lightening and scarring within the treated area has been predicted by either: (*a*) pretreatment punch biopsy (Fig. 75.5) or (*b*) test patching (Fig. 75.6). Initial investigation by Apfelberg and Noe based treatment predictions upon punch biopsy (Fig. 75.7). Their studies concluded that vascular lesions with large caliber vessels, more vessels per high-power field, a high red cell volume, and low flow rate respond better than other lesions (Fig. 75.8). These biopsy results correlate well with the clinical appearance observed in our patients, i.e., the clinical equivalent of an optimal biopsy is a superficial vascular lesion that is darker in color and blanches easily with pressure. Port wine stains in the older age group (age 17 or older) contain larger caliber vessels, which produce a darker hemangioma. These too are ideal lesions for argon laser therapy.

We prefer to test patch the majority of our patients prior to extensive treatment (Fig. 75.9). Initially, a small inconspicuous part of the face is mapped out. Variable intensities of laser are applied within this region. After approximately 1 month, the decision is made as to which intensity will produce the best result.

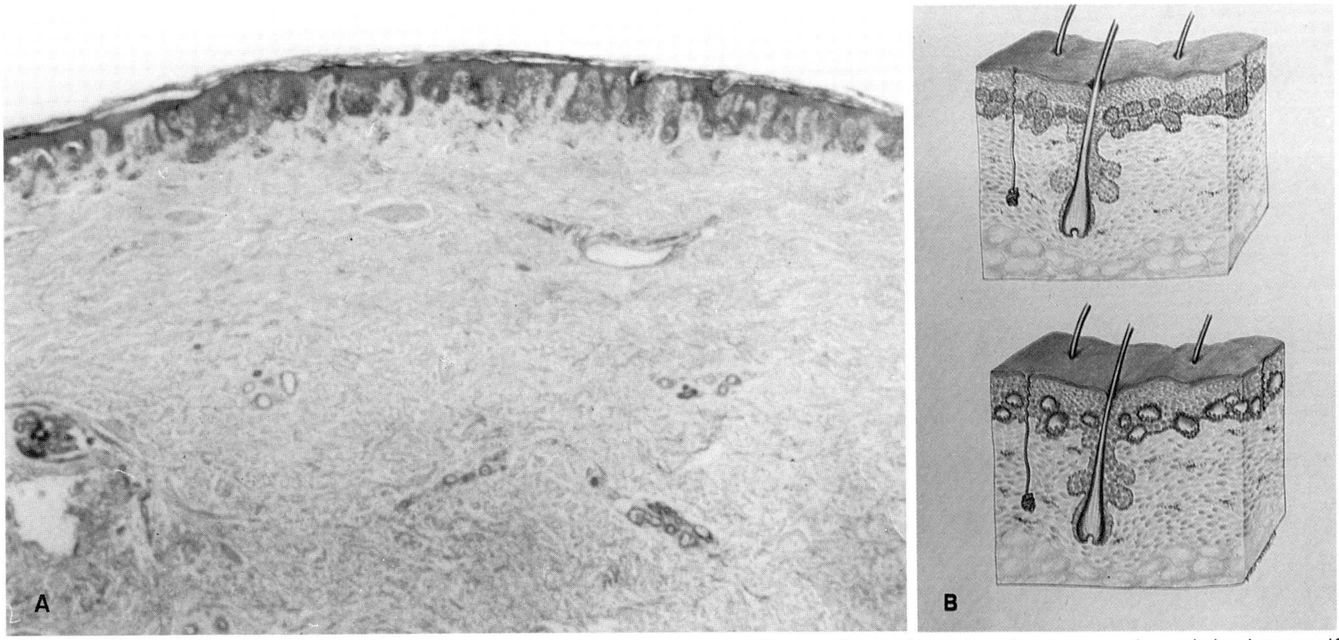

Figure 75.7. *A,* Posttreatment biopsy shows reduced number of vessels and vessels of smaller caliber. Remaining vessels are crowded out by fibrous tissue. Overlying epidermis subsequently transmits a lighter color. Compare with Figure 75.4. Hematoxylin and eosin; original magnification ×60. *B,* Artists diagram of pretreatment biopsy (*top*) and posttreatment biopsy (*bottom*). Note reduction of vessels with fewer red blood cells per high-power field.

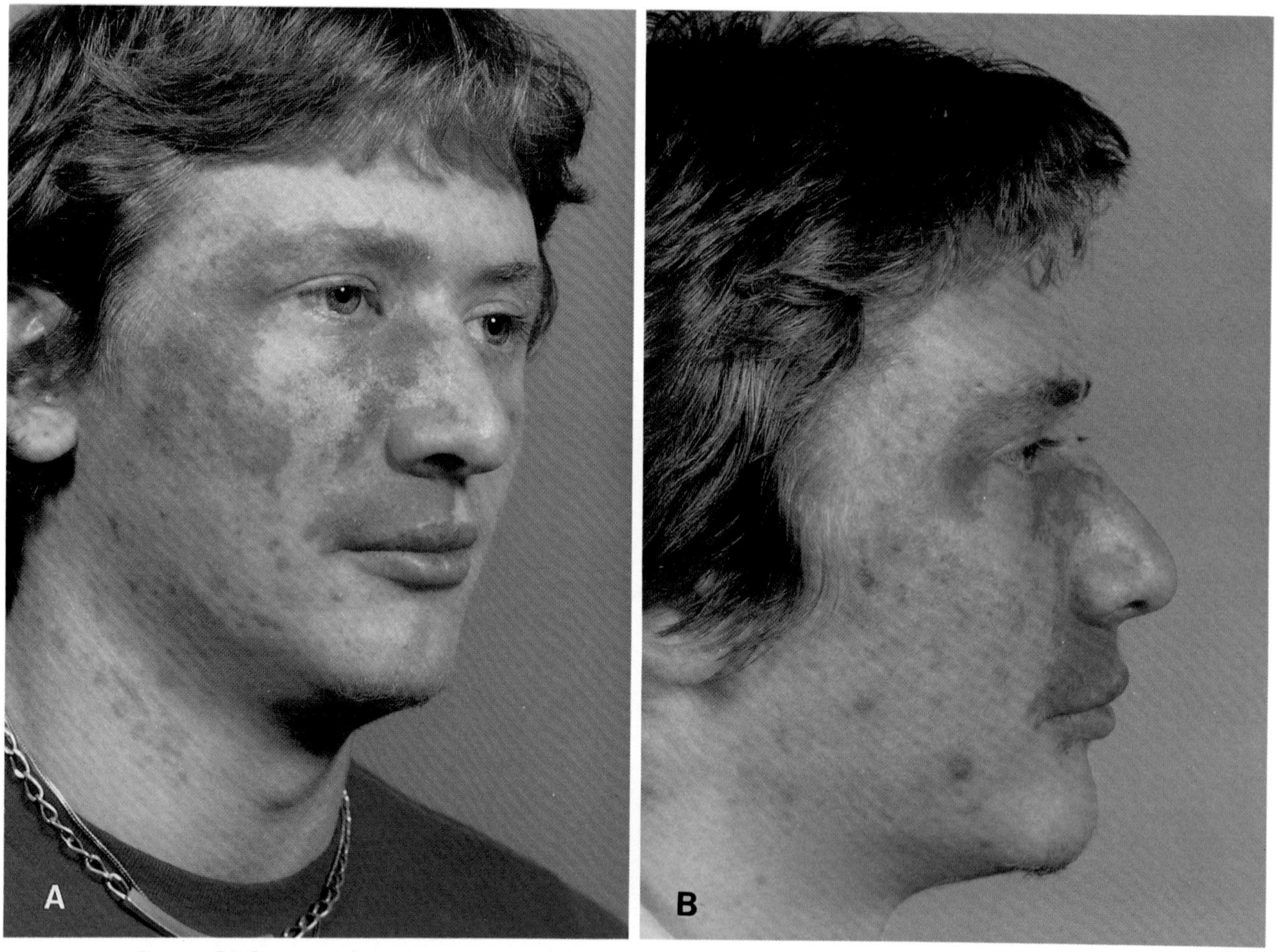

Figure 75.8. *A,* Pretreatment nevus flammeus. *B,* Lightened stain after three treatments.

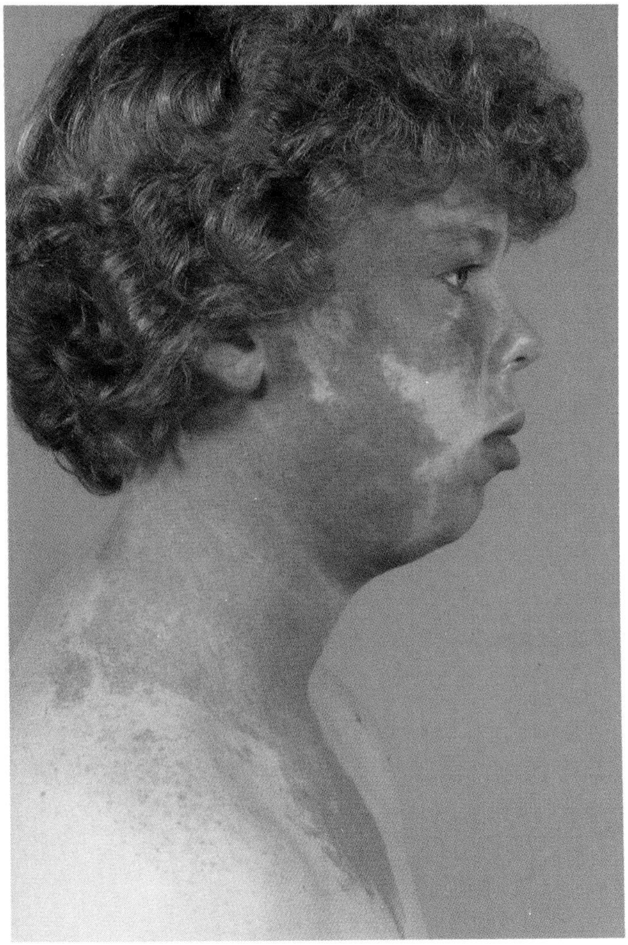

Figure 75.9. Extensive hemangioma, which is best treated in the operating room and with intravenous administration of analgesia. Cutaneous handpiece can be used on a "continuous" laser mode.

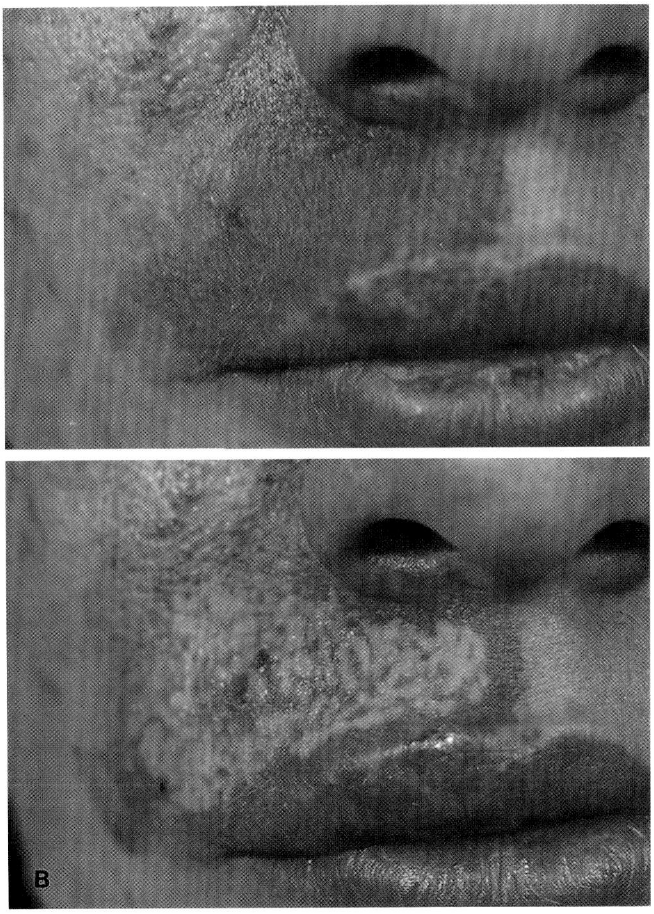

Figure 75.10. *A*, Lip and nasolabial fold must be treated lightly with multiple treatments to avoid scarring. *B*, Appearance immediately after receiving one laser treatment.

Following the above regimen, treatment is completed either during multiple outpatient visits or during a single inpatient stay. Outpatient therapy is performed either with local anesthesia (lidocaine) or without anesthesia. The treatments are scheduled at least 4 to 6 weeks apart. Posttreatment care is minimal; cleansing the treated areas with water and mild soap is sufficient. Antibiotics, either parenteral or topical, are unnecessary unless infection is evident. Sun exposure during this time must be avoided. If an inpatient regimen is chosen, therapy is performed in the operating room with intravenous analgesia.

Clinically, the lesion blanches immediately upon the application of the argon laser. In the first 48 hours, there is extensive epidermal and dermal necrosis. This is evidenced by erythema of the treated area. During the next week to 10 days, an eschar forms and falls off. At this time, the lesion reaches its peak of erythema. In 4–6 weeks there is vessel closure; recanalization by smaller vessels occurs in 2–4 months. Lightening of the lesion occurs because of both fibrosis of the lesion and recanalization of the region with smaller caliber vessels (Figs. 75.10 and 75.11).

MANAGEMENT OF OTHER CUTANEOUS LESIONS

EYELID OR FACIAL TELANGIECTASIA

Argon laser has been used to treat patients with cherry angioma, spider telangiectasia, and essential telangiectasia of the eyelid and periorbital region (Figs. 75.12 and 75.13). Large angiomas are very amenable to therapy and blanch immediately with laser application. Since the skin in the periorbital region is very thin, however, the superficial 2 mm of epidermis and dermis undergo extensive thermal damage. These regions remain very erythematous 6–8 weeks after treatment; although vessel closure and fibrosis occur late, cosmetic results are excellent.

Poor results have been noted in a small percentage of patients. These have had hyperpigmentation of the lower lids secondary to pigment dispersion and a dilated periorbital venous plexus (Fig. 75.14). The treated vessels were noted to be thick-walled and of small caliber. In general, these types of vessels are resistant to laser ablation.

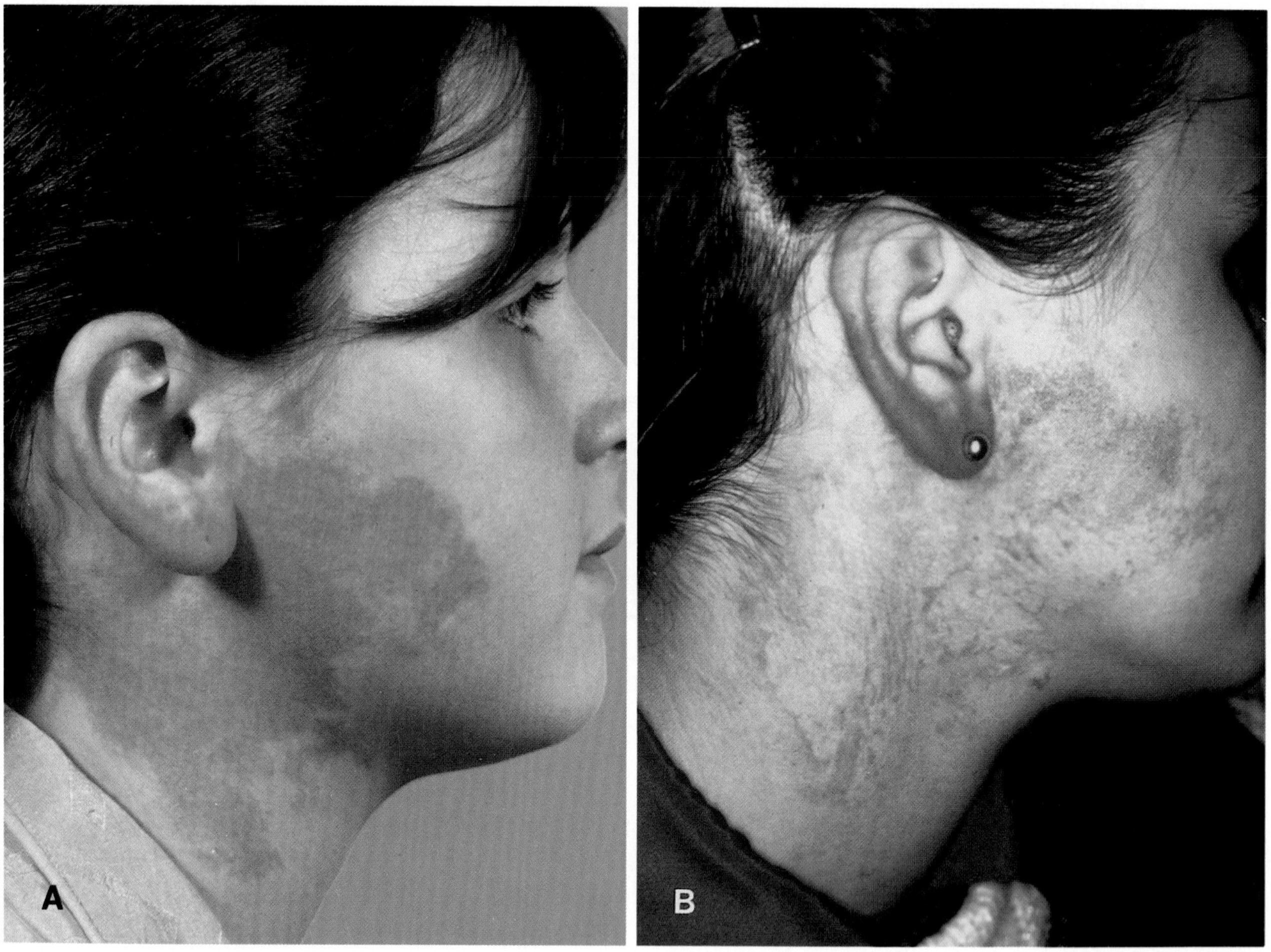

Figure 75.11. *A,* Pretreatment appearance of pale stain in 14-year-old patient. *B,* Unsatisfactory result shows mottling and thickening of dermis after laser treatment. Pale stains in patients under 17 years of age are no longer treated. Patients wait for treatment until stain darkens or vessels dilate.

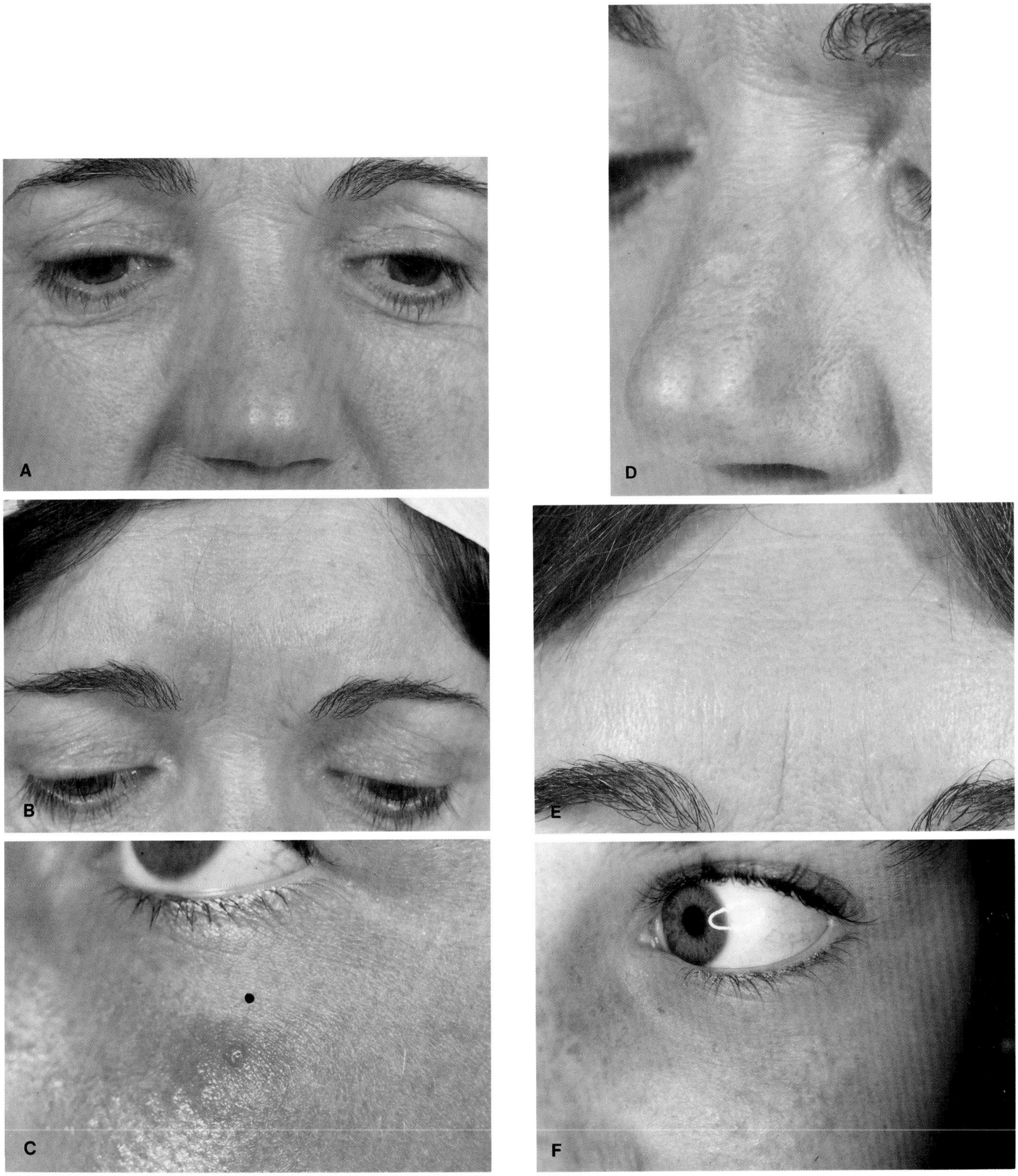

Figure 75.12. *A,* Angioma of nose, pretreatment appearance. *B,* Angioma of forehead, pretreatment appearance. *C,* Angioma of lower eyelid, pretreatment appearance. *D–F,* Closure of angiomas with less than 10 burns in each lesion.

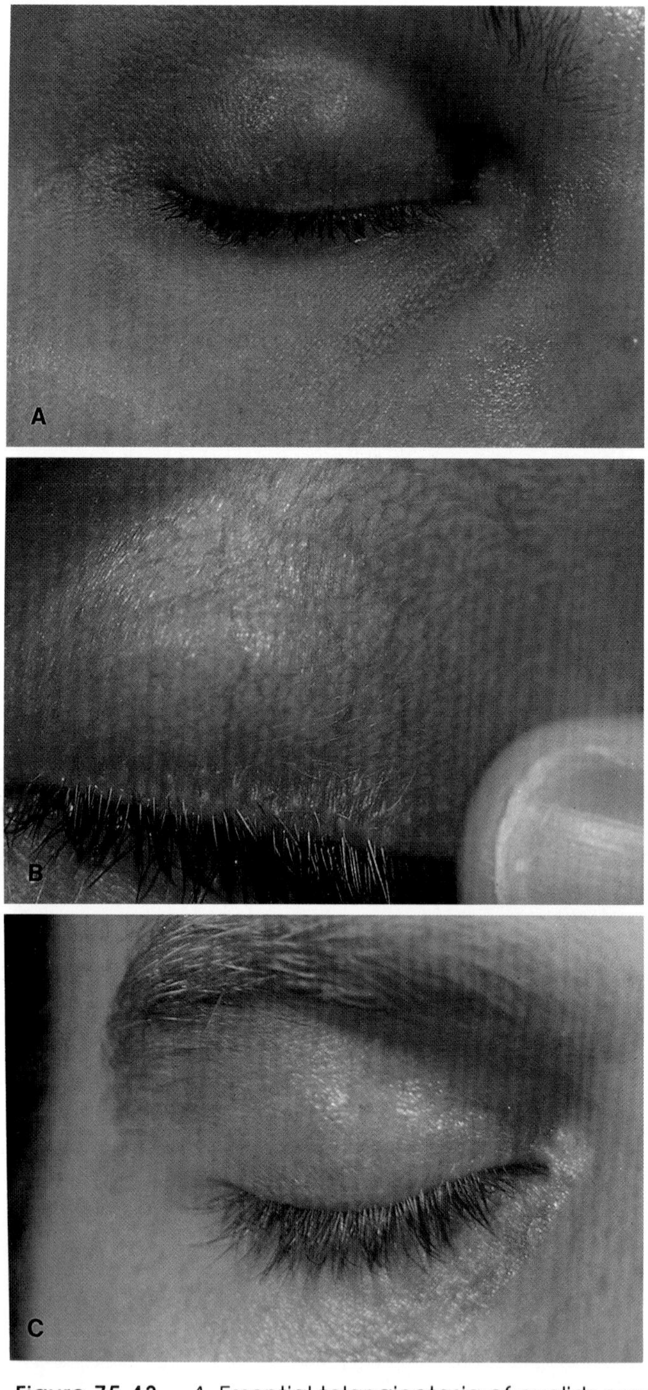

Figure 75.13. *A,* Essential telangiectasia of eyelids previously treated as "chronic blepharitis," pretreatment appearance. *B,* Close-up of panel *A. C,* After laser closure of telangiectatic vessels of eyelids with lightening of eyelids. Patient is a male model.

VIRAL OR FUNGAL DERMATITIS

Treatment of viral-induced (herpes simplex and herpes zoster) dermatitis is generally reserved for those patients who have undergone unsuccessful conventional treatment. Those with fungal dermatitis have undergone laser therapy because of medical contraindications to systemic antifungal therapy. In this group of patients test patches are usually unnecessary. Each lesion is treated separately with 0.5-second bursts, 1 to 2 watts of power, and a 1-mm diameter spot size. The endpoint of treatment is clinical destruction of the epidermal portion of the lesion.

DECORATIVE TATTOOS

Tattoos located outside the periorbital region can be thermally dermabraded with the argon laser. Prior to the use of laser ablation, tattoo removal was performed with cryosurgery, dermabrasion, excision with skin grafting, and chemical cauterization. None of these methods produced cosmetically acceptable results and all were associated with scarring and discomfort (Figs. 75.15 and 75.16).

Since professional tattoos are placed within the superficial dermis, pigment removal requires burning of the papillary and reticular dermis after epidermal ablation by the argon beam. This is most effectively performed with hydrogen peroxide scrubs between burns. Although the end result is flat, white scarring, the cosmetic results are good.

HYPERTROPHIC OR KELOID SCARS

Hypertrophic and keloid scars (Fig. 75.17) are treated by laser ablation alone or in combination with dermabra-

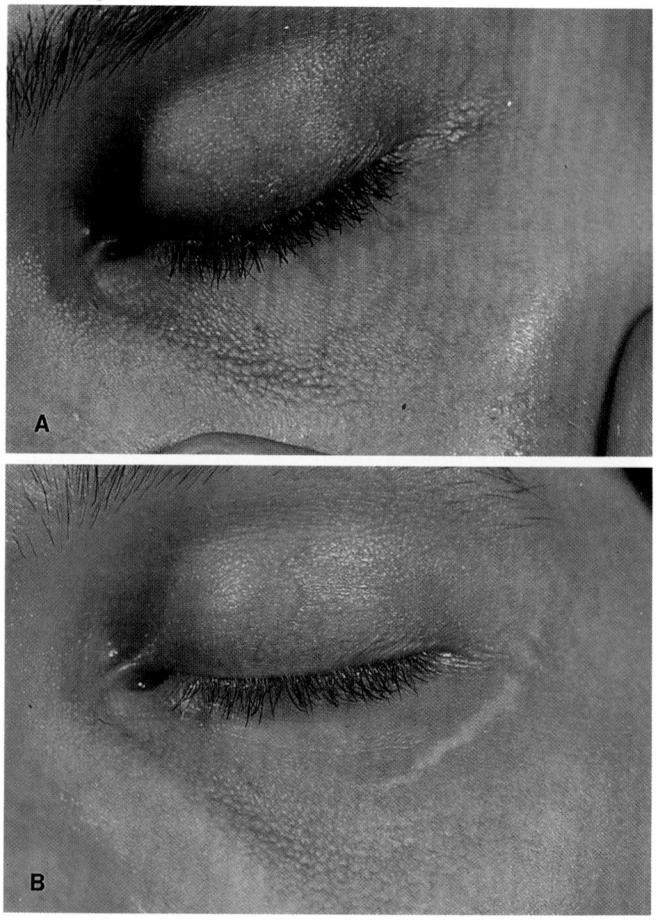

Figure 75.14. *A,* Patient with dilated periorbital venous plexus who desired a lightening of periorbital "dark circles." *B,* Poor cosmetic result. Venous channels have thick walls, few red blood cells per high-power field, and high vessel flow. These lesions are poor candidates for laser closure.

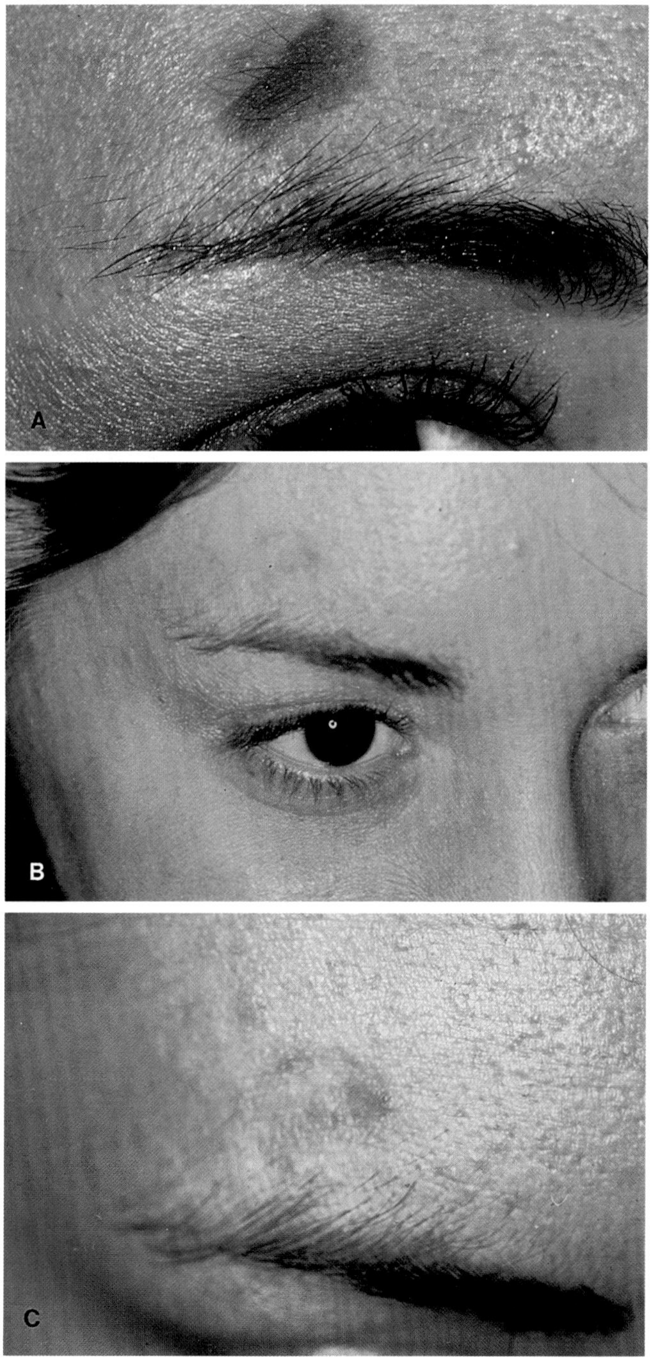

Figure 75.15. *A,* Appearance of nevus of brow before laser treatment. *B,* Five weeks after argon-laser lightening of nevus. Thermal injury to dermis lightens and "shaves" the nevus. *C,* Close-up of posttreatment appearance in panel *B. D,* Nevus of left midface, pretreatment appearance. *E,* Lightened nevus, 8 weeks posttreatment.

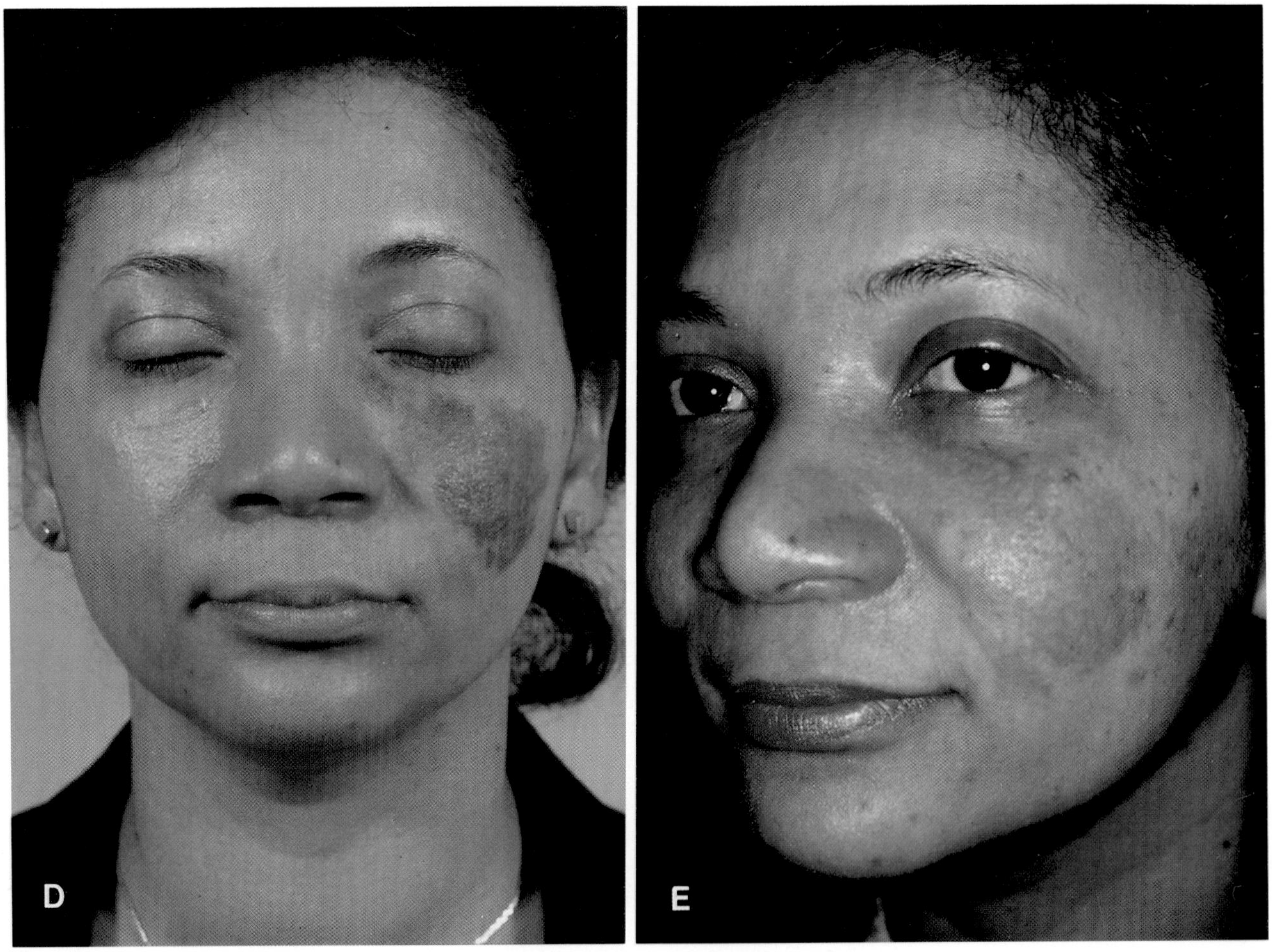

Figure 75.15. *D* and *E*.

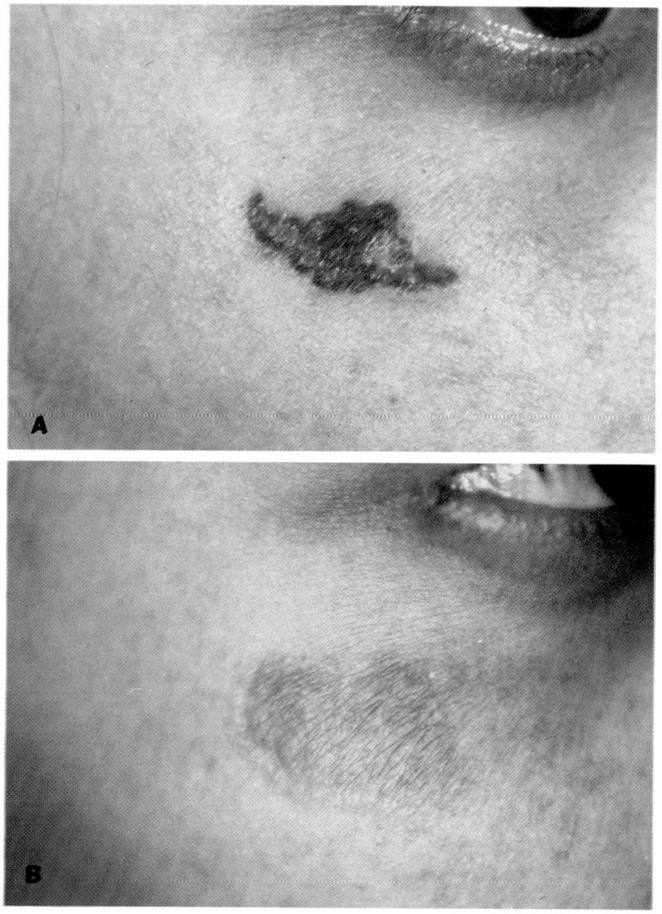

Figure 75.16. *A,* Tattoo of right malar eminence. *B,* Green and red pigments are thermally dermabraided with cutaneous argon laser, 4 weeks posttreatment.

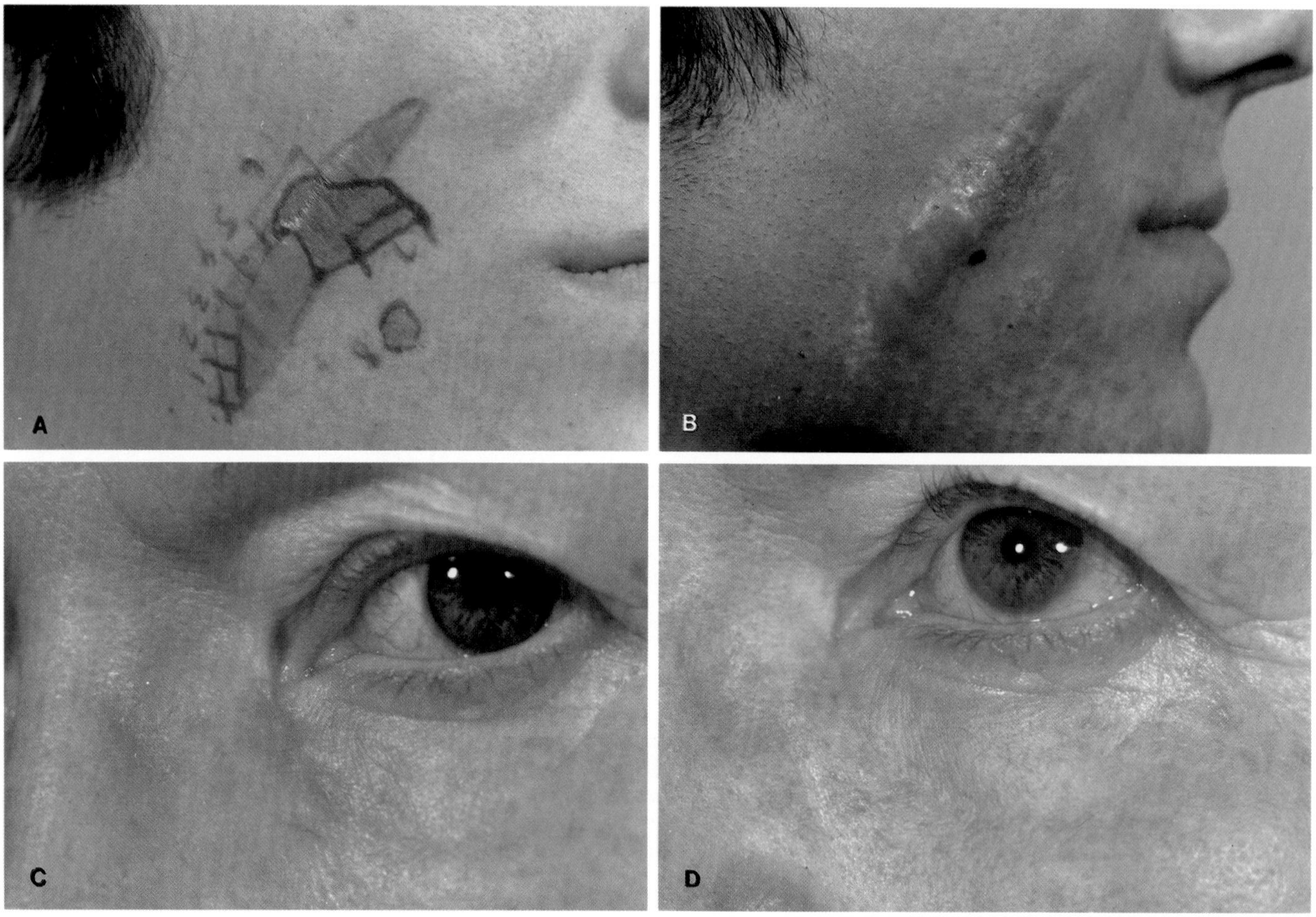

Figure 75.17. *A,* Erythematous hypertrophic scar of cheek. *B,* Argon lightens and mildly flattens scar, 6 weeks posttreatment. *C,* Erythematous DCR incisional scar, postoperative appearance. *D,* Two weeks after argon laser treatment. Scars will lighten with time, but argon laser can produce an immediate lightening if the patient desires it.

sion (preceding laser treatment) or surgical excision (following laser therapy). In addition to lightening the scar, laser treatment induces a flattening. The major complication observed is depigmentation of dark-skinned individuals.

Test patches are performed outside the facial region. After determining the optimal laser parameters, the facial scars are treated, usually along with dermabrasion or surgical excision. Excision is utilized in white patients only.

Theoretically, the argon laser disrupts new fibroblast activity. In vitro studies are being conducted to substantiate this hypothesis.

SUGGESTED READINGS

Apfelberg DB, Maser MR, Lash H: Argon laser management of cutaneous vascular deformities: a preliminary report. *West J Med* 124: 99–101, 1978.

Apfelberg D, Maser MR, Lash H: Argon laser treatment of decorative tattoos. *Br J Plast Surg* 32: 141–144, 1979.

Apfelberg D, Maser M, Lash H: Extended clinical use of the argon laser for cutaneous lesions. *Arch Dermatol* 115: 719–721, 1979.

Apfelberg D, Kosek J, Maser M, Lash H: Histology of port wine stains following argon laser treatment. *Br J Plast Surg* 32: 232–237, 1979.

Apfelberg DB, Taub DR, Maser MR, Lash H: Pathophysiology and treatment of decorative tattoos with reference to argon laser treatment. *Clin Plast Surg* 7: 369–377, 1980.

Cosman B: Experience in the argon laser therapy of port wine stains. *Plast Reconstr Surg* 65: 119–129, 1980.

Finley J, Barsky S, Geer D, et al: Healing of port wine stains after argon laser therapy. *Arch Dermatol* 117: 486–489, 1981.

Goldman L: Laser surgery for melanoma. *J Derm Surg Oncol* 5: 2, 1979.

Goldman L, Rockwell RJ, Meyer R, et al: Laser treatment of decorative tattoos. *Br J Plast Surg* 32: 141–144, 1979.

Goldman L, Dreffer R, Rockwell RJ, Perry E: Treatment of port wine marks by an argon laser. *J Dermatol Surg* 2: 385–388, 1976.

Jacobs HA, Walton RG: The incidence of birthmarks in the neonate. *Pediatrics* 58 (2): 218–222, 1978.

Lisman RD, Smith B, Rodriquez-Sains R, Jelks G: The use of cutaneous argon laser in ophthalmic plastic surgery. In Jakobiec F, Sigelman J, (eds): *Advanced Techniques. Ocular Surgery.* Philadelphia, WB Saunders, 1984.

Noe JM, Barsky SH, Geer DE, Rosen S: Port wine stains and the response to argon laser therapy: successful treatment and the predictive role of color, age, and biopsy. *Plast Reconst Surg*, in press.

CHAPTER 76

Pterygium

ROBERT G. SMALL, M.D.

The term "pterygium" is from the Greek *pterygion*, meaning wing. *Ocular pterygium* is a triangular wedge of fibrous tissue covered by conjunctiva that grows onto the cornea. The base is usually nasal in the interpalpebral fissure, and the apex is directed toward the center of the cornea. The term "pterygium," familiar to ophthalmologists, is also applied to abnormalities of the fingernail, neck, axilla, elbow, and knee (1). No relationship exists between ocular pterygium and pterygia elsewhere in the body except for the wing-like shape common to these lesions.

Ocular pterygium is a common problem for ophthalmologists practicing in warm, dry climates where there is high exposure to ultraviolet solar radiation. There is a voluminous literature on the subject, but no generally accepted surgical technique. Opinion is divided on the efficacy of postoperative radiation.

HISTORY

Pterygium has been known from ancient times. Susruta of India, in the 2nd century BC, may have been the first to mention pterygium (2). He noted various types of pterygium and recommended excision of the lesion. The Ebers papyrus contains writings on pterygium (1553 BC). Other ancient descriptions are found in the *Corpus Hippocraticum* (460 BC); in Celcus' *De Re Medica* in the 1st century AD, and in the works of Galen (AD 138–201).

From the middle of the 19th century through the early 1900s are articles by Chelius, Arlt, Winther, Shreitr, Mannhardt, and Fuchs (3). In his textbook of ophthalmology, Fuchs describes pterygium crassum, vasculosum, carnosum, sarcomatosum, and membranaceum (4). These terms refer to the color, thickness, vascularity, and clinical aggressiveness of the lesion. Arlt recommended excision of the pterygium with simple closure of the conjunctival defect. McReynolds described his transplant operation in 1902 (5). Cameron in 1965 reviewed 223 cases in his monograph *Pterygium Throughout the World* (6). He stressed the etiologic importance of ultraviolet light. There was a high recurrence rate after surgery in his series that was reduced by postsurgical radiation to 20%.

Duke-Elder reviewed the literature up to 1965 in the *System of Ophthalmology* (7). Since then, hundreds of articles have appeared in the world literature, indicating the continued interest in this subject. One reviewer said "As usual, there are almost as many ophthalmological articles describing the treatment of pterygium as there are recurrent pterygia.... The thoughtful student of ophthalmology might conclude that pterygium seems to advance and persist principally unhampered by ophthalmologists" (8).

DESCRIPTION

A pterygium is a triangular wedge of fibrous tissue covered by conjunctiva, which grows from the nasal limbus, slightly below the midline, onto the cornea, beneath the basement membrane of the corneal epithelium. The pterygium destroys Bowman's membrane as it advances toward the center of the cornea. Stratified conjunctival epithelium covers the body of the pterygium while cylindrical epithelium envelops its folds, where there are numerous goblet cells. Cysts form when epithelial cells grow into the body of the pterygium.

ETIOLOGY

There is a high incidence of pterygium and epibulbar corneal lesions in the sunny, hot, dusty, dry regions of the world near the equator, where there is direct exposure to the sun (6, 9, 10–13). In equatorial areas with high humidity and solar protection by thick vegetation, the incidence of pterygium is low (14). There is strong evidence that ultraviolet light is important in its etiology (6, 15–20). It has been proposed that ultraviolet light alters deoxyribonucleic acid in fibroblasts, which then multiply and invade the cornea (21). Ultraviolet light, wind, and cold produce degenerative conjunctival and corneal lesions in the Arctic (22, 23). Pterygium is more common in male outdoor workers (11), but the incidence is probably the same in females, when outside exposure is equal to that of males. Pterygium is frequent in indoor workers with high exposure to irritants (24–26). Pterygium also occurs in damp northern climates with strong ultraviolet radiation even when dust, heat, and dryness are absent. When the eyes are squeezed in sunlight there is less complete closure of the eyelids nasally. This may account for the nasal location of pterygium. It is suggested that since the eyes tend to move away from direct sunlight, pterygia almost never cross the apex of the cornea. Perspiration, shading of the eyes with a hand, occurrence in the dominant eye (since the nondominant eye tends to be closed in sunlight) are of possible etiologic importance (27, 28). Low vitamin A levels and delayed dark adaptation have been recorded in patients with pterygium (29). Other possible etiological factors are protein breakdown causing corneal vascularization (30) and abnormal blinking (31).

Pterygium is rare in youth (10) and less common in women. Heredity is also important (11, 32, 33). Evidence suggests the tendency for the development of pterygium, rather than the lesion itself, is inherited. The occurrence of pterygium in twins further suggests the importance of heredity (34).

True pterygia are limited to the interpalpebral fissure, usually on the nasal side. Bilateral lesions are relatively common and temporal pterygia are not infrequent. Bilateral nasal and temporal pterygia have been reported (35–38).

Normally the bulbar conjunctiva glides smoothly over the palpebral conjunctiva when the globe and eyelids move. Pseudopterygium, symblepharon, and complicated recurrent pterygium are related in that abnormal adhesions or bands occur between the bulbar, corneal, or palpebral conjunctiva.

Pseudopterygium occurs when conjunctival epithelium becomes attached to a corneal ulcer following any kind of inflammation. Usually a probe can be passed under a pseudopterygium unlike a true pterygium, which is adherent to the cornea throughout its entire extent. Pseudopterygia occur anywhere around the circumference of the cornea. True pterygia occur only medially and laterally. Pseudopterygium may be associated with Terrien's marginal degeneration (39).

Symblepharon occurs in this manner: After inflammation or injury to the bulbar, palpebral, or corneal epithelium, two opposing raw surfaces may heal so that one or more strands or surfaces of palpebral conjunctiva become attached to the adjacent bulbar or corneal epithelium. (Figs. 76.1 and 76.2). Symblepharon is often present in complicated recurrent pterygium.

Other lesions occur in the same location and under the same conditions present with the development of pterygium:

1. Spheroidal degeneration of the cornea and conjunctiva (40, 41);
2. Pinguecula (42, 43);
3. Solar keratosis and squamous carcinoma (44).

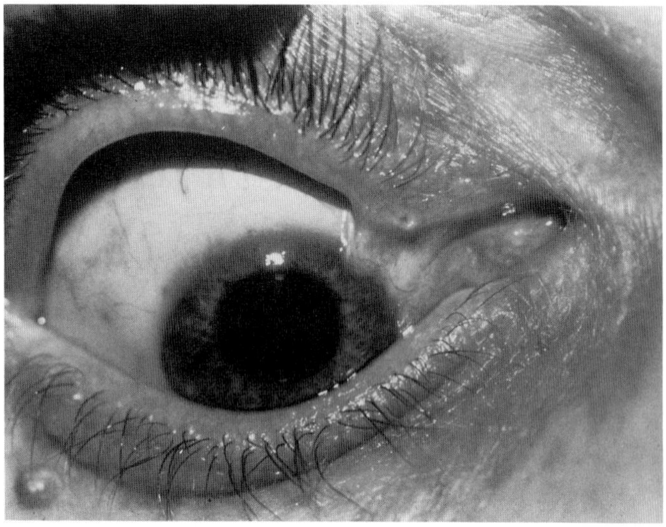

Figure 76.1. A symblepharon and pseudopterygium followed drainage of a fungal orbital abscess. The surgical problem is similar to that of complicated recurrent pterygium.

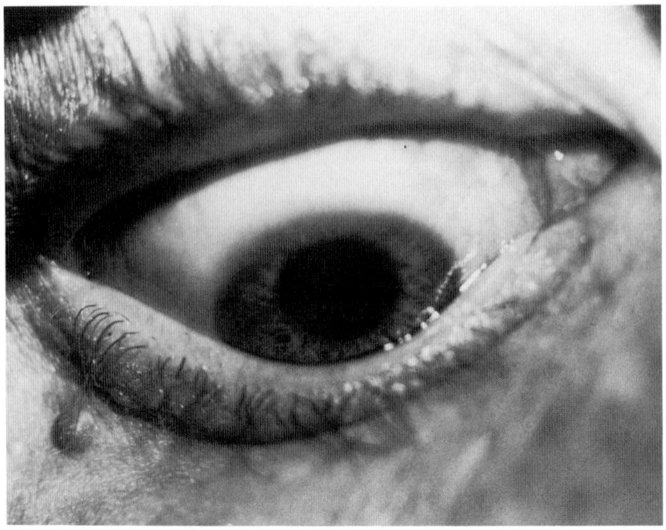

Figure 76.2. The result following the author's technique of conjunctival grafting and fixation of the eye in abduction.

Some authors suggest that pinguecula, pterygium, solar keratosis and squamous carcinoma are a spectrum of entities related to ultraviolet light exposure (14, 44, 45). Others think they are unrelated except for their association with solar radiation (15, 42, 43).

Pyogenic granuloma (46) and, less commonly, ligneous conjunctivitis (47) sometimes occur after pterygium removal.

PATHOLOGY

The light- and electron-microscopic appearance of pterygium has been well described (7, 21, 48–50). The first microscopic changes are vesicles in Bowman's membrane at the site where fibroblasts grow over the corneal surface at the apex of the advancing pterygium. This fibrous mass insinuates itself under the corneal epithelium and destroys Bowman's membrane as it advances across the cornea. The pterygium is covered by conjunctival epithelium. Just in front of the advancing head of the pterygium a pigmented line from deposition of hemosiderin often occurs (Stocker line). A small area of cornea at the apex of the advancing pterygium stains with fluorescein. Goblet cells are distributed through pterygia (51).

An important clinical classification of pterygium according to type is based on its bulk and the amount of vascular tissue present. A proliferative or progressive pterygium with a rich vascular supply visible both clinically and histologically tends to advance more rapidly over the cornea. Histochemical examination shows there are more collagen and elastic fibers present in the rapidly growing pterygium (52). The number of mast cells is greatest in pterygia with abundant collagen and blood vessels.

The intermediate fibromatous, or mildly progressive pterygium contains the same fibrous component as the proliferative type, but with less vascularity and less tendency to advance.

The atrophic, or regressive pterygium is thin with few vessels and little fibrous tissue, and may remain stationary for years (53–55).

CLINICAL ASPECTS

The patient with a pterygium notices a growth in the corner of the eye, which is usually associated with eye irritation and in more advanced cases astigmatism (56–59). Visual loss, except from astigmatism, is not common when the patient is first seen.

Untreated pterygia move toward the center of the cornea but rarely cross the apex. In a report of 1352 cases only 0.2% crossed the center of the cornea (56). The infrequency of central corneal involvement may be related to the natural tendency of individuals to direct their eyes away from sunlight. Thus, while pterygium is common, central corneal involvement is rare.

The corneascope can be utilized to follow the progress of a pterygium by a simple technique (J.J. Rowsey, M.D., personal communication). The corneascope is centered on the visual axis. As the pterygium traverses the cornea from the limbus toward the visual axis, it causes optical distortion, subepithelial fibrosis, and scar tissue on the surface of the cornea (Fig. 76.3). Most pterygia, when first seen, touch the ninth ring on the corneascope photograph. When the pterygium approaches the third or fourth ring, counting from the center outward, excision is recommended. The amount of induced astigmatism can be measured by observing the chord length of the central rings. The distance from the visual axis can be measured by placing a ruler on the center of the photograph and measuring to the most central disturbed ring. This is divided by 4.81, which is the magnification of the original corneascope photograph, to give the distance of the pterygium from the optical center of the cornea in millimeters. The thickness of the pterygium can also be measured. As the pterygium elevates the corneal surface, the convex corneal mirror effect is closer to the examiner and the flattened cornea is measured as a lower dioptric power in the quadrant involved by the pterygium. This alteration permits an objective measurement of the thickness of the pterygium.

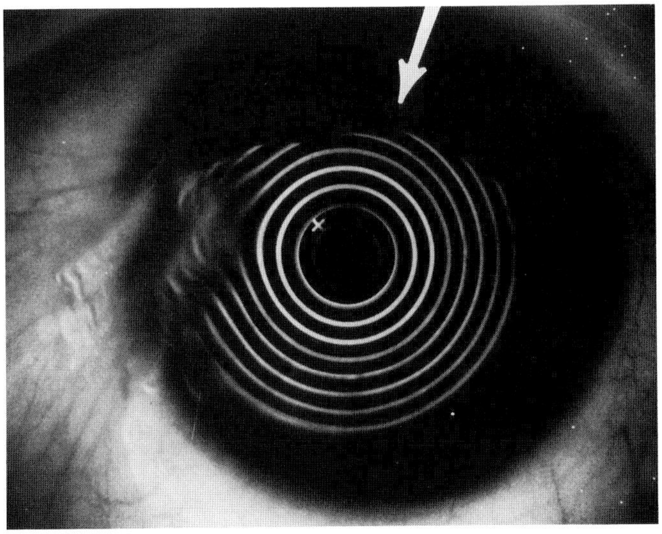

Figure 76.3. Corneascope photograph showing astigmatism induced by a pterygium. *Arrow* is at right angles to the corneal meridian flattened by the pterygium.

The patient is often anxious for surgery even without astigmatism or visual loss. The cosmetic blemish, eye irritation, and potential threat to vision tend to make patients want surgery.

GENERAL CONSIDERATIONS FOR TREATMENT

Nonsurgical treatment includes prophylactic measures, periodic observation, reassurance, and topical medication. Surgery includes any of various operative techniques with or without adjunct treatment with radiation, steroids, and cytotoxic agents such as triethylene thiophosphoramide.

NONSURGICAL TREATMENT

If the pterygium is small and inactive, ultraviolet light-blocking sunglasses are worn. Conditions known to favor progression of pterygia are avoided (sunlight, exposure to dust, etc). The patient is reassured that although slight growth of the pterygium may be evident, there is no threat to vision.

A sketch is made. The pterygium is accurately measured under the slitlamp. Photographs are taken. Reexamination at appropriate intervals establishes whether the pterygium is growing. Surgery is recommended for significant growth, eye irritation, and induced astigmatism.

SURGICAL TECHNIQUES

Before surgery, the patient is advised of possible complications such as recurrence, persistent redness, and irritation. As in any eye operation, loss of vision or even the eye itself is possible, but the patient is reassured this is very unlikely.

In the past, authors recommended "fitting the operation to the pterygium" (60, 61). One atlas of ophthalmic surgery describes 17 operations (62). Another states "the fact that there are so many proposed techniques for pterygium removal attests to the lack of uniformity of excellent results with any one technique" (63). Various surgical procedures for primary pterygium are discussed next.

Dissection of the Pterygium from the Cornea

Methods of removal of the pterygium include knife dissection lamellar keratectomy, avulsion (64), scissor dissection, and microdissection. Most recommend careful lamellar dissection of the pterygium from the cornea. The object is to remove the pterygium in its entirety and leave the smoothest possible corneoscleral surface for reepithelialization. The operating microscope is preferred by many surgeons for this dissection.

Polishing of the Dissected Cornea, Sclera and Limbus with a Diamond Burr

This technique has been recommended by several authors (65–67). Evidence suggests that recurrence is less likely if the dissected surfaces of the cornea, limbus, and sclera are polished mirror smooth.

Transplantation

This technique is not recommended. The dissected head of the pterygium is directed away from the corneal limbus by suturing it under a tunnel in the adjacent conjunctiva. Transplantation, popularized by McReynolds in the early 1900s (5), is associated with a high rate of recurrence.

Bare Sclera Technique

In the bare sclera technique, the denuded sclera is left to epithelialize after the pterygium is removed. Like transplantation, the bare sclera technique is associated with a high recurrence rate (68). This is reduced by the adjunct use of radiation. (This technique is not recommended unless radiation is used.)

Use of a Limbic Groove

Recurrence is uncommon when a pterygium is removed at the time of cataract surgery. The cataract incision may be a barrier to recurrent growth. This led some to use a limbic groove or gutter in pterygium surgery (69–71). Although this technique may have some value, it is not generally used.

Simple Closure of the Adjacent Conjunctiva or Mobilization and Closure of Adjacent Conjunctiva

There is evidence that closure of the adjacent conjunctiva with sliding or other conjunctival flaps tends to prevent recurrence (28, 66, 69, 70, 72–75). Evidence suggests the use of a free conjunctival graft is a better technique.

Free Conjunctival Grafts

This procedure is now recommended by most authorities. The upper bulbar conjunctiva of the same or fellow eye is ballooned up by saline injection. A thin conjunctival graft is cut free and sutured in the bed of the dissected pterygium. Old and recent evidence suggests the efficacy of free conjunctival grafts (66, 76, 77). Barraquer (66) suggests a sliding or free conjunctival graft in pterygium surgery so that radiation may be avoided. Vastine and associates (76) report 14 patients who had free conjunctival grafts after removal of a variety of periocular lesions. Four of these patients were operated for pterygia; two of the four were operated for recurrent pterygia. The results in all 14 patients were excellent. They conclude autologous conjunctival transplantation is the preferred method of periocular mucous membrane replacement after excision of epibulbar lesions. In another report good results were obtained in 48 of 50 patients operated for pterygium with the use of free conjunctival grafts without sutures (77).

Mucous membrane can be obtained from the lip when the bulbar conjunctiva is scarred from xerosis or trachoma. In one series there were 28 recurrences in 100 cases of primary pterygium without a mucous membrane graft. There were no recurrences in 100 cases when a mucous membrane graft was used (78).

RADIATION THERAPY

Pterygium, though not a tumor, has some of the characteristics of a neoplasm: progressive growth, invasion of normal tissue, and recurrence after removal. Since radiation inhibits tissue growth it has been used to prevent recurrence after surgery for primary and recurrent pterygium. Statistics show radiation of the dissected sclera after pterygium excision significantly reduces recurrences. Enthusiasm for radiation is tempered by two facts: (*a*) There are recurrences after radiation; (*b*) Early and late complications may follow radiation.

A stream of electrons from the radiation source penetrates the treated tissue and disrupts its metabolism by ionization and disorganization of various cellular components. Growing cells are most vulnerable to this effect, which is always destructive. The radiotherapist selects the dose, penetration depth, and other variables to quantitate this destructive biologic action in an attempt to benefit the host tissue.

Surgery, to some extent, is of secondary importance when radiation is used since this use is a tacit assumption that surgery alone is inadequate to prevent recurrence. The usual technique employed with radiation is simple excision ("bare sclera" technique). No attempt is made to cover the radiated sclera, which is left to epithelialize.

The strontium-90 applicator is the most useful source of β-radiation for pterygia. Radioactive strontium decomposes to yttrium and then to zirconium with emission of a measurable electron dose per unit time. The electron barrage is concentrated at and just below the surface of the eye so that undesirable effects on intraocular structures, such as the lens and iris, are minimized. The device is safe to handle. The tip size is convenient for ocular use. Different shields vary the area radiated for lesions of different size.

Radiation units include the radiation-absorbed dose (rad) and Gray units (Gy). One Gy = 100 rad. The term Roentgen equivalent physical (Rep) is now less often used. One Rep = 0.89 rad.

While each radiotherapist accurately regulates the dose, area, penetration and other conditions, there is no generally accepted treatment protocol. Published reports note dosage from 1000 to 6000 rad. The usual dose is 2500–3000 rad; above this, complications are more likely. Each manufacturer supplies an applicator with a unique design, size, and effective treatment area. Tip sizes vary from about 5 to 10 mm; treatment areas vary from about 4 to 8 mm.

Some radiotherapists recommend radiation for all pterygia; others recommend it only for recurrent lesions. There is no uniformity in indications, methods, and protocols for radiation treatment of primary or recurrent pterygium.

RESULTS

The literature on radiation therapy of pterygium is extensive. A sampling of reported results indicates an average of about 6% recurrence after radiation of primary pterygia (79–85). Other authors report lower (86–88) or higher recurrence rates (56, 89). Recurrence after radiation of recurrent pterygium is significantly higher than after primary pterygium (56, 84, 90).

COMPLICATIONS

The reported frequency and seriousness of complications following radiation for primary and recurrent pterygium varies widely (80, 81, 91–96). Early complications include eye irritation, photophobia, lacrimation, redness, pain, and formation of granulomas. Late complications are epithelial telangiectasis and keratinization, scleral thinning, scleral necrosis (97), perforation of the eye, endophthalmitis, cataract, iritis, and glaucoma. As one might expect, the more radiation, the more frequent and more serious the complications. With less radiation there are fewer complications but more recurrences. Some complications occur even with low radiation dosage. If radiation is used, the patient must be informed of possible early and late complications.

A cooperative effort might make possible standardization of radiation dosage, equipment, treatment protocols, and follow-up data. This would more accurately define the place of radiation in the treatment of pterygium and the risk of complications following its use.

OTHER ADJUNCTS TO PTERYGIUM SURGERY

There is evidence that thiotepa eye drops after surgery tend to prevent the development of recurrent pterygium (98–105). A review of thiotepa in the treatment of pterygium concluded that more data are needed to determine its usefulness (99). Poliosis and skin depigmentation are important complications of thiotepa treatment (106, 107).

Topical steroid drops tend to prevent recurrence of pterygium after surgery (108–110). Steroid eye drops increase the susceptibility of the eye to herpes simplex and fungus infection. The potential complications of glaucoma and cataract with long-term topical steroids are well known.

Caldwell reports success with laser obliteration of neovascular fronds after pterygium excision in 187 patients (111).

SUGGESTED TREATMENT FOR PRIMARY PTERYGIUM

Radiation therapy is omitted from the following suggested treatment for primary and recurrent pterygium, although it is recognized that some authors make a strong argument for its use.

1. Surgery is avoided for inactive pterygia that demonstrate no growth. One author says "most pterygia are benign lesions that need no treatment" (112). The pterygium is measured. Surgery is not recommended when the pterygium is not bulky or vascular and is more than 2 mm from the center of the cornea with no induced astigmatism. A sketch is made. The pterygium is photographed. The patient is observed at appropriate intervals. Ultraviolet screening sunglasses are worn. Conditions known to favor development of pterygia are avoided.

2. When surgery is elected, the pterygium is microsurgically dissected from the cornea, limbus, and adjacent sclera and removed.

3. The bed of the dissected cornea, limbus, and sclera is polished with a 5 mm diamond burr (Storz E0814) designed for that purpose (65).

4. The area of bare sclera is covered by a thin conjunctival graft obtained from the upper bulbar conjunctiva of the same eye, which is then sutured to the sclera with interrupted 8-0 collagen sutures. The graft should be free of all remnants of Tenon's capsule. If Tenon's capsule is left on the conjunctival graft, it will remain elevated, red, and vascularized.

It is important that the epithelial side of the graft be kept uppermost. This can be done by placing a small suture with a knot tied on the upper side before removal of the graft. Fluorescein can also be used to orient the graft since the smooth surface of the graft does not stain (113). The conjunctival donor site heals rapidly without symblepharon.

Evidence suggests that free conjunctival grafting is the best method for the surgical treatment of primary pterygium (66, 69, 70, 76, 77, 114, 115). Grafts of skin are bulky and unsatisfactory. Mucous membrane from the lip or mouth is an alternative when there is scarring of the bulbar conjunctiva (78) but is less desireable than a conjunctival graft.

TECHNIQUES FOR RECURRENT PTERYGIUM

Recurrent pterygium is often associated with dense scar tissue at the inner canthus, which obliterates the adjacent conjunctival fornices and prevents abduction of the eye. Double vision occurs with attempted abduction secondary to conjunctival contracture and medial rectus muscle immobilization in dense scar tissue. A similar surgical problem exists in patients with symblepharon and pseudopterygium (Figs. 76.1 and 76.2), complicated strabismus, and other conditions with conjunctival scarring and fibrosis. These entities have varying degrees of encroachment of scar tissue on the cornea, conjunctival contracture, scarring of ocular muscles, obliteration of the conjunctival fornices, and restriction of ocular motility with diplopia on attempted lateral gaze. The technique suggested below is applicable to these related conditions (Figs. 76.4–76.10).

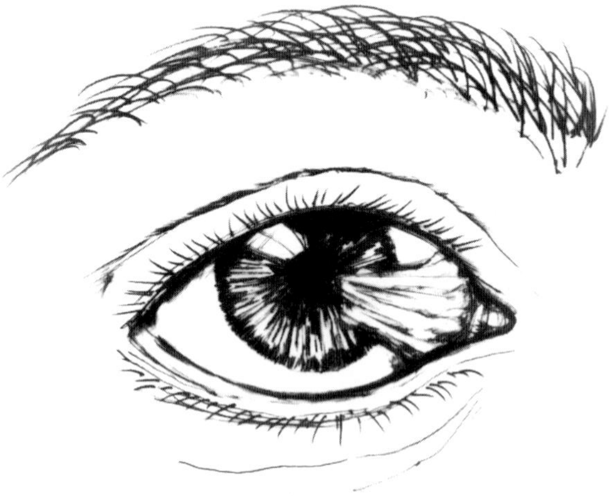

Figure 76.4. A recurrent pterygium. The eye is fixed. The patient has diplopia on attempted right gaze. Symblepharon and entrapment of the medial rectus muscle with dense scar tissue are present.

SUGGESTED PROCEDURE

1. The recurrent pterygium is carefully dissected from the cornea (Fig. 76.5). All scar tissue is removed from the adjacent sclera, eyelids, and medial rectus muscle. The medial rectus muscle is dissected free of all scar tissue so the eye can be fully abducted (Fig. 76.6).

2. The pterygium is excised and the resulting bared area of cornea, limbus and sclera is polished with a diamond burr as in the technique for primary pterygium (Fig. 76.7).

3. A conjunctival graft is taken from the upper bulbar conjunctiva of the same eye as described in the treatment of primary pterygium. The sclera bared by the dissection may require a large graft. The entire upper bulbar conjunctiva of the same eye can be used. If more is needed, the upper bulbar conjunctiva of the fellow eye is used. The graft is sutured to the sclera with interrupted 8-0 collagen sutures. When bulbar conjunctiva is not available because of scarring, mucous membrane from the lip can be used. In one series there were no recurrences in 40 cases of recurrent pterygium treated with mucous membrane graft from the lip.

4. When there is medial canthal scarring and restriction of abduction of the eye, immobilization of the eye in abduction is a useful addition to conjunctival grafting. This is done with a "pullover" suture suggested by the author. This suture is passed under the medial rectus muscle and brought laterally beneath Tenon's capsule

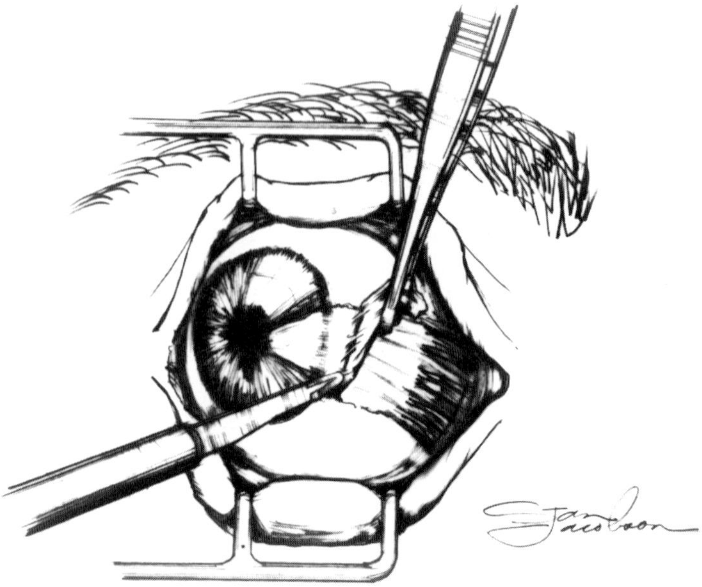

Figure 76.5. Microdissection of the pterygium from the cornea, limbus, and adjacent sclera.

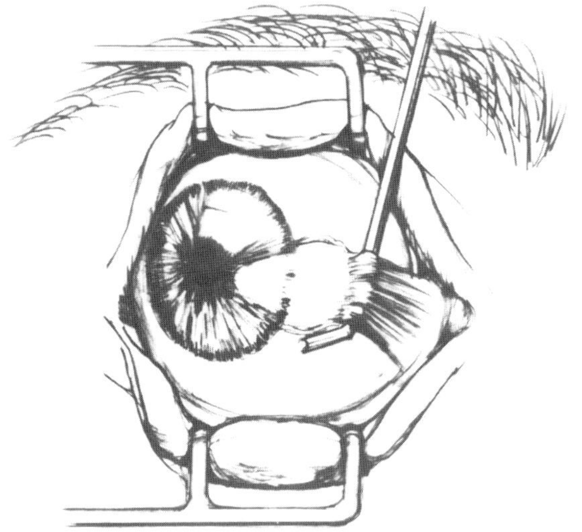

Figure 76.6. The medial rectus muscle is completely dissected so that the eye can be freely abducted.

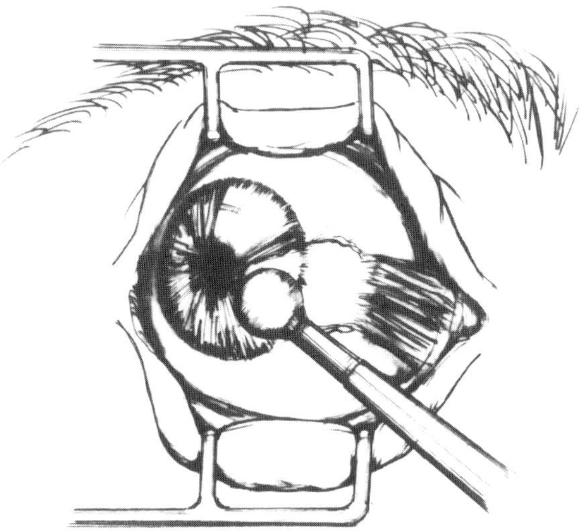

Figure 76.7. Cornea, limbus, and adjacent sclera are polished with a 5-mm diamond burr.

above and below the limbus (pullover fixation technique) (Figs. 76.8 and 76.9). A Supramyd suture swaged on to a ski needle designed for frontalis suspension for ptosis is used. The sharp tip is blunted slightly with a wire cutter so the needle will slide under Tenon's capsule without engaging the tissues as it is passed, but will still pass through the skin at the lateral canthus. The suture exits at the lateral canthus and is tied over a bolster (Fig. 76.10).

Previous inflammation may cause scarring and fixation of the bulbar conjunctiva to the globe. This prevents passing the pullover suture above and below the limbus. In this situation the eye is immobilized in abduction by a lateral rectus muscle suture. A 5-0 monofilament nylon suture passed under the lateral rectus muscle, exits through the skin of the lateral canthus close to the margin of the orbital rim and is tied over a bolster. This is effective, but less so than the medial rectus fixation suture.

Fixation of the eye in abduction adds to the operation in two ways: (*a*) the eye is immobilized while the conjunctival graft is healing; (*b*) the abducted eye presents the maximum area of the globe bared by dissection for application of the conjunctival graft. There is less chance of postoperative fibrosis and contracture at the medial canthus. The fixation technique is used only when there is conjunctival scarring, fibrosis, and immobilization of the medial rectus muscle at the medial canthus, with secondary limitation of abduction and diplopia in attempted lateral gaze.

As noted, in pseudopterygium, symblepharon, and similar conditions with conjunctival scarring, fixation of the eye in abduction is similarly useful as an adjunct to conjunctival grafting.

After surgery the patient is instructed to turn the head slightly away from the operated side to reduce pull on the fixation suture. The pullover suture is removed in 1 week. With very severe scarring at the medial canthus it can be left in 2 weeks. Cheese-wire cutting of the suture through

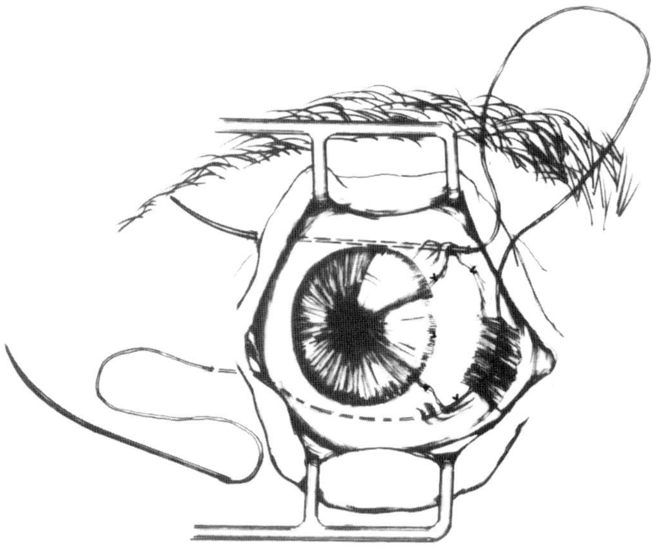

Figure 76.8. A conjunctival graft has been sutured to the sclera bared by the dissection. The "pullover" suture is placed beneath the medial rectus muscle and passed under Tenon's capsule above and below the limbus to exit at the lateral canthus.

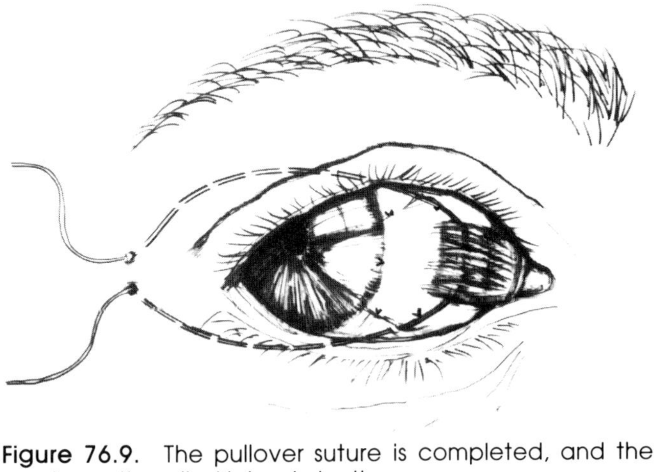

Figure 76.9. The pullover suture is completed, and the eye is gently pulled into abduction.

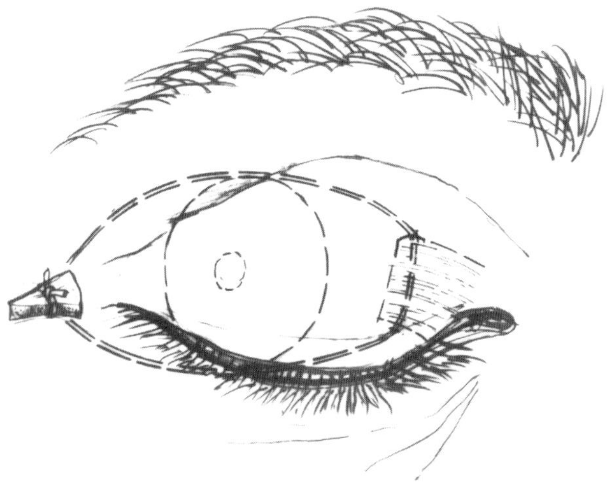

Figure 76.10. The pullover suture is tied over a bolster and kept in place for 1 week with the eye patched.

the medial rectus muscle insertion has not occurred. Restriction of adduction or abduction of the eye after removal of the fixation suture has not occurred.

The eye is patched until the pullover fixation suture is removed. Antibiotic drops are instilled three times a day and the patch is changed twice a day. In 1 week when the fixation suture is removed, there is good preliminary healing of the graft. The patient is examined every few weeks. Topical steroid medication is used if redness in the grafted area is slow to resolve.

Fixation sutures have been previously reported for strabismus complicated by conjunctival contracture. Bedrossian (117) reported two cases of lateral rectus palsy treated by fixation of the eye in abduction. Conjunctival contraction and shortening in his cases is similar to the problem of recurrent pterygium. (The illustration in his paper is similar to Fig. 76.10). Callahan (118) recommended fixation in abduction with conjunctival grafting in two cases of paralytic esotropia. His use of both fixation in abduction and conjunctival grafts is similar to the technique suggested here for recurrent pterygium.

Figures 76.11 and 76.12 show a typical recurrent pterygium before and after the author's technique of careful dissection of the pterygium, polishing with a diamond burr, conjunctiva grafting, and fixation of the eye in abduction. Other authors report similar success with conjunctival grafting in recurrent pterygium (116, 120), and as noted, fixation of the eye in abduction has been successfully used in complicated strabismus with scarring at the medial canthus similar to that of recurrent pterygium.

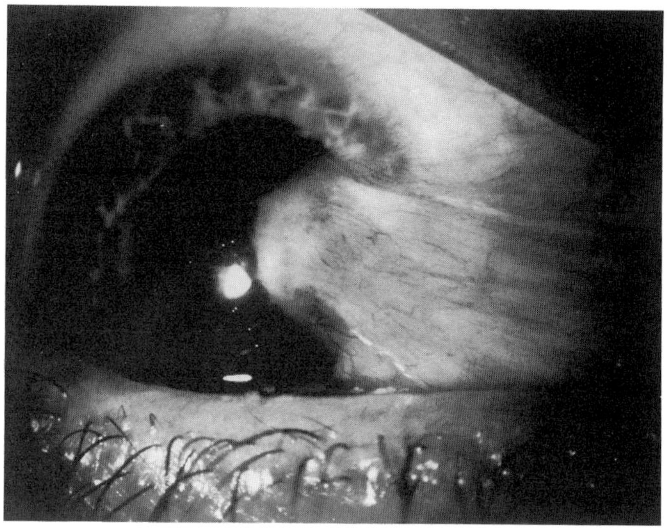

Figure 76.11. A typical recurrent pterygium from the author's series. These patients had up to seven previous surgical procedures, and one-third had previous radiation therapy.

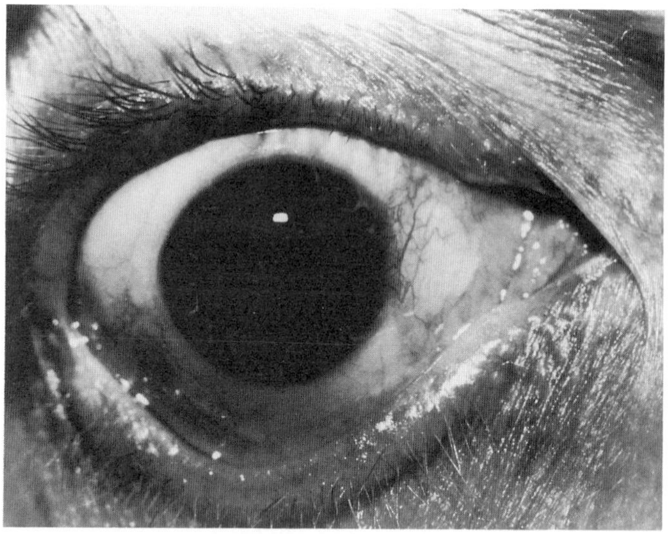

Figure 76.12. Result after removing the recurrent pterygium, freeing the medial rectus muscle, polishing with a diamond burr, conjunctival grafting, and fixating the eye in abduction.

LAMELLAR KERATOPLASTY IN RECURRENT PTERYGIUM

Uniformly good results are reported following lamellar keratoplasty for recurrent pterygium (119–126).

If the cornea under the pterygium is of near-normal thickness, a free conjunctival graft is easier, heals more rapidly, and is as effective as lamellar keratoplasty.

PENETRATING KERATOPLASTY IN RECURRENT PTERYGIUM

This has been reported by a number of authors (121–125, 127–130). Penetrating keratoplasty is recommended as a last resort in threatened or actual perforation of the cornea in complicated recurrent pterygium.

AUTHOR'S SERIES

Primary Pterygium

In a previously reported series of 50 cases, simply polishing the cornea, limbus, and sclera with a diamond burr after removal of the pterygium resulted in a recurrence rate of 5% (65). A conjunctival graft is now used in all pterygia (primary and recurrent), after removal of the pterygium and polishing with a diamond burr.

Recurrent Pterygium

In 28 patients with recurrent pterygia, the fixation or "pullover" technique was used. The 28 patients had one to seven previous surgical procedures. One-third had previous radiation. Originally the pullover fixation technique was used without a conjunctival graft. There were two recurrences. In the last 2 years conjunctival grafts have been used in all cases with no recurrences. Conjunctival grafts are now used in all operations for pterygium, both primary and recurrent. The pullover fixation technique is now recommended only in patients with medial canthal scarring and limitation of abduction. Fixation of the eye in abduction is unnecessary when the eye is freely movable. Most recurrent pterygia in this series, however, were associated with conjunctival scarring and limitation of abduction.

SUMMARY

Irritation of the eye by ultraviolet light in sunny, dry, dusty areas leads to the development of pterygium in susceptible individuals. Heredity is a factor. Irritants should be avoided. Ultraviolet-blocking sunglasses are important for prevention.

Pterygia vary from indolent, intermediate, to vascular rapidly growing lesions. Surgical treatment is reserved for symptomatic lesions that grow, distort, or threaten vision.

The most effective surgical technique for pterygium is careful microdissection of the pterygium, polishing the dissected corneal limbus and sclera with a diamond burr, and the use of a free conjunctival graft. For recurrent pterygium, removal of scar tissue at the medial canthus, freeing the medial rectus muscle, conjunctival grafting, and fixation of the eye in abduction during healing of the conjunctival grafts are recommended. Lamellar or penetrating keratoplasty is used when there is marked corneal thinning, with threatened or actual perforation of the cornea.

Adjunct treatment with radiation, topical administration of corticosteroids, and/or thiotepa eye drops are used according to the preference and experience of the surgeon with due regard to possible complications.

Past and recent evidence suggests that of all techniques, a free, thin conjunctival graft carefully sutured in the sclera bed of the dissected pterygium, is the most important factor in the cure of primary and recurrent pterygium.

ACKNOWLEDGMENT

The author acknowledges the assistance of Stephen E. Acker, M.D., who reviewed the manuscript's section on radiation therapy.

REFERENCES

1. Rossi E, Caflisch A: Le syndome du pterygium Status Bonnevie—Ullrich, dystrophia brevicolli congenita, syndome de Turner et arthromyodysplasia. *Helvet Paediatr Acta* 6: 119–148, 1951.
2. Arrington GE: *A History of Ophthalmology.* New York, MD Publications, 1959.
3. Duke-Elder WS: *Textbook of Ophthalmology.* St. Louis, CV Mosby, 1946.
4. Fuchs E: *Textbooks of Ophthalmology*, ed 4. Duane A, Philadelphia, JB Lippincott, 196–201, 1911.
5. McReynolds JO: The nature and treatment of pterygia. *JAMA* 39: 296–299, 1902.
6. Cameron ME: *Pterygium Throughout the World.* Springfield, IL, Charles C Thomas, 1965.
7. Duke-Elder S: Pterygium. In Duke-Elder S (ed): *System of Ophthalmology.* St. Louis, CV Mosby, 1965, vol 8, p 573–585.
8. Burns RP: Eyelids, lacrimal apparatus and conjunctiva. *Arch Ophthalmol* 79: 211–225, 1968.
9. Maertens K, Blodi FC: Epibulbar lesions among bantus. *Am J Ophthalmol* 74: 680–687, 1972.
10. Miller D: Optical features of the ocular surface. In Thoft RA, Friend J (eds): *The Ocular Surface.* Boston, Little Brown & Co, 1979, p 37–51.
11. Hilgers JH: Pterygium: its incidence heredity and etiology. *Am J Ophthalmol* 50: 635–644, 1960.
12. Ayanru JO: Affections of conjunctiva and cornea in Bendel State of Nigeria. *Trop Geogr Med* 30: 69–74, 1978.
13. Peckar CO: The aetiology and histo-pathogenesis of pterygium. A review of the literature and a hypothesis. *Doc Ophthalmol* 31: 141–157, 1972.
14. Sivasubramanism P: Pterygium in Ceylon. *Br J Ophthalmol* 55: 5–9, 1971.
15. Norn MS: Prevalence of pinguecula in Greenland and in Copenhagen, and its relation to pterygium and spheroid degeneration. *Acta Ophthalmol* 57: 96–105, 1979.
16. Darrell RW, Bachrach CA: Pterygium among veterans. *Arch Ophthalmol* 70: 158–169, 1963.
17. Newsome DA, Milton RC, Frederique G: High prevalence of eye disease in a Haitian locale. *J Trop Med Hygiene* 86: 37–46, 1983.
18. Hosni FA: Pterygium in Qatar. *Ophthalmologica* 174: 81–87, 1977.
19. Taylor HR: Aetiology of climatic droplet keratopathy and pterygium. *Br J Ophthalmol* 64: 154–163, 1980.
20. Elliott R: The aetiology and pathology of pterygium. *Trans Ophthalmol Soc Aust* 25: 71–74, 1966.
21. Cameron ME: Histology of pterygium: an electron microscopic study. *Br J Ophthalmol* 67: 604–608, 1983.
22. Forsius H: Climatic changes in the eyes of Eskimos, Lapps, and Cheremisses. *Acta Ophthalmol* 50: 532–538, 1972.
23. Young JDH, Finlay RD: Primary spheroidal degeneration of the cornea in Labrador and northern Newfoundland. *Am J Ophthalmol* 79: 129–134, 1975.
24. Youngson RM: Pterygium in Israel. *Am J Ophthalmol* 74: 954–959, 1972.
25. Wesley RE, Collins JW: Pseudopterygium from exposure to selenium dioxide. *Ann Ophthalmol* 14: 588–589, 1982.
26. Dhir SP, Detels R, Alexander ER: The role of environmental factors in cataract, pterygium, and trachoma. *Am J Ophthalmol* 64: 128–135, 1967.
27. Jenson OL: Pterygium, the dominant eye and the habit of closing one eye in sunlight. *Acta Ophthalmol* 60: 568–574, 1982.
28. Dolezalova V: Kotazce drazdeni v. eiologii pterygia. *Cesk Oftalmol* 30: 127–131, 1974.
29. Rankov BG: Vitamin-A und Carotinkonzentrationen im Serum bei Personen mit chronischer Conjunctivitis und Pterygium. *Int J Vitam Nutr Res* 46: 454–457, 1976.
30. Wong WW: A hypothesis on the pathogenesis of pterygiums. *Ann Ophthalmol* 10: 303–308, 1978.
31. Mackie IA: Localized corneal drying in association with dellen pterygia and related lesions. *Trans Ophthalmol Soc UK* 91: 129–145, 1971.
32. Jacklin HN: Familial predisposition to pterygium formation. Report of a family. *Am J Ophthalmol* 57: 481–482, 1964.
33. Murken JD, Dannheim R: Zue genetik des pterygium corneae. *Kin Monatsbl Augenheilkd* 147: 574–579, 1965.
34. Faraldi NC, Gracis GP: Pterygium on twins. *Ophthalmologica* 172: 361–366, 1976.
45. Dolezalova V: Is the occurrence of a temporal pterygium really so rare? *Ophthalmologica* 174: 88–91, 1977.
36. Awan KJ: The clinical significance of a single unilateral temporal pterygium. *Can J Ophthalmol* 10: 222–225, 1975.

37. Mamo JG: Multiple bilateral pterygia. *Am J Ophthalmol* 66: 343–345, 1968.
38. Heriot WJ, Crock GW, Taylor R, Zimmet P: Ophthalmic findings among one thousand inhabitants of Rarotonga, Cook Islands. *Aust J Ophthalmol* 11: 81–94, 1983.
39. Goldman KN, Kaufman HE: Atypical pterygium. *Arch Ophthalmol* 96: 1027–1029, 1978.
40. Norn MS: Spheroid degeneration, pinguecula and pterygium among Arabs in the Red Sea Territory, Jordan. *Acta Ophthalmol* 60: 949–954, 1982.
41. Bartholomew RS: Spheroidal degeneration of the cornea. *Doc Ophthalmol* 43: 325–340, 1977.
42. Forsius H, Eriksson A: Pterygium and its relation to arcus senilis, pinguecula and other similar conditions. *Acta Ophthalmol* 40: 402–410, 1962.
43. Norn MS: Spheroid degeneration of the cornea and conjunctiva. *Acta Ophthalmol* 56: 551–562, 1978.
44. Clear AS, Chirambo MC, Hutt MSR: Solar keratosis, pterygium, and squamous cell carcinoma of the conjunctiva in Malawi. *Br J Ophthalmol* 63: 102–109, 1979.
45. Seel D, Sealy R: Pterygia and carcinoma of the conjunctiva. *Trans Ophthalmol Soc UK* 88: 567–578, 1969.
46. Boockvar W, Wessely Z, Ballen P: Recurrent granuloma pyogenicum of limbus. *Arch Ophthalmol* 91: 42–44, 1974.
47. Wesinstock WM, Kielar RA: Bulbar ligneous conjunctivitis after pterygium removal in an elderly man. *Am J Ophthalmol* 6: 913–915, 1975.
48. Yanoff M, Fine BS: *The Ocular Pathology*, ed 2. New York, Harper & Row, 1982, p 332.
49. Menzell EJ, Egerer I, Kulnig W, Smolen JS: Elektronenmikroskopische und biochemische charakteristika von pterygia. *Klin Monatsbl Augenheilkd* 179: 438–441, 1981.
50. van der Zypen F, van der Zypen E, Daicker B: Zur Ultrastruktur des pterygium. *Graefes Arch Klin Ophthalmol* 193: 161–175, 1975.
51. English FP, Yates WHB, Kirkwood R, Slu S: The conjunctival goblet cell in pterygium formation. *Aust J Ophthalmol* 8: 53–54, 1980.
52. Vass Z, Tapaszto I: The histochemical examination of the fibers of pterybium by elastase. *Acta Ophthalmol* 42: 849–854, 1964.
53. Zauberman H: Pterygium and its recurrence. *Am J Ophthalmol* 63: 1780–1786, 1967.
54. Raizada IN, Goswami AP, Bhatnagar NK: Histopathology of pterygium. *Eye Ear Nose Throat Monthly* 47: 340–343, 1968.
55. Raizada IN, Bhatnagar NK: Pinguecula and pterygium (a histopathological study). *Indian J Ophthalmol* 24: 16–18, 1976.
56. Wilson B: Beta irradiation of pterygia. *Trans Ophthal Soc Aust* 23: 96–100, 1963.
57. Bedrossian RH: The effects of pterygium surgery on refraction and corneal curvature. *Arch Ophthalmol* 64: 553–557, 1960.
58. Hochbaum DR: Moskowitz SE, Wirtschafter JD: A quantitative analysis of astigmatism induced by pterygium. *J Biomech* 10: 735–746, 1977.
59. Hansen A, Norn M: Astigmatism and surface phenomena in pterygium. *Acta Ophthalmol* 58: 174–181, 1980.
60. King JH. The pterygium. Brief review and evaluation of certain methods of treatment. *Arch Ophthalmol* 44: 854–869, 1950.
61. Ehrlich D: The management of pterygium. *Ophthal Surg* 8: 23–29, 1977.
62. King JH, Wadsworth JAC (eds): *An Atlas of Ophthalmic Surgery*, ed 3. Philadelphia, JB Lippincott, 1981, p 216.
63. Spaeth GL (ed): *Ophthalmic Surgery Principles and Practice.* Philadelphia, WB Saunders, 1982.
64. Rich AM, Kietzman B, Payne T, McPherson SD: A simplified way to remove pterygia. *Ann Ophthalmol* 6: 739–742, 1974.
65. Small RG: A technique for removal of pterygium. *Ann Ophthalmol* 9: 349–350, 1977.
66. Barraquer JI: Etiology, pathogenesis, and treatment of the pterygium. *Symposium on Medical and Surgical Diseases of the Cornea.* St. Louis, CV Mosby, 1980, chap 9, p 167–178.
67. Rizzuti AB: A simplified corneoabrasion unit. *Trans Am Acad Ophthalmol Otolaryngol* 73: 328, 1969.
68. Youngson RM: Recurrence of pterygium after excision. *Br J Ophthalmol* 2: 120–125, 1972.
69. Walter WL: Pterygium surgery. *Eye Ear Nose Throat Monthly* 43: 41–49, 1964.
70. Walter WL: Pterygium surgery. *Am J Ophthalmol* 51: 441–450, 1961.
71. Newton FH: Operation for recurrent pterygium. *Am J Ophthalmol* 44: 258–259, 1957.
72. Aratoon V: Surgery of pterygium by conjunctival pedicle flap. *Am J Ophthalmol* 63: 1778–1779, 1967.
73. Fouad AR: A sliding conjunctiva flap for pterygium. *Bull Ophthalmol Soc Egypt* 65: 41–44, 1972.
74. Dolezalova V, Zmolikova J: Das rezidivierende pterygium. *Klin Monatsbl Augenheilkd* 174: 68–72, 1979.
75. Sato T: A new approach to the pterygium operation. *Am J Ophthalmol* 37: 903–904, 1954.
76. Vastine DW, Stewart WB, Schwab IR: Reconstruction of the periocular mucous membrane by autologous conjunctival transplantation. *Am Acad Ophthalmol* 89: 1072–1081, 1982.
77. Majoros J: Conjunctival transplant for the treatment of pterygium. *Am J Ophthalmol* 33: 1289, 1950.
78. Trivedi LK, Massey DB, Rohatgi R: Management of pterygium and its recurrence by grafting with mucous membrane from the mouth. *Am J Ophthalmol* 68: 353–354, 1969.
79. Bernstein M, Unger SM: Experiences with surgery and strontium-90 in the treatment of pterygium. *Am J Ophthalmol* 49: 1024–1029, 1960.
80. Pinkerton OD: Strontium 90 (Yttrium 90) in pterygium surgery. *Pac Coast Ophthalmol Soc* 43: 121–127, 1962.
81. Pinkerton OD: Surgical and strontium treatment of pterygium. *Ophthal Surg* 10: 45–47, 1979.
82. Thommy CP, Abiose A: Beta-irradiation in the management of pterygium. *J Ocul Ther Surg* 2: 236–241, 1983.
83. Lentino W, Zaret MM, Rossignol B, Rubenfeld S: Treatment of pterygium by surgery followed by beta radiation. *Am J Roentg* 81: 93–98, 1959.
84. Bahrassa F, Datta R: Postoperative beta radiation treatment of pterygium. *Int J Radiat Oncol Biol Phys* 9: 679–684, 1983.
85. Hilberg AW, Telles NC: A review of the use of ionizing radiation for the treatment of benign diseases. Washington, DC, US Department of Health, Education and Welfare, 1977, FDA Publication 78-8043, p 35.
86. Ozarda AT: Evaluation of postexcisional strontium-90 beta ray therapy for pterygium. *South Med J* 70: 1304, 1977.
87. Haik GM: The management of pterygia. A third report on a combined surgical-irradiation technique. *Am J Ophthalmol* 61: 1128–1134, 1966.
88. Van Den Brenk HAS: Results of prophylactic postoperative irradiation in 1300 cases of pterygium. *Am J Roent Rad Ther Nuc Med* 103: 723–733, 1968.
89. Cooper JS, Lerch IA: Postoperative irradiation of pterygia. *Radiology* 135: 743–745, 1980.
90. Pearlman G, Susal AL, Hushaw J, Bartlett RE: Recurrent pterygium and treatment with lamellar keratoplasty with presentation of a technique to limit recurrences. *Ann Ophthalmol* 2: 763–771, 1970.
91. Thommy CP: A rare complication of pterygium. *Indian J Ophthalmol* 30: 61–62, 1982.
92. Tong ECK, Zaret MM, Rubenfeld S: Cellular changes in the conjunctiva after strontium-90 treatment for pterygium. *Ann J Roent Rad Ther Nuc Med* 106: 848–853, 1969.
93. Cameron ME: Preventable complications of pterygium excision with beta-irradiation. *Br J Ophthalmol* 1: 52–56, 1972.
94. Tarr KH, Constable IJ: Pseudomonas endophthalmitis associated with scleral necrosis. *Br J Ophthalmol* 64: 676–679, 1980.
95. Tarr KH, Constable IJ: Late complications of pterygium treatment. *Br J Ophthalmol* 64: 496–505, 1980.
96. Tarr KH, Constable IJ: Radiation damage after pterygium treatment. *Aust J Ophthalmol* 9: 97–101, 1981.
97. Cappin JM: Radiation scleral necrosis simulating early scleromalacia perforans. *Br J Ophthalmol* 16: 425–428, 1973.
98. Colvin C: Treatment of pterygia with and without thiotepa. *Trans Ophthalmol Soc NZ* 25: 67–69, 1973.
99. Vitali G: La Recidiva nel trattamento dello pterigio. Nostri resultati con l'uso locale di un antimitotico. *Ann Ottalmol Clin Ocul* 94: 753–769, 1968.
100. Choon LK: Topical thio-tepa in the prevention of pterygium recurrence after surgery. *Med J Malaysia* 24: 58–61, 1969.
101. Asregadoo ER: Surgery, thio-tepa, and corticosteroid in the treat-

ment of pterygium. *Am J Ophthalmol* 74: 960–963, 1972.
102. Kleis W, Pico G: Thio-tepa therapy to prevent postoperative pterygium occurrence and neovascularization. *Am J Ophthalmol* 76: 371–373, 1973.
103. Cooper JC: Pterygium: prevention of recurrence by excision and postoperative thio-tepa. *Eye Ear Nose Throat Monthly* 45: 59–62, 1966.
104. Harrison M, Kelly A., Ohlrich J: Pterygium "thiotepa" versus beta radiation in a double-blind trial. *Trans Aust Coll Ophthalmol* 1: 64–66, 1969.
105. Meacham CT: Triethylene thiophosphoramide in the prevention of pterygium recurrence. *Am J Ophthalmol* 54: 751–753, 1962.
106. Howitt D, Karp EJ: Side effect of topical thio-tepa. *Am J Ophthalmol* 68: 473–474, 1969.
107. Hornblass A, Adler RI, Vukcevich WM, Gombos GM: A delayed side effect of topical thiotepa. *Ann Ophthalmol* 6: 1155–1157, 1974.
108. Goldberg B, Kara GB, Zavell S: Topical use of triamcinolone acetonide in inflammatory conditions of the eye. *Am J Ophthalmol* 61: 150–155, 1966.
109. Portney GL: Bare sclera, scleral cautery and corticosteroid therapy of endemic pterygium in the Navajo Indian. *Am J Ophthalmol* 67: 759–761, 1969.
110. Sabiston DW: "Medrysone": a new topical steroid. *Trans Aust Coll Ophthalmol* 2: 49–53, 1970.
111. Caldwell D: Laser treatment of pterygium. In Boyd BF: *Highlights of Ophthalmology* vol 11, No. 11, 1983. Highlights of Ophthalmology, P.O. Box 1189, Panama 1, Republic of Panama.
112. Paton D: Pterygium management based upon a theory of pathogenesis. *Trans Amer Acad Ophthal Otolaryng* 79: 603–612, 1975.
113. Fox SA: Conjunctival repairs. In Fox SA: *Ophthalmic Plastic Surgery*, ed 5. New York, Grune & Stratton, 1976, p 446–466.
114. Morozova OD: Corneal-conjunctival plastic surgery in the treatment of symblepharon and recurrent pterygium. *Vestn Oftalmol* 2: 24–27, 1971.
115. Naib K: Conjunctival graft following excision of recurrent pterygium. *Am J Ophthalmol* 58: 861–862, 1964.
116. Wong WW: Behavior of skin grafts in treatment of recurrent pterygium. *Ann Ophthalmol* 9: 352–356, 1977.
117. Bedrossian EH: Traction sutures in the treatment of paralytic esotropia. *Ann Ophthalmol* 253–256, 1969.
118. Callahan A: The arrangement of the conjunctiva in surgery for oculomotor paralysis and strabismus. *Arch Ophthalmol* 66: 117–122, 1961.
119. Dowlut MS, Laflamme MY: Les pterygions recidivants: frequence et correction par autogreffe conjonctivale. *Can J Ophthalmol* 16: 119–120, 1981.
120. Castroviejo R: Plastic and reconstructive surgery of the conjunctiva. *Plast Reconstr Surg* 24: 1–12, 1959.
121. Dake CL, Crone RA, De Keizer JW: Treatment of (recurrent) pterygium oculi by lamellar keratoplasty. *Doc Ophthalmol* 48: 223–230, 1979.
122. Durant L, Magnard G: Resultats du traitement des pterygions graves et recidivants par greffe cornea-conjonctivale. *Ann Ocul* 204: 1047–1057, 1971.
123. Anseth A, Palm E: Surgical treatment of corneal disorders. *Acta Ophthalmol* 49: 552–564, 1971.
124. Poirier RH, Fish JR: Lamellar keratoplasty for recurrent pterygium. *Ophthal Surg* 7: 38–41, 1976.
125. Beran K: Simutane lamellare und extrakorneale keratoplastik bi rezidivierenden pterygien. *Klin Monatsbl Augenheilkd* 183: 142–144, 1983.
126. Pierse D, Casey TA: Lamellar keratoplasty. *Br J Ophthalmol* 45: 733–743, 1959.
127. Reeh MJ: Corneoscleral lamellar transplant for recurrent pterygium. *Arch Ophthalmol* 86: 296–297, 1971.
128. Buxton JN, Chambers CF: Indication for surgery. *Int Ophthalmol Clin* 10: 197–213, 1970.
129. Bourne RA: Visual improvement with lamellar keratoplasty. *Can J Ophthalmol* 3: 43–45, 1968.
130. Louw JG: Some techniques in corneal grafting. *South Afr Med J* 408–412, 1971.

Index

Page numbers in *italics* denote figures; those followed by "*t*" denote tables.